KAPLAN & SADOCK'S

Concise Textbook of
Clinical Psychiatry

Second Edition

KAPLAN & SADOCK'S

Concise Textbook of Clinical Psychiatry

SECOND EDITION

Benjamin James Sadock, M.D.

Menas S. Gregory Professor of Psychiatry and Vice Chairman,
Department of Psychiatry, New York University School of Medicine;
Attending Psychiatrist, Tisch Hospital;
Attending Psychiatrist, Bellevue Hospital Center;
Consulting Psychiatrist, Lenox Hill Hospital,
New York, New York

Virginia Alcott Sadock, M.D.

Professor of Psychiatry, Department of Psychiatry,
New York University School of Medicine;
Attending Psychiatrist, Tisch Hospital;
Attending Psychiatrist, Bellevue Hospital Center,
New York, New York

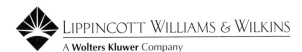
LIPPINCOTT WILLIAMS & WILKINS
A **Wolters Kluwer** Company
Philadelphia · Baltimore · New York · London
Buenos Aires · Hong Kong · Sydney · Tokyo

Acquisitions Editor: Charles W. Mitchell
Managing Editor: Joyce A. Murphy
Developmental Editor: Lisa R. Kairis
Supervising Editor: Melanie Bennitt
Production Editor: Alyson Langlois, Silverchair Science + Communications
Manufacturing Manager: Benjamin Rivera
Compositor: Silverchair Science + Communications
Printer: Quebecor World, Dubuque

© 2004 by LIPPINCOTT WILLIAMS & WILKINS
530 Walnut Street
Philadelphia, PA 19106 USA
LWW.com

Library of Congress Cataloging-in-Publication Data
Sadock, Benjamin J., 1933-
  Kaplan & Sadock's concise textbook of clinical psychiatry / Benjamin James Sadock, Virginia Alcott Sadock.-- 2nd ed.
    p. ; cm.
Rev. ed. of: Concise textbook of clinical psychiatry / Harold I. Kaplan, Benjamin J. Sadock. c1996.
Includes bibliographical references and index.
  ISBN 0-7817-5033-4
  1. Mental illness. 2. Psychiatry.
  [DNLM: 1. Mental Disorders. WM 140 S126ka 2003] I. Title: Kaplan and Sadock's concise textbook of clinical psychiatry. II. Title: Concise textbook of clinical psychiatry. III. Sadock, Virginia A. IV. Kaplan, Harold I., 1927-. Concise textbook of clinical psychiatry. V. Title.
RC454.K349 2003
616.89--dc22

                                    2003060571

Care has been taken to confirm the accuracy of the information presented and to describe generally accepted practices. However, the authors, editors, and publisher are not responsible for errors or omissions or for any consequences from application of the information in this book and make no warranty, expressed or implied, with respect to the currency, completeness, or accuracy of the contents of the publication. Application of this information in a particular situation remains the professional responsibility of the practitioner.

The authors, editors, and publisher have exerted every effort to ensure that drug selection and dosage set forth in this text are in accordance with current recommendations and practice at the time of publication. However, in view of ongoing research, changes in government regulations, and the constant flow of information relating to drug therapy and drug reactions, the reader is urged to check the package insert for each drug for any change in indications and dosage and for added warnings and precautions. This is particularly important when the recommended agent is a new or infrequently employed drug.

Some drugs and medical devices presented in this publication have Food and Drug Administration (FDA) clearance for limited use in restricted research settings. It is the responsibility of the physician or health care provider to ascertain the FDA status of each drug or device planned for use in their clinical practice.

10 9 8 7 6 5 4 3 2 1

Dedicated to all those persons who work with
and care for the mentally ill

Preface

This textbook is published as the clinical psychiatry portion of a larger volume, *Kaplan & Sadock's Synopsis of Psychiatry*, Ninth Edition, that covers both the basic behavioral sciences and all of the clinical psychiatric disorders. This new smaller volume covers the clinical psychiatric disorders alone, with some modification. We have added fresh material in this special concise edition since the publication of the larger *Synopsis* in 2003. Updated information about clinical syndromes and new data about recently introduced pharmacological agents are included. The larger format provides the student with a book that can be used throughout the entire 4 years of medical school. This smaller one is of use to the student who requires a textbook covering clinical psychiatry alone. We believe such flexibility in choice will also meet the needs of a variety of readers from psychiatry, psychology, psychiatric social work, psychiatric nursing, occupational and recreational therapy, and other mental health professions.

NEW AND REVISED AREAS

The mental disorders discussed in this textbook are consistent with nosology of the fourth revised edition of the American Psychiatric Association's *Diagnostic and Statistical Manual of Mental Disorders* (DSM-IV-TR). The inclusion of the DSM-IV-TR nosology and diagnostic criteria means that almost every section has undergone a thorough and extensive revision. Several chapters appear for the first time. "End-of-Life Care and Palliative Medicine" reflects our belief that psychiatrists have a unique role to play in the emerging clinical specialty of palliative care and pain control. Too little time—especially in medical school—is provided in training students to care for the dying patient with sensitivity and compassion. A new chapter, "Psychiatry and Reproductive Medicine," was written to keep pace with the rapid advances in women's health issues, including the controversial role of hormone replacement therapy in the treatment of mental and other disorders.

The chapter "Ethics in Psychiatry" was completely revised and updated and includes an extensive discussion of the role of euthanasia and physician-assisted suicide and their impact on the practice of medicine. In the section "Mental Disorders Due to a General Medical Condition," there is a new discussion of prion disorders and "mad cow disease." The section on "Posttraumatic Stress Disorder" includes a discussion of the psychological sequelae of the tragic events of September 11, 2001, involving the World Trade Center in New York and the Pentagon in Washington, DC. The reader will also find a new discussion on the psychiatric aspects of torture and survivors of torture.

Finally, every section on clinical psychiatry has been updated to include the latest information about diagnosing and treating mental disorders.

Psychopharmacology

Drugs used to treat mental disorders are classified according to their pharmacological activity and mechanism of action to replace such categories as antidepressants, antipsychotics, anxiolytics, and mood stabilizers, which are overly broad and do not reflect the clinical use of psychotropic medication. For example, many antidepressant drugs are used to treat anxiety disorders; some anxiolytics are used to treat depression and bipolar disorders; and drugs from all categories are used to treat other clinical disorders, such as eating disorders, panic disorders, and impulse-control disorders. There are also many drugs used to treat a variety of disorders that do not fit into any broad classification. Information about all pharmacological agents used in psychiatry, including pharmacodynamics, pharmacokinetics, dosages, adverse effects, and drug–drug interactions, was thoroughly updated and includes all drugs approved since the last edition was published.

Childhood Disorders

The chapter "Adolescent Substance Abuse" was expanded for this edition to reflect the epidemic of illicit drug use among youth and the problems of violence and dependency. New data about posttraumatic stress disorders in children have been added, including discussions of false memory syndrome and the psychological sequelae for children of terrorist activities. Every clinical disorder section was updated and revised, especially those that deal with the use of pharmacological agents in children, which is rapidly increasing.

TEACHING SYSTEM

This textbook forms one part of a comprehensive teaching system we have developed to facilitate the teaching of psychiatry and the behavioral sciences. At the head of the system is the *Comprehensive Textbook of Psychiatry*, which is global in depth and scope; it is designed for and used by psychiatrists, behavioral scientists, and all workers in the mental health field. *Kaplan & Sadock's Synopsis of Psychiatry* is a relatively brief, highly modified, original, and current version useful for medical students, psychiatric residents, practicing psychiatrists, and mental health professionals. Another part of the system is *Study Guide and Self-Examination Review in Psychiatry*, which consists of multiple-choice questions and answers; it is designed for students of psychiatry in preparation for a variety of examinations. Other parts of the system are the pocket handbooks: *Pocket Handbook of Clinical Psychiatry*, *Pocket Handbook of Psychiatric Drug Treatment*, and *Pocket Handbook of Emergency Psychiatric Medicine*. Those books cover the diagnosis and the treatment of psychiatric disorders, psychopharmacology, and psychiatric emergencies, respectively, and are concisely written and compactly designed to be carried in the pocket by clinical clerks and practicing physicians, whatever their specialty, to provide a quick reference. Finally, *Comprehensive Glossary of Psychiatry and Psychology* provides simply written definitions for psychiatrists and other physicians, psychologists, students, other mental health professionals, and the general public. Taken together, these books create a multipronged approach to the teaching, study, and learning of psychiatry.

Case Histories

Case histories make clinical disorders more vital for the student and are an integral part of this book. All cases in this edition are new, derived from various sources: *ICD-10 Casebook*, *The DSM Casebooks*, from contributors to the *Comprehensive Textbook of Psychiatry*, and from the authors' clinical experience at New York's Bellevue Hospital Center. We especially wish to thank the American Psychiatric Press and the World Health Organization for permission to use many of their cases. Cases appear in tinted type to help the reader find them easily.

Format

The interested reader is referred to either *Synopsis of Psychiatry* or the *Comprehensive Textbook of Psychiatry* for an in-depth, thorough, and detailed discussion of the topics in this book. In addition, to conserve space, references were not included at the end of each section. A complete bibliography for each section can be found in either of the above-mentioned texts. We find also that modern-day readers make extensive use of online data banks, such as Medline or PsychInfo, available on the Internet to stay abreast of the most recent literature in a particular area. As both educators and authors, we strongly encourage that trend.

Finally, although this book is intended for medical students and others in the medical profession, we are fully aware of its wide use by professionals from other fields who care for and work with the mentally ill. Accordingly, those mental health professionals should feel free, as appropriate, to substitute their own discipline into the subject of the sentence when the term *psychiatrist* or *physician* is used.

Acknowledgments

As mentioned above, this book is derived from the ninth edition of *Kaplan & Sadock's Synopsis of Psychiatry*, and we deeply appreciate the work of the consulting editors, who gave generously of their time and expertise to that edition. They include the following persons: Glen Gabbard, M.D., James Edmondson, M.D., Caroly Pataki, M.D., Myrl Manley, M.D., and Jack Grebb, M.D. We especially want to thank Norman Sussman, M.D., who, in addition to serving as consulting editor to *Synopsis*, was also contributing editor to *Concise*, helping us update the section on psychopharmacology. Dr. Sussman directs the psychopharmacology consultation service at Bellevue Hospital Center and is a highly skilled clinician and educator.

Yande McMillan played a key and invaluable role as project editor, as she has in many of our previous books. She was ably assisted by Nitza Jones, who helped remarkably in the editing of this book. We also thank Phyllis Coyne Proofreading Service.

We especially wish to acknowledge the contributions of James Sadock, M.D., and Victoria Sadock, M.D., for help in their areas of expertise—emergency adult and emergency pediatric medicine, respectively.

The staff at Lippincott Williams & Wilkins was most efficient. We wish to thank Lisa Kairis, Developmental Editor, who encouraged us throughout the project and who was of enormous help.

Finally, we want to express our deepest thanks to Robert Cancro, M.D., Professor and Chairman of the Department of Psychiatry at New York University School of Medicine. Dr. Cancro's commitment to psychiatric education and psychiatric research is recognized throughout the world. He is a much valued and highly esteemed colleague and friend. Our collaboration and association with this outstanding American educator has been a source of great inspiration.

B.J.S.
V.A.S.

Contents

Preface

1 Clinical Examination of the Psychiatric Patient 1

2 Psychiatric Report 11

3 Medical Assessment of the Psychiatric Patient 15

4 Laboratory Tests in Psychiatry 21

5 Signs and Symptoms in Psychiatry 26

6 Classification in Psychiatry and Psychiatric Rating Scales 33

7 Delirium, Dementia, and Amnestic and Other Cognitive Disorders and Mental Disorders Due to a General Medical Condition 45

7.1	Overview	45
7.2	Delirium	46
7.3	Dementia	50
7.4	Amnestic Disorder	58
7.5	Mental Disorders Due to a General Medical Condition	62

8 Neuropsychiatric Aspects of HIV Infection and AIDS 73

9 Substance-Related Disorders 77

9.1	Introduction and Overview	77
9.2	Alcohol-Related Disorders	80
9.3	Amphetamine (or Amphetamine-like)-Related Disorders	92
9.4	Caffeine-Related Disorders	97
9.5	Cannabis-Related Disorders	100
9.6	Cocaine-Related Disorders	102
9.7	Hallucinogen-Related Disorders	107
9.8	Inhalant-Related Disorders	111
9.9	Nicotine-Related Disorders	114
9.10	Opioid-Related Disorders	117
9.11	Phencyclidine (or Phencyclidine-like)-Related Disorders	122
9.12	Sedative-, Hypnotic-, or Anxiolytic-Related Disorders	125
9.13	Anabolic Steroid Abuse	131
9.14	Other Substance-Related Disorders	132

10 Schizophrenia 134

11 Other Psychotic Disorders 154

11.1	Schizophreniform Disorder	154
11.2	Schizoaffective Disorder	155
11.3	Delusional Disorder and Shared Psychotic Disorder	157
11.4	Brief Psychotic Disorder, Psychotic Disorder Not Otherwise Specified, and Secondary Psychotic Disorders	164
11.5	Culture-Bound Syndromes	169

12 Mood Disorders 173

12.1	Major Depression and Bipolar Disorder	173
12.2	Dysthymia and Cyclothymia	199
12.3	Other Mood Disorders	204

13 Anxiety Disorders   211

  13.1 Overview   211
  13.2 Panic Disorder and Agoraphobia   214
  13.3 Specific Phobia and Social Phobia   221
  13.4 Obsessive-Compulsive Disorder   227
  13.5 Posttraumatic Stress Disorder and
            Acute Stress Disorder   232
  13.6 Generalized Anxiety Disorder   238
  13.7 Anxiety Disorder Due to a General
            Medical Condition   242

14 Somatoform and Pain Disorders   247

**15 Chronic Fatigue Syndrome and
     Neurasthenia   259**

16 Factitious Disorders   261

17 Dissociative Disorders   266

18 Human Sexuality   275

  18.1 Normal Sexuality   275
  18.2. Abnormal Sexuality and Sexual
            Dysfunctions   277
  18.3 Sexual Disorder Not Otherwise
            Specified and Paraphilias   290

19 Gender Identity Disorders   297

20 Eating Disorders   302

  20.1 Anorexia Nervosa   302
  20.2 Bulimia Nervosa and Eating
            Disorder Not Otherwise Specified   305

21 Normal Sleep and Sleep Disorders   309

  21.1 Normal Sleep   309
  21.2 Sleep Disorders   311

**22 Impulse-Control Disorders Not
     Elsewhere Classified   323**

23 Adjustment Disorders   332

24 Personality Disorders   336

**25 Psychological Factors Affecting
     Medical Condition and
     Psychosomatic Medicine   355**

**26 Psychiatry and Reproductive
     Medicine   364**

27 Relational Problems   367

**28 Problems Related to Abuse
     or Neglect   370**

**29 Additional Conditions That May
     Be a Focus of Clinical Attention   377**

30 Emergency Psychiatric Medicine   382

  30.1 Psychiatric Emergencies   382
  30.2 Suicide   389

31 Psychotherapies   396

  31.1 Psychoanalysis and Psychoanalytic
            Psychotherapy   396
  31.2 Brief Psychotherapy   401
  31.3 Group Psychotherapy, Combined
            Individual and Group Psychotherapy,
            and Psychodrama   404
  31.4 Family Therapy and Couples Therapy 407
  31.5 Biofeedback   409
  31.6 Behavior Therapy   410
  31.7 Cognitive Therapy   413
  31.8 Hypnosis   414
  31.9 Psychosocial Treatment and
            Rehabilitation   415

32 Biological Therapies   418

  32.1 General Principles of
            Psychopharmacology   418

32.2	Medication-Induced Movement Disorders	422
32.3.1	α$_2$-Adrenergic Receptor Agonists: Clonidine and Guanfacine	425
32.3.2	β-Adrenergic Receptor Antagonists	427
32.3.3	Amantadine	429
32.3.4	Anticholinergics	430
32.3.5	Antihistamines	431
32.3.6	Barbiturates and Similarly Acting Drugs	433
32.3.7	Benzodiazepines	435
32.3.8	Bupropion	440
32.3.9	Buspirone and Gepirone	442
32.3.10	Calcium Channel Inhibitors	443
32.3.11	Carbamazepine	444
32.3.12	Chloral Hydrate	448
32.3.13	Cholinesterase Inhibitors	448
32.3.14	Dantrolene	450
32.3.15	Disulfiram	451
32.3.16	Dopamine Receptor Agonists and Precursors: Bromocriptine, Levodopa, Pergolide, Pramipexole, and Ropinirole	452
32.3.17	Dopamine Receptor Antagonists: Typical Antipsychotics	454
32.3.18	Lithium	458
32.3.19	Mirtazapine	463
32.3.20	Monoamine Oxidase Inhibitors	464
32.3.21	Nefazodone	467
32.3.22	Opioid Receptor Agonists: Methadone, Levomethadyl, and Buprenorphine	468
32.3.23	Opioid Receptor Antagonists: Naltrexone and Nalmefene	471
32.3.24	Other Anticonvulsants: Gabapentin, Lamotrigine, Pregabalin, Tiagabine, and Topiramate	473
32.3.25	Reboxetine	476
32.3.26	Selective Serotonin Reuptake Inhibitors	476
32.3.27	Serotonin-Dopamine Antagonists: Second-Generation Antipsychotics	483
32.3.28	Sympathomimetics and Related Drugs	487
32.3.29	Trazodone	492
32.3.30	Tricyclics and Tetracyclics	493
32.3.31	Valproate	497
32.3.32	Venlafaxine	499
32.4	Electroconvulsive Therapy	500
32.5	Other Biological and Pharmacological Therapies	504

33	**Child Psychiatry: Assessment, Examination, and Psychological Testing**	**507**
34	**Mental Retardation**	**512**
35	**Learning Disorders**	**521**
36	**Motor Skills Disorder: Developmental Coordination Disorder**	**526**
37	**Communication Disorders**	**528**
38	**Pervasive Developmental Disorders**	**535**
39	**Attention-Deficit Disorders**	**544**
40	**Disruptive Behavior Disorders**	**548**
41	**Feeding and Eating Disorders of Infancy or Early Childhood**	**553**
42	**Tic Disorders**	**557**
43	**Elimination Disorders**	**562**
44	**Other Disorders of Infancy, Childhood, and Adolescence**	**566**
44.1	Separation Anxiety Disorder	566
44.2	Selective Mutism	569

44.3   Reactive Attachment Disorder of Infancy or Early Childhood   570

44.4   Stereotypic Movement Disorder and Disorder of Infancy, Childhood, or Adolescence Not Otherwise Specified   572

45   **Mood Disorders and Suicide in Children and Adolescents**   575

46   **Early-Onset Schizophrenia**   579

47   **Adolescent Substance Abuse**   582

48   **Child Psychiatry: Additional Conditions That May Be a Focus of Clinical Attention**   585

49   **Psychiatric Treatment of Children and Adolescents**   589

49.1   Individual Psychotherapy   589

49.2   Group Psychotherapy   591

49.3   Residential, Day, and Hospital Treatment   593

49.4   Biological Therapies   595

49.5   Psychiatric Treatment of Adolescents   597

50   **Geriatric Psychiatry**   599

51   **End-of-Life Care and Palliative Medicine**   603

52   **Forensic Psychiatry**   609

53   **Ethics in Psychiatry**   615

Index   619

KAPLAN† & SADOCK TEXTBOOKS
Published by Lippincott Williams & Wilkins

Comprehensive Textbook of Psychiatry
1st edition, 1967 (with A.M. Freedman)
2nd edition, 1975 (with A.M. Freedman)
3rd edition, 1980 (with A.M. Freedman)
4th edition, 1985
5th edition, 1989
6th edition, 1995
7th edition, 1998 (with V.A. Sadock)

Synopsis of Psychiatry
1st edition, 1972 (with A.M. Freedman)
2nd edition, 1976
3rd edition, 1981
4th edition, 1985
5th edition, 1988
6th edition, 1991
7th edition, 1994 (with J. Grebb)
8th edition, 1998
9th edition, 2003 (with V.A. Sadock)

Study Guide and Self-Examination Review of Psychiatry
1st edition, 1983
2nd edition, 1985
3rd edition, 1989
4th edition, 1991
5th edition, 1994
6th edition, 1999 (with V.A. Sadock)
7th edition, 2003 (with V.A. Sadock and R.M. Jones)

Comprehensive Group Psychotherapy
1st edition, 1971
2nd edition, 1983
3rd edition, 1993

The Sexual Experience
1976 (with A.M. Freedman)

Clinical Psychiatry
1988

Concise Textbook of Clinical Psychiatry
1996

Pocket Handbook of Clinical Psychiatry
1st edition, 1990
2nd edition, 1996
3rd edition, 2001 (with V.A. Sadock)

Comprehensive Glossary of Psychiatry and Psychology
1991

Pocket Handbook of Psychiatric Drug Treatment
1st edition, 1993
2nd edition, 1996
3rd edition, 2001 (with V.A. Sadock)

Pocket Handbook of Emergency Psychiatric Medicine
1993

Pocket Handbook of Primary Care Psychiatry
1996

Various editions of the above books have been translated and published in Croatian, French, German, Greek, Indonesian, Italian, Japanese, Polish, Portuguese, Russian, Spanish, and Turkish. In addition, an International Asian edition has been published in English.

By Other Publishers

Studies in Human Behavior, 1–5
1972 (with A.M. Freedman)
Athenaeum
  1. Diagnosing Mental Illness: Evaluation in Psychiatry and Psychology
  2. Interpreting Personality: A Survey of Twentieth-Century Views
  3. Human Behavior: Biological, Psychological, and Sociological
  4. Treating Mental Illness: Aspects of Modern Therapy
  5. The Child: His Psychological and Cultural Development
Vol. 1: Normal Development and Psychological Assessment
Vol. 2: The Major Psychological Disorders and Their Treatment

Modern Group Books I–VI
1972
E.P. Dutton
  I Origins of Group Analysis
  II Evolution of Group Therapy
  III Groups and Drugs
  IV Sensitivity Through Encounter and Motivation
  V New Models for Group Therapy
  VI Group Treatment of Mental Illness

The Human Animal
1974 (with A.M. Freedman)
K.F.S. Publications
Vol. 1: Man and His Mind
Vol. 2: The Disordered Personality

†Harold I. Kaplan, M.D., 1927–1998

About the Authors

BENJAMIN JAMES SADOCK, M.D., is the Menas S. Gregory Professor of Psychiatry and Vice Chairman of the Department of Psychiatry at the New York University (NYU) School of Medicine. He is a graduate of Union College, received his M.D. degree from New York Medical College, and completed his internship at Albany Hospital. He completed his residency at Bellevue Psychiatric Hospital and then entered military service, where he served as Acting Chief of Neuropsychiatry at Sheppard Air Force Base in Texas. He has held faculty and teaching appointments at Southwestern Medical School and Parkland Hospital in Dallas and at New York Medical College, St. Luke's Hospital, the New York State Psychiatric Institute, and Metropolitan Hospital in New York City. Dr. Sadock joined the faculty of the NYU School of Medicine in 1980 and served in various positions: Director of Medical Student Education in Psychiatry, Co-Director of the Residency Training Program in Psychiatry, and Director of Graduate Medical Education. Currently, Dr. Sadock is Director of Student Mental Health Services, Psychiatric Consultant to the Admissions Committee, and Co-Director of Continuing Education in Psychiatry at the NYU School of Medicine. He is on the staff of Bellevue Hospital and Tisch Hospital and is a Consulting Psychiatrist at Lenox Hill Hospital. Dr. Sadock is a Diplomate of the American Board of Psychiatry and Neurology and served as an Associate Examiner for the Board for more than a decade. He is a Distinguished Life Fellow of the American Psychiatric Association, a Fellow of the American College of Physicians, a Fellow of the New York Academy of Medicine, and a member of Alpha Omega Alpha Honor Society. He is active in numerous psychiatric organizations and is president and founder of the NYU-Bellevue Psychiatric Society. Dr. Sadock was a member of the National Committee in Continuing Education in Psychiatry of the American Psychiatric Association, served on the Ad Hoc Committee on Sex Therapy Clinics of the American Medical Association, was a Delegate to the Conference on Recertification of the American Board of Medical Specialists, and was a representative of the American Psychiatric Association Task Force on the National Board of Medical Examiners and the American Board of Psychiatry and Neurology. In 1985, he received the Academic Achievement Award from New York Medical College and was appointed Faculty Scholar at NYU School of Medicine in 2000. He is the author or editor of more than 100 publications, a book reviewer for psychiatric journals, and lectures on a broad range of topics in general psychiatry. Dr. Sadock maintains a private practice for diagnostic consultations and psychiatric treatment. He has been married to Virginia Alcott Sadock, M.D., Professor of Psychiatry at NYU School of Medicine, since completing his residency. Dr. Sadock enjoys opera, golf, skiing, traveling, and is an enthusiastic fly fisherman.

VIRGINIA ALCOTT SADOCK, M.D., joined the faculty of the New York University (NYU) School of Medicine in 1980, where she is currently Professor of Psychiatry. She is an Attending Psychiatrist at the Tisch Hospital and Bellevue Hospital. She is Director of the Program in Human Sexuality and Sex Therapy at the NYU Medical Center, one of the largest treatment and training programs of its kind in the United States. She is the author of more than 50 articles and chapters on sexual behavior and was the developmental editor of *The Sexual Experience*, one of the first major textbooks on human sexuality, published by Williams & Wilkins. She serves as a referee and book reviewer for several medical journals, including the *American Journal of Psychiatry* and the *Journal of the American Medical Association.* She has long been interested in the role of women in medicine and psychiatry and was a founder of the Committee on Women in Psychiatry of the New York County District Branch of the American Psychiatric Association. She is active in academic matters, has served as an Assistant and Associate Examiner for the American Board of Psychiatry and Neurology for more than 15 years, and was also a member of the Test Committee in Psychiatry for both the American Board of Psychiatry and the Psychiatric Knowledge and Self-Assessment Program (PKSAP) of the American Psychiatric Association. She has chaired the Committee on Public Relations of the New York County District Branch of the American Psychiatric Association and has participated in the National Medical Television Network series *Women in Medicine* and the Emmy Award–winning PBS television documentary *Women and Depression.* She has been Vice-President of the Society of Sex Therapy and Research and a regional council member of the American Association of Sex Education Counselors and Therapists, and she is currently President of the Alumni Association of Sex Therapists. She lectures extensively both in this country and abroad on sexual dysfunction, relational problems, and depression and anxiety disorders. She is a Distinguished Fellow of the American Psychiatric Association, a Fellow of the New York Academy of Medicine, and a Diplomate of the American Board of Psychiatry and Neurology. Dr. Sadock is a graduate of Bennington College, received her M.D. degree from New York Medical College, and trained in psychiatry at Metropolitan Hospital. She lives in Manhattan with her husband, Dr. Benjamin Sadock, where she maintains an active practice that includes individual psychotherapy, couples and marital therapy, sex therapy, psychiatric consultation, and pharmacotherapy. She and her husband have two children, James and Victoria, both emergency physicians. In her leisure time, Dr. Sadock enjoys theater, film, golf, reading fiction, and travel.

Clinical Examination of the Psychiatric Patient

The psychiatric evaluation comprises two sections. The first, a section of histories (for example, psychiatric, medical, family), includes the patient's description of how symptoms of the current episode have evolved, a review of past episodes and treatments, a description of current and past medical conditions, a summary of family members' psychiatric problems and treatments, and the patient's personal history, which reveals interpersonal and adaptive functioning over time. Information for the history will come from the patient but may be supplemented by collateral information from family members, social referral agencies, previous treating physicians, and old hospital records. The second section of the psychiatric evaluation, the mental status examination, systematically reviews the patient's emotional and cognitive functioning at the time the interview is conducted.

THE PSYCHIATRIC HISTORY

The psychiatric history is the record of the patient's life; it allows a psychiatrist to understand who the patient is, where the patient has come from, and where the patient is likely to go in the future. The history is the patient's life story told to the psychiatrist in the patient's own words from his or her own point of view. Many times, the history also includes information about the patient obtained from other sources, such as a parent, or, if necessary, a spouse. Obtaining a comprehensive history from a patient and, if necessary, from informed sources is essential to making a correct diagnosis and formulating a specific and effective treatment plan. As mentioned above, a psychiatric history differs slightly from histories taken in medicine or surgery. In addition to gathering the concrete and factual data related to the chronology of symptom formation and to psychiatric and medical history, a psychiatrist strives to derive from the history the elusive picture of the patient's individual personality characteristics, including both strengths and weaknesses. The psychiatric history provides insight into the nature of relationships with those closest to the patients and includes all the important people in their lives. A reasonably comprehensive picture of the patient's development, from the earliest formative years until the present, can usually be elicited.

The most important technique for obtaining a psychiatric history is to allow patients to tell their own stories in their own words in the order that they feel is most important. Skillful interviewers recognize the points, as patients relate their stories, at which they

can introduce relevant questions about the areas described in the outline of the history and mental status examination.

The structure presented in this section is not intended as a rigid plan for interviewing a patient; it is intended as a guide for organizing the patient's history when it is written up. Several acceptable and standard formats for a psychiatric history are available; one such format is presented in Table 1–1.

Identifying Data

The identifying data provide a succinct demographic summary of the patient by name, age, marital status, sex, occupation, language if other than English, ethnic background and religion insofar as they are pertinent, and current circumstances of living. The information can also include in what place or situation the current interview took place, the sources of the information, the reliability of the source, and whether the current disorder is the first episode for the patient. The psychiatrist should indicate whether the patient came in on his or her own, was referred by someone else, or was brought in by someone else. The identifying data are meant to provide a thumbnail sketch of potentially important patient characteristics that may affect diagnosis, prognosis, treatment, and compliance.

An example of the written report of the identifying data is as follows:

> Mr. Jones is a 25-year-old-white, single, Catholic man, currently unemployed and homeless, living in public shelters and on the street. The current interview occurred in the emergency room (ER), with the patient in four-point restraints in the presence of two clinical staff members and one police officer. It was the tenth such visit to the ER for Mr. Jones in the past year. The sources of information on Mr. Jones included the patient himself and the police officer who brought him to the ER. The police officer had witnessed the patient on the street and knew him from previous episodes.

Chief Complaint

The chief complaint, in the patient's own words, states why he or she has come or been brought in for help. It should be

Table 1–1
Outline of Psychiatric History

I. Identifying data
II. Chief complaint
III. History of present illness
   A. Onset
   B. Precipitating factors
IV. Past illnesses
   A. Psychiatric
   B. Medical
   C. Alcohol and other substance history
V. Family history
VI. Personal history (anamnesis)
   A. Prenatal and perinatal
   B. Early childhood (through age 3)
   C. Middle childhood (ages 3–11)
   D. Late childhood (puberty through adolescence)
   E. Adulthood
      1. Occupational history
      2. Marital and relationship history
      3. Military history
      4. Educational history
      5. Religion
      6. Social activity
      7. Current living situation
      8. Legal history
   F. Sexual history
   G. Fantasies and dreams
   H. Values

recorded even if the patient is unable to speak, and a description of the person who provided the information should be included. The patient's explanation, regardless of how bizarre or irrelevant, should be recorded verbatim in the section on the chief complaint. The other individuals present as sources of information can then give their versions of the presenting events in the section on the history of the present illness.

History of Present Illness

The history of present illness provides a comprehensive and chronological picture of the events leading up to the current moment in the patient's life. This part of the history is probably the most helpful in making a diagnosis: When was the onset of the current episode, and what were the immediate precipitating events or triggers? An understanding of the history of the present illness helps answer the question, "Why now?" Why did the patient come to the doctor at this time? What were the patient's life circumstances at the onset of the symptoms or behavioral changes, and how did they affect the patient so that the presenting disorder became manifest? Knowing the previously well patient's personality also helps give perspective on the currently ill patient.

The evolution of the patient's symptoms should be determined and summarized in an organized and systematic way. Symptoms not present should also be delineated. The more detailed the history of the present illness, the more likely the cli-

nician is to make an accurate diagnosis. What past precipitating events were part of the chain leading up to the immediate events? In what ways has the patient's illness affected his or her life activities (for example, work, important relationships)? What is the nature of the dysfunction (for example, details about changes in such factors as personality, memory, speech)? Are there psychophysiological symptoms? If so, they should be described in terms of location, intensity, and fluctuation. Any relation between physical and psychological symptoms should be noted. A description of the patient's current anxieties, whether they are generalized and nonspecific (free floating) or are specifically related to particular situations, is helpful. How does the patient handle these anxieties? Frequently, a relatively open-ended question—such as, "How did this all begin?"—leads to an adequate unfolding of the history of the present illness. A well organized patient is generally able to present a chronological account of the history, but a disorganized patient is difficult to interview, as the chronology of events is confused. In this case, contacting other informants, such as family members and friends, can be a valuable aid in clarifying the patient's story.

Past Illness

This section of the psychiatric history is a transition between the story of the present illness and the patient's personal history (anamnesis). Past episodes of both psychiatric and medical illnesses are described. Ideally, a detailed account of the patient's preexisting and underlying psychological and biological substrates is given at this point, and important clues and evidence of vulnerable areas in the patient's functioning are provided. The patient's symptoms, extent of incapacity, type of treatment received, names of hospitals, length of each illness, effects of previous treatments, and degree of compliance should all be explored and recorded chronologically. Particular attention should be paid to the first episodes that signaled the onset of illness, because first episodes can often provide crucial data about precipitating events, diagnostic possibilities, and coping capabilities.

With regard to medical history, the psychiatrist should obtain a medical review of symptoms and note any major medical or surgical illnesses and major traumas, particularly those requiring hospitalization. Episodes of craniocerebral trauma, neurological illness, tumors, and seizure disorders are especially relevant to psychiatric histories, and so is a history of having tested positive for the human immunodeficiency virus (HIV) or having acquired immune deficiency syndrome (AIDS). Specific questions need to be asked about the presence of a seizure disorder, episodes of loss of consciousness, changes in usual headache patterns, changes in vision, and episodes of confusion and disorientation. A history of infection with syphilis is critical and relevant.

Cause, complaint, and treatment of any illness and the effects of the illness on the patient should be noted. Specific questions about psychosomatic disorders should be asked and noted. Included in this category are hay fever, rheumatoid arthritis, ulcerative colitis, asthma, hyperthyroidism, gastrointestinal upsets, recurrent colds, and skin conditions. All patients must be asked about alcohol and other substance use, including details about the quantity and frequency of use. It is often advisable to frame the question in the form of an assumption of use, such as, "How much alcohol would you say you drink in a day?" rather than, "Do you drink?" The latter question may put the patient on the defensive, concerned about what the physician will think if the answer is yes. If the physician assumes that drinking is a fact, the patient is likely to feel comfortable admitting use.

Family History

A brief statement about any psychiatric illnesses, hospitalization, and treatments of the patient's immediate family members should be placed in this part of the report. Is there a family history of alcohol and other substance abuse or of antisocial behavior? In addition, the family history should provide a description of the personalities and intelligence of the various people living in the patient's home, from childhood to the present, as well as a description of the various households in which the patient lived. The psychiatrist should also define the role each person has played in the patient's upbringing and this person's current relationship with the patient. What were and are the family ethnic, national, and religious traditions? Informants other than the patient may be available to contribute to the family history, and the source should be cited in the written record. Various members of the family often give different descriptions of the family's attitude toward and insight into the patient's illness. Does the patient feel that the family members are supportive, indifferent, or destructive? What is the role of illness in the family?

Other questions that provide useful information in this section include the following: What are the patient's attitudes toward his or her parents and siblings? The psychiatrist should ask the patient to describe each family member. Whom does the patient mention first? Whom does the patient leave out? What do the siblings do? How do siblings' occupations compare with the patient's work, and how does the patient feel about it? Whom does the patient feel he or she is most like in the family and why?

Personal History (Anamnesis)

In addition to studying the patient's present illness and current life situation, the psychiatrist needs a thorough understanding of the patient's past and its relation to the present emotional problem. The anamnesis, or personal history, is usually divided into the major developmental period, late childhood, and adulthood. The predominant emotions associated with the different life periods (for example, painful, stressful, conflictual) should be noted. Depending on time and situation, the psychiatrist may go into detail with regard to each of those areas.

Prenatal and Perinatal History.
The psychiatrist considers the nature of the home situation into which the patient was born and whether the patient was planned and wanted. Were there any problems with the mother's pregnancy and delivery? What was the mother's emotional and physical state at the time of the patient's birth? Were there any maternal health problems during pregnancy? Was the mother abusing alcohol or other substances during her pregnancy?

Early Childhood (Birth through Age 3 Years).
The early childhood period consists of the first 3 years of the patient's life. The quality of the mother–child interaction during feeding and toilet training is important. It is frequently possible to learn whether the child presented problems in these areas. Early disturbances in sleep patterns and signs of unmet needs, such as head banging and body rocking, provide clues about possible maternal deprivation or developmental disability. In addition, the psychiatrist should obtain a history of human constancy during the first 3 years. Was there psychiatric or medical illness present in the parents that may have interfered with parent–child interactions? Did persons other than the mother care for the patient? Did the patient exhibit excessive problems at an early period with stranger anxiety or separation anxiety? The patient's siblings and the details of his or her relationship to them should be explored. The emerging personality of the child is also a topic of crucial importance. Was the child shy, restless, overactive, withdrawn, studious, outgoing, timid, athletic, friendly? The clinician should seek data about the child's ability to concentrate, tolerate frustration, and postpone gratification. The child's preference for active or passive roles in physical play should also be noted. What were the child's favorite games or toys? Did the child prefer to play alone, with others, or not at all? What is the patient's earliest memory? Were there any recurrent dreams or fantasies during this period? A summary of the important areas to be covered follows:

Feeding Habits. Breast fed or bottle fed, eating problems.
Early Development. Walking, talking, teething, language development, motor development, signs of unmet needs, sleep pattern, object constancy, stranger anxiety, maternal deprivation, separation anxiety, other caretakers in the home.
Toilet Training. Age, attitude of parents, feelings about it.
Symptoms of Behavior Problems. Thumb sucking, temper tantrums, tics, head bumping, rocking, night terrors, fears, bed-wetting or bed-soiling, nail biting, excessive masturbation.
Personality as a Child. Shy, restless, overactive, withdrawn, persistent, outgoing, timid, athletic, friendly; patterns of play.
Early or Recurrent Dreams or Fantasies.

Middle Childhood (Ages 3 to 11 Years).
In this section, the psychiatrist can address such important subjects as gender identification, punishments used in the home, and the people who provided the discipline and influenced early conscience formation. The psychiatrist must inquire about the patient's early school experiences, especially how the patient first tolerated being separated from his or her mother. Data about the patient's earliest friendships and personal relationships are valuable. The psychiatrist should identify and define the number and the closeness of the patient's friends, describe whether the patient took the role of a leader or a follower, and describe the patient's social popularity and participation in group or gang activities. Was the child able to cooperate with peers, to be fair, to understand and comply with rules, and to develop an early conscience? Early patterns of assertion, impulsiveness, aggression, passivity, anxiety, or antisocial behavior emerge in the context of school relationships. A history of the patient's learning to read and of the development of other intellectual and motor skills is important. A history of learning disabilities, their management, and their effects on the child are of particular significance. The presence of nightmares, phobias,

bed-wetting, fire setting, cruelty to animals, and excessive masturbation should also be explored.

Late Childhood (Puberty through Adolescence).

During late childhood, people begin to develop independence from their parents through relationships with peers and in group activities. The psychiatrist should attempt to define the values of the patient's social groups and to determine who were the patient's idealized figures. This information provides useful clues about the patient's emerging idealized self-image.

It is helpful to explore the patient's school history, relationships with teachers, and favorite studies and interests, both in school and in extracurricular areas. The psychiatrist should ask about the patient's participation in sports and hobbies and inquire about any emotional or physical problems that may have first appeared during this phase. Examples of the types of questions that are commonly asked include the following: What was the patient's sense of personal identity? How extensive was the use of alcohol and other substances? Was the patient sexually active, and what was the quality of the sexual relationships? Was the patient interactive and involved with school and peers, or was he or she isolated, withdrawn, perceived as odd by others? Did the patient have a generally intact self-esteem, or was there evidence of excessive self-loathing? What was the patient's body image? Were there suicidal episodes? Were there problems in school, including excessive truancy? How did the patient use private time? What was the relationship with the parents? What were the feelings about the development of secondary sex characteristics? What was the response to menarche? What were the attitudes about dating, petting, crushes, parties, and sex games? One way to organize the diverse and large amount of information is to break late childhood into subsets of behavior (for example, social relationships, school history, cognitive and motor development, emotional and physical problems, and sexuality), as described next.

> *Social Relationships.* Attitudes toward sibling(s) and playmates, number and closeness of friends, leader or follower, social popularity, participation in group or gang activities, idealized figures, patterns of aggression, passivity, anxiety, antisocial behavior.
>
> *School History.* How far the patient progressed, adjustment to school, relationships with teachers—teacher's pet versus rebel—favorite studies or interests, particular abilities or assets, extracurricular activities, sports, hobbies, relation of problems or symptoms to any social period.
>
> *Cognitive and Motor Development.* Learning to read and other intellectual and motor skills, minimal cerebral dysfunctions, learning disabilities—their management and effects on the child.
>
> *Emotional and Physical Problems.* Nightmares, phobias, masturbation, bed-wetting, running away, delinquency, smoking, alcohol or other substance use, anorexia, bulimia, weight problems, feelings of inferiority, depression, suicidal ideas and acts.

Adulthood

OCCUPATIONAL HISTORY. The psychiatrist should describe the patient's choice of occupation, the requisite training and preparation, any work-related conflicts, and the long-term ambitions and goals. The interviewer should also explore the patient's feelings about his or her current job and relationships at work (with authorities, peers, and, if applicable, subordinates) and describe the job history (for example, number and duration of jobs, reasons for job changes, and changes in job status). What would the patient do for work if he or she could freely choose?

A 40-year-old physician in a successful general practice also had many business ventures in which he invested a great deal of the money he had earned from property development. The ventures frequently entangled him in legal disputes. He spent 12 to 14 hours in his medical office each day seeing patients, completed his charting and paperwork on weekends, and snatched odd moments to conduct complicated business transactions with his attorney. He was snappy and irritable with his family; he expected them to be at his beck and call and to notice his "self-sacrificing" on their behalf. Reducing his practice, taking on an associate, and limiting his business activities were all unacceptable to him.

MARITAL AND RELATIONSHIP HISTORY. In this section, the psychiatrist describes the history of each marriage, legal or common law. Significant relationships with persons with whom the patient has lived for a protracted period are also included. The story of the marriage or long-term relationship should give a description of the evolution of the relationship, including the age of the patient at the beginning of the marriage or the long-term relationship. The areas of agreement and disagreement—including the management of money, housing difficulties, roles of the in-laws, and attitudes toward raising children—should be described. Other questions include: Is the patient currently in a long-term relationship? How long is the longest relationship that the patient has had? What is the quality of the patient's sexual relationship (for example, is the patient's sexual life experienced as satisfactory or inadequate)? What does the patient look for in a partner? Is the patient able to initiate a relationship or to approach someone he or she feels attracted to or compatible with? How does the patient describe the current relationship in terms of its positive and negative qualities? How does the patient perceive failures of past relationships in terms of understanding what went wrong and who was or was not to blame?

A 32-year-old woman had a series of relationships in which she was ultimately abused, always emotionally and often physically and sexually. Despite her conscious intent to find a caring man with whom she could have a less abusive relationship, the pattern repeated itself. Her mother had been chronically beaten by her abusive father. She recalled that her mother warned her repeatedly, "A woman's role is to give in to her husband and put up with the crap as best we can."

MILITARY HISTORY. The psychiatrist should inquire about the patient's general adjustment to the military, whether he or she saw combat or sustained an injury, and the nature of the discharge. Was the patient ever referred for psychiatric consultation, and did he or she suffer any disciplinary action during the period of service?

> A 22-year-old soldier returning from Vietnam claimed to have no memory of his last month in combat. He had been assigned to a squad conducting a long-range patrol; only three of eight soldiers returned alive. Through repeated amobarbital interviews conducted in a supportive setting, gradually and with much emotion he recalled that his squad had been ambushed, that early in the firefight he had killed two or three 12- or 13-year-old Vietnamese boys who were in the attacking group, and that at a certain point he turned and ran away, leaving one or two of his wounded buddies behind, pleading with him to help them.

EDUCATION HISTORY.   The psychiatrist needs to have a clear picture of the patient's educational background. This information can provide clues about the patient's social and cultural background, intelligence, motivation, and any obstacles to achievement. For instance, a patient from an economically deprived background who never had the opportunity to attend the best schools and whose parents never graduated from high school shows strength of character, intelligence, and tremendous motivation by graduating from college. A patient who dropped out of high school because of violence and substance use displays creativity and determination by going to school at night to obtain a high school diploma while working during the day as a drug counselor. How far did the patient go in school? What was the highest grade or graduate level attained? What did the patient like to study, and what was the level of academic performance? How far did the other members of the patient's family go in school, and how do they compare with the patient's progress? What is the patient's attitude toward academic achievement?

RELIGION.   The psychiatrist should describe the religious background of both parents and the details of the patient's religious instruction. Was the family's attitude toward religion strict or permissive, and were there any conflicts between the parents over the child's religious education? The psychiatrist should trace the evolution of the patient's adolescent religious practices to present beliefs and activities. Does the patient have a strong religious affiliation, and, if so, how does this affiliation affect the patient's life? What does the patient's religion say about the treatment of psychiatric or medical illness? What is the religious attitude toward suicide?

SOCIAL ACTIVITY.   The psychiatrist should describe the patient's social life and the nature of friendships, with an emphasis on the depth, duration, and quality of human relationships. What social, intellectual, and physical interests does the patient share with friends? What relationships does the patient have with people of the same sex and the opposite sex? Is the patient essentially isolated and asocial? Does the patient prefer isolation, or is the patient isolated because of anxieties and fears about other people? Who visits the patient in the hospital and how frequently?

> An attractive, successful 32-year-old woman reported having a long string of admiring suitors and a series of intimate sexual relationships since the age of 17. Although several of the suitors to whom she was strongly attracted had proposed marriage, she felt unable to commit herself; she was never sufficiently in love with any of them and hoped that she would someday meet "Mr. Perfect."

CURRENT LIVING SITUATION.   The psychiatrist should ask the patient to describe where he or she lives in terms of the neighborhood and the residence. He or she should include the number of rooms, the number of family members living in the home, and the sleeping arrangements. The psychiatrist should inquire as to how issues of privacy are handled, with particular emphasis on parental and sibling nudity and bathroom arrangements. He or she should ask about the sources of family income and any financial hardships. If applicable, the psychiatrist may inquire about public assistance and the patient's feelings about it. If the patient has been hospitalized, have provisions been made so that he or she will not lose a job or an apartment? The psychiatrist should ask who is caring for the children at home, who visits the patient in the hospital, and how frequently.

LEGAL HISTORY.   Has the patient ever been arrested and, if so, for what? How many times? Was the patient ever in jail? For how long? Is the patient on probation, or are charges pending? Is the patient mandated to be in treatment as part of a stipulation of probation? Does the patient have a history of assault or violence? Against whom? Using what? What is the patient's attitude toward the arrests or prison terms? An extensive legal history, as well as the patient's attitude toward it, may indicate an antisocial personality disorder. An extensive history of violence may alert the psychiatrist to the potential for violence in the future.

Sexual History.   Much of the history of infantile sexuality is not recoverable, although many patients are able to recall curiosities and sexual games played from the ages of 3 to 6 years. The psychiatrist should ask how the patient learned about sex and what he or she felt were parents' attitudes about sexual development. The interviewer can also inquire whether the patient was sexually abused in childhood. It is not important where in the history it is covered, as long as it is included.

The onset of puberty and the patient's feelings about this milestone are important. Adolescent masturbatory history, including the nature of the patient's fantasies and feelings about them, is of significance. Attitudes toward sex should be described in detail. Is the patient shy, timid, aggressive? Or does the patient need to impress others and boast of sexual conquests? Did the patient experience anxiety in the sexual setting? Was there promiscuity? What is the patient's sexual orientation?

The sexual history should include any sexual symptoms, such as anorgasmia, vaginismus, erectile disorder, impotence, premature or retarded ejaculation, lack of sexual desire, and paraphilias (for example, sexual sadism, fetishism, voyeurism). Attitudes toward fellatio, cunnilingus, and coital techniques may be discussed. The topic of sexual adjustment should include a description of how sexual activity is usually initiated; the frequency of sexual relations; and sexual preferences, variations, and techniques. It is usually appropriate to inquire whether the patient has engaged in extramarital relationships and, if so, under what circumstances and whether the spouse knew of the affair. If the spouse did learn of the affair, the psychiatrist should ask the patient to describe what happened. The reasons underlying an extramarital affair are just as important as an understanding of its effect on the marriage. Attitudes toward contraception and family planning are important. What form of contraception does the patient use? The psychiatrist, however, should not assume that the patient uses birth control. If an interviewer asks a lesbian patient to describe what type of birth control she uses (on the assumption that she is heterosexual), the patient may surmise that the interviewer will not be understanding or accepting of her sexual orientation. A more helpful question is, "Do you need to use birth control?" or "Is contraception something that is part of your sexuality?"

The psychiatrist should ask whether the patient wants to mention other areas of sexual functioning and sexuality. Is the patient aware of the issues involved in safe sex? Does the patient have a sexually transmitted disease, such as herpes or AIDS? Does the patient worry about being HIV positive?

Fantasies and Dreams.   Sigmund Freud stated that dreams are the royal road to the unconscious. Repetitive dreams are of particular value. If the patient has nightmares, what are their repetitive themes? Some of the most common dream themes are food, examinations, sex, helplessness, and impotence. Can the patient describe a recent dream and discuss its possible meanings? Fantasies and daydreams are another valuable source of unconscious material. As with dreams, the psychiatrist can explore and record all manifest details and attendant feelings.

What are the patient's fantasies about the future? If the patient could make any change in his or her life, what would it be? What are the patient's most common or favorite current fantasies? Does the patient experience daydreams? Are the patient's fantasies grounded in reality, or is the patient unable to tell the difference between fantasy and reality?

Values.   The psychiatrist may inquire about the patient's system of values—both social and moral—including values about work, money, play, children, parents, friends, sex, community concerns, and cultural issues. For instance, are children a burden or a joy? Is work a necessary evil, an avoidable chore, or an opportunity? What is the patient's concept of right and wrong?

MENTAL STATUS EXAMINATION

The mental status examination is the part of the clinical assessment that describes the sum total of the examiner's observations and impressions of the psychiatric patient at the time of the interview. Whereas the patient's history remains stable, the patient's mental status can change from day to day or hour to hour. The mental status examination is the description of the patient's appearance, speech, actions, and thoughts during the interview. Even when a patient is mute, incoherent, or refusing to answer questions, the clinician can obtain a wealth of information through careful observation. Although practitioners' organizational formats for writing up the mental

Table 1–2
Outline for the Mental Status Examination

1. Appearance
2. Speech
3. Mood
   a. Subjective
   b. Objective
4. Thinking
   a. Form
   b. Content
5. Perceptions
6. Sensorium
   a. Alertness
   b. Orientation (person, place, time)
   c. Concentration
   d. Memory (immediate, recent, long term)
   e. Calculations
   f. Fund of knowledge
   g. Abstract reasoning
7. Insight
8. Judgment

status examination vary slightly, the format must contain certain categories of information. One such format is outlined in Table 1–2.

General Description

Appearance.   In this category, the psychiatrist describes the patient's appearance and overall physical impression, as reflected by posture, poise, clothing, and grooming. If the patient appears particularly bizarre, the clinician may ask, "Has anyone ever commented on how you look?" "How would you describe how you look?" "Can you help me understand some of the choices you make in how you look?"

Common terms used to describe appearance are healthy, sickly, ill at ease, poised, old looking, young looking, disheveled, childlike, and bizarre. Signs of anxiety are noted: moist hands, perspiring forehead, tense posture, wide eyes.

Overt Behavior and Psychomotor Activity.   This category refers to both the quantitative and qualitative aspects of the patient's motor behavior. Included are mannerisms, tics, gestures, twitches, stereotyped behavior, echopraxia, hyperactivity, agitation, combativeness, flexibility, rigidity, gait, and agility. Restlessness, wringing of hands, pacing, and other physical manifestations are described. Psychomotor retardation or generalized slowing down of body movements should be noted. Any aimless, purposeless activity should be described.

Attitude Toward Examiner.   The patient's attitude toward the examiner can be described as cooperative, friendly, attentive, interested, frank, seductive, defensive, contemptuous, perplexed, apathetic, hostile, playful, ingratiating, evasive, or guarded; any number of other adjectives can be used. The level of rapport established should be recorded.

Mood and Affect

Mood.   *Mood* is defined as a pervasive and sustained emotion that colors the person's perception of the world. The psychiatrist is interested in whether the patient remarks voluntarily about feelings or whether it is necessary to ask the patient how he or she feels. Statements about the patient's mood should include depth, intensity, duration, and fluctuations. Common adjectives used to describe mood include depressed, despairing, irritable, anxious, angry, expansive, euphoric, empty, guilty, awed, futile, self-contemptuous, frightened, and perplexed. Mood may be labile, fluctuating, or alternating rapidly between extremes (for example, laughing loudly and expansively one moment, tearful and despairing the next).

Affect.   Affect may be defined as the patient's present emotional responsiveness, inferred from the patient's facial expression, including the amount and the range of expressive behavior. Affect may or may not be congruent with mood. Affect can be described as within normal range, constricted, blunted, or flat. In the normal range of affect, there is variation in facial expression, tone of voice, use of hands, and body movements. When affect is constricted, the range and intensity of expression are reduced. Similarly, in blunted affect, emotional expression is further reduced. To diagnose flat affect, there should be virtually no signs of affective expression; the patient's voice should be monotonous, and the face should be immobile. *Blunted*, *flat*, and *constricted* are terms used to refer to the apparent depth of emotion; depressed, proud, angry, fearful, anxious, guilty, euphoric, and expansive are terms used to refer to particular moods. The psychiatrist should note the patient's difficulty in initiating, sustaining, or terminating an emotional response.

Appropriateness of Affect.   The psychiatrist can consider the appropriateness of the patient's emotional responses in the context of the subject the patient is discussing. Delusional patients who are describing a delusion of persecution should be angry or frightened about the experiences they believe are happening to them. Anger or fear in this context is an appropriate expression. Some psychiatrists have reserved the term *inappropriateness of affect* for a quality of response found in some schizophrenic patients, in which the patient's affect is incongruent with what the patient is saying (for example, flattened affect when speaking about murderous impulses).

Speech Characteristics

This part of the report describes the physical characteristics of speech. Speech can be described in terms of its quantity, rate of production, and quality. The patient may be described as talkative, garrulous, voluble, taciturn, unspontaneous, or normally responsive to cues from the interviewer. Speech may be rapid or slow, pressured, hesitant, emotional, dramatic, monotonous, loud, whispered, slurred, staccato, or mumbled. Impairments of speech, such as stuttering, are included in this section. Unusual rhythms (termed *dysprosody*) and any accent that may be present should be noted. Is the patient's speech spontaneous or not?

Perception

Perceptual disturbances, such as hallucinations and illusions, may be experienced in reference to the self or the environment. The sensory system involved (for example, auditory, visual, olfactory, or tactile) and the content of the illusion or the hallucinatory experience should be described. The circumstances of the occurrence of any hallucinatory experience are important; hypnagogic hallucinations (occurring as a person falls asleep) and hypnopompic hallucinations (occurring as a person awakens) are of much less serious significance than are other types of hallucinations. Hallucinations may also occur in particular times of stress for individual patients. Feelings of depersonalization and derealization (extreme feelings of detachment from the self or the environment) are other examples of perceptual disturbance. Formication, the feeling of bugs crawling on or under the skin, is seen in cocainism.

Examples of questions used to elicit the experience of hallucinations include the following: Have you ever heard voices or other sounds that no one else could hear or when no one else was around? Have you experienced any strange sensations in your body that others do not seem to experience? Have you ever had visions or seen things that other people do not seem to see?

> A terrified 37-year-old man in acute delirium tremens glanced agitatedly about the room. He pointed out the window and said: "My God, the Spanish armada is on the lawn. They're about to attack." He experienced the hallucination as real, and it persisted intermittently for 3 days before abating. Subsequently, the patient had no memory of the experience.

Thought Content and Mental Trends

Thought can be divided into process (or form) and content. *Process* refers to the way in which a person puts together ideas and associations, the form in which a person thinks. Process or form of thought may be logical and coherent or completely illogical and even incomprehensible. *Content* refers to what a person is actually thinking about: ideas, beliefs, preoccupations, obsessions.

Thought Process (Form of Thinking).   The patient may have either an overabundance or a poverty of ideas. There may be rapid thinking, which, if carried to the extreme, is called a *flight of ideas*. A patient may exhibit slow or hesitant thinking.

Thought may be vague or empty. Do the patient's replies really answer the questions asked, and does the patient have the capacity for goal-directed thinking? Are the responses relevant or irrelevant? Is there a clear cause-and-effect relation in the patient's explanations? Does the patient have *loose associations* (for example, do the ideas expressed appear to be unrelated and idiosyncratically connected)? Disturbances of the continuity of thought include statements that are tangential, circumstantial, rambling, evasive, and perseverative.

Blocking is an interruption of the train of thought before an idea has been completed; the patient may indicate an inability to recall what was being said or intended to be said. *Circumstantiality* indicates the loss of capacity for goal-directed thinking; in the process of explaining an idea, the patient brings in many irrelevant details and parenthetical comments but eventually does get back to the original point. *Tangentiality* is a disturbance in which the patient loses the thread of the conversation and pursues tangential thoughts stimulated by various external or internal irrelevant stimuli and never returns to the original point. Thought process impairments may be reflected by *word salad* (incoherent or incomprehensible connections of thoughts), *clang associations* (association by rhyming), *punning* (association by double meaning), and *neologisms* (new words created by the patient through the combination or condensation of other words).

Thought Content. Disturbances in content of thought include delusions, preoccupations (which may involve the patient's illness), obsessions ("Do you have ideas that are intrusive and repetitive?"), compulsions ("Are there things you do over and over, in a repetitive manner?" "Are there things you must do in a particular way or order?" "If you do not do them that way, must you repeat them?" "Do you know why you do things that way?"), phobias, plans, intentions, recurrent ideas about suicide or homicide, hypochondriacal symptoms, and specific antisocial urges.

> A 32-year-old woman with a mild viral syndrome picked up a carton of milk in the supermarket and then returned it to its shelf, after deciding not to buy it. Over the next few days, she spent increasing amounts of time thinking about the act. She could not stop herself from thinking that the mother of a young child picked up the same container, contracted the patient's virus, and gave it to her child, who may then have become ill and died as a result of a fulminant infection. Despite knowing that this sequence of events was extremely unlikely, the woman could not stop replaying the scenario in her mind.

Does the patient have thoughts of doing harm to himself or herself? Is there a plan? A major category of disturbances of thought content involves delusions. Delusions—fixed, false beliefs out of keeping with the patient's cultural background—may be mood congruent (in keeping with a depressed or elated mood) or mood incongruent. The content of any delusional system should be described, and the psychiatrist should attempt to evaluate its organization and the patient's conviction as to its validity. The manner in which it affects the patient's life is appropriately described in the history of the present illness. Delusions may be bizarre and may involve beliefs about external control. Delusions may have themes that are persecutory or paranoid, grandiose, jealous, somatic, guilty, nihilistic, or erotic. Ideas of reference and of influence should also be described. Examples of ideas of reference include a person's belief that the television or radio is speaking to or about him or her. Examples of ideas of influence are beliefs about another person or force controlling some aspect of a person's behavior.

> A young man with schizophrenia heard an insistent voice repeatedly telling him to stop his antipsychotic medication. After resisting the command for many weeks, the patient felt that he could no longer fight the voice, and he discontinued treatment. Two months later, he was hospitalized involuntarily and near cardiovascular collapse. He later said that once he stopped the medication, the voice further insisted that he should stop eating and drinking to purify himself.

Sensorium and Cognition

The sensorium and cognition portion of the mental status examination seeks to assess organic brain function and the patient's intelligence, capacity for abstract thought, and level of insight and judgment.

Consciousness. Disturbances of consciousness usually indicate organic brain impairment. Clouding of consciousness is an overall reduced awareness of the environment. A patient may be unable to sustain attention to environmental stimuli or to maintain goal-directed thinking or behavior. Clouding or obtunding of consciousness is frequently not a fixed mental state. A patient typically manifests fluctuations in the level of awareness of the surrounding environment. The patient who has an altered state of consciousness often shows some impairment of orientation as well, although the reverse is not necessarily true. Some terms used to describe the patient's level of consciousness are clouding, somnolence, stupor, coma, lethargy, alertness, and fugue state.

Orientation and Memory. Disorders of orientation are traditionally separated according to time, place, and person. Any impairment usually appears in this order (that is, sense of time is impaired before sense of place); similarly, as the patient improves, the impairment clears in the reverse order. The psychiatrist must determine whether patients can give the approximate date and time of day. In addition, if patients are in a hospital, do they know how long they have been there? Do the patients behave as though they are oriented to the present? In questions about patients' orientation to place, it is not sufficient that they be able to state the name and the location of the hospital correctly; they should also behave as though they know where they are. In assessing orientation for person, the psychiatrist asks patients whether they know the names of the people around them and whether they understand their roles in relationship to them. Do they know who the examiner is? It is only in the most severe instances that patients do not know who they themselves are.

> A 42-year-old alcoholic man in delirium tremens, examined in a California hospital in 1995, was asked the date and where he was. He replied: "I'm standing on a street corner in Kansas City in 1966 minding my own business. Why don't you mind yours?"

Memory functions have traditionally been divided into four areas: remote memory, recent past memory, recent memory, and immediate retention and recall. Recent memory may be checked by asking patients about their appetite and then about what they had for breakfast or for dinner the previous evening. Patients may be asked at this point if they recall the interviewer's name. Asking patients to repeat six digits forward and then backward is a test for immediate retention. Remote memory can be tested by asking patients for information about their childhoods that can be later verified. Asking patients to recall important news events from the past few months checks recent past memory. Often in cognitive disorders, recent or short-term memory is impaired first, and remote or long-term memory is impaired later. If there is impairment, what are the efforts made to cope with it or to conceal it? Is denial, confabulation, catastrophic reaction, or circumstantiality used to conceal a deficit? Reactions to the loss of memory can give important clues to underlying disorders and coping mechanisms. For instance, a patient who appears to have memory impairment but, in fact, is depressed is more likely to be concerned about memory loss than is someone with memory loss secondary to dementia.

A 40-year-old chronically alcoholic man, whose memory on the mental status examination was markedly impaired, frantically demanded to be released from the hospital, saying that his wife had just been in an automobile accident and that he had to rush to another hospital to see her. He said it with sincere conviction and appropriate fearful concern; for the patient, at least, the story was real. In fact, his wife had been dead for 15 years. The patient told the same story over and over again, always with evident conviction, in spite of the fact that staff members confronted him with the reality that his wife had been dead for years. The patient was never influenced by their assertions, because he could not register new memories. Although his past memory was patchy at best, he could repeatedly recall the story of his wife's emergency.

Confabulation (unconsciously making up false answers when memory is impaired) is most closely associated with cognitive disorders.

Concentration and Attention.

A patient's concentration may be impaired for many reasons. A cognitive disorder, anxiety, depression, and internal stimuli, such as auditory hallucinations—all may contribute to impaired concentration. Subtracting serial 7s from 100 is a simple task that requires intact concentration and cognitive capacities. Was the patient able to subtract 7 from 100 and keep subtracting 7s? If the patient could not subtract 7s, could 3s be subtracted? Were easier tasks accomplished—4×9, 5×4? The examiner must always assess whether anxiety, some disturbance of mood or consciousness, or a learning deficit is responsible for the difficulty.

Attention is assessed by calculations or by asking the patient to spell the word *world* (or others) backward. The patient can also be asked to name five things that start with a particular letter.

During his most recent manic episode, a 48-year-old man with bipolar disorder had intense, grandiose, psychotic ideas. He was convinced that he could control the traffic in Los Angeles by driving on certain freeways at specified times and willing others to leave the road. After the manic episode ended and during the depressive episode that immediately followed, he could recall virtually no details of his previous thought content while he was manic. Later, when euthymic, he remembered only a few hazy images. A year later, the beginning of a new hypomanic period was heralded by the patient's spontaneously remembering and describing in great detail the psychotic plans of the previous episode.

Reading and Writing.

The patient should be asked to read a sentence (for example, "Close your eyes") and then do what the sentence says. The patient should also be asked to write a simple but complete sentence.

Visuospatial Ability.

The patient should be asked to copy a figure, such as a clock face or interlocking pentagons.

Abstract Thought.

Abstract thinking is the ability to deal with concepts. Patients may have disturbances in the manner in which they conceptualize or handle ideas. Can patients explain similarities, such as those between an apple and a pear or those between truth and beauty? Are the meanings of simple proverbs, such as "A rolling stone gathers no moss," understood? Answers may be concrete (giving specific examples to illustrate the meaning) or overly abstract (giving too generalized an explanation). Appropriateness of answers and the manner in which answers are given should be noted. In a catastrophic reaction, brain-damaged patients become extremely emotional and cannot think abstractly.

Information and Intelligence.

If a possible cognitive impairment is suspected, does the patient have trouble with mental tasks, such as counting the change from $10 after a purchase of $6.37? If this task is too difficult, are easy problems (such as how many nickels are in $1.35) solved? The patient's intelligence is related to vocabulary and general fund of knowledge (for example, the distance from New York to Paris, Presidents of the United States). The patient's education level (both formal and self-education) and socioeconomic status must be taken into account. Handling of difficult or sophisticated concepts can reflect intelligence, even in the absence of formal education or an extensive fund of information. Ultimately, the psychiatrist estimates the patient's intellectual capability and capacity to function at the level of basic endowment.

Impulsivity

Is the patient capable of controlling sexual, aggressive, and other impulses? An assessment of impulse control is critical in ascertaining the patient's awareness of socially appropriate behavior and is a measure of the patient's potential danger to self and others. Patients may be unable to control impulses secondary to cognitive and psychotic disorders or resulting from chronic characterological defects, as observed in the personality disorders. Impulse control can be estimated from information in the patient's recent history and from behavior observed during the interview.

Judgment and Insight

Judgment.   During the course of history taking, the psychiatrist should be able to assess many aspects of the patient's capability for social judgment. Does the patient understand the likely outcome of his or her behavior, and is he or she influenced by this understanding? Can the patient predict what he or she would do in imaginary situations? For instance, what would the patient do if he or she smelled smoke in a crowded movie theater?

Insight.   Insight is a patient's degree of awareness and understanding about being ill. Patients may exhibit a complete denial of their illness or may show some awareness that they are ill but place the blame on others, on external factors, or even on organic factors. They may acknowledge that they have an illness but ascribe it to something unknown or mysterious in themselves.

An 18-year-old man went to an emergency room with the belief that he was controlled by a computer on an Enterprise-like starship, an elaboration from the television series "Star Trek." He was convinced that all his thoughts, actions, and feelings were being programmed on board the starship, which was located light years away and, therefore, could never be detected by anyone else.

Intellectual insight is present when patients can admit that they are ill and acknowledge that their failures to adapt are, in part, due to their own irrational feelings. Patients' inability to apply their knowledge to alter future experiences, however, is the major limitation to intellectual insight. True emotional insight is present when patients' awareness of their own motives and deep feelings leads to a change in their personality or behavior patterns.

A summary of levels of insight follows:

1. Complete denial of illness.
2. Slight awareness of being sick and needing help but denying it at the same time.
3. Awareness of being sick but blaming it on others, on external factors, or on organic factors.
4. Awareness that illness is due to something unknown in the patient.
5. Intellectual insight: admission that the patient is ill and that symptoms or failures in social adjustment are due to the patient's own particular irrational feelings or disturbances without applying this knowledge to future experiences.
6. True emotional insight: emotional awareness of the motives and feelings within the patient and the important people in his or her life, which can lead to basic changes in behavior.

Reliability

The mental status part of the report concludes with the psychiatrist's impressions of the patient's reliability and capacity to report his or her situation accurately. It includes an estimate of the psychiatrist's impression of the patient's truthfulness or veracity. For instance, if the patient is open about significant active substance abuse or about circumstances that the patient knows may reflect badly (for example, trouble with the law), the psychiatrist may estimate the patient's reliability to be good.

2 △

Psychiatric Report

The psychiatric report is a written document that details the findings obtained from the psychiatric history and mental status examination. The report may follow the outline described below or it may also be formatted in other ways, providing all the pertinent data are recorded.

The psychiatric report includes a final summary of both positive and negative findings and an interpretation of the data. It has more than descriptive value; it has meaning that helps provide an understanding of the case. The examiner addresses critical questions in the report: Are future diagnostic studies needed and, if so, which ones? Is a consultant needed? Is a comprehensive neurological workup needed, including an electroencephalogram or computerized tomography scan? Are psychological tests indicated? Are psychodynamic factors relevant? The report includes a diagnosis made according to the fourth revised edition of *Diagnostic and Statistical Manual of Mental Disorders* (DSM-IV-TR). A prognosis is also discussed in the report, with both good and bad prognostic factors listed. Finally, a treatment plan discusses and makes firm recommendations about management issues.

I. Psychiatric history

A. Identification: name, age, marital status, sex, occupation, language if other than English, race, nationality, and religion if pertinent; previous admissions to a hospital for the same or a different condition; with whom the patient lives

B. Chief complaint: exactly why the patient came to the psychiatrist, preferably in the patient's own words; if that information does not come from the patient, note who supplied it

C. History of present illness: chronological background and development of the symptoms or behavioral changes that culminated in the patient's seeking assistance; patient's life circumstances at the time of onset; personality when well; how illness has affected life activities and personal relations—changes in personality, interests, mood, attitudes toward others, dress, habits, level of tenseness, irritability, activity, attention, concentration, memory, speech; psychophysiological symptoms—nature and details of dysfunction; pain—location, intensity, fluctuation; level of anxiety—generalized and nonspecific (free floating) or specifically related to particular situations, activities, or objects; how anxieties are handled—avoidance, repetition of feared situation, use of drugs or other activities for alleviation

D. Past psychiatric and medical history: (1) emotional or mental disturbances—extent of incapacity, type of treatment, names of hospitals, length of illness, effect of treatment; (2) psychosomatic disorders: hay fever arthritis, colitis, rheumatoid arthritis, recurrent colds, skin conditions; (3) medical conditions: follow customary review of systems; sexually transmitted diseases; alcohol or other substance abuse; at risk for acquired immune deficiency syndrome (AIDS); (4) neurological disorders: headache, craniocerebral trauma, loss of consciousness, seizures or tumors

E. Family history: Elicited from patient and from someone else, since quite different descriptions may be given of the same people and events; ethnic, national, and religious traditions; other people in the home, descriptions of them—personality and intelligence—and what has become of them since patient's childhood; descriptions of different households lived in; present relationships between patient and those who were in family; role of illness in the family; family history of mental illness; where does patient live—neighborhood and particular residence of the patient; is home crowded; privacy of family members from each other and from other families; sources of family income and difficulties in obtaining it; public assistance (if any) and attitude about it; will patient lose job or apartment by remaining in the hospital; who is caring for children

F. Personal history (anamnesis): history of the patient's life from infancy to the present to the extent it can be recalled; gaps in history as spontaneously related by the patient; emotions associated with different life periods (painful, stressful, conflictual) or with phases of life cycle

1. Early childhood (through age 3)
   a. Prenatal history and mother's pregnancy and delivery: length of pregnancy, spontaneity and normality of delivery, birth trauma, whether patient was planned and wanted, birth defects
   b. Feeding habits: breast-fed or bottle-fed, eating problems
   c. Early development: maternal deprivation, language development, motor development, signs of unmet needs, sleep pattern, object constancy, stranger anxiety, separation anxiety
   d. Toilet training: age, attitude of parents, feelings about it

e. Symptoms of behavior problems: thumb sucking, temper tantrums, tics, head bumping, rocking, night terrors, fears, bed-wetting or bed-soiling, nail biting, masturbation

f. Personality and temperament as a child: shy, restless, overactive, withdrawn, studious, outgoing, timid, athletic, friendly patterns of play, reactions to siblings

g. Early or recurrent dreams or fantasies

2. Middle childhood (ages 3 to 11): early school history—feelings about going to school, early adjustment, gender identification, conscience development, punishment; social relationships, attitudes toward siblings and playmates

3. Later childhood (prepuberty through adolescence)

a. Peer relationships: number and closeness of friends, leader or follower, social popularity, participation in group or gang activities, idealized figures; patterns of aggression, passivity, anxiety, antisocial behavior

b. School history: how far the patient went, adjustment to school, relationships with teachers—teacher's pet or rebellious—favorite studies or interests, particular abilities or assets, extracurricular activities, sports, hobbies, relationships of problems or symptoms to any school period

c. Cognitive and motor development: learning to read and other intellectual and motor skills, minimal cerebral dysfunction, learning disabilities—their management and effects on the child

d. Particular adolescent emotional or physical problems: nightmares, phobias, masturbation, bed-wetting, running away, delinquency, smoking, drug or alcohol use, weight problems, feelings of inferiority

e. Psychosexual history

i. Early curiosity, infantile masturbation, sex play

ii. Acquiring of sexual knowledge, attitude of parents toward sex, sexual abuse

iii. Onset of puberty, feelings about it, kind of preparation, feelings about menstruation, development of secondary sexual characteristics

iv. Adolescent sexual activity: crushes, parties, dating, petting, masturbation, wet dreams and attitudes toward them

v. Attitudes toward same and opposite sex: timid, shy, aggressive, need to impress, seductive, sexual conquests, anxiety

vi. Sexual practices: sexual problems, homosexual and heterosexual experiences, paraphilias, promiscuity

f. Religious background: strict, liberal, mixed (possible conflicts), relationship of background to current religious practices

4. Adulthood

a. Occupational history: choice of occupation, training, ambitions, conflicts; relations with authority, peers, and subordinates; number of jobs and duration; changes in job status; current job and feelings about it

b. Social activity: whether patient has friends or not; is he or she withdrawn or socializing well; social, intellectual, and physical interests; relationships with same sex and opposite sex; depth, duration, and quality of human relations

c. Adult sexuality

i. Premarital sexual relationships, age of first coitus, sexual orientation

ii. Marital history: common-law marriages, legal marriages, description of courtship and role played by each partner, age at marriage, family planning and contraception, names and ages of children, attitudes toward raising children, problems of any family members, housing difficulties if important to the marriage, sexual adjustment, extramarital affairs, areas of agreement and disagreement, management of money, role of in-laws

iii. Sexual symptoms: anorgasmia, impotence, premature ejaculation, lack of desire

iv. Attitudes toward pregnancy and having children; contraceptive practices and feelings about them

v. Sexual practices: paraphilias such as sadism, fetishes, voyeurism; attitude toward fellatio, cunnilingus; coital techniques, frequency

d. Military history: general adjustment, combat, injuries, referral to psychiatrists, type of discharge, veteran status

e. Value systems: whether children are seen as a burden or a joy; whether work is seen as a necessary evil, an avoidable chore, or an opportunity; current attitude about religion; belief in heaven and hell

II. Mental status

Sum total of the examiner's observations and impressions derived from the initial interview

A. Appearance

1. Personal identification: may include a brief non-technical description of the patient's appearance and behavior as a novelist might write it; attitude toward examiner: cooperative, attentive, interested, frank, seductive, defensive, hostile, playful, ingratiating, evasive, guarded

2. Behavior and psychomotor activity: gait, mannerisms, tics, gestures, twitches, stereotypes, picking, touching examiner, echopraxia, clumsy, agile, limp, rigid, retarded, hyperactive, agitated, combative, waxy

3. General description: posture, bearing, clothes, grooming, hair, nails; healthy, sickly, angry, frightened, apathetic, perplexed, contemptuous, ill at ease, poised, old looking, young looking, effeminate, masculine; signs of anxiety—moist hands, perspiring forehead, restlessness, tense posture, strained voice, wide eyes; shifts in level of anxiety during interview or with particular topic

B. Speech: rapid, slow, pressured, hesitant, emotional, monotonous, loud, whispered, slurred, mumbled, stuttering, echolalia, intensity, pitch, ease, spontaneity, productivity, manner, reaction time, vocabulary, prosody

C. Mood and affect
1. Mood (a pervasive and sustained emotion that colors the person's perception of the world): how does patient say he or she feels; depth, intensity, duration, and fluctuations of mood—depressed, despairing, irritable, anxious, terrified, angry, expansive, euphoric, empty, guilty, awed, futile, self-contemptuous, anhedonic, alexithymic
2. Affect (the outward expression of the patient's inner experiences): how examiner evaluates patient's affects—broad, restricted, blunted or flat, shallow, amount and range of expression; difficulty in initiating, sustaining, or terminating an emotional response; is the emotional expression appropriate to the thought content, culture, and setting of the examination; give examples if emotional expression is not appropriate
D. Thinking and perception
1. Form of thinking
a. Productivity: overabundance of ideas, paucity of ideas, flight of ideas, rapid thinking, slow thinking, hesitant thinking; does patient speak spontaneously or only when questions are asked, stream of thought, quotations from patient
b. Continuity of thought: whether patient's replies really answer questions and are goal directed, relevant, or irrelevant; loose associations; lack of cause-and-effect relationships in patient's explanations; illogical, tangential, circumstantial, rambling, evasive, perseverative statements; blocking or distractibility
c. Language impairments: impairments that reflect disordered mentation, such as incoherent or incomprehensible speech (word salad), clang associations, neologisms
2. Content of thinking
Preoccupations: about the illness, environmental problems; obsessions, compulsions, phobias; obsessions or plans about suicide, homicide; hypochondriacal symptoms, specific antisocial urges or impulses
3. Thought disturbances
a. Delusions: content of any delusional system, its organization, the patient's convictions as to its validity, how it affects his or her life; persecutory delusions—isolated or associated with pervasive suspiciousness; mood-congruent or mood-incongruent
b. Ideas of reference and ideas of influence: how ideas began, their content, and the meaning the patient attributes to them
4. Perceptual disturbances
a. Hallucinations and illusions: whether patient hears voices or sees visions; content, sensory system involvement, circumstances of the occurrence; hypnagogic or hypnopompic hallucinations; thought broadcasting
b. Depersonalization and derealization: extreme feelings of detachment from self or from the environment

5. Dreams and fantasies
a. Dreams: prominent ones, if patient will tell them; nightmares
b. Fantasies: recurrent, favorite, or unshakable daydreams
E. Sensorium
1. Alertness: awareness of environment, attention span, clouding of consciousness, fluctuations in levels of awareness, somnolence, stupor, lethargy, fugue state, coma
2. Orientation
a. Time: whether patient identifies the day correctly; or approximate date, time of day; if in a hospital, knows how long he or she has been there; behaves as though oriented to the present
b. Place: whether patient knows where he or she is
c. Person: whether patient knows who the examiner is and the roles or names of the persons with whom in contact
3. Concentration and calculation: subtracting 7 from 100 and keep subtracting 7s; if patient cannot subtract 7s, can easier tasks be accomplished—4×9; 5×4; how many nickels are in $1.35; whether anxiety or some disturbance of mood or concentration seems to be responsible for difficulty
4. Memory: impairment, efforts made to cope with impairment—denial, confabulation, catastrophic reaction, circumstantiality used to conceal deficit; whether the process of registration, retention, or recollection of material is involved
a. Remote memory: childhood data, important events known to have occurred when the patient was younger or free of illness, personal matters, neutral material
b. Recent past memory: past few months
c. Recent memory: past few days; what did patient do yesterday, the day before; have for breakfast, lunch, dinner
d. Immediate retention and recall: ability to repeat six figures after examiner dictates them—first forward, then backward, then after a few minutes' interruption; other test questions; did same questions, if repeated, call forth different answers at different times
e. Effect of defect on patient: mechanisms patient has developed to cope with defect
5. Fund of knowledge: level of formal education and self-education; estimate of the patient's intellectual capability and whether capable of functioning at the level of his or her basic endowment; counting, calculation, general knowledge; questions should have relevance to the patient's educational and cultural background
6. Abstract thinking: disturbances in concept formation; manner in which the patient conceptualizes or handles his or her ideas; similarities (e.g., between apples and pears), differences, absurdities; meanings of simple proverbs, such as, "A rolling stone gathers no moss"; answers may be concrete (giving specific examples to illustrate the

meaning) or overly abstract (giving generalized explanation); appropriateness of answers

    7. Insight: degree of personal awareness and understanding of illness

      a. Complete denial of illness

      b. Slight awareness of being sick and needing help but denying it at the same time

      c. Awareness of being sick but blaming it on others, on external factors, on medical or unknown organic factors

      d. Intellectual insight: admission of illness and recognition that symptoms or failures in social adjustment are due to irrational feelings or disturbances, without applying that knowledge to future experiences

      e. True emotional insight: emotional awareness of the motives and feelings within, of the underlying meaning of symptoms; does the awareness lead to changes in personality and future behavior; openness to new ideas and concepts about self and the important people in his or her life

    8. Judgment

      a. Social judgment: subtle manifestations of behavior that are harmful to the patient and contrary to acceptable behavior in the culture; does the patient understand the likely outcome of personal behavior and is the patient influenced by that understanding

      b. Test judgment: patient's prediction of what he or she would do in imaginary situations; for instance, what patient would do with a stamped, addressed letter found in the street

III. Further diagnostic studies

  A. Physical examination

  B. Neurological examination

  C. Additional psychiatric diagnostic interviews

  D. Interviews with family members, friends, or neighbors by a social worker

  E. Psychological, neurological, or laboratory tests as indicated: electroencephalogram, computed tomography scan, magnetic resonance imaging, tests of other medical conditions, reading comprehension and writing tests, test for aphasia, projective or objective psychological tests, dexamethasone-suppression test, 24-hour urine test for heavy metal intoxication, urine screen for drugs of abuse

IV. Summary of findings

Mental symptoms, medical and laboratory findings, and psychological and neurological test results, if available, are summarized. Include medications patient has been taking, dosage, and duration.

Clarity of thinking is reflected in clarity of writing. When summarizing the mental status, for example, the phrase "Patient denies hallucinations and delusions" is not as precise as "Patient denies hearing voices or thinking that he is being followed." The latter indicates the specific question asked and the specific response given. Similarly, in the conclusion of the report, one would write, "Hallucinations and delusions were not elicited."

V. Diagnosis

Diagnostic classification is made according to DSM-IV-TR, which uses a multiaxial classification scheme consisting of five axes, each of which should be covered in the diagnosis.

    Axis I: clinical syndromes (e.g., mood disorders, schizophrenia, generalized anxiety disorder) and other conditions that may be a focus of clinical attention

    Axis II: personality disorders, mental retardation, and defense mechanisms

    Axis III: any general medical conditions (e.g., epilepsy, cardiovascular disease, endocrine disorders)

    Axis IV: psychosocial and environmental problems (e.g., divorce, injury, death of a loved one) relevant to the illness

    Axis V: global assessment of functioning exhibited by the patient during the interview (e.g., social, occupational, and psychological functioning); a rating scale with a continuum from 100 (superior functioning) to 1 (grossly impaired functioning) is used

VI. Prognosis

Opinion about the probable future course, extent, and outcome of the disorder; good and bad prognostic factors; specific goals of therapy

VII. Psychodynamic formulation

Causes of the patient's psychodynamic breakdown—influences in the patient's life that contributed to the present disorder; environmental, genetic, and personality factors relevant to determining the patient's symptoms; primary and secondary gains; outline of the major defense mechanism used by the patient

VIII. Comprehensive treatment plan

Modalities of treatment recommended, role of medication, inpatient or outpatient treatment, frequency of sessions, probable duration of therapy; type of psychotherapy; individual, group, or family therapy; symptoms or problems to be treated. Initially, treatment must be directed toward any life-threatening situations, such as suicidal risk or risk of danger to others, that require psychiatric hospitalization. Danger to self or others is an acceptable reason (both legally and medically) for involuntary hospitalization. In the absence of the need for confinement, a variety of outpatient treatment alternatives are available: day hospitals, supervised residences, outpatient psychotherapy or pharmacotherapy, among others. In some cases, treatment planning must attend to vocational and psychosocial skills training and even legal or forensic issues. Comprehensive treatment planning requires a therapeutic team approach using the skills of psychologists, social workers, nurses, activity and occupational therapists, and a variety of other mental health professionals, with referral to self-help groups (e.g., Alcoholics Anonymous [AA]) if needed. If either the patient or family members are unwilling to accept the recommendations of treatment, and the clinician thinks that the refusal of the recommendations may have serious consequences, the patient, parent, or guardian should sign a statement to the effect that the recommended treatment was refused.

Medical Assessment of the Psychiatric Patient

Although psychiatrists do not perform routine physical examinations on their patients, a knowledge and understanding of physical signs and symptoms are parts of their training that enable them to recognize signs and symptoms of possible medical or surgical illness. For example, palpitations may be associated with mitral valve prolapse, which is diagnosed by cardiac auscultation.

Some psychiatrists insist that every patient have a complete medical workup; others may not. Whatever their policy, psychiatrists should consider patients' medical status at the outset of a psychiatric evaluation. Psychiatrists must often decide whether a patient needs a medical examination and, if so, what it should include—most commonly, a thorough medical history, including a review of systems, a physical examination, and relevant diagnostic laboratory studies. In a recent study of 1,000 medical patients, it was found that, in 75 percent of cases, the causes of their subjective complaints could not be found, and a psychological basis was assumed in 10 percent of cases.

HISTORY OF MEDICAL ILLNESS

In the course of conducting a psychiatric evaluation, information should be gathered about known bodily diseases or dysfunctions, hospitalizations and operative procedures, medications taken recently or at present, personal habits and occupational history, family history of illnesses, and specific physical complaints. Information about medical illnesses should be gathered from the patient, the referring physician, and the family, if necessary.

Information about previous episodes of illness may provide valuable clues about the nature of the present disorder. For example, if the present disorder is distinctly delusional, the patient has a history of several similar episodes, and each responded promptly to diverse forms of treatment, the possibility of substance-induced psychotic disorder is strongly suggested. To pursue this lead, the psychiatrist should order a drug screen. The history of a surgical procedure may also be useful; for instance, a thyroidectomy suggests hypothyroidism as the cause of depression.

Depression is a side effect of several medications prescribed for hypertension. Medication taken in a therapeutic dosage occasionally reaches high blood concentrations. Digitalis intoxication, for example, may occur under such circumstances and result in impaired mental functioning. Proprietary drugs may cause or contribute to an anticholinergic delirium. Therefore, the psychiatrist must inquire about over-the-counter remedies,

as well as prescribed medications. A history of herbal intake and alternative therapy use is essential in view of their increased use.

An occupational history may also provide essential information. Exposure to mercury may result in complaints suggesting a psychosis, and exposure to lead, as in smelting, may produce a cognitive disorder. The latter clinical picture can also result from imbibing "moonshine" whiskey with a high lead content.

In eliciting information about specific symptoms, the psychiatrist brings medical and psychological knowledge into full play. For example, the psychiatrist should elicit sufficient information from the patient complaining of headache to predict, with considerable certainty, whether the pain is the result of intracranial disease. Also, the psychiatrist should be able to recognize that the pain in the right shoulder of a hypochondriacal patient with abdominal discomfort may be the classic referred pain of gallbladder disease.

REVIEW OF SYSTEMS

An inventory by systems should follow the open-ended inquiry. The review may be organized according to organ systems (for example, liver, pancreas), functional systems (for example, gastrointestinal), or a combination of the two, as in the following sections. In all cases, the review should be comprehensive and thorough. Even if a psychiatric component is suspected, a complete workup is still indicated.

Head

Many patients give a history of headache; its duration, frequency, character, location, and severity should be ascertained. Headaches often result from substance abuse, including alcohol, nicotine, and caffeine. Vascular (migraine) headaches are precipitated by stress. Temporal arteritis causes unilateral throbbing headaches and may lead to blindness. Brain tumors are associated with headaches as a result of increases in intracranial pressure; a history of head injury may result in subdural hematoma and in boxers can cause progressive dementia with extrapyramidal symptoms. The headache of subarachnoid hemorrhage is sudden, severe, and associated with changes in the sensorium. Normal pressure hydrocephalus may follow a head injury or encephalitis and may be associated with dementia, shuffling gait, and urinary incontinence. Dizziness occurs in up

Table 3–1
Approach to the Differentiation of Dizziness Subtypes

Dizziness Subtype	Type of Sensation	Temporal Characteristics	Other Specifications
Vertigo	A feeling that one or one's surroundings are moving (typically, spinning)	Episodic vertigo occurs in attacks that last seconds to days Continuous vertigo is present all or most of the time for at least a week	Descriptions of episodic vertigo should include the characteristics, duration, and date of the first episode; length of episodes; and exacerbating factors
Presyncope	A lightheaded, faint feeling, as though one were about to pass out	Typically occurs in episodes lasting seconds to hours	The following questions should be answered: (1) Has syncope ever occurred during an episode? (2) Do episodes occur only when the patient is upright, or do they occur in other positions? (3) Are episodes associated with palpitations, medication, meals, bathing, dyspnea, or chest discomfort?
Disequilibrium	A sense of unsteadiness that is (1) primarily felt in the lower extremities, (2) most prominent when standing or walking, and (3) relieved by sitting or lying down	Usually present, although it may fluctuate in intensity	Identify whether symptom occurs in isolation or accompanies another dizziness subtype; describe exacerbating factors
Other dizziness: anxiety-related, ocular, tilting environment, other	A feeling not covered by the above definitions. May include swimming or floating sensations, vague lightheadedness, or feelings of dissociation. May be difficult for the patient to describe	Usually present all or most of the time for days or weeks, sometimes years	The following questions should be answered: (1) Is dizziness associated with anxiety or hyperventilation? (2) Was change in vision connected with dizziness onset? (3) Is dizziness a sensation that the environment is tilting sideways (suggests an otolith problem)?

From Sloane PD, Coeytaux RR, Beck RS, Dallara J. Dizziness. State of the science. *Ann Intern Med.* 2001;134:825.

to 30 percent of persons, and determining its etiology is challenging (Table 3–1).

Eye, Ear, Nose, and Throat

Visual acuity, diplopia, hearing problems, tinnitus, glossitis, and bad taste are covered in this area. A patient taking antipsychotics who gives a history of twitching about the mouth or disturbing movements of the tongue may be in the early and potentially reversible stage of tardive dyskinesia. Impaired vision may occur with thioridazine (Mellaril) in high dosages (over 800 mg a day). A history of glaucoma contraindicates drugs with anticholinergic effects. Aphonia may be hysterical in nature. The late stage of cocaine abuse can result in perforations of the nasal septum and difficulty in breathing. A transitory episode of diplopia may herald multiple sclerosis. Delusional disorder is more common in hearing-impaired people than in those with normal hearing.

Respiratory System

Cough, asthma, pleurisy, hemoptysis, dyspnea, and orthopnea are considered in this section. Hyperventilation is suggested if the patient's symptoms include all or a few of the following: onset at rest, sighing respirations, apprehension, anxiety, depersonalization, palpitations, inability to swallow, numbness of the feet and hands, and carpopedal spasm. Dyspnea and breathlessness may occur in depression. In pulmonary or obstructive airway disease, the onset of symptoms is usually insidious, whereas in depression, it is sudden. In depression, breathlessness is experienced at rest, shows little change with exertion,

and may fluctuate within a matter of minutes; the onset of breathlessness coincides with the onset of a mood disorder and is often accompanied by attacks of dizziness, sweating, palpitations, and paresthesias.

In obstructive airway disease, patients with the most advanced respiratory incapacity experience breathlessness at rest. Most striking and of greatest assistance in making a differential diagnosis is the emphasis placed on the difficulty in inspiration experienced by patients with depression and on the difficulty in expiration experienced by patients with pulmonary disease. Bronchial asthma has sometimes been associated with childhood histories of extreme dependence on the mother. Patients with bronchospasm should not receive propranolol (Inderal) because it may block catecholamine-induced bronchodilation; propranolol is specifically contraindicated for patients with bronchial asthma because epinephrine given to such patients in an emergency will not be effective. Patients taking ACE inhibitors (angiotensin-converting enzyme) may develop a dry cough as a side effect of the drug.

Cardiovascular System

Tachycardia, palpitations, and cardiac arrhythmia are among the most common signs of anxiety about which the patient may complain. Pheochromocytoma usually produces symptoms that mimic anxiety disorders, such as rapid heartbeat, tremors, and pallor. Increased urinary catecholamines are diagnostic of pheochromocytoma. Patients taking guanethidine (Micronase) for hypertension should not receive tricyclic drugs, which reduce or eliminate the antihypertensive effect of guanethidine. A history of hypertension may preclude the use of monoamine oxidase inhibitors (MAOIs) because of the risk of a hypertensive crisis if such hypertensive patients inadvertently ingest foods high in tyramine. Patients with a suspected cardiac disease should have an electrocardiogram before tricyclics or lithium (Eskalith) is prescribed. A history of substernal pain should be evaluated, and the clinician should keep in mind that psychological stress can precipitate angina-type chest pain in the presence of normal coronary arteries. Patients taking opioids should never receive monoamine oxidase inhibitors, a combination that can cause cardiovascular collapse.

Gastrointestinal System

This area covers such topics as appetite, distress before or after meals, food preferences, diarrhea, vomiting, constipation, laxative use, and abdominal pain. A history of weight loss is common in depressive disorders; but depression may accompany the weight loss caused by ulcerative colitis, regional enteritis, and cancer. Anorexia nervosa is accompanied by severe weight loss in the presence of normal appetite. Avoidance of certain foods may be a phobic phenomenon or part of an obsessive ritual. Laxative abuse and induced vomiting are common in bulimia nervosa. Constipation can be caused by opioid dependence and by psychotropic drugs with anticholinergic side effects. Cocaine or amphetamine abuse causes a loss of appetite and weight loss. Weight gain can occur under stress or in association with atypical depression. Polyphagia, polyuria, and polydipsia are the triad of diabetes mellitus. Polyuria, polydipsia, and diarrhea are signs of lithium toxicity.

Genitourinary System

Urinary frequency, nocturia, pain or burning on urination, and changes in the size and force of the stream are some of the signs and symptoms in this area. Anticholinergic side effects associated with antipsychotics and tricyclic drugs may cause urinary retention in men with prostate hypertrophy. Erectile difficulty and retarded ejaculation are also common side effects of these drugs, and retrograde ejaculation occurs with thioridazine. A baseline level of sexual responsiveness before using pharmacological agents should be obtained. A history of sexually transmitted diseases—for example, gonorrheal discharge, chancre, herpes, and pubic lice—may indicate sexual promiscuity or unsafe sexual practices. In some cases, the first symptom of acquired immune deficiency syndrome is the gradual onset of mental confusion leading to dementia. Incontinence should be evaluated carefully, and if it persists, further investigation for more extensive disease should include a workup for human immunodeficiency virus infection (HIV). Drugs with anticholinergic side effects should be avoided in patients with prostatism.

Menstrual History

A menstrual history should include the age of the onset of menarche and menopause; the interval, regularity, duration, and amount of flow of periods; irregular bleeding; dysmenorrhea; and abortions. Amenorrhea is characteristic of anorexia nervosa and also occurs in women who are psychologically stressed. Women who are afraid of becoming pregnant or who have a wish to be pregnant may have delayed periods. Pseudocyesis is false pregnancy with complete cessation of the menses. Peri-menstrual mood changes (for example, irritability, depression, and dysphoria) should be noted. Painful menstruation can result from uterine disease (for example, myomata), from psychological conflicts about the menses, or from a combination of the two. Some women report a premenstrual increase in sexual desire. The emotional distress associated with abortion should be explored since it can be mild or severe.

GENERAL OBSERVATION

An important part of the medical examination is subsumed under the broad heading of general observation—visual, auditory, and olfactory. Such nonverbal clues as posture, facial expression, and mannerisms should also be noted.

Vision

Scrutiny of the patient begins at the first encounter. When the patient goes from the waiting room to the interview room, the psychiatrist should observe the patient's gait. Is the patient unsteady? Ataxia suggests diffuse brain disease, alcohol or other substance intoxication, chorea, spinocerebellar degeneration, weakness based on a debilitating process, and an underlying disorder, such as myotonic dystrophy. Does the patient walk without the usual associated arm movements and turn in a rigid fashion, like a toy soldier, as is seen in early Parkinson's disease? Does the patient have an asymmetry of gait, such as turning one foot outward, dragging a leg, or not swinging one arm, suggesting a focal brain lesion?

As soon as the patient is seated, the psychiatrist should direct attention to grooming. Is the patient's hair combed, are the nails clean, and are the teeth brushed? Has clothing been chosen with care, and is it appropriate? Although inattention to dress and hygiene is common in mental disorders—in particular, depressive disorders—it is also a hallmark of cognitive disorders. Lapses—such as mismatching socks, stockings, or shoes—may suggest a cognitive disorder.

The patient's posture and automatic movements or the lack of them should be noted. A stooped, flexed posture with a paucity of automatic movements may be due to Parkinson's disease, diffuse cerebral hemispheric disease, or the side effects of antipsychotics. An unusual tilt of the head may be adopted to avoid eye contact, but it can also result from diplopia, a visual field defect, or focal cerebellar dysfunction. Frequent quick, purposeless movements are characteristic of anxiety disorders, but they are equally characteristic of chorea and hyperthyroidism. Tremors, although commonly seen in anxiety disorders, may point to Parkinson's disease, essential tremor, or side effects of psychotropic medication. Patients with essential tremor sometimes seek psychiatric treatment because they believe the tremor must be due to unrecognized fear or anxiety, as others often suggest. Unilateral paucity or excess of movement suggests focal brain disease.

The patient's appearance is then scrutinized to assess general health. Does the patient appear to be robust, or is there a sense of ill health? Does looseness of clothing indicate recent weight loss? Is the patient short of breath or coughing? Does the patient's general physiognomy suggest a specific disease? Men with Klinefelter's syndrome have a feminine fat distribution and lack the development of secondary male sex characteristics. Acromegaly is usually immediately recognizable by the large head and jaw.

What is the patient's nutritional status? Recent weight loss, although often seen in depressive disorders and schizophrenia, may be due to gastrointestinal disease, diffuse carcinomatosis, Addison's disease, hyperthyroidism, and many other somatic disorders. Obesity may result from either emotional distress or organic disease. Moon facies, truncal obesity, and buffalo hump are striking findings in Cushing's syndrome. The puffy, bloated appearance seen in hypothyroidism and the massive obesity and periodic respiration seen in Pickwickian syndrome are easily recognized in patients referred for psychiatric help.

The skin frequently provides valuable information. The yellow discoloration of hepatic dysfunction and the pallor of anemia are reasonably distinctive. Intense reddening may be due to carbon monoxide poisoning or to photosensitivity resulting from porphyria or phenothiazines. Eruptions may be manifestations of such disorders as systemic lupus erythematosus, tuberous sclerosis with adenoma sebaceum, and sensitivity to drugs. A dusky purplish cast to the face, plus telangiectasia, is almost pathognomonic of alcohol abuse.

> A young woman, complaining of depression and listlessness, mentioned in an off-hand manner that she had a rash. An on-the-spot examination of her skin revealed petechial hemorrhages on both arms and both legs. Further inquiry disclosed information about bleeding from several sites. Her blood platelet count was 4,000/mm³. The diagnosis was thrombocytopenia.

Careful observation may reveal clues that lead to the correct diagnosis in patients who create their own skin lesions. For example, the location and shape of the lesions and the time of their appearance may be characteristic of dermatitis factitia.

The patient's face and head should be scanned for evidence of disease. Premature whitening of the hair occurs in pernicious anemia, and thinning and coarseness of the hair occur in myxedema. Pupillary changes are produced by various drugs—constriction by opioids and dilation by anticholinergic agents and hallucinogens. The combination of dilated and fixed pupils and dry skin and mucous membranes should immediately suggest the likelihood of atropine use or atropine-like toxicity. Diffusion of the conjunctiva suggests alcohol abuse, cannabis abuse, or obstruction of the superior vena cava. Flattening of the nasolabial fold on one side or weakness of one side of the face—as manifested in speaking, smiling, and grimacing—may be the result of focal dysfunction of the contralateral cerebral hemisphere.

The patient's state of alertness and responsiveness should be carefully evaluated. Drowsiness and inattentiveness may be due to a psychological problem, but they are more likely to result from an organic brain dysfunction, whether secondary to an intrinsic brain disease or to an exogenous factor, such as substance intoxication.

Hearing

Listening intently is just as important as looking intently for evidence of somatic disorders. Slowed speech is characteristic not only of depression but also of diffuse brain dysfunction and subcortical dysfunction; unusually rapid speech is characteristic not only of manic episodes and anxiety disorders but also of hyperthyroidism. A weak voice with monotony of tone may be a clue to Parkinson's disease in patients who complain mainly of depression. A slow, low-pitched, hoarse voice should suggest the possibility of hypothyroidism; this voice quality has been described as sounding like a drowsy, slightly intoxicated person with a bad cold and a plum in the mouth.

Difficulty in initiating speech may be due to anxiety or stuttering or may indicate Parkinson's disease or aphasia. Easy fatigability of speech may sometimes be a manifestation of an emotional problem, but it is also characteristic of myasthenia gravis. Patients with these complaints are likely to be seen by a psychiatrist before the correct diagnosis is made.

Word production, as well as the quality of speech, is important. When words are mispronounced or incorrect words are used, the possibility of aphasia caused by a lesion of the dominant hemisphere should be entertained. The same possibility exists when the patient perseverates, has trouble finding a name or a word, or describes an object or an event in an indirect fashion (paraphasia). When not consonant with patients' socioeconomic and educational levels, coarseness, profanity, or inappropriate disclosures may indicate loss of inhibition caused by dementia.

Smell

Much less is learned through the sense of smell than through the senses of sight and hearing, but smell occasionally provides useful information. The unpleasant odor of a patient who fails to bathe suggests a cognitive disorder or a depressive disorder. The odor of alcohol or of substances used to hide it is revealing in a patient who attempts to conceal a drinking problem. Occasionally, a uriniferous odor calls attention to bladder dysfunction secondary to a nervous system disease. Characteristic odors are also noted in patients with diabetic acidosis, uremia, and hepatic coma. Precocious puberty can be associated with the smell of adult sweat produced by mature apocrine glands.

PHYSICAL EXAMINATION

Patient Selection

The nature of the patient's complaints is critical to determine whether a complete physical examination is required. Complaints fall into the three categories of body, mind, and social interactions.

Bodily symptoms—such as headaches and palpitations—call for a thorough medical examination to determine what part, if any, somatic processes play in causing the distress. The same can be said for mental symptoms—such as depression, anxiety, hallucinations, and persecutory delusions—that can be expressions of somatic processes. If the problem is clearly limited to the social sphere—as in long-standing difficulties in interactions with teachers, employers, parents, or a spouse—there may be no special indication for a physical examination.

Psychological Factors

Even a routine physical examination may evoke adverse reactions; instruments, procedures, and the examining room may be frightening. A simple running account of what is being done can prevent much needless anxiety. Moreover, if the patient is consistently forewarned of what will be done, the dread of being suddenly and painfully surprised recedes. Comments such as, "There's nothing to this" and "You don't have to be afraid because this won't hurt" leave the patient in the dark and are much less reassuring than a few words about what actually will be done.

Although the physical examination is likely to engender or intensify a reaction of anxiety, it can also stir up sexual feelings. Some women with fears or fantasies of being seduced may misinterpret an ordinary movement in the physical examination as a sexual advance. Similarly, a delusional man with homosexual fears may perceive a rectal examination as a sexual attack. Lingering over the examination of a particular organ because an unusual but normal variation has aroused the physician's scientific curiosity is likely to raise concern in the patient that a serious pathological process has been discovered. Such a reaction in an anxious or hypochondriacal patient may be profound.

The physical examination occasionally serves a psychotherapeutic function. An anxious patient may be relieved to learn that, in spite of troublesome symptoms, there is no evidence of the serious illness that is feared. The young person who complains of chest pain and is certain that the pain heralds a heart attack can usually be reassured by the report of normal findings after a physical examination and electrocardiogram. The reassurance relieves only the worry occasioned by the immediate episode, however. Unless psychiatric treatment succeeds in dealing with the determinants of the reaction, recurrent episodes are likely.

Sending a patient who has a deeply rooted fear of malignancy for still another test that is intended to be reassuring is usually unrewarding. Some patients may have a false fixed belief that a disorder is present.

> In spite of repeated examinations, a patient who was a physician was convinced that he had carcinoma of the pharynx. A colleague, in an effort to produce positive proof, performed a biopsy of the area of complaint. When the patient was shown a microscopic section of normal tissue, he immediately declared that the normal section had been substituted for one showing malignant cells.

During the performance of the physical examination, an observant physician may note indications of emotional distress. For instance, during genital examinations, a patient's behavior may reveal information about sexual attitudes and problems, and these reactions may be used later to open this area for exploration.

Timing of the Physical Examination

Circumstances occasionally make it desirable or necessary to defer a complete medical assessment. For example, a delusional or manic patient may be combative or resistive or both. In this instance, a medical history should be elicited from a family member if possible, but, unless there is a pressing reason to proceed with the examination, it should be deferred until the patient is tractable.

For psychological reasons, it may be ill advised to recommend a medical assessment at the time of an initial office visit. In view of today's increased sensitivity and openness about sex-

ual matters and a proneness to turn quickly to psychiatric help, young men may complain about their failure to consummate their first coital attempt. After taking a detailed history, the psychiatrist may conclude that the failure was due to situational anxiety. If so, neither a physical examination nor psychotherapy should be recommended; they would have the undesirable effect of reinforcing the notion of pathology. Should the problem be recurrent, further evaluation would be warranted.

Neurological Examination

If the psychiatrist suspects that the patient has an underlying somatic disorder, such as diabetes mellitus or Cushing's syndrome, referral is usually made to a medical physician for diagnosis and treatment. The situation is different when a cognitive disorder is suspected. The psychiatrist often chooses to assume responsibility in these cases. At some point, however, a thorough neurological evaluation may be indicated.

During the history-taking process in such cases, the patient's level of awareness, attentiveness to the details of the examination, understanding, facial expression, speech, posture, and gait are noted. It is also assumed that a thorough mental status examination will be performed. The neurological examination is carried out with two objectives in mind: to elicit signs pointing to focal, circumscribed cerebral dysfunction and to elicit signs suggesting diffuse, bilateral cerebral disease. The first objective is met by the routine neurological examination, which is designed primarily to reveal asymmetries in the motor, perceptual, and reflex functions of the two sides of the body caused by focal hemispheric disease. The second objective is met by seeking to elicit signs that have been attributed to diffuse brain dysfunction and to frontal lobe disease. These signs include the sucking, snout, palmomental, and grasp reflexes and the persistence of the glabella tap response. Regrettably, with the exception of the grasp reflex, such signs do not correlate strongly with the presence of underlying brain pathology.

Other Findings

Psychiatrists should be able to evaluate the significance of findings uncovered by consultants. With a patient who complains of a lump in the throat (globus hystericus) and who is found on examination to have hypertrophied lymphoid tissue, it is tempting to wonder about a cause-and-effect relation. How can a clinician be sure that the finding is not incidental? Has the patient been known to have hypertrophied lymphoid tissue at a time when no complaint was made? Do many people with hypertrophied lymphoid tissue never experience the sensation of a lump in the throat?

With a patient with multiple sclerosis who complains of an inability to walk but, on neurological examination, has only mild spasticity and a unilateral Babinski sign, it is tempting to ascribe the symptom to the neurological disorder; but the neurological abnormality may be aggravated by emotional distress. The same holds true for a patient with profound dementia in whom a small frontal meningioma is seen on a computed tomography scan. Dementia is not always correlated to the findings. Significant brain atrophy could cause very mild dementia, and minimal brain atrophy could cause significant dementia.

A lesion is often found that can account for a symptom, but the psychiatrist should make every effort to separate an incidental finding from a causative one, to separate a lesion merely found in the area of the symptom from a lesion producing the symptom.

PATIENTS UNDERGOING PSYCHIATRIC TREATMENT

While patients are being treated for psychiatric disorders, psychiatrists should be alert to the possibility of intercurrent illnesses that call for diagnostic studies. Patients in psychotherapy, particularly those in psychoanalysis, may be all too willing to ascribe their new symptoms to emotional causes. Attention should be given to the possible use of denial, especially if the symptoms seem to be unrelated to the conflicts currently in focus.

> At a time of increased psychological stress, a patient had urinary frequency, which she ascribed to her current situation. Only after much urging did she agree to see a urologist, who diagnosed and treated her cystitis.

Not only may patients in psychotherapy be prone to attribute new symptoms to emotional causes, but sometimes their therapists do so as well. The danger of providing psychodynamic explanations for physical symptoms is ever present.

> A disturbed young woman in a psychiatric unit, who would curl up in a clothes basket and remain there for long periods, was described as regressing and assuming the fetal position. Later, when the diagnosis of meningoencephalitis was confirmed, it seemed that a better explanation for her behavior was the need to relieve pressure on nerve roots.

Symptoms such as drowsiness and dizziness and signs such as a skin eruption and a gait disturbance, common side effects of psychotropic medication, call for a medical reevaluation if the patient fails to respond in a reasonable time to changes in the dosage or the kind of medication prescribed. If patients who are receiving tricyclic or antipsychotic drugs complain of blurred vision (usually an anticholinergic side effect), and if the condition does not recede with a reduction in dosage or a change in medication, they should be evaluated to rule out other causes. In one case, the diagnosis proved to be *Toxoplasma* chorioretinitis. The absence of other anticholinergic side effects, such as a dry mouth and constipation, is an additional clue alerting the psychiatrist to the possibility of a concomitant medical illness.

Early in an illness, there may be few, if any, positive physical or laboratory results. In such instances, especially if the evidence of psychic trauma or emotional conflicts is glaring, all symptoms are likely to be regarded as psychosocial in origin and new symptoms also seen in this light. Indications for repeating portions of the medical workup may be missed unless the psychiatrist is alert to clues suggesting that some symptoms do not fit the original diagnosis and point, instead, to a medical illness. Occasionally, a patient with an acute illness, such as encephalitis, is hospitalized with the diagnosis of schizophrenia; or a patient with a subacute illness, such as carcinoma of the pancreas, is treated in a private office or clinic with the diagnosis of a depressive disorder.

Although it may not be possible to make the correct diagnosis at the time of the initial psychiatric evaluation, continued surveillance and attention to clinical details usually provide clues leading to the recognition of the cause.

The likelihood of intercurrent illness is greater with some psychiatric disorders than with others. Substance abusers, for example, because of their life patterns, are susceptible to infection and are likely to suffer from the adverse effects of trauma, dietary deficiencies, and poor hygiene. Depression decreases the immune response.

When somatic and psychological dysfunctions are known to coexist, the psychiatrist should be thoroughly conversant with the patient's medical status. In cases of cardiac decompensation, peripheral neuropathy, and other disabling disorders, the nature and the degree of the impairment that can be attributed to the physical disorder should be assessed. It is important to answer the question: Does the patient exploit a disability, or is it ignored or denied with resultant overexertion? To answer this question, the psychiatrist must assess the patient's capabilities and limitations, rather than make sweeping judgments based on a diagnostic label.

Special vigilance about medical status is required for some patients in treatment for somatoform and eating disorders. Such is the case for patients with ulcerative colitis who are bleeding profusely and for patients with anorexia nervosa who are losing appreciable weight. These disorders can become life threatening.

IMPORTANCE OF MEDICAL ILLNESS

Numerous articles have called attention to the need for thorough medical screening of patients seen in psychiatric inpatient services and clinics. (A similar need has been shown to exist for the psychiatric evaluation of patients seen in medical inpatient services and clinics). The concept of *medical clearance* remains ambiguous and has meaning in the context of psychiatric admission or clearance for transfers from different settings or institutions.

Among identified psychiatric patients, anywhere from 24 to 60 percent have been shown to suffer from associated physical disorders. In a survey of 2,090 psychiatric clinic patients, 43 percent were found to have associated physical disorders; of these, almost half the physical disorders had not been diagnosed by the referring sources. (In this study, 69 patients were found to have diabetes mellitus, but only 12 of the cases of diabetes had been diagnosed before referral.)

Expecting all psychiatrists to be experts in internal medicine is unrealistic, but expecting them to recognize or have high suspicion of physical disorders when present is realistic. Moreover, they should make appropriate referrals and collaborate in treating patients who have both physical and mental disorders.

Psychiatric symptoms are nonspecific; they can herald medical as well as psychiatric illness. Moreover, psychiatric symptoms often precede the appearance of definitive medical symptoms. Some psychiatric symptoms—such as visual hallucinations, distortions, and illusions—should call forth a high level of suspicion.

The medical literature abounds with case reports of patients whose disorders were initially considered emotional but ultimately proved to be secondary to medical conditions. The data in most of the reports revealed features pointing toward organicity. Diagnostic errors arose because such features were accorded too little weight.

Laboratory Tests in Psychiatry

Laboratory testing is an integral part of psychiatric assessment and treatment. Compared to other medical specialists, however, psychiatrists depend more on clinical examinations and patients' signs and symptoms than on laboratory tests. For example, no test can establish or rule out a diagnosis of schizophrenia, bipolar I disorder, or major depressive disorder. Nevertheless, advances in neuropsychiatry and biological psychiatry have made laboratory tests more and more useful to psychiatrists as well as to biological researchers.

NEUROENDOCRINE TESTS

Thyroid Function Tests

Several thyroid function tests are available, including tests for thyroxine (T_4) by competitive protein binding (T_4D) and by radioimmunoassay (T_4RIA) involving a specific antigen-antibody reaction. More than 90 percent of T_4 is bound to serum protein and is responsible for thyroid-stimulating hormone (TSH) secretion and for cellular metabolism. Other thyroid measures include the free T_4 index (FT_4I), triiodothyronine uptake, and total serum triiodothyronine measured by radioimmunoassay (T_3RIA). These tests are used to rule out hypothyroidism, which can appear with symptoms of depression. In some studies, up to 10 percent of patients complaining of depression and associated fatigue had incipient hypothyroid disease. Other associated signs and symptoms common to both depression and hypothyroidism include weakness, stiffness, poor appetite, constipation, menstrual irregularities, slowed speech, apathy, impaired memory, and even hallucinations and delusions. Lithium can cause hypothyroidism and, more rarely, hyperthyroidism. Table 4–1 outlines the suggested monitoring of thyroid function for patients taking lithium. Neonatal hypothyroidism results in mental retardation and is preventable if the diagnosis is made at birth.

The thyrotropin-releasing hormone (TRH) stimulation test is indicated in patients whose marginally abnormal thyroid test results suggest subclinical hypothyroidism, which may account for clinical depression. The test is also used for patients with possible lithium-induced hypothyroidism. The procedure entails an intravenous (IV) injection of 500 mg of TRH, which produces a sharp rise in serum TSH when measured at 15, 30, 60, and 90 minutes. An increase in serum TSH of from 5 to 25 μIU/mL above the baseline is normal. An increase of less than 7 μIU/mL is considered a blunted response, which may correlate with a diagnosis of a depressive disorder. Eight percent of all patients with depressive disorders have some thyroid illness.

Dexamethasone-Suppression Test

Dexamethasone is a long-acting synthetic glucocorticoid with a long half-life. Approximately 1 mg of dexamethasone is equivalent to 25 mg of cortisol. The dexamethasone-suppression test (DST) is used to help confirm a diagnostic impression of major depressive disorder.

Procedure

The patient is given 1 mg of dexamethasone by mouth at 11 p.m., and plasma cortisol is measured at 8 a.m., 4 p.m., and 11 p.m. Plasma cortisol above 5 μg/dL (known as *nonsuppression*) is considered abnormal (that is, positive). Suppression of cortisol indicates that the hypothalamic-adrenal-pituitary axis is functioning properly. Since the 1930s, dysfunction of this axis has been known to be associated with stress.

The DST can be used to follow a depressed person's response to treatment. Normalization of the DST, however, is not an indication to stop antidepressant treatment, because the DST may normalize before the depression resolves.

Reliability

The problems associated with the DST include varying reports of sensitivity and specificity. False-positive and false-negative results are common. The sensitivity of the DST is considered to be 45 percent in major depressive disorders and 70 percent in major depressive episodes with psychotic features. The specificity is 90 percent compared with controls and 77 percent compared with other psychiatric diagnoses. Some evidence indicates that patients with a positive DST result (especially 10 μg/dL) will have a good response to somatic treatment, such as electroconvulsive therapy or cyclic antidepressant therapy.

Other Endocrine Tests

Many other hormones affect behavior. Exogenous hormonal administration has been shown to affect behavior, and known endocrine diseases have been associated mental disorders.

In addition to thyroid hormones, these hormones include the anterior pituitary hormone prolactin, growth hormone, somatostatin, gonadotrophin-releasing hormone, and the sex steroids—luteinizing hormone, follicle-stimulating hormone, testosterone, and estrogen. Melatonin from the pineal gland has been implicated in seasonal affective disorder (called *mood disorder with seasonal pattern* in the fourth revised edition of the *Diagnostic and Statistical Manual of Mental Disorders* [DSM-IV-TR]).

Symptoms of anxiety or depression may be explained in some patients on the basis of unspecified changes in endocrine function or homeostasis.

Table 4–1
Thyroid Monitoring for Patients Taking Lithium

Evaluation	Before Treatment	Repeat at 6 Months	Repeat Yearly
Medical			
1. Careful medical and family history to detect family history of thyroid disease	x		
2. Review of symptoms of hyperthyroidism and hypothyroidism	x	x	x
3. Physical examination, including palpation of thyroid	x		x
Laboratory			
T$_3$RU	x		x
T$_4$RIA	x		x
T$_2$I (free thyroxine index)	x		x
TSH	x	x	x
Antithyroid antibodies	x		x

Reprinted with permission from MacKinnon RA, Yudofsky SC. *Principles of the Psychiatric Evaluation.* Philadelphia: JB Lippincott; 1991:104.

Catecholamines

The level of serotonin metabolite 5-hydroxyindoleacetic acid (5-HIAA) is elevated in the urine of patients with carcinoid tumors. Elevated levels are noted at times in patients who take phenothiazine medication and in those who eat foods high in serotonin (for example, walnuts, bananas, and avocados). The amount of 5-HIAA in cerebrospinal fluid (CSF) is low in some people who are in a suicidal depression and in postmortem studies of those who have committed suicide in particularly violent ways. Low CSF 5-HIAA levels are associated with violence in general. Norepinephrine and its metabolic products—metanephrine, normetanephrine, and vanillylmandelic acid—can be measured in the urine, the blood, and the plasma. Plasma catecholamine levels are markedly elevated in pheochromocytoma, which is associated with anxiety, agitation, and hypertension. Some cases of chronic anxiety may share elevated blood norepinephrine and epinephrine levels. Some depressed patients have a low urinary norepinephrine to epinephrine ratio.

High levels of urinary norepinephrine and epinephrine have been found in some patients with posttraumatic stress disorder. The norepinephrine metabolic 3-methoxy-4-hydroxyphenylglycol level is decreased in patients with severe depressive disorders, especially in those patients who attempt suicide.

Renal Function Tests

Creatinine clearance detects early kidney damage and can be serially monitored to follow the course of renal disease. Blood urea nitrogen (BUN) is also elevated in renal disease and is excreted by way of the kidneys; the serum BUN and creatinine are monitored in patients taking lithium (Eskalith). If the serum BUN or creatinine is abnormal, the patient's 2-hour creatinine clearance and, ultimately, the 24-hour creatinine clearance are

Table 4–2
Other Laboratory Testing for Patients Taking Lithium

Test	Frequency
1. Complete blood count	Before treatment and yearly
2. Serum electrolytes	Before treatment and yearly
3. Fasting blood glucose	Before treatment and yearly
4. Electrocardiogram	Before treatment and yearly
5. Pregnancy testing for women of childbearing age[a]	Before treatment

[a]Test more frequently when compliance with treatment plan is uncertain.
Reprinted with permission from MacKinnon RA, Yudofsky SC. *Principles of the Psychiatric Evaluation.* Philadelphia: JB Lippincott; 1991:106.

tested. Table 4–2 summarizes other laboratory testing for patients taking lithium.

Liver Function Tests

Total bilirubin and direct bilirubin values are elevated in hepatocellular injury and intrahepatic bile stasis, which can occur with phenothiazine or tricyclic medication and with alcohol and other substance abuse. Certain drugs—for example, phenobarbital (Luminal)—may decrease serum bilirubin concentration. Liver damage or disease, which is reflected by abnormal findings in liver function tests (LFTs), may manifest with signs and symptoms of a cognitive disorder, including disorientation and delirium. Impaired hepatic function may increase the elimination half-lives of certain drugs, including some benzodiazepines, so that the drug may stay in a patient's system longer than it would under normal circumstances. LFTs must be monitored routinely when using certain drugs, such as carbamazepine (Tegretol) and valproate (Depakene).

BLOOD TEST FOR SEXUALLY TRANSMITTED DISEASES

The Venereal Disease Research Laboratory (VDRL) test is used as a screening test for syphilis. If positive, the result is confirmed by using the specific fluorescent treponemal antibody-absorption test (FTA-ABS test), in which the spirochete *Treponema pallidum* is used as the antigen. Central nervous system VDRL is measured in patients with suspected neurosyphilis. A positive human immunodeficiency virus test result indicates that a person has been exposed to infection with the virus that causes acquired immune deficiency syndrome.

TESTS RELATED TO PSYCHOTROPIC DRUGS

In caring for patients receiving psychotropic medication, there is a trend to take regular measurements of their plasma levels of the prescribed drug. For some drugs, such as lithium, the monitoring is essential; for other drugs, such as antipsychotics, it is mainly of academic or research interest. A clinician need not practice defensive medicine by insisting that all patients receiving psychotropic drugs have blood levels taken for medicolegal purposes. The current status of psychopharmacological treatment is such that a psychiatrist's clinical judgment and experience, except in rare instances, is a better indication of a drug's therapeutic efficacy than is a plasma-level determination. Moreover, the reliance on plasma levels cannot replace clinical skills and the need to maintain the humanitarian aspects of patient care. The major classes of drugs and the suggested guidelines are outlined in the following discussion.

Benzodiazepines

No special tests are needed for patients taking benzodiazepines. Among the benzodiazepines metabolized in the liver by oxidation, impaired hepatic function increases the half-life. Baseline LFTs are indicated in patients with suspected liver damage. Urine testing for benzodiazepines is used routinely in cases of substance abuse.

Antipsychotics

No special tests are needed, although it is good to obtain baseline values for liver function and a complete blood cell count. Antipsychotics are metabolized primarily in the liver, with metabolites excreted primarily in urine. Many metabolites are active. Peak plasma concentration usually is reached 2 to 3 hours after an oral dose. Elimination half-life is 12 to 30 hours but may be much longer. Steady state requires at least 1 week at a constant dose (months at a constant dose of depot antipsychotics). With the exception of clozapine (Clozaril), all antipsychotics acutely cause an elevation in serum prolactin (secondary to tuberoinfundibular activity). A normal prolactin level often indicates either noncompliance or nonabsorption. Side effects include leukocytosis, leukopenia, impaired platelet function, mild anemia (both aplastic and hemolytic), and agranulocytosis. Bone marrow and blood element side effects can occur abruptly, even when the dosage has remained constant. Low-potency antipsychotics are most likely to cause agranulocytosis, which is the most common bone marrow side effect. These agents may cause hepatocellular injury and intrahepatic biliary stasis (indicated by elevated total and direct bilirubin and elevated transaminases). They also can cause electrocardiographic changes (not as frequently as with tricyclic antidepressants), including a prolonged QT interval; flattened, inverted, or bifid T waves; and U waves. Dose–plasma concentration relations differ widely among patients.

Clozapine.
Because of the risk of agranulocytosis (1 to 2 percent), patients who are being treated with clozapine must have a baseline white blood cell (WBC) and differential count before the initiation of treatment, a WBC count every week throughout treatment, and a WBC count for 4 weeks after the discontinuation of clozapine. Physicians and pharmacists who provide clozapine are required to be registered through the Clozaril National Registry (1-800-448-5938).

Tricyclic and Tetracyclic Drugs

An electrocardiogram (ECG) should be given before starting a regimen of cyclic drugs to assess for conduction delays, which may lead to heart blocks at therapeutic levels. Some clinicians believe that all patients receiving prolonged cyclic drug therapy should have an annual ECG. At therapeutic levels, the drugs suppress arrhythmias through a quinidine-like effect.

Blood levels should be tested routinely when using imipramine (Tofranil), desipramine (Norpramin), or nortriptyline (Pamelor) in the treatment of depressive disorders. Taking blood levels may also be of use in patients with a poor response at normal dosage ranges and in high-risk patients for whom there is an urgent need to know whether a therapeutic or toxic plasma level of the drug has been reached. Blood level tests should also include the measurement of active metabolites (for example, imipramine is converted to desipramine, amitriptyline [Elavil] to nortriptyline). Some characteristics of tricyclic drug plasma levels are described as follows.

Imipramine (Tofranil).
The percentage of favorable responses to imipramine correlates with plasma levels in a linear manner between 200 and 250 ng/mL, but some patients may respond at a lower level. At levels that exceed 250 ng/mL, there is no improved favorable response, and side effects increase.

Nortriptyline (Pamelor).
The therapeutic window (the range within which a drug is most effective) of nortriptyline is between 50 and 150 ng/mL. There is a decreased response rate at levels greater than 150 ng/mL.

Desipramine (Norpramin).
Levels of desipramine greater than 125 ng/mL correlate with a higher percentage of favorable responses.

Amitriptyline (Elavil).
Different studies have produced conflicting results with regard to blood levels of amitriptyline, but they range from 75 to 175 ng/mL.

Procedure for Determining Blood Concentrations.
The blood specimen should be drawn 10 to 14 hours after the last dose, usually in the morning after a bedtime dose. Patients must be receiving stable daily dosage for at least 5 days for the test to be valid. Some patients are unusually poor metabolizers of cyclic drugs and may have levels as high as 2,000 ng/mL while taking normal dosages and before showing a favorable clinical response. Such patients must be monitored closely for cardiac side effects. Patients with levels greater than 1,000 ng/mL are generally at risk for cardiotoxicity.

Monoamine Oxidase Inhibitors

Patients taking monoamine oxidase inhibitors (MAOIs) are instructed to avoid tyramine-containing foods because of the danger of a potential hypertensive crisis. A baseline normal blood pressure (BP) must be recorded, and the BP must be monitored during treatment. MAOIs may also cause orthostatic hypotension as a direct drug side effect unrelated to diet. Other than their potential for causing elevated BP when taken with certain foods, MAOIs are relatively free of other side effects. A test used both in a research setting and in current clinical practice involves correlating the therapeutic response with the degree of platelet MAO inhibition.

Lithium

Patients receiving lithium should have baseline thyroid function tests, electrolyte monitoring, a WBC, renal function tests (specific gravity, BUN, and creatinine), and a baseline ECG. The rationale for these tests is that lithium can cause renal concentrating defects, hypothyroidism, and leukocytosis; sodium depletion can cause toxic lithium levels; and approximately 95 percent of lithium is excreted in the urine. Lithium has also been shown to cause ECG changes, including various conduction defects.

Lithium is most clearly indicated in the prophylactic treatment of manic episodes (its direct antimanic effect may take up to 2 weeks) and is commonly coupled with antipsychotics for the treatment of acute manic episodes. Lithium itself may also have antipsychotic activity.

Table 4–3
Substances of Abuse That Can Be Tested in Urine

Substance	Length of Time Detected in Urine
Alcohol	7–12 hrs
Amphetamine	48 hrs
Barbiturate	24 hrs (short-acting)
	3 wks (long-acting)
Benzodiazepine	3 days
Cannabis	3 days to 4 wks (depending on use)
Cocaine	6–8 hrs (metabolites 2–4 days)
Codeine	48 hrs
Heroin	36–72 hrs
Methadone	3 days
Methaqualone	7 days
Morphine	48–72 hrs
Phencyclidine (PCP)	8 days
Propoxyphene	6–48 hrs

The maintenance level is 0.6 to 1.2 mEq/L, although acutely manic patients can tolerate up to 1.5 to 1.8 mEq/L. Some patients may respond at lower levels, whereas others may require higher levels. A response below 0.4 mEq/L is probably a placebo. Toxic reactions may occur with levels over 2.0 mEq/L. Regular lithium monitoring is essential; there is a narrow therapeutic range beyond which cardiac problems and central nervous system effects can occur.

Lithium levels are drawn 8 to 12 hours after the last dose, usually in the morning after the bedtime dose. The level should be measured at least twice a week while stabilizing the patient and may be drawn monthly thereafter.

Carbamazepine

A pretreatment complete blood count, including platelet count, should be done. Reticulocyte count and serum iron tests are also desirable. These tests should be repeated weekly during the first 3 months of treatment and monthly thereafter. Carbamazepine can cause aplastic anemia, agranulocytosis, thrombocytopenia, and leukopenia. Because of the minor risk of hepatotoxicity, LFTs should be done every 3 to 6 months. The medication should be discontinued if the patient shows any signs of bone marrow suppression as measured with periodic complete blood counts. The therapeutic level of carbamazepine is 8 to 12 ng/mL, with toxicity most often reached at levels of 15 ng/mL. Most clinicians report that levels as high as 12 ng/mL are hard to achieve.

Valproate

Serum levels of valproic acid (Depakene) and divalproex (Depakote) are therapeutic in the range of 45 to 50 ng/mL. Above 125 ng/mL, side effects occur, including thrombocytopenia. Serum levels should be obtained periodically, and LFTs should be obtained every 6 to 12 months.

Tacrine

Tacrine (Cognex) may cause liver damage. A baseline of liver function should be established, and follow-up serum transaminase levels should be obtained every other week for approximately 5 months. Patients who develop jaundice or who have bilirubin levels higher than 3 mg/dL must be withdrawn from the drug.

Table 4–4
Biochemical Markers in Psychiatry

A. Monoamines
1. Plasma homovanillic acid (pHVA), a major dopamine metabolite, may have value in identifying schizophrenic patients who respond to antipsychotics
2. 3-Methoxy-4-hydroxyphenylglycol (MHPG) is a norepinephrine metabolite
3. 5-Hydroxyindoleacetic acid (5-HIAA) is associated with suicidal behavior, aggression, poor impulse control, and depression; elevated levels may be associated with anxious, obsessional, and inhibited behaviors
B. Alzheimer's disease
1. Apolipoprotein E allele—associated with increased risk for Alzheimer's disease; some asymptomatic middle-aged persons exhibit reduced glucose metabolism on positron emission tomography (PET), similar to findings in Alzheimer's patients
2. Neural thread protein—reported to be increased in patients with Alzheimer's disease; CSF neural thread protein is marketed as a diagnostic test
3. Other potential CSF tests include CSF tau (increased), CSF amyloid (decreased), ratio of CSF albumin to serum albumin (normal in Alzheimer's disease, elevated in vascular dementia), and inflammatory markers (e.g., CSF acute-phase reactive proteins); the gene for the amyloid precursor protein is considered to have possible etiological significance, but further research is needed

PROVOCATION OF PANIC ATTACKS WITH SODIUM LACTATE

Up to 72 percent of patients with panic disorder have a panic attack when administered an IV injection of sodium lactate. Therefore, lactate provocation is used to confirm a diagnosis of panic disorder. Lactate provocation has also been used to trigger flashbacks in patients with posttraumatic stress disorder. Hyperventilation, another known trigger of panic attacks in predisposed persons, is not as sensitive as lactate provocation in inducing panic attacks. Carbon dioxide inhalation also precipitates panic attacks in those so predisposed. Panic attacks triggered by sodium lactate are not inhibited by peripherally acting β-blockers but are inhibited by alprazolam (Xanax) and tricyclic drugs.

DRUG-ASSISTED INTERVIEW

Interviews with amobarbital (Amytal) have both diagnostic and therapeutic indications. Diagnostically, the interviews are helpful in differentiating nonorganic and organic conditions, particularly in patients with symptoms of catatonia, stupor, and muteness. Organic conditions tend to worsen with infusions of amobarbital, but nonorganic or psychogenic conditions tend to get better because of disinhibition, decreased anxiety, or increased relaxation. Therapeutically, amobarbital interviews are useful in disorders of repression and dissociation—for example, in the recovery of memory in psychogenic amnestic disorders and fugue, in the recovery of function in conversion disorder, and in the facilitation of emotional expression in posttraumatic stress disorder. Benzodiazepines can be substituted for amobarbital in the infusion.

LUMBAR PUNCTURE

Lumbar puncture is of use in patients who have a sudden manifestation of new psychiatric symptoms, especially changes in cognition. The clinician should be especially vigilant if there is fever or neurological symptoms such as seizures. Lumbar puncture is of use in diagnosing central nervous system infection (for example, meningitis).

URINE TESTING FOR SUBSTANCE ABUSE

A number of substances may be detected in a patient's urine if the urine is tested within a specific (and variable) period after ingestion. Knowledge of urine substance testing is becoming crucial for practicing physicians in view of the controversial issue of mandatory or random substance testing. Table 4–3 provides a summary of substances of abuse that can be tested in urine.

Laboratory tests are also used in the detection of substances that may be contributing to cognitive disorders.

Biochemical Markers

Many potential biochemical markers, including neurotransmitters and their metabolites, may help in the diagnosis and treatment of psychiatric disorders. Research in this area is still evolving. Table 4–4 summarizes some new developments.

Signs and Symptoms in Psychiatry

The language of psychiatry is precise, which allows clinicians to reliably articulate their observations. This facilitates accurate diagnosis, which informs effective treatment. Accuracy in language enables psychiatrists and other clinicians to communicate fruitfully, not only with one another, but also with their patients. *Signs* are observations and objective findings elicited by the clinician, such as a patient's constricted affect or psychomotor retardation. *Symptoms* are the subjective experiences described by the patient, often expressed as the chief complaints, such as depressed mood or lack of energy. A *syndrome* is a group of signs and symptoms that together make up a recognizable condition, which can be more equivocal than a specific disorder or disease.

Many of the signs and symptoms listed below can be understood as various points on a spectrum of behavior ranging from normal to abnormal. It is extremely rare to have a pathognomonic sign or symptom in psychiatry. In internal medicine, by contrast, one is more likely to find signs indicative of a specific disorder, for example, the Kayser-Fleischer ring of Wilson's disease.

SIGNS AND SYMPTOMS OF PSYCHIATRIC ILLNESS

I. **Consciousness:** state of awareness.
  A. **Disturbances of consciousness:** apperception is perception modified by a person's own emotions and thoughts; sensorium is the state of cognitive functioning of the special senses (sometimes used as a synonym for consciousness); disturbances of consciousness are most often associated with brain pathology.
    1. Disorientation: disturbance of orientation in time, place, or person.
    2. Clouding of consciousness: incomplete clear-mindedness with disturbances in perception and attitudes.
    3. Stupor: lack of reaction to and unawareness of surroundings.
    4. Delirium: bewildered, restless, confused, disoriented reaction associated with fear and hallucinations.
    5. Coma: profound degree of unconsciousness.
    6. Coma vigil: coma in which a patient appears to be asleep but ready to be aroused (also known as *akinetic mutism*).
    7. Twilight state: disturbed consciousness with hallucinations.
    8. Dream-like state: often used as a synonym for complex partial seizure or psychomotor epilepsy.
    9. Somnolence: abnormal drowsiness.

    10. Confusion: disturbance of consciousness in which reactions to environmental stimuli are inappropriate; manifested by a disordered orientation in relation to time, place, or person.
    11. Drowsiness: a state of impaired awareness associated with a desire or inclination to sleep.
    12. Sundowning: syndrome in older people that usually occurs at night and is characterized by drowsiness, confusion, ataxia, and falling as the result of being overly sedated with medications; also called *sundowner's syndrome*.
  B. **Disturbances of attention:** attention is the amount of effort exerted in focusing on certain portions of an experience; ability to sustain a focus on one activity; ability to concentrate.
    1. Distractibility: inability to concentrate attention; state in which attention is drawn to unimportant or irrelevant external stimuli.
    2. Selective inattention: blocking out only those things that generate anxiety.
    3. Hypervigilance: excessive attention and focus on all internal and external stimuli, usually secondary to delusional or paranoid states; similar to hyperpragia: excessive thinking and mental activity.
    4. Trance: focused attention and altered consciousness, usually seen in hypnosis, dissociative disorders, and ecstatic religious experiences.
    5. Disinhibition: removal of an inhibitory effect that permits persons to lose control of impulses as occurs in alcohol intoxication.
  C. **Disturbances in suggestibility:** compliant and uncritical response to an idea or influence.
    1. *Folie à deux* (or *folie à trois*): communicated emotional illness between two (or three) persons.
    2. Hypnosis: artificially induced modification of consciousness characterized by a heightened suggestibility.

II. **Emotion:** complex feeling state with psychic, somatic, and behavioral components that is related to affect and mood.
  A. **Affect:** observed expression of emotion, possibly inconsistent with patient's description of emotion.
    1. Appropriate affect: condition in which the emotional tone is in harmony with the accompanying idea, thought, or speech; also further described as broad or full affect in which a full range of emotions is appropriately expressed.
    2. Inappropriate affect: disharmony between the emotional feeling tone and the idea, thought, or speech accompanying it.

3. Blunted affect: disturbance in affect manifested by a severe reduction in the intensity of externalized feeling tone.
4. Restricted or constricted affect: reduction in intensity of feeling tone less severe than blunted affect but clearly reduced.
5. Flat affect: absence or near absence of any signs of affective expression; voice monotonous, face immobile.
6. Labile affect: rapid and abrupt changes in emotional feeling tone, unrelated to external stimuli.

B. Mood: a pervasive and sustained emotion subjectively experienced and reported by a patient and observed by others; examples include depression, elation, and anger.
1. Dysphoric mood: an unpleasant mood.
2. Euthymic mood: normal range of mood, implying absence of depressed or elevated mood.
3. Expansive mood: a person's expression of feelings without restraint, frequently with an overestimation of their significance or importance.
4. Irritable mood: a state in which a person is easily annoyed and provoked to anger.
5. Mood swings (labile mood): oscillations between euphoria and depression or anxiety.
6. Elevated mood: air of confidence and enjoyment; a mood more cheerful than usual.
7. Euphoria: intense elation with feelings of grandeur.
8. Ecstasy: feeling of intense rapture.
9. Depression: psychopathological feeling of sadness.
10. Anhedonia: loss of interest in and withdrawal from all regular and pleasurable activities, often associated with depression.
11. Grief or mourning: sadness appropriate to a real loss; also called *bereavement*.
12. Alexithymia: a person's inability to describe or difficulty in describing or being aware of emotions or mood.
13. Suicidal ideation: thoughts or act of taking one's own life.
14. Elation: feelings of joy, euphoria, triumph, intense self-satisfaction, or optimism.
15. Hypomania: mood abnormality with the qualitative characteristics of mania, but somewhat less intense.
16. Mania: mood state characterized by elation, agitation, hyperactivity, hypersexuality, and accelerated thinking and speaking.
17. Melancholia: severe depressive state; used in the term *involutional melancholia* both descriptively and also in reference to a distinct diagnostic entity.
18. *La belle indifférence*: inappropriate attitude of calm or lack of concern about one's disability.

C. Other emotions.
1. Anxiety: feeling of apprehension caused by anticipation of danger, which may be internal or external.
2. Free-floating anxiety: pervasive, unfocused fear not attached to any idea.
3. Fear: anxiety caused by consciously recognized and realistic danger.
4. Agitation: severe anxiety associated with motor restlessness; similar to irritability characterized by excessive excitability with easily triggered anger or annoyance.
5. Tension: increased and unpleasant motor and psychological activity.

6. Panic: acute, episodic, intense attack of anxiety associated with overwhelming feelings of dread and autonomic discharge.
7. Apathy: dulled emotional tone associated with detachment or indifference.
8. Ambivalence: coexistence of two opposing impulses toward the same thing in the same person at the same time.
9. Abreaction: emotional release or discharge after recalling a painful experience.
10. Shame: failure to live up to self-expectations.
11. Guilt: emotion secondary to doing what is perceived as wrong.
12. Impulse control: ability to resist an impulse, drive, or temptation to perform an action.
13. Ineffability: ecstatic state in which person states it is indescribable, inexpressible, and impossible to convey to another person.
14. Acathexis: lack of feeling associated with an ordinarily emotionally charged subject; in *cathexis* the feeling is connected.
15. Decathexis: detaching emotions from thoughts, ideas, or persons.

D. Physiological disturbances associated with mood: signs of somatic (usually autonomic) dysfunction, most often associated with depression (also called *vegetative signs*).
1. Anorexia: loss of or decrease in appetite.
2. Hyperphagia: increase in intake of food.
3. Insomnia: lack of or diminished ability to sleep.
   a. Initial: difficulty in falling asleep.
   b. Middle: difficulty in sleeping through the night without waking up and difficulty in going back to sleep.
   c. Terminal: early morning awakening.
4. Hypersomnia: excessive sleeping.
5. Diurnal variation: mood is regularly worst in the morning, immediately after awakening, and improves as the day progresses.
6. Diminished libido: decreased sexual interest, drive, and performance (increased libido is often associated with manic states).
7. Constipation: inability to defecate or difficulty in defecating.
8. Fatigue: a feeling of weariness, sleepiness, or irritability following a period of mental or bodily activity.
9. Pica: craving and eating of nonfood substances, such as paint and clay.
10. Pseudocyesis: rare condition in which a patient has the signs and symptoms of pregnancy, such as abdominal distention, breast enlargement, pigmentation, cessation of menses, and morning sickness.
11. Bulimia: insatiable hunger and voracious eating; seen in *bulimia nervosa* and atypical depression.
12. Adynamia: weakness and fatigability.

III. Motor behavior (conation): aspect of the psyche that includes impulses, motivations, wishes, drives, instincts, and cravings, as expressed by a person's behavior or motor activity.
1. Echopraxia: pathological imitation of movements of one person by another.
2. Catatonia and postural abnormalities: seen in catatonic schizophrenia and some cases of brain diseases, such as encephalitis.

a. Catalepsy: general term for an immobile position that is constantly maintained.

b. Catatonic excitement: agitated, purposeless motor activity, uninfluenced by external stimuli.

c. Catatonic stupor: markedly slowed motor activity, often to a point of immobility and seeming unawareness of surroundings.

d. Catatonic rigidity: voluntary assumption of a rigid posture, held against all efforts to be moved.

e. Catatonic posturing: voluntary assumption of an inappropriate or bizarre posture, generally maintained for long periods.

f. *Cerea flexibilitas* (waxy flexibility): condition of a person who can be molded into a position that is then maintained; when an examiner moves the person's limb, the limb feels as if it were made of wax.

g. Akinesia: lack of physical movement, as in the extreme immobility of catatonic schizophrenia; may also occur as an extrapyramidal side effect of antipsychotic medication.

3. Negativism: motiveless resistance to all attempts to be moved or to all instructions.

4. Cataplexy: temporary loss of muscle tone and weakness precipitated by a variety of emotional states.

5. Stereotypy: repetitive fixed pattern of physical action or speech.

6. Mannerism: ingrained, habitual involuntary movement.

7. Automatism: automatic performance of an act or acts generally representative of unconscious symbolic activity.

8. Command automatism: automatic following of suggestions (also *automatic obedience*).

9. Mutism: voicelessness without structural abnormalities.

10. Overactivity.

a. Psychomotor agitation: excessive motor and cognitive overactivity, usually nonproductive and in response to inner tension.

b. Hyperactivity (hyperkinesis): restless, aggressive, destructive activity, often associated with some underlying brain pathology.

c. Tic: involuntary, spasmodic motor movement.

d. Sleepwalking (somnambulism): motor activity during sleep.

e. Akathisia: subjective feeling of muscular tension secondary to antipsychotic or other medication, which can cause restlessness, pacing, repeated sitting and standing; can be mistaken for psychotic agitation.

f. Compulsion: uncontrollable impulse to perform an act repetitively.

i. Dipsomania: compulsion to drink alcohol.

ii. Kleptomania: compulsion to steal.

iii. Nymphomania: excessive and compulsive need for coitus in a woman.

iv. Satyriasis: excessive and compulsive need for coitus in a man

v. Trichotillomania: compulsion to pull out hair.

vi. Ritual: automatic activity, compulsive in nature, anxiety reducing in origin.

g. Ataxia: failure of muscle coordination; irregularity of muscle action.

h. Polyphagia: pathological overeating.

i. Tremor: rhythmical alteration in movement, which is usually faster than one beat a second; typically, tremors decrease during periods of relaxation and sleep and increase during periods of anger and increased tension.

j. Floccillation: aimless picking usually at clothing or bedclothes, commonly seen in delirium.

11. Hypoactivity (hypokinesis): decreased motor and cognitive activity, as in psychomotor retardation; visible slowing of thought, speech, and movements.

12. Mimicry: simple, imitative motor activity of childhood.

13. Aggression: forceful, goal-directed action that may be verbal or physical; the motor counterpart of the affect of rage, anger, or hostility.

14. Acting out: direct expression of an unconscious wish or impulse in action; living out unconscious fantasy impulsively in behavior.

15. Abulia: reduced impulse to act and think, associated with indifference about consequences of action; a result of neurological deficit.

16. Anergia: lack of energy (anergy).

17. Astasia abasia: the inability to stand or walk in a normal manner, even though normal leg movements can be performed in a sitting or lying down position. The gait is bizarre and is not suggestive of a specific organic lesion; seen in conversion disorder.

18. Coprophagia: eating of filth or feces.

19. Dyskinesia: difficulty in performing voluntary movements, as in extrapyramidal disorders.

20. Muscle rigidity: state in which the muscles remain immovable; seen in schizophrenia.

21. Twirling: a sign present in autistic children who continually rotate in the direction in which their head is turned.

22. Bradykinesia: slowness of motor activity with a decrease in normal spontaneous movement.

23. Chorea: random and involuntary quick, jerky, purposeless movements.

24. Convulsion: An involuntary, violent muscular contraction or spasm.

a. Clonic convulsion: convulsion in which the muscles alternately contract and relax.

b. Tonic convulsion: convulsion in which the muscle contraction is sustained.

25. Seizure: an attack or sudden onset of certain symptoms, such as convulsions, loss of consciousness, and psychic or sensory disturbances; seen in epilepsy and can be substance-induced.

a. Generalized tonic-clonic seizure: generalized onset of tonic-clonic movements of the limbs, tongue biting, and incontinence followed by slow, gradual recovery of consciousness and cognition; also called *grand mal seizure* and *psychomotor seizure*.

b. Simple partial seizure: localized ictal onset of seizure without alterations in consciousness.

c. Complex partial seizure: localized ictal onset of seizure with alterations in consciousness.

26. Dystonia: slow, sustained contractions of the trunk or limbs; seen in medication-induced dystonia.

27. Aminia: inability to make gestures or to comprehend those made by others.

IV. **Thinking:** goal-directed flow of ideas, symbols, and associations initiated by a problem or task and leading toward a reality-oriented conclusion; when a logical sequence occurs, thinking is normal; parapraxis (unconsciously motivated lapse from logic is also called a *freudian slip*) considered part of normal thinking. Abstract thinking is the ability to grasp the essentials of a whole, to break a whole into its parts, and to discern common properties.

A. General disturbances in form or process of thinking.

1. Mental disorder: clinically significant behavior or psychological syndrome associated with distress or disability, not just an expected response to a particular event or limited to relations between a person and society.

2. Psychosis: inability to distinguish reality from fantasy; impaired reality testing, with the creation of a new reality (as opposed to neurosis: mental disorder in which reality testing is intact; behavior may not violate gross social norms, but is relatively enduring or recurrent without treatment).

3. Reality testing: objective evaluation and judgment of the world outside the self.

4. Formal thought disorder: disturbance in the form of thought rather than the content of thought; thinking characterized by loosened associations, neologisms, and illogical constructs; thought process is disordered, and the person is defined as psychotic.

5. Illogical thinking: thinking containing erroneous conclusions or internal contradictions; psychopathological only when it is marked and when not caused by cultural values or intellectual deficit.

6. Dereism: mental activity not concordant with logic or experience.

7. Autistic thinking: preoccupation with inner, private world; term used somewhat synonymously with dereism.

8. Magical thinking: a form of dereistic thought; thinking similar to that of the preoperational phase in children (Jean Piaget), in which thoughts, words, or actions assume power (for example, to cause or prevent events).

9. Primary process thinking: general term for thinking that is dereistic, illogical, magical; normally found in dreams, abnormally in psychosis.

10. Emotional insight: deep level of understanding or awareness that is likely to lead to positive changes in personality and behavior.

B. Specific disturbances in form of thought.

1. Neologism: new word created by a patient, often by combining syllables of other words, for idiosyncratic psychological reasons.

2. Word salad: incoherent mixture of words and phrases.

3. Circumstantiality: indirect speech that is delayed in reaching the point but eventually gets from original point to desired goal; characterized by an overinclusion of details and parenthetical remarks.

4. Tangentiality: inability to have goal-directed associations of thought; speaker never gets from desired point to desired goal.

5. Incoherence: thought that generally is not understandable; running together of thoughts or words with no logical or grammatical connection, resulting in disorganization.

6. Perseveration: persisting response to a previous stimulus after a new stimulus has been presented; often associated with cognitive disorders.

7. Verbigeration: meaningless repetition of specific words or phrases.

8. Echolalia: psychopathological repeating of words or phrases of one person by another; tends to be repetitive and persistent; may be spoken with mocking or staccato intonation.

9. Condensation: fusion of various concepts into one.

10. Irrelevant answer: answer that is not in harmony with the question asked (person appears to ignore or not attend to the question).

11. Loosening of associations: flow of thought in which ideas shift from one subject to another in a completely unrelated way; when severe, speech may be incoherent.

12. Derailment: gradual or sudden deviation in train of thought without blocking; sometimes used synonymously with loosening of associations.

13. Flight of ideas: rapid, continuous verbalizations or plays on words produce constant shifting from one idea to another; ideas tend to be connected, and in the less severe form a listener may be able to follow them.

14. Clang association: association of words similar in sound but not in meaning; words have no logical connection; may include rhyming and punning.

15. Blocking: abrupt interruption in train of thinking before a thought or idea is finished; after a brief pause, person indicates no recall of what was being said or was going to be said (also known as *thought deprivation*).

16. Glossolalia: expression of a revelatory message through unintelligible words (also known as *speaking in tongues*); not considered a disturbance in thought if associated with practices of specific Pentecostal religions; also known as *cryptolalia*, a private spoken language.

C. Specific disturbances in content of thought.

1. Poverty of content: thought that gives little information because of vagueness, empty repetitions, or obscure phrases.

2. Overvalued idea: unreasonable, sustained false belief maintained less firmly than a delusion.

3. Delusion: false belief, based on incorrect inference about external reality, not consistent with patient's intelligence and cultural background; cannot be corrected by reasoning.

   a. Bizarre delusion: an absurd, totally implausible, strange false belief (for example, invaders from space have implanted electrodes in a person's brain).

   b. Systematized delusion: false belief or beliefs united by a single event or theme (for example, a person is being persecuted by the CIA, the FBI, or the Mafia).

   c. Mood-congruent delusion: delusion with mood-appropriate content (for example, a depressed patient believes that he or she is responsible for the destruction of the world).

   d. Mood-incongruent delusion: delusion with content that has no association to mood or is mood neutral (for example, a depressed patient has delusions of thought control or thought broadcasting).

   e. Nihilistic delusion: false feeling that self, others, or the world is nonexistent or coming to an end.

   f. Delusion of poverty: a person's false belief that he or she is bereft or will be deprived of all material possessions.

   g. Somatic delusion: false belief involving functioning of the body (for example, belief that the brain is rotting or melting).

h. Paranoid delusions: includes persecutory delusions and delusions of reference, control, and grandeur (distinguished from paranoid ideation, which is suspiciousness of less than delusional proportions).

   i. Delusion of persecution: a person's false belief that he or she is being harassed, cheated, or persecuted; often found in litigious patients who have a pathological tendency to take legal action because of imagined mistreatment.

   ii. Delusion of grandeur: a person's exaggerated conception of his or her importance, power, or identity.

   iii. Delusion of reference: a person's false belief that the behavior of others refers to himself or herself; that events, objects, or other people have a particular and unusual significance, usually of a negative nature; derived from idea of reference, in which a person falsely feels that others are talking about him or her (for example, belief that people on television or radio are talking to or about the person).

i. Delusion of self-accusation: false feeling of remorse and guilt.

j. Delusion of control: false feeling that a person's will, thoughts, or feelings are being controlled by external forces.

   i. Thought withdrawal: delusion that thoughts are being removed from a person's mind by other people or forces.

   ii. Thought insertion: delusion that thoughts are being implanted in a person's mind by other people or forces.

   iii. Thought broadcasting: delusion that a person's thoughts can be heard by others, as though they were being broadcast over the air.

   iv. Thought control: delusion that a person's thoughts are being controlled by other people or forces.

k. Delusion of infidelity (delusional jealousy): false belief derived from pathological jealousy about a person's lover being unfaithful.

l. Erotomania: delusional belief, more common in women than in men, that someone is deeply in love with them (also known as *Clérambault-Kandinsky complex*).

m. Pseudologia phantastica: a type of lying in which a person appears to believe in the reality of his or her fantasies and acts on them; associated with Munchausen syndrome, repeated feigning of illness.

4. Trend or preoccupation of thought: centering of thought content on a particular idea, associated with a strong affective tone, such as a paranoid trend or a suicidal or homicidal preoccupation.

5. Egomania: pathological self-preoccupation.

6. Monomania: preoccupation with a single object.

7. Hypochondria: exaggerated concern about health that is based not on real organic pathology but, rather, on unrealistic interpretations of physical signs or sensations as abnormal.

8. Obsession: pathological persistence of an irresistible thought or feeling that cannot be eliminated from consciousness by logical effort; associated with anxiety.

9. Compulsion: pathological need to act on an impulse that, if resisted, produces anxiety; repetitive behavior in response to an obsession or performed according to certain rules, with no true end in itself other than to prevent something from occurring in the future.

10. Coprolalia: compulsive utterance of obscene words.

11. Phobia: persistent, irrational, exaggerated, and invariably pathological dread of a specific stimulus or situation; results in a compelling desire to avoid the feared stimulus.

a. Specific phobia: circumscribed dread of a discrete object or situation (for example, dread of spiders or snakes).

b. Social phobia: dread of public humiliation, as in fear of public speaking, performing, or eating in public.

c. Acrophobia: dread of high places.

d. Agoraphobia: dread of open places.

e. Algophobia: dread of pain.

f. Ailurophobia: dread of cats.

g. Erythrophobia: dread of red (refers to a fear of blushing).

h. Panphobia: dread of everything.

i. Claustrophobia: dread of closed places.

j. Xenophobia: dread of strangers.

k. Zoophobia: dread of animals.

l. Needle phobia: the persistent, intense, pathological fear of receiving an injection; also called *blood injection phobia*.

12. Noesis: a revelation in which immense illumination occurs in association with a sense that a person has been chosen to lead and command.

13. *Unio mystica*: an oceanic feeling of mystic unity with an infinite power; not considered a disturbance in thought content if congruent with person's religious or cultural milieu.

V. Speech: ideas, thoughts, feelings as expressed through language; communication through the use of words and language.

  A. Disturbances in speech.

1. Pressure of speech: rapid speech that is increased in amount and difficult to interrupt.

2. Volubility (logorrhea): copious, coherent, logical speech.

3. Poverty of speech: restriction in the amount of speech used; replies may be monosyllabic.

4. Nonspontaneous speech: verbal responses given only when asked or spoken to directly; no self-initiation of speech.

5. Poverty of content of speech: speech that is adequate in amount but conveys little information because of vagueness, emptiness, or stereotyped phrases.

6. Dysprosody: loss of normal speech melody (called *prosody*).

7. Dysarthria: difficulty in articulation, not in word finding or in grammar.

8. Excessively loud or soft speech: loss of modulation of normal speech volume; may reflect a variety of pathological conditions ranging from psychosis to depression to deafness.

9. Stuttering: frequent repetition or prolongation of a sound or syllable, leading to markedly impaired speech fluency.

10. Cluttering: erratic and dysrhythmic speech, consisting of rapid and jerky spurts.

11. Aculalia: nonsense speech associated with marked impairment of comprehension.

12. Bradylalia: abnormally slow speech.
13. Dysphonia: difficulty or pain in speaking.

B. Aphasic disturbances: disturbances in language output.

1. Motor aphasia: disturbance of speech caused by a cognitive disorder in which understanding remains but the ability to speak is grossly impaired; halting, laborious, and inaccurate speech (also known as *Broca's, nonfluent,* and *expressive aphasia*).

2. Sensory aphasia: organic loss of the ability to comprehend the meaning of words; fluid and spontaneous but incoherent and nonsensical speech (also known as *Wernicke's, fluent,* and *receptive aphasia*).

3. Nominal aphasia: difficulty in finding correct name for an object (also termed *anomia* and *amnestic aphasia*).

4. Syntactical aphasia: inability to arrange words in proper sequence.

5. Jargon aphasia: words produced are totally neologistic; nonsense words repeated with various intonations and inflections.

6. Global aphasia: combination of a grossly nonfluent aphasia and a severe fluent aphasia.

7. Alogia: inability to speak because of a mental deficiency or an episode of dementia.

8. Coprophrasia: involuntary use of vulgar or obscene language; seen in Tourette's disorder and some cases of schizophrenia.

VI. Perception: process of transferring physical stimulation into psychological information; mental process by which sensory stimuli are brought to awareness.

A. Disturbances of perception.

1. Hallucination: false sensory perception not associated with real external stimuli; there may or may not be a delusional interpretation of the hallucinatory experience.

   a. Hypnagogic hallucination: false sensory perception occurring while falling asleep; generally considered a nonpathological phenomenon.

   b. Hypnopompic hallucination: false perception occurring while awakening from sleep; generally considered nonpathological.

   c. Auditory hallucination: false perception of sound, usually voices but also other noises, such as music; most common hallucination in psychiatric disorders.

   d. Visual hallucination: false perception involving sight consisting of both formed images (for example, people) and unformed images (for example, flashes of light); most common in medically determined disorders.

   e. Olfactory hallucination: false perception of smell; most common in medical disorders.

   f. Gustatory hallucination: false perception of taste, such as unpleasant taste, caused by an uncinate seizure; most common in medical disorders.

   g. Tactile (haptic) hallucination: false perception of touch or surface sensation, as from an amputated limb (phantom limb); crawling sensation on or under the skin (formication).

   h. Somatic hallucination: false sensation of things occurring in or to the body, most often visceral in origin (also known as *cenesthesic hallucination*).

   i. Lilliputian hallucination: false perception in which objects are seen as reduced in size (also termed *micropsia*).

   j. Mood-congruent hallucination: hallucination in which the content is consistent with either a depressed or a manic mood (for example, a depressed patient hears voices saying that the patient is a bad person; a manic patient hears voices saying that the patient is of inflated worth, power, and knowledge).

   k. Mood-incongruent hallucination: hallucination in which the content is not consistent with either depressed or manic mood (for example, in depression, hallucinations not involving such themes as guilt, deserved punishment, or inadequacy; in mania, hallucinations not involving such themes as inflated worth or power).

   l. Hallucinosis: hallucinations, most often auditory, that are associated with chronic alcohol abuse and that occur within a clear sensorium, as opposed to delirium tremens, hallucinations that occur in the context of a clouded sensorium.

   m. Synesthesia: sensation or hallucination caused by another sensation (for example, an auditory sensation accompanied by or triggering a visual sensation; a sound experienced as being seen or a visual event experienced as being heard).

   n. Trailing phenomenon: perceptual abnormality associated with hallucinogenic drugs in which moving objects are seen as a series of discrete and discontinuous images.

   o. Command hallucination: false perception of orders that a person may feel obliged to obey or unable to resist.

2. Illusion: misperception or misinterpretation of real external sensory stimuli.

B. Disturbances associated with cognitive disorder and medical conditions.

1. Agnosia: an inability to recognize and interpret the significance of sensory impressions.

2. Anosognosia (ignorance of illness): a person's inability to recognize a neurological deficit as occurring to himself or herself.

3. Somatopagnosia (ignorance of the body): a person's inability to recognize a body part as his or her own (also called *autotopagnosia*).

4. Visual agnosia: inability to recognize objects or persons.

5. Astereognosis: inability to recognize objects by touch.

6. Prosopagnosia: inability to recognize faces.

7. Apraxia: inability to carry out specific tasks.

8. Simultagnosia: inability to comprehend more than one element of a visual scene at a time or to integrate the parts into a whole.

9. Adiadochokinesia: inability to perform rapid alternating movements.

10. Aura: warning sensations such as automatisms, fullness in the stomach, blushing, and changes in respiration, cognitive sensations, and affective states usually experienced before a seizure; a sensory prodrome that precedes a classic migraine headache.

C. Disturbances associated with conversion and dissociative phenomena: somatization of repressed material or the development of physical symptoms and distortions involving the voluntary muscles or special sense organs; not under voluntary control and not explained by any physical disorder.

1. Hysterical anesthesia: loss of sensory modalities resulting from emotional conflicts.
2. Macropsia: state in which objects seem larger than they are.
3. Micropsia: state in which objects seem smaller than they are (both macropsia and micropsia can also be associated with clear organic conditions, such as complex partial seizures).
4. Depersonalization: a person's subjective sense of being unreal, strange, or unfamiliar.
5. Derealization: a subjective sense that the environment is strange or unreal; a feeling of changed reality.
6. Fugue: taking on a new identity with amnesia for the old identity; often involves travel or wandering to new environments.
7. Multiple personality: one person who appears at different times to be two or more entirely different personalities and characters (called *dissociative identity disorder* in the fourth revised edition of *Diagnostic and Statistical Manual of Mental Disorders* [DSM-IV-TR]).
8. Dissociation: unconscious defense mechanism involving the segregation of any group of mental or behavioral processes from the rest of the person's psychic activity; may entail the separation of an idea from its accompanying emotional tone, as seen in dissociative and conversion disorders.

VII. **Memory:** function by which information stored in the brain is later recalled to consciousness. Orientation is the normal state of oneself and one's surroundings in terms of time, place, and person.

   A. Disturbances of memory.
   1. Amnesia: partial or total inability to recall past experiences; may be organic or emotional in origin.
      a. Anterograde: amnesia for events occurring after a point in time.
      b. Retrograde: amnesia for events occurring before a point in time.
   2. Paramnesia: falsification of memory by distortion of recall.
      a. *Fausse reconnaissance*: false recognition.
      b. Retrospective falsification: memory becomes unintentionally (unconsciously) distorted by being filtered through a person's present emotional, cognitive, and experiential state.
      c. Confabulation: unconscious filling of gaps in memory by imagined or untrue experiences that a person believes but that have no basis in fact; most often associated with organic pathology.
      d. *Déjà vu*: illusion of visual recognition in which a new situation is incorrectly regarded as a repetition of a previous memory.
      e. *Déjà entendu*: illusion of auditory recognition.
      f. *Déjà pensé*: illusion that a new thought is recognized as a thought previously felt or expressed.
      g. *Jamais vu*: false feeling of unfamiliarity with a real situation that a person has experienced.
      h. False memory: a person's recollection and belief by the patient of an event that did not actually occur.
   3. Hypermnesia: exaggerated degree of retention and recall.

4. Eidetic image: visual memory of almost hallucinatory vividness.
5. Screen memory: a consciously tolerable memory covering for a painful memory.
6. Repression: a defense mechanism characterized by unconscious forgetting of unacceptable ideas or impulses.
7. Lethologica: temporary inability to remember a name or a proper noun.
8. Blackout: amnesia experienced by alcoholics about behavior during drinking bouts; usually indicates that reversible brain damage has occurred.

   B. Levels of memory.
   1. Immediate: reproduction or recall of perceived material within seconds to minutes.
   2. Recent: recall of events over past few days.
   3. Recent past: recall of events over past few months.
   4. Remote: recall of events in distant past.

VIII. **Intelligence:** ability to understand, recall, mobilize, and constructively integrate previous learning in meeting new situations.

   A. Mental retardation: lack of intelligence to a degree in which there is interference with social and vocational performance: mild (IQ of 50 or 55 to approximately 70), moderate (IQ of 35 or 40 to 50 or 55), severe (IQ of 20 or 25 to 35 or 40), or profound (IQ below 20 or 25); obsolete terms are *idiot* (mental age less than 3 years), *imbecile* (mental age of 3 to 7 years), and *moron* (mental age of approximately 8 years).

   B. Dementia: organic and global deterioration of intellectual functioning without clouding of consciousness.
   1. Dyscalculia (acalculia): loss of ability to do calculations; not caused by anxiety or impairment in concentration.
   2. Dysgraphia (agraphia): loss of ability to write in cursive style; loss of word structure.
   3. Alexia: loss of a previously possessed reading facility; not explained by defective visual acuity.

   C. Pseudodementia: clinical features resembling a dementia not caused by an organic condition; most often caused by depression (dementia syndrome of depression).

   D. Concrete thinking: literal thinking; limited use of metaphor without understanding of nuances of meaning; one-dimensional thought.

   E. Abstract thinking: ability to appreciate nuances of meaning; multidimensional thinking with ability to use metaphors and hypotheses appropriately.

IX. **Insight:** a person's ability to understand the true cause and meaning of a situation (such as a set of symptoms).

   A. Intellectual insight: understanding of the objective reality of a set of circumstances without the ability to apply the understanding in any useful way to master the situation.

   B. True insight: understanding of the objective reality of a situation, coupled with the motivation and the emotional impetus to master the situation.

   C. Impaired insight: diminished ability to understand the objective reality of a situation.

X. **Judgment:** ability to assess a situation correctly and to act appropriately in the situation.

   A. Critical judgment: ability to assess, discern, and choose among various options in a situation.

   B. Automatic judgment: reflex performance of an action.

   C. Impaired judgment: diminished ability to understand a situation correctly and to act appropriately.

Classification in Psychiatry and Psychiatric Rating Scales

Advances in scientific psychiatry are to a great extent shaped by its system of classification. Systems of classification are fundamental to all sciences, containing the concepts on which theory is based and influencing what can and cannot be seen. The classification of illnesses (*nosology*) has always been an integral part of the theory and practice of medicine.

Systems of classification for psychiatric diagnoses have several purposes: to distinguish one psychiatric diagnosis from another, so that clinicians can offer the most effective treatment; to provide a common language among health care professionals; and to explore the causes of the many mental disorders that are still unknown. The two most important psychiatric classifications are the *Diagnostic and Statistical Manual of Mental Disorders* (DSM) (Table 6–1), developed by the American Psychiatric Association in collaboration with other groups of mental health professionals, and the *International Classification of Diseases* (ICD), developed by the World Health Organization.

DSM-IV-TR'S RELATION TO ICD-10

The fourth revised edition of the DSM (DSM-IV-TR) was designed to correspond with ICD-10, developed in 1992. There was a strong consensus that diagnostic systems used in the United States must be compatible with the ICD to ensure uniform reporting of national and international health statistics. In addition, Medicare requires that billing codes for reimbursement follow ICD.

ICD-10 is the official classification system used in Europe and many other parts of the world. All categories used in DSM-IV-TR are found in ICD-10, but not all ICD-10 categories are in DSM-IV-TR. Also, some terms and diagnostic categories used in ICD-10 are not used in DSM-IV-TR. This textbook uses the official DSM-IV-TR terminology.

Basic Features in DSM-IV-TR

Descriptive Approach. The approach to DSM-IV-TR is atheoretical with regard to causes. Thus, DSM-IV-TR attempts to describe the manifestations of the mental disorders and only rarely attempts to account for how the disturbances come about. The definitions of the disorders usually consist of descriptions of clinical features.

Diagnostic Criteria. Specified diagnostic criteria are provided for each specific mental disorder. These criteria include a list of features that must be present for the diagnosis to be made. Such criteria increase the reliability of clinicians' process of diagnosis.

Multiaxial Evaluation

DSM-IV-TR is a multiaxial system that evaluates patients along several variables and contains five axes. Axis I and Axis II make up the entire classification of mental disorder: 17 major classifications and more than 300 specific disorders. In many instances, patients have disorders on both axes. For example, a patient may have major depressive disorder noted on Axis I and obsessive-compulsive personality disorder on Axis II.

Axis I. Axis I consists of clinical disorders and other conditions that may be a focus of clinical attention (Table 6–2).

Axis II. Axis II consists of personality disorders and mental retardation (Table 6–3). The habitual use of a particular defense mechanism can be indicated on Axis II.

Axis III. Axis III lists any physical disorder or general medical condition that is present in addition to the mental disorder. The physical condition may be causative (for example, kidney failure causing delirium), the result of a mental disorder (for example, alcohol gastritis secondary to alcohol dependence), or unrelated to the mental disorder.

Axis IV. Axis IV is used to code the psychosocial and environmental problems that significantly contribute to the development or exacerbation of the current disorder. The evaluation of stressors is based on a clinician's assessment of the stress that an average person with similar sociocultural values and circumstances would experience from the psychosocial stressors. This judgment is based on the amount of change that the stressor causes in the person's life, the degree to which the event is desired and under the person's control, and the number of stressors. Stressors may be positive (such as a job promotion) or negative (such as the loss of a loved one). Information about stressors may be important in formulating a treatment plan that includes attempts to remove the psychosocial stressors or to help the patient cope with them.

Axis V. Axis V is a Global Assessment of Functioning (GAF) Scale in which clinicians judge patients' overall levels of functioning during a particular time (for example, the patient's level of functioning at the time of the evaluation or the patient's highest level of functioning for at least a few months during the past year). Functioning is consid-

Table 6–1.
DSM-IV-TR Classification (with ICD-10 Codes)

NOS = Not Otherwise Specified.

An *x* appearing in a diagnostic code indicates that a specific code number is required.

An ellipsis (. . .) is used in the names of certain disorders to indicate that the name of a specific mental disorder or general medical condition should be inserted when recording the name (e.g., F05.0 Delirium Due to Hypothyroidism).

Numbers in parentheses are page numbers.

If criteria are currently met, one of the following severity specifiers may be noted after the diagnosis:
Mild
Moderate
Severe

If criteria are no longer met, one of the following specifiers may be noted:
In Partial Remission
In Full Remission
Prior History

Disorders Usually First Diagnosed in Infancy, Childhood, or Adolescence (39)

MENTAL RETARDATION (41)
Note: These are coded on Axis II.

F70.9	Mild Mental Retardation (43)
F71.9	Moderate Mental Retardation (43)
F72.9	Severe Mental Retardation (43)
F73.9	Profound Mental Retardation (44)
F79.9	Mental Retardation, Severity Unspecified (44)

LEARNING DISORDERS (49)

F81.0	Reading Disorder (51)
F81.2	Mathematics Disorder (53)
F81.8	Disorder of Written Expression (54)
F81.9	Learning Disorder NOS (56)

MOTOR SKILLS DISORDER (56)

F82	Developmental Coordination Disorder (56)

COMMUNICATION DISORDERS (58)

F80.1	Expressive Language Disorder (58)
F80.2	Mixed Receptive-Expressive Language Disorder (62)
F80.0	Phonological Disorder (65)
F98.5	Stuttering (67)
F80.9	Communication Disorder NOS (69)

PERVASIVE DEVELOPMENTAL DISORDERS (69)

F84.0	Autistic Disorder (70)
F84.2	Rett's Disorder (76)
F84.3	Childhood Disintegrative Disorder (77)
F84.5	Asperger's Disorder (80)
F84.9	Pervasive Developmental Disorder NOS (84)

ATTENTION-DEFICIT AND DISRUPTIVE BEHAVIOR DISORDERS (85)

__.__	Attention-Deficit/Hyperactivity Disorder (85)
F90.0	Combined Type
F98.8	Predominantly Inattentive Type
F90.0	Predominantly Hyperactive-Impulsive Type
F90.9	Attention-Deficit/Hyperactivity Disorder NOS (93)
F91.8	Conduct Disorder (93)
	Specify type: Childhood-Onset Type/Adolescent-Onset Type
F91.3	Oppositional Defiant Disorder (100)
F91.9	Disruptive Behavior Disorder NOS (103)

FEEDING AND EATING DISORDERS OF INFANCY OR EARLY CHILDHOOD (103)

F98.3	Pica (103)
F98.2	Rumination Disorder (105)
F98.2	Feeding Disorder of Infancy or Early Childhood (107)

TIC DISORDERS (108)

F95.2	Tourette's Disorder (111)
F95.1	Chronic Motor or Vocal Tic Disorder (114)
F95.0	Transient Tic Disorder (115)
	Specify if: Single Episode/Recurrent
F95.9	Tic Disorder NOS (116)

ELIMINATION DISORDERS (116)

__.__	Encopresis (116)
R15	With Constipation and Overflow Incontinence *(also code K59.0 constipation on Axis III)*
F98.1	Without Constipation and Overflow Incontinence
F98.0	Enuresis (Not Due to a General Medical Condition) (118)
	Specify type: Nocturnal Only/Diurnal Only/Nocturnal and Diurnal

OTHER DISORDERS OF INFANCY, CHILDHOOD, OR ADOLESCENCE (121)

F93.0	Separation Anxiety Disorder (121)
	Specify if: Early Onset
F94.0	Selective Mutism (125)
F94.x	Reactive Attachment Disorder of Infancy or Early Childhood (127)
.1	Inhibited type
.2	Disinhibited type
F98.4	Stereotypic Movement Disorder (131)
	Specify if: With Self-Injurious Behavior
F98.9	Disorder of Infancy, Childhood, or Adolescence NOS (134)

Delirium, Dementia, and Amnestic and Other Cognitive Disorders (135)

DELIRIUM (136)

F05.0	Delirium Due to ... *[Indicate the General Medical Condition] (code F05.1 if superimposed on Dementia)* (141)
__.__	Substance Intoxication Delirium *(refer to Substance-Related Disorders for substance-specific codes)* (143)
__.__	Substance Withdrawal Delirium *(refer to Substance-Related Disorders for substance-specific codes)* (143)
__.__	Delirium Due to Multiple Etiologies *(code each of the specific etiologies)* (146)
F05.9	Delirium NOS (147)

(continued)

Table 6–1 (continued)

DEMENTIA (147)

F00.xx	Dementia of the Alzheimer's Type, With Early Onset *(also code G30.0 Alzheimer's Disease, With Early Onset, on Axis III)* (154)
.00	Uncomplicated
.01	With Delusions
.03	With Depressed Mood
	Specify if: With behavioral disturbance
F00.xx	Dementia of the Alzheimer's Type, With Late Onset *(also code G30.1 Alzheimer's Disease, With Late Onset, on Axis III)* (154)
.10	Uncomplicated
.11	With Delusions
.13	With Depressed Mood
	Specify if: With Behavioral Disturbance
F01.xx	Vascular Dementia (158)
.80	Uncomplicated
.81	With Delusions
.83	With Depressed Mood
	Specify if: With Behavioral Disturbance
F02.4	Dementia Due to HIV Disease *(also code B22.0 HIV disease resulting in encephalopathy on Axis III)* (163)
F02.8	Dementia Due to Head Trauma *(also code S06.9 Intracranial injury on Axis III)* (164)
F02.3	Dementia Due to Parkinson's Disease *(also code G20 Parkinson's disease on Axis III)* (164)
F02.2	Dementia Due to Huntington's Disease *(also code G10 Huntington's disease on Axis III)* (165)
F02.0	Dementia Due to Pick's Disease *(also code G31.0 Pick's disease on Axis III)* (165)
F02.1	Dementia Due to Creutzfeldt-Jakob Disease *(also code A81.0 Creutzfeldt-Jakob disease on Axis III)* (166)
F02.8	Dementia Due to ... *[Indicate the General Medical Condition not listed above] (also code the general medical condition on Axis III)* (167)
—.—	Substance-Induced Persisting Dementia *(refer to Substance-Related Disorders for substance-specific codes)* (168)
F02.8	Dementia Due to Multiple Etiologies *(instead code F00.2 for mixed Alzheimer's and Vascular Dementia)* (170)
F03	Dementia NOS (171)

AMNESTIC DISORDERS (172)

F04	Amnestic Disorder Due to ... *[Indicate the General Medical Condition]* (175)
	Specify if: Transient/Chronic
—.—	Substance-Induced Persisting Amnestic Disorder *(refer to Substance-Related Disorders for substance-specific codes)* (177)
R41.3	Amnestic Disorder NOS (179)

OTHER COGNITIVE DISORDERS (179)

F06.9	Cognitive Disorder NOS (179)

Mental Disorders Due to a General Medical Condition Not Elsewhere Classified (181)

F06.1	Catatonic Disorder Due to ... *[Indicate the General Medical Condition]* (185)
F07.0	Personality Change Due to ... *[Indicate the General Medical Condition]* (187)
	Specify type: Labile Type/Disinhibited Type/ Aggressive Type/Apathetic Type/Paranoid Type/Other Type/Combined Type/Unspecified Type

F09	Mental Disorder NOS Due to ... *[Indicate the General Medical Condition]* (190)

Substance-Related Disorders (191)

[a]The following specifiers may be applied to Substance Dependence:
Specify if: With Physiological Dependence/Without Physiological Dependence
Code course of Dependence in fifth character:
0 = Early Full Remission/Early Partial Remission
0 = Sustained Full Remission/Sustained Partial Remission
1 = In a Controlled Environment
2 = On Agonist Therapy
4 = Mild/Moderate/Severe
The following specifiers apply to Substance-Induced Disorders as noted:
[I]With Onset During Intoxication/[W]With Onset During Withdrawal

ALCOHOL-RELATED DISORDERS (212)

Alcohol Use Disorders (213)

F10.2x	Alcohol Dependence[a] (213)
F10.1	Alcohol Abuse (214)

Alcohol-Induced Disorders (214)

F10.00	Alcohol Intoxication (214)
F10.3	Alcohol Withdrawal (215)
	Specify if: With Perceptual Disturbances
F10.03	Alcohol Intoxication Delirium (143)
F10.4	Alcohol Withdrawal Delirium (143)
F10.73	Alcohol-Induced Persisting Dementia (168)
F10.6	Alcohol-Induced Persisting Amnestic Disorder (177)
F10.xx	Alcohol-Induced Psychotic Disorder (338)
.51	With Delusions[I,W]
.52	With Hallucinations[I,W]
F10.8	Alcohol-Induced Mood Disorder[I,W] (405)
F10.8	Alcohol-Induced Anxiety Disorder[I,W] (479)
F10.8	Alcohol-Induced Sexual Dysfunction[I] (562)
F10.8	Alcohol-Induced Sleep Disorder[I,W] (655)
F10.9	Alcohol-Related Disorder NOS (223)

AMPHETAMINE (OR AMPHETAMINE-LIKE)–RELATED DISORDERS (223)

Amphetamine Use Disorders (224)

F15.2x	Amphetamine Dependence[a] (224)
F15.1	Amphetamine Abuse (225)

Amphetamine-Induced Disorders (226)

F15.00	Amphetamine Intoxication (226)
F15.04	Amphetamine Intoxication, With Perceptual Disturbances (226)
F15.3	Amphetamine Withdrawal (227)
F15.03	Amphetamine Intoxication Delirium (143)
F15.xx	Amphetamine-Induced Psychotic Disorder (338)
.51	With Delusions[I]
.52	With Hallucinations[I]
F15.8	Amphetamine-Induced Mood Disorder[I,W] (405)
F15.8	Amphetamine-Induced Anxiety Disorder[I] (479)
F15.8	Amphetamine-Induced Sexual Dysfunction[I] (562)
F15.8	Amphetamine-Induced Sleep Disorder[I,W] (655)
F15.9	Amphetamine-Related Disorder NOS (231)

CAFFEINE-RELATED DISORDERS (231)

Caffeine-Induced Disorders (232)

F15.00	Caffeine Intoxication (232)
F15.8	Caffeine-Induced Anxiety Disorder[I] (479)
F15.8	Caffeine-Induced Sleep Disorder[I] (655)
F15.9	Caffeine-Related Disorder NOS (234)

(continued)

Table 6–1 (continued)

CANNABIS-RELATED DISORDERS (234)

Cannabis Use Disorders (236)

F12.2x   Cannabis Dependence[a] (236)
F12.1   Cannabis Abuse (236)

Cannabis-Induced Disorders (237)

F12.00   Cannabis Intoxication (237)
F12.04   Cannabis Intoxication With Perceptual Disturbances (237)
F12.03   Cannabis Intoxication Delirium (143)
F12.xx   Cannabis-Induced Psychotic Disorder (338)
.51   With Delusions[I]
.52   With Hallucinations[I]
F12.8   Cannabis-Induced Anxiety Disorder[I] (479)
F12.9   Cannabis-Related Disorder NOS (241)

COCAINE-RELATED DISORDERS (241)

Cocaine Use Disorders (242)

F14.2x   Cocaine Dependence[a] (242)
F14.1   Cocaine Abuse (243)

Cocaine-Induced Disorders (244)

F14.00   Cocaine Intoxication (244)
F14.04   Cocaine Intoxication, With Perceptual Disturbances (244)
F14.3   Cocaine Withdrawal (245)
F14.03   Cocaine Intoxication Delirium (143)
F14.xx   Cocaine-Induced Psychotic Disorder (338)
.51   With Delusions[I]
.52   With Hallucinations[I]
F14.8   Cocaine-Induced Mood Disorder[I,W] (405)
F14.8   Cocaine-Induced Anxiety Disorder[I,W] (479)
F14.8   Cocaine-Induced Sexual Dysfunction[I] (562)
F14.8   Cocaine-Induced Sleep Disorder[I,W] (655)
F14.9   Cocaine-Related Disorder NOS (250)

HALLUCINOGEN-RELATED DISORDERS (250)

Hallucinogen Use Disorders (251)

F16.2x   Hallucinogen Dependence[a] (251)
F16.1   Hallucinogen Abuse (252)

Hallucinogen-Induced Disorders (252)

F16.00   Hallucinogen Intoxication (252)
F16.70   Hallucinogen Persisting Perception Disorder (Flashbacks) (253)
F16.03   Hallucinogen Intoxication Delirium (143)
F16.xx   Hallucinogen-Induced Psychotic Disorder (338)
.51   With Delusions[I]
.52   With Hallucinations[I]
F16.8   Hallucinogen-Induced Mood Disorder[I] (405)
F16.8   Hallucinogen-Induced Anxiety Disorder[I] (479)
F16.9   Hallucinogen-Related Disorder NOS (256)

INHALANT-RELATED DISORDERS (257)

Inhalant Use Disorders (258)

F18.2x   Inhalant Dependence[a] (258)
F18.1   Inhalant Abuse (259)

Inhalant-Induced Disorders (259)

F18.00   Inhalant Intoxication (259)
F18.03   Inhalant Intoxication Delirium (143)
F18.73   Inhalant-Induced Persisting Dementia (168)
F18.xx   Inhalant-Induced Psychotic Disorder (338)
.51   With Delusions[I]
.52   With Hallucinations[I]
F18.8   Inhalant-Induced Mood Disorder[I] (405)

F18.8   Inhalant-Induced Anxiety Disorder[I] (479)
F18.9   Inhalant-Related Disorder NOS (263)

NICOTINE-RELATED DISORDERS (264)

Nicotine Use Disorder (264)

F17.2x   Nicotine Dependence[a] (264)

Nicotine-Induced Disorder (265)

F17.3   Nicotine Withdrawal (265)
F17.9   Nicotine-Related Disorder NOS (269)

OPIOID-RELATED DISORDERS (269)

Opioid Use Disorders (270)

F11.2x   Opioid Dependence[a] (270)
F11.1   Opioid Abuse (271)

Opioid-Induced Disorders (271)

F11.00   Opioid Intoxication (271)
F11.04   Opioid Intoxication, With Perceptual Disturbances (272)
F11.3   Opioid Withdrawal (272)
F11.03   Opioid Intoxication Delirium (143)
F11.xx   Opioid-Induced Psychotic Disorder (338)
.51   With Delusions[I]
.52   With Hallucinations[I]
F11.8   Opioid-Induced Mood Disorder[I] (405)
F11.8   Opioid-Induced Sexual Dysfunction[I] (562)
F11.8   Opioid-Induced Sleep Disorder[I,W] (655)
F11.9   Opioid-Related Disorder NOS (277)

PHENCYCLIDINE (OR PHENCYCLIDINE-LIKE)–RELATED DISORDERS (278)

Phencyclidine Use Disorders (279)

F19.2x   Phencyclidine Dependence[a] (279)
F19.1   Phencyclidine Abuse (279)

Phencyclidine-Induced Disorders (280)

F19.00   Phencyclidine Intoxication (280)
F19.04   Phencyclidine Intoxication, With Perceptual Disturbances (280)
F19.03   Phencyclidine Intoxication Delirium (143)
F19.xx   Phencyclidine-Induced Psychotic Disorder (338)
.51   With Delusions[I]
.52   With Hallucinations[I]
F19.8   Phencyclidine-Induced Mood Disorder[I] (405)
F19.8   Phencyclidine-Induced Anxiety Disorder[I] (479)
F19.9   Phencyclidine-Related Disorder NOS (283)

SEDATIVE-, HYPNOTIC-, OR ANXIOLYTIC-RELATED DISORDERS (284)

Sedative, Hypnotic, or Anxiolytic Use Disorders (285)

F13.2x   Sedative, Hypnotic, or Anxiolytic Dependence[a] (285)
F13.1   Sedative, Hypnotic, or Anxiolytic Abuse (286)

Sedative-, Hypnotic-, or Anxiolytic-Induced Disorders (286)

F13.00   Sedative, Hypnotic, or Anxiolytic Intoxication (286)
F13.3   Sedative, Hypnotic, or Anxiolytic Withdrawal (287)
           Specify if: With Perceptual Disturbances
F13.03   Sedative, Hypnotic, or Anxiolytic Intoxication Delirium (143)
F13.4   Sedative, Hypnotic, or Anxiolytic Withdrawal Delirium (143)
F13.73   Sedative-, Hypnotic-, or Anxiolytic-Induced Persisting Dementia (168)
F13.6   Sedative-, Hypnotic-, or Anxiolytic-Induced Persisting Amnestic Disorder (177)

(continued)

F13.xx	Sedative-, Hypnotic-, or Anxiolytic-Induced Psychotic Disorder (338)
.51	With Delusions[I,W]
.52	With Hallucinations[I,W]
F13.8	Sedative-, Hypnotic-, or Anxiolytic-Induced Mood Disorder[I,W] (405)
F13.8	Sedative-, Hypnotic-, or Anxiolytic-Induced Anxiety Disorder[W] (479)
F13.8	Sedative-, Hypnotic-, or Anxiolytic-Induced Sexual Dysfunction[I] (562)
F13.8	Sedative-, Hypnotic-, or Anxiolytic-Induced Sleep Disorder[I,W] (655)
F13.9	Sedative-, Hypnotic-, or Anxiolytic-Related Disorder NOS (293)

POLYSUBSTANCE-RELATED DISORDER (293)

F19.2x	Polysubstance Dependence[a] (293)

OTHER (OR UNKNOWN) SUBSTANCE-RELATED DISORDERS (294)

Other (or Unknown) Substance Use Disorders (294)

F19.2x	Other (or Unknown) Substance Dependence[a] (192)
F19.1	Other (or Unknown) Substance Abuse (198)

Other (or Unknown) Substance-Induced Disorders (295)

F19.00	Other (or Unknown) Substance Intoxication (199)
F19.04	Other (or Unknown) Substance Intoxication, With Perceptual Disturbances (199)
F19.3	Other (or Unknown) Substance Withdrawal (201)
	Specify if: With Perceptual Disturbances
F19.03	Other (or Unknown) Substance-Induced Delirium *(code F19.4 if onset during withdrawal)* (143)
F19.73	Other (or Unknown) Substance-Induced Persisting Dementia (168)
F19.6	Other (or Unknown) Substance-Induced Persisting Amnestic Disorder (177)
F19.xx	Other (or Unknown) Substance-Induced Psychotic Disorder (338)
.51	With Delusions[I,W]
.52	With Hallucinations[I,W]
F19.8	Other (or Unknown) Substance-Induced Mood Disorder[I,W] (405)
F19.8	Other (or Unknown) Substance-Induced Anxiety Disorder[I,W] (479)
F19.8	Other (or Unknown) Substance-Induced Sexual Dysfunction[I] (562)
F19.8	Other (or Unknown) Substance-Induced Sleep Disorder[I,W] (655)
F19.9	Other (or Unknown) Substance-Related Disorder NOS (295)

Schizophrenia and Other Psychotic Disorders (297)

F20.xx	Schizophrenia (298)
.0x	Paranoid Type (313)
.1x	Disorganized Type (314)
.2x	Catatonic Type (315)
.3x	Undifferentiated Type (316)
.5x	Residual Type (316)

Code course of Schizophrenia in fifth character:

2 = Episodic With Interepisode Residual Symptoms (*specify if:* With Prominent Negative Symptoms)

3 = Episodic With No Interepisode Residual Symptoms

0 = Continuous (*specify if:* With Prominent Negative Symptoms)

4 = Single Episode In Partial Remission (*specify if:* With Prominent Negative Symptoms)

5 = Single Episode In Full Remission

8 = Other or Unspecified Pattern

9 = Less than 1 year since onset of initial active-phase symptoms

F20.8	Schizophreniform Disorder (317)
	Specify if: Without Good Prognostic Features/ With Good Prognostic Features
F25.x	Schizoaffective Disorder (319)
.0	Bipolar Type
.1	Depressive Type
F22.0	Delusional Disorder (323)
	Specify type: Erotomanic Type/Grandiose Type/Jealous Type/Persecutory Type/Somatic Type/Mixed Type/Unspecified Type
F23.xx	Brief Psychotic Disorder (329)
.81	With Marked Stressor(s)
.80	Without Marked Stressor(s)
	Specify if: With Postpartum Onset
F24	Shared Psychotic Disorder (332)
F06.x	Psychotic Disorder Due to ... *[Indicate the General Medical Condition]* (334)
.2	With Delusions
.0	With Hallucinations
__.__	Substance-Induced Psychotic Disorder *(refer to Substance-Related Disorders for substance-specific codes)* (338)
	Specify if: With Onset During Intoxication/With Onset During Withdrawal
F29	Psychotic Disorder NOS (343)

Mood Disorders (345)

The following specifiers apply (for current or most recent episode) to Mood Disorders as noted:

[a]Severity/Psychotic/Remission Specifiers/[b]Chronic/[c]With Catatonic Features/[d]With Melancholic Features/[e]With Atypical Features/[f]With Postpartum Onset

The following specifiers apply to Mood Disorders as noted:

[g]With or Without Full Interepisode Recovery/[h]With Seasonal Pattern/[i]With Rapid Cycling

DEPRESSIVE DISORDERS (369)

F32.x	Major Depressive Disorder, Single Episode[a,b,c,d,e,f] (369)
F33.x	Major Depressive Disorder, Recurrent[a,b,c,d,e,f,g,h] (369)

Code current state of Major Depressive Episode in fourth character:

0 = Mild

1 = Moderate

2 = Severe Without Psychotic Features

3 = Severe With Psychotic Features

   Specify: Mood-Congruent Psychotic Features/ Mood-Incongruent Psychotic Features

4 = In Partial Remission

4 = In Full Remission

9 = Unspecified

F34.1	Dysthymic Disorder (376)
	Specify if: Early Onset/Late Onset
	Specify: With Atypical Features
F32.9	Depressive Disorder NOS (381)

BIPOLAR DISORDERS (382)

F30.x	Bipolar I Disorder, Single Manic Episode[a,c,f] (382)
	Specify if: Mixed

Code current state of Manic Episode in fourth character:

1 = Mild, Moderate, or Severe Without Psychotic Features

2 = Severe With Psychotic Features

(continued)

Table 6–1 (continued)

8 = In Partial or Full Remission

F31.0   Bipolar I Disorder, Most Recent Episode
           Hypomanic[g,h,i] (382)

F31.x   Bipolar I Disorder, Most Recent Episode Manic[a,c,f,g,h,i]
           (382)

Code current state of Manic Episode in fourth character:
1 = Mild, Moderate, or Severe Without Psychotic Features
2 = Severe With Psychotic Features
7 = In Partial or Full Remission

F31.6   Bipolar I Disorder, Most Recent Episode Mixed[a,c,f,g,h,i]
           (382)

F31.x   Bipolar I Disorder, Most Recent Episode
           Depressed[a,b,c,d,e,f,g,h,i] (382)

Code current state of Major Depressive Episode in fourth character:
3 = Mild or Moderate
4 = Severe Without Psychotic Features
5 = Severe With Psychotic Features
7 = In Partial or Full Remission

F31.9   Bipolar I Disorder, Most Recent Episode Unspeci-
           fied[g,h,i] (382)

F31.8   Bipolar II Disorder[a,b,c,d,e,f,g,h,i] (392)
           Specify (current or most recent episode): Hypomanic/
           Depressed

F34.0   Cyclothymic Disorder (398)

F31.9   Bipolar Disorder NOS (400)

F06.xx   Mood Disorder Due to ... *[Indicate the General Medi-
           cal Condition]* (401)

    .32   With Depressive Features
    .32   With Major Depressive—Like Episode
    .30   With Manic Features
    .33   With Mixed Features

—.—   Substance-Induced Mood Disorder *(refer to Sub-
           stance-Related Disorders for substance-specific
           codes)* (405)
           Specify type: With Depressive Features/With Manic
           Features/With Mixed Features
           Specify if: With Onset During Intoxication/With Onset
           During Withdrawal

F39   Mood Disorder NOS (410)

Anxiety Disorders (429)

F41.0   Panic Disorder Without Agoraphobia (433)
F40.01   Panic Disorder With Agoraphobia (433)
F40.00   Agoraphobia Without History of Panic Disorder (441)
F40.2   Specific Phobia (443)
           Specify type: Animal Type/Natural Environment Type/Blood-
           Injection-Injury Type/Situational Type/Other Type
F40.1   Social Phobia (450)
           Specify if: Generalized
F42.8   Obsessive-Compulsive Disorder (456)
           Specify if: With Poor Insight
F43.1   Posttraumatic Stress Disorder (463)
           Specify if: Acute/Chronic
           Specify if: With Delayed Onset
F43.0   Acute Stress Disorder (469)
F41.1   Generalized Anxiety Disorder (472)
F06.4   Anxiety Disorder Due to ... *[Indicate the General
           Medical Condition]* (476)
           Specify if: With Generalized Anxiety/With Panic
           Attacks/With Obsessive-Compulsive Symptoms

—.—   Substance-Induced Anxiety Disorder *(refer to Sub-
           stance-Related Disorders for substance-specific
           codes)* (479)
           Specify if: With Generalized Anxiety/With Panic
           Attacks/With Obsessive-Compulsive Symptoms/
           With Phobic Symptoms
           Specify if: With Onset During Intoxication/With
           Onset During Withdrawal

F41.9   Anxiety Disorder NOS (484)

Somatoform Disorders (485)

F45.0   Somatization Disorder (486)
F45.1   Undifferentiated Somatoform Disorder (490)
F44.x   Conversion Disorder (492)
    .4   With Motor Symptom or Deficit
    .5   With Seizures or Convulsions
    .6   With Sensory Symptom or Deficit
    .7   With Mixed Presentation
F45.4   Pain Disorder (498)
           Specify type: Associated With Psychological Fac-
           tors/Associated With Both Psychological Factors
           and a General Medical Condition
           Specify if: Acute/Chronic
F45.2   Hypochondriasis (504)
           Specify if: With Poor Insight
F45.2   Body Dysmorphic Disorder (507)
F45.9   Somatoform Disorder NOS (511)

Factitious Disorders (513)

F68.1   Factitious Disorder (513)
           Specify type: With Predominantly Psychological
           Signs and Symptoms/With Predominantly Physi-
           cal Signs and Symptoms/With Combined Psy-
           chological and Physical Signs and Symptoms
F68.1   Factitious Disorder NOS (517)

Dissociative Disorders (519)

F44.0   Dissociative Amnesia (520)
F44.1   Dissociative Fugue (523)
F44.81   Dissociative Identity Disorder (526)
F48.1   Depersonalization Disorder (530)
F44.9   Dissociative Disorder NOS (532)

Sexual and Gender Identity Disorders (535)

SEXUAL DYSFUNCTIONS (535)
The following specifiers apply to all primary Sexual Dysfunctions:
Lifelong Type/Acquired Type/Generalized Type/Situational
   Type/Due to Psychological Factors/Due to Combined Factors

Sexual Desire Disorders (539)

F52.0   Hypoactive Sexual Desire Disorder (539)
F52.10   Sexual Aversion Disorder (541)

Sexual Arousal Disorders (543)

F52.2   Female Sexual Arousal Disorder (543)
F52.2   Male Erectile Disorder (545)

Orgasmic Disorders (547)

F52.3   Female Orgasmic Disorder (547)
F52.3   Male Orgasmic Disorder (550)
F52.4   Premature Ejaculation (552)

Sexual Pain Disorders (554)

F52.6   Dyspareunia (Not Due to a General Medical Con-
           dition) (554)
F52.5   Vaginismus (Not Due to a General Medical Con-
           dition) (556)

(continued)

Table 6–1 (continued)

Sexual Dysfunction Due to a General Medical Condition (558)

N94.8	Female Hypoactive Sexual Desire Disorder Due to ... *[Indicate the General Medical Condition]* (558)
N50.8	Male Hypoactive Sexual Desire Disorder Due to ... *[Indicate the General Medical Condition]* (558)
N48.4	Male Erectile Disorder Due to ... *[Indicate the General Medical Condition]* (558)
N94.1	Female Dyspareunia Due to ... *[Indicate the General Medical Condition]* (558)
N50.8	Male Dyspareunia Due to ... *[Indicate the General Medical Condition]* (558)
N94.8	Other Female Sexual Dysfunction Due to ... *[Indicate the General Medical Condition]* (558)
N50.8	Other Male Sexual Dysfunction Due to ... *[Indicate the General Medical Condition]* (558)
—.—	Substance-Induced Sexual Dysfunction *(refer to Substance-Related Disorders for substance-specific codes)* (562)
	Specify if: With Impaired Desire/With Impaired Arousal/With Impaired Orgasm/With Sexual Pain
	Specify if: With Onset During Intoxication
F52.9	Sexual Dysfunction NOS (565)

PARAPHILIAS (566)

F65.2	Exhibitionism (569)
F65.0	Fetishism(569)
F65.8	Frotteurism (570)
F65.4	Pedophilia (571)
	Specify if: Sexually Attracted to Males/Sexually Attracted to Females/Sexually Attracted to Both
	Specify if: Limited to Incest
	Specify type: Exclusive Type/Nonexclusive Type
F65.5	Sexual Masochism (572)
F65.5	Sexual Sadism (573)
F65.1	Transvestic Fetishism (574)
	Specify if: With Gender Dysphoria
F65.3	Voyeurism (575)
F65.9	Paraphilia NOS (576)

GENDER IDENTITY DISORDERS (576)

F64.x	Gender Identity Disorder (576)
.2	in Children
.0	in Adolescents or Adults
	Specify if: Sexually Attracted to Males/Sexually Attracted to Females/Sexually Attracted to Both/Sexually Attracted to Neither
F64.9	Gender Identity Disorder NOS (582)
F52.9	Sexual Disorder NOS (582)

Eating Disorders (583)

F50.0	Anorexia Nervosa (583)
	Specify type: Restricting Type; Binge-Eating/Purging Type
F50.2	Bulimia Nervosa (589)
	Specify type: Purging Type/Nonpurging Type
F50.9	Eating Disorder NOS (594)

Sleep Disorders (597)

PRIMARY SLEEP DISORDERS (598)

Dyssomnias (598)

F51.0	Primary Insomnia (599)
F51.1	Primary Hypersomnia (604)
	Specify if: Recurrent
G47.4	Narcolepsy (609)
G47.3	Breathing-Related Sleep Disorder (615)
F51.2	Circadian Rhythm Sleep Disorder (622)
	Specify type: Delayed Sleep Phase Type/Jet Lag Type/Shift Work Type/Unspecified Type
F51.9	Dyssomnia NOS (629)

Parasomnias (630)

F51.5	Nightmare Disorder (631)
F51.4	Sleep Terror Disorder (634)
F51.3	Sleepwalking Disorder (639)
F51.8	Parasomnia NOS (644)

SLEEP DISORDERS RELATED TO ANOTHER MENTAL DISORDER (645)

F51.0	Insomnia Related to ... *[Indicate the Axis I or Axis II Disorder]* (645)
F51.1	Hypersomnia Related to ... *[Indicate the Axis I or Axis II Disorder]* (645)

OTHER SLEEP DISORDERS (651)

G47.x	Sleep Disorder Due to ... *[Indicate the General Medical Condition]* (651)
.0	Insomnia Type
.1	Hypersomnia Type
.8	Parasomnia Type
.8	Mixed Type
—.—	Substance-Induced Sleep Disorder *(refer to Substance-Related Disorders for substance-specific codes)* (655)
	Specify type: Insomnia Type/Hypersomnia Type/Parasomnia Type/Mixed Type
	Specify if: With Onset During Intoxication/With Onset During Withdrawal

Impulse-Control Disorders Not Elsewhere Classified (663)

F63.8	Intermittent Explosive Disorder (663)
F63.2	Kleptomania (667)
F63.1	Pyromania (669)
F63.0	Pathological Gambling (671)
F63.3	Trichotillomania (674)
F63.9	Impulse-Control Disorder NOS (677)

Adjustment Disorders (679)

F43.xx	Adjustment Disorder (679)
.20	With Depressed Mood
.28	With Anxiety
.22	With Mixed Anxiety and Depressed Mood
.24	With Disturbance of Conduct
.25	With Mixed Disturbance of Emotions and Conduct
.9	Unspecified
	Specify if: Acute/Chronic

Personality Disorders (685)

Note: *These are coded on Axis II.*

F60.0	Paranoid Personality Disorder (690)
F60.1	Schizoid Personality Disorder (694)
F21	Schizotypal Personality Disorder (697)
F60.2	Antisocial Personality Disorder (701)
F60.31	Borderline Personality Disorder (706)
F60.4	Histrionic Personality Disorder (711)
F60.8	Narcissistic Personality Disorder (714)
F60.6	Avoidant Personality Disorder (718)
F60.7	Dependent Personality Disorder (721)
F60.5	Obsessive-Compulsive Personality Disorder (725)
F60.9	Personality Disorder NOS (729)

(continued)

Table 6–1 (continued)

Other Conditions That May Be a Focus of Clinical Attention (731)	

PSYCHOLOGICAL FACTORS AFFECTING MEDICAL CONDITION (731)

F54   ... [Specified Psychological Factor]
Affecting ... [Indicate the General Medical Condition]
Choose name based on nature of factors: (731)
Mental Disorder Affecting Medical Condition
Psychological Symptoms Affecting Medical Condition
Personality Traits or Coping Style Affecting Medical Condition
Maladaptive Health Behaviors Affecting Medical Condition
Stress-Related Physiological Response Affecting Medical Condition
Other or Unspecified Psychological Factors Affecting Medical Condition

MEDICATION-INDUCED MOVEMENT DISORDERS (734)

G21.0	Neuroleptic-Induced Parkinsonism (735)
G21.0	Neuroleptic Malignant Syndrome (735)
G24.0	Neuroleptic-Induced Acute Dystonia (735)
G21.1	Neuroleptic-Induced Acute Akathisia (735)
G24.0	Neuroleptic-Induced Tardive Dyskinesia (736)
G25.1	Medication-Induced Postural Tremor (736)
G25.9	Medication-Induced Movement Disorder NOS (736)

OTHER MEDICATION-INDUCED DISORDER (736)

T88.7	Adverse Effects of Medication NOS (736)

RELATIONAL PROBLEMS (736)

Z63.7	Relational Problem Related to a Mental Disorder or General Medical Condition (737)
Z63.8	Parent-Child Relational Problem *(code Z63.1 if focus of attention is on child)* (737)

Z63.0	Partner Relational Problem (737)
F93.3	Sibling Relational Problem (737)
Z63.9	Relational Problem NOS (737)

PROBLEMS RELATED TO ABUSE OR NEGLECT (738)

T74.1	Physical Abuse of Child (738)
T74.2	Sexual Abuse of Child (738)
T74.0	Neglect of Child (738)
T74.1	Physical Abuse of Adult (738)
T74.2	Sexual Abuse of Adult (738)

ADDITIONAL CONDITIONS THAT MAY BE A FOCUS OF CLINICAL ATTENTION (739)

Z91.1	Noncompliance With Treatment (739)
Z76.5	Malingering (739)
Z72.8	Adult Antisocial Behavior (740)
Z72.8	Child or Adolescent Antisocial Behavior (740)
R41.8	Borderline Intellectual Functioning (740)
R41.8	Age-Related Cognitive Decline (740)
Z63.4	Bereavement (740)
Z55.8	Academic Problem (741)
Z56.7	Occupational Problem (741)
F93.8	Identity Problem (741)
Z71.8	Religious or Spiritual Problem (741)
Z60.3	Acculturation Problem (741)
Z60.0	Phase of Life Problem (742)

Additional Codes (743)	
F99	Unspecified Mental Disorder (nonpsychotic) (743)
Z03.2	No Diagnosis or Condition on Axis I (743)
R69	Diagnosis or Condition Deferred on Axis I (743)
Z03.2	No Diagnosis on Axis II (743)
R46.8	Diagnosis Deferred on Axis II (743)

From American Psychiatric Association. *Diagnostic and Statistical Manual of Mental Disorders.* 4th ed. Text rev. Washington, DC: American Psychiatric Association; copyright 2000, with permission.

Table 6–2
DSM-IV-TR Axis I: Clinical Disorders and Other Disorders That May Be a Focus of Clinical Attention

Disorders usually first diagnosed in infancy, childhood, or adolescence (excluding mental retardation)
Delirium, dementia, and amnestic and other cognitive disorders
Mental disorders due to a general medical condition not elsewhere classified
Substance-related disorders
Schizophrenia and other psychotic disorders
Mood disorders
Anxiety disorders
Somatoform disorders
Factitious disorders
Dissociative disorders
Sexual and gender identity disorders
Eating disorders
Sleep disorders
Impulse-control disorders not elsewhere classified
Adjustment disorders
Other conditions that may be a focus of clinical attention

From American Psychiatric Association. *Diagnostic and Statistical Manual of Mental Disorders.* 4th ed. Text rev. Washington, DC: American Psychiatric Association; copyright 2000, with permission.

ered a composite of three major areas: social functioning, occupational functioning, and psychological functioning. The GAF Scale, based on a continuum of mental health and mental illness, is a 100-point scale, 100 representing the highest level of functioning in all areas (Table 6–4).

People who had a high level of functioning before an episode of illness generally have a better prognosis than do those who had a low level of functioning.

DSM-IV-TR CLASSIFICATION OF MENTAL DISORDERS

Table 6–1 presents the DSM-IV-TR classification of mental disorders (Axis I and Axis II).

PSYCHIATRIC RATING SCALES

Psychiatric rating scales, also called *rating instruments*, provide a way to quantify aspects of a patient's psyche, behavior, and relationships with individuals and society. The measurement of pathology in these areas of a person's life may initially seem to be less straightforward than is the measurement of pathology—hypertension, for example—by other medical specialists. Nevertheless, many psychiatric rating scales are able to measure carefully chosen features of well-formulated concepts. Moreover, psychiatrists who do not use these rating scales are left

Table 6–3
DSM-IV-TR Axis II: Personality Disorders and Mental Retardation

Paranoid personality disorder
Schizoid personality disorder
Schizotypal personality disorder
Antisocial personality disorder
Borderline personality disorder
Histrionic personality disorder
Narcissistic personality disorder
Avoidant personality disorder
Dependent personality disorder
Obsessive-compulsive personality disorder
Personality disorder not otherwise specified
Mental retardation

From American Psychiatric Association. *Diagnostic and Statistical Manual of Mental Disorders.* 4th ed. Text rev. Washington, DC: American Psychiatric Association; copyright 2000, with permission.

with only their clinical impressions, which are difficult to record in a manner that allows for reliable future comparison and communication. Without psychiatric rating scales, quantitative data in psychiatry are crude (for example, length of hos-

pitalization or other treatment, discharge and readmission to hospital, length of relationships or employment, and presence of legal troubles). A description of the four major scales used in DSM-IV-TR follows.

GAF Scale

Axis V in DSM-IV-TR uses the GAF Scale (Table 6–4). This axis is used for reporting a clinician's judgment of a patient's overall level of functioning. The information is used to decide on a treatment plan and later to measure the plan's effect.

Social and Occupational Functioning Assessment Scale

The Social and Occupational Functioning Assessment Scale can be used to track a patient's progress in social and occupational areas (Table 6–5). It is independent of the psychiatric diagnosis and of the severity of the patient's psychological symptoms.

Other Scales

Two other scales that may be useful are the Global Assessment of Relational Functioning (GARF) Scale and the Defensive Functioning Scale (Tables 6–6 and 6–7).

Table 6–4
Global Assessment of Functioning (GAF) Scale

Consider psychological, social, and occupational functioning on a hypothetical continuum of mental health–illness. Do not include impairment in functioning due to physical (or environmental) limitations.

Code (**Note:** Use intermediate codes when appropriate, e.g., 45, 68, 72.)

Code	Description
100–91	Superior functioning in a wide range of activities, life's problems never seem to get out of hand, is sought out by others because of his or her many positive qualities. No symptoms.
90–81	Absent or minimal symptoms (e.g., mild anxiety before an exam), good functioning in all areas, interested and involved in a wide range of activities, socially effective, generally satisfied with life, no more than everyday problems or concerns (e.g., an occasional argument with family members).
80–71	If symptoms are present, they are transient and expectable reactions to psychosocial stressors (e.g., difficulty concentrating after family argument): no more than slight impairment in social, occupational, or school functioning (e.g., temporarily falling behind in schoolwork).
70–61	Some mild symptoms (e.g., depressed mood and mild insomnia) OR some difficulty in social, occupational, or school functioning (e.g., occasional truancy, or theft within the household), but generally functioning pretty well, has some meaningful interpersonal relationships.
60–51	Moderate symptoms (e.g., flat affect and circumstantial speech, occasional panic attacks) OR moderate difficulty in social, occupational, or school functioning (e.g., few friends, conflicts with peers or coworkers).
50–41	Serious symptoms (e.g., suicidal ideation, severe obsessional rituals, frequent shoplifting) OR any serious impairment in social, occupational, or school functioning (e.g., no friends, unable to keep a job).
40–31	Some impairment in reality testing or communication (e.g., speech is at times illogical, obscure, or irrelevant) OR major impairment in several areas, such as work or school, family relations, judgment, thinking, or mood (e.g., depressed man avoids friends, neglects family, and is unable to work; child frequently beats up younger children, is defiant at home, and is failing at school).
30–21	Behavior is considerably influenced by delusions or hallucinations OR serious impairment in communication or judgment (e.g., sometimes incoherent, acts grossly inappropriately, suicidal preoccupation) OR inability to function in almost all areas (e.g., stays in bed all day; no job, home, or friends).
20–11	Some danger of hurting self or others (e.g., suicide attempts without clear expectation of death, frequently violent, manic excitement) OR occasionally fails to maintain minimal personal hygiene (e.g., smears feces) OR gross impairment in communication (e.g., largely incoherent or mute).
10–1	Persistent danger of severely hurting self or others (e.g., recurrent violence) OR persistent inability to maintain minimal personal hygiene OR serious suicidal act with clear expectation of death.
0	Inadequate information.

The GAF Scale is a revision of the GAS (Endicott J, Spitzer RL, Fleiss JL, Cohen I. The Global Assessment Scale: a procedure for measuring overall severity of psychiatric disturbance. *Arch Gen Psychiatry.* 1976;33:766) and CGAS (Shaffer D, Gould MS, Brasio J, et al. Children's Global Assessment Scale (CGAS). *Arch Gen Psychiatry.* 1983;40:1228). They are revisions of the Global Scale of the Health-Sickness Rating Scale (Luborsky I. Clinicians' judgments of mental health. *Arch Gen Psychiatry.* 1962;7:407).
From American Psychiatric Association. *Diagnostic and Statistical Manual of Mental Disorders.* 4th ed. Text rev. Washington, DC: American Psychiatric Association; copyright 2000, with permission.

Table 6–5
Social and Occupational Functioning Assessment Scale (SOFAS)

Consider social and occupational functioning on a continuum from excellent functioning to grossly impaired functioning. Include impairments in functioning due to physical limitations, as well as those due to mental impairments. To be counted, impairment must be a direct consequence of mental and physical health problems; the effects of lack of opportunity and other environmental limitations are not to be considered.

Code   (**Note:** Use intermediate codes when appropriate, e.g., 45, 68, 72.)

100   Superior functioning in a wide range of activities.

91
90   Good functioning in all areas, occupationally and socially effective.

81

80   No more than a slight impairment in social, occupational, or school functioning (e.g., infrequent interpersonal conflict, temporarily falling behind in schoolwork).
71
70   Some difficulty in social, occupational, or school functioning, but generally functioning well, has some meaningful interpersonal relationships.

61
60   Moderate difficulty in social, occupational, or school functioning (e.g., few friends, conflicts with peers or coworkers).

51

50   Serious impairment in social, occupational, or school functioning (e.g., no friends, unable to keep a job).

41
40   Major impairment in several areas, such as work or school, family relations (e.g., depressed man avoids friends, neglects family, and is unable to work; child frequently beats up younger children, is defiant at home, and is failing at school).
31

30   Inability to function in almost all areas (e.g., stays in bed all day; no job, home, or friends).

21
20   Occasionally fails to maintain minimal personal hygiene; unable to function independently.

11
10   Persistent inability to maintain minimal personal hygiene. Unable to function without harming self or others or without considerable external support (e.g., nursing care and supervision).
1

0   Inadequate information.

Note: The rating of overall psychological functioning on a scale of 0–100 was operationalized by Luborsky in the Health-Sickness Rating Scale. Luborsky L. Clinicians' judgments of mental health. *Arch Gen Psychiatry.* 1962;7:407. Spitzer and colleagues developed a revision of the Health-Sickness Rating Scale called the Global Assessment Scale (GAS) (Endicott J, Spitzer RL, Fleiss JL, et al. The Global Assessment Scale: a procedure for measuring overall severity of psychiatric disturbance. *Arch Gen Psychiatry.* 1976;33:766). The SOFAS is derived from the GAS and its development is described in Goldman HH, Skodol AE, Lave TR. Revising Axis V for DSM-IV: a review of measures of social functioning. *Am J Psychiatry.* 1992;149:1148.
From American Psychiatric Association. *Diagnostic and Statistical Manual of Mental Disorders.* 4th ed. Text rev. Washington, DC: American Psychiatric Association; copyright 2000, with permission.

Table 6–6
Global Assessment of Relational Functioning (GARF)

INSTRUCTIONS: The GARF Scale can be used to indicate an overall judgment of the functioning of a family or other ongoing relationship on a hypothetical continuum ranging from competent, optimal relational functioning to a disrupted, dysfunctional relationship. It is analogous to Axis V (Global Assessment of Functioning Scale) provided for individuals in DSM-IV. The GARF Scale permits the clinician to rate the degree to which a family or other ongoing relational unit meets the affective and/or instrumental needs of its members in the following areas:

A. *Problem solving*—skills in negotiating goals, rules, and routines; adaptability to stress; communication skills; ability to resolve conflict.

B. *Organization*—maintenance of interpersonal roles and subsystem boundaries; hierarchical functioning, coalitions and distribution of power, control and responsibility.

C. *Emotional climate*—tone and range of feelings; quality of caring, empathy, involvement and attachment/commitment; sharing of values; mutual affective responsiveness, respect, and regard; quality of sexual functioning.

In most instances, the GARF Scale should be used to rate functioning during the current period (i.e., the level of relational functioning at the time of the evaluation). In some settings, the GARF Scale may also be used to rate functioning for other time periods (i.e., the highest level of relational functioning for at least a few months during the past year). **Note:** Use specific, intermediate codes when possible, for example, 45, 68, 72. If detailed information is not adequate to make specific ratings, use midpoints of the five ranges, that is, 90, 70, 50, 30, or 10.

(81–100) Overall: Relational unit is functioning satisfactorily from self-report of participants and from perspectives of observers.

Agreed-on patterns or routines exist that help meet the usual needs of each family/couple member; there is flexibility for change in response to unusual demands or events; occasional conflicts and stressful transitions are resolved through problem-solving communication and negotiation.

There is a shared understanding and agreement about roles and appropriate tasks; decision making is established for each functional area, and there is recognition of the unique characteristics and merit of each subsystem (e.g., parents/spouses, siblings, and individuals).

There is a situationally appropriate, optimistic atmosphere in the family; a wide range of feelings is freely expressed and managed within the family; there is a general atmosphere of warmth, caring, and sharing of values among all family members. Sexual relations of adult members are satisfactory.

(61–80) Overall: Functioning of relational unit is somewhat unsatisfactory. Over a period of time, many but not all difficulties are resolved without complaints.

Daily routines are present but there is some pain and difficulty in responding to the unusual. Some conflicts remain unresolved, but do not disrupt family functioning.

Decision making is usually competent, but efforts at control of one another quite often are greater than necessary or are ineffective. Individuals and relationships are clearly demarcated but sometimes a specific subsystem is depreciated or scapegoated.

A range of feeling is expressed, but instances of emotional blocking or tension are evident. Warmth and caring are present but are marred by a family member's irritability and frustrations. Sexual activity of adult members may be reduced or problematic.

(41–60) Overall: Relational unit has occasional times of satisfying and competent functioning together, but clearly dysfunctional, unsatisfying relationships tend to predominate.

Communication is frequently inhibited by unresolved conflicts that often interfere with daily routines; there is significant difficulty in adapting to family stress and transitional change.

Decision making is only intermittently competent and effective; either excessive rigidity or significant lack of structure is evident at these times. Individual needs are quite often submerged by a partner or coalition.

Pain or ineffective anger or emotional deadness interferes with family enjoyment. Although there is some warmth and support for members, it is usually unequally distributed. Troublesome sexual difficulties between adults are often present.

(21–40) Overall: Relational unit is obviously and seriously dysfunctional; forms and time periods of satisfactory relating are rare.

Family/couple routines do not meet the needs of members; they are grimly adhered to or blithely ignored. Life cycle changes, such as departures or entries into the relational unit, generate painful conflict and obviously frustrating failures of problem solving.

Decision making is tyrannical or quite ineffective. The unique characteristics of individuals are unappreciated or ignored by either rigid or confusingly fluid coalitions.

There are infrequent periods of enjoyment of life together; frequent distancing or open hostility reflect significant conflicts that remain unresolved and quite painful. Sexual dysfunction among adult members is commonplace.

(1–20) Overall: Relational unit has become too dysfunctional to retain continuity of contact and attachment.

Family/couple routines are negligible (e.g., no mealtime, sleeping, or waking schedule); family members often do not know where others are or when they will be in or out; there is little effective communication among family members.

Family/couple members are not organized in such a way that personal or generational responsibilities are recognized. Boundaries of relational unit as a whole and subsystems cannot be identified or agreed upon. Family members are physically endangered or injured or sexually attacked.

Despair and cynicism are pervasive; there is little attention to the emotional needs of others; there is almost no sense of attachment, commitment, or concern about one another's welfare.

0 Inadequate information.

From American Psychiatric Association. *Diagnostic and Statistical Manual of Mental Disorders.* 4th ed. Text rev. Washington, DC: American Psychiatric Association; copyright 2000, with permission.

Table 6-7
Defensive Functioning Scale

High adaptive level. This level of defensive functioning results in optimal adaptation in the handling of stressors. These defenses usually maximize gratification and allow the conscious awareness of feelings, ideas, and their consequences. They also promote an optimum balance among conflicting motives. Examples of defenses characteristically at this level are
- affiliation
- altruism
- anticipation
- humor
- self-assertion
- self-observation
- sublimation
- suppression

Mental inhibitions (compromise formation) level. Defensive functioning at this level keeps potentially threatening ideas, feelings, memories, wishes, or fears out of awareness. Examples are
- displacement
- dissociation
- intellectualization
- isolation of affect
- reaction formation
- repression
- undoing

Minor image-distorting level. This level is characterized by distortions in the image of the self, body, or others that may be employed to regulate self-esteem. Examples are
- devaluation
- idealization
- omnipotence

Disavowal level. This level is characterized by keeping unpleasant or unacceptable stressors, impulses, ideas, affect, or responsibility out of awareness with or without a misattribution of these to external causes. Examples are
- denial
- projection
- rationalization

Major image-distorting level. This level is characterized by gross distortion or misattribution of the image of self or others. Examples are
- autistic fantasy
- projective identification
- splitting of self-image or image of others

Action level. This level is characterized by defensive functioning that deals with internal or external stressors by action or withdrawal. Examples are
- acting out
- apathetic withdrawal
- help-rejecting complaining
- passive aggression

Level of defensive dysregulation. This level is characterized by failure of defensive regulation to contain the individual's reaction to stressors, leading to a pronounced break with objective reality. Examples are
- delusional projection
- psychotic denial
- psychotic distortion

From American Psychiatric Association. *Diagnostic and Statistical Manual of Mental Disorders.* 4th ed. Text rev. Washington, DC: American Psychiatric Association; copyright 2000, with permission.

7

Delirium, Dementia, and Amnestic and Other Cognitive Disorders and Mental Disorders Due to a General Medical Condition

▲ 7.1 Overview

In the text revision of the fourth edition of *Diagnostic Statistical Manual of Mental Disorders* (DSM-IV-TR), three groups of disorders—delirium, dementia, and the amnestic disorders—are characterized by the primary symptoms common to all the disorders: an impairment in cognition (as in memory, language, or attention). Although DSM-IV-TR acknowledges that other psychiatric disorders can exhibit a degree of cognitive impairment as a symptom, cognitive impairment is the cardinal symptom in delirium, dementia, and the amnestic disorders. Within each of these diagnostic categories, DSM-IV-TR delimits specific types (Table 7.1–1).

In the past, these conditions were classified under the heading *organic mental disorders*. Traditionally, organic brain disorders were defined as disorders for which there is an identifiable pathologic condition, such as brain tumor, cerebrovascular disease, or drug intoxication. Those brain disorders with no generally accepted organic basis (such as depression) were called *functional disorders*. Historically, the field of neurology has been associated with the treatment of organic disorders, and psychiatry has been associated with the treatment of functional disorders.

This century-old distinction between organic and functional disorders is outdated and has been deleted from the nomenclature. The only unbiased conclusion to be made from evaluation of the available data is that every psychiatric disorder has an organic (that is, biological) component. Because of this reassessment of the data, the concept of functional disorders has been determined to be misleading, and both the term *functional* and its historical opposite, *organic*, are no longer used in that context in DSM-IV-TR.

A further indication that the dichotomy is no longer valid is the revival of the term *neuropsychiatry*. As defined in the seventh edition of *Campbell's Psychiatric Dictionary*, neuropsychiatry emphasizes the somatic substructure on which mental operations and emotions are based; it is concerned with the psy-

chopathologic accompaniments of brain dysfunction as observed in seizure disorders, for example. Neuropsychiatry focuses on the psychiatric aspects of neurological disorders and the role of brain dysfunction in psychiatric disorders.

CLASSIFICATION

For each of the three major groups—delirium, dementia, and amnestic disorders—there are subcategories based on etiology. They are defined and summarized as follows.

Delirium

Delirium is marked by short-term confusion and changes in cognition. There are four subcategories based on several causes: (1) general medical condition, such as infection; (2) substance induced, such as cocaine, opioids, phencyclidine; (3) multiple etiologies, such as head trauma and kidney disease; and (4) delirium not otherwise specified, such as sleep deprivation.

Dementia

Dementia is marked by severe impairment in memory, judgment, orientation, and cognition. There are six subcategories: (1) dementia of the Alzheimer's type—usually occurs in persons older than 65 years and is manifested by progressive intellectual disorientation and dementia, delusions, or depression; (2) vascular dementia—caused by vessel thrombosis or hemorrhage; (3) other medical conditions, such as human immunodeficiency virus (HIV) disease, head trauma, Pick's disease, Creutzfeldt-Jakob disease (caused by slow-growing transmittable virus); (4) substance-induced—caused by toxin or medication, such as from gasoline fumes, atropine; (5) multiple etiologies; and (6) not otherwise specified (if unknown).

Amnestic Disorder

Amnestic disorder is marked by memory impairment and forgetfulness. There are three subcategories: (1) caused by medical

**Table 7.1–1
DSM-IV-TR Cognitive Disorders**

Delirium
  Delirium due to a general medical condition
  Substance-induced delirium
  Delirium due to multiple etiologies
  Delirium not otherwise specified
Dementia
  Dementia of the Alzheimer's type
  Vascular dementia
  Dementia due to other general medical conditions
    Dementia due to HIV disease
    Dementia due to head trauma
    Dementia due to Parkinson's disease
    Dementia due to Huntington's disease
    Dementia due to Pick's disease
    Dementia due to Creutzfeldt-Jakob disease
    Dementia due to other general medical conditions
  Substance-induced persisting dementia
  Dementia due to multiple etiologies
  Dementia not otherwise specified
Amnestic disorders
  Amnestic disorder due to a general medical condition
  Substance-induced persisting amnestic disorder
  Amnestic disorder not otherwise specified
  Cognitive disorder not otherwise specified

condition (hypoxia); (2) caused by toxin, or medication, such as marijuana, diazepam; and (3) not otherwise specified.

Cognitive Disorder Not Otherwise Specified

Cognitive disorder not otherwise specified is a DSM-IV-TR category that allows for the diagnosis of cognitive disorders

**Table 7.1–2
DSM-IV-TR Diagnostic Criteria for Cognitive Disorder Not Otherwise Specified**

This category is for disorders that are characterized by cognitive dysfunction presumed to be due to the direct physiological effect of a general medical condition that do not meet criteria for any of the specific deliriums, dementias, or amnestic disorders listed in this section and that are not better classified as delirium not otherwise specified, dementia not otherwise specified, or amnestic disorder not otherwise specified. For cognitive dysfunction due to a specific or unknown substance, the specific substance-related disorder not otherwise specified category should be used.

Examples include

1. Mild neurocognitive disorder: impairment in cognitive functioning as evidenced by neuropsychological testing or quantified clinical assessment, accompanied by objective evidence of a systemic general medical condition or central nervous system dysfunction
2. Postconcussional disorder: following a head trauma, impairment in memory or attention with associated symptoms

From American Psychiatric Association. *Diagnostic and Statistical Manual of Mental Disorders*. 4th ed. Text rev. Washington, DC: American Psychiatric Association; copyright 2000, with permission.

that do not meet the criteria for delirium, dementia, or amnestic disorders. These disorders fit into the not otherwise specified category (Table 7.1–2). The cause of these syndromes is presumed to involve a specific general medical condition, a pharmacologically active agent, or possibly both.

CLINICAL EVALUATION OF COGNITION

When testing cognitive functions, the clinician should evaluate memory, visuospatial and constructional abilities, and reading, writing, and mathematical abilities. Abstraction ability is also valuable to assess, although a patient's performance on tasks, such as proverb interpretation, may be a useful bedside projective test in some patients, but the specific interpretation may result from a variety of factors, such as poor education, low intelligence, and failure to understand the concept of proverbs, as well as a broad array of primary and secondary psychopathological disturbances.

Although formal evaluation of cognitive impairment requires time-consuming consultation with an expert in psychological testing, one practical and clinically useful test for practitioners is the Mini-Mental State examination (MMSE). MMSE is a screening test that can be used during a patient's clinical examination. The test, devised by M.F. Goldstein, S. Folstein, and P.R. McHugh, consists of five categories: (1) orientation (e.g., time, place, and person), (2) registration (e.g., subtract 7 from 100 serially, naming three objects), (3) recall (e.g., recalling objects named), (4) language (e.g., naming objects, repetition of words, writing a sentence), and (5) construction (e.g., copying a design). Points are given for each correrct answer in each category, with a maximum score of 30 indicating no impairment (Folstein MF, Folstein S, McHugh PR. Mini-mental state: a practical method for grading the cognitive state of patients for the clinician. *J Psychiatr Res* 1975;12:189.) The reader is referred to *Synopsis of Psychiatry*, 9th ed., page 321, for further information about the Mini-Mental State Examination.

▲ 7.2 Delirium

Delirium

Delirium is a syndrome, not a disease, and it has many causes, all of which result in a similar pattern of symptoms relating to the patient's level of consciousness and cognitive impairment. Most of the causes of delirium arise outside the central nervous system, for example, in renal or hepatic failure. Delirium remains an underrecognized and underdiagnosed clinical disorder. Part of the problem is that the syndrome has a variety of other names, for example, acute confusional state, acute brain syndrome, metabolic encephalopathy, toxic psychosis, and acute brain failure. The intent of the new classification system has been to help consolidate the myriad of terms into a single diagnostic label.

In the text revision of the fourth edition of the *Diagnostic and Statistical Manual of Mental Disorders* (DSM-IV-TR), delirium is "characterized by a disturbance of consciousness and a change in cognition that develop over a short time." The hallmark symptom of delirium is an impairment of consciousness, usually occurring in association with global impairments of cognitive functions. Abnormalities of mood, perception, and behavior are common psychiatric symptoms; tremor, asterixis, nystagmus, incoordination, and urinary incontinence are common neurological symptoms. Classically, delirium has a sudden onset (hours or days), a brief and fluctuating course, and a rapid improvement when the causative factor is identified and eliminated, but each of these characteristic features can vary in individual patients.

Physicians must recognize delirium to identify and treat the underlying cause and to avert the development of delirium-related complications. Such complications include accidental injury because of the patient's clouded consciousness or impaired coordination or because of the unnecessary use of restraints. The disruption of ward routine is an especially troubling problem on nonpsychiatric units, such as intensive care units and general medical and surgical wards.

EPIDEMIOLOGY

Delirium is a common disorder. According to the DSM-IV-TR, the point prevalence of delirium in the general population is 0.4 percent for people 18 years and older and 1.1 percent for people 55 and older. Approximately 10 to 30 percent of medically ill patients who are hospitalized exhibit delirium. Approximately 30 percent of patients in surgical intensive care units and cardiac intensive care units and 40 to 50 percent of patients who are recovering from surgery for hip fractures have an episode of delirium. The highest rate of delirium is found in postcardiotomy patients—more than 90 percent in some studies. An estimated 20 percent of patients with severe burns and 30 to 40 percent of patients with acquired immune deficiency syndrome have episodes of delirium while they are hospitalized. Delirium develops in 80 percent of terminally ill patients. The causes of postoperative delirium include the stress of surgery, postoperative pain, insomnia, pain medication, electrolyte imbalances, infection, fever, and blood loss.

Advanced age is a major risk factor for the development of delirium. Approximately 30 to 40 percent of hospitalized patients older than age 65 have an episode of delirium, and another 10 to 15 percent of elderly persons exhibit delirium on admission to the hospital. Sixty percent of nursing home residents over age 75 have repeated episodes of delirium. Other predisposing factors for the development of delirium are young age (that is, children), preexisting brain damage (such as dementia, cerebrovascular disease, tumor), a history of delirium, alcohol dependence, diabetes, cancer, sensory impairment (such as blindness), and malnutrition. Male gender is an independent risk factor for delirium, according to DSM-IV-TR.

The presence of delirium is a poor prognostic sign. Rates of institutionalization are increased by three times for patients 65 years and older who exhibit delirium while in the hospital. The 3-month mortality rate of patients who have an episode of delirium is estimated to be 23 to 33 percent. The 1-year mortality rate for patients who have an episode of delirium may be as high as 50 percent. Elderly patients who experience delirium while hospitalized have a 20 to 75 percent mortality rate during that hospitalization. After discharge, up to 15 percent of these persons die within a 1-month period, and 25 percent die within 6 months.

ETIOLOGY

The major causes of delirium are central nervous system disease (such as epilepsy), systemic disease (such as cardiac failure), and either intoxication or withdrawal from pharmacological or toxic agents. When evaluating patients with delirium, clinicians should assume that any drug that a patient has taken may be causatively relevant to the delirium.

DIAGNOSIS AND CLINICAL FEATURES

The syndrome of delirium is almost always caused by one or more systemic or cerebral derangements that affect brain function.

A 74-year-old African-American woman, Ms. Richardson, was brought to a city hospital emergency room by the police. She is unkempt, dirty, and foul smelling. She does not look at the interviewer and is apparently confused and unresponsive to most of his questions. She knows her name and address but not the day or the month. She is unable to describe the events that led to her admission.

The police reported that they were called by neighbors because Ms. Richardson had been wandering around the neighborhood and not taking care of herself. The medical center mobile crisis unit went to her house twice but could not get in and presumed she was not home. Finally, the police came and broke into the apartment, where they were met by a snarling German shepherd. They shot the dog with a tranquilizing gun and then found Ms. Richardson hiding in the corner, wearing nothing but a bra. The apartment was filthy; the floor was littered with dog feces. The police found a gun, which they took into custody.

The following day, while Ms. Richardson was awaiting transfer to a medical unit for treatment of her out-of-control diabetes, the supervising psychiatrist attempted to interview her. Her facial expression was still mostly unresponsive, and she still didn't know the month and couldn't say what hospital she was in. She reported that the neighbors had called the police because she was "sick," and indeed she had felt sick and weak, with pains in her shoulder; in addition, she had not eaten for 3 days. She remembered that the dog was not in "the shop" and would be returned to her when she got home. She refused to give the name of a neighbor who was a friend, saying, "He's got enough troubles of his own." She denied ever being in a psychiatric hospital or hearing voices, but acknowledged that she had at one point seen a psychiatrist "near Lincoln Center" because she couldn't sleep. He had prescribed medication that was too strong, so she didn't take it. She didn't remember the name so the interviewer asked if it was Thorazine. She said no, it was "allal." "Haldol?" asked the interviewer. She nodded. The interviewer was convinced that was the drug, but other observers thought she might have said yes to anything that sounded remotely like it, such as "Elavil." When asked about the gun, she denied, with some annoyance, that it was real and said it was a toy gun that had been brought to the house by her brother, who had died 8 years ago. She was still feeling weak and sick, complained of pain in her shoulder, and apparently had trouble swallowing. She did manage to smile as the team left her bedside. (Reprinted with permission from *DSM-IV Casebook.*)

Table 7.2–1
DSM-IV-TR Diagnostic Criteria for 293.0 Delirium Due to General Medical Condition

A. Disturbance of consciousness (i.e., reduced clarity of awareness of the environment) with reduced ability to focus, sustain, or shift attention.

B. A change in cognition (such as memory deficit, disorientation, language disturbance) or the development of a perceptual disturbance that is not better accounted for by a preexisting, established, or evolving dementia.

C. The disturbance develops over a short period of time (usually hours to days) and tends to fluctuate during the course of the day.

D. There is evidence from the history, physical examination, or laboratory findings that the disturbance is caused by the direct physiological consequences of a general medical condition.

Coding note: If delirium is superimposed on a preexisting vascular dementia, indicate the delirium by coding vascular dementia, with delirium.

Coding note: Include the name of the general medical condition on Axis I, e.g., Delirium due to hepatic encephalopathy; also code the general medical condition on Axis III.

Table 7.2–2
DSM-IV-TR Diagnostic Criteria for Substance Intoxication Delirium

A. Disturbance of consciousness (i.e., reduced clarity of awareness of the environment) with reduced ability to focus, sustain, or shift attention.

B. A change in cognition (such as memory deficit, disorientation, language disturbance) or the development of a perceptual disturbance that is not better accounted for by a preexisting, established, or evolving dementia.

C. The disturbance develops over a short period of time (usually hours to days) and tends to fluctuate during the course of the day.

D. There is evidence from the history, physical examination, or laboratory findings of either (1) or (2):

(1) the symptoms in Criteria A and B developed during substance intoxication

(2) medication use is etiologically related to the disturbance*

Note: This diagnosis should be made instead of a diagnosis of substance intoxication only when the cognitive symptoms are in excess of those usually associated with the intoxication syndrome and when the symptoms are sufficiently severe to warrant independent clinical attention.

*Note: The diagnosis should be recorded as substance-induced delirium if related to medication use.

Code (Specific substance) intoxication delirium:

(Alcohol; Amphetamine [or amphetaminelike substance]; Cannabis; Cocaine; Hallucinogen; Inhalant; Opioid; Phencyclidine [or phencyclidinelike substance]; Sedative, hypnotic, or anxiolytic; Other [or unknown] substance [e.g., cimetidine, digitalis, benztropine])

Table 7.2–3
DSM-IV-TR Diagnostic Criteria for Substance Withdrawal Delirium

A. Disturbance of consciousness (i.e., reduced clarity of awareness of the environment) with reduced ability to focus, sustain, or shift attention.

B. A change in cognition (such as memory deficit, disorientation, language disturbance) or the development of a perceptual disturbance that is not better accounted for by a preexisting, established, or evolving dementia.

C. The disturbance develops over a short period of time (usually hours to days) and tends to fluctuate during the course of the day.

D. There is evidence from the history, physical examination, or laboratory findings that the symptoms in Criteria A and B developed during, or shortly after, a withdrawal syndrome.

Note: This diagnosis should be made instead of a diagnosis of substance withdrawal only when the cognitive symptoms are in excess of those usually associated with the withdrawal syndrome and when the symptoms are sufficiently severe to warrant independent clinical attention.

Code (Specific substance) withdrawal delirium:

(Alcohol; Sedative, hypnotic, or anxiolytic; Other [or unknown] substance)

DSM-IV-TR gives separate diagnostic criteria for delirium due to a general medical condition (Table 7.2–1), for delirium related to systemic medical conditions or primary cerebral conditions, substance intoxication delirium (Table 7.2–2), substance withdrawal delirium (Table 7.2–3), delirium due to multiple etiologies (Table 7.2–4), and delirium not otherwise specified (Table 7.2–5) for a delirium of unknown cause or due

Table 7.2–4
DSM-IV-TR Diagnostic Criteria for Delirium Due to Multiple Etiologies

A. Disturbance of consciousness (i.e., reduced clarity of awareness of the environment) with reduced ability to focus, sustain, or shift attention.

B. A change in cognition (such as memory deficit, disorientation, language disturbance) or the development of a perceptual disturbance that is not better accounted for by a preexisting, established, or evolving dementia.

C. The disturbance develops over a short period of time (usually hours to days) and tends to fluctuate during the course of the day.

D. There is evidence from the history, physical examination, or laboratory findings that the delirium has more than one etiology (e.g., more than one etiological general medical condition, a general medical condition plus substance intoxication or medication side effect).

Coding note: Use multiple codes reflecting specific delirium and specific etiologies, e.g., Delirium due to viral encephalitis; Alcohol withdrawal delirium.

Table 7.2–5
DSM-IV-TR Diagnostic Criteria for Delirium Not Otherwise Specified

This category should be used to diagnose a delirium that does not meet criteria for any of the specific types of delirium described in this section.

Examples include

1. A clinical presentation of delirium that is suspected to be due to a general medical condition or substance use but for which there is insufficient evidence to establish a specific etiology
2. Delirium due to causes not listed in this section (e.g., sensory deprivation)

From American Psychiatric Association. *Diagnostic and Statistical Manual of Mental Disorders*. 4th ed. Text rev. Washington, DC: American Psychiatric Association; copyright 2000, with permission.

to causes not listed, such as sensory deprivation. However, the core syndrome is the same, regardless of cause.

The core features of delirium include altered consciousness, such as decreased level of consciousness; altered attention, which may include diminished ability to focus, sustain, or shift attention; impairment in other realms of cognitive function, which may manifest as disorientation (especially to time and space) and decreased memory; relatively rapid onset (usually hours to days); brief duration (usually days to weeks); and often marked, unpredictable fluctuations in severity and other clinical manifestations during the course of the day, sometimes worse at night (sundowning), which may range from periods of lucidity to quite severe cognitive impairment and disorganization.

Associated clinical features are often present and may be prominent. They may include disorganization of thought processes (ranging from mild tangentiality to frank incoherence), perceptual disturbances such as illusions and hallucinations, psychomotor hyperactivity and hypoactivity, disruption of the sleep–wake cycle (often manifested as fragmented sleep at night, with or without daytime drowsiness), mood alterations (from subtle irritability to obvious dysphoria, anxiety, or even euphoria), and other manifestations of altered neurological function (e.g., autonomic hyperactivity or instability, myoclonic jerking, and dysarthria). The electroencephalogram (EEG) usually shows diffuse slowing of background activity, although patients with delirium due to alcohol or sedative-hypnotic withdrawal have low-voltage fast activity.

PHYSICAL AND LABORATORY EXAMINATIONS

Delirium is usually diagnosed at the bedside and is characterized by the sudden onset of symptoms. A bedside mental status examination—such as the Mini-Mental State Examination (MMSE)—can be used to document the cognitive impairment and to provide a baseline from which to measure the patient's clinical course. The physical examination often reveals clues to the cause of the delirium. The presence of a known physical illness or a history of head trauma or alcohol or other substance dependence increases the likelihood of the diagnosis.

The laboratory workup of a patient with delirium should include standard tests and additional studies indicated by the clinical situation. In delirium, the EEG characteristically shows a generalized slowing of activity and may be useful in differentiating delirium from depression or psychosis. The EEG of a delirious patient sometimes shows focal areas of hyperactivity. In rare cases, it may be difficult to differentiate delirium related to epilepsy from delirium related to other causes.

DIFFERENTIAL DIAGNOSIS

Delirium versus Dementia

A number of clinical features help distinguish delirium from dementia. In contrast to the sudden onset of delirium, the onset of dementia is usually insidious. Although both conditions include cognitive impairment, the changes in dementia are more stable over time and, for example, do not fluctuate over the course of a day. A patient with dementia is usually alert; a patient with delirium has episodes of decreased consciousness. Occasionally, delirium occurs in a patient with dementia, a condition known as *beclouded dementia*. A diagnosis of delirium can be made when there is a definite history of preexisting dementia.

Delirium versus Schizophrenia or Depression

Delirium must also be differentiated from schizophrenia and depressive disorder. Patients with factitious disorders may attempt to simulate the symptoms of delirium but usually reveal the factitious nature of their symptoms by inconsistencies on their mental status examinations, and an EEG can easily separate the two diagnoses. Some patients with psychotic disorders, usually schizophrenia or manic episodes, may have periods of extremely disorganized behavior that are difficult to distinguish from delirium. In general, however, the hallucinations and delusions of patients with schizophrenia are more constant and better organized than are those of patients with delirium. Patients with schizophrenia usually experience no change in their level of consciousness or in their orientation. Patients with hypoactive symptoms of delirium may appear somewhat similar to severely depressed patients but can be distinguished on the basis of an EEG. Other psychiatric diagnoses to consider in the differential diagnosis of delirium are brief psychotic disorder, schizophreniform disorder, and dissociative disorders.

COURSE AND PROGNOSIS

Although the onset of delirium is usually sudden, prodromal symptoms (such as restlessness and fearfulness) may occur in the days preceding the onset of florid symptoms. The symptoms of delirium usually persist as long as the causally relevant factors are present, although delirium generally lasts less than a week. After identification and removal of the causative factors, the symptoms of delirium usually recede over a 3- to 7-day period, although some symptoms may take up to 2 weeks to resolve completely. The older the patient and the longer the patient has been delirious, the longer the delirium takes to resolve. Recall of what transpired during a delirium, once it is over, is characteristically spotty; a patient may refer to the episode as a bad dream or a nightmare only vaguely remembered.

As stated in the discussion on epidemiology, the occurrence of delirium is associated with a high mortality rate in the ensuing year, primarily because of the serious nature of the associated medical conditions that lead to delirium.

Whether delirium progresses to dementia has not been demonstrated in carefully controlled studies, although many clinicians believe that they have seen such a progression. A clinical observation that has been validated by some studies, however, is that periods of delirium are sometimes followed by depression or posttraumatic stress disorder.

TREATMENT

In treating delirium, the primary goal is to treat the underlying cause. When the underlying condition is anticholinergic toxicity, the use of physostigmine salicylate (Antilirium), 1 to 2 mg intravenously or intramuscularly, with repeated doses in 15 to 30 minutes may be indicated. The other important goal of treatment is to provide physical, sensory, and environmental support. Physical support is necessary so that delirious patients do not get into situations in which they may have accidents. Patients with delirium should be neither sensory deprived nor overly stimulated by the environment. They are usually helped by having a friend or relative in the room or by the presence of a regular sitter. Familiar pictures and decorations, the presence of a clock or a calendar, and regular orientations to person, place, and time help make patients with delirium be comfortable. Delirium can sometimes occur in older patients wearing eye patches after cataract surgery (black-patch delirium). Such patients can be helped by placing pinholes in the patches to let in some stimuli or by occasionally removing one patch at a time during recovery.

Pharmacotherapy

The two major symptoms of delirium that may require pharmacological treatment are psychosis and insomnia. The drug of choice for psychosis is haloperidol (Haldol), a butyrophenone antipsychotic drug. Depending on a patient's age, weight, and physical condition, the initial dose may range from 2 to 10 mg intramuscularly, repeated in an hour if the patient remains agitated. As soon as the patient is calm, oral medication in liquid concentrate or tablet form should begin. Two daily oral doses should suffice, with two-thirds of the dose being given at bedtime. To achieve the same therapeutic effect, the oral dose should be approximately 1.5 times higher than the parenteral dose. The effective total daily dosage of haloperidol may range from 5 to 50 mg for most patients with delirium. Droperidol (Inapsine) is a butyrophenone available as an alternative intravenous formulation, although careful monitoring of the electrocardiogram may be prudent with this treatment. Phenothiazines should be avoided in delirious patients: These drugs are associated with significant anticholinergic activity.

Insomnia is best treated with benzodiazepines with short half-lives. Benzodiazepines with long half-lives and barbiturates should be avoided unless they are being used as part of the treatment for the underlying disorder (such as alcohol withdrawal). There have been case reports of improvements in or remission of delirious states due to intractable medical illnesses with electroconvulsive therapy (ECT). Although electroconvulsive therapy may rarely be advised by a consultant

with expertise in the procedures, routine consideration of electroconvulsive therapy for delirium is not advised. If delirium is due to severe pain or dyspnea, physicians should not hesitate to prescribe opioids for both their analgesic and sedative effects.

▲ 7.3 Dementia

Dementia is a diminution in cognition in the setting of a stable level of consciousness. The persistent and stable nature of the impairment distinguishes dementia from the altered consciousness and fluctuating deficits of delirium. In the text revision of the fourth edition of *Diagnostic and Statistical Manual of Mental Disorders* (DSM-IV-TR), dementia is "characterized by multiple cognitive defects that include impairment in memory," without impairment in consciousness. The cognitive functions that can be affected in dementia include general intelligence, learning and memory, language, problem solving, orientation, perception, attention and concentration, judgment, and social abilities. A person's personality is also affected. A person with an impairment of consciousness probably fits the diagnostic criteria for delirium. In addition, a diagnosis of dementia, according to DSM-IV-TR, requires that the symptoms result in a significant impairment in social or occupational functioning and that they represent a significant decline from a previous level of functioning.

The critical clinical points of dementia are the identification of the syndrome and the clinical workup of its cause. The disorder may be progressive or static, permanent or reversible. An underlying cause is always assumed, although in rare cases it is impossible to determine a specific cause. The potential reversibility of dementia is related to the underlying pathological condition and to the availability and application of effective treatment. Approximately 15 percent of people with dementia have reversible illnesses if treatment is initiated before irreversible damage takes place.

EPIDEMIOLOGY

Dementia is essentially a disease of older people. According to the American Psychiatric Association's (APA) *Practice Guideline for the Treatment of Patients with Alzheimer's Disease and other Dementias of Late Life*, the onset of the disease generally occurs most commonly in the 60s, 70s, and 80s and beyond, but in rare instances the disorder appears in the 40s and 50s (known as *early-onset dementia*). The incidence of Alzheimer's disease also increases with age, and it is estimated at 0.5 percent per year from age 65 to 69, 1 percent per year from age 70 to 74, 2 percent per year from age 75 to 79, 3 percent per year from age 80 to 84, and 8 percent per year from age 85 onward. Progression is gradual but steadily downward. Previous estimates of death from onset of symptoms was from 5 to 9 years; however, in a 2001 study of patients with Alzheimer's disease, the median survival was only 3 years after onset of symptoms.

The second most common type of dementia is vascular dementia, which is causally related to cerebrovascular diseases. Hypertension predisposes a person to the disease. Vascular dementias account for 15 to 30 percent of all dementia cases. Vascular dementia is most common in people between the ages of 60 and 70 years and is more common in men than in women. Approximately 10 to 15 percent of patients have coexisting vascular dementia and dementia of the Alzheimer's type.

Other common causes of dementia, each representing 1 to 5 percent of all cases, include head trauma, alcohol-related dementias, and various movement disorder–related dementias, such as Huntington's disease and Parkinson's disease. Because dementia is a fairly general syndrome, it has many causes, and clinicians must embark on a careful clinical workup of a patient with dementia to establish its cause.

ETIOLOGY

Dementia has many causes, but dementia of the Alzheimer's type and vascular dementia together represent as many as 75 percent of all cases. Other causes of dementia specified in DSM-IV-TR are Pick's disease, Creutzfeldt-Jakob disease, Huntington's disease, Parkinson's disease, human immunodeficiency virus (HIV), and head trauma.

Dementia of the Alzheimer's Type

In 1907, Alois Alzheimer first described the condition that later assumed his name. He described a 51-year-old woman with a 4 1/2-year course of progressive dementia. The final diagnosis of Alzheimer's disease is based on a neuropathological examination of the brain; nevertheless, dementia of the Alzheimer's type is commonly diagnosed in the clinical setting after other causes of dementia have been excluded from diagnostic consideration.

Genetic Factors.   Although the cause of dementia of the Alzheimer's type remains unknown, progress has been made in understanding the molecular basis of the amyloid deposits that are a hallmark of the disorder's neuropathology. Some studies have indicated that as many as 40 percent of patients have a family history of dementia of the Alzheimer's type; thus, genetic factors are presumed to play a part in the development of the disorder, at least in some cases. Additional support for a genetic influence is the concordance rate for monozygotic twins, which is higher than the rate for dizygotic twins (43 percent versus 8 percent, respectively). In several well-documented cases, the disorder has been transmitted in families through an autosomal dominant gene, although such transmission is rare. Alzheimer's-type dementia has shown linkage to chromosomes 1, 14, and 21.

AMYLOID PRECURSOR PROTEIN.   The gene for amyloid precursor protein is on the long arm of chromosome 21. Through the process of differential splicing, there are four forms of amyloid precursor protein. The β/A4 protein, the major constituent of senile plaques, is a 42–amino acid peptide that is a breakdown product of amyloid precursor protein. In Down syndrome (trisomy 21), there are three copies of the amyloid precursor protein gene, and in a disease in which there is a mutation at codon 717 in the amyloid precursor protein gene, a pathological process results in the excessive deposition of β/A4 protein. Whether the processing of abnormal amyloid precursor protein is of primary causative significance in Alzheimer's disease is unknown, but many research groups are studying both the normal metabolic processing of amyloid precursor protein and its processing in patients with dementia of the Alzheimer's type in an attempt to answer this question.

MULTIPLE E4 GENES.   In one study, gene E4 was implicated in the etiological origin of Alzheimer's disease. People with one copy of the gene have Alzheimer's disease three times more frequently than do those with no E4 gene, and people with two E4 genes have the disease eight times more frequently than do those with no E4 gene. Diagnostic testing for this gene is not currently recommended because it is found in persons without dementia and not found in all cases of dementia.

Neuropathology.   The classic gross neuroanatomical observation of a brain from a patient with Alzheimer's disease is diffuse atrophy with flattened cortical sulci and enlarged cerebral ventricles. The classic and pathognomonic microscopic findings are senile plaques, neurofibrillary tangles, neuronal loss (particularly in the cortex and the hippocampus), synaptic loss (perhaps as much as 50 percent in the cortex), and granulovacuolar degeneration of the neurons. Neurofibrillary tangles are composed of cytoskeletal elements, primarily phosphorylated tau protein, although other cytoskeletal proteins are also present. Neurofibrillary tangles are not unique to Alzheimer's disease, but also occur in Down syndrome, dementia pugilistica (punch-drunk syndrome), Parkinson-dementia complex of Guam, Hallervorden-Spatz disease, and the brains of normal people as they age. Neurofibrillary tangles are commonly found in the cortex, the hippocampus, the substantia nigra, and the locus ceruleus.

Senile plaques, also referred to as *amyloid plaques*, are much more indicative of Alzheimer's disease, although they are also seen in Down syndrome and, to some extent, in normal aging. Senile plaques are composed of a particular protein, β/A4, and astrocytes, dystrophic neuronal processes, and microglia. The number and the density of senile plaques present in postmortem brains have been correlated with the severity of the disease that affected the person.

Neurotransmitters.   The neurotransmitters that are most often implicated in the pathophysiological condition of Alzheimer's disease are acetylcholine and norepinephrine, both of which are hypothesized to be hypoactive in Alzheimer's disease. Several studies have reported data consistent with the hypothesis that a specific degeneration of cholinergic neurons is present in the nucleus basalis of Meynert in people with Alzheimer's disease. Other data in support of a cholinergic deficit in Alzheimer's disease are those that demonstrate decreases in acetylcholine and choline acetyltransferase concentrations in the brain. Choline acetyltransferase is the key enzyme for the synthesis of acetylcholine, and a reduction in choline acetyltransferase concentrations suggests a decrease in the number of cholinergic neurons present. Additional support for the cholinergic deficit hypothesis comes from the observation that cholinergic antagonists, such as scopolamine and atropine, impair cognitive abilities, whereas cholinergic agonists, such as physostigmine and arecoline, enhance cognitive abilities. The decrease in norepinephrine activity in Alzheimer's disease is suggested by the decrease in norepinephrine-containing neurons in the locus ceruleus found in some pathological examinations of brains from people with Alzheimer's disease. Three other neurotransmitters implicated in the pathophysiological condition of Alzheimer's disease are glutamate and the neuroactive peptides somatostatin and corticotropin; decreased concentrations of each have been reported in persons with Alzheimer's disease.

Other Causes.   Other causative theories have been proposed to explain the development of Alzheimer's disease. One theory is that an abnormality in the regulation of membrane phospholipid metabolism results in membranes that are less fluid—that is, more rigid—than normal. Several investigators are using molecular resonance spectroscopic imaging to assess this hypothesis directly in patients with dementia of the Alzheimer's type. Aluminum toxicity has also been hypothesized to be a causative factor, because high levels of aluminum have been found in the brains of some patients with Alzheimer's disease; but this is not considered a significant etiological factor.

Familial Multiple System Taupathy with Presenile Dementia.   A recently discovered type of dementia, familial multiple system taupathy, shares some brain abnormalities found in people with Alzheimer's disease. The gene that causes the disorder is thought to be carried on chromosome 17. The symptoms of the disorder include short-term memory problems and difficulty maintaining balance and walking. The onset of disease occurs in the 40s and 50s, and people with the disease live an average of 11 years after the onset of symptoms.

As in Alzheimer's disease patients, tau protein builds up in neurons and glial cells of people with familial multiple system taupathy. Eventually, the protein buildup kills brain cells. The disorder is not associated with the senile plaques associated with Alzheimer's disease.

Vascular Dementia

The primary cause of vascular dementia, formerly referred to as *multi-infarct dementia*, is presumed to be multiple cerebral vascular disease, resulting in a symptom pattern of dementia. Vascular dementia is most common in men, especially those with preexisting hypertension or other cardiovascular risk factors. The disorder affects primarily small and medium-sized cerebral vessels, which undergo infarction and produce multiple parenchymal lesions spread over wide areas of the brain. The causes of the infarctions may include occlusion of the vessels by arteriosclerotic plaque or thromboemboli from distant origins (such as heart valves). An examination of a patient may reveal carotid bruits, funduscopic abnormalities, or enlarged cardiac chambers.

Binswanger's Disease.   Binswanger's disease, also known as *subcortical arteriosclerotic encephalopathy*, is characterized by the presence of many small infarctions of the white matter that spare the cortical regions. Although Binswanger's disease was previously considered a rare condition, the advent of sophisticated and powerful imaging techniques, such as magnetic resonance imaging (MRI), has revealed that the condition is more common than was previously thought.

Pick's Disease

In contrast to the parietal-temporal distribution of pathological findings in Alzheimer's disease, Pick's disease is characterized by a preponderance of atrophy in the frontotemporal regions. These regions also have neuronal loss, gliosis, and the presence of neuronal Pick's bodies, which are masses of cytoskeletal elements. Pick's bodies are seen in some postmortem specimens but are not necessary for the diagnosis. The cause of Pick's disease is unknown, but the disease constitutes approximately 5 percent of all irreversible dementias. It is most common in men, especially those who have a first-degree relative with the condition. Pick's disease is difficult to distinguish from dementia of the Alzheimer's type, although the early stages of Pick's disease are more often characterized by personality and behavioral changes, with a relative preservation of other cognitive functions. Features of Klüver-Bucy syndrome (such as hypersexuality, placidity, hyperorality) are much more common in Pick's disease than in Alzheimer's disease.

Lewy Body Disease

Lewy body disease is a dementia clinically similar to Alzheimer's disease and often characterized by hallucinations, parkinsonian features, and extrapyramidal signs. Lewy inclusion bodies are found in the cerebral cortex. The exact incidence is unknown. These patients show marked adverse effects when given antipsychotic medications.

Huntington's Disease

Huntington's disease is classically associated with the development of dementia. The dementia seen in this disease is the subcortical type of dementia, characterized by more motor abnormalities and fewer language abnormalities than in the cortical type of dementia. The dementia of Huntington's disease exhibits psychomotor slowing and difficulty with complex tasks, but memory, language, and insight remain relatively intact in the early and middle stages of the illness. As the disease progresses, however, the dementia becomes complete; the features distinguishing it from dementia of the Alzheimer's type are the high incidence of depression and psychosis, in addition to the classic choreoathetoid movement disorder.

Parkinson's Disease

Like Huntington's disease, parkinsonism is a disease of the basal ganglia commonly associated with dementia and depression. An estimated 20 to 30 percent of patients with Parkinson's disease have dementia, and an additional 30 to 40 percent have a measurable impairment in cognitive abilities. The slow movements of people with Parkinson's disease are paralleled in the slow thinking of some affected patients, a feature that clinicians may refer to as *bradyphrenia*.

Human Immunodeficiency Virus–Related Dementia

Infection with HIV commonly leads to dementia and other psychiatric symptoms. Patients infected with HIV experience dementia at an annual rate of approximately 14 percent. An estimated 75 percent of patients with acquired immune deficiency syndrome (AIDS) have involvement of the central nervous system at the time of autopsy. The development of dementia in people infected with HIV is often paralleled by the appearance of parenchymal abnormalities in MRI scans. Other infectious dementias are caused by *Cryptococcus*.

Head Trauma–Related Dementia

Dementia can be a sequela of head trauma, as can a wide range of neuropsychiatric syndromes, including neurosyphilis.

DIAGNOSIS AND CLINICAL FEATURES

The dementia diagnoses in DSM-IV-TR are dementia of the Alzheimer's type (Table 7.3–1), vascular dementia (Table 7.3–2), dementia due to other general medical conditions (Table 7.3–3), substance-induced persisting dementia (Table 7.3–4), dementia due to multiple etiologies (Table 7.3–5), and dementia not otherwise specified (Table 7.3–6).

The diagnosis of dementia is based on a patient's clinical examination, including a mental status examination, and on information from the patient's family, friends, and employers. Complaints of a personality change in a patient older than age 40 suggest that a diagnosis of dementia should be carefully considered.

Clinicians should note patients' complaints about intellectual impairment and forgetfulness as well as evidence of patients' evasion, denial, or rationalization aimed at concealing cognitive deficits. Excessive orderliness, social withdrawal, or a tendency to relate events in minute detail can be characteristic, and sudden outbursts of anger or sarcasm may occur. Patients' appearance and behavior should be observed. Lability of emotions, sloppy grooming, uninhibited remarks, silly jokes, or a dull, apathetic, or vacuous facial expression and manner suggest the presence of dementia, especially when coupled with memory impairment.

Memory impairment is typically an early and prominent feature in dementia, especially in dementias involving the cortex, such as dementia of the Alzheimer's type. Early in the course of dementia, memory impairment is mild and is usually most marked for recent events; people forget telephone numbers, conversations, and events of the day. As the course of dementia progresses, memory impairment becomes severe, and only the earliest learned information (such as a person's place of birth) is retained.

Inasmuch as memory is important for orientation to person, place, and time, orientation can be progressively affected during the course of a dementing illness. For example, patients with dementia may forget how to get back to their rooms after going to the bathroom. No matter how severe the disorientation seems, however, patients show no impairment in their level of consciousness.

Dementing processes that affect the cortex, primarily dementia of the Alzheimer's type and vascular dementia, can affect patients' language abilities. DSM-IV-TR includes aphasia as one of the diagnostic criteria. The language difficulty may be characterized by a vague, stereotyped, imprecise, or circumstantial locution, and patients may also have difficulty in naming objects.

Table 7.3–1
DSM-IV-TR Diagnostic Criteria for Dementia of the Alzheimer's Type

A. The development of multiple cognitive deficits manifested by both
  (1) memory impairment (impaired ability to learn new information or to recall previously learned information)
  (2) one (or more) of the following cognitive disturbances:
    (a) aphasia (language disturbance)
    (b) apraxia (impaired ability to carry out motor activities despite intact motor function)
    (c) agnosia (failure to recognize or identify objects despite intact sensory function)
    (d) disturbance in executive functioning (i.e., planning, organizing, sequencing, abstracting)
B. The cognitive deficits in Criteria A1 and A2 each cause significant impairment in social or occupational functioning and represent a significant decline from a previous level of functioning.
C. The course is characterized by gradual onset and continuing cognitive decline.
D. The cognitive deficits in Criteria A1 and A2 are not due to any of the following:
  (1) other central nervous system conditions that cause progressive deficits in memory and cognition (e.g., cerebrovascular disease, Parkinson's disease, Huntington's disease, subdural hematoma, normal-pressure hydrocephalus, brain tumor)
  (2) systemic conditions that are known to cause dementia (e.g., hypothyroidism, vitamin B_{12} or folic acid deficiency, niacin deficiency, hypercalcemia, neurosyphilis, HIV infection)
  (3) substance-induced conditions
E. The deficits do not occur exclusively during the course of a delirium.
F. The disturbance is not better accounted for by another Axis I disorder (e.g., major depressive disorder, schizophrenia).
Code based on presence or absence of a clinically significant behavioral disturbance:
  Without behavioral disturbance: if the cognitive disturbance is not accompanied by any clinically significant behavioral disturbance.
  With behavioral disturbance: if the cognitive disturbance is accompanied by a clinically significant behavioral disturbance (e.g., wandering, agitation).
Specify subtype:
  With early onset: if onset is at age 65 years or below
  With late onset: if onset is after age 65 years
Coding note: Also code Alzheimer's disease on Axis III. Indicate other prominent clinical features related to the Alzheimer's disease on Axis I (e.g., Mood disorder due to Alzheimer's disease, with depressive features, and Personality change due to Alzheimer's disease, aggressive type).

Personality

Preexisting personality traits may be accentuated during the development of a dementia. Patients with dementia may also

Table 7.3–2
DSM-IV-TR Diagnostic Criteria for Vascular Dementia

A. The development of multiple cognitive deficits manifested by both

(1) memory impairment (impaired ability to learn new information or to recall previously learned information)

(2) one (or more) of the following cognitive disturbances:

(a) aphasia (language disturbance)

(b) apraxia (impaired ability to carry out motor activities despite intact motor function)

(c) agnosia (failure to recognize or identify objects despite intact sensory function)

(d) disturbance in executive functioning (i.e., planning, organizing, sequencing, abstracting)

B. The cognitive deficits in Criteria A1 and A2 each cause significant impairment in social or occupational functioning and represent a significant decline from a previous level of functioning.

C. Focal neurological signs and symptoms (e.g., exaggeration of deep tendon reflexes, extensor plantar response, pseudobulbar palsy, gait abnormalities, weakness of an extremity) or laboratory evidence indicative of cerebrovascular disease (e.g., multiple infarctions involving cortex and underlying white matter) that are judged to be etiologically related to the disturbance.

D. The deficits do not occur exclusively during the course of a delirium.

Code based on predominant features:

With delirium: if delirium is superimposed on the dementia

With delusions: if delusions are the predominant feature

With depressed mood: if depressed mood (including presentations that meet full symptom criteria for a major depressive episode) is the predominant feature. A separate diagnosis of mood disorder due to a general medical condition is not given.

Uncomplicated: if none of the above predominates in the current clinical presentation

Specify if:

With behavioral disturbance

Coding note: Also code cerebrovascular condition on Axis III.

Table 7.3–3
DSM-IV-TR Diagnostic Criteria for Dementia Due to Other General Medical Conditions

A. The development of multiple cognitive deficits manifested by both

(1) memory impairment (impaired ability to learn new information or to recall previously learned information)

(2) one (or more) of the following cognitive disturbances:

(a) aphasia (language disturbance)

(b) apraxia (impaired ability to carry out motor activities despite intact motor function)

(c) agnosia (failure to recognize or identify objects despite intact sensory function)

(d) disturbance in executive functioning (i.e., planning, organizing, sequencing, abstracting)

B. The cognitive deficits in Criteria A1 and A2 each cause significant impairment in social or occupational functioning and represent a significant decline from a previous level of functioning.

C. There is evidence from the history, physical examination, or laboratory findings that the disturbance is the direct physiological consequence of a general medical condition other than Alzheimer's disease or cerebrovascular disease (e.g., HIV infection, traumatic brain injury, Parkinson's disease, Huntington's disease, Pick's disease, Creutzfeldt-Jakob disease, normal-pressure hydrocephalus, hypothyroidism, brain tumor, or vitamin B_{12} deficiency).

D. The deficits do not occur exclusively during the course of a delirium.

Code based on presence or absence of a clinically significant behavioral disturbance:

Without behavioral disturbance: if the cognitive disturbance is not accompanied by any clinically significant behavioral disturbance.

With behavioral disturbance: if the cognitive disturbance is accompanied by a clinically significant behavioral disturbance (e.g., wandering, agitation).

Coding note: Also code the general medical condition on Axis III (e.g., HIV infection, head injury, Parkinson's disease, Huntington's disease, Pick's disease, Creutzfeldt-Jakob disease).

become introverted and may seem to be less concerned than they previously were about the effects of their behavior on others. People with dementia who have paranoid delusions are generally hostile to family members and caretakers. Patients with frontal and temporal involvement are likely to have marked personality changes and may be irritable and explosive.

Hallucinations and Delusions

An estimated 20 to 30 percent of patients with dementia, primarily patients with dementia of the Alzheimer's type, have hallucinations, and 30 to 40 percent have delusions, primarily of a paranoid or persecutory and unsystematized nature, although complex, sustained, and well-systematized delusions are also reported by these patients. Physical aggression and

other forms of violence are common in demented patients who also have psychotic symptoms.

Mood

In addition to psychosis and personality changes, depression and anxiety are major symptoms in an estimated 40 to 50 percent of patients with dementia, although the full syndrome of depressive disorder may be present in only 10 to 20 percent. Patients with dementia may also exhibit pathological laughter or crying—that is, extremes of emotions—with no apparent provocation.

Cognitive Change

In addition to the aphasias in patients with dementia, apraxias and agnosias are common, and they are included as potential diagnostic criteria in DSM-IV-TR. Other neurological signs

Table 7.3–4
DSM-IV-TR Diagnostic Criteria for Substance-Induced Persisting Dementia

A. The development of multiple cognitive deficits manifested by both

(1) memory impairment (impaired ability to learn new information or to recall previously learned information)

(2) one (or more) of the following cognitive disturbances:

(a) aphasia (language disturbance)

(b) apraxia (impaired ability to carry out motor activities despite intact motor function)

(c) agnosia (failure to recognize or identify objects despite intact sensory function)

(d) disturbance in executive functioning (i.e., planning, organizing, sequencing, abstracting)

B. The cognitive deficits in Criteria A1 and A2 each cause significant impairment in social or occupational functioning and represent a significant decline from a previous level of functioning.

C. The deficits do not occur exclusively during the course of a delirium and persist beyond the usual duration of substance intoxication or withdrawal.

D. There is evidence from the history, physical examination, or laboratory findings that the deficits are etiologically related to the persisting effects of substance use (e.g., a drug of abuse, a medication).

Code (Specific substance)-induced persisting dementia:

(Alcohol; Inhalant; Sedative, hypnotic, or anxiolytic; Other [or unknown] substance)

From American Psychiatric Association. *Diagnostic and Statistical Manual of Mental Disorders.* 4th ed. Text rev. Washington, DC: American Psychiatric Association; copyright 2000, with permission.

Table 7.3–5
DSM-IV-TR Diagnostic Criteria for Dementia Due to Multiple Etiologies

A. The development of multiple cognitive deficits manifested by both

(1) memory impairment (impaired ability to learn new information or to recall previously learned information)

(2) one (or more) of the following cognitive disturbances:

(a) aphasia (language disturbance)

(b) apraxia (impaired ability to carry out motor activities despite intact motor function)

(c) agnosia (failure to recognize or identify objects despite intact sensory function)

(d) disturbance in executive functioning (i.e., planning, organizing, sequencing, abstracting)

B. The cognitive deficits in Criteria A1 and A2 each cause significant impairment in social or occupational functioning and represent a significant decline from a previous level of functioning.

C. There is evidence from the history, physical examination, or laboratory findings that the disturbance has more than one etiology (e.g., head trauma plus chronic alcohol use, dementia of the Alzheimer's type with the subsequent development of vascular dementia).

D. The deficits do not occur exclusively during the course of a delirium.

Coding note: Use multiple codes based on specific dementias and specific etiologies, e.g., Dementia of the Alzheimer's type, with late onset, without behavioral disturbance; Vascular dementia, uncomplicated.

From American Psychiatric Association. *Diagnostic and Statistical Manual of Mental Disorders.* 4th ed. Text rev. Washington, DC: American Psychiatric Association; copyright 2000, with permission.

that can be associated with dementia are seizures, seen in approximately 10 percent of patients with dementia of the Alzheimer's type and in 20 percent of patients with vascular dementia, and atypical neurological presentations, such as nondominant parietal lobe syndromes. Primitive reflexes—such as the grasp, snout, suck, tonic-foot, and palmomental reflexes—may be present on neurological examination, and myoclonic jerks are present in 5 to 10 percent of patients.

Patients with vascular dementia may have additional neurological symptoms, such as headaches, dizziness, faintness, weakness, focal neurological signs, and sleep disturbances, possibly attributable to the location of the cerebrovascular disease. Pseudobulbar palsy, dysarthria, and dysphagia are also more common in vascular dementia than in other dementing conditions.

Catastrophic Reaction

Patients with dementia also exhibit a reduced ability to apply what Kurt Goldstein called *the abstract attitude*. Patients have difficulty in generalizing from a single instance, in forming concepts, and in grasping similarities and differences among concepts. Furthermore, the ability to solve problems, to reason logically, and to make sound judgments is compromised. Goldstein also described a catastrophic reaction, marked by agitation secondary to the subjective awareness of intellectual deficits under stressful circumstances. People usually attempt to compensate for defects by using strategies to avoid demonstrating failures in intellectual performance; they may change the subject, make jokes, or

otherwise divert the interviewer. Lack of judgment and poor impulse control commonly appear, particularly in dementias that primarily affect the frontal lobes. Examples of these impairments include coarse language, inappropriate jokes, the neglect of personal appearance and hygiene, and a general disregard for the conventional rules of social conduct.

Sundowner Syndrome

Sundowner syndrome is characterized by drowsiness, confusion, ataxia, and accidental falls. It occurs in older people who are overly sedated and in patients with dementia who react adversely to even a small dose of a psychoactive drug. The syndrome also occurs in

Table 7.3–6
DSM-IV-TR Diagnostic Criteria for Dementia Not Otherwise Specified

This category should be used to diagnose a dementia that does not meet criteria for any of the specific types described in this section.

An example is a clinical presentation of dementia for which there is insufficient evidence to establish a specific etiology.

From American Psychiatric Association. *Diagnostic and Statistical Manual of Mental Disorders.* 4th ed. Text rev. Washington, DC: American Psychiatric Association; copyright 2000, with permission.

demented patients when external stimuli, such as light and interpersonal orienting cues, are diminished. It most commonly occurs as a result of benzodiazepines.

PATHOLOGY, PHYSICAL FINDINGS, AND LABORATORY EXAMINATION

A comprehensive laboratory workup must be performed when evaluating a patient with dementia. The purposes of the workup are to detect reversible causes of dementia and to provide the patient and family with a definitive diagnosis. The range of possible causes of dementia mandates selective use of laboratory tests. The evaluation should follow informed clinical suspicion, based on the history and physical and mental status examination results. The continued improvements in brain imaging techniques, particularly MRI, have, in some cases, made the differentiation between dementia of the Alzheimer's type and vascular dementia somewhat more straightforward than in the past. An active area of research is the use of single photon emission computed tomography (SPECT) to detect patterns of brain metabolism in various types of dementia; the use of SPECT images may soon help in the clinical differential diagnosis of dementing illnesses.

A general physical examination is a routine component of the workup for dementia. It may reveal evidence of systemic disease causing brain dysfunction, such as an enlarged liver and hepatic encephalopathy, or it may demonstrate systemic disease related to particular central nervous system processes. The detection of Kaposi's sarcoma, for example, should alert the clinician to the probable presence of AIDS and the associated possibility of AIDS dementia complex. Focal neurological findings, such as asymmetrical hyperreflexia or weakness, are seen more often in vascular than in degenerative disease. Frontal lobe signs and primitive reflexes are present in many disorders and often point to a greater extent of progression.

DIFFERENTIAL DIAGNOSIS

Dementia of the Alzheimer's Type versus Vascular Dementia

Classically, vascular dementia has been distinguished from dementia of the Alzheimer's type by the decremental deterioration that may accompany cerebrovascular disease over time. Although the discrete, stepwise deterioration may not be apparent in all cases, focal neurological symptoms are more common in vascular dementia than in dementia of the Alzheimer's type, as are the standard risk factors for cerebrovascular disease.

Vascular Dementia versus Transient Ischemic Attacks

Transient ischemic attacks (TIAs) are brief episodes of focal neurological dysfunction lasting less than 24 hours (usually 5 to 15 minutes). Although a variety of mechanisms may be responsible, the episodes are frequently the result of microembolization from a proximal intracranial arterial lesion that produces transient brain ischemia, and the episodes usually resolve without significant pathological alteration of the parenchymal tis-

sue. Approximately one-third of people whose TIAs were untreated experienced a brain infarction later; therefore, recognition of TIAs is an important clinical strategy to prevent brain infarction.

Clinicians should distinguish episodes involving the vertebrobasilar system from those involving the carotid arterial system. In general, symptoms of vertebrobasilar disease reflect a transient functional disturbance in either the brain stem or the occipital lobe; carotid distribution symptoms reflect unilateral retinal or hemispheric abnormality. Anticoagulant therapy, antiplatelet agglutinating drugs such as aspirin, and extracranial and intracranial reconstructive vascular surgery are effective in reducing the risk of infarction in patients with TIAs.

Delirium

Differentiating between delirium and dementia can be more difficult than the DSM-IV-TR classification indicates. In general, delirium is distinguished by rapid onset, brief duration, fluctuation of cognitive impairment during the course of the day, nocturnal exacerbation of symptoms, marked disturbance of the sleep–wake cycle, and prominent disturbances in attention and perception.

Depression

Some patients with depression have symptoms of cognitive impairment that are difficult to distinguish from symptoms of dementia. The clinical picture is sometimes referred to as *pseudodementia*, although the term *depression-related cognitive dysfunction* is preferable and more descriptive. Patients with depression-related cognitive dysfunction generally have prominent depressive symptoms, have more insight into their symptoms than do demented patients, and often have a history of depressive episodes.

Factitious Disorder

Persons who attempt to simulate memory loss, as in factitious disorder, do so in an erratic and inconsistent manner. In true dementia, memory for time and place is lost before memory for person, and recent memory is lost before remote memory.

Schizophrenia

Although schizophrenia may be associated with some degree of acquired intellectual impairment, its symptoms are much less severe than are the related symptoms of psychosis and thought disorder seen in dementia.

Normal Aging

Aging is not necessarily associated with any significant cognitive decline, but a minor degree of memory problems can occur as a normal part of aging. These normal occurrences are sometimes referred to as *benign senescent forgetfulness* or *age-associated memory impairment*. They are distinguished from dementia by their minor severity and by the fact that they do not significantly interfere with a person's social or occupational behavior.

Other Disorders

Mental retardation does not include memory impairment and occurs in childhood. Amnestic disorder is characterized by circumscribed loss of memory and no deterioration. Major depression in which there is impaired memory responds to medication. Malingering and pituitary disorder must be ruled out but are unlikely.

COURSE AND PROGNOSIS

The classic course of dementia is an onset in a patient's 50s or 60s, with gradual deterioration over 5 to 10 years, leading eventually to death. The age of onset and the rapidity of deterioration vary among different types of dementia and within individual diagnostic categories. The average survival expectation for patients with dementia of the Alzheimer's type is approximately 8 years, with a range of 1 to 20 years. Data suggest that people with an early onset of dementia or with a family history of dementia are likely to have a rapid course. In a recent study of 821 persons with Alzheimer's disease, the median survival time was 3.5 years. Once dementia is diagnosed, patients must undergo a complete medical and neurological workup, because 10 to 15 percent of all patients with dementia have a potentially reversible condition if treatment is initiated before permanent brain damage occurs.

The most common course of dementia begins with a number of subtle signs that may, at first, be ignored by both the patient and the people closest to the patient. A gradual onset of symptoms is most commonly associated with dementia of the Alzheimer's type, vascular dementia, endocrinopathies, brain tumors, and metabolic disorders. Conversely, the onset of dementia resulting from head trauma, cardiac arrest with cerebral hypoxia, or encephalitis may be sudden. Although the symptoms of the early phase of dementia are subtle, the symptoms become conspicuous as the dementia progresses, and family members may then bring a patient to a physician's attention. People with dementia may be sensitive to the use of benzodiazepines or alcohol, which can precipitate agitated, aggressive, or psychotic behavior. In the terminal stages of dementia, patients become empty shells of their former selves—profoundly disoriented, incoherent, amnestic, and incontinent of urine and feces.

With psychosocial and pharmacological treatments, and possibly because of self-healing properties of the brain, the symptoms of dementia may progress slowly for a time or may even recede somewhat. The regression of symptoms is certainly a possibility in reversible dementias (dementias caused by hypothyroidism, normal pressure hydrocephalus, and brain tumors) once treatment is initiated. The course of the dementia varies from a steady progression (commonly seen with dementia of the Alzheimer's type) to an incrementally worsening dementia (commonly seen with vascular dementia) to a stable dementia (as may be seen in dementia related to head trauma).

Psychosocial Determinants

The severity and course of dementia can be affected by psychosocial factors. The greater a person's premorbid intelligence and education, the better the ability to compensate for intellectual deficits. People who have a rapid onset of dementia use fewer defenses than do those who experience an insidious onset. Anxiety and depression may intensify and aggravate the symptoms. Pseudodementia occurs in depressed people who complain of impaired memory but who do, in fact, have a depressive disorder. When the depression is treated, the cognitive defects disappear.

TREATMENT

The first step in the treatment of dementia is verification of the diagnosis. Accurate diagnosis is imperative, for the progression may be halted or even reversed if appropriate therapy is provided. Preventive measures are important, particularly in vascular dementia. Such measures might include changes in diet, exercise, and control of diabetes and hypertension. Pharmacological agents might include antihypertensive, anticoagulant, or antiplatelet agents. Blood pressure control should aim for the higher end of the normal range, as that has been demonstrated to improve cognitive function in patients with vascular dementia. Blood pressure below the normal range has been demonstrated to result in further impairment of cognitive function in the patient with dementia. The choice of antihypertensive agent can be significant in that β-blocking agents have been associated with exaggeration of cognitive impairment. Angiotensin-converting enzyme inhibitors and diuretics have not been linked to the exaggeration of cognitive impairment and are thought to lower blood pressure without affecting cerebral blood flow (cerebral blood flow is presumed to correlate with cognitive function). Surgical removal of carotid plaques may prevent subsequent vascular events in carefully selected patients. The general treatment approach to patients with dementia is to provide supportive medical care, emotional support for the patients and their families, and pharmacological treatment for specific symptoms, including disruptive behavior.

Psychosocial Therapies

The deterioration of mental faculties has significant psychological meaning for patients with dementia. The experience of a person's having continuity over time depends on memory. Recent memory is lost before remote memory in most cases of dementia, and many patients are highly distressed by clearly recalling how they used to function while observing their obvious deterioration. At the most fundamental level, the self is a product of brain functioning. Patients' identities begin to fade as the illness progresses, and they can recall less and less of their past. Emotional reactions ranging from depression to severe anxiety to catastrophic terror can stem from the realization that the sense of self is disappearing.

Patients often benefit from a supportive and educational psychotherapy in which the nature and course of their illness are clearly explained. They may also benefit from assistance in grieving and accepting the extent of their disability and from attention to self-esteem issues. Any areas of intact functioning should be maximized by helping patients identify activities in which successful functioning is possible. A psychodynamic assessment of defective ego functions and cognitive limitations can also be useful. Clinicians can assist patients to find ways to deal with the defective ego functions, such as keeping calendars for orientation problems, making schedules to help structure activities, and taking notes for memory problems.

Psychodynamic interventions with family members of patients with dementia may be of great assistance. Those who take care of a patient struggle with feelings of guilt, grief, anger, and exhaustion as they watch a family member gradually deteriorate. A common problem that develops among caregivers involves their self-sacrifice in caring for a patient. The gradually developing resentment from this self-sacrifice is often suppressed because of the guilt feelings it produces. Clinicians can help caregivers understand the complex mixture of feelings associated with seeing a loved one decline and can provide understanding as well as permission to express these feelings. Clinicians must also be aware of the caregivers' tendencies to blame themselves or others for patients' illnesses and must appreciate the role that patients with dementia play in the lives of family members.

Pharmacotherapy

Clinicians may prescribe benzodiazepines for insomnia and anxiety, antidepressants for depression, and antipsychotic drugs for delusions and hallucinations, but they should be aware of possible idiosyncratic drug effects in older people (such as paradoxical excitement, confusion, and increased sedation). In general, drugs with high anticholinergic activity should be avoided.

Donepezil (Aricept), rivastigmine (Exelon), galantamine (Reminyl), and tacrine (Cognex) are cholinesterase inhibitors used for the treatment of mild-to-moderate cognitive impairment in Alzheimer's disease. They reduce the inactivation of the neurotransmitter acetylcholine and thus potentiate cholinergic neurotransmitter, which in turn produces a modest improvement in memory and goal-directed thought. These drugs are most useful for persons with mild-to-moderate memory loss who have enough preservation of their basal forebrain cholinergic neurons to benefit from augmentation of cholinergic neurotransmission.

Donepezil is well tolerated and widely used. Tacrine is rarely used because of its potential for hepatotoxicity. There are fewer clinical data available for rivastigmine and galantamine, which appear more likely to cause gastrointestinal and neuropsychiatric adverse effects than is donepezil. None of these medications prevents the progressive neuronal degeneration of the disorder. A new agent, memantine, influences glutamate metabolism and is a promising new agent.

Other Treatment Approaches

A wide variety of other pharmacological treatments for the cognitive decline of dementia are being studied, most of which are designed to enhance the functioning of the cholinergic neurotransmitter system. Other drugs that are being tested for cognitive-enhancing activity include general cerebral metabolic enhancers, calcium channel inhibitors, and serotonergic agents. Some studies have shown that selegiline (Eldepryl), a selective monoamine oxidase-B inhibitor, and

nonsteroidal antiinflammatory drugs may slow the advance of this disease.

Estrogen replacement therapy may reduce the risk of cognitive decline in postmenopausal women; however, more studies are needed to confirm this effect. Complementary medicine studies are examining ginkgo biloba and other phytomedicinals to see if they have a positive effect on cognition.

▲ 7.4 Amnestic Disorder

The essential feature of amnestic disorders is the acquired impaired ability to learn and recall new information, coupled with the inability to recall previously learned knowledge or past events. The impairment must be sufficiently severe to compromise personal, social, or occupational functioning. The diagnosis is not made if the memory impairment exists in the context of reduced ability to maintain and shift attention, as encountered in delirium, or in association with significant functional problems due to the compromise of multiple intellectual abilities, as seen in dementia. Amnestic disorders are secondary syndromes caused by systemic medical or primary cerebral disease, substance use disorders, or medication adverse effects, as evidenced by findings from clinical history, physical examination, and/or laboratory examination.

EPIDEMIOLOGY

No adequate studies have reported on the incidence or prevalence of amnestic disorders. Amnesia is most commonly found in alcohol use disorders and in head injury. In general practice and hospital settings, there has been a decrease in the frequency of amnesia related to chronic alcohol abuse and an increase in the frequency of amnesia related to head trauma.

ETIOLOGY

The major neuroanatomical structures involved in memory and in the development of an amnestic disorder are particular diencephalic structures such as the dorsomedial and midline nuclei of the thalamus and midtemporal lobe structures such as the hippocampus, the mamillary bodies, and the amygdala. Although amnesia is usually the result of bilateral damage to these structures, some cases of unilateral damage result in an amnestic disorder, and evidence indicates that the left hemisphere may be more critical than the right hemisphere in the development of memory disorders. Many studies of memory and amnesia in animals have suggested that other brain areas may also be involved in the symptoms accompanying amnesia. Frontal lobe involvement may result in such symptoms as confabulation and apathy, which can be seen in patients with amnestic disorders.

Amnestic disorders have many potential causes. Thiamine deficiency, hypoglycemia, hypoxia (including carbon monoxide poisoning), and herpes simplex encephalitis all have a predilection to damage the temporal lobes, particularly the hippocampi, and thus can be associated with the development of amnestic disorders. Similarly, when tumors, cerebrovascular diseases, surgical procedures, or multiple sclerosis plaques involve the diencephalic or temporal regions of the brain, the symptoms of an amnestic disorder may develop. General insults to the brain such as seizures, electroconvulsive therapy (ECT), and head trauma may also result in memory impairments. Transient global amnesia is presumed to be a cerebrovascular disorder involving transient impairment in blood flow through the vertebrobasilar arteries.

Many drugs have been associated with the development of amnesia, and clinicians should review all drugs taken, including nonprescription drugs, in the diagnostic workup of a patient with amnesia. The benzodiazepines are the most commonly used prescription drugs associated with amnesia. One benzodiazepine in particular, the short-acting hypnotic triazolam (Halcion), has inaccurately been singled out as being associated with anterograde amnesia. A review of the scientific data has concluded that all benzodiazepines can be associated with amnesia and that the association is related to dosage. When triazolam is used in doses (generally less than or equal to 0.25 mg) equivalent to standard doses of other benzodiazepines, amnesia is no more common than with other benzodiazepines. With alcohol and higher doses, however, anterograde amnesia has been reported.

DIAGNOSIS

For the diagnosis of amnestic disorder, the text revision of the fourth edition of *Diagnostic and Statistical Manual of Mental Disorders* (DSM-IV-TR) requires the "development of memory impairment as manifested by impairment in the ability to learn new information or the inability to recall previously learned information," and the "memory disturbance [must cause] . . . significant impairment in social or occupational functioning." A diagnosis of amnestic disorder due to a general medical condition (Table 7.4–1) is made when there is evidence of a causatively relevant specific medical condition (including physical trauma). DSM-IV-TR further categorizes the diagnosis as being transient or chronic. A diagnosis of substance-induced persisting amnestic disorder is made when there is evidence that the symptoms are causatively related to the use of a substance (Table 7.4–2). DSM-IV-TR refers clinicians to specific diagnoses within substance-related disorders: alcohol-induced persisting amnestic disorder; sedative, hypnotic, or anxiolytic-induced persisting amnestic disorder; and other (or unknown) substance-induced persisting amnestic disorder. DSM-IV-TR also provides for the diagnosis of amnestic disorder not otherwise specified (Table 7.4–3).

CLINICAL FEATURES AND SUBTYPES

The central symptom of amnestic disorders is the development of a memory disorder characterized by impairment in the ability to learn new information (anterograde amnesia) and the inability to recall previously remembered knowledge (retrograde amnesia). The symptom must result in significant prob-

Table 7.4–1
DSM-IV-TR Diagnostic Criteria for Amnestic Disorder Due to a General Medical Condition

A. The development of memory impairment as manifested by impairment in the ability to learn new information or the inability to recall previously learned information.

B. The memory disturbance causes significant impairment in social or occupational functioning and represents a significant decline from a previous level of functioning.

C. The memory disturbance does not occur exclusively during the course of a delirium or a dementia.

D. There is evidence from the history, physical examination, or laboratory findings that the disturbance is the direct physiological consequence of a general medical condition (including physical trauma).

Specify if:

Transient: if memory impairment lasts for 1 month or less

Chronic: if memory impairment lasts for more than 1 month

Coding note: Include the name of the general medical condition on Axis I, e.g., Amnestic disorder due to head trauma; also code the general medical condition on Axis III.

From American Psychiatric Association. *Diagnostic and Statistical Manual of Mental Disorders.* 4th ed. Text rev. Washington, DC: American Psychiatric Association; copyright 2000, with permission.

lems for patients in their social or occupational functioning. The time for which a patient is amnestic may begin directly at the point of trauma or may include a period before the trauma. Memory for the time during the physical insult (as during a cerebrovascular event) may also be lost.

Short-term and recent memory are usually impaired. Patients cannot remember what they had for breakfast or lunch,

Table 7.4–2
DSM-IV-TR Diagnostic Criteria for Substance-Induced Persisting Amnestic Disorder

A. The development of memory impairment as manifested by impairment in the ability to learn new information or the inability to recall previously learned information.

B. The memory disturbance causes significant impairment in social or occupational functioning and represents a significant decline from a previous level of functioning.

C. The memory disturbance does not occur exclusively during the course of a delirium or a dementia and persists beyond the usual duration of substance intoxication or withdrawal.

D. There is evidence from the history, physical examination, or laboratory findings that the memory disturbance is etiologically related to the persisting effects of substance use (e.g., a drug of abuse, a medication).

Code (Specific substance)-induced persisting amnestic disorder:

(Alcohol; Sedative, hypnotic, or anxiolytic; Other [or unknown] substance)

From American Psychiatric Association. *Diagnostic and Statistical Manual of Mental Disorders.* 4th ed. Text rev. Washington, DC: American Psychiatric Association; copyright 2000, with permission.

Table 7.4–3
DSM-IV-TR Diagnostic Criteria for Amnestic Disorder Not Otherwise Specified

This category should be used to diagnose an amnestic disorder that does not meet criteria for any of the specific types described in this section.

An example is a clinical presentation of amnesia for which there is insufficient evidence to establish a specific etiology (i.e., dissociative, substance induced, or due to a general medical condition).

the name of the hospital, or their doctors. In some patients, the amnesia is so profound that they cannot orient themselves to city and time, although orientation to person is seldom lost in amnestic disorders. Memory for overlearned information or events from the remote past, such as childhood experiences, is good; but memory for events from the less remote past (over the past decade) is impaired. Immediate memory (tested, for example, by asking a patient to repeat six numbers) remains intact. With improvement, patients may experience a gradual shrinking of the time for which memory has been lost, although some patients experience a gradual improvement in memory for the entire period.

The onset of symptoms may be sudden, as in trauma, cerebrovascular events, and neurotoxic chemical assaults, or gradual, as in nutritional deficiency and cerebral tumors. The amnesia can be of short duration (specified by DSM-IV-TR as transient if lasting 1 month or less) or of long duration (specified by DSM-IV-TR as persistent if lasting longer than 1 month).

A variety of other symptoms can be associated with amnestic disorders. For patients with other cognitive impairments, a diagnosis of dementia or delirium is more appropriate than a diagnosis of an amnestic disorder. Both subtle and gross changes in personality can accompany the symptoms of memory impairment in amnestic disorders. Patients may be apathetic, lack initiative, have unprovoked episodes of agitation, or appear to be overly friendly or agreeable. Patients with amnestic disorders may also appear bewildered and confused and may attempt to cover their confusion with confabulatory answers to questions. Characteristically, patients with amnestic disorders do not have good insight into their neuropsychiatric conditions.

Ms. R is a 48-year-old woman who is divorced and has three teenage children. Until 3 years earlier, Ms. R worked as a buyer for a department store. At that time, she experienced fatigue, forgetfulness, a sense of apathy, and headaches, which she attributed to a preexisting migraine condition. She visited a psychiatrist who prescribed an antidepressant to which she did not respond. The headaches worsened, and Ms. R visited a neurologist who found nothing on neurological examination but recommended a CT scan as a precautionary measure. The CT scan revealed a large, grade II of IV right frontal glioma. This was resected surgically followed by

7,500 rads of radiotherapy focused on the right frontal quadrant. Ms. R recovered well from the surgery and radiation, with no focal neurological deficits. She had a surprisingly benign course and was able to return to work. The only medication she was taking was carbamazepine as a prophylactic against seizures, which she has never had.

Three years after her surgery, the patient and her family began to notice a problem in her short-term memory, which began with forgetting appointments and losing objects. On one occasion, she was unable to find her car in the airport parking lot because she forgot its make and where she had parked it. With time, this forgetfulness progressed and became severe enough to interfere with her work. For example, she would forget she had placed orders and would repeat them. At first, Ms. R became irritable about these incidents and often blamed others for her problems (e.g., her secretary for losing her papers, her children for misplacing things at home). Ms. R's memory problems were especially distressing to her because she had always prided herself on her memory and had been the one to find things for others in the household. With time, however, she developed insight and accepted that this memory problem was a result of the radiation she had received. Her long-term memory is intact as are her other cognitive abilities, except for some reduced ability to plan ahead, but because this had been very well developed before, the patient can still function better than average. Ms. R eventually began to make so many mistakes at work that it was obvious she could no longer continue in her job. She is able to function reasonably well at home, however, with the assistance of "things to do" lists and cuing bulletin boards in many rooms of the house.

DSM-IV-TR DIAGNOSIS

Axis I: Amnestic disorder due to central nervous system radiation, chronic
Axis II: No diagnosis
Axis III: Postradiation for brain tumor
Axis IV: Inability to work causing financial stress
Axis V: GAF = 55

Cerebrovascular Diseases

Cerebrovascular diseases affecting the hippocampus involve the posterior cerebral and basilar arteries and their branches. Infarctions are rarely limited to the hippocampus; they often involve the occipital or parietal lobes. Thus, common accompanying symptoms of cerebrovascular diseases in this region are focal neurological signs involving vision or sensory modalities. Cerebrovascular diseases affecting the bilateral medial thalamus, particularly the anterior portions, are often associated with symptoms of amnestic disorders. A few case studies report amnestic disorders from ruptures of an aneurysm of the anterior communicating artery, resulting in an infarction of the basal forebrain region.

Korsakoff's Syndrome

Korsakoff's syndrome is an amnestic syndrome caused by thiamine deficiency, most commonly associated with the poor nutritional habits of people with chronic alcohol abuse. Other causes of poor nutrition (such as starvation), gastric carcinoma, hemodialysis, hyperemesis gravidarum, prolonged intravenous hyperalimentation, and gastric plication may also result in thiamine deficiency. Korsakoff's syndrome is often associated with Wernicke's encephalopathy, which is the associated syndrome of confusion, ataxia, and ophthalmoplegia. In patients with these thiamine deficiency–related symptoms, the neuropathological findings include hyperplasia of the small blood vessels with occasional hemorrhages, hypertrophy of astrocytes, and subtle changes in neuronal axons. Although the delirium clears up within a month or so, the amnestic syndrome either accompanies or follows untreated Wernicke's encephalopathy in approximately 85 percent of all cases.

The onset of Korsakoff's syndrome may be gradual. Recent memory tends to be affected more than remote memory, but this feature is variable. Confabulation, apathy, and passivity are often prominent symptoms in the syndrome. With treatment, patients may remain amnestic for up to 3 months and then gradually improve over the ensuing year. The administration of thiamine may prevent the development of additional amnestic symptoms, but rarely is the treatment able to reverse severe amnestic symptoms once they are present. Approximately one-third to one-fourth of all patients recover completely, and approximately one-fourth of all patients have no improvement of their symptoms.

Alcoholic Blackouts

In some people with severe alcohol abuse, the syndrome commonly referred to as an *alcoholic blackout* may occur. Characteristically, the person awakens in the morning with a conscious awareness of being unable to remember a time the night before during which the person was intoxicated. Sometimes, specific behaviors (hiding money in a secret place and provoking fights) are associated with the blackouts.

Electroconvulsive Therapy

ECT treatments are usually associated with a retrograde amnesia for a period of several minutes before the treatment and an anterograde amnesia after the treatment. The anterograde amnesia usually resolves within 5 hours. Mild memory deficits may remain for 1 to 2 months after a course of ECT treatments, but the symptoms are usually completely resolved 6 to 9 months after treatment.

Head Injury

Head injuries (both closed and penetrating) can result in a wide range of neuropsychiatric symptoms, including dementia, depression, personality changes, and amnestic disorders. Amnestic disorders caused by head injuries are commonly associated with a period of retrograde amnesia leading up to the traumatic incident and amnesia for the traumatic incident itself. The severity of the brain injury is somewhat correlated with the duration and severity of the amnestic syndrome, but the best correlate of eventual improvement is the degree of clinical improvement of the amnesia during the first week after the patient regains consciousness.

Transient Global Amnesia

Transient global amnesia is characterized by the abrupt loss of the ability to recall recent events or to remember new information. The syndrome is often characterized by a lack of insight into the problem, a clear sensorium, a mild degree of confusion, and, occasionally, the ability to perform some well-learned complex tasks. Episodes last from 6 to 24 hours. Studies suggest that transient global amnesia occurs in 5 to 10 cases per 100,000 people per year, although, for patients older than age 50, the rate may be as high as 30 cases per 100,000 people per year. The pathophysiology is unknown, but it is likely to involve ischemia of the temporal lobe and the diencephalic brain regions. Several studies of patients with single photon emission computed tomography (SPECT) have shown decreased blood flow in the temporal and parietal-temporal regions, particularly in the left hemisphere. Patients with transient global amnesia almost universally experience complete improvement, although one study found that approximately 20 percent of patients may have a recurrence of the episode, and another study found that approximately 7 percent of patients may have epilepsy. Patients with transient global amnesia have been differentiated from patients with transient ischemic attacks in that fewer patients have diabetes, hypercholesterolemia, and hypertriglyceridemia, but more have hypertension and migrainous episodes.

PATHOLOGY AND LABORATORY EXAMINATION

Laboratory findings diagnostic of the disorder may be obtained using quantitative neuropsychological testing. Standardized tests also are available to assess recall of well-known historical events or public figures to characterize the nature of an individual's inability to remember previously learned information. Performance on such tests varies among individuals with amnestic disorder. Subtle deficits in other cognitive functions may be noted in individuals with amnestic disorder. However, memory deficits constitute the predominant feature of the mental status examination and account largely for any functional deficits. No specific or diagnostic features are detectable on imaging studies such as MRI or CT. However, damage of middle-temporal lobe structures is common and may be reflected in enlargement of third ventricle or temporal horns or in structural atrophy detected on MRI.

DIFFERENTIAL DIAGNOSIS

To make the diagnosis, clinicians must obtain a patient's history, conduct a complete physical examination, and order all appropriate laboratory tests. Other diagnoses can be confused with the amnestic disorders.

Dementia and Delirium

Clinicians must differentiate amnestic disorders from dementia and delirium. Memory impairment is commonly present in dementia but is accompanied by other cognitive deficits. Memory impairment is also commonly present in delirium but occurs in the setting of an impairment in attention and consciousness.

Normal Aging

Some minor impairment in memory may accompany normal aging, but the DSM-IV-TR requirement that the memory impairment cause significant impairment in social or occupational functioning should exclude normal aging in patients from the diagnosis.

Dissociative Disorders

The dissociative disorders can sometimes be difficult to differentiate from the amnestic disorders. Patients with dissociative disorders, however, are more likely to have lost their orientation to self and may have more selective memory deficits than do patients with amnestic disorders. For example, patients with dissociative disorders may not know their names or home addresses but may still be able to learn new information and remember selected past memories. Dissociative disorders are also often associated with emotionally stressful life events involving money, the legal system, or troubled relationships.

Factitious Disorders

Patients with factitious disorders who are mimicking an amnestic disorder often have inconsistent results on memory tests and have no evidence of an identifiable cause. These findings, coupled with evidence of primary or secondary gain for a patient, should suggest a factitious disorder.

COURSE AND PROGNOSIS

The specific cause of the amnestic disorder determines the course and the prognosis for a patient. The onset may be sudden or gradual, the symptoms may be transient or persistent, and the outcome can range from no improvement to complete recovery. Transient amnestic disorder with full recovery is common in temporal lobe epilepsy, ECT, the intake of such drugs as benzodiazepines and barbiturates, and resuscitation from cardiac arrest. Permanent amnestic syndromes may follow a head trauma, carbon monoxide poisoning, a cerebral infarction, a subarachnoid hemorrhage, and herpes simplex encephalitis.

TREATMENT

The primary approach to treating amnestic disorders is to treat the underlying cause. Although a patient is amnestic, supportive prompts about the date, the time, and the patient's location can be helpful and can reduce the patient's anxiety. After the resolution of the amnestic episode, psychotherapy of some type (cognitive, psychodynamic, or supportive) may help patients incorporate the amnestic experience into their lives.

Most patients who are amnestic because of brain injury engage in denial. Clinicians must respect and empathize with the patient's need to deny the reality of what has happened. Insensitive and blunt confrontations destroy any developing therapeutic alliance and may cause patients to feel attacked. In a sensitive approach, clinicians help patients accept their cognitive limitations by exposing them to these deficits bit by bit over time. Clinicians must also be wary of being seduced into thinking that all of the patient's symptoms are directly related to the brain insult. An evaluation of preexisting personality disorders, such as borderline, antisocial, and narcissistic personality disorders, must be part of the overall assessment; many patients with personality disorders place themselves in situations that predispose them to injuries. These personality features may become a crucial part of the psychodynamic psychotherapy.

▲ 7.5 Mental Disorders Due to a General Medical Condition

MOOD DISORDERS DUE TO A GENERAL MEDICAL CONDITION

Also known as *secondary mood disorders*, mood disorders due to a general medical condition are characterized by a prominent mood alteration that is thought to be the direct physiological effect of a specific medical illness or agent. These disorders are often difficult to define and have not been extensively researched; however, the key feature is prominent, persistent, distressing, or functionally impairing depressed mood (anhedonia) or elevated, expansive, or irritable mood, judged to be caused by either medical or surgical illness or by substance intoxication or withdrawal. Cognitive impairment is not the predominant clinical feature; otherwise, the mood disturbance would be viewed as part of delirium, dementia, or other cognitive deficit disorder. The diagnostician is asked to specify if the mood syndrome is manic, depressed, or mixed, and if criteria for a fully symptomatic major depressive or manic syndrome are fulfilled.

Epidemiology

The incidence and prevalence of secondary mood disorders is unknown. Depression in the medically ill appears to be equally prevalent by sex, or possibly slightly higher in men than in women. Major and minor depressive episodes are common after certain illnesses such as strokes, Parkinson's disease, Huntington's disease, human immunodeficiency virus (HIV) infection and multiple sclerosis (MS). Secondary mania is less prevalent in neurological disease than is depression; however, many experienced clinicians report a high rate of euphoria in patients with MS.

Table 7.5–1
Causes of Secondary Mood Disorders

Drug intoxication
Alcohol or sedative-hypnotics
Antipsychotics
Antidepressants
Metoclopramide, H$_2$-receptor blockers
Antihypertensives (especially centrally acting agents, e.g., methyldopa, clonidine, reserpine)
Sex steroids (e.g., oral contraceptives, anabolic steroids)
Glucocorticoids
Levodopa
Bromocriptine

Drug withdrawal
Nicotine, caffeine, alcohol or sedative-hypnotics, cocaine, amphetamines

Tumor
Primary cerebral
Systemic neoplasm

Trauma
Cerebral contusion
Subdural hematoma

Infection
Cerebral (e.g., meningitis, encephalitis, HIV, syphilis)
Systemic (e.g., sepsis, urinary tract infection, pneumonia)

Cardiac and vascular
Cerebrovascular (e.g., infarcts, hemorrhage, vasculitis)
Cardiovascular (e.g., low-output states, congestive heart failure, shock)

Physiological or metabolic
Hypoxemia, electrolyte disturbances, renal or hepatic failure, hypo- or hyperglycemia, postictal states

Endocrine
Thyroid or glucocorticoid disturbances

Nutritional
Vitamin B$_{12}$, folate deficiency

Demyelinating
Multiple sclerosis

Neurodegenerative
Parkinson's disease, Huntington's disease

Courtesy of Eric D. Caine, M.D., and Jeffrey M. Lyness, M.D.

Etiology

The list of potential causes for both depressive and manic syndromes is long. Table 7.5–1 lists some of the causes most commonly considered.

Diagnosis and Clinical Features

The depressive or manic symptoms found in secondary mood disorders are phenomenologically similar to those found in primary (idiopathic) mood disorders (see Table 12.3–7 in Section 12.3). It is not known if certain symptoms occur more commonly in the secondary disorders; presumably, the prevalence may vary depending on the specific etiology of the secondary disorder. For example, anxiety has been described as prominent in major depressive syndromes seen in patients with Parkinson's disease.

Differential Diagnosis

There are two broad domains of differential diagnosis to consider when establishing the presence of a secondary mood disorder. The first is phenomenological: Does the patient have clinically significant manic or depressive symptoms in the absence of evidence of a predominant cognitive deficit? That assessment requires attention to symptoms and function in the history and mental status examination. As part of the process, the clinician is also establishing whether there is a clearly defined mood syndrome sufficient to warrant an empirical treatment trial with antidepressant medications.

The second domain is etiological: Does the patient have an Axis III condition or a state of substance intoxication or withdrawal that is causing the mood disturbance? Establishing the presence of the relevant condition depends on standard psychiatric and medical–neurological assessments. Establishing the causal relation to the mood disorder may be difficult.

Course and Prognosis

Depressive conditions that are comorbid with general medical illnesses or substance-related disorders have poorer prognoses than those that have no demonstrated associations. Secondary depressive illness is most often a chronic disease that is sometimes characterized by periods of remission followed by recurrences and sometimes by continuous illness. The prognosis varies, depending on the etiological disease state; depression secondary to a readily treatable disease (e.g., hypothyroidism) has a better outcome than depression associated with a terminal, essentially untreatable condition (e.g., metastatic pancreatic carcinoma).

Treatment

Standard antidepressant medications (including tricyclic antidepressants, monoamine oxidase inhibitors (MAOIs), selective serotonin reuptake inhibitors (SSRIs), and psychostimulants) are effective in many depressed patients with medical and neurological illnesses or substance use disorders. Electroconvulsive therapy (ECT) may be useful in those patients who do not respond to medication.

The clinician treating a patient with a secondary mood disorder should treat the underlying medical cause as effectively as possible. Standard treatment approaches as used for the corresponding primary mood disorder should be used, although the risk of toxic effects from psychotropic drugs may require more gradual dosage increases. At a minimum, psychotherapy should focus on psychoeducational issues. The concept of a secondary behavioral disturbance secondary to medical illness may be new or difficult for many patients and families to understand and support. More specific intrapsychic, interpersonal, and family issues are addressed as indicated in psychotherapy.

PSYCHOTIC DISORDER DUE TO A GENERAL MEDICAL CONDITION

To establish the diagnosis of psychotic disorder due to a general medical condition, the clinician first must exclude syndromes in which psychotic symptoms may be present in association with cognitive impairment (e.g., delirium and dementia of the Alzheimer's type). Disorders in this category are not associated usually with changes in the sensorium.

Epidemiology

The incidence and prevalence of secondary psychotic disorders in the general population are unknown. The prevalence of psychotic symptoms is increased in selected clinical populations, such as nursing home residents, but it is unclear how to extrapolate these findings to other patient groups.

Etiology

Virtually any cerebral or systemic disease that affects brain function can produce psychotic symptoms. Degenerative disorders, such as Alzheimer's disease or Huntington's disease, may present initially with new-onset psychosis, with minimal evidence of cognitive impairment at the earliest stages.

Diagnosis and Clinical Features

To establish the diagnosis of a secondary psychotic syndrome, the clinician first determines that the patient is not delirious, as evidenced by a stable level of consciousness. A careful mental status assessment is conducted to exclude significant cognitive impairments, such as those encountered in dementia or amnestic disorder. The next step is to search for systemic or cerebral diseases that might be causally related to the psychosis. Psychotic symptomatology per se is not helpful in distinguishing a secondary from a primary (idiopathic) cause.

A systematic physical and neurological examination should be performed. The examiner should bear in mind, however, that nonlocalizing, soft neurological signs and a variety of dyskinesias can be present in schizophrenia. A neuroimaging evaluation with magnetic resonance imaging for any new-onset psychosis, irrespective of patient age, is recommended. The detection of a systemic or cerebral abnormality such as a brain tumor may lead to the determination of secondary psychosis; however, establishing a diagnosis of secondary psychotic syndrome requires thoughtful clinical reasoning.

Course and Prognosis

The course and prognosis of secondary psychotic syndromes depend on their etiology. Vivid psychotic symptoms arising from head trauma may improve dramatically during recovery. Delusions associated with degenerative diseases may diminish as the disease worsens, for the capacity to generate those more complex cognitions is gradually lost. Some secondary psychotic disorders improve with treatment of the underlying disorder, such as the interictal psychosis of epilepsy, which often improves with the pharmacological or surgical control of seizures. Psychotic disorders secondary to infectious disease may not improve, despite eradication of the infectious organism, because of irreversible tissue damage sustained during the acute infection.

Treatment

The principles of treatment for a secondary psychotic disorder are similar to those for any secondary neuropsychiatric disorder, namely, rapid identification of the etiological agent and treatment of the underlying cause. Antipsychotic medication may provide symptomatic relief.

ANXIETY DISORDER DUE TO A GENERAL MEDICAL CONDITION

Definition

The key feature of anxiety disorder due to a general medical condition is the presence of prominent anxiety symptoms, which may include generalized anxiety, panic attacks, obsessions, compulsions, or phobias, and which are judged to be caused by either a medical or surgical Axis III condition or by substance intoxication or withdrawal.

Epidemiology

The prevalence of anxiety symptoms is high in general medical patients and in patients with many of the specific medical illnesses that are putative potential causes for secondary anxiety syndromes.

Etiology

Causes most commonly described in anxiety syndromes include substance-related states (intoxication with caffeine, cocaine, amphetamines, and other sympathomimetic agents; withdrawal from nicotine, sedative-hypnotics, and alcohol), endocrinopathies (especially pheochromocytoma, hyperthyroidism, hypercortisolemic states, and hyperparathyroidism), metabolic derangements (e.g., hypoxemia, hypercalcemia, and hypoglycemia), and neurological disorders (including vascular, trauma, and degenerative). Many of these conditions are either inherently transient or easily remediable. Whether that reflects the pathophysiology of secondary anxiety or is an artifact of reporting (e.g., anxiety with subacute onset and complete resolution after removal of a pheochromocytoma is more likely to be reported as an example of anxiety due to a medical illness than is chronic anxiety in the context of chronic obstructive pulmonary disease) is not known. Much attention has been paid to the association of panic attacks and mitral valve prolapse. The nature of that association is unknown, and, therefore, the diagnosis of panic attacks secondary to mitral valve prolapse currently is premature. Interestingly, several recent reports have sought to tie obsessive-compulsive symptoms to the development of pathology in the basal ganglia.

Diagnosis and Clinical Features

The symptoms of secondary anxiety disorders are by definition phenomenologically similar to those found in the corresponding primary anxiety disorder (e.g., panic attacks and obsessions) (see Table 13.7–1 in Section 13.7).

Course and Prognosis

The outcome presumably depends on the specific etiology; thus, anxiety due to hyperthyroidism may well remit with treatment of the hyperthyroid state, whereas anxiety due to cardiomyopathy with a low-output state may run a more chronic course.

Treatment

Aside from treating the underlying causes, clinicians have found benzodiazepines to be helpful in decreasing anxiety symptoms; supportive psychotherapy (including psychoeducational issues focusing on the diagnosis and prognosis) may also be useful. The efficacy of other, more specific therapies in secondary syndromes (e.g., antidepressant medications for panic attacks, selective serotonin reuptake inhibitors for obsessive-compulsive symptoms, behavior therapy for simple phobias) is unknown, but they may be of use.

SLEEP DISORDER DUE TO A GENERAL MEDICAL CONDITION

Sleep disorders can manifest in four ways: by an excess of sleep (hypersomnia), by a deficiency of sleep (insomnia), by abnormal behavior or activity during sleep (parasomnia), and by a disturbance in the timing of sleep (circadian rhythm sleep disorders). Primary sleep disorders occur unrelated to any other medical or psychiatric illness.

The diagnosis of a secondary sleep disorder hinges on the identification of an active disease process known to exert the observed effect on sleep. Treatment first addresses the underlying neurological or medical disease. Symptomatic treatments focus on behavior modifications, such as improvement of sleep hygiene. Pharmacological options may also be used, such as benzodiazepines for restless legs syndrome or nocturnal myoclonus, stimulants for hypersomnia, and tricyclic antidepressant medications for manipulation of rapid eye movement (REM) sleep.

SEXUAL DYSFUNCTION DUE TO A GENERAL MEDICAL CONDITION

Specific syndromes characterized by sexual dysfunction thought to be physiologically caused by a general medical condition are female or male hypoactive sexual desire disorder, male erectile disorder, dyspareunia, and other male or female sexual dysfunction.

Although surveys have repeatedly demonstrated a high prevalence of sexual dysfunctions in the general population, valid data on secondary dysfunctions are lacking. Similarly, certain medications may be associated with specific rates of sexual symptoms, but the percentage of patients with truly secondary syndromes is not known.

The type of sexual dysfunction is affected by the etiology, but specificity is rare; that is, a given etiology may manifest as one (or more than one) of several syndromes. General categories include medications and drugs of abuse, local disease processes that affect the primary or secondary sexual organs, and systemic illnesses that affect sexual organs via neurological, vascular, or endocrinological routes.

The course and prognosis of secondary sexual dysfunctions vary widely, depending on the etiology. Drug-induced syn-

dromes generally remit with discontinuation (or dosage reduction) of the offending agent. Endocrine-based dysfunctions also generally improve with restoration of normal physiology. By contrast, dysfunctions due to neurological disease may run protracted, even progressive, courses.

The treatment approach varies widely, depending on the etiology. When reversal of the underlying cause is not possible, supportive and behaviorally oriented psychotherapy with the patient (and perhaps the partner) may minimize distress and increase sexual satisfaction (for example, by developing sexual interactions that are not limited by the specific dysfunction). Support groups for people with specific types of dysfunction are available. Other symptom-based treatments may be used in certain conditions; for example, sildenafil (Viagra) administration or surgical implantation of a penile prosthesis may be used in the treatment of male erectile dysfunction.

MENTAL DISORDERS DUE TO A GENERAL MEDICAL CONDITION NOT ELSEWHERE CLASSIFIED

The text revision of the fourth edition of *Diagnostic and Statistical Manual of Mental Disorders* (DSM-IV-TR) has three additional diagnostic categories for clinical presentations of mental disorders due to a general medical condition that do not meet the diagnostic criteria for specific diagnoses. The first of the diagnoses is catatonic disorder due to a general medical condition (Table 7.5–2). The second is personality change due to a general medical condition. The third diagnosis is mental disorder not otherwise specified due to a general medical condition (Table 7.5–3).

Catatonia Due to a Medical Condition

Catatonia may be caused by a variety of medical or surgical conditions. It is characterized usually by fixed posture and

Table 7.5–2
DSM-IV-TR Diagnostic Criteria for Catatonic Disorder Due to General Medical Condition

A. The presence of catatonia as manifested by motoric immobility, excessive motor activity (that is apparently purposeless and not influenced by external stimuli), extreme negativism or mutism, peculiarities of voluntary movement, or echolalia or echopraxia.

B. There is evidence from the history, physical examination, or laboratory findings that the disturbance is the direct physiological consequence of a general medical condition.

C. The disturbance is not better accounted for by another mental disorder (e.g., a manic episode).

D. The disturbance does not occur exclusively during the course of a delirium.

Coding note: Include the name of the general medical condition on Axis I, e.g., Catatonic disorder due to hepatic encephalopathy; also code the general medical condition on Axis III.

From American Psychiatric Association. *Diagnostic and Statistical Manual of Mental Disorders.* 4th ed. Text rev. Washington, DC: American Psychiatric Association; copyright 2000, with permission.

Table 7.5–3
DSM-IV-TR Diagnostic Criteria for Mental Disorder Not Otherwise Specified Due to a General Medical Condition

This residual category should be used for situations in which it has been established that the disturbance is caused by the direct physiological effects of a general medical condition, but the criteria are not met for a specific mental disorder due to a general medical condition (e.g., dissociative symptoms due to complex partial seizures).

Coding note: Include the name of the general medical condition on Axis I, e.g., Mental disorder not otherwise specified due to HIV disease; also code the general medical condition on Axis III.

From American Psychiatric Association. *Diagnostic and Statistical Manual of Mental Disorders.* 4th ed. Text rev. Washington, DC: American Psychiatric Association; copyright 2000, with permission.

Table 7.5–4
DSM-IV-TR Diagnostic Criteria for Personality Change Due to General Medical Condition

A. A persistent personality disturbance that represents a change from the individual's previous characteristic personality pattern. (In children, the disturbance involves a marked deviation from normal development or a significant change in the child's usual behavior patterns lasting at least 1 year.)

B. There is evidence from the history, physical examination, or laboratory findings that the disturbance is the direct physiological consequence of a general medical condition.

C. The disturbance is not better accounted for by another mental disorder (including other mental disorders due to a general medical condition).

D. The disturbance does not occur exclusively during the course of a delirium.

E. The disturbance causes clinically significant distress or impairment in social, occupational, or other important areas of functioning.

Specify type:

    Labile type: if the predominant feature is affective lability

    Disinhibited type: if the predominant feature is poor impulse control as evidenced by sexual indiscretions, etc.

    Aggressive type: if the predominant feature is aggressive behavior

    Apathetic type: if the predominant feature is marked apathy and indifference

    Paranoid type: if the predominant feature is suspiciousness or paranoid ideation

    Other type: if the presentation is not characterized by any of the above subtypes

    Combined type: if more than one feature predominates in the clinical picture

    Unspecified type

Coding note: Include the name of the general medical condition on Axis I, e.g., Personality change due to temporal lobe epilepsy; also code the general medical condition on Axis III.

From American Psychiatric Association. *Diagnostic and Statistical Manual of Mental Disorders.* 4th ed. Text rev. Washington, DC: American Psychiatric Association; copyright 2000, with permission.

waxy flexibility. Mutism, negativism, and echolalia may be associated features. The incidence of catatonia due to a general medical condition is unknown. Catatonia symptoms are more likely to be associated with schizophrenia than with other disorders.

Peculiarities of movement are the most characteristic feature; rigidity being the most common. Hyperactivity and psychomotor agitation may also occur. The course and prognosis is intimately related to etiology. Neoplasms, encephalitic, head trauma, diabetes, and other metabolic disorders may present with catatonic features. If the underlying disorder is treatable, the catatonic syndrome will resolve. Treatment must be directed to the underlying etiology. Antipsychotic medication may improve postural abnormalities even though they have no effect on the underlying disorder. ECT has been used successfully in intractable cases.

Personality Change Due to a General Medical Condition

Personality change means that the person's fundamental means of interacting and behaving have been altered. When a true personality change occurs in adulthood, the clinician should always suspect brain injury. Almost every medical disorder can cause personality change, however.

There is no one particular type of behavior or change in personality trait that is diagnostic. Diseases that preferentially affect the frontal lobes or subcortical structures are more likely to manifest with prominent personality change. Head trauma is a common cause. Frontal lobe tumors, such as meningiomas and gliomas, can grow to considerable size before coming to medical attention, as they may be neurologically silent (i.e., without focal signs). Progressive dementia syndromes, especially those with a subcortical pattern of degeneration, such as acquired immune deficiency syndrome (AIDS) dementia complex, Huntington's disease, or progressive supranuclear palsy, often cause significant personality disturbance. MS can impinge on the personality, reflecting subcortical white matter degeneration. Exposures to toxins with a predilection for white matter, such as irradiation, may also produce significant personality change disproportionate to the cognitive or motor impair-

ment. The DSM-IV-TR diagnostic criteria for personality change due to a general medical condition are listed in Table 7.5–4.

Treatment for secondary personality syndromes is first directed toward correcting the underlying etiology. Lithium carbonate, carbamazepine, and valproic acid have been used for the control of affective lability and impulsivity. Aggression or explosiveness may be treated with lithium (Eskalith), anticonvulsant medications, or a combination of lithium and an anticonvulsant agent. Centrally active β-adrenergic receptor antagonists, such as propranolol (Inderal), have some efficacy as well. Apathy and inertia have occasionally improved with psychostimulant agents. Because cognition and verbal skills may be preserved in patients with secondary personality changes, they may be candidates for psychotherapy. Families should be involved in the therapy process, with a focus on education and understanding the origins of the patient's inappropriate behaviors. Issues such as competency, disability, and advocacy are frequently of clinical concern in those patients in light of the unpredictable and pervasive behavior change.

SPECIFIC DISORDERS

Epilepsy

Epilepsy is the most common chronic neurological disease in the general population and affects approximately 1 percent of the population in the Unites States. For psychiatrists, the major concerns about epilepsy are consideration of an epileptic diagnosis in psychiatric patients, the psychosocial ramifications of a diagnosis of epilepsy for a patient, and the psychological and cognitive effects of commonly used anticonvulsant drugs. With regard to the first of these concerns, 30 to 50 percent of all people with epilepsy have psychiatric difficulties sometime during the course of their illness. The most common behavioral symptom of epilepsy is a change in personality. Psychosis and violence occur much less commonly than was previously believed.

Symptoms

PREICTAL SYMPTOMS. Preictal events (auras) in complex partial epilepsy include autonomic sensations (such as fullness in the stomach, blushing, and changes in respiration), cognitive sensations (such as *déjà vu*, *jamais vu*, forced thinking, and dreamy states), affective states (such as fear, panic, depression, and elation), and, classically, automatisms (such as lip smacking, rubbing, and chewing).

ICTAL SYMPTOMS. Brief, disorganized, and uninhibited behavior characterizes the ictal event. Although some defense attorneys may claim otherwise, rarely does a person exhibit organized, directed violent behavior during an epileptic episode. The cognitive symptoms include amnesia for the time during the seizure and a period of resolving delirium after the seizure. In patients with complex partial epilepsy, a seizure focus can be found on an electroencephalogram (EEG) in 25 to 50 percent of all patients. The use of sphenoidal or anterior temporal electrodes and of sleep-deprived EEGs may increase the likelihood of finding an EEG abnormality. Multiple normal EEGs are often obtained for a patient with complex partial epilepsy; therefore, normal EEGs cannot be used to exclude a diagnosis of complex partial epilepsy. The use of long-term EEG recordings (usually 24 to 72 hours) can help clinicians detect a seizure focus in some patients. Most studies show that the use of nasopharyngeal leads does not add much to the sensitivity of an EEG, but they do add to the discomfort of the procedure for the patient.

INTERICTAL SYMPTOMS

Personality Disturbances. The most frequent psychiatric abnormalities reported in epileptic patients are personality disorders, and they are especially likely to occur in patients with epilepsy of temporal lobe origin. The most common features are religiosity, a heightened experience of emotions—a quality usually called *viscosity of personality*—and changes in sexual behavior. The syndrome in its complete form is relatively rare, even in those with complex partial seizures of temporal lobe origin. Many patients are not affected by personality disturbances; others suffer from a variety of disturbances that differ strikingly from the classic syndrome.

Psychotic Symptoms. The onset of psychotic symptoms in epilepsy is variable. Classically, psychotic symptoms appear in patients who have had epilepsy for a long time, and the onset of psychotic symptoms is preceded by the development of personality changes related to the epileptic brain activity. The most characteristic symptoms of the psychoses are hallucinations and paranoid delusions.

Violence. Episodic violence has been a problem in some patients with epilepsy, especially epilepsy of temporal and frontal lobe origin. Whether the violence is a manifestation of the seizure itself or is of interictal psychopathological origin is uncertain. Most evidence points to the extreme rarity of violence as an ictal phenomenon. Only in rare cases should an epileptic patient's violence be attributed to the seizure itself.

Mood Disorder Symptoms. Mood disorder symptoms, such as depression and mania, are seen less often in epilepsy than are schizophrenia-like symptoms. The mood disorder symptoms that do occur tend to be episodic and appear most often when the epileptic foci affect the temporal lobe of the nondominant cerebral hemisphere. The importance of mood disorder symptoms may be attested to by the increased incidence of attempted suicide in people with epilepsy.

Anticonvulsant drugs are the mainstay of treatments. First-line drugs for generalized seizures are valproate and phenytoin. First-line drugs for partial seizures include carbamazepine, oxcarbazepine, and phenytoin. Ethosuximide and valproate are first-line drugs for absence (petit mal) seizures. Psychotherapy, family counseling, and group therapy are useful in addressing the psychosocial issues associated with epilepsy. In addition, clinicians should be aware that many antiepileptic drugs cause a mild to moderate degree of cognitive impairment, and an adjustment of the dosage or a change in medications should be considered if symptoms of cognitive impairment are a problem in a patient.

Brain Tumors

Brain tumors and cerebrovascular diseases can cause virtually any psychiatric symptom or syndrome. In general, tumors are associated with much less psychopathological affectations than are cerebrovascular diseases affecting a similar volume of brain tissue. The two key approaches to the diagnosis of either condition are a comprehensive clinical history and a complete neurological examination. Performance of the appropriate brain imaging technique is usually the final diagnostic procedure; the imaging should confirm the clinical diagnosis, not discover an unsuspected cause.

Mental symptoms are experienced at some time during the course of illness in approximately 50 percent of patients with brain tumors. In approximately 80 percent of these patients with mental symptoms, the tumors are located in frontal or limbic brain regions rather than in parietal or temporal regions. Meningiomas are likely to cause focal symptoms by compressing a limited region of the cortex, whereas gliomas are likely to cause diffuse symptoms. Delirium is most often a component of rapidly growing, large, or metastatic tumors. If a patient's history and a physical examination reveal bowel or bladder incontinence, a frontal lobe tumor should be suspected; if the history and examination reveal abnormalities in memory and speech, a temporal lobe tumor should be suspected. Impaired cognition often accompanies the presence of a brain tumor, regardless of its type or location.

Head Trauma

Head trauma can result in an array of mental symptoms and can lead to a diagnosis of dementia due to head trauma or to mental

Table 7.5–5
DSM-IV-TR Research Criteria for Postconcussional Disorder

A. A history of head trauma that has caused significant cerebral concussion.

   Note: The manifestations of concussion include loss of consciousness, posttraumatic amnesia, and, less commonly, posttraumatic onset of seizures. The specific method of defining this criterion needs to be established by further research.

B. Evidence from neuropsychological testing or quantified cognitive assessment of difficulty in attention (concentrating, shifting focus of attention, performing simultaneous cognitive tasks) or memory (learning or recalling information).

C. Three (or more) of the following occur shortly after the trauma and last at least 3 months:

   (1) becoming fatigued easily
   (2) disordered sleep
   (3) headache
   (4) vertigo or dizziness
   (5) irritability or aggression on little or no provocation
   (6) anxiety, depression, or affective lability
   (7) changes in personality (e.g., social or sexual inappropriateness)
   (8) apathy or lack of spontaneity

D. The symptoms in Criteria B and C have their onset following head trauma or else represent a substantial worsening of preexisting symptoms.

E. The disturbance causes significant impairment in social or occupational functioning and represents a significant decline from a previous level of functioning. In school-age children, the impairment may be manifested by a significant worsening in school or academic performance dating from the trauma.

F. The symptoms do not meet criteria for dementia due to head trauma and are not better accounted for by another mental disorder (e.g., amnestic disorder due to head trauma, personality change due to head trauma).

From American Psychiatric Association. *Diagnostic and Statistical Manual of Mental Disorders.* 4th ed. Text rev. Washington, DC: American Psychiatric Association; copyright 2000, with permission.

disorder not otherwise specified due to a general medical condition (such as postconcussional disorder). The postconcussive syndrome remains controversial, because it focuses on the wide range of psychiatric symptoms, some serious, that can follow what seem to be minor head traumas. DSM-IV-TR includes a set of research criteria for postconcussional disorder in an appendix (Table 7.5–5).

Pathophysiology. Head trauma is a common clinical situation; an estimated 2 million incidents involve head trauma each year. Head trauma most commonly occurs in people 15 to 25 years of age and has a male-to-female predominance of approximately 3 to 1. Gross estimates based on the severity of the head trauma suggest that virtually all patients with serious head trauma, more than half of patients with moderate head trauma, and approximately 10 percent of patients with mild head trauma have ongoing neuropsychiatric sequelae resulting from the head trauma. Head trauma can be divided grossly into penetrating head trauma (such as trauma produced by a bullet) and blunt trauma, in which there is no physical penetration of the skull. Blunt trauma is far more common than penetrating head

trauma. Motor vehicle accidents account for more than half of all the incidents of blunt central nervous system trauma, and falls, violence, and sports-related head trauma account for most of the remaining cases.

Whereas brain injury from penetrating wounds is usually localized to the areas directly affected by the missile, brain injury from blunt trauma involves several mechanisms. During the actual head trauma, the head usually moves back and forth violently, so that the brain crashes repeatedly against the skull as it and the skull are mismatched in their rapid deceleration and acceleration. This crashing results in focal contusions, and the stretching of the brain parenchyma produces diffuse axonal injury. Later-developing processes, such as edema and hemorrhaging, may result in further damage to the brain.

Symptoms. The two major clusters of symptoms related to head trauma are those of cognitive impairment and of behavioral sequelae. After a period of posttraumatic amnesia, there is usually a 6- to 12-month period of recovery, after which the remaining symptoms are likely to be permanent. The most common cognitive problems are a decreased speed in information processing, decreased attention, increased distractibility, deficits in problem solving and in the ability to sustain effort, and problems with memory and learning new information. A variety of language disabilities may also be present.

Behaviorally, the major symptoms involve depression, increased impulsivity, increased aggression, and changes in personality. These symptoms may be further exacerbated by the use of alcohol, which is often involved in the head trauma event itself. A debate has ensued about how preexisting character and personality traits affect the development of behavioral symptoms after a head trauma. The critical studies needed to answer the question definitively have not yet been done, but the weight of opinion is leaning toward a biologically and neuroanatomically based association between the head trauma and the behavioral sequelae.

Treatment. The treatment of the cognitive and behavioral disorders in head trauma patients is basically similar to the treatment approaches used in other patients with these symptoms. One difference is that head trauma patients may be particularly susceptible to the side effects associated with psychotropic drugs; therefore, these agents should be initiated in lower dosages than usual and should be titrated upward more slowly than usual. Standard antidepressants can be used to treat depression, and either anticonvulsants or antipsychotics can be used to treat aggression and impulsivity. Other approaches to the symptoms include lithium, calcium channel blockers, and β-adrenergic antagonists.

Clinicians must support patients through individual or group psychotherapy and should support the major caretakers through couples and family therapy. Especially with minor and moderate head traumas, the patients rejoin their families and restart their jobs; therefore, all involved parties need help to adjust to any changes in the affected patient's personality and mental abilities.

Demyelinating Disorders

MS is the major demyelinating disorder. Other demyelinating disorders include amyotrophic lateral sclerosis, metachromatic leukodystrophy, adrenoleukodystrophy, gangliosidoses, subacute sclerosing panencephalitis, and Kufs' disease. All these disorders can be associated with neurological, cognitive, and behavioral symptoms.

Multiple Sclerosis.   MS is characterized by multiple episodes of symptoms pathophysiologically related to multifocal lesions in the white matter of the central nervous system. The cause remains unknown, but studies have focused on slow viral infections and disturbances in the immune system. The estimated prevalence of MS in the Western Hemisphere is 50 per 100,000 people. The disease is much more frequent in cold and temperate climates than in the tropics and subtropics and more common in women than in men; it is predominantly a disease of young adults. In most patients, the onset occurs between the ages of 20 and 40 years.

The neuropsychiatric symptoms of MS can be divided into cognitive and behavioral types. Research reports have found that 30 to 50 percent of patients with MS have some cognitive impairment and that 20 to 30 percent of MS patients have serious cognitive impairments. Although evidence indicates that MS patients experience a decline in their general intelligence, memory is the most commonly affected cognitive function. The severity of the memory impairment does not seem to be correlated with the severity of the neurological symptoms or the duration of the illness.

The behavioral symptoms associated with MS are euphoria, depression, and personality changes. Psychosis is a rare complication. Approximately 25 percent of people with MS exhibit a euphoric mood that is not hypomanic in severity but, rather, somewhat more cheerful than their situation warrants and not necessarily in character with their disposition before the onset of MS. Only 10 percent of MS patients have a sustained and elevated mood, although it is still not truly hypomanic in severity. Depression, however, is common; it affects 25 to 50 percent of patients with MS and results in a higher rate of suicide than is seen in the general population. Risk factors for suicide in MS patients are male gender, onset of MS before age 30, and a relatively recent diagnosis of the disorder. Personality changes are also common in MS patients; they affect 20 to 40 percent of patients and are often characterized by increased irritability or apathy.

Amyotrophic Lateral Sclerosis.   Amyotrophic lateral sclerosis is a progressive, noninherited disease of asymmetrical muscle atrophy. It begins in adult life and progresses over months or years to involve all the striated muscles except the cardiac and ocular muscles. In addition to muscle atrophy, patients have signs of pyramidal tract involvement. The illness is rare and occurs in approximately 1.6 persons per 100,000 a year. A few patients have concomitant dementia. The disease progresses rapidly, and death generally occurs within 4 years of onset.

Infectious Diseases

Herpes Simplex Encephalitis.   Herpes simplex encephalitis is the most common type of focal encephalitis and most commonly affects the frontal and temporal lobes. The symptoms often include anosmia, olfactory and gustatory hallucinations, and personality changes and can also involve bizarre or psychotic behaviors. Complex partial epilepsy may also

develop in patients with herpes simplex encephalitis. Although the mortality rate for the infection has decreased, many patients exhibit personality changes, symptoms of memory loss, and psychotic symptoms.

Rabies Encephalitis.   The incubation period for rabies ranges from 10 days to 1 year, after which symptoms of restlessness, overactivity, and agitation can develop. Hydrophobia, present in up to 50 percent of patients, is characterized by an intense fear of drinking water. The fear develops from the severe laryngeal and diaphragmatic spasms that the patients experience when they drink water. Once rabies encephalitis develops, the disease is fatal within days or weeks.

Neurosyphilis.   Neurosyphilis (also known as *general paresis*) appears 10 to 15 years after the primary *Treponema* infection. Since the advent of penicillin, neurosyphilis has become a rare disorder, although AIDS is associated with reintroducing neurosyphilis into medical practice in some urban settings. Neurosyphilis generally affects the frontal lobes and results in personality changes, the development of poor judgment, irritability, and decreased care for self. Delusions of grandeur develop in 10 to 20 percent of affected patients. The disease progresses with the development of dementia and tremor, until patients are paretic. The neurological symptoms include Argyll-Robertson pupils, which are small, irregular, and unequal; tremor; dysarthria; and hyperreflexia. A cerebrospinal fluid examination shows lymphocytosis, increased protein, and a positive result on a Venereal Disease Research Laboratory (VDRL) test.

Chronic Meningitis.   Chronic meningitis is also seen more often than it was in the recent past because of the immunocompromised condition of people with AIDS. The most usual causative agents are *Mycobacterium tuberculosis*, *Cryptococcus*, and *Coccidioides*. The usual symptoms are headache, memory impairment, confusion, and fever.

Subacute Sclerosing Panencephalitis.   Subacute sclerosing panencephalitis is a disease of childhood and early adolescence, with a 3 to 1 male-to-female ratio. The onset usually follows either an infection with measles or a vaccination for measles. The initial symptoms may be behavioral change, temper tantrums, sleepiness, and hallucinations, but the classic symptoms of myoclonus, ataxia, seizures, and intellectual deterioration eventually develop. The disease relentlessly progresses to coma and death in 1 to 2 years.

Prion Disease.   Prion disease is a group of related disorders caused by a transmissible infectious protein known as a *prion*. Included in this group are Creutzfeldt-Jakob disease (CJD), Gerstmann-Sträussler-Scheinker syndrome (GSS); fatal familial insomnia (FFI), and kuru. A variant of CJD (vCJD) also called *mad cow disease* appeared in 1995 in the United Kingdom and is attributed to the transmission of bovine spongiform encephalopathy (BSE) from cattle to humans. Collectively, these disorders are also known as *subacute spongiform encephalopathy* because of shared neuropathologic changes that consist of (1) spongiform vacuolization, (2) neuronal loss, and (3) astrocyte proliferation in the cerebral cortex. Amyloid plaques may or may not be present.

ETIOLOGY. Prions are transmissible agents but differ from viruses in that they lack nucleic acid. Prions are mutated proteins generated from the human prion protein gene (PrP), which is located on the short arm of chromosome 20. There is no direct link between prion disease and Alzheimer's disease, which has been traced to chromosome 21.

PrP mutates into a disease-related isoform PrP–Super–C (PrP^{Sc}) that can replicate and is infectious. The neuropathological changes that occur in prion disease are presumed to be caused by direct neurotoxic effects of PrP^{Sc}.

The specific prion disease that develops depends on the mutation of PrP that occurs. Mutations at PrP 178N/129V cause CJD; mutations at 178N/129M cause FFI; mutations at 102L/129M cause GSS and kuru. Other mutations of PrP have been described, and research continues in this important area of genomic identification.

Some mutations are both fully penetrant and autosomal dominant and account for inherited forms of prion disease. For example, both GSS and FFI are inherited disorders, and approximately 10 percent of cases of CJD are also inherited. Prenatal testing for the abnormal PrP gene is available; whether such testing should be routinely done is open to question at this time.

Creutzfeldt-Jakob Disease.   First described in 1920, this is an invariably fatal, rapidly progressive disorder that occurs mainly in middle-aged or older adults. It is manifested initially by fatigue, flu-like symptoms, and cognitive impairment. As the disease progresses, focal neurological findings such as aphasia and apraxia occur. Psychiatric manifestations are protean and include emotional liability, anxiety, euphoria, depression, delusions, hallucinations, or marked personality changes. Progression of disease occurs over months, leading to dementia, akinetic mutism, coma, and death.

The rates of CJD range from 1 to 2 cases per million persons a year worldwide. The infectious agent self-replicates and can be transmitted to humans by inoculation with infected tissue and sometimes by ingestion of contaminated food. Iatrogenic transmission has been reported via transplantation of contaminated cornea or dura mater or to children via contaminated supplies of human growth hormone derived from infected persons. Neurosurgical transmission has also been reported. Household contacts are not at greater risk for developing the disease than the general population, unless there is direct inoculation.

Diagnosis requires pathological examination of the cortex, which reveals the classic triad of spongiform vacuolation, loss of neurons, and astrocyte cell proliferation. The cortex and basal ganglia are most affected. An immunoassay test for CJD in the cerebrospinal fluid shows promise in supporting the diagnosis; however, this needs to be tested more extensively. EEG abnormalities, although not specific for CJD, are present in nearly all patients, consisting of a slow and irregular background rhythm with periodic complex discharges. Computed tomography (CT) and magnetic resonance imaging (MRI) studies may reveal cortical atrophy later in the course of disease. Single photon emission computed tomography (SPECT) and positron emission tomography (PET) reveal heterogeneously decreased uptake throughout the cortex.

There is no known treatment for CJD. Death usually occurs within 6 months after diagnosis.

Variant Creutzfeldt-Jakob Disease.   In 1995, vCJP, a variant of CJD, appeared in the United Kingdom. The patients affected all died; they were young (younger than 40), and none had risk factors of CJD. At autopsy, prion disease was found. The disease was attributed to the transmission in the United Kingdom of BSE between cattle and from cattle to humans in the 1980s. BSE appears to have had its origins from sheep scrapie–contaminated feed given to cattle. Scrapie is a spongiform encephalopathy found in sheep and goats that has not been shown to cause human disease; however, it is transmissible to other animal species.

To date, approximately 100 cases have been reported with a mean age of onset of 29 years of age. Clinicians must be alert to the diagnosis in young people with behavioral and psychiatric abnormalities in association with cerebellar signs, such as ataxia or myoclonus. The psychiatric presentation of CJD is not specific. Most patients reported depression, withdrawal, anxiety, and sleep disturbance. Paranoid delusions have occurred.

Neuropathological changes are similar to those in CJD with the addition of amyloid plaques.

Epidemiologic data are still being gathered. The incubation period for vCJD and the amount of infected meat product required to cause infection are unknown. One patient was reported to have been a vegetarian for 5 years before his disease was diagnosed. vCJD can be diagnosed antemortem by examining the tonsils with Western blot immunostains to detect PrP^{Sc} that is present in lymphoid tissue. Diagnosis relies on the development of progressive neurodegenerative features in persons who have ingested contaminated meat or brains. There is no cure, and death usually occurs within 2 to 3 years after diagnosis.

Kuru

Kuru is an epidemic prion disease found in New Guinea that is caused by cannibalistic funeral rituals in which the brains of the deceased are eaten. Women are more affected by the disorder than men presumably because they participate in the ceremony to a greater extent. Death usually occurs within 2 years after symptoms develop. Neuropsychiatric signs and symptoms consist of ataxia, chorea, strabismus, delirium, and dementia. Pathologic changes are similar to other prion disease consisting of neuronal loss, spongiform lesions, and astrocytic proliferation. The cerebellum is most affected. Iatrogenic transmission of kuru has occurred when cadaveric material such as dura mater and cornea were transplanted into normal recipients. Since the cessation of cannibalism in New Guinea, the incidence of the disease has decreased drastically.

Gerstmann-Sträussler-Scheinker Disease

First described in 1928, GSS disease is a neurodegenerative syndrome characterized by ataxia, chorea, and cognitive decline leading to dementia. It is caused by a mutation in the PrP gene, which is fully penetrant and autosomal dominant; thus, the disease is inherited and affected families have been identified over several generations. Genetic testing can confirm the presence of the abnormal genes before onset. Pathological changes characteristic of prion disease are present: spongiform lesions, neuronal loss, and astrocyte proliferation. Amyloid plaques have been found in the cerebellum. Onset of the disease occurs between 30 and 40 years of age. The disease is fatal within 5 years of onset.

Fatal Familial Insomnia

FFI is an inherited prion disease that primarily affects the thalamus. A syndrome of insomnia, and autonomic nervous system dysfunction consisting of fever, sweating, labile blood pressure, and tachycardia occurs that is debilitating. Onset is in middle adulthood, and death usually occurs in 1 year. There is no treatment.

Immune Disorders

The major immune disorder in contemporary society is AIDS, but other immune disorders can also present diagnostic and treatment challenges to mental health clinicians.

Systemic Lupus Erythematosus.
Systemic lupus erythematosus (SLE) is an autoimmune disease that involves an inflammation of multiple organ systems. The officially accepted diagnosis of SLE requires a patient to have 4 of 11 criteria that have been defined by the American Rheumatism Association. Between 5 and 50 percent of SLE patients have mental symptoms at the initial presentation, and approximately 50 percent of patients eventually show neuropsychiatric manifestations. The major symptoms are depression, insomnia, emotional lability, nervousness, and confusion. Treatment with steroids commonly induces further psychiatric complications, including mania and psychosis.

Endocrine Disorders

Thyroid Disorders.
Hyperthyroidism is characterized by confusion, anxiety, and an agitated depressive syndrome. Patients may also complain of being easily fatigued and of feeling generally weak. Insomnia, weight loss despite increased appetite, tremulousness, palpitations, and increased perspiration are also common symptoms. Serious psychiatric symptoms include impairments in memory, orientation, and judgment; manic excitement; delusions; and hallucinations.

In 1949, Irvin Asher named hypothyroidism *myxedema madness*. In its most severe form, hypothyroidism is characterized by paranoia, depression, hypomania, and hallucinations. Slowed thinking and delirium can also be symptoms. The physical symptoms include weight gain, a deep voice, thin and dry hair, loss of the lateral eyebrow, facial puffiness, cold intolerance, and impaired hearing. Approximately 10 percent of all patients have residual neuropsychiatric symptoms after hormone replacement therapy.

Parathyroid Disorders.
Dysfunction of the parathyroid gland results in the abnormal regulation of calcium metabolism. Excessive secretion of the parathyroid hormone causes hypercalcemia, which can result in delirium, personality changes, and apathy in 50 to 60 percent of patients and cognitive impairments in approximately 25 percent of patients. Neuromuscular excitability, which depends on proper calcium ion concentration, is reduced, and muscle weakness may appear.

Hypocalcemia can occur with hypoparathyroid disorders and can result in neuropsychiatric symptoms of delirium and personality changes. If the calcium level decreases gradually, clinicians may see the psychiatric symptoms without the characteristic tetany of hypocalcemia. Other symptoms of hypocalcemia are cataract formation, seizures, extrapyramidal symptoms, and increased intracranial pressure.

Adrenal Disorders.
Adrenal disorders disturb the normal secretion of hormones from the adrenal cortex and produce significant neurological and psychological changes. Patients with chronic adrenocortical insufficiency (Addison's disease), which is most frequently the result of adrenocortical atrophy or granulomatous invasion caused by tuberculous or fungal infection, exhibit mild mental symptoms, such as apathy, easy fatigability, irritability, and depression. Occasionally, confusion or psychotic reactions develop. Cortisone or one of its synthetic derivatives is effective in correcting such abnormalities.

Excessive quantities of cortisol produced endogenously by an adrenocortical tumor or hyperplasia (Cushing's syndrome) lead to a secondary mood disorder, a syndrome of agitated depression, and, often, suicide. Decreased concentration and memory deficits may also be present. Psychotic reactions, with schizophrenia-like symptoms, are seen in a small number of patients. The administration of high doses of exogenous corticosteroids typically leads to a secondary mood disorder similar to mania. Severe depression may follow the termination of steroid therapy.

Pituitary Disorders.
Patients with total pituitary failure can exhibit psychiatric symptoms, particularly postpartum women who have hemorrhaged into the pituitary, a condition known as Sheehan's syndrome. Patients have a combination of symptoms, especially of thyroid and adrenal disorders, and can show virtually any psychiatric symptom.

Metabolic Disorders

A common cause of organic brain dysfunction, metabolic encephalopathy is capable of producing alterations in mental processes, behavior, and neurological functions. The diagnosis should be considered whenever recent and rapid changes in behavior, thinking, and consciousness have occurred. The earliest signals are likely to be impairment of memory, particularly recent memory, and impairment of orientation. Some patients become agitated, anxious, and hyperactive; others become quiet, withdrawn, and inactive. As metabolic encephalopathies progress, confusion or delirium gives way to decreased responsiveness, stupor, and, eventually, death.

Hepatic Encephalopathy.
Severe hepatic failure can result in hepatic encephalopathy, characterized by asterixis, hyperventilation, EEG abnormalities, and alterations in consciousness. The alterations in consciousness can range from apathy to drowsiness to coma. Associated psychiatric symptoms are changes in memory, general intellectual skills, and personality.

Uremic Encephalopathy.
Renal failure is associated with alterations in memory, orientation, and consciousness. Restlessness, crawling sensations on the limbs, muscle twitching, and persistent hiccups are also associated symptoms. In young people with brief episodes of uremia, the neuropsychiatric symptoms tend to be reversible; in elderly people with long episodes of uremia, the neuropsychiatric symptoms can be irreversible.

Hypoglycemic Encephalopathy.
Hypoglycemic encephalopathy can be caused either by the excessive endogenous production of insulin or by excessive exogenous insulin administration. The premonitory symptoms, which do not occur in every patient, include nausea, sweating, tachycardia, and feelings of hunger, apprehension, and restlessness. As the disorder progresses, disorientation, confusion, and hallucinations, as well as other neurological and medical symptoms, can develop. Stupor and coma may occur, and a residual and persistent dementia can sometimes be a serious neuropsychiatric sequela of the disorder.

Diabetic Ketoacidosis. Diabetic ketoacidosis begins with feelings of weakness, easy fatigability, and listlessness and with increasing polyuria and polydipsia. Headache and sometimes nausea and vomiting appear. Patients with diabetes mellitus have an increased likelihood of chronic dementia with general arteriosclerosis.

Acute Intermittent Porphyria. The porphyrias are disorders of heme biosynthesis that result in the excessive accumulation of porphyrins. The triad of symptoms is acute, colicky abdominal pain, motor polyneuropathy, and psychosis. Acute intermittent porphyria is an autosomal dominant disorder that affects more women than men and that has its onset between ages 20 and 50. The psychiatric symptoms include anxiety, insomnia, lability of mood, depression, and psychosis. Some studies have found that between 0.2 and 0.5 percent of chronic psychiatric patients may have undiagnosed porphyrias. Barbiturates precipitate or aggravate the attacks of acute porphyria, and the use of barbiturates for any reason is absolutely contraindicated in a person with acute intermittent porphyria and in anyone who has a relative with the disease.

Nutritional Disorders

Niacin Deficiency. Dietary insufficiency of niacin (nicotinic acid) and its precursor, tryptophan, is associated with pellagra, a globally occurring nutritional deficiency disease seen in association with alcohol abuse, vegetarian diets, and extreme poverty and starvation. The neuropsychiatric symptoms of pellagra include apathy, irritability, insomnia, depression, and delirium; the medical symptoms include dermatitis, peripheral neuropathies, and diarrhea. The course of pellagra has traditionally been described as five Ds: dermatitis, diarrhea, delirium, dementia, and death. The response to treatment with nicotinic acid is rapid; but dementia from prolonged illness may improve only slowly and incompletely.

Thiamine Deficiency. Thiamine (vitamin B_1) deficiency leads to beriberi, characterized chiefly by cardiovascular and neurological changes, and to Wernicke-Korsakoff syndrome, which is most often associated with chronic alcohol abuse. Beriberi occurs primarily in Asia and in areas of famine and poverty. The psychiatric symptoms include apathy, depression, irritability, nervousness, and poor concentration; severe memory disorders can develop with prolonged deficiencies.

Cobalamin Deficiency. Deficiencies in cobalamin (vitamin B_{12}) arise because of the failure of the gastric mucosal cells to secrete a specific substance, intrinsic factor, required for the normal absorption of vitamin B_{12} in the ileum. The deficiency state is characterized by the development of a chronic macrocytic megaloblastic anemia (pernicious anemia) and by neurological manifestations resulting from degenerative changes in the peripheral nerves, the spinal cord, and the brain. Neurological changes are seen in approximately 80 percent of all patients. These changes are commonly associated with megaloblastic anemia, but they occasionally precede the onset of hematological abnormalities.

Mental changes such as apathy, depression, irritability, and moodiness are common. In a few patients, encephalopathy and its associated delirium, delusions, hallucinations, dementia, and sometimes paranoid features are prominent and are sometimes called *megaloblastic madness*. The neurological manifestations of vitamin B_{12} deficiency can be completely and rapidly arrested by the early and continued administration of parenteral vitamin therapy.

Toxins

Environmental toxins are becoming an increasingly serious threat to physical and mental health in contemporary society.

Mercury. Mercury poisoning can be caused by either inorganic or organic mercury. Inorganic mercury poisoning results in the Mad Hatter syndrome (previously seen in workers in the hat industry who softened mercury by putting it in their mouths), with depression, irritability, and psychosis. Associated neurological symptoms are headache, tremor, and weakness. Organic mercury poisoning can be caused by contaminated fish or grain and can result in depression, irritability, and cognitive impairments. Associated symptoms are sensory neuropathies, cerebellar ataxia, dysarthria, paresthesias, and visual field defects. Mercury poisoning in pregnant women causes abnormal fetal development. No specific therapy is available, although chelation therapy with dimercaprol has been used in acute poisoning.

Lead. Lead poisoning occurs when the amount of lead ingested exceeds the body's ability to eliminate it. It takes several months for toxic symptoms to appear.

The signs and symptoms of lead poisoning depend on the level of lead in the blood. When lead reaches levels above 200 mg/mL, symptoms of severe lead encephalopathy occur, with dizziness, clumsiness, ataxia, irritability, restlessness, headache, and insomnia. Later, an excited delirium occurs, with associated vomiting and visual disturbances, progressing to convulsions, lethargy, and coma.

Treatment of lead encephalopathy should be instituted as rapidly as possible, even without laboratory confirmation, because of the high mortality. The treatment of choice to facilitate lead excretion is the intravenous administration of calcium disodium edetate (calcium disodium versenate) daily for 5 days.

Manganese. Early manganese poisoning produces manganese madness, with symptoms of headache, irritability, joint pains, and somnolence. An eventual picture appears of emotional lability, pathological laughter, nightmares, hallucinations, and compulsive and impulsive acts associated with periods of confusion and aggressiveness. Lesions involving the basal ganglia and pyramidal system result in gait impairment, rigidity, monotonous or whispering speech, tremors of the extremities and tongue, masked facies (manganese mask), micrographia, dystonia, dysarthria, and loss of equilibrium. The psychological effects tend to clear 3 or 4 months after the patient's removal from the site of exposure, but neurological symptoms tend to remain stationary or to progress. There is no specific treatment for manganese poisoning, other than removal from the source of poisoning.

Arsenic. Chronic arsenic poisoning most commonly results from prolonged exposure to herbicides containing arsenic or from drinking water contaminated with arsenic. Arsenic is also used in the manufacture of silicon-based computer chips. Early signs of toxicity are skin pigmentation, gastrointestinal complaint, renal and hepatic dysfunction, hair loss, and a characteristic garlic odor to the breath. Encephalopathy eventually occurs with generalized sensory and motor loss. Chelation therapy with dimercaprol has been used successfully to treat arsenic poisoning.

Neuropsychiatric Aspects of HIV Infection and AIDS

Acquired immune deficiency syndrome (AIDS) is a lethal neuromedical disorder associated with infection by viruses of the *Retroviridae* family known as human immunodeficiency viruses (HIV). Although the central feature of HIV infection involves gradual collapse of the body's ability to mount an appropriate cell-mediated immune response with attendant medical complications, neuropsychiatric phenomena can also be prominent.

The first case of AIDS was reported in 1981. Analysis of specimens retained from persons who died before 1981, however, has shown that HIV infections were present as early as 1959. This suggests that in the 1960s and 1970s, HIV-related disorders and AIDS were increasingly common but unrecognized, particularly in Africa and North America. According to the Centers for Disease Control and Prevention, in 2001 an estimated 500,000 to 600,000 Americans were infected with HIV infection, and another 320,000 persons have full-blown AIDS. New infections, which peaked at more than 150,000 annually in the mid-1980s, were reduced to an estimated 40,000 a year in the early 1990s. The World Health Organization estimates that, worldwide, 2.5 million adults and 1 million children have AIDS, and approximately 30 million persons are infected with HIV.

HIV AND ITS TRANSMISSION

HIV is a retrovirus related to the human T-cell leukemia viruses and to retroviruses that infect animals, including nonhuman primates. At least two types of HIV have been identified, HIV-1 and HIV-2. HIV-1 is the causative agent for most HIV-related diseases; HIV-2, however, seems to be causing an increasing number of infections in Africa. There may be other subtypes of HIV, which are now classified as HIV-O. HIV is present in blood, semen, cervical and vaginal secretions, and, to a lesser extent, in saliva, tears, breast milk, and the cerebrospinal fluid of those who are infected. HIV is most often transmitted through sexual intercourse or the transfer of contaminated blood from one person to another. Unprotected anal and vaginal sex are the sexual activities most likely to transmit the virus. Oral sex has also been implicated, but rarely. Health providers should be aware of the guideline for safe sexual practices and should advise their patients to practice safe sex.

Children can be infected *in utero* or through breast-feeding when their mothers are infected with HIV. Zidovudine (Retrovir) and protease inhibitors taken by the HIV-infected pregnant woman prevent perinatal transmission in more than 95 percent of cases. Health workers are theoretically at risk because of potential contact with bodily fluids from HIV-infected patients. In practice, however, the incidence of such transmission is very low, and almost all reported cases have been traced to accidental needle punctures with contaminated hypodermic needles. No evidence has been found that HIV can be contracted through casual contact, such as by sharing a living space or a classroom with a person who is infected, although direct and indirect contact with an infected person's bodily fluids, such as blood and semen, should be avoided (Table 8–1).

Diagnosis

Two assay techniques are now widely available to detect the presence of anti-HIV antibodies in human serum. Both health care workers and their patients must understand that the presence of HIV antibodies indicates infection, not immunity to infection. Those with a positive finding on an HIV test have been exposed to the virus, have the virus within their bodies, have the potential to transmit the virus to another person, and will almost certainly eventually develop AIDS. Those with a negative HIV test result either have not been exposed to the HIV virus and are not infected or were exposed to the HIV virus but have not yet developed antibodies, a possibility if the exposure occurred less than a year before the testing.

The two assay techniques used are the enzyme-linked immunosorbent assay (ELISA) and the Western blot assay. The ELISA is used as an initial screening test because it is less expensive than the Western blot assay and better suited for large-scale screening. The ELISA is sensitive and reasonably specific; it is unlikely to report a false-negative result, but it may indicate a false-positive one. For this reason, positive results from an ELISA are confirmed by using the more expensive and cumbersome Western blot assay, which is sensitive and specific.

Seroconversion is the change, after infection with HIV, from a negative HIV antibody test result to a positive one. Seroconversion most commonly occurs 6 to 12 weeks after infection, although in rare cases seroconversion can take 6 to 12 months.

Counseling

Counseling both before and after testing should be done and should cover the significance of the test results and their implications for behavioral changes. During pretest counseling, counselors should review past practices that may have put the testee at risk for HIV infection and should discuss safe sexual practices. During posttest counseling, counselors should explain that a negative test finding implies that safe sexual

Table 8–1
Centers for Disease Control and Prevention (CDC) Guidelines for the Prevention of HIV Transmission from Infected to Uninfected Persons

Infected persons should be counseled to prevent the further transmission of HIV by:

1. Informing prospective sex partners of their infection with HIV, so they can take appropriate precautions. Abstention from sexual activity with another person is one option that would eliminate any risk of sexually transmitted HIV infection.

2. Protecting a partner during any sexual activity by taking appropriate precautions to prevent that person's coming into contact with the infected person's blood, semen, urine, feces, saliva, cervical secretions, or vaginal secretions. Although the efficacy of using condoms to prevent infections with HIV is still under study, the consistent use of condoms should reduce the transmission of HIV by preventing exposure to semen and infected lymphocytes.

3. Informing previous sex partners and any persons with whom needles were shared of their potential exposure to HIV and encouraging them to seek counseling and testing.

4. For IV drug abusers, enrolling or continuing in programs to eliminate the abuse of IV substances. Needles, other apparatus, and drugs must never be shared.

5. Never sharing toothbrushes, razors, or other items that could become contaminated with blood.

6. Refraining from donating blood, plasma, body organs, other tissue, or semen.

7. Avoiding pregnancy until more is known about the risks of transmitting HIV from the mother to the fetus or newborn.

8. Cleaning and disinfecting surfaces on which blood or other body fluids have spilled, in accordance with previous recommendations.

9. Informing physicians, dentists, and other appropriate health professionals of antibody status when seeking medical care, so that the patient can be appropriately evaluated.

Reprinted from *MMWR Morb Mortal Wkly Rep.* 1986;35:152.

behavior and the avoidance of shared hypodermic needles are recommended for the person to remain free of HIV infection. A positive test result indicates that the person is infected with HIV and can spread the disease. Those with positive results must receive counseling about safe practices and potential treatment options. They may need additional psychotherapeutic interventions if anxiety or depressive disorders develop after they discover that they are infected.

Couples who are considering taking the HIV antibody test must decide who will be tested and whether to go alone or together. The therapist should ask why they are considering taking the test; partners often for the first time discuss issues of commitment, honesty, and trust, such as sexual contacts outside the relationship. They need to be prepared for the possibility that one or both are infected and must discuss what effect this will have on their relationship.

Confidentiality

Confidentiality is a key issue in serum testing. No one should be given an HIV test without previous knowledge and consent, although various jurisdictions and organizations, such as the military, now require HIV testing for all inhabitants or members. The results of an HIV test can be shared with other members of a medical team, although the information should be

provided to no one else except in the special circumstances discussed below. The patient should be advised against disclosing the results of HIV testing too readily to employers, friends, and family members; the information could result in discrimination in employment, housing, and insurance.

The major exception to restriction of disclosure is the need to notify potential and past sexual or intravenous substance partners. Most HIV-positive patients act responsibly. If, however, a treating physician knows that an HIV-infected patient is putting another person at risk of becoming infected, the physician may try either to hospitalize the infected person involuntarily (to prevent danger to others) or to notify the potential victim. Clinicians should be aware of the laws about such issues, which vary among the states. These guidelines also apply to inpatient psychiatric wards when an HIV-infected patient is believed to be sexually active with other patients.

PSYCHIATRIC SYNDROMES

HIV-Associated Dementia

The text revision of the fourth edition of the *Diagnostic and Statistical Manual of Mental Disorders* (DSM-IV-TR) allows the diagnosis of dementia due to HIV disease when there is "the presence of a dementia that is judged to be the direct pathophysiological consequence of human immunodeficiency virus (HIV) disease."

Although HIV-associated dementia is found in a large proportion of patients infected with HIV, other causes of dementia in these patients must be considered. These causes include central nervous system (CNS) infections, CNS neoplasms, CNS abnormalities caused by systemic disorders and endocrinopathies, and adverse CNS responses to drugs. The development of dementia is generally a poor prognostic sign, and 50 to 75 percent of patients with dementia die within 6 months.

Mild Neurocognitive Disorder

A less severe form of brain involvement is called *HIV-associated neurocognitive disorder*, also known as *HIV encephalopathy*. It is characterized by impaired cognitive functioning and reduced mental activity that interferes with work, homemaking, or social functioning. There are no laboratory findings specific to the disorder, and it occurs independently of depression and anxiety. Progression to HIV-associated dementia usually occurs but may be prevented by early treatment.

Delirium

Delirium can result from the same causes that lead to dementia in patients infected with HIV. Clinicians have classified delirious states characterized by both increased and decreased activity. Delirium in HIV-infected patients is probably underdiagnosed, but it should always precipitate a medical workup of an HIV-infected patient to determine whether a new CNS-related process has begun.

Anxiety Disorders

Patients with HIV infection may have any of the anxiety disorders, but generalized anxiety disorder, posttraumatic stress disorder, and obsessive-compulsive disorder are particularly common.

Adjustment Disorder

Adjustment disorder with anxiety or depressed mood has been reported to occur in 5 to 20 percent of patients infected with HIV. The incidence of adjustment disorder in persons infected with HIV is higher than usual in some special populations, such as military recruits and prison inmates.

Depressive Disorders

A range of 4 to 40 percent of HIV-infected patients have been reported to meet the diagnostic criteria for depressive disorders. The pre-HIV infection prevalence of depressive disorders may be higher than usual in some groups who are at risk for contracting HIV. Another reason for the reported variation in prevalence rates is the variable application of the diagnostic criteria; some of the criteria for depressive disorders (poor sleep and weight loss) can also be caused by the HIV infection itself. Depression is higher in women than in men.

Mania

Mood disorder with manic features, with or without hallucinations, delusions, or a disorder of thought process, can complicate any stage of HIV infection, but most commonly occurs in late-stage disease complicated by neurocognitive impairment.

Substance Abuse

Substance abuse is a problem not only for intravenous substance abusers who contract HIV-related diseases but also for other patients with HIV, who may have used illegal substances only occasionally in the past but may now be tempted to use them regularly to deal with depression or anxiety.

Suicide

Suicidal ideation and suicide attempts may increase in patients with HIV infection and AIDS. The risk factors for suicide among persons infected with HIV are having friends who died from AIDS, recent notification of HIV seropositivity, relapses, difficult social issues relating to homosexuality, inadequate social and financial support, and the presence of dementia or delirium.

Psychotic Disorder

Psychotic symptoms are usually later-stage complications of HIV infection. They require immediate medical and neurological evaluation and often require management with antipsychotic medications.

Worried Well

The so-called worried well are those in high-risk groups who, although seronegative and disease free, are anxious about contracting the virus. Some are reassured by repeated negative serum test results, but others cannot be reassured. Their worried well status can progress to generalized anxiety, panic attacks, obsessive-compulsive disorder, and hypochondriasis.

TREATMENT

Prevention is the primary approach to HIV infection. Primary prevention involves protecting persons from getting the disease; secondary prevention involves modification of the disease's course. All persons with any risk of HIV infection should be informed about safe-sex practices and about the necessity to avoid sharing contaminated hypodermic needles. Preventive strategies, however, are complicated by the complex societal values surrounding sexual acts, sexual orientation, birth control, and substance abuse. Many public health officials have advocated condom distribution in schools and the distribution of clean needles to drug addicts. These issues remain controversial, although condom use has been shown to be a fairly (although not completely) safe and effective preventive strategy against HIV infection. Those who are conservative and religious argue that the educational message should be sexual abstinence. A vaccine to protect persons from infection by HIV is being tested; however, the results are currently inconclusive about its success.

Pharmacotherapy

A growing list of agents that act at different points in viral replication has raised for the first time the hope that HIV might be permanently suppressed or actually eradicated from the body. At the time of this writing, the active agents were in two general classes: reverse transcriptase inhibitors and protease inhibitors. The reverse transcriptase inhibitors are further subdivided into the nucleoside reverse transcriptase inhibitor group and the nonnucleoside reverse transcriptase inhibitor group. Current recommendations are that treatment should be initiated with triple therapy—that is, a combination of two reverse transcriptase inhibitors plus one protease inhibitor.

Triple therapy may be used for persons who have had an unexpected sexual encounter with a potentially infected partner. It is also used in health care workers who have been pricked by a needle from an infected patient. In both instances, triple therapy is started immediately after the event and is usually continued for 3 months.

The antiretroviral agents have many adverse effects, too numerous to describe. Of importance to psychiatrists is that protease inhibitors are metabolized by the hepatic cytochrome P450 oxidase system and can therefore increase levels of certain psychotropic drugs that are similarly metabolized. These include bupropion (Wellbutrin), meperidine (Demerol), various benzodiazepines, and selective serotonin reuptake inhibitors (SSRIs). Therefore, one must exercise caution in prescribing psychotropic drugs to persons taking protease inhibitors.

If neurological damage is present, then the usual supportive measures for neurocognitively impaired persons are indicated. These include identifying areas of cognitive strength and deficit, reducing emphasis on areas that are now impaired (e.g., divided attention, speeded processing), emphasizing efforts to maintain good orientation and reality testing, and avoiding medications that might further compromise cognitive function, in particular, benzodiazepine drugs. If they must be used, such medications should be given at lower-than-usual doses. Antidepressant and antipsychotic agents, if indicated, may also have to be prescribed in much lower dosages (for example, 25 percent of the usual recommended dosage).

Psychotherapy

Approaches. Major psychodynamic themes for HIV-infected patients involve self-blame, self-esteem, and issues regarding death. The psychiatrist can help patients deal with feelings of guilt regarding behaviors that contributed to infection or AIDS. Some HIV and AIDS patients feel that they are being punished. Difficult health care decisions, such as whether to initiate or continue taking antiretroviral medication and terminal care and life-support systems, should be explored, and here denial of illness may be evident. Major practical themes involve employment, medical benefits, life insurance, career plans, dating and sex, and relationships with families and friends. The entire range of psychotherapeutic approaches may be appropriate for patients with HIV-related disorders. Both individual therapy and group therapy can be effective. Individual therapy may be either short-term or long-term and may be supportive, cognitive, behavioral, or psychodynamic. Group therapy techniques can range from psychodynamic to completely supportive in nature.

9 △

Substance-Related Disorders

▲ 9.1 Introduction and Overview

The phenomenon of substance abuse has many implications for brain research and for clinical psychiatry. Some substances can affect both internally perceived mental states, such as mood, and externally observable activities, such as behavior. Substances can cause neuropsychiatric symptoms indistinguishable from those of common psychiatric disorders with no known causes (for example, schizophrenia and mood disorders), and, thus, primary psychiatric disorders and disorders involving the use of substances are possibly related. If the depressive symptoms seen in some persons who have not taken a brain-altering substance are indistinguishable from the depressive symptoms in a person who has taken a brain-altering substance, there may be a brain-based commonality between substance-taking behavior and depression. The very existence of brain-altering substances is a fundamental clue to the ways in which the brain works in both normal and abnormal states.

TERMINOLOGY

The complexity of the subject of illicit substance use is reflected in the associated terminology, which seems to change regularly as various professional and governmental committees convene to discuss the problem. One question is what to call the brain-altering substances. The text revision of the fourth edition of *Diagnostic and Statistical Manual of Mental Disorders* (DSM-IV-TR) refers to brain-altering substances as *substances* and to the related disorders as *substance-related disorders*. In DSM-IV-TR, the concept of *psychoactive substance* does not include chemicals with brain-altering properties such as organic solvents, which may be ingested either on purpose or by accident. Legal substances cannot be separated from illegal substances; many legal substances, such as morphine, are often obtained by illegal means and used for nonprescribed purposes. The word *substance* is generally preferable to the word *drug*, because *drug* implies a manufactured chemical, whereas many substances associated with abuse patterns occur naturally (for example, opium) or are not meant for human consumption (for example, airplane glue).

Although all substances considered by DSM-IV-TR in the substance-related disorders category are associated with a pathological intoxication state, the substances vary as to whether the pathological state is associated with withdrawal or persists after the elimination of the substance from the body. Within the DSM-IV-TR system, patients who are experiencing substance intoxication or withdrawal accompanied by psychiatric symptoms but who do not meet the criteria for a specific syndromal pattern of symptoms (for example, depression) receive the diagnosis of substance intoxication (Table 9.1–1) or substance withdrawal (Table 9.1–2), possibly along with dependence or abuse.

Substance Dependence and Abuse

In 1964, the World Health Organization concluded that the term *addiction* is no longer a scientific term and recommended substituting the term *drug dependence*. The concept of substance dependence has had many officially recognized and commonly used meanings over the decades. Two concepts have been used to define aspects of dependence: behavioral and physical. In behavioral dependence, substance-seeking activities and related evidence of pathological use patterns are emphasized, whereas *physical dependence* refers to the physical (physiological) effects of multiple episodes of substance use. In definitions stressing physical dependence, ideas of tolerance or withdrawal appear in the classification criteria.

Somewhat related to *dependence* are the related words *addiction* and *addict*. The word *addict* has acquired a distinctive, unseemly, and pejorative connotation that ignores the concept of substance abuse as a medical disorder. *Addiction* has also been trivialized in popular usage, as in the phrases *TV addiction* and *money addiction*. Although these connotations have helped the officially sanctioned nomenclature to avoid use of the word *addiction*, there may be common neurochemical and neuroanatomical substrates among all the addictions, whether to substances or to gambling, sex, stealing, or eating. These various addictions may have similar effects on the activities of specific reward areas of the brain, such as the ventral tegmental area, the locus ceruleus, and the nucleus accumbens.

DSM-IV-TR allows clinicians to specify whether symptoms of physiological abuse dependence are present (Table 9.1–3 or 9.1–4). The presence or absence of physiological dependence need not be distinguished from physical and psychological dependence, respectively. Such a distinction parallels the flawed organic–functional distinction; psychological or behavioral dependence undoubtedly reflects physiological changes in the behavioral centers of the brain. DSM-IV-TR also allows clinicians to assess the current state of the substance dependence by providing a list of course modifiers. *Psychological dependence*, also referred to as *habituation*, is characterized by a continuous or intermittent craving for the substance to avoid a

Table 9.1–1
DSM-IV-TR Criteria for Substance Intoxication

A. The development of a reversible substance-specific syndrome due to recent ingestion of (or exposure to) a substance. **Note:** Different substances may produce similar or identical syndromes.

B. Clinically significant maladaptive behavioral or psychological changes that are due to the effect of the substance on the central nervous system (e.g., belligerence, mood lability, cognitive impairment, impaired judgment, impaired social or occupational functioning) and develop during or shortly after use of the substance.

C. The symptoms are not due to a general medical condition and are not better accounted for by another mental disorder.

From American Psychiatric Association. *Diagnostic and Statistical Manual of Mental Disorders*. 4th ed. Text rev. Washington, DC: American Psychiatric Association; copyright 2000, with permission.

Table 9.1–3
DSM-IV-TR Criteria for Substance Abuse

A. A maladaptive pattern of substance use leading to clinically significant impairment or distress, as manifested by one (or more) of the following, occurring within a 12-month period:

(1) recurrent substance use resulting in a failure to fulfill major role obligations at work, school, or home (e.g., repeated absences or poor work performance related to substance use; substance-related absences, suspensions, or expulsions from school; neglect of children or household)

(2) recurrent substance use in situations in which it is physically hazardous (e.g., driving an automobile or operating a machine when impaired by substance use)

(3) recurrent substance-related legal problems (e.g., arrests for substance-related disorderly conduct)

(4) continued substance use despite having persistent or recurrent social or interpersonal problems caused or exacerbated by the effects of the substance (e.g., arguments with spouse about consequences of intoxication, physical fights)

B. The symptoms have never met the criteria for Substance Dependence for this class of substance.

From American Psychiatric Association. *Diagnostic and Statistical Manual of Mental Disorders*. 4th ed. Text rev. Washington, DC: American Psychiatric Association; copyright 2000, with permission.

dysphoric state. DSM-IV-TR defines substance abuse as characterized by the presence of a least one specific symptom indicating that substance use has interfered with the person's life (Table 9.1–3). Persons cannot meet the diagnosis of substance abuse for a particular substance if they have ever met the criteria for dependence on the same substance.

Codependence

The terms *coaddiction, coalcoholism*, or, more commonly, *codependency* or *codependence* are used to designate the behavioral patterns of family members who have been significantly affected by another family member's substance use or addiction. Enabling was one of the first, and more agreed on, characteristics of codependence or coaddiction. Characteristics of enabling include unwillingness to accept the notion of addiction as a disease. The family members continue to behave as if the substance-using behavior were voluntary and willful (if not actually spiteful) and as if the user cares more for alcohol and drugs than for the members of the family.

The 2000 National Household Survey on Drug Abuse Data found that rates of illicit drug use in the U.S. population remained largely unchanged from those in 1999. A slight decrease in drug use was noted among the youngest teenagers. The survey also showed that current cigarette use declined among youths aged 12 to 17 years and young adults aged 18 to 25 years.

Table 9.1–2
DSM-IV-TR Criteria for Substance Withdrawal

A. The development of a substance-specific syndrome due to the cessation of (or reduction in) substance use that has been heavy and prolonged.

B. The substance-specific syndrome causes clinically significant distress or impairment in social, occupational, or other important areas of functioning.

C. The symptoms are not due to a general medical condition and are not better accounted for by another mental disorder.

From American Psychiatric Association. *Diagnostic and Statistical Manual of Mental Disorders*. 4th ed. Text rev. Washington, DC: American Psychiatric Association; copyright 2000, with permission.

An estimated 14 million Americans, or 6.3 percent of the population 12 years old and older, reported that they had used an illicit drug at least once during the 30 days before the 2000 survey interview. Among 12- to 17-year-olds, 9.7 percent were illicit drug users in 2000, compared with 9.8 percent in 1999.

A leading indicator of drug use—the rate of use in the youngest age group—suggests that rates may decline in the future. Among youths 12 and 13 years old, a key target audience of the National Youth Anti-Drug Media Campaign, the rate of past-month illicit drug use declined from 3.9 percent in 1999 to 3 percent in 2000.

Marijuana is the most commonly used illicit drug. In 2000 it was used by 76 percent of current illicit drug users. Approximately 59 percent of illicit drug users consumed only marijuana, 17 percent used marijuana and another illicit drug, and the remaining 24 percent reported use of an illicit drug other than marijuana.

An estimated 65.5 million Americans aged 12 and older—29.3 percent—reported current use of a tobacco product in 2000. Of these, 55.7 million (24.9 percent) smoked cigarettes, 10.7 million (4.8 percent) smoked cigars, 7.6 million (1.0 percent) smoked pipes.

The rates of alcohol use among youths aged 12 to 20 and the general population have remained relatively flat for the past several years. In 2000, almost half of Americans 12 years old and older—46.6 percent, or 104 million persons—reported being current drinkers. The prevalence of current alcohol use increased with age, from 2.4 percent at age 12 to a peak of 65.2 percent for 21-year-olds. About 9.7 million persons in the 12- to 20-year age group, or 27.5 percent, reported drinking alcohol in the past month. Of these, 6.6 million, or 18.7 percent, were binge drinkers, and 2.1 million, or 6 percent, were heavy drinkers.

ETIOLOGY

Psychodynamic Factors

The range of psychodynamic theories about substance abuse reflects the various popular theories during the past 100 years.

**Table 9.1–4
DSM-IV-TR Diagnostic Criteria for
Substance Dependence**

A maladaptive pattern of substance use, leading to clinically
significant impairment or distress, as manifested by three
(or more) of the following, occurring at any time in the
same 12-month period:

(1) tolerance, as defined by either of the following:

(a) a need for markedly increased amounts of the substance to achieve intoxication or desired effect

(b) markedly diminished effect with continued use of
the same amount of the substance

(2) withdrawal, as manifested by either of the following:

(a) the characteristic withdrawal syndrome for the substance (refer to Criteria A and B of the criteria sets for
Withdrawal from the specific substances)

(b) the same (or a closely related) substance is taken to
relieve or avoid withdrawal symptoms

(3) the substance is often taken in larger amounts or over a
longer period than was intended

(4) there is a persistent desire or unsuccessful efforts to cut
down or control substance use

(5) a great deal of time is spent in activities necessary to
obtain the substance (e.g., visiting multiple doctors or
driving long distances), use the substance (e.g.,
chain-smoking), or recover from its effects

(6) important social, occupational, or recreational activities are given up or reduced because of substance use

(7) the substance use is continued despite knowledge of
having a persistent or recurrent physical or psychological problem that is likely to have been caused or exacerbated by the substance (e.g., current cocaine use
despite recognition of cocaine-induced depression, or
continued drinking despite recognition that an ulcer
was made worse by alcohol consumption)

Specify if:

With Physiological Dependence: evidence of tolerance or
withdrawal (i.e., either Item 1 or 2 is present)

Without Physiological Dependence: no evidence of tolerance or withdrawal (i.e., neither Item 1 nor 2 is present)

Course specifiers (see Table 12.1–7 for definitions):

Early Full Remission
Early Partial Remission
Sustained Full Remission
Sustained Partial Remission
On Agonist Therapy
In a Controlled Environment

From American Psychiatric Association. *Diagnostic and Statistical
Manual of Mental Disorders.* 4th ed. Text rev. Washington, DC:
American Psychiatric Association; copyright 2000, with permission.

According to classic theories, substance abuse is a masturbatory equivalent (i.e., the need for orgasm), a defense against
anxious impulses, or a manifestation of oral regression (i.e.,
dependency). Recent psychodynamic formulations relate substance use to depression or treat substance use as a reflection of
disturbed ego functions (i.e., the inability to deal with reality).

Behavioral Theories

Some behavioral models of substance abuse have focused on
substance-seeking behavior rather than on the symptoms of

physical dependence. Most substances of abuse produce a positive experience after their first use, and, thus, the substance acts
as a positive reinforcer for substance-seeking behavior.

Genetic Factors

Strong evidence from studies of twins, adoptees, and siblings
brought up separately indicates that the cause of alcohol abuse
has a genetic component. Other types of substance abuse or
substance dependence also may have a genetic pattern in their
development. Researchers recently have used restriction fragment length polymorphism in the study of substance abuse and
substance dependence, and a few reports of restriction fragment
length polymorphism associations have been published.

Neurochemical Factors

Receptors and Receptor Systems. With the exception
of alcohol, researchers have identified particular neurotransmitters or neurotransmitter receptors involved with most substances
of abuse. Some researchers base their studies on such hypotheses. The opioids, for example, act on opioid receptors. A person
with too little endogenous opioid activity (for example, low concentrations of endorphins) or with too much activity of an endogenous opioid antagonist may be at risk for developing opioid
dependence. Even in a person with completely normal endogenous receptor function and neurotransmitter concentration, the
long-term use of a particular substance of abuse may eventually
modulate receptor systems in the brain so that the presence of the
exogenous substance is needed to maintain homeostasis. Such a
receptor-level process may be the mechanism for developing tolerance within the central nervous system. Demonstrating modulation of neurotransmitter release and neurotransmitter receptor
function has proved difficult, however, and recent research
focuses on the effects of substances on the second-messenger
system and on gene regulation.

Pathways and Neurotransmitters. The major neurotransmitters possibly involved in developing substance abuse
and substance dependence are the opioid, catecholamine (particularly dopamine), and γ-aminobutyric acid systems. The
dopaminergic neurons in the ventral tegmental area are particularly important. These neurons project to the cortical and limbic
regions, especially the nucleus accumbens. This pathway is
probably involved in the sensation of reward and may be the
major mediator of the effects of such substances as amphetamine and cocaine. The locus ceruleus, the largest group of
adrenergic neurons, probably mediates the effects of the opiates
and the opioids. These pathways have collectively been called
the *brain-reward circuitry*.

COMORBIDITY

Comorbidity is the cooccurrence of two or more psychiatric disorders in a single patient. A high prevalence of additional psychiatric disorders is found among persons seeking treatment for
alcohol, cocaine, or opioid dependence. Although opioid,
cocaine, and alcohol abusers with current psychiatric problems
are more likely to seek treatment, those who do not seek treatment are not necessarily free of comorbid psychiatric problems;

such persons may have social supports that enable them to deny the impact that drug use is having on their lives. Two large epidemiological studies have shown that, even among representative samples of the population, those who meet the criteria for alcohol or drug abuse and dependence (excluding tobacco dependence) are far more likely to meet the criteria for other psychiatric disorders such as antisocial personality disorders and depression. Substance use is also a major precipitating factor for suicide.

TREATMENT AND REHABILITATION

Some persons who develop substance-related problems recover without formal treatment, especially as they age. For those patients with less severe disorders, such as nicotine addiction, relatively brief interventions are often as effective as more-intensive treatments. Since these brief interventions do not change the environment, alter drug-induced brain changes, or provide new skills, a change in the patient's motivation (cognitive change) probably best explains their impact on the drug-using behavior. For those individuals who do not respond or whose dependence is more severe, a variety of interventions appear to be effective.

It is useful to distinguish among specific procedures or techniques (e.g., individual therapy, family therapy, group therapy, relapse prevention, and pharmacotherapy) and treatment programs. Most programs use a number of specific procedures and involve several professional disciplines as well as nonprofessionals who have special skills or personal experience with the substance problem being treated. The best treatment programs combine specific procedures and disciplines to meet the needs of the individual patient after a careful assessment.

Programs are often broadly grouped on the basis of one or more of their salient characteristics: whether the program is aimed at merely controlling acute withdrawal and consequences of recent drug use (detoxification) or is focused on longer-term behavioral change; whether the program makes extensive use of pharmacological interventions; and the degree to which the program is based on individual psychotherapy, Alcoholics Anonymous (AA), or other 12-step principles, or therapeutic community principles.

Treatment of Comorbidity—Integrated versus Concurrent

The treatment of the severely mentally ill (primarily those with schizophrenia and schizoaffective disorders) who are also drug dependent continues to pose problems for clinicians. Although some special facilities have been developed that use both antipsychotic drugs and therapeutic community principles, for the most part, specialized addiction agencies have difficulty treating these patients. Generally, integrated treatment in which the same staff can treat both the psychiatric disorder and the addiction is more effective than either parallel treatment (a mental health and a specialty addiction program providing care concurrently) or sequential treatment (treating either the addiction or the psychiatric disorder first and then dealing with the comorbid condition).

The sections that follow deal with substances of abuse according to the particular drug (e.g., alcohol, caffeine) and discuss their diagnosis, etiology, pharmacology, and treatment in depth.

▲ 9.2 Alcohol-Related Disorders

Although alcohol abuse and dependency are commonly called *alcoholism*, the text revision of the fourth edition of the *Diagnostic and Statistical Manual of Mental Disorders* (DSM-IV-TR) does not use the term because it lacks a precise definition. Table 9.2–1 lists various categories and definitions of alcohol use.

EPIDEMIOLOGY

Approximately 30 to 45 percent of all adults in the United States have had at least one transient episode of an alcohol-related problem, usually an alcohol-induced amnestic episode like a blackout, driving a motor vehicle while intoxicated (DWI), or missing school or work because of excessive drinking. Approximately 10 percent of women and 20 percent of men have met the diagnostic criteria for alcohol abuse during their lifetimes, and 3 to 5 percent of women and 10 percent of men have met the diagnostic criteria for the more serious diagnosis of alcohol dependence during their lifetimes. Approximately 200,000 deaths each year are directly related to alcohol abuse. The common causes of death among persons with the alcohol-related disorders are suicide, cancer, heart disease, and

Table 9.2–1
Categories and Definitions for Patterns of Alcohol Use

Category	Definition
Moderate drinking	Men, ≤2 drinks/d
	Women, ≤1 drink/d
	Persons >65 years of age, ≤1 drink/d
At-risk drinking	Men, >14 drinks/wk or >4 drinks per occasion
	Women, >7 drinks/wk or >3 drinks per occasion
Hazardous drinking	At risk for adverse consequences from alcohol
Harmful drinking	Alcohol causing physical or psychological harm
Alcohol abuse	≤1 of the following events in a year: recurrent use resulting in failure to fulfill major role obligations, recurrent use in hazardous situations, recurrent alcohol-related legal problems (e.g., citations for driving under the influence), continued use despite social or interpersonal problems caused or exacerbated by alcohol
Alcohol dependence	≤3 of the following events in a year: tolerance; increased amounts to achieve effect; diminished effects from same amount; withdrawal; a great deal of time spent obtaining alcohol, using it, or recovering from its effects; important activities given up or reduced because of alcohol; drinking more or longer than intended; persistent desire or unsuccessful efforts to cut down or control alcohol use; continued use despite knowledge of a psychological problem caused or exacerbated by alcohol

From Fiellin DA, Reid C, O'Connor PG. Outpatient management of patients with alcohol problems. *Ann Intern Med.* 2000;133:815.

hepatic disease. Although persons involved in automotive fatalities do not always meet the diagnostic criteria for an alcohol-related disorder, drunken drivers are involved in approximately 50 percent of all automotive fatalities, and this percentage increases to approximately 75 percent when only accidents occurring in the late evening are considered. Alcohol use and alcohol-related disorders are also associated with approximately 50 percent of all homicides and 25 percent of all suicides. Alcohol abuse reduces life expectancy by approximately 10 years, and alcohol leads all other substance in substance-related deaths.

Race and Ethnicity

Compared with other groups, whites have the highest rate of alcohol use—56 percent. Rates for Hispanics and blacks are similar. The rate of binge use is lower among blacks than among whites and Hispanics. Heavy use shows no statistically significant differences by race or ethnicity (5.7 percent for whites, 6.3 percent for Hispanics, and 4.6 percent for blacks).

Gender

Sixty percent of men are past-month alcohol users, compared with 45 percent of women. Men are much more likely than women to be binge drinkers (23.8 and 8.5 percent, respectively) and heavy drinkers (9.4 and 2.0 percent, respectively).

Region and Urbanicity

The rate of current alcohol use was 59 percent in the North Central region, 54 percent in the Northeast region, 53 percent in the West, and 47 percent in the South in 1995. Rates of binge use were 20 percent in the North Central region, 16 percent in the West, and 14 percent in the South and Northeast. Heavy alcohol use rates were 7 percent in the North Central region, 5.6 percent in the West, 4.9 percent in the Northeast, and 4.8 percent in the South. The rate of past-month alcohol use was 56 percent in large metropolitan areas, 52 percent in small metropolitan areas, and 46 percent in nonmetropolitan areas. There was little variation in binge and heavy alcohol use rates by population density.

Education

In contrast to the pattern for illicit drugs, the higher the educational attainment, the more likely is the current use of alcohol. Approximately 70 percent of adults with college degrees are current drinkers, compared with only 40 percent of those with less than a high school education. Binge alcohol use rates are similar across different levels of education. The rate of heavy alcohol use, however, is 4 percent among adults who had completed college and 7 percent among adults who had not completed high school.

Socioeconomic Class

Alcohol-related disorders appear among persons of all socioeconomic classes. In fact, persons who are stereotypical skid-row alcoholics constitute less than 5 percent of those with alcohol-related disorders in the United States. Moreover, these disorders are particularly frequent in persons with advanced academic degrees and upper socioeconomic standing.

Among high school students, alcohol-related problems are correlated with a history of school difficulties. High school dropouts and persons with a record of frequent truancy and delinquency appear to be at particularly high risk for alcohol abuse. These epidemiological data are consistent with the high comorbidity between alcohol-related disorders and antisocial personality disorder.

COMORBIDITY

The psychiatric diagnoses most commonly associated with the alcohol-related disorders are other substance-related disorders, antisocial personality disorder, mood disorders, and anxiety disorders. Although the data are somewhat controversial, most suggest that persons with alcohol-related disorders have a markedly higher suicide rate than the general population.

Antisocial Personality Disorder

A relation between antisocial personality disorder and alcohol-related disorders has frequently been reported. Some studies have suggested that antisocial personality disorder is particularly common in men with an alcohol-related disorder and can precede the development of the alcohol-related disorder. Other studies, however, have suggested that antisocial personality disorder and alcohol-related disorders are completely distinct entities that are not causally related.

Mood Disorders

Approximately 30 to 40 percent of persons with an alcohol-related disorder meet the diagnostic criteria for major depressive disorder sometime during their lifetimes. Depression is more common in women than in men with these disorders. Several studies reported that depression is likely to occur in patients with alcohol-related disorders who have a high daily consumption of alcohol and a family history of alcohol abuse. Persons with alcohol-related disorders and major depressive disorder are at great risk for attempting suicide and are likely to have other substance-related disorders. Some clinicians recommend that depressive symptoms that remain after 2 to 3 weeks of sobriety be treated with antidepressant drugs. Patients with bipolar I disorder are thought to be at risk for developing an alcohol-related disorder; they may use alcohol to self-medicate their manic episodes. Some studies have shown that persons with both alcohol-related disorder and depressive disorder diagnoses have concentrations of dopamine metabolites (homovanillic acid) and γ-aminobutyric acid (GABA) in their cerebrospinal fluid.

Anxiety Disorders

Many persons use alcohol for its efficacy in alleviating anxiety. Although the comorbidity between alcohol-related disorders and mood disorders is fairly widely recognized, it is less well known that perhaps 25 to 50 percent of all persons with alcohol-related disorders also meet the diagnostic criteria for an anxiety disorder. Phobias and panic disorder are particularly frequent comorbid diagnoses in these patients. Some data indicate that alcohol may be used in an attempt to self-medicate symptoms of agoraphobia or social phobia, but an alcohol-related disorder is likely to precede the development of panic disorder or generalized anxiety disorder.

Suicide

Most estimates of the prevalence of suicide among persons with alcohol-related disorders range from 10 to 15 percent, although alcohol use itself may be involved in a much higher percentage of suicides. Some investigators have questioned whether the suicide rate among persons with alcohol-related disorders is as high as the numbers suggest. Factors that have been associated with suicide among persons with alcohol-related disorders include the presence of a major depressive episode, weak psychosocial support systems, a serious coexisting medical condition, unemployment, and living alone.

ETIOLOGY

Alcohol-related disorders, like virtually all other psychiatric conditions, probably represent a heterogeneous group of disease processes. In any individual case, psychosocial, genetic, or behavioral factors may be more important than other factors. Within any single set of factors, such as biological factors, one element, such as a neurotransmitter receptor gene, may be more critically involved than another element, such as a neurotransmitter uptake pump. Except for research purposes, it is not necessary to identify the single causative factor; treating alcohol-related disorders requires taking whatever approaches are effective, regardless of theory.

Childhood History

Researchers have identified several factors in the childhood histories of persons with later alcohol-related disorders and in children at high risk for having an alcohol-related disorder because one or both of their parents are affected. In experimental studies, children at high risk for alcohol-related disorders have been found to possess, on average, a range of deficits on neurocognitive testing, low amplitude of the P300 wave on evoked potential testing, and a variety of abnormalities on electroencephalogram (EEG) recordings. These findings suggest that a heritable biological brain function may predispose a person to an alcohol-related disorder. A childhood history of attention-deficit/hyperactivity disorder or conduct disorder or both increases a child's risk for an alcohol-related disorder as an adult. Personality disorders, especially antisocial personality disorder, as noted above, also predispose a person to an alcohol-related disorder.

Psychodynamic Theories

Psychodynamic theories of alcohol-related disorders have centered on hypotheses about overly punitive superegos and fixation at the oral stage of psychosexual development. According to psychoanalytic theory, persons with harsh superegos who are self-punitive turn to alcohol as a way of diminishing unconscious stress. Anxiety in persons fixated at the oral stage may be reduced by taking substances, such as alcohol, by mouth. Some psychodynamic psychiatrists describe the general personality of a person with an alcohol-related disorder as shy, isolated, impatient, irritable, anxious, hypersensitive, and sexually repressed. According to a common psychoanalytic aphorism, the superego is soluble in alcohol. On a less theoretical level, alcohol may be abused by some persons to reduce tension, anxiety, and psychic pain. Alcohol consumption can also lead to a sense of power and increased self-worth.

Sociocultural Theories

Some social settings commonly lead to excessive drinking. College dormitories and military bases are two such examples; in these settings, excessive and frequent drinking is often completely normal and socially expected. Colleges and universities have recently tried to educate students about the health risks of drinking large quantities of alcohol. Some cultural and ethnic groups are more restrained than others about alcohol consumption. For example, Asians and conservative Protestants use alcohol less frequently than do liberal Protestants and Catholics.

Behavioral and Learning Factors

Just as cultural factors can affect drinking habits, so can the habits within a family, specifically, parental drinking habits. Some evidence indicates, however, that familial drinking habits that affect children's drinking habits are less directly linked to development of alcohol-related disorders than was previously thought. From a behavioral viewpoint, the positive reinforcing aspects of alcohol can induce feelings of well-being and euphoria and can reduce fear and anxiety, which may further encourage drinking.

Genetic Theories

The best-supported biological theory of alcoholism centers on genetics. One finding supporting the genetic conclusion is the three- to fourfold higher risk for severe alcohol problems in close relatives of alcoholic persons. The rate of alcohol problems increases with the number of alcoholic relatives, the severity of their illness, and the closeness of their genetic relationship to the person under study. Family investigations do little to separate the importance of genetics and environment, but twin studies take the data a step further. The rate of similarity, or concordance, for severe alcohol-related problems is enhanced in the offspring of alcoholic parents, even when the children were separated from their biological parents close to birth and raised without any knowledge of the problems within the biological family. The risk for severe alcohol-related difficulties is not further enhanced by being raised by an alcoholic adoptive family.

These data not only support the importance of genetic factors in alcoholism, but also highlight the complexity of the phenomenon. The absence of evidence of a single major locus indicates the possibility that a limited number of genes operate with incomplete penetrance or that a combination of genes is required before the disorder expresses itself (a polygenic mode of inheritance). Making matters even more complex is the likelihood that the disorder is solely an expression of environmental events in some families and that different genetic factors operate in different families to produce a picture of genetic heterogeneity.

Some evidence indicates that the brains of children with parents who have alcohol-related disorders exhibit unusual qualities in terms of electrophysiological measures—for example, evoked potentials and EEGs—and response to alcohol infusions. Neurotransmitter receptors such as the dopamine type 2 (D_2) receptors may be factors in the inheritance of alcohol-related disorders. Some studies have found abnormal concentrations of neurotransmitters and neurotransmitter metabolites in the cerebrospinal fluid of patients with alcohol-related disorders. Results of many of these studies demonstrated low concentrations of neurotransmitters and neurotransmitter metabolites in the cerebrospinal fluid of patients with alcohol-related disorders. Results of many of these studies demonstrated low concentrations of serotonin, dopamine, and GABA or their metabolites.

EFFECTS OF ALCOHOL

The term *alcohol* refers to a large group of organic molecules that have a hydroxyl group (–OH) attached to a saturated carbon atom. Ethyl alcohol, also called *ethanol*, is the common form of alcohol; sometimes referred to as *beverage alcohol*, ethyl alcohol is used for drinking. The chemical formula for ethanol is $CH_3–CH_2–OH$.

Absorption

Approximately 10 percent of consumed alcohol is absorbed from the stomach, the remainder from the small intestine. Peak blood concentration alcohol is reached in 30 to 90 minutes and usually in 45 to 60 minutes, depending on whether the alcohol was taken on an empty stomach (which enhances absorption) or with food (which delays absorption). The time to peak blood concentration also depends on the time during which the alcohol was consumed; rapid drinking reduces the time to peak concentration, slower drinking increases it. Absorption is most rapid with beverages containing 15 to 30 percent alcohol (30 to 60 proof). There is some dispute about whether carbonation (for example, in champagne and in drinks mixed with seltzer) enhances the absorption of alcohol.

The body has protective devices against inundation by alcohol. For example, if the concentration of alcohol in the stomach becomes too high, mucus is secreted, and the pyloric valve closes. These actions slow the absorption and keep the alcohol from passing into the small intestine, where there are no significant restraints to absorption. Thus, a large amount of alcohol can remain unabsorbed in the stomach for hours. Furthermore, pylorospasm often results in nausea and vomiting.

Once alcohol is absorbed into the bloodstream, it is distributed to all body tissues. Because alcohol is uniformly dissolved in the body's water, tissues containing a high proportion of water receive a high concentration of alcohol. The intoxicating effects are greater when the blood alcohol concentration is rising than when it is falling (the Mellanby effects). For this reason, the rate of absorption bears directly on the intoxication response.

Metabolism

Approximately 90 percent of absorbed alcohol is metabolized through oxidation in the liver; the remaining 10 percent is excreted unchanged by the kidneys and lungs. The rate of oxidation by the liver is constant and independent of the body's energy requirements. The body can metabolize approximately 15 mg/dL per hour, with a range of 10 to 34 mg/dL per hour. Stated another way, the average person oxidizes three-fourths of an ounce of 40 percent (80 proof) alcohol in an hour. In persons with a history of excessive alcohol consumption, upregulation of the necessary enzymes results in rapid alcohol metabolism.

Alcohol is metabolized by two enzymes: alcohol dehydrogenase (ADH) and aldehyde dehydrogenase. ADH catalyzes the conversion of alcohol into acetaldehyde, which is a toxic compound; aldehyde dehydrogenase catalyzes the conversion of acetaldehyde into acetic acid. Aldehyde dehydrogenase is inhibited by disulfiram (Antabuse), often used in the treatment of alcohol-related disorders. Some studies have shown that women have a lower ADH blood content than men; this fact may account for women's tendency to become more intoxicated than men after drinking the same amount of alcohol. The decreased function of alcohol-metabolizing enzymes in some Asian persons can also lead to easy intoxication and toxic symptoms.

Effects on the Brain

Biochemistry. In contrast to most other substances of abuse with identified receptor targets—such as the *N*-methyl-D-aspartate (NMDA) receptor of phencyclidine—no single molecular target has been identified as the mediator for the effects of alcohol. The long-standing theory about the biochemical effects of alcohol concerns its effects on the membranes of neurons. Data support the hypothesis that alcohol produces its effects by intercalating itself into membranes and thus increasing fluidity of the membranes with short-term use. With long-term use, however, the theory hypothesizes that the membranes become rigid or stiff. The fluidity of the membranes is critical to normal functioning of receptors, ion channels, and other membrane-bound functional proteins. In recent studies, researchers have attempted to identify specific molecular targets for the effects of alcohol. Most attention has been focused on the effects of alcohol at ion channels. Specifically, studies have found that alcohol ion channel activities associated with the nicotinic acetylcholine, serotonin 5-HT_3, and GABA type A ($GABA_A$) receptors are enhanced by alcohol, whereas ion channel activities associated with glutamate receptors and voltage-gated calcium channels are inhibited.

Behavioral Effects. As the net result of the molecular activities, alcohol functions as a depressant much like the barbiturates and the benzodiazepines, with which alcohol has some cross-tolerance and cross-dependence. At a level of 0.05 percent alcohol in the blood, thought, judgment, and restraint are loosened and sometimes disrupted. At a concentration of 0.1 percent, voluntary motor actions usually become perceptibly clumsy. In most states, legal intoxication ranges from 0.1 to 0.15 percent blood alcohol level. At 0.2 percent, the function of the entire motor area of the brain is measurably depressed, and the parts of the brain that control emotional behavior are also affected. At 0.3 percent, a person is commonly confused or may become stuporous; at 0.4 to 0.5 percent, the person falls into a coma. At higher levels, the primitive centers of the brain that control breathing and heart rate are affected, and death ensues secondary to direct respiratory depression or the aspiration of vomitus. Persons with long-term histories of alcohol abuse, however, can tolerate much higher concentrations of alcohol than can alcohol-naïve persons; their alcohol tolerance may cause them to falsely appear less intoxicated than they really are.

Sleep Effects. Although alcohol consumed in the evening usually increases the ease of falling asleep (decreased sleep latency), alcohol also has adverse effects on sleep architecture. Specifically, alcohol use is associated with a decrease in rapid eye movement sleep (REM or dream sleep) and deep sleep (stage 4) and more sleep fragmentation, with more and longer episodes of awakening. Therefore, the idea that drinking alcohol helps persons fall asleep is a myth.

Other Physiological Effects

Liver.   The major adverse effects of alcohol use are related to liver damage. Alcohol use, even as short as week-long episodes of increased drinking, can result in an accumulation of fats and proteins, which produce the appearance of a fatty liver, sometimes found on physical examination as an enlarged liver. The association between fatty infiltration of the liver and serious liver damage remains unclear. Alcohol use, however, is associated with the development of alcoholic hepatitis and hepatic cirrhosis.

Gastrointestinal System.   Long-term heavy drinking is associated with developing esophagitis, gastritis, achlorhydria, and gastric ulcers. The development of esophageal varices can accompany particularly heavy alcohol abuse; the rupture of the varices is a medical emergency often resulting in death by exsanguination. Disorders of the small intestine occasionally occur, and pancreatitis, pancreatic insufficiency, and pancreatic cancer are also associated with heavy alcohol use. Heavy alcohol intake may interfere with the normal processes of food digestion and absorption; as a result, consumed food is inadequately digested. Alcohol abuse also appears to inhibit the intestine's capacity to absorb various nutrients, such as vitamins and amino acids. This effect, coupled with the often poor dietary habits of those with alcohol-related disorders, can cause serious vitamin deficiencies, particularly of the B vitamins.

Other Bodily Systems.   Significant intake of alcohol has been associated with increased blood pressure, dysregulation of lipoprotein and triglyceride metabolism, and increased risk for myocardial infarctions and cerebrovascular diseases. Alcohol has been shown to affect the hearts of nonalcoholic persons who do not usually drink, increasing the resting cardiac output, the heart rate, and the myocardial oxygen consumption. Evidence indicates that alcohol intake can adversely affect the hematopoietic system and can increase the incidence of cancer, particularly head, neck, esophageal, stomach, hepatic, colonic, and lung cancer. Acute intoxication may also be associated with hypoglycemia, which, when unrecognized, may be responsible for some of the sudden deaths of persons who are intoxicated. Muscle weakness is another side effect of alcoholism. Recent evidence shows that alcohol intake raises the blood concentration of estradiol in women. The increase in estradiol correlates with the blood alcohol level.

Laboratory Tests.   The adverse effects of alcohol appear in common laboratory tests, which can be useful diagnostic aids in identifying persons with alcohol-related disorders. The γ-glutamyl transpeptidase levels are high in approximately 80 percent of those with alcohol-related disorders, and the mean corpuscular volume is high in approximately 60 percent, more so in women than in men. Other laboratory test values that may be high in association with alcohol abuse are those of uric acid, triglycerides, aspartate aminotransferase, and aminotransferase.

Drug Interactions

The interaction between alcohol and other substances can be dangerous, even fatal. Certain substances such as alcohol and

phenobarbital (Luminal) are metabolized by the liver, and their prolonged use may lead to acceleration of their metabolism. When persons with alcohol-related disorders are sober, this accelerated metabolism makes them unusually tolerant to many drugs such as sedatives and hypnotics; when they are intoxicated, however, these drugs compete with the alcohol for the same detoxification mechanisms, and potentially toxic concentrations of all involved substances can accumulate in the blood.

The effects of alcohol and other central nervous system (CNS) depressants are usually synergistic. Sedatives, hypnotics, and drugs that relieve pain, motion sickness, head colds, and allergy symptoms must be used with caution by persons with alcohol-related disorders. Narcotics depress the sensory areas of the cerebral cortex and can produce pain relief, sedation, apathy, drowsiness, and sleep; high doses can result in respiratory failure and death. Increasing the dosages of sedative-hypnotic drugs such as chloral hydrate (Noctec) and benzodiazepines, especially when they are combined with alcohol, produces a range of effects from sedation to motor and intellectual impairment to stupor, coma, and death. Because sedatives and other psychotropic drugs can potentiate the effects of alcohol, patients should be instructed about the dangers of combining CNS depressants and alcohol, particularly when they are driving or operating machinery.

DISORDERS

DSM-IV-TR lists the alcohol-related disorders (Table 9.2–2) and specifies the diagnostic criteria for alcohol intoxication (Table 9.2–3) and alcohol withdrawal (Table 9.2–4). The diagnostic criteria for the other alcohol-related disorders are listed in DSM-IV-TR under the major symptom. For example, the diagnostic criteria for alcohol-induced anxiety disorder are found in the anxiety disorders category, under the heading "Substance-Induced Anxiety Disorder."

Alcohol Intoxication

DSM-IV-TR establishes formal criteria for diagnosing alcohol intoxication (Table 9.2–3): sufficient alcohol consumption, specific maladaptive behavioral changes, signs of neurological impairment, and the absence of other confounding diagnoses or conditions. Alcohol intoxication is not a trivial condition and, in extreme cases, can lead to coma, respiratory depression, and death from respiratory arrest or because of aspiration of vomitus. Treatment for severe alcohol intoxication requires mechanical ventilatory support in an intensive care unit, with attention to the patient's acid-base balance, electrolytes, and temperature. Some studies of cerebral blood flow (CBF) during alcohol intoxication have found a modest increase in CBF after the ingestion of small amounts of alcohol, but CBF decreases with continued drinking.

The severity of alcohol intoxication symptoms correlates roughly with the blood concentration of alcohol, which reflects the alcohol concentration in the brain. With the onset of intoxication, some persons become talkative and gregarious; others become withdrawn and sullen or belligerent. Some patients show lability of mood with intermittent episodes of laughing and crying. The person may show a short-term tolerance to

Table 9.2–2
DSM-IV-TR Alcohol-Related Disorders

Alcohol use disorders
Alcohol dependence
Alcohol abuse
Alcohol-induced disorders
Alcohol intoxication
Alcohol withdrawal
   Specify if:
      With perceptual disturbances
Alcohol intoxication delirium
Alcohol withdrawal delirium
Alcohol-induced persisting dementia
Alcohol-induced persisting amnestic disorder
Alcohol-induced psychotic disorder, with delusions
   Specify if:
      With onset during intoxication
      With onset during withdrawal
Alcohol-induced psychotic disorder, with hallucinations
   Specify if:
      With onset during intoxication
      With onset during withdrawal
Alcohol-induced mood disorder
   Specify if:
      With onset during intoxication
      With onset during withdrawal
Alcohol-induced anxiety disorder
   Specify if:
      With onset during intoxication
      With onset during withdrawal
Alcohol-induced sexual dysfunction
   Specify if:
      With onset during intoxication
Alcohol-induced sleep disorder
   Specify if:
      With onset during intoxication
      With onset during withdrawal
Alcohol disorder not otherwise specified

From American Psychiatric Association. *Diagnostic and Statistical Manual of Mental Disorders.* 4th ed. Text rev. Washington, DC: American Psychiatric Association; copyright 2000, with permission.

Table 9.2–3
DSM-IV-TR Diagnostic Criteria for Alcohol Intoxication

A. Recent ingestion of alcohol.
B. Clinically significant maladaptive behavioral or psychological changes (e.g., inappropriate sexual or aggressive behavior, mood lability, impaired judgment, impaired social or occupational functioning) that developed during, or shortly after, alcohol ingestion.
C. One (or more) of the following signs, developing during, or shortly after, alcohol use:
   (1) slurred speech
   (2) incoordination
   (3) unsteady gait
   (4) nystagmus
   (5) impairment in attention or memory
   (6) stupor or coma
D. The symptoms are not due to a general medical condition and are not better accounted for by another mental disorder.

From American Psychiatric Association. *Diagnostic and Statistical Manual of Mental Disorders.* 4th ed. Text rev. Washington, DC: American Psychiatric Association; copyright 2000, with permission.

include fatigue, malnutrition, physical illness, and depression. The DSM-IV-TR criteria for alcohol withdrawal (Table 9.2–4) require the cessation or reduction of alcohol use that was heavy and prolonged as well as the presence of specific physical or neuropsychiatric symptoms. The diagnosis also allows for the specification "with perceptual disturbances." One recent positron emission tomographic (PET) study of blood flow during alcohol withdrawal in otherwise healthy persons with alcohol depen-

Table 9.2–4
DSM-IV-TR Diagnostic Criteria for Alcohol Withdrawal

A. Cessation of (or reduction in) alcohol use that has been heavy and prolonged.
B. Two (or more) of the following, developing within several hours to a few days after Criterion A:
   (1) autonomic hyperactivity (e.g., sweating or pulse rate greater than 100)
   (2) increased hand tremor
   (3) insomnia
   (4) nausea or vomiting
   (5) transient visual, tactile, or auditory hallucinations or illusions
   (6) psychomotor agitation
   (7) anxiety
   (8) grand mal seizures
C. The symptoms in Criterion B cause clinically significant distress or impairment in social, occupational, or other important areas of functioning.
D. The symptoms are not due to a general medical condition and are not better accounted for by another mental disorder.
Specify if:
   With perceptual disturbances

From American Psychiatric Association. *Diagnostic and Statistical Manual of Mental Disorders.* 4th ed. Text rev. Washington, DC: American Psychiatric Association; copyright 2000, with permission.

alcohol and seem to be less intoxicated after many hours of drinking than after only a few hours.

The medical complications of intoxication include those that result from falls such as subdural hematomas and fractures. Telltale signs of frequent bouts of intoxication are facial hematomas, particularly about the eyes, the result of falls or fights while drunk. In cold climates, hypothermia and death may occur when a person is exposed to the elements. A person with alcohol intoxication may also be predisposed to infections secondary to a suppressed immune system.

Alcohol Withdrawal

Alcohol withdrawal, even without delirium, can be serious and can include seizures and autonomic hyperactivity. Conditions that may predispose to, or aggravate, withdrawal symptoms

dence reported a globally low rate of metabolic activity, although, with further inspection of the data, the authors concluded that activity was especially low in the left parietal and right frontal areas.

The classic sign of alcohol withdrawal is tremulousness, although the spectrum of symptoms can expand to include psychotic and perceptual symptoms (for example, delusions and hallucinations), seizures, and the symptoms of delirium tremens (DTs), called *alcohol withdrawal delirium* in DSM-IV-TR. Tremulousness (commonly called the "shakes" or the "jitters") develops 6 to 8 hours after cessation of drinking, and DTs during 72 hours, although physicians should watch for the development of DTs for the first week of withdrawal. The syndrome of withdrawal sometimes skips the usual progression and, for example, goes directly to DTs.

The tremor of alcohol withdrawal can be similar to either physiological tremor, with a continuous tremor of great amplitude and of more than 8 Hz, or familial tremor, with bursts of tremor activity slower than 8 Hz. Other symptoms of withdrawal include general irritability, gastrointestinal symptoms (for example, nausea and vomiting), and sympathetic autonomic hyperactivity, including anxiety, arousal, sweating, facial flushing, mydriasis, tachycardia, and mild hypertension. Patients experiencing alcohol withdrawal are generally alert but may startle easily.

> A 23-year-old computer consultant with alcohol dependence was unable to establish even 24 hours of sobriety as an outpatient. Therefore, reflecting his continued drinking, he was referred for inpatient care. Following approximately 10 hours of abstinence and with a documented blood alcohol concentration of 0 mg/dL, he was noted to be mildly diaphoretic, with a respiratory rate of 25 breaths per minute, blood pressure of 130/90, a mild bilateral tremor of the hands, and a pulse rate of 85 beats per minute. He had a history of jogging 2 to 5 miles a day, and these figures represented moderate elevation of his usual vital signs. Treated with multiple vitamins, good nutrition, oral fluids, and benzodiazepines, the symptoms rapidly improved, and his vital signs were close to normal by day 4 of abstinence. (Courtesy of Marc A. Schuckit, M.D.)

Withdrawal Seizures. Seizures associated with alcohol withdrawal are stereotyped, generalized, and tonic-clonic in character. Patients often have more than one seizure 3 to 6 hours after the first seizure. Status epilepticus is relatively rare and occurs in less than 3 percent of patients. Although anticonvulsant medications are not required in the management of alcohol withdrawal seizures, the cause of the seizures is difficult to establish when a patient is first assessed in the emergency room; thus, many patients with withdrawal seizures receive anticonvulsant medications, which are then discontinued once the cause of the seizures is recognized. Seizure activity in patients with known alcohol abuse histories should still prompt clinicians to consider other causative factors, such as head injuries, CNS infections, CNS neoplasms, and other cerebrovascular diseases; long-term severe alcohol abuse can result in hypoglycemia, hyponatremia, and hypomagnesemia—all of which can also be associated with seizures.

Treatment. The primary medications for the control of alcohol withdrawal symptoms are the benzodiazepines. Many studies have found that benzodiazepines help control seizure activity, delirium, anxiety, tachycardia, hypertension, diaphoresis, and tremor associated with alcohol withdrawal. Benzodiazepines can be given either orally or parenterally: neither diazepam (Valium) nor chlordiazepoxide (Librium), however, should be given intramuscularly (IM) because of their erratic absorption by this route. Clinicians must titrate the dosage of the benzodiazepine, starting with a high dosage and lowering the dosage as the patient recovers. Enough benzodiazepines should be given to keep patients calm and sedated but not so sedated that they cannot be aroused for clinicians to perform appropriate procedures, including neurological examinations.

Although benzodiazepines are the standard treatment for alcohol withdrawal, studies have shown that carbamazepine (Tegretol) in daily doses of 800 mg is as effective as benzodiazepines and has the added benefit of minimal abuse liability. Carbamazepine use is gradually becoming common in the United States and Europe. The β-adrenergic receptor antagonists and clonidine (Catapres) have also been used to block the symptoms of sympathetic hyperactivity, but neither drug is an effective treatment for seizures or delirium.

Delirium

Diagnosis and Clinical Features. DSM-IV-TR contains the diagnostic criteria for alcohol intoxication delirium in the category of substance intoxication delirium and the diagnostic criteria for alcohol withdrawal delirium in the category of substance withdrawal delirium (see Tables 7.2–3 and 7.2–4 in Chapter 7, Section 7.2). Patients with recognized alcohol withdrawal symptoms should be carefully monitored to prevent progression to alcohol withdrawal delirium, the most severe form of the withdrawal syndrome, also known as *DTs*. Alcohol withdrawal delirium is a medical emergency that can result in significant morbidity and mortality. Patients with delirium are a danger to themselves and to others. Because of the unpredictability of their behavior, patients with delirium may be assaultive or suicidal or may act on hallucinations or delusional thoughts as if they were genuine dangers. Untreated, DTs has a mortality rate of 20 percent, usually as a result of an intercurrent medical illness such as pneumonia, renal disease, hepatic insufficiency, or heart failure. Although withdrawal seizures commonly precede the development of alcohol withdrawal delirium, delirium can also appear unheralded. The essential feature of the syndromes is delirium occurring within 1 week after a person stops drinking or reduces the intake of alcohol. In addition to the symptoms of delirium, the features of alcohol intoxication delirium include autonomic hyperactivity such as tachycardia, diaphoresis, fever, anxiety, insomnia, and hypertension; perceptual distortions, most frequently visual or tactile hallucinations; and fluctuating levels of psychomotor activity, ranging from hyperexcitability to lethargy.

Approximately 5 percent of persons with alcohol-related disorders who are hospitalized have DTs. Because the syndrome usually develops on the third hospital day, a patient admitted for an unrelated condition may unexpectedly have an episode of delirium, the first sign of a previously undiagnosed alcohol-related disorder. Episodes of DTs usually begin in a patient's 30s or 40s after 5 to 15 years of heavy drinking, typically of the binge type. Physical illness (for example, hepatitis or pancreatitis) predisposes to the syndrome; a person in good physical health rarely has DTs during alcohol withdrawal.

Treatment. The best treatment for DTs is prevention. Patients withdrawing from alcohol who exhibit withdrawal phenomena should receive a benzodiazepine, such as 25 to 50 mg of chlordiazepoxide every 2 to 4 hours until they seem to be out of danger. Once the delirium appears, however, 50 to 100 mg of chlordiazepoxide should be given every 4 hours orally, or lorazepam (Ativan) should be given intravenously (IV) if oral medication is not possible. Antipsychotic medications that may reduce the seizure threshold in patients should be avoided. A high-calorie, high-carbohydrate diet supplemented by multivitamins is also important.

Physically restraining patients with the DTs is risky; they may fight against the restraints to a dangerous level of exhaustion. When patients are disorderly and uncontrollable, a seclusion room can be used. Dehydration, often exacerbated by diaphoresis and fever, can be corrected with fluids given by mouth or IV. Anorexia, vomiting, and diarrhea often occur during withdrawal. Antipsychotic medications should be avoided because they may reduce the seizure threshold in the patient. The emergence of focal neurological symptoms, lateralizing seizures, increased intracranial pressure, or evidence of skull fractures or other indications of CNS pathology should prompt clinicians to examine a patient for additional neurological disease. Nonbenzodiazepine anticonvulsant medication is not useful in preventing or treating alcohol withdrawal convulsions, although benzodiazepines are generally effective.

Warm, supportive psychotherapy in the treatment of DTs is essential. Patients are often bewildered, frightened, and anxious because of their tumultuous symptoms, and skillful verbal support is imperative.

Alcohol-Induced Persisting Dementia

The legitimacy of the concept of alcohol-induced persisting dementia remains controversial; some clinicians and researchers believe that it is difficult to separate the toxic effects of alcohol abuse from the CNS damage done by poor nutrition and multiple trauma and that following the malfunctioning of other bodily organs such as the liver, pancreas, and kidneys. Although several studies have found enlarged ventricles and cortical atrophy in persons with dementia and a history of alcohol dependence, the studies do not help clarify the cause of the dementia. Nonetheless, DSM-IV-TR includes the diagnosis of alcohol-induced persisting dementia. The controversy about the diagnosis should encourage clinicians to complete a diagnostic assessment of the dementia before concluding that it was caused by alcohol.

Alcohol-Induced Persisting Amnestic Disorder

Diagnosis and Clinical Features. The diagnostic criteria of alcohol-induced persisting amnestic disorder are contained in the DSM-IV-TR category of substance-induced persisting amnestic disorder. The essential feature of alcohol-induced persisting amnestic disorder is a disturbance in short-term memory caused by prolonged heavy use of alcohol. Because the disorder usually

occurs in persons who have been drinking heavily for many years, the disorder is rare in persons younger than age 35.

Wernicke-Korsakoff Syndrome. The classic names for alcohol-induced persisting amnestic disorder are *Wernicke's encephalopathy* (a set of acute symptoms) and *Korsakoff's syndrome* (a chronic condition). Whereas Wernicke's encephalopathy is completely reversible with treatment, only approximately 20 percent of patients with Korsakoff's syndrome recover. The pathophysiological connection between the two syndromes is thiamine deficiency, caused either by poor nutritional habits or by malabsorption problems. Thiamine is a cofactor for several important enzymes and may also be involved in conduction of the axon potential along the axon and in synaptic transmission. The neuropathological lesions are symmetrical and paraventricular, involving the mammillary bodies, the thalamus, hypothalamus, midbrain, pons, medulla, fornix, and cerebellum.

Wernicke's encephalopathy, also called *alcoholic encephalopathy*, is an acute neurological disorder characterized by ataxia (affecting primarily the gait), vestibular dysfunction, confusion, and a variety of ocular motility abnormalities, including horizontal nystagmus, lateral rectal palsy, and gaze palsy. These eye signs are usually bilateral but not necessarily symmetrical. Other eye signs may include a sluggish reaction to light and anisocoria. Wernicke's encephalopathy may clear spontaneously in a few days or weeks or may progress into Korsakoff's syndrome.

Treatment. In the early stages, Wernicke's encephalopathy responds rapidly to large doses of parenteral thiamine, which is believed to be effective in preventing the progression into Korsakoff's syndrome. The dosage of thiamine is usually initiated at 100 mg by mouth two to three times daily and is continued for 1 to 2 weeks. In patients with alcohol-related disorders who are receiving IV administration of glucose solution, it is good practice to include 100 mg of thiamine in each liter of the glucose solution. Korsakoff's syndrome is the chronic amnestic syndrome that can follow Wernicke's encephalopathy, and the two syndromes are believed to be pathophysiologically related. The cardinal features of Korsakoff's syndrome are impaired mental syndrome (especially recent memory) and anterograde amnesia in an alert and responsive patient. The patient may or may not have the symptom of confabulation. Treatment of Korsakoff's syndrome is also thiamine given 100 mg by mouth two to three times daily; the treatment regimen should continue for 3 to 12 months. Few patients who progress to Korsakoff's syndrome ever fully recover, although a substantial proportion have some improvement in their cognitive abilities with thiamine and nutritional support.

Blackouts. Alcohol-related blackouts are not included in DSM-IV-TR's diagnostic classification, although the symptom of alcohol intoxication is common. Blackouts are similar to episodes of transient global amnesia (see Chapter 7, Section 7.4) in that they are discrete episodes of anterograde amnesia that occur in association with alcohol intoxication. The periods of amnesia can be particularly distressing when persons fear that they have unknowingly harmed someone or behaved imprudently while intoxicated. During a blackout, persons have relatively intact remote memory but experience a specific short-term memory deficit in which they are unable to recall events that happened in the previous 5 or 10 minutes. Because their other intellectual faculties are well preserved, they can perform complicated tasks and appear normal to casual observers. The neurobiological mechanisms for alcoholic blackouts are now known at the molecular level; alcohol blocks the consolidation of new memories into old memories, a process that is thought to involve the hippocampus and related temporal lobe structures.

Alcohol-Induced Psychotic Disorder

Diagnosis and Clinical Features.   The diagnostic criteria for alcohol-induced psychotic disorders, such as delusions and hallucinations, are found in the DSM-IV-TR category of substance-induced psychotic disorder (see Table 11.4–5). DSM-IV-TR further allows the specification of onset (during intoxication or withdrawal) and whether hallucinations or delusions are present. The most common hallucinations are auditory, usually voices, but they are often unstructured. The voices are characteristically maligning, reproachful, or threatening, although some patients report that the voices are pleasant and nondisruptive. The hallucinations usually last less than a week, but during that week impaired reality testing is common. After the episode, most patients realize the hallucinatory nature of the symptoms.

Hallucinations after alcohol withdrawal are considered rare, and the syndrome is distinct from alcohol withdrawal delirium. The hallucinations can occur at any age but usually appear in persons abusing alcohol for a long time. Although the hallucinations usually resolve within a week, some may linger; in these cases, clinicians must consider other psychotic disorders in the differential diagnosis. Alcohol withdrawal-related hallucinations are differentiated from the hallucinations of schizophrenia by the temporal association with alcohol withdrawal, the absence of a classic history of schizophrenia, and their usually short-lived duration. Alcohol withdrawal-related hallucinations are differentiated from the DTs by the presence of a clear sensorium in patients.

A 39-year-old male letter carrier was brought to an emergency room by the police after he behaved in an unusual fashion at home and complained that his neighbors were trying to kill him. The history obtained from the patient and his wife revealed that his psychotic thinking developed slowly over the preceding 3 weeks; he began with feelings that persons were looking at him at work, progressed to vague feelings that persons were against him, and went on to frank auditory hallucinations that persons at work and in the neighboring houses were talking about their plans to kill him. He had no insight into those paranoid delusions and auditory hallucinations. The relatively abrupt onset of the syndrome—he was in his late 30s—pointed to a potential organic cause, and further probing documented that he had been drinking between 6 and 18 beers daily for at least the preceding 10 weeks. A diagnosis of alcohol-induced psychotic disorder with onset during intoxication was made, and both hallucinations and delusions disappeared after 3 weeks of abstinence. After alcohol treatment, the man stayed sober for the next 8 months. Unfortunately, he later resumed heavy drinking and had a recurrence of both hallucinations and delusions. (Courtesy of Marc A. Schuckit, M.D.)

Treatment.   The treatment of alcohol withdrawal-related hallucinations is much like the treatment of DTs—benzodiazepines, adequate nutrition, and fluids if necessary. If this regimen fails or for long-term cases, antipsychotics may be used.

Alcohol-Induced Mood Disorder

DSM-IV-TR allows for the diagnosis of alcohol-induced mood disorder with manic, depressive, or mixed features (see Table 12.3–8 in Chapter 12, Section 12.3) and also for the specification of onset during either intoxication or withdrawal. As with all the secondary and substance-induced disorders, clinicians must consider whether the abused substance and the symptoms have a causal relation.

A consultation was requested on a 42-year-old woman with alcohol dependence who complained of persisting severe depressive symptoms despite 5 days of abstinence. In the initial stage of the interview she noted that she had "always been depressed" and felt that she "drank to cope with the depressive symptoms." Her current complaint included a prominent sadness that had persisted for several weeks, difficulties concentrating, initial and terminal insomnia, and a feeling of hopelessness and guilt. In an effort to distinguish between an alcohol-induced mood disorder and an independent major depressive episode, a time-line–based history was obtained. This focused on the age of onset of alcohol dependence, periods of abstinence that extended for several months or more since the onset of dependence, and the ages of occurrence of clear major depressive episodes lasting several weeks or more at a time. Despite this patient's original complaints, it became clear that there had been no major depressive episodes prior to her mid-20s when alcohol dependence began, and that during a 1-year period of abstinence related to the gestation and neonatal period of her son, her mood had significantly improved. A provisional diagnosis of an alcohol-induced mood disorder was made. The patient was offered education, reassurance, and cognitive therapy to help her to deal with the depressive symptoms, but no antidepressant medications were prescribed. The depressive symptoms remained at their original intensity for several additional days and then began to improve. By approximately 3 weeks abstinent the patient no longer met criteria for a major depressive episode, although she demonstrated mood swings similar to dysphemia for several additional weeks. This case is a fairly typical example of an alcohol-induced mood disorder in an individual with alcohol dependence. (Courtesy of Marc A. Shuckit, M.D.)

Alcohol-Induced Anxiety Disorder

DSM-IV-TR allows for the diagnosis of alcohol-induced anxiety disorder and suggests that the diagnosis specify whether the symptoms are those of generalized anxiety, panic attacks, obsessive-compulsive symptoms, or phobic symptoms and whether the onset was during intoxication or during withdrawal. The association between alcohol use and anxiety symptoms is discussed above; deciding whether the anxiety symptoms are primary or secondary can be difficult.

Alcohol-Induced Sexual Dysfunction

In DSM-IV-TR, the formal diagnosis of symptoms of sexual dysfunction associated with alcohol intoxication is alcohol-induced sexual dysfunction (see Table 18.2–11 in Section 18.2 of Chapter 18).

Alcohol-Induced Sleep Disorder

In DSM-IV-TR, the diagnostic criteria for alcohol-induced sleep disorders with an onset during either alcohol intoxication or alcohol withdrawal are found in the sleep disorders section (see Table 21.2–14 in Section 21.2 of Chapter 21).

Alcohol-Related Use Disorder Not Otherwise Specified

DSM-IV-TR allows for the diagnosis of alcohol-related disorder not otherwise specified for alcohol-related disorders that do not meet the diagnostic criteria for any of the other diagnoses (Table 9.2–5).

Idiosyncratic Alcohol Intoxication.   Whether there is such a diagnostic entity as idiosyncratic alcohol intoxication is under debate; DSM-IV-TR does not recognize this category as an official diagnosis. Several well-controlled studies of persons who supposedly have the disorder have raised questions about the validity of the designation. The condition has been variously called *pathologic, complicated, atypical,* and *paranoid alcohol intoxication*; all these terms indicate that a severe behavioral syndrome develops rapidly after a person consumes a small amount of alcohol that would have minimal behavioral effects on most persons. The diagnosis is important in the forensic arena because alcohol intoxication is not generally accepted as a reason for judging persons not responsible for their activities. Idiosyncratic alcohol intoxication, however, can be used in a person's defense if a defense lawyer can argue successfully that the defendant has an unexpected, idiosyncratic, pathological reaction to a minimal amount of alcohol.

In anecdotal reports, persons with idiosyncratic alcohol intoxication have been described as confused and disoriented and as experiencing illusions, transitory delusions, and visual hallucinations. Persons may display greatly increased psychomotor activity and impulsive, aggressive behavior. They may be dangerous to others and may also exhibit suicidal ideation and make suicide attempts. The disorder, usually described as lasting for a few hours, terminates in prolonged sleep, and those affected cannot recall the episodes on awakening. The cause of the condition is unknown, but it is reported to be most common in persons with high levels of anxiety. According to one hypothesis, alcohol causes sufficient disorganization and loss of control to release aggressive impulses. Another suggestion is that brain damage, particularly encephalitic or traumatic damage, predisposes some persons to an intolerance for alcohol and thus to abnormal behavior after they ingest only small amounts. Other predisposing factors may include advancing age, using sedative-hypnotic drugs, and feeling fatigued. A person's behavior while intoxicated tends to be atypical; after one weak drink, a quiet, shy person becomes belligerent and aggressive.

In treating idiosyncratic alcohol intoxication, clinicians must help protect patients from harming themselves and others. Physical restraint may be necessary but is difficult because of the abrupt onset of the condition. Once a patient has been restrained, injection of an antipsychotic drug, such as haloperidol (Haldol), is useful for controlling assaultiveness. This condition must be differentiated from other causes of abrupt behavioral change, such as complex partial epilepsy. Some persons with the disorder reportedly showed temporal lobe spiking on an EEG after ingesting small amounts of alcohol.

Other Alcohol-Related Neurological Disorders

Only the major neuropsychiatric syndromes associated with alcohol use are discussed here. *Alcoholic pellagra encephalopathy* is one diagnosis of potential interest to psychiatrists presented with a patient who appears to be afflicted with Wernicke-Korsakoff syndrome but does not respond to thiamine treatment. The symptoms of alcoholic pellagra encephalopathy include confusion, clouding of consciousness, myoclonus, oppositional hypertonias, fatigue, apathy, irritability, anorexia, insomnia, and sometimes delirium. Patients suffer from a deficiency of niacin (nicotinic acid), and the specific treatment is 50 mg of niacin by mouth four times daily or 25 mg parenterally two to three times daily.

Fetal Alcohol Syndrome

Data indicate that women who are pregnant or are breast-feeding should not drink alcohol. Fetal alcohol syndrome, the leading cause of mental retardation in the United States, occurs when mothers drinking alcohol expose fetuses to alcohol in utero. The alcohol inhibits intrauterine growth and postnatal development. Microcephaly, craniofacial malformations, and limb and heart defects are common in affected infants. Short adult stature and development of a range of adult maladaptive behaviors have also been associated with fetal alcohol syndrome.

Women with alcohol-related disorders have a 35 percent risk of having a child with defects. Although the precise mechanism of the damage to the fetus is unknown, the damage seems to result from exposure in utero to ethanol or to its metabolites; alcohol may also cause hormone imbalances that increase the risk of abnormalities.

Prognosis

Between 10 and 40 percent of alcoholic persons enter some kind of formal treatment program during the course of their alcohol

Table 9.2–5
DSM-IV-TR Diagnostic Criteria for Alcohol-Related Disorder Not Otherwise Specified

The alcohol-related disorder not otherwise specified category is for disorders associated with the use of alcohol that are not classifiable as alcohol dependence, alcohol abuse, alcohol intoxication, alcohol withdrawal, alcohol intoxication delirium, alcohol withdrawal delirium, alcohol-induced persisting dementia, alcohol-induced persisting amnestic disorder, alcohol-induced psychotic disorder, alcohol-induced mood disorder, alcohol-induced anxiety disorder, alcohol-induced sexual dysfunction, or alcohol-induced sleep disorder.

From American Psychiatric Association. *Diagnostic and Statistical Manual of Mental Disorders.* 4th ed. Text rev. Washington, DC: American Psychiatric Association; copyright 2000, with permission.

problems. A number of prognostic signs are favorable. First is the absence of preexisting antisocial personality disorder or a diagnosis of other substance abuse or dependence. Second, evidence of general life stability with a job, continuing close family contacts, and the absence of severe legal problems also bodes well for the patient. Third, if the patient stays for the full course of the initial rehabilitation (perhaps 2 to 4 weeks), the chances of maintaining abstinence are good. The combination of these three attributes predicts at least a 60 percent chance for 1 or more years of abstinence. Few studies have documented the long-term course, but researchers agree that 1 year of abstinence is associated with a good chance for continued abstinence over an extended period. However, alcoholic persons with severe drug problems (especially IV drug use or cocaine or amphetamine dependence) and those who are homeless may have only a 10 to 15 percent or so chance of achieving 1 year of abstinence.

Accurately predicting whether any specific person will achieve or maintain abstinence is impossible, but the prognostic factors listed above are associated with an increased likelihood of abstinence. However, the factors reflecting life stability probably explain only 20 percent or less of the course of alcohol use disorders. Many forces that are difficult to measure affect the clinical course significantly; they are likely to include such intangibles as motivational level and the quality of the patient's social support system.

In general, alcoholic persons with preexisting independent major psychiatric disorders—such as antisocial personality disorder, schizophrenia, and bipolar I disorder—are likely to run the course of their independent psychiatric illness. Thus, for example, clinicians must treat the patient with bipolar I disorder who has secondary alcoholism with appropriate psychotherapy and lithium (Eskalith), use relevant psychological and behavioral techniques for the patient with antisocial personality disorder, and offer appropriate antipsychotic medications on a long-term basis to the patient with schizophrenia. The goal is to minimize the symptoms of the independent psychiatric disorder in the hope that greater life stability will be associated with a better prognosis for the patient's alcohol problems.

TREATMENT AND REHABILITATION

Intervention

The goal in this step, which has also been called *confrontation*, is to break through feelings of denial and help the patient recognize the adverse consequences likely to occur if the disorder is not treated. Intervention is, as a process, aimed at maximizing the motivation for treatment and continued abstinence.

The family can be of great help in the intervention. Family members must learn not to protect the patient from the problems caused by alcohol; otherwise, the patient may not be able to gather the energy and the motivation necessary to stop drinking. During the intervention stage, the family can also suggest that the patient meet with persons who are recovering from alcoholism, perhaps through Alcoholics Anonymous (AA), and they can meet with groups, such as Alanon, that reach out to family members. Those support groups for families meet many times a week and help family members and friends see that they are not alone in their fears, worries, and feelings of guilt. Members share coping strategies and help each other find community resources. The

groups can be most useful in helping family members rebuild their lives, even if the alcoholic person refuses to seek help.

Detoxification

Most persons with alcohol dependence have relatively mild symptoms when they stop drinking. If the patient is in relatively good health, is adequately nourished, and has a good social support system, the depressant withdrawal syndrome usually resembles a mild case of the flu. Even intense withdrawal syndromes rarely approach the severity of symptoms described by some early textbooks in the field.

The essential first step in detoxification is a thorough physical examination. In the absence of a serious medical disorder or combined drug abuse, severe alcohol withdrawal is unlikely. The second step is to offer rest, adequate nutrition, and multiple vitamins, especially those containing thiamine.

Mild or Moderate Withdrawal

Withdrawal develops because the brain has physically adapted to the presence of a brain depressant and cannot function adequately in the absence of the drug. Giving enough brain depressant on the first day to diminish symptoms and then weaning the patient off the drug over the next 5 days offers most patients optimal relief and minimizes the possibility that severe withdrawal will develop. Any depressant—including alcohol, barbiturates, or any of the benzodiazepines—can work, but most clinicians choose a benzodiazepine for its relative safety. Adequate treatment can be given with either short-acting drugs (for example, lorazepam) or long-acting substances (for example, chlordiazepoxide and diazepam).

An example of treatment is the administration of 25 mg of chlordiazepoxide by mouth three or four times a day on the first day, with a notation to skip a dose if the patient is asleep or feeling sleepy. An additional one or two 25-mg doses can be given during the first 24 hours if the patient is jittery or shows signs of increasing tremor or autonomic dysfunction. Whatever benzodiazepine dosage is required on the first day can be decreased by 20 percent each subsequent day, with a resulting need for no further medication after 4 or 5 days. When giving a long-acting agent, such as chlordiazepoxide, the clinician must avoid producing excessive sleepiness through overmedication; if the patient is sleepy, the next scheduled dose should be omitted. When taking a short-acting drug, such as lorazepam, the patient must not miss any dose because rapid changes in benzodiazepine concentrations in the blood may precipitate severe withdrawal.

A social model program of detoxification saves money by avoiding medications while using social supports. This less-expensive regimen can be helpful for mild or moderate withdrawal syndromes. Some clinicians have also recommended β-adrenergic receptor antagonists (for example, clonidine), although these medications do not appear to be superior to the benzodiazepines. Unlike the brain depressants, these other agents do little to decrease the risk of seizures or delirium.

Severe Withdrawal

For the approximately 1 to 3 percent of alcoholic patients with extreme autonomic dysfunction, agitation, and confusion—that is, those with alcoholic withdrawal delirium, or DTs—no optimal treatment has yet been developed. The first step is to ask why such a severe and relatively uncommon withdrawal syndrome has occurred; the answer often relates to a severe concomitant medical problem that needs immediate treatment. The withdrawal symptoms can then be minimized through the use of either benzodiazepines (in which case high doses are sometimes required) or antipsychotic agents, such as haloperidol (Haldol). Once again, on the first or second day, doses are used to control behavior, and the patient can be weaned off the medication by about the fifth day.

Another 1 to 3 percent of patients may have a single grand mal convulsion; the rare person has multiple fits, with the peak incidence on the second day of withdrawal. Such patients require neurological evaluation, but in the absence of evidence of a seizure disorder, they do not benefit from anticonvulsant drugs.

Rehabilitation

For most patients, rehabilitation includes three major components: (1) continued efforts to increase and maintain high levels of motivation for abstinence, (2) work to help the patient readjust to a lifestyle free of alcohol, and (3) relapse prevention. Because these steps are carried out in the context of acute and protracted withdrawal syndromes and life crises, treatment requires repeated presentations of similar materials that remind the patient how important abstinence is and that help the patient develop new day-to-day support systems and coping styles.

No single major life event, traumatic life period, or identifiable psychiatric disorder is known to be a unique cause of alcoholism. In addition, the effects of any causes of alcoholism are likely to have been diluted by the effects of alcohol on the brain and the years of an altered lifestyle, so that the alcoholism has developed a life of its own. This is true even though many alcoholic persons believe that the cause was depression, anxiety, life stress, or pain syndromes. Research, data from records, and resource persons usually reveal that alcohol contributed to the mood disorder, accident, or life stress, not vice versa.

The same general treatment approach is used in inpatient and outpatient settings. Selection of the more expensive and intensive inpatient mode often depends on evidence of additional severe medical or psychiatric syndromes, the absence of appropriate nearby outpatient groups and facilities, and the patient's history of having failed in outpatient care. The treatment process in either setting involves intervention, optimizing physical and psychological functioning, enhancing motivation, reaching out to family, and using the first 2 to 4 weeks of care as an intensive period of help. Those efforts must be followed by at least 3 to 6 months of less-frequent outpatient care. Outpatient care uses a combination of individual and group counseling, judicious avoidance of psychotropic medications unless needed for independent disorders, and involvement in such self-help groups as AA.

Counseling

Counseling efforts in the first several months should focus on day-to-day life issues to help patients maintain a high level of motivation for abstinence and to enhance their functioning.

Psychotherapy techniques that provoke anxiety or that require deep insights have not been shown to be of benefit during the early months of recovery and, at least theoretically, may actually impair efforts at maintaining abstinence. Thus, this discussion focuses on the efforts likely to characterize the first 3 to 6 months of care.

Counseling or therapy can be carried out in an individual or group setting; few data indicate that either approach is superior. The technique used is not likely to matter greatly and usually boils down to simple day-to-day counseling or almost any behavioral or psychotherapeutic approach focusing on the here and now. To optimize motivation, treatment sessions should explore the consequences of drinking, the likely future course of alcohol-related life problems, and the marked improvement that can be expected with abstinence. Whether in an inpatient or an outpatient setting, individual or group counseling is usually offered a minimum of three times a week for the first 2 to 4 weeks, followed by less intense efforts, perhaps once a week, for the subsequent 3 to 6 months.

Much time in counseling deals with how to build a lifestyle free of alcohol. Discussions cover the need for a sober peer group, a plan for social and recreational events without drinking, and approaches for reestablishing communication with family members and friends.

The third major component, relapse prevention, first identifies situations in which the risk for relapse is high. The counselor must help the patient develop modes of coping to be used when the craving for alcohol increases or when any event or emotional state makes a return to drinking likely. An important part of relapse prevention is reminding the patient about the appropriate attitude toward slips. Short-term experiences with alcohol can never be used as an excuse for returning to regular drinking. The efforts to achieve and maintain a sober lifestyle are not a game in which all benefits are lost with that first sip. Rather, recovery is a process of trial and error; patients use slips that occur to identify high-risk situations and to develop more appropriate coping techniques.

Medications

If detoxification has been completed and the patient is not one of the 10 to 15 percent of alcoholic persons who have an independent mood disorder, schizophrenia, or anxiety disorder, little evidence favors prescribing psychotropic medications for the treatment of alcoholism. Lingering levels of anxiety and insomnia as part of a reaction to life stresses and protracted abstinence should be treated with behavior modification approaches and reassurance. Medications for these symptoms (including benzodiazepines) are likely to lose their effectiveness much faster than the insomnia disappears; thus, the patient may increase the dose and have subsequent problems. Similarly, sadness and mood swings can linger at low levels for several months. However, controlled clinical trials indicate no benefit in prescribing antidepressant medications or lithium to treat the average alcoholic person who has no independent or long-lasting psychiatric disorder. The mood disorder will clear before the medications can take effect, and patients who resume drinking while on the medications face significant potential dangers. With little or no evidence that the medications are effective, the dangers significantly outweigh any potential benefits from their routine use.

One possible exception to the proscription against the use of medications is the alcohol-sensitizing agent disulfiram. Disulfiram is given in daily doses of 250 mg before the patient is discharged from the intensive first phase of outpatient rehabilitation or from inpatient care. The goal is to place the patient in a condition in which drinking alcohol precipitates an uncomfortable physical reaction, including nausea, vomiting, and a burning sensation in the face and stomach. Unfortunately, few data prove that disulfiram is more effective than a placebo, probably because most persons stop taking the disulfiram when they resume drinking. Many clinicians have stopped routinely prescribing the agent, partly in recognition of the dangers associated with the drug itself: mood swings, rare instances of psychosis, the possibility of increased peripheral neuropathies, the relatively rare occurrence of other significant neuropathies, and potentially fatal hepatitis. Moreover, patients with preexisting heart disease, cerebral thrombosis, diabetes, and a number of other conditions cannot be given disulfiram because an alcohol reaction to the disulfiram could be fatal.

Two additional promising pharmacological interventions have recently been studied. The first involves the opioid antagonist naltrexone (ReVia), which is at least theoretically believed to possibly decrease the craving for alcohol or blunt the rewarding effects of drinking. In any event, two relatively small (approximately 90 patients on the active drug across the studies) and short-term (3 months of active treatment) investigations using 50 mg per day of this drug had potentially promising results.

The second medication of interest, acamprosate (Campral), has been tested in more than 5,000 alcohol-dependent patients in Europe; this drug is not yet available in the United States. Used in dosages of approximately 2,000 mg per day, this medication was associated with approximately 10 to 20 percent more positive outcomes than placebo when used in the context of the usual psychological and behavioral treatment regimen for alcoholism. The mechanism of action of acamprosate is not known, but it may act directly or indirectly at GABA receptors or N-methyl-D-aspartate sites, the effects of which alter the development of tolerance or physical dependence on alcohol.

Another medication with potential promise in the treatment of alcoholism is the nonbenzodiazepine antianxiety drug buspirone (BuSpar), although the effect of this drug on alcohol rehabilitation is inconsistent between studies. However, no evidence exists that antidepressant medications such as the selective serotonin reuptake inhibitors (SSRIs), lithium, or antipsychotic medications are significantly effective in the treatment of alcoholism.

Self-Help Groups

Clinicians must recognize the potential importance of self-help groups like AA. Members of AA have help available 24 hours a day, associate with a sober peer group, learn that it is possible to participate in social functions without drinking, and are given a model of recovery by observing the accomplishments of sober members of the group. Learning about AA usually begins during inpatient or outpatient rehabilitation. The clinician can play a major role in helping patients understand the differences between specific groups. Some groups are composed of only men or only women; others are mixed. Some meetings are mostly for blue-collar men and women; others are mostly for professionals. Some groups place great emphasis on religion; others are eclectic.

Al-Anon is an organization for the spouses of persons with alcohol-related disorders; it is structured along the same lines as AA. The aims of Al-Anon are, through group support, to assist the efforts of the spouses to regain self-esteem, to refrain from feeling responsible for the spouse's drinking, and to develop a rewarding life for themselves and their families. Alateen is directed toward the children of alcohol-dependent persons to help them understand their parent's alcohol dependence.

▲ 9.3 Amphetamine (or Amphetamine-like)-Related Disorders

Amphetamines are one of the most widely used illicit drugs, second to cannabis in Great Britain, Australia, and several countries of Western Europe. In the United States, lifetime and current cocaine use still exceeds the nonmedical use of amphetamines; some studies report up to 600,000 abusers; in addition, methamphetamine (a congener of amphetamine) has also become a major drug of abuse.

The current Food and Drug Administration (FDA)–approved indications for amphetamine are limited to attention-deficit/hyperactivity disorder and narcolepsy. Amphetamines are also used in the treatment of obesity, depression, dysthymia, chronic fatigue syndrome, acquired immune deficiency syndrome, and neurasthenia and as adjunctive therapy for depression resistant to drug treatment.

PREPARATIONS

The major amphetamines currently available and used in the United States are dextroamphetamine (Dexedrine), methamphetamine (Desoxyn), a mixed dextroamphetamine-amphetamine salt (Adderall), and methylphenidate (Ritalin). These drugs go by such street names as ice, crystal, crystal meth, and speed. As a general class, the amphetamines are also referred to as *analeptics*, *sympathomimetics*, *stimulants*, and *psychostimulants*. The typical amphetamines are used to increase performance and to induce a euphoric feeling, for example, by students studying for examinations, by long-distance truck drivers on trips, by business people with important deadlines, and by athletes in competition. Although not as addictive as cocaine, amphetamines are nonetheless addictive drugs.

Other amphetamine-like substances are ephedrine and pseudoephedrine, which are available over the counter in the United States as nasal decongestants. Phenylpropanolamine (PPA) is a psychostimulant, which, although less potent than the classic amphetamines, and ephedrine, is subject to abuse, partly because of its easy availability and low price. These drugs, PPA in particular, can dangerously exacerbate hypertension, precipitate a toxic psychosis, or result in death. The safety margin for PPA is particularly narrow, and three to four times the normal dose can result in life threatening hypertension.

Methamphetamine

Methamphetamine (also called "ice") is a pure form that abusers of the substance inhale, smoke, or inject intravenously. Its psychological effects last for hours and are described as particularly powerful. Unlike crack cocaine (see Section 9.6), which must be imported, methamphetamine is a synthetic drug that can be manufactured domestically in illicit laboratories.

Amphetamine-like Substances

The classic amphetamine drugs (i.e., dextroamphetamine, methamphetamine, and methylphenidate) exert their major effects through the dopaminergic system. Substituted, so-called designer amphetamines (discussed below) have neurochemical effects on both the serotonergic and the dopaminergic systems and have behavioral effects that reflect a combination of amphetamine-like and hallucinogen-like activities. Some psychopharmacologists classify the substituted amphetamines as hallucinogens; in this textbook, however, they are classified with the amphetamines to which they are closely related structurally. Examples of the substituted amphetamines include 3,4-methylenedioxymethamphetamine (MDMA), also referred to as "ecstasy," "XTC," and "Adam"; N-ethyl-3,4-methylene-dioxyamphetamine (MDEA), also referred to as "Eve"; 5-methoxy-3,4-methylenedioxy-amphetamine (MMDA); and 2,5-dimethoxy-4-methylamphetamine (DOM), also referred to as "STP." Of these drugs, MDMA has been studied most closely and is perhaps the most widely available. These drugs are discussed in greater detail below.

EPIDEMIOLOGY

In 2000, approximately 4 percent of the U.S. population used psychostimulants. The 18- to 25-year-old age group reported the highest level of use, followed by the 12- to 17-year-old group. Amphetamine use occurs in all socioeconomic groups, and amphetamine use is increasing among white professionals. Because amphetamines are available by prescription for specific indications, prescribing physicians must be aware of the risk of amphetamine use by others, including friends and family members of the patient receiving the amphetamine. No reliable data are available on the epidemiology of designer amphetamine use, but they are greatly abused. According to the text revision of the fourth edition of *Diagnostic and Statistical Manual of Mental Disorders* (DSM-IV-TR), the lifetime prevalence of amphetamine dependence and abuse is 1.5 percent, and the male to female ratio is 1.

NEUROPHARMACOLOGY

All the amphetamines are rapidly absorbed orally and have a rapid onset of action, usually within 1 hour when taken orally. The classic amphetamines are also taken intravenously and have an almost immediate effect by this route. Nonprescribed amphetamines and designer amphetamines are also inhaled ("snorting"). Tolerance develops with both classic and designer amphetamines, although amphetamine users often overcome the tolerance by taking more of the drug. Amphetamine is less addictive than cocaine, as evidenced by experiments on rats in which not all animals spontaneously self-administered low doses of amphetamine.

The classic amphetamines (i.e., dextroamphetamine, methamphetamine, and methylphenidate) produce their primary effects by causing the release of catecholamines, particularly dopamine, from presynaptic

terminals. The effects are particularly potent for the dopaminergic neurons projecting from the ventral tegmental area to the cerebral cortex and the limbic areas. This pathway has been termed the *reward circuit pathway*, and its activation is probably the major addicting mechanism for the amphetamines.

The designer amphetamines (e.g., MDMA, MDEA, MMDA, and DOM) cause the release of catecholamines (dopamine and norepinephrine) and of serotonin, the neurotransmitter implicated as the major neurochemical pathway for hallucinogens. Therefore, the clinical effects of designer amphetamines are a blend of the effects of classic amphetamines and those of hallucinogens. The pharmacology of MDMA is the best understood of this group. MDMA is taken up in serotonergic neurons by the serotonin transporter responsible for serotonin reuptake. Once in the neuron, MDMA causes rapid release of a bolus of serotonin and inhibits the activity of serotonin-producing enzymes.

DIAGNOSIS

DSM-IV-TR lists many amphetamine (or amphetamine-like)-related disorders (Table 9.3–1) but specifies diagnostic criteria

Table 9.3–1
DSM-IV-TR Amphetamine (or Amphetamine-like)-Related Disorders

Amphetamine use disorders
Amphetamine dependence
Amphetamine abuse
Amphetamine-induced disorders
Amphetamine intoxication
  Specify if:
    With perceptual disturbances
Amphetamine withdrawal
Amphetamine intoxication delirium
Amphetamine-induced psychotic disorder, with delusions
  Specify if:
    With onset during intoxication
Amphetamine-induced psychotic disorder, with hallucinations
  Specify if:
    With onset during intoxication
Amphetamine-induced mood disorder
  Specify if:
    With onset during intoxication
    With onset during withdrawal
Amphetamine-induced anxiety disorder
  Specify if:
    With onset during intoxication
Amphetamine-induced sexual dysfunction
  Specify if:
    With onset during intoxication
Amphetamine-induced sleep disorder
  Specify if:
    With onset during intoxication
    With onset during withdrawal
Amphetamine-related disorder not otherwise specified

From American Psychiatric Association. *Diagnostic and Statistical Manual of Mental Disorders.* 4th ed. Text rev. Washington, DC: American Psychiatric Association; copyright 2000, with permission.

Table 9.3–2
DSM-IV-TR Diagnostic Criteria for Amphetamine Intoxication

A. Recent use of amphetamine or a related substance (e.g., methylphenidate).

B. Clinically significant maladaptive behavioral or psychological changes (e.g., euphoria or affective blunting; changes in sociability; hypervigilance; interpersonal sensitivity; anxiety, tension, or anger; stereotyped behaviors; impaired judgment; or impaired social or occupational functioning) that developed during, or shortly after, use of amphetamine or a related substance.

C. Two (or more) of the following, developing during, or shortly after, use of amphetamine or a related substance:

　(1) tachycardia or bradycardia

　(2) pupillary dilation

　(3) elevated or lowered blood pressure

　(4) perspiration or chills

　(5) nausea or vomiting

　(6) evidence of weight loss

　(7) psychomotor agitation or retardation

　(8) muscular weakness, respiratory depression, chest pain, or cardiac arrhythmias

　(9) confusion, seizures, dyskinesias, dystonias, or coma

D. The symptoms are not due to a general medical condition and are not better accounted for by another mental disorder.

Specify if:

With perceptual disturbances

From American Psychiatric Association. *Diagnostic and Statistical Manual of Mental Disorders.* 4th ed. Text rev. Washington, DC: American Psychiatric Association; copyright 2000, with permission.

only for amphetamine intoxication (Table 9.3–2), amphetamine withdrawal (Table 9.3–3), and amphetamine-related disorder not otherwise specified (Table 9.3–4) in the section on amphetamine (or amphetamine-like)-related disorders. The diagnostic criteria for the other amphetamine (or amphetamine-like)-

Table 9.3–3
DSM-IV-TR Diagnostic Criteria for Amphetamine Withdrawal

A. Cessation of (or reduction in) amphetamine (or a related substance) use that has been heavy and prolonged.

B. Dysphoric mood and two (or more) of the following physiological changes, developing within a few hours to several days after Criterion A:

　(1) fatigue

　(2) vivid, unpleasant dreams

　(3) insomnia or hypersomnia

　(4) increased appetite

　(5) psychomotor retardation or agitation

C. The symptoms in Criterion B cause clinically significant distress or impairment in social, occupational, or other important areas of functioning.

D. The symptoms are not due to a general medical condition and are not better accounted for by another mental disorder.

From American Psychiatric Association. *Diagnostic and Statistical Manual of Mental Disorders.* 4th ed. Text rev. Washington, DC: American Psychiatric Association; copyright 2000, with permission.

Table 9.3–4
DSM-IV-TR Diagnostic Criteria for Amphetamine-Related Disorder Not Otherwise Specified

The amphetamine-related disorder not otherwise specified category is for disorders associated with the use of amphetamine (or a related substance) that are not classifiable as amphetamine dependence, amphetamine abuse, amphetamine intoxication, amphetamine withdrawal, amphetamine intoxication delirium, amphetamine-induced psychotic disorder, amphetamine-induced mood disorder, amphetamine-induced anxiety disorder, amphetamine-induced sexual dysfunction, or amphetamine-induced sleep disorder.

From American Psychiatric Association. *Diagnostic and Statistical Manual of Mental Disorders.* 4th ed. Text rev. Washington, DC: American Psychiatric Association; copyright 2000, with permission.

related disorders are contained in the DSM-IV-TR sections dealing with the primary phenomenological symptom (for example, psychosis).

Amphetamine Dependence and Amphetamine Abuse

The DSM-IV-TR criteria for dependence and abuse are applied to amphetamine and its related substances (see Tables 9.1–3 and 9.1–4 in Section 9.1). Amphetamine dependence can result in a rapid down-spiral of a person's abilities to cope with work- and family-related obligations and stresses. A person who abuses amphetamines requires increasingly high doses of amphetamine to obtain the usual high, and physical signs of amphetamine abuse (for example, decreased weight and paranoid ideas) almost always develop with continued abuse.

Amphetamine Intoxication

The intoxication syndromes of cocaine (which blocks dopamine reuptake) and amphetamines (which cause the release of dopamine) are similar. Because more rigorous, in-depth research has been done on cocaine abuse and intoxication than on amphetamines, the clinical literature on amphetamines has been strongly influenced by the clinical findings of cocaine abuse. In DSM-IV-TR, the diagnostic criteria for amphetamine intoxication (Table 9.3–2) and cocaine intoxication (see Table 9.6–2 in Section 9.6) are separated but are virtually the same. DSM-IV-TR specifies perceptual disturbances as a symptom of amphetamine intoxication. If intact reality testing is absent, a diagnosis of amphetamine-induced psychotic disorder with onset during intoxication is indicated. The symptoms of amphetamine intoxication are mostly resolved after 24 hours and are generally completely resolved after 48 hours.

Amphetamine Withdrawal

After amphetamine intoxication, a crash occurs with symptoms of anxiety, tremulousness, dysphoric mood, lethargy, fatigue, nightmares (accompanied by rebound rapid eye movement sleep), headache, profuse sweating, muscle cramps, stomach cramps, and insatiable hunger. The withdrawal symptoms generally peak in 2 to 4 days and are resolved in 1 week. The most serious withdrawal symptom is depression, which can be particularly severe after the sustained use of high doses of amphetamine and which can be associated with suicidal ideation or behavior. The DSM-IV-TR diagnostic criteria for amphetamine withdrawal (Table 9.3–3) specify that a dysphoric mood and physiological changes are necessary for the diagnosis.

Amphetamine Intoxication Delirium

Under substance-related disorder, DSM-IV-TR includes a diagnosis of amphetamine intoxication delirium (see Table 7.2–3). Delirium associated with amphetamine use generally results from high doses of amphetamine or from sustained use, and so sleep deprivation affects the clinical presentation. The combination of amphetamines with other substances and the use of amphetamines by a person with preexisting brain damage can also cause development of delirium. It is not uncommon for university students using amphetamines to cram for examinations to exhibit this type of delirium.

Amphetamine-Induced Psychotic Disorder

The clinical similarity of amphetamine-induced psychosis to paranoid schizophrenia has prompted extensive study of the neurochemistry of amphetamine-induced psychosis to elucidate the pathophysiology of paranoid schizophrenia. The hallmark of amphetamine-induced psychotic disorder is the presence of paranoia. Amphetamine-induced psychotic disorder can be distinguished from paranoid schizophrenia by several differentiating characteristics associated with the former, including a predominance of visual hallucinations, generally appropriate affects, hyperactivity, hypersexuality, confusion and incoherence, and little evidence of disordered thinking (such as looseness of associations). In several studies, investigators also noted that although the positive symptoms of amphetamine-induced psychotic disorder and schizophrenia are similar, amphetamine-induced psychotic disorder generally lacks the affective flattening and alogia of schizophrenia. Clinically, however, acute amphetamine-induced psychotic disorder can be completely indistinguishable from schizophrenia, and only the resolution of the symptoms in a few days or a positive finding in a urine drug screen test eventually reveals the correct diagnosis. The treatment of choice for amphetamine-induced psychotic disorder is the short-term use of an antipsychotic medication such as haloperidol (Haldol).

Amphetamine-Induced Mood Disorder

The onset of amphetamine-induced mood disorder can occur during intoxication or withdrawal. In general, intoxication is associated with manic or mixed mood features, whereas withdrawal is associated with depressive mood features.

Amphetamine-Induced Anxiety Disorder

Amphetamine, like cocaine, can induce symptoms similar to those seen in obsessive-compulsive disorder, panic disorder, and phobic disorders, in particular. The onset of amphetamine-induced anxiety disorder can also occur during intoxication or withdrawal.

Amphetamine-Induced Sexual Dysfunction

Amphetamine is often used to enhance sexual experiences; however, high doses and long-term use are associated with erectile disorder and other sexual dysfunctions. These dysfunctions are classified in DSM-IV-TR as amphetamine-induced sexual dysfunction.

Amphetamine-Induced Sleep Disorder

Amphetamine intoxication can produce insomnia and sleep deprivation, whereas persons undergoing amphetamine withdrawal can experience hypersomnolence and nightmares.

Disorder Not Otherwise Specified

If an amphetamine (or amphetamine-like)-related disorder does not meet the criteria of one or more of the categories discussed above, it can be diagnosed as an amphetamine-related disorder not otherwise specified (Table 9.3–4).

CLINICAL FEATURES

In persons who have not previously used amphetamines, a single 5-mg dose increases the sense of well-being and induces elation, euphoria, and friendliness. Small doses generally improve attention and increase performance on written, oral, and performance tasks. There is also an associated decrease in fatigue, induction of anorexia, and heightening of the pain threshold. Undesirable effects result from the use of high doses for long periods.

Adverse Effects

Amphetamines

PHYSICAL. Amphetamine abuse can produce adverse effects, the most serious of which include cerebrovascular, cardiac, and gastrointestinal effects. Among the specific life-threatening conditions are myocardial infarction, severe hypertension, cerebrovascular disease, and ischemic colitis. A continuum of neurological symptoms, from twitching to tetany to seizures to coma and death, is associated with increasingly high amphetamine doses. Intravenous use of amphetamines can transmit human immunodeficiency virus and hepatitis and further the development of lung abscesses, endocarditis, and necrotizing angiitis. Several studies have shown that abusers of amphetamines knew little—or did not care—about safe-sex practices and the use of condoms. The non-life-threatening adverse effects of amphetamine abuse include flushing, pallor, cyanosis, fever, headache, tachycardia, palpitations, nausea, vomiting, bruxism (teeth grinding), shortness of breath, tremor, and ataxia. Pregnant women who use amphetamines often have babies with low birth weight, small head circumference, early gestational age, and growth retardation.

PSYCHOLOGICAL. The adverse psychological effects associated with amphetamine use include restlessness, dysphoria, insomnia, irritability, hostility, and confusion. Amphetamine use can also induce symptoms of anxiety disorders, such as generalized anxiety disorder and panic disorder as well as ideas of reference, paranoid delusions, and hallucinations.

Other Agents

Substituted Amphetamines.

MDMA is one of a series of substituted amphetamines that also includes 3,4-methylenedioxyamphetamine (MDA), 2,5-dimethoxy-4-bromoamphetamine (DOB), paramethoxyamphetamine (PMA), and others. These drugs produce subjective effects resembling those of amphetamine and lysergic acid diethylamide (LSD), and in that sense, MDMA and similar analogues may represent a distinct category of drugs.

A methamphetamine derivative that came into use in the 1980s, MDMA was not technically subject to legal regulation at the time. Although it has been labeled a "designer drug" in the belief that it was deliberately synthesized to evade legal regulation, it was actually synthesized and patented in 1914. Several psychiatrists used it as an adjunct to psychotherapy and concluded that it had value. At one time it was advertised as legal and was used in psychotherapy for its subjective effects. However, it was never approved by the FDA. Its use raised questions of both safety and legality, since the related amphetamine derivatives MDA, DOB, and PMA had caused a number of overdose deaths, and MDA was known to cause extensive destruction of serotonergic nerve terminals in the central nervous system. Using emergency scheduling authority, the Drug Enforcement Agency made MDMA a Schedule I drug, along with LSD, heroin, and marijuana. Despite its illegal status, MDMA continues to be manufactured, distributed, and used in the United States, Europe, and Australia. Its use is common in Australia and Great Britain at extended dances ("raves") popular with adolescents and young adults.

Mechanisms of Action. The unusual properties of the drugs may be a consequence of the different actions of the optical isomers: the $R(-)$ isomers produce LSD-like actions, which, in turn, may be linked to the capacity to release serotonin. The various derivatives may exhibit significant differences in subjective effects and toxicity. Animals in laboratory experiments will self-administer the drugs, suggesting prominent amphetamine-like effects.

Subjective Effects. After taking usual doses (100 to 150 mg), MDMA users experience elevated mood and, according to various reports, increased self-confidence and sensory sensitivity; peaceful feelings coupled with insight, empathy, and closeness to persons; and decreased appetite. Difficulty concentrating and an increased capacity to focus have both been reported. Dysphoric reactions, psychotomimetic effects, and psychosis have also been reported. Higher doses seem more likely to produce psychotomimetic effects. Sympathomimetic effects of tachycardia, palpitation, increased blood pressure, sweating, and bruxism are common. The subjective effects are reported to be prominent for about 4 to 8 hours, but they may not last as long or may last longer, depending on the dose and route of administration. The drug is usually taken orally but is also snorted and injected. Both tachyphylaxis and some tolerance are reported by users.

Toxicity. Although it is not as toxic as MDA, various somatic toxicities have been attributed to MDMA use as well as fatal overdoses. It does not appear to be neurotoxic when injected into the brains of animals, but it is metabolized to MDA in both animals and humans. In animals, MDMA produces selective, long-lasting damage to serotonergic nerve terminals. It is not certain if the levels of the MDA metabolite reached in humans after the usual doses of MDMA suffice to produce lasting damage. Nonhuman primates are more sensitive than rodents to MDMA's toxic effects and show more prolonged or permanent neurotoxicity at doses not much higher than those used by humans. Users of MDMA show differences in neuroendocrine responses to serotonergic probes, and studies of former MDMA users show global and regional decreases in serotonin transporter binding, as measured by positron emission tomography (PET). There are currently no established clinical uses for MDMA, although, before its regulation, there were several reports of its beneficial effects as an adjunct to psychotherapy.

Khat.

The fresh leaves of *Catha edulis*, a bush native to East Africa, have been used as a stimulant in the Middle East, Africa, and the Arabian Peninsula for at least 1,000 years. Khat is still widely used in Ethiopia, Kenya, Somalia, and Yemen. The amphetamine-like effects of khat have long been recognized, and although efforts to isolate the active ingredient were first undertaken in the 19th century, only since the 1970s has cathinone ($S[-]\alpha$-aminopropiophenone or $S[-]$2-amino-1-propanone) been identified as the substance responsible. Cathinone has most of the central nervous system and peripheral actions of amphetamine and appears to have the same mechanism of action. In humans it elevates mood, decreases hunger, and alleviates fatigue. At high doses it can induce an amphetamine-like psychosis in humans.

In the 1990s, several clandestine laboratories began synthesizing methcathinone, a drug with actions quite similar to those of cathinone. Known by a number of street names (e.g., "CAT," "goob," and "crank"), its popularity is due primarily to its ease of synthesis from ephedrine or pseudoephedrine, which were readily available until placed under special controls. Methcathinone has been moved to Schedule (Control Level) I of the Controlled Substances Act. The patterns of use, adverse effects, and complications closely resemble those reported for amphetamine.

TREATMENT AND REHABILITATION

The treatment of amphetamine (or amphetamine-like)-related disorders shares with cocaine-related disorders the difficulty of helping patients remain abstinent from the drug, which is powerfully reinforcing and induces craving. An inpatient setting and the use of multiple therapeutic methods (individual, family, and group psychotherapy) are usually necessary to achieve lasting abstinence. The treatment of specific amphetamine-induced disorders (for example, amphetamine-induced psychotic disorder and amphetamine-induced anxiety disorder) with specific drugs (for example, antipsychotic and anxiolytics) may be necessary on a short-term basis. Antipsychotics may be prescribed for the first few days. In the absence of psychosis, diazepam (Valium) is useful to treat patients' agitation and hyperactivity.

Physicians should establish a therapeutic alliance with patients to deal with the underlying depression or personality disorder or both. Because many patients are heavily dependent on the drug, however, psychotherapy may be especially difficult.

Comorbid conditions such as depression may respond to antidepressant medication. Bupropion (Wellbutrin) may be of use after patients have withdrawn from amphetamine. It has the effect of producing feelings of well-being as these patients cope with the dysphoria that may accompany abstinence.

▲ 9.4 Caffeine-Related Disorders

The most widely consumed psychoactive substance in the world is caffeine. It is estimated that more than 80 percent of adults in the United States consume caffeine regularly, and throughout the world, caffeine consumption is well integrated into daily cultural practices (for example, the coffee break in the United States, tea time in the United Kingdom, and kola nut chewing in Nigeria). Because caffeine use is so pervasive and widely accepted, disorders associated with caffeine use may be overlooked. However, one must recognize that caffeine is a psychoactive compound that can produce a wide variety of syndromes.

EPIDEMIOLOGY

Caffeine is contained in drinks, foods, prescription medicines, and over-the-counter medicines. An adult in the United States consumes about 200 mg of caffeine per day on average, although 20 to 30 percent of all adults consume more than 500 mg per day. The per capita use of coffee in the United States is 10.2 pounds per year. A cup of coffee generally contains 100 to 150 mg of caffeine; tea contains approximately one-third as much. Many over-the-counter medications contain one-third to one-half as much caffeine as a cup of coffee, and some migraine medications and over-the-counter stimulants contain more caffeine than a cup of coffee. Cocoa, chocolate, and soft drinks contain significant amounts of caffeine, enough to cause some symptoms of caffeine intoxication in small children when they ingest a candy bar and a 12-ounce cola drink.

According to the text revision of the fourth edition of the *Diagnostic and Statistical Manual of Mental Disorders* (DSM-IV-TR), the actual prevalence of caffeine-related disorders is unknown, but up to 85 percent of adults consume caffeine in any given year.

COMORBIDITY

Persons with caffeine-related disorders are more likely to have additional substance-related disorders than are those without diagnoses of caffeine-related disorders. Approximately two-thirds of those who consume large amounts of caffeine daily also use sedative and hypnotic drugs.

NEUROPHARMACOLOGY

Caffeine, a methylxanthine, is more potent than another commonly used methylxanthine, theophylline (Primatene). The half-life of caffeine in the human body is 3 to 10 hours, and the time of peak concentration is 30 to 60 minutes. Caffeine readily crosses the blood–brain barrier. Caffeine acts primarily as an antagonist of the adenosine receptors. Activation of adenosine receptors activates an inhibitory G protein (G_i) and thus inhibits the formation of the second-messenger cyclic adenosine monophosphate (cAMP). Caffeine intake, therefore, results in an increase in intraneuronal cAMP concentrations in neurons with adenosine receptors. Three cups of coffee are estimated to deliver so much caffeine to the brain that approximately 50 percent of the adenosine receptors are occupied by caffeine. Several experiments indicate that caffeine, especially at high doses or concentrations, can affect dopamine and noradrenergic neurons. Specifically, dopamine activity may be enhanced by caffeine, a hypothesis that could explain clinical reports associating caffeine intake with an exacerbation of psychotic symptoms in patients with schizophrenia. Activation of noradrenergic neurons has been hypothesized to be involved in the mediation of some symptoms of caffeine withdrawal.

Genetics and Caffeine Use

Several investigations comparing coffee use in monozygotic and dizygotic twins have shown higher concordance rates for monozygotic twins, suggesting that there may be some genetic predisposition to continued coffee use after exposure to coffee.

Caffeine as a Substance of Abuse

Caffeine evidences all the traits associated with commonly accepted substances of abuse. First, caffeine can act as a positive reinforcer, particularly at low doses. Caffeine doses of approximately 100 mg induce a mild euphoria in humans and repeated substance-seeking behavior effects in other animals. Caffeine doses of 300 mg, however, do not act as positive reinforcers and can produce increased anxiety and mild dysphoria. Second, studies in animals and humans have reported that caffeine can be discriminated from a placebo in blind experimental conditions. Third, both animal and human studies have shown that physical tolerance develops to some effects of caffeine and that withdrawal symptoms occur.

Effect on Cerebral Blood Flow

Most studies have found that caffeine results in global cerebral vasoconstriction, with a resultant decrease in cerebral blood flow, although this effect may not occur in persons over 65 years of age. According to one recent study, tolerance does not develop to these vasoconstrictive effects, and the cerebral blood flow shows a rebound increase after withdrawal from caffeine. Some clinicians believe that caffeine use can cause a similar constriction in the coronary arteries.

DIAGNOSIS

The diagnosis of caffeine intoxication or other caffeine-related disorders depends primarily on a comprehensive history of a patient's intake of caffeine-containing products. The history should cover whether a patient has experienced any symptoms of caffeine withdrawal during periods when caffeine consumption was either stopped or severely reduced. The differential diagnosis for caffeine-related disorders should include the following psychiatric diagnoses: generalized anxiety disorder, panic disorder with or without agoraphobia, bipolar II disorder, attention-deficit/hyperactivity disorder, and sleep disorders. The differential diagnosis should include the abuse of caffeine-containing over-the-counter medications, anabolic steroids, and other stimulants, such as amphetamines and cocaine. A urine sample may be needed to screen for these substances. The differential diagnosis should also include hyperthyroidism and pheochromocytoma.

Table 9.4–1
DSM-IV-TR Caffeine-Related Disorders

Caffeine-induced disorders
  Caffeine intoxication
  Caffeine-induced anxiety disorder
    Specify if:
      With onset during intoxication
  Caffeine-induced sleep disorder
    Specify if:
      With onset during intoxication
  Caffeine-related disorder not otherwise specified

From American Psychiatric Association. *Diagnostic and Statistical Manual of Mental Disorders*. 4th ed. Text rev. Washington, DC: American Psychiatric Association; copyright 2000, with permission.

DSM-IV-TR lists the caffeine-related disorders (Table 9.4–1) and provides diagnostic criteria for caffeine intoxication (Table 9.4–2) but does not formally recognize a diagnosis of caffeine withdrawal (discussed below), which is classified as a caffeine-related disorder not otherwise specified (Table 9.4–3).

Caffeine Intoxication

DSM-IV-TR specifies the diagnostic criteria for caffeine intoxication (Table 9.4–2), including the recent consumption of caffeine, usually in excess of 250 mg. The annual incidence of caffeine intoxication is an estimated 10 percent,

Table 9.4–2
DSM-IV-TR Diagnostic Criteria for Caffeine Intoxication

A. Recent consumption of caffeine, usually in excess of 250 mg (e.g., more than 2–3 cups of brewed coffee).
B. Five (or more) of the following signs, developing during, or shortly after, caffeine use:
  (1) restlessness
  (2) nervousness
  (3) excitement
  (4) insomnia
  (5) flushed face
  (6) diuresis
  (7) gastrointestinal disturbance
  (8) muscle twitching
  (9) rambling flow of thought and speech
  (10) tachycardia or cardiac arrhythmia
  (11) periods of inexhaustibility
  (12) psychomotor agitation
C. The symptoms in Criterion B cause clinically significant distress or impairment in social, occupational, or other important areas of functioning.
D. The symptoms are not due to a general medical condition and are not better accounted for by another mental disorder (e.g., an Anxiety Disorder).

From American Psychiatric Association. *Diagnostic and Statistical Manual of Mental Disorders*. 4th ed. Text rev. Washington, DC: American Psychiatric Association; copyright 2000, with permission.

Table 9.4–3
DSM-IV-TR Diagnostic Criteria for Caffeine-Related Disorder Not Otherwise Specified

The caffeine-related disorder not otherwise specified category is for disorders associated with the use of caffeine that are not classifiable as caffeine intoxication, caffeine-induced anxiety disorder, or caffeine-induced sleep disorder. An example is caffeine withdrawal.

From American Psychiatric Association. *Diagnostic and Statistical Manual of Mental Disorders*. 4th ed. Text rev. Washington, DC: American Psychiatric Association; copyright 2000, with permission.

although some clinicians and investigators suspect that the actual incidence is much higher. The common symptoms associated with caffeine intoxication include anxiety, psychomotor agitation, restlessness, irritability, and psychophysiological complaints such as muscle twitching, flushed face, nausea, diuresis, gastrointestinal distress, excessive perspiration, tingling in the fingers and toes, and insomnia. Consumption of more than 1g of caffeine can produce rambling speech, confused thinking, cardiac arrhythmias, inexhaustibleness, marked agitation, tinnitus, and mild visual hallucinations (light flashes). Consumption of more than 10 g of caffeine can cause generalized tonic-clonic seizures, respiratory failure, and death.

Caffeine Withdrawal

In spite of the fact that DSM-IV-TR does not include a diagnosis of caffeine withdrawal, several well-controlled studies indicate that caffeine withdrawal is a real phenomenon, and DSM-IV-TR gives research criteria for caffeine withdrawal (Table 9.4–4). The appearance of withdrawal symptoms reflects the tolerance and physiological dependence that develop with continued caffeine use. Several epidemiological studies have reported symptoms of caffeine withdrawal in 50 to

Table 9.4–4
DSM-IV-TR Research Criteria for Caffeine Withdrawal

A. Prolonged daily use of caffeine.
B. Abrupt cessation of caffeine use, or reduction in the amount of caffeine used, closely followed by headache and one (or more) of the following symptoms:
  (1) marked fatigue or drowsiness
  (2) marked anxiety or depression
  (3) nausea or vomiting
C. The symptoms in Criterion B cause clinically significant distress or impairment in social, occupational, or other important areas of functioning.
D. The symptoms are not due to the direct physiological effects of a general medical condition (e.g., migraine, viral illness) and are not better accounted for by another mental disorder.

From American Psychiatric Association. *Diagnostic and Statistical Manual of Mental Disorders*. 4th ed. Text rev. Washington, DC: American Psychiatric Association; copyright 2000, with permission.

75 percent of all caffeine users studied. The most common symptoms are headache and fatigue; other symptoms include anxiety, irritability, mild depressive symptoms, impaired psychomotor performance, nausea, vomiting, craving for caffeine, and muscle pain and stiffness. The number and severity of the withdrawal symptoms are correlated with the amount of caffeine ingested and the abruptness of the withdrawal. Caffeine withdrawal symptoms have their onset 12 to 24 hours after the last dose; the symptoms peak in 24 to 48 hours and resolve within 1 week.

The induction of caffeine withdrawal can sometimes be iatrogenic. Physicians often ask their patients to discontinue caffeine intake before certain medical procedures, such as endoscopy, colonoscopy, and cardiac catheterization. Physicians also often recommend that patients with anxiety symptoms, cardiac arrhythmias, esophagitis, hiatal hernias, fibrocystic disease of the breast, and insomnia stop caffeine intake. Some persons simply decide that it would be good for them to stop using caffeine-containing products over a 7- to 14-day period rather than stop abruptly.

Ms. E was a 32-year-old single white woman employed full-time at a local factory. She occasionally used nonsteroidal antiinflammatory drugs, but was taking no regular prescription medications. She had a history of alcohol dependence, in remission for 9 years, and was otherwise in good health.

She first began consuming caffeine when she started college, and her current beverage of choice was coffee. She typically drank 4 to 5 mugs of coffee each day and preferred to drink it without cream, milk, or sugar. She estimated that 5 minutes elapsed between the time she got up in the morning and the time she had her first cup of coffee; her roommate made a pot before Ms. E got up, and Ms. E immediately poured a mug when she got out of bed. She spaced her mugs over the course of the day, with her last mug either after lunch or with dinner.

Physicians had recommended that she cut down or stop her coffee use because of complaints of mild indigestion, but she had been unable to do so. Her roommate had also complained about her coffee use at times. Ms. E routinely drank hot coffee in her car, and had spilled it and burned herself on one occasion.

When she stopped caffeine abruptly, Ms. E experienced marked irritability; poor concentration; and a severe, generalized headache. When asked to rate the severity of the headache, she replied that "on a scale of 1 to 10 it's a 12." She also had muscle aches, low energy, lethargy, and a craving to drink a mug of coffee. On the day she had stopped coffee use abruptly, she left work 2 hours early because of problems concentrating on the job and went to bed several hours earlier than usual. She then returned to her usual pattern of coffee use. (Courtesy of Eric C. Strain, M.D., and Roland R. Griffiths, Ph.D.)

Caffeine-Induced Anxiety Disorder

Caffeine-induced anxiety disorder, which can occur during caffeine intoxication, is a DSM-IV-TR diagnosis. The anxiety related to caffeine use can resemble that of generalized anxiety disorder. Patients with the disorder may be perceived as "wired," overly talkative, and irritable; they may complain of not sleeping well and of having energy to burn. Caffeine may induce and exacerbate panic attacks in persons with a panic disorder, and although a causative association between caffeine and a panic disorder has not yet been demonstrated, patients with panic disorder should avoid caffeine.

Caffeine-Induced Sleep Disorder

Caffeine-induced sleep disorder, which can occur during caffeine intoxication, is a DSM-IV-TR diagnosis. Caffeine is associated with delay in falling asleep, inability to remain asleep, and early morning awakening.

Caffeine-Related Disorder Not Otherwise Specified

DSM-IV-TR contains a residual category for caffeine-related disorders that do not meet the criteria for caffeine intoxication, caffeine-induced anxiety disorder, or caffeine-induced sleep disorder (Table 9.4–3).

CLINICAL FEATURES

Signs and Symptoms

After the ingestion of 50 to 100 mg of caffeine, common symptoms include increased alertness, a mild sense of well-being, and a sense of improved verbal and motor performance. Caffeine ingestion is also associated with diuresis, cardiac muscle stimulation, increased intestinal peristalsis, increased gastric acid secretion, and (usually mildly) increased blood pressure.

Adverse Effects

Although caffeine is not associated with cardiac-related risks in healthy persons, those with preexisting cardiac disease are often advised to limit their caffeine intake because of a possible association between cardiac arrhythmias and caffeine. Caffeine is clearly associated with increased gastric acid secretion, and clinicians usually advise patients with gastric ulcers not to ingest any caffeine-containing products. Limited data suggest that caffeine is associated with fibrocystic disease of the breasts in women. Although the question of whether caffeine is associated with birth defects remains controversial, women who are pregnant or breast-feeding should probably avoid caffeine-containing products. No solid data link caffeine intake with cancer.

TREATMENT

Analgesics, such as aspirin, almost always suffice to control the headaches and muscle aches that may accompany caffeine withdrawal. Rarely do patients require benzodiazepines to relieve withdrawal symptoms. If benzodiazepines are used for this purpose, they should be used in small dosages for a brief time, approximately 7 to 10 days at the longest.

The first step in reducing or eliminating caffeine use is to have patients determine their daily consumption of caffeine. This can best be accomplished by having the patient keep a daily food diary. The patient must recognize all sources of caffeine in the diet, including forms of caffeine (e.g., beverages, medications) and accurately record the amount consumed. After several days of keeping such a diary, the clinician can meet with the patient, review the diary, and determine the average daily caffeine dose in milligrams.

The patient and clinician should then decide on a fading schedule for caffeine consumption. Such a schedule could involve a decrease in increments of 10 percent every few days. Since caffeine is typically consumed in beverage form, the patient can use a substitution procedure in which decaffeinated beverages are gradually used in place of caffeinated beverages. The diary should be maintained during this time so that the patient's progress can be monitored. The fading should be individualized for each patient so that the rate of decrease in caffeine consumption minimizes withdrawal symptoms. One should probably avoid stopping all caffeine use abruptly, because withdrawal symptoms are likely to develop with sudden discontinuation of all caffeine use.

▲ 9.5 Cannabis-Related Disorders

Known in central Asia and China for at least 4,000 years, the Indian hemp plant *Cannabis sativa* is a hardy, aromatic annual herb. The bioactive substances derived from it are collectively referred to as *cannabis*. By most estimates, cannabis remains one of the world's most commonly used illicit drug.

All parts of *Cannabis sativa* contain psychoactive cannabinoids, of which (–)-Δ9-tetrahydrocannabinol (Δ9-THC) is most abundant. The most potent forms of cannabis come from the flowering tops of the plants or from the dried, black-brown, resinous exudates from the leaves, which is referred to as *hashish* or *hash*. The cannabis plant is usually cut, dried, chopped, and rolled into cigarettes (commonly called "joints"), which are then smoked. The common names for cannabis are *marijuana*, *grass*, *pot*, *weed*, *tea*, and *Mary Jane*. Other names, which describe cannabis types of various strengths, are *hemp*, *chasra*, *bhang*, *ganja*, *dagga*, and *sinsemilla*.

EPIDEMIOLOGY

Prevalence and Recent Trends

The *Monitoring the Future* survey of adolescents in school indicates recent increases in lifetime, annual, current (within the past 30 days), and daily use of marijuana by eighth and tenth graders, continuing a trend that began in the early 1990s.

Another measure of the prevalence of marijuana use comes from the National Household Survey on Drug Abuse, a population-based random sample of households throughout the United States. Marijuana was the most commonly used illicit drug in the study. Lifetime prevalence of marijuana use increased with each age group until age 34 years, then decreased gradually. Those aged 18 to 21 were the most likely to have used marijuana in the past year (25 percent) or the past month (14 percent), and use was lowest among those aged 50 or older, where

it was 1 percent or less. According to the text revision of the fourth edition of the *Diagnostic and Statistical Manual of Mental Disorders* (DSM-IV-TR), there is a 5 percent lifetime rate of cannabis abuse of dependence.

Race and ethnicity were also related to marijuana use, but the relationships varied by age group. Among those ages 12 to 17, whites had higher rates of lifetime and past-year marijuana use than blacks. Among 17- to 34-year-old adults, whites reported higher levels of lifetime use than blacks and Hispanics. But among those 35 and older, whites and blacks reported the same levels of use. The lifetime rates for black adults were significantly higher than those for Hispanics.

NEUROPHARMACOLOGY

As stated above, the principal component of cannabis is Δ9-THC; however, the cannabis plant contains more than 400 chemicals, of which approximately 60 are chemically related to Δ9-THC. In humans, Δ9-THC is rapidly converted into 11-hydroxy-9-THC, the metabolite that is active in the central nervous system.

A specific receptor for the cannabinols has been identified, cloned, and characterized. The cannabinoid receptor, a member of the G protein–linked family of receptors, is linked to the inhibitory G protein (Gi), which is linked to adenylyl cyclase in an inhibitory fashion. The cannabinoid receptor is found in highest concentrations in the basal ganglia, the hippocampus, and the cerebellum, with lower concentrations in the cerebral cortex. It is not found in the brainstem, a fact consistent with cannabis's minimal effects on respiratory and cardiac functions. Studies in animals have shown that the cannabinoids affect the monoamine and γ-aminobutyric acid neurons.

According to most studies, animals do not self-administer cannabinoids as they do most other substances of abuse. Moreover, there is some debate about whether the cannabinoids stimulate the so-called reward centers of the brain, such as the dopaminergic neurons of the ventral tegmental area. Tolerance to cannabis does develop, however, and psychological dependence has been found, although the evidence for physiological dependence is not strong. Withdrawal symptoms in humans are limited to modest increases in irritability, restlessness, insomnia, and anorexia and mild nausea; all these symptoms appear only when a person abruptly stops taking high doses of cannabis.

When cannabis is smoked, the euphoric effects appear within minutes, peak in approximately 30 minutes, and last 2 to 4 hours. Some motor and cognitive effects last 5 to 12 hours. Cannabis can also be taken orally when it is prepared in food, such as brownies and cakes. About two to three times as much cannabis must be taken orally to be as potent as cannabis taken by inhaling its smoke. Many variables affect the psychoactive properties of cannabis, including the potency of the cannabis used, the route of administration, the smoking technique, the effects of pyrolysis on the cannabinoid content, the dose, the setting, the user's past experience, the user's expectations, and the user's unique biological vulnerability to the effects of cannabinoids.

DIAGNOSIS AND CLINICAL FEATURES

The most common physical effects of cannabis are dilation of the conjunctival blood vessels (red eye) and mild tachycardia. At high doses, orthostatic hypotension may appear. Increased appetite—often referred to as "the munchies"—and dry mouth are common effects of cannabis intoxication. The fact that there has never been a clearly documented case of death caused by cannabis intoxication alone reflects the substance's lack of effect on the respiratory rate. The most serious potential adverse effects of cannabis use are those caused by inhaling the same carcinogenic hydrocarbons present in conventional tobacco, and some data indicate that heavy cannabis users are at risk for chronic respiratory disease and lung cancer. The practice of smoking cannabis-containing cigarettes to their very ends, so-called roaches, further increases the intake of tar (particulate matter). Many reports indicate that long-term cannabis use is associated with cerebral atrophy, seizure susceptibility, chromosomal damage, birth defects, impaired immune reactivity, alterations in testosterone concentrations, and dysregulation of menstrual cycles; these reports, however, have not been conclusively replicated, and the association between these findings and cannabis use is uncertain.

DSM-IV-TR lists the cannabis-related disorders (Table 9.5–1) but has specific criteria within the cannabis-related disorders section only for cannabis intoxication (Table 9.5–2).

Cannabis Dependence and Cannabis Abuse

DSM-IV-TR includes the diagnoses of cannabis dependence and cannabis abuse. The experimental data clearly show tolerance to many of the effects of cannabis, but the data are less supportive of the existence of physical dependence. Psychological dependence on cannabis use does develop in long-term users.

Cannabis Intoxication

DSM-IV-TR formalizes the diagnostic criteria for cannabis intoxication (Table 9.5–2). These criteria state that the diagno-

Table 9.5–1
DSM-IV-TR Cannabis-Related Disorders

Cannabis use disorders
Cannabis dependence
Cannabis abuse
Cannabis-induced disorders
Cannabis intoxication
  Specify if:
    With perceptual disturbances
Cannabis intoxication delirium
Cannabis-induced psychotic disorder, with delusions
  Specify if:
    With onset during intoxication
Cannabis-induced psychotic disorder, with hallucinations
  Specify if:
    With onset during intoxication
Cannabis-induced anxiety disorder
  Specify if:
    With onset during intoxication
Cannabis-related disorder not otherwise specified

From American Psychiatric Association. *Diagnostic and Statistical Manual of Mental Disorders.* 4th ed. Text rev. Washington, DC: American Psychiatric Association; copyright 2000, with permission.

Table 9.5–2
DSM-IV-TR Diagnostic Criteria for Cannabis Intoxication

A. Recent use of cannabis.
B. Clinically significant maladaptive behavioral or psychological changes (e.g., impaired motor coordination, euphoria, anxiety, sensation of slowed time, impaired judgment, social withdrawal) that developed during, or shortly after, cannabis use.
C. Two (or more) of the following signs, developing within 2 hours of cannabis use:
   (1) conjunctival injection
   (2) increased appetite
   (3) dry mouth
   (4) tachycardia
D. The symptoms are not due to a general medical condition and are not better accounted for by another mental disorder.
Specify if:
   With perceptual disturbances

From American Psychiatric Association. *Diagnostic and Statistical Manual of Mental Disorders.* 4th ed. Text rev. Washington, DC: American Psychiatric Association; copyright 2000, with permission.

sis can be augmented with the phrase "with perceptual disturbances." If intact reality testing is not present, the diagnosis is cannabis-induced psychotic disorder.

Cannabis intoxication commonly heightens users' sensitivities to external stimuli, reveals new details, makes colors seem brighter and richer than in the past, and subjectively slows the appreciation of time. In high doses, users may experience depersonalization and derealization. Motor skills are impaired by cannabis use, and the impairment in motor skills remains after the subjective, euphoriant effects have resolved. For 8 to 12 hours after using cannabis, users' impaired motor skills interfere with the operation of motor vehicles and other heavy machinery. Moreover, these effects are additive to those of alcohol, which is commonly used in combination with cannabis.

Cannabis Intoxication Delirium

Cannabis intoxication delirium is a DSM-IV-TR diagnosis. The delirium associated with cannabis intoxication is characterized by marked impairment on cognition and performance tasks. Even modest doses of cannabis impair memory, reaction time, perception, motor coordination, and attention. High doses that also impair users' levels of consciousness have marked effects on cognitive measures.

Cannabis-Induced Psychotic Disorder

Cannabis-induced psychotic disorder is diagnosed in the presence of a cannabis-induced psychosis. Cannabis-induced psychotic disorder is rare; transient paranoid ideation is more common. Florid psychosis is somewhat common in countries in which some persons have long-term access to cannabis of particularly high potency. The psychotic episodes are sometimes referred to as "hemp insanity." Cannabis use rarely causes a "bad-trip" experience, which is often associated with hallucinogen intoxication. When cannabis-induced psychotic disorder

Table 9.5–3
DSM-IV-TR Diagnostic Criteria for Cannabis-Related Disorder Not Otherwise Specified

The cannabis-related disorder not otherwise specified category is for disorders associated with the use of cannabis that are not classifiable as cannabis dependence, cannabis abuse, cannabis intoxication, cannabis intoxication delirium, cannabis-induced psychotic disorder, or cannabis-induced anxiety disorder.

From American Psychiatric Association. *Diagnostic and Statistical Manual of Mental Disorders*. 4th ed. Text rev. Washington, DC: American Psychiatric Association; copyright 2000, with permission.

does occur, it may be correlated with a preexisting personality disorder in the affected person.

Cannabis-Induced Anxiety Disorder

Cannabis-induced anxiety disorder is a common diagnosis for acute cannabis intoxication, which in many persons induces short-lived anxiety states often provoked by paranoid thoughts. In such circumstances, panic attacks may be induced, based on ill-defined and disorganized fears. The appearance of anxiety symptoms is correlated with the dose and is the most frequent adverse reaction to the moderate use of smoked cannabis. Inexperienced users are much more likely to experience anxiety symptoms than are experienced users.

Cannabis-Related Disorder Not Otherwise Specified

DSM-IV-TR does not formally recognize cannabis-induced mood disorders; therefore, such disorders are classified as cannabis-related disorders not otherwise specified (Table 9.5–3). Cannabis intoxication can be associated with depressive symptoms, although such symptoms may suggest long-term cannabis use. Hypomania, however, is a common symptom in cannabis intoxication.

When either sleep disorder or sexual dysfunction symptoms are related to cannabis use, they almost always resolve within days or a week after cessation of cannabis use. They are both classified as cannabis-related disorders not otherwise specified in DSM-IV-TR.

Flashbacks.   Persisting perceptual abnormalities after cannabis use are not formally classified in DSM-IV-TR, although there are case reports of persons who have experienced—at times significantly—sensations related to cannabis intoxication after the short-term effects of the substance have disappeared. Continued debate concerns whether flashbacks are related to cannabis use alone or to the concomitant use of hallucinogens or of cannabis tainted with phencyclidine.

Amotivational Syndrome.   Another controversial cannabis-related syndrome is amotivational syndrome. Whether the syndrome is related to cannabis use or reflects characterological traits in a subgroup of persons regardless of cannabis use is under debate. Traditionally, the amotivational syndrome has been associated with long-term heavy use and has been characterized by a person's unwillingness to persist in a task—be it at school, at work, or in any setting that requires prolonged attention or tenac-

ity. Persons are described as becoming apathetic and anergic, usually gaining weight, and appearing slothful.

TREATMENT AND REHABILITATION

Treatment of cannabis use rests on the same principles as treatment of other substances of abuse—abstinence and support. Abstinence can be achieved through direct interventions, such as hospitalization, or through careful monitoring on an outpatient basis by the use of urine drug screens, which can detect cannabis for up to 4 weeks after use. Support can be achieved through the use of individual, family, and group psychotherapies. Education should be a cornerstone for both abstinence and support programs. A patient who does not understand the intellectual reasons for addressing a substance-abuse problem has little motivation to stop. For some patients, an antianxiety drug may be useful for short-term relief of withdrawal symptoms. For other patients, cannabis use may be related to an underlying depressive disorder that may respond to specific antidepressant treatment.

Medical Use of Marijuana

Marijuana has been used as a medicinal herb for centuries, and cannabis was listed in the U.S. pharmacopeia until the end of the 19th century as a remedy for anxiety, depression, and gastrointestinal disorders, among others. Currently, cannabis is a controlled substance with a high potential for abuse and no medical use recognized by the Drug Enforcement Agency; however, it is used to treat various disorders such as the nausea from chemotherapy, leukemia, multiple sclerosis, chronic pain, acquired immune deficiency syndrome, and glaucoma. In 1996, California residents approved the California Compensation Use Act that allowed state residents to grow and use marijuana for these disorders, but in 2001 the U.S. Supreme Court ruled 8 to 0 that the manufacture and distribution of marijuana are illegal under any circumstances. It is unclear how that ruling will affect California, but in 2003, a federal court convicted a grower of medical marijuana in that state. Dronabinol, a synthetic form of THC, has been approved by the Food and Drug Administration; however, taken orally, it is not considered as effective as smoking the entire plant product.

In 1996, an expert report by the Institute of Medicine suggested that marijuana be converted to a Schedule II drug with established controls on medical use. This would allow more controlled scientific drug trials to determine if there is unequivocal therapeutic efficacy in different conditions. The opposition to this is based on the illicit recreational use of marijuana, which obscures its legitimate medical use.

▲ 9.6 Cocaine-Related Disorders

Cocaine is an alkaloid derived from the shrub *Erythroxylon coca*, which is indigenous to South America, where the leaves of the shrub are chewed by local inhabitants to obtain the stimulation effects. The cocaine alkaloid was first isolated in 1860 and first used as a local anesthetic in 1880. It is still used as a local anesthetic, especially for eye, nose, and throat surgery, for which its vasoconstrictive and analgesic effects are helpful. In 1884, Sigmund Freud made a study of cocaine's general pharmacological effects and, for a period of time, according to his biographers, was addicted to the drug. In the 1880s and 1890s, cocaine was widely touted as a cure for many ills and was listed in the 1899 *Merck Manual*. In 1914, however, once its addictive and adverse effects had been recognized, cocaine was classified as a narcotic, along with morphine and heroin.

EPIDEMIOLOGY

According to DSM-IV-TR, approximately 10 percent of the U.S. population has tried cocaine, with 2 percent reporting use in the last year, 0.8 percent reporting use in the past month, and a lifetime rate of cocaine abuse or dependence of approximately 2 percent. Cocaine use is highest among persons aged 18 to 25 years (1.3 percent) and ages 26 to 34 (1.2 percent). Current cocaine use, however, is on the decline, primarily because of increased awareness of cocaine's risks as well as a comprehensive public campaign about cocaine and its effects. The societal effects of the decrease in cocaine use, however, have been somewhat offset by the frequent use over the past years of crack, a highly potent form of cocaine. Crack use is most common in persons aged 18 to 25, who are particularly attracted to the low street price of a single 50- to 100-mg dose. Males are twice as likely to be cocaine abusers than females, and all races and socioeconomic groups are equally affected.

COMORBIDITY

Like other substance-related disorders, cocaine-related disorders are often accompanied by additional psychiatric disorders. The development of mood disorders and alcohol-related disorders usually follows the onset of cocaine-related disorders, whereas anxiety disorders, antisocial personality disorder, and attention-deficit/hyperactivity disorder are thought to precede the development of cocaine-related disorders. Most studies of comorbidity in patients with cocaine-related disorders have shown that major depressive disorder, bipolar II disorder, cyclothymic disorder, anxiety disorders, and antisocial personality disorder are the most commonly associated psychiatric diagnoses.

ETIOLOGY

Genetic Factors

Laboratory animal strains differ greatly in their willingness to self-administer psychoactive drugs, including cocaine, and strains can be developed that differ even more markedly. The most convincing evidence to date of a genetic influence on cocaine dependence comes from studies of twins. Monozygotic twins have higher concordance rates for stimulant dependence (cocaine, amphetamines, and amphetamine-like drugs) than dizygotic twins. The analyses indicate that genetic factors and unique (unshared) environmental factors contribute about equally to the development of stimulant dependence.

Sociocultural Factors

Social, cultural, and economic factors are powerful determinants of initial use, continuing use, and relapse. Excessive use is far more likely in countries where cocaine is readily available. Different economic opportunities may influence certain groups more than others to engage in selling illicit drugs, and selling is more likely to be carried out in familiar communities than in those where the seller runs a high risk of arrest.

Learning and Conditioning

Learning and conditioning are also considered important in perpetuating cocaine use. Each inhalation or injection of cocaine yields a "rush" and a euphoric experience that reinforce the antecedent drug-taking behavior. In addition, the environmental cues associated with substance use become associated with the euphoric state so that long after a period of cessation, such cues (e.g., white powder and paraphernalia) can elicit memories of the euphoric state and reawaken craving for cocaine.

In cocaine abusers (but not in normal controls), cocaine-related stimuli activate brain regions subserving episodic and working memory and produce electroencephalographic arousal (desynchronization). Increased metabolic activity in the limbic-related regions such as amygdala, parahippocampal gyrus, and dorsolateral prefrontal cortex reportedly correlate with reports of craving for cocaine, but the degree of electroencephalographic arousal does not.

Pharmacological Factors

As a result of actions in the central nervous system (CNS), cocaine can produce a sense of alertness, euphoria, and well-being. There may be decreased hunger and less need for sleep. Performance impaired by fatigue is usually improved. Some users believe that cocaine enhances sexual performance.

NEUROPHARMACOLOGY

Cocaine's primary pharmacodynamic action related to its behavioral effects is competitive blockade of dopamine reuptake by the dopamine transporter. This blockade increases the concentration of dopamine in the synaptic cleft and results in increased activation of both dopamine type 1 (D_1) and type 2 (D_2) receptors. The effects of cocaine on the activity mediated by D_3, D_4, and D_5 receptors are not yet well understood, but at least one preclinical study has implicated the D_3 receptor. Although the behavioral effects are attributed primarily to the blockade of dopamine reuptake, cocaine also blocks the reuptake of the other major catecholamine, norepinephrine, and that of serotonin. The behavioral effects related to these activities are receiving increased attention in the scientific literature. The effects of cocaine on cerebral blood flow and cerebral glucose use have also been studied. Results in most studies generally showed that cocaine is associated with decreased cerebral blood flow and possibly with the development of patchy areas of decreased glucose use.

The behavioral effects of cocaine are felt almost immediately and last for a relatively brief time (30 to 60 minutes); thus, users require repeated doses of the drug to maintain the feelings of intoxication. Despite the short-lived behavioral effects, metabolites of cocaine may be present in the blood and urine for up to 10 days.

Cocaine has powerful addictive qualities. Because of its potency as a positive reinforcer of behavior, psychological dependence on cocaine can develop after a single use. With repeated administration, both tolerance and sensitivity to various effects of cocaine can arise, although the development of tolerance or sensitivity is apparently due to many factors and is not easily predicted. Physiological dependence on cocaine does occur, although cocaine withdrawal is mild compared with a withdrawal from opiates and opioids.

METHODS OF USE

Because drug dealers often dilute cocaine powder with sugar or procaine, street cocaine varies greatly in purity. Cocaine is sometimes cut with amphetamine. The most common method of using cocaine is inhaling the finely chopped powder into the nose, a practice referred to as "snorting" or "tooting." Other methods of ingesting cocaine are subcutaneous or intravenous (IV) injection and smoking (freebasing). Freebasing involves mixing street cocaine with chemically extracted pure cocaine alkaloid (the freebase) to get an increased effect. Smoking is also the method used for ingesting crack cocaine. Inhaling is the least dangerous method of cocaine use; IV injection and smoking are the most dangerous. The most direct methods of ingestion are often associated with cerebrovascular diseases, cardiac abnormalities, and death. Although cocaine can be taken orally, it is rarely ingested via this, the least effective, route.

Crack

Crack, a freebase form of cocaine, is extremely potent. It is sold in small, ready-to-smoke amounts, often called "rocks." Crack cocaine is highly addictive; even one or two experiences with the drug can cause intense craving for more. Users have been known to resort to extremes of behavior to obtain the money to buy more crack. Reports from urban emergency rooms have also associated extremes of violence with crack abuse.

DIAGNOSIS AND CLINICAL FEATURES

DSM-IV-TR lists many cocaine-related disorders (Table 9.6–1) but only specifies the diagnostic criteria for cocaine intoxication (Table 9.6–2) and cocaine withdrawal (Table 9.6–3) within the cocaine-related disorders section. The diagnostic criteria for the other cocaine-related disorders are in the DSM-IV-TR sections that focus on the principal symptom—for example, cocaine-induced mood disorder in the mood disorders section (see Chapter 12).

Cocaine Dependence and Abuse

DSM-IV-TR uses the general guidelines for substance dependence and substance abuse to diagnose cocaine dependence and cocaine abuse (see Tables 9.1–3 and 9.1–4). Clinically and practically, cocaine dependence or cocaine abuse can be suspected in patients who evidence unexplained changes in personality. Common changes associated with cocaine use are

Table 9.6–1
DSM-IV-TR Cocaine-Related Disorders

Cocaine use disorders
Cocaine dependence
Cocaine abuse
Cocaine-induced disorders
Cocaine intoxication
   Specify if:
      With perceptual disturbances
Cocaine withdrawal
Cocaine intoxication delirium
Cocaine-induced psychotic disorder, with delusions
   Specify if:
      With onset during intoxication
Cocaine-induced psychotic disorder, with hallucinations
   Specify if:
      With onset during intoxication
Cocaine-induced mood disorder
   Specify if:
      With onset during intoxication
      With onset during withdrawal
Cocaine-induced anxiety disorder
   Specify if:
      With onset during intoxication
      With onset during withdrawal
Cocaine-induced sexual dysfunction
   Specify if:
      With onset during intoxication
Cocaine-induced sleep disorder
   Specify if:
      With onset during intoxication
      With onset during withdrawal
Cocaine-related disorder not otherwise specified

From American Psychiatric Association. *Diagnostic and Statistical Manual of Mental Disorders.* 4th ed. Text rev. Washington, DC: American Psychiatric Association; copyright 2000, with permission.

irritability, impaired ability to concentrate, compulsive behavior, severe insomnia, and weight loss. Colleagues at work and family members may notice a person's general and increasing inability to perform the expected tasks associated with work and family life. The patient may show new evidence of increased debt or inability to pay bills on time because of the large sums used to buy cocaine. Cocaine abusers often excuse themselves from work or social situations every 30 to 60 minutes to find a secluded place to inhale more cocaine. Because of the vasoconstricting effect of cocaine, users almost always develop nasal congestion, which they may attempt to self-medicate with decongestant sprays.

Cocaine Intoxication

DSM-IV-TR specifies the diagnostic criteria for cocaine intoxication (Table 9.6–2), which emphasizes the behavioral and physical signs and symptoms of cocaine use. The DSM-IV-TR diagnostic criteria allow for specification of the presence of perceptual disturbances. If hallucinations are present in the

Table 9.6–2
DSM-IV-TR Diagnostic Criteria for Cocaine Intoxication

A. Recent use of cocaine.

B. Clinically significant maladaptive behavioral or psychological changes (e.g., euphoria or affective blunting; changes in sociability; hypervigilance; interpersonal sensitivity; anxiety, tension, or anger; stereotyped behaviors; impaired judgment; or impaired social or occupational functioning) that developed during, or shortly after, use of cocaine.

C. Two (or more) of the following, developing during, or shortly after, cocaine use:

(1) tachycardia or bradycardia

(2) pupillary dilation

(3) elevated or lowered blood pressure

(4) perspiration or chills

(5) nausea or vomiting

(6) evidence of weight loss

(7) psychomotor agitation or retardation

(8) muscular weakness, respiratory depression, chest pain, or cardiac arrhythmias

(9) confusion, seizures, dyskinesias, dystonias, or coma

D. The symptoms are not due to a general medical condition and are not better accounted for by another mental disorder.

Specify if:

With perceptual disturbances

From American Psychiatric Association. *Diagnostic and Statistical Manual of Mental Disorders.* 4th ed. Text rev. Washington, DC: American Psychiatric Association; copyright 2000, with permission.

absence of intact reality testing, the appropriate diagnosis is cocaine-induced psychotic disorder, with hallucinations.

Persons use cocaine for its characteristic effects of elation, euphoria, heightened self-esteem, and perceived improvement on mental and physical tasks. Some studies have indicated that low doses of cocaine can actually be associated with improved performance on some cognitive tasks. With high doses, however, the

Table 9.6–3
DSM-IV-TR Diagnostic Criteria for Cocaine Withdrawal

A. Cessation of (or reduction in) cocaine use that has been heavy and prolonged.

B. Dysphoric mood and two (or more) of the following physiological changes, developing within a few hours to several days after Criterion A:

(1) fatigue

(2) vivid, unpleasant dreams

(3) insomnia or hypersomnia

(4) increased appetite

(5) psychomotor retardation or agitation

C. The symptoms in Criterion B cause clinically significant distress or impairment in social, occupational, or other important areas of functioning.

D. The symptoms are not due to a general medical condition and are not better accounted for by another mental disorder.

From American Psychiatric Association. *Diagnostic and Statistical Manual of Mental Disorders.* 4th ed. Text rev. Washington, DC: American Psychiatric Association; copyright 2000, with permission.

symptoms of intoxication include agitation, irritability, impaired judgment, impulsive and potentially dangerous sexual behavior, aggression, a generalized increase in psychomotor activity, and, potentially, symptoms of mania. The major associated physical symptoms are tachycardia, hypertension, and mydriasis.

Cocaine Withdrawal

After cessation of cocaine use or after acute intoxication, postintoxication depression ("crash") may be associated with symptoms of dysphoria, anhedonia, anxiety, irritability, fatigue, hypersomnolence, and sometimes agitation. With mild-to-moderate cocaine use, these withdrawal symptoms end within 18 hours. With heavy use, as in cocaine dependence, withdrawal symptoms can last up to a week but usually peak in 2 to 4 days. Some patients and some anecdotal reports have described cocaine withdrawal syndromes that have lasted for weeks or months. The withdrawal symptoms can also be associated with suicidal ideation in affected persons. A person in the state of withdrawal can experience powerful and intense cravings for cocaine, especially because taking cocaine can eliminate the unpleasant withdrawal symptoms. Persons experiencing cocaine withdrawal often attempt to self-medicate with alcohol, sedatives, hypnotics, or antianxiety agents such as diazepam (Valium). The DSM-IV-TR diagnostic criteria for cocaine withdrawal are listed in Table 9.6–3.

Cocaine Intoxication Delirium

DSM-IV-TR has specified a diagnosis for cocaine intoxication delirium. Cocaine intoxication delirium is most common when high doses of cocaine are used; when cocaine has been used over a short time, so that cocaine blood concentrations rapidly increase; or when cocaine is mixed with other psychoactive substances (e.g., amphetamine, opiates, opioids, and alcohol). Persons with preexisting brain damage (often resulting from previous episodes of cocaine intoxication) are also at increased risk for cocaine intoxication delirium.

Cocaine-Induced Psychotic Disorder

Paranoid delusions and hallucinations may occur in up to 50 percent of all persons who use cocaine. The occurrence of these psychotic symptoms depends on the dose, the duration of use, and the individual user's sensitivity to the substance. Cocaine-induced psychotic disorders are most common with IV users and crack users. Men are much more likely to have psychotic symptoms than are women. Paranoid delusions are the most frequent psychotic symptoms. Auditory hallucinations are also common, but visual and tactile hallucinations may be less common than paranoid delusions. The sensation of bugs crawling just beneath the skin (formication) has been reported to be associated with cocaine use. Psychotic disorders can develop with grossly inappropriate sexual and generally bizarre behavior and homicidal or other violent actions related to the content of the paranoid delusions or hallucinations.

Cocaine-Induced Mood Disorder

DSM-IV-TR allows for the diagnosis of cocaine-induced mood disorder, which can begin during either intoxication or withdrawal. Classically, the mood disorder symptoms associated

Table 9.6–4
DSM-IV-TR Diagnostic Criteria for Cocaine-Related Disorder Not Otherwise Specified

The cocaine-related disorder not otherwise specified category is for disorders associated with the use of cocaine that are not classifiable as cocaine dependence, cocaine abuse, cocaine intoxication, cocaine withdrawal, cocaine intoxication delirium, cocaine-induced psychotic disorder, cocaine-induced mood disorder, cocaine-induced anxiety disorder, cocaine-induced sexual dysfunction, or cocaine-induced sleep disorder.

From American Psychiatric Association. *Diagnostic and Statistical Manual of Mental Disorders.* 4th ed. Text rev. Washington, DC: American Psychiatric Association; copyright 2000, with permission.

with intoxication are hypomanic or manic; the mood disorder symptoms associated with withdrawal are characteristic of depression.

Cocaine-Induced Anxiety Disorder

DSM-IV-TR also allows for the diagnosis of cocaine-induced anxiety disorder. Common anxiety disorder symptoms associated with cocaine intoxication or withdrawal are those of obsessive-compulsive disorder, panic disorders, and phobias.

Cocaine-Induced Sexual Dysfunction

DSM-IV-TR allows for the diagnosis of cocaine-induced sexual dysfunction, which can begin when a person is intoxicated with cocaine. Although cocaine is used as an aphrodisiac and as a way to delay orgasm, its repeated use can result in impotence.

Cocaine-Induced Sleep Disorder

Cocaine-induced sleep disorder, which can begin during either intoxication or withdrawal, is described under substance-induced sleep disorders (see Chapter 21). Cocaine intoxication is associated with the inability to sleep; cocaine withdrawal is associated with disrupted sleep or hypersomnolence.

Cocaine-Related Disorder Not Otherwise Specified

DSM-IV-TR provides a diagnosis of cocaine-related disorder not otherwise specified for cocaine-related disorders that cannot be classified into one of the previously discussed diagnoses (Table 9.6–4).

Adverse Effects

A common adverse effect associated with cocaine use is nasal congestion; serious inflammation, swelling, bleeding, and ulceration of the nasal mucosa can also occur. Long-term use of cocaine can also lead to perforation of the nasal septa. Freebasing and smoking crack can damage the bronchial passages and the lungs. The IV use of cocaine can result in infection, embolisms, and the transmission of human immunodeficiency virus. Minor neurological complications with cocaine use include the development of acute dystonia, tics, and migraine-like headaches. The major complications of cocaine use, however, are cere-

brovascular, epileptic, and cardiac. Approximately two-thirds of these acute toxic effects occur within 1 hour of intoxication, approximately one-fifth occur in 1 to 3 hours, and the remainder occur up to several days later.

Cerebrovascular Effects.   The most common cerebrovascular diseases associated with cocaine use are nonhemorrhagic cerebral infarctions. When hemorrhagic infarctions do occur, they can include subarachnoid, intraparenchymal, and intraventricular hemorrhages. Transient ischemic attacks have also been associated with cocaine use. Although these vascular disorders usually affect the brain, spinal cord hemorrhages have also been reported. The obvious pathophysiological mechanism for these vascular disorders is vasoconstriction, but other pathophysiological mechanisms have also been proposed.

Seizures.   Seizures have been reported to account for 3 to 8 percent of cocaine-related emergency room visits. Cocaine is the substance of abuse most commonly associated with seizures; the second most common substance is amphetamine. Cocaine-induced seizures are usually single events, although multiple seizures and status epilepticus are also possible. A rare and easily misdiagnosed complication of cocaine use is partial complex status epilepticus, which should be considered as a diagnosis in a patient who seems to have cocaine-induced psychotic disorder with an unusually fluctuating course. The risk of having cocaine-induced seizures is highest in patients with a history of epilepsy who use high doses of cocaine as well as crack.

Cardiac Effects.   Myocardial infarctions and arrhythmias are perhaps the most common cocaine-induced cardiac abnormalities. Cardiomyopathies can develop with long-term use of cocaine, and cardioembolic cerebral infarctions can be a further complication of cocaine-induced myocardial dysfunction.

Death.   High doses of cocaine are associated with seizures, respiratory depression, cerebrovascular diseases, and myocardial infarctions—all of which can lead to death in persons who use cocaine. Users may experience warning signs of syncope or chest pain but may ignore these signs because of the irrepressible desire to take more cocaine. Deaths have also been reported with the ingestion of "speedballs," which are combinations of opioids and cocaine.

TREATMENT AND REHABILITATION

Most cocaine users do not come to treatment voluntarily. Their experience with the substance is too positive, and the negative effects are perceived as too minimal, to warrant seeking treatment. Those who do not seek treatment often have polysubstance-related disorder, fewer negative consequences associated with cocaine use, fewer work-related or family-related obligations, and increased contact with the legal system and with illegal activities.

The major hurdle to overcome in the treatment of cocaine-related disorders is the user's intense craving for the drug. Although animal studies have shown that cocaine is a powerful inducer of self-administration, these studies have also shown that animals limit their use of cocaine when negative reinforcers are experimentally linked to the cocaine intake. In humans, negative reinforcers may take the form of work and family-related problems brought on by cocaine use. Therefore, clinicians must take a broad treatment approach and include social, psychological, and perhaps biological strategies in the treatment program.

Attaining abstinence from cocaine in their patients may require complete or partial hospitalization to remove patients from the usual social settings in which they had obtained or used cocaine. Frequent, unscheduled urine testing is almost always necessary to monitor patients' continued abstinence, especially in the first weeks and months of treatment. Relapse prevention therapy is a therapy that relies on cognitive and behavioral techniques in addition to hospitalization and outpatient therapy to achieve the goal of abstinence.

Psychological intervention usually involves individual, group, and family modalities. In individual therapy, therapists should focus on the dynamics leading to cocaine use, the perceived positive effects of the cocaine, and other ways to achieve these effects. Group therapy and support groups, such as Narcotics Anonymous, often focus on discussions with other persons who use cocaine and on sharing past experiences and effective coping methods. Family therapy is often an essential component of the treatment strategy. Common issues discussed in family therapy are the ways the patient's past behavior has harmed the family and the response of family members to these behaviors. Therapy should also focus, however, on the future and on changes in the family's activities that may help the patient stay off the drug and direct energies in different directions. This approach can be used on an outpatient basis.

Pharmacological Adjuncts

Presently, no pharmacological treatments produce decreases in cocaine use comparable to the decreases in opioid use seen when heroin users are treated with methadone, levomethadyl acetate (ORLAAM) (commonly called L-α-acetylmethadol [LAAM]), or buprenorphine (Buprenex). However, a variety of pharmacological agents, most of which are approved for other uses, have been, and are being, tested clinically for the treatment of cocaine dependence and relapse.

Cocaine users presumed to have preexisting attention-deficit/hyperactivity disorder or mood disorders have been treated with methylphenidate (Ritalin) and lithium (Eskalith), respectively. Those drugs are of little or no benefit in patients without the disorders, and clinicians should adhere strictly to maximal diagnostic criteria before using either of them in the treatment of cocaine dependence. In patients with attention-deficit/hyperactivity disorder, slow-release forms of methylphenidate may be less likely to trigger cocaine craving, but the impact of such pharmacotherapy on cocaine use remains to be demonstrated.

Many pharmacological agents have been explored on the premise that chronic cocaine use alters the function of multiple neurotransmitter systems, especially the dopaminergic and serotonergic transmitters regulating hedonic tone, and that cocaine induces a state of relative dopaminergic deficiency. Although the evidence for such alterations in dopaminergic function has been growing, it has been difficult to demonstrate that agents theoretically capable of modifying dopamine function can alter the course of treatment. The following agents are among those that have not been found to reduce cocaine use: neurotransmitter precursors (e.g., dopa, tyrosine), dopaminergic agonists (e.g., bromocriptine [Parlodel], lisuride [Dopergin], pergolide [Permax]), and antiparkinson drugs that may also affect the dopaminergic system (amantadine [Symmetrel]).

Tricyclic antidepressant drugs such as desipramine (Norpramin) and imipramine (Tofranil) have also been tried. Although some double-blind studies that relied heavily on self-reports of drug use yielded some posi-

tive results, other studies did not find them significantly beneficial in inducing abstinence or preventing relapse. Used early in treatment, however, they may have some transient benefit for patients who are not severely dependent.

Also tried but not confirmed effective in controlled studies are other antidepressants, such as bupropion (Wellbutrin), monoamine oxidase inhibitors (selegiline [Eldepryl]), selective serotonin uptake inhibitors (e.g., fluoxetine [Prozac], mazindol [Sanorex], pemoline [Cylert]), antipsychotics (e.g., flupenthixol [Depixol]), lithium, several different calcium channel inhibitors, and anticonvulsants (e.g., carbamazepine [Tegretol] and valproic acid [Depakene]). One study found that 300 mg a day of phenytoin (Dilantin) reduced cocaine use; this study requires further replication.

Several agents are being developed that have not been tried in human studies. These include agents that would selectively block or stimulate dopamine receptor subtypes (e.g., selective D_1 agonists) and drugs that can selectively block the access of cocaine to the dopamine transports but still permit the transporters to remove cocaine from the synapse. Another approach is aimed at preventing cocaine from reaching the brain by using antibodies to bind cocaine in the bloodstream (a so-called cocaine vaccine). Such cocaine-binding antibodies do reduce the reinforcing effects of cocaine in animal models. Also under study are catalytic antibodies that accelerate the hydrolysis of cocaine; and butyrylcholinesterase (pseudocholinesterase), which appear to hydrolyze cocaine selectively and is normally present in the body.

Detoxification

The cocaine withdrawal syndrome is distinct from that of opioids, alcohol, or sedative-hypnotic agents, since there are no physiological disturbances that necessitate inpatient or residential drug withdrawal. Thus, it is generally possible to engage in a therapeutic trial of outpatient withdrawal before deciding whether a more intensive or controlled setting is required for patients unable to stop without help in limiting their access to cocaine. Patients withdrawing from cocaine typically experience fatigue, dysphoria, disturbed sleep, and some craving; some may experience depression. No pharmacological agents reliably reduce the intensity of withdrawal, but recovery over a week or two is generally uneventful. It may take longer, however, for sleep, mood, and cognitive function to recover fully.

▲ 9.7 Hallucinogen-Related Disorders

Hallucinogens are natural and synthetic substances that are variously called *psychedelics* or *psychotomimetics* because, besides inducing hallucinations, they produce a loss of contact with reality and an experience of expanded and heightened consciousness. The hallucinogens are classified as Schedule I drugs; the U.S. Food and Drug Administration has decreed that they have no medical use and a high abuse potential.

The classic, naturally occurring hallucinogens are *psilocybin* (from some mushrooms) and *mescaline* (from peyote cactus); others are harmine, harmaline, ibogaine, and dimethyltryptamine. The classic synthetic hallucinogen is *lysergic acid diethylamide* (LSD), synthesized in 1938 by Albert Hoffman, who later accidentally ingested some of the drug and experienced the first LSD-induced hallucinogenic episode. Some researchers classify the substituted or so-called designer amphetamines, such as 3,4-methylenedioxymethamphetamine (MDMA), as hallucinogens. However, because these drugs are structurally related to amphetamines, this textbook classifies them as amphetamine-like substances, and they are covered in Section 9.3.

EPIDEMIOLOGY

According to the text revision of the fourth edition of the *Diagnostic and Statistical Manual of Mental Disorders* (DSM-IV-TR), 10 percent of persons in the United States had used a hallucinogen at least once. Hallucinogen use is most common among young (15 to 35 years of age) white men. The ratio of whites to blacks that have used a hallucinogen is 2 to 1; the white to Hispanic ratio is approximately 1.5 to 1. Men represent 62 percent of those who have used a hallucinogen at some time and 75 percent of those who have used a hallucinogen in the preceding month. Persons 26 to 34 years of age show the highest use of hallucinogens, with 15.5 percent having used a hallucinogen at least once. Persons 18 to 25 years of age have the highest recent use of a hallucinogen.

Cultural factors influence the use of hallucinogens; their use in the western United States is significantly higher than in the southern United States. Hallucinogen use is associated with less morbidity and less mortality than that of some other substances. For example, one study found that only 1 percent of substance-related emergency room visits were related to hallucinogens, compared with 40 percent for cocaine-related problems. Of persons visiting the emergency room for hallucinogen-related reasons, however, more than 50 percent were younger than 20 years of age. Resurgence in the popularity of hallucinogens has been reported. According to DSM-IV-TR, the lifetime rate of hallucinogen abuse is approximately 0.6 percent, with a 12-month prevalence of approximately 0.1 percent.

NEUROPHARMACOLOGY

Although most hallucinogenic substances vary in their pharmacological effects, LSD can serve as a hallucinogenic prototype. The pharmacodynamic effect of LSD remains controversial, although it is generally agreed that the drug acts on the serotonergic system, whether as an antagonist or as an agonist. Data at this time suggest that LSD acts as a partial agonist at postsynaptic serotonin receptors.

Most hallucinogens are well absorbed after oral ingestion, although some are ingested by inhalation, smoking, or intravenous injection. Tolerance for LSD and other hallucinogens develops rapidly and is virtually complete after 3 or 4 days of continuous use. Tolerance also reverses quickly, usually in 4 to 7 days. Neither physical dependence nor withdrawal symptoms occur with hallucinogens, but a user can develop a psychological dependence on the insight-inducing experiences of episodes of hallucinogen use.

DIAGNOSIS

DSM-IV-TR lists a number of hallucinogen-related disorders (Table 9.7–1) but contains specific diagnostic criteria

Table 9.7–1
DSM-IV-TR Hallucinogen-Related Disorders

Hallucinogen use disorders
Hallucinogen dependence
Hallucinogen abuse
Hallucinogen-induced disorders
Hallucinogen intoxication
Hallucinogen persisting perception disorder (flashbacks)
Hallucinogen intoxication delirium
Hallucinogen-induced psychotic disorder, with delusions
Specify if:
With onset during intoxication
Hallucinogen-induced psychotic disorder, with hallucinations
Specify if:
With onset during intoxication
Hallucinogen-induced mood disorder
Specify if:
With onset during intoxication
Hallucinogen-induced anxiety disorder
Specify if:
With onset during intoxication
Hallucinogen-related disorder not otherwise specified

From American Psychiatric Association. *Diagnostic and Statistical Manual of Mental Disorders.* 4th ed. Text rev. Washington, DC: American Psychiatric Association; copyright 2000, with permission.

only for hallucinogen intoxication (Table 9.7–2) and hallucinogen persisting perception disorder (flashbacks) (Table 9.7–3).

Hallucinogen Dependence and Hallucinogen Abuse

Long-term hallucinogen use is not common. As stated above, there is no physical addiction. Although psychological dependence occurs, it is rare, in part because each LSD experience is different and in part because there is no reliable euphoria. Nonetheless, hallucinogen dependence and hallucinogen abuse are genuine syndromes, defined by DSM-IV-TR criteria (see Section 9.1).

Hallucinogen Intoxication

Intoxication with hallucinogens is defined in DSM-IV-TR as characterized by maladaptive behavioral and perceptual changes and by certain physiological signs (Table 9.7–2). The differential diagnosis for hallucinogen intoxication includes anticholinergic and amphetamine intoxication and alcohol withdrawal. The preferred treatment for hallucinogen intoxication is talking down the patient; during this process, guides can reassure patients that the symptoms are drug induced, that they are not going crazy, and that the symptoms will resolve shortly. In the most severe cases, dopaminergic antagonists—for example, haloperidol (Haldol)—or benzodiazepine—for example, diazepam (Valium)—can be used for a limited time. Hallucinogen intoxication usually lacks a withdrawal syndrome.

**Table 9.7–2
DSM-IV-TR Diagnostic Criteria for
Hallucinogen Intoxication**

A. Recent use of a hallucinogen.

B. Clinically significant maladaptive behavioral or psychological changes (e.g., marked anxiety or depression, ideas of reference, fear of losing one's mind, paranoid ideation, impaired judgment, or impaired social or occupational functioning) that developed during, or shortly after, hallucinogen use.

C. Perceptual changes occurring in a state of full wakefulness and alertness (e.g., subjective intensification of perceptions, depersonalization, derealization, illusions, hallucinations, synesthesias) that developed during, or shortly after, hallucinogen use.

D. Two (or more) of the following signs, developing during, or shortly after, hallucinogen use:

  (1) pupillary dilation
  (2) tachycardia
  (3) sweating
  (4) palpitations
  (5) blurring of vision
  (6) tremors
  (7) incoordination

E. The symptoms are not due to a general medical condition and are not better accounted for by another mental disorder.

From American Psychiatric Association. *Diagnostic and Statistical Manual of Mental Disorders.* 4th ed. Text rev. Washington, DC: American Psychiatric Association; copyright 2000, with permission.

Hallucinogen Persisting Perception Disorder

Long after ingesting a hallucinogen, a person can experience a flashback of hallucinogenic symptoms. This syndrome is diagnosed as hallucinogen persisting perception disorder (Table 9.7–3) in DSM-IV-TR. According to studies, from 15 to 80 percent of users of hallucinogens report having experienced flash-

**Table 9.7–3
DSM-IV-TR Diagnostic Criteria for Hallucinogen Persisting Perception Disorder (Flashbacks)**

A. The reexperiencing, following cessation of use of a hallucinogen, of one or more of the perceptual symptoms that were experienced while intoxicated with the hallucinogen (e.g., geometric hallucinations, false perceptions of movement in the peripheral visual fields, flashes of color, intensified colors, trails of images of moving objects, positive afterimages, halos around objects, macropsia, and micropsia).

B. The symptoms in Criterion A cause clinically significant distress or impairment in social, occupational, or other important areas of functioning.

C. The symptoms are not due to a general medical condition (e.g., anatomical lesions and infections of the brain, visual epilepsies) and are not better accounted for by another mental disorder (e.g., delirium, dementia, schizophrenia) or hypnopompic hallucinations.

From American Psychiatric Association. *Diagnostic and Statistical Manual of Mental Disorders.* 4th ed. Text rev. Washington, DC: American Psychiatric Association; copyright 2000, with permission.

backs. The differential diagnosis for flashbacks includes migraine, seizures, visual system abnormalities, and posttraumatic stress disorder. The following can trigger a flashback: emotional stress; sensory deprivation, such as monotonous driving; or use of another psychoactive substance, such as alcohol or marijuana.

Flashbacks are spontaneous, transitory recurrences of the substance-induced experience. Most flashbacks are episodes of visual distortion, geometric hallucinations, hallucinations of sounds or voices, false perceptions of movement in peripheral fields, flashes of color, trails of images from moving objects, positive afterimages and halos, macropsia, micropsia, time expansion, physical symptoms, or relived intense emotion. The episodes usually last a few seconds to a few minutes but can sometimes last longer. Most often, even in the presence of distinct perceptual disturbances, the person has insight into the pathological nature of the disturbance. Suicidal behavior, major depressive disorder, and panic disorders are potential complications.

Hallucinogen Intoxication Delirium

DSM-IV-TR allows for the diagnosis of hallucinogen intoxication delirium, a relatively rare disorder beginning during intoxication in those who have ingested pure hallucinogens. Hallucinogens are often mixed with other substances, however, and the other components of their interactions with the hallucinogens can produce clinical delirium.

Hallucinogen-Induced Psychotic Disorders

If psychotic symptoms are present in the absence of retained reality testing, a diagnosis of hallucinogen-induced psychotic disorder may be warranted. DSM-IV-TR also allows clinicians to specify whether hallucinations or delusions are the prominent symptoms. The most common adverse effect of LSD and related substances is a "bad trip," an experience resembling the acute panic reaction to cannabis but sometimes more severe; a bad trip can occasionally produce true psychotic symptoms. The bad trip generally ends when the immediate effects of the hallucinogen wear off, but its course is variable. Occasionally, a protracted psychotic episode is difficult to distinguish from a nonorganic psychotic disorder. Whether a chronic psychosis after drug ingestion is the result of the drug ingestion, is unrelated to the drug ingestion, or is a combination of both the drug ingestion and predisposing factors is currently unanswerable.

Occasionally, the psychotic disorder is prolonged, a reaction thought to be most common in persons with preexisting schizoid personality disorder and prepsychotic personalities, an unstable ego balance, or much anxiety. Such persons cannot cope with the perceptual changes, body-image distortions, and symbolic unconscious material stimulated by the hallucinogen. The rate of previous mental instability in persons hospitalized for LSD reactions is high. Adverse reactions occurred in the late 1960s when LSD was being promoted as a self-prescribed psychotherapy for emotional crises in the lives of seriously disturbed persons. Now that this practice is less frequent, prolonged adverse reactions are less common.

A 22-year-old female photography student presented to the hospital with inappropriate mood and bizarre thinking. She had no prior psychiatric history. Nine days prior to admission she ingested one or two psilocybin mushrooms. Following the immediate ingestion, the patient began to giggle. She then described euphoria, which progressed to auditory hallucinations and belief in the ability to broadcast her thoughts on the media. Two days later she repeated the ingestion, and continued to exhibit psychotic symptoms to the day of admission. When examined she heard voices telling her she could be president, and reported the sounds of "lambs crying." She continued to giggle inappropriately, bizarrely turning her head from side to side ritualistically. She continued to describe euphoria, but with an intermittent sense of hopelessness in a context of thought blocking. Her self-description was "feeling lucky." She was given haloperidol, 10 mg twice a day, along with benztropine (Cogentin) 1 mg three times a day and lithium carbonate (Eskalith) 300 mg twice a day. On this regimen her psychosis abated after 5 days.

Hallucinogen-Induced Mood Disorder

DSM-IV-TR provides a diagnostic category for hallucinogen-induced mood disorder. Unlike cocaine-induced mood disorder and amphetamine-induced mood disorder, in which the symptoms are somewhat predictable, mood disorder symptoms accompanying hallucinogen abuse can vary. Abusers may experience manic-like symptoms with grandiose delusions or depression-like feelings and ideas or mixed symptoms. As with the hallucinogen-induced psychotic disorder symptoms, the symptoms of hallucinogen-induced mood disorder usually resolve once the drug has been eliminated from the person's body.

Hallucinogen-Induced Anxiety Disorder

Hallucinogen-induced anxiety disorder varies in its symptom pattern, but few data about symptom patterns are available. Anecdotally, emergency room physicians who treat patients with hallucinogen-related disorders frequently report panic disorder with agoraphobia.

A 20-year-old man had a 7-year history of polysubstance abuse, including having used LSD an estimated 400 times. While driving with his girlfriend he ingested an unknown quantity of LSD and became intoxicated; he reported using no other drugs at this time. Within minutes after ingestion, he began to experience visual hallucinations that intensified as he drove. When he attempted to speak to his girlfriend, he saw that she had become a giant lizard. He became terrified and attempted to kill her by crashing the car, injuring himself and his passenger. By the time of discharge from the hospital 3 days later, his panic had resolved.

Table 9.7–4
DSM-IV-TR Diagnostic Criteria for Hallucinogen-Related Disorder Not Otherwise Specified

The hallucinogen-related disorder not otherwise specified category is for disorders associated with the use of hallucinogens that are not classifiable as hallucinogen dependence, hallucinogen abuse, hallucinogen intoxication, hallucinogen persisting perception disorder, hallucinogen intoxication delirium, hallucinogen-induced psychotic disorder, hallucinogen-induced mood disorder, or hallucinogen-induced anxiety disorder.

From American Psychiatric Association. *Diagnostic and Statistical Manual of Mental Disorders.* 4th ed. Text rev. Washington, DC: American Psychiatric Association; copyright 2000, with permission.

Hallucinogen-Related Disorder Not Otherwise Specified

When a patient with a hallucinogen-related disorder does not meet the diagnostic criteria for any of the standard hallucinogen-related disorders, the patient may be classified as having hallucinogen-related disorder not otherwise specified (Table 9.7–4). DSM-IV-TR does not have a diagnostic category of hallucinogen withdrawal, but some clinicians anecdotally report a syndrome with depression and anxiety after cessation of frequent hallucinogen use. Such a syndrome may best fit the diagnosis of hallucinogen-related disorder not otherwise specified.

CLINICAL FEATURES

The onset of action of LSD occurs within an hour, peaks in 2 to 4 hours, and lasts 8 to 12 hours. The sympathomimetic effects of LSD include tremors, tachycardia, hypertension, hyperthermia, sweating, blurring of vision, and mydriasis. Death caused by cardiac or cerebrovascular pathology related to hypertension or hyperthermia can occur with hallucinogenic use. A syndrome similar to neuroleptic malignant syndrome has reportedly been associated with LSD. Death can also be caused by a physical injury when LSD use impairs judgment about, for example, traffic or a person's ability to fly. The psychological effects are usually well tolerated, but when persons cannot recall experiences or appreciate that the experiences are substance induced, they may fear the onset of insanity.

With hallucinogen use, perceptions become unusually brilliant and intense. Colors and textures seem to be richer than in the past, contours sharpened, music more emotionally profound, and smells and tastes heightened. Synesthesia is common; colors may be heard or sounds seen. Changes in body image and alterations of time and space perception also occur. Hallucinations are usually visual, often of geometric forms and figures, but auditory and tactile hallucinations are sometimes experienced. Emotions become unusually intense and may change abruptly and often; two seemingly incompatible feelings may be experienced at the same time. Suggestibility is greatly heightened, and sensitivity or detachment from other persons may arise. Other common features are a seeming awareness of internal organs, the recovery of lost early memories, the release of unconscious material in symbolic form, and regression and the apparent reliving of past events, including birth. Introspective reflection and feelings of religious and philosophical insight are common. The sense of self is greatly changed, sometimes to the point of depersonalization, merging with the external world, separation of self from body, or total dissolution of the ego in mystical ecstasy.

There is no clear evidence of drastic personality change or chronic psychosis produced by long-term LSD use by moderate users not otherwise predisposed to these conditions. Some heavy users of hallucinogens, however, may experience chronic anxiety or depression and may benefit from a psychological or pharmacological approach that addresses the underlying problem.

TREATMENT

Hallucinogen Intoxication

Persons have historically been treated for hallucinogen intoxication by psychological support for the remainder of the trip, so-called talking down. This is a time-consuming and potentially hazardous undertaking given the lability of a patient with hallucinogen-related delusions. Accordingly, treatment of hallucinogen intoxication is the oral administration of 20 mg of diazepam. This medication brings the LSD experience and any associated panic to a halt within 20 minutes and should be considered superior to "talking down" the patient over a period of hours or to administering antipsychotic agents. The marketing of lower doses of LSD and a more sophisticated approach to treatment of casualties by drug users themselves have combined to reduce the appearance of this once-common disorder in psychiatric treatment facilities.

Hallucinogen Persisting Perception Disorder

Treatment for hallucinogen persisting perception disorder is palliative. The first step in the process is correct identification of the disorder; it is not uncommon for the patient to consult a number of specialists before the diagnosis is made. Pharmacological approaches include long-lasting benzodiazepines such as clonazepam (Klonopin) and, to a lesser extent, anticonvulsants including valproic acid (Depakene) and carbamazepine (Tegretol). Currently, no drug is completely effective in ablating symptoms. Comorbid conditions associated with hallucinogen persisting perception disorder include panic disorder, major depression, and alcohol dependence. Each of these conditions requires primary prevention and early intervention.

Hallucinogen-Induced Psychosis

Treatment of hallucinogen-induced psychosis does not differ from conventional treatment for other psychoses. However, in addition to antipsychotic medications, a number of agents are reportedly effective, including lithium carbonate, carbamazepine, and electroconvulsive therapy. Antidepressant drugs, benzodiazepines, and anticonvulsant agents may each have a role in treatment as well. One hallmark of this disorder is that, as opposed to schizophrenia, in which negative symptoms and poor interpersonal relatedness may commonly be found, patients with hallucinogen-induced psychosis exhibit the positive symptoms of hallucinations and delusions while retaining the ability to relate to the psychiatrist. Medical therapies are best applied in a context of supportive, educational, and family therapies. The goals of treatment are the control of symptoms, a minimal use of hospitals, daily work, the development and preservation of social relationships, and the management of comorbid illnesses such as alcohol dependence.

▲ 9.8 Inhalant-Related Disorders

The category of inhalant-related disorders includes the psychiatric syndromes resulting from the use of solvents, glues, adhesives, aerosol propellants, paint thinners, and fuels. Among specific examples of these substances are gasoline, varnish remover, lighter fluid, airplane glue, rubber cement, cleaning fluid, spray paint, shoe conditioner, and typewriter correction fluid. A resurgence of inhalants' popularity among young persons has been reported. The active compounds in these inhalants include toluene, acetone, benzene, trichloroethane, perchlorethylene, trichloroethylene, 1,2-dichloropropane, and halogenated hydrocarbons.

The text revision of the fourth edition of the *Diagnostic and Statistical Manual of Mental Disorders* (DSM-IV-TR) specifically excludes anesthetic gases (e.g., nitrous oxide and ether) and short-acting vasodilators (e.g., amyl nitrite) from the inhalant-related disorders, which are classified as other (or unknown) substance-related disorders and are discussed in Section 9.14.

EPIDEMIOLOGY

Inhalant substances are easily available, legal, and inexpensive. These three factors contribute to the high use of inhalants among poor persons and young persons. According to DSM-IV-TR, approximately 6 percent of persons in the United States had used inhalants at least once, and approximately 1 percent were current users. Among young adults 18 to 25 years old, 11 percent had used inhalants at least once, and 2 percent were current users. Among adolescents 12 to 17 years old, 7 percent had used inhalants at least once, and 2 percent were current users. In one study of high school seniors, 18 percent reported having used inhalants at least once, and 2.7 percent reported having used inhalants within the preceding month. White users of inhalants are more common than either black or Hispanic users. Most users (up to 80 percent) are male. Some data suggest that inhalant use may be more common in suburban communities in the United States than in urban communities.

Inhalant use accounts for 1 percent of all substance-related deaths and fewer than 0.5 percent of all substance-related emergency room visits. Approximately 20 percent of the emergency room visits for inhalant use involve persons younger than 18 years of age. Inhalant use among adolescents may be most common in those whose parents or older siblings use illegal substances. Inhalant use among adolescents is also associated with an increased likelihood of conduct disorder or antisocial personality disorder.

Table 9.8–1
DSM-IV-TR Inhalant-Related Disorders

Inhalant use disorders
Inhalant dependence
Inhalant abuse
Inhalant-induced disorders
Inhalant intoxication
Inhalant intoxication delirium
Inhalant-induced persisting dementia
Inhalant-induced psychotic disorder, with delusions
   Specify if:
      With onset during intoxication
Inhalant-induced psychotic disorder, with hallucinations
   Specify if:
      With onset during intoxication
Inhalant-induced mood disorder
   Specify if:
      With onset during intoxication
Inhalant-induced anxiety disorder
   Specify if:
      With onset during intoxication
Inhalant-related disorder not otherwise specified

From American Psychiatric Association. *Diagnostic and Statistical Manual of Mental Disorders.* 4th ed. Text rev. Washington, DC: American Psychiatric Association; copyright 2000, with permission.

Table 9.8–2
DSM-IV-TR Diagnostic Criteria for Inhalant Intoxication

A. Recent intentional use or short-term, high-dose exposure to volatile inhalants (excluding anesthetic gases and short-acting vasodilators).
B. Clinically significant maladaptive behavioral or psychological changes (e.g., belligerence, assaultiveness, apathy, impaired judgment, impaired social or occupational functioning) that developed during, or shortly after, use of or exposure to volatile inhalants.
C. Two (or more) of the following signs, developing during, or shortly after, inhalant use or exposure:
   (1) dizziness
   (2) nystagmus
   (3) incoordination
   (4) slurred speech
   (5) unsteady gait
   (6) lethargy
   (7) depressed reflexes
   (8) psychomotor retardation
   (9) tremor
   (10) generalized muscle weakness
   (11) blurred vision or diplopia
   (12) stupor or coma
   (13) euphoria
D. The symptoms are not due to a general medical condition and are not better accounted for by another mental disorder.

From American Psychiatric Association. *Diagnostic and Statistical Manual of Mental Disorders.* 4th ed. Text rev. Washington, DC: American Psychiatric Association; copyright 2000, with permission.

NEUROPHARMACOLOGY

Persons usually use inhalants with a tube, a can, a plastic bag, or an inhalant-soaked rag, through or from which a user can sniff the inhalant through the nose or "huff" it through the mouth. Inhalants generally act as a central nervous system depressant. Tolerance for inhalants can develop, although withdrawal symptoms are usually fairly mild and are not classified as a disorder in DSM-IV-TR.

Inhalants are rapidly absorbed through the lungs and rapidly delivered to the brain. The effects appear within 5 minutes and may last for 30 minutes to several hours, depending on the inhalant substance and the dose. For example, 15 to 20 breaths of a 1 percent solution of gasoline may result in a high of several hours. The concentrations of many inhalant substances in blood are increased when used in combination with alcohol, perhaps because of competition for hepatic enzymes. Although approximately one-fifth of an inhalant substance is excreted unchanged by the lungs, the remainder is metabolized by the liver. Inhalants are detectable in the blood for 4 to 10 hours after use, and blood samples should be taken in the emergency room when inhalant use is suspected.

Much like alcohol, inhalants have specific pharmacodynamic effects that are not well understood. Because their effects are generally similar and additive to the effects of other central nervous system depressants (e.g., ethanol, barbiturates, and benzodiazepines), some investigators have suggested that inhalants operate by enhancing the γ-aminobutyric acid system. Other investigators have suggested that inhalants work through membrane fluidization, which has also been hypothesized to be a pharmacodynamic effect of ethanol.

DIAGNOSIS

DSM-IV-TR lists a number of inhalant-related disorders (Table 9.8–1) but contains specific diagnostic criteria only for inhalant intoxication (Table 9.8–2) within the inhalant-related disorders section. The diagnostic criteria of other inhalant-related disorders are specified in the DSM-IV-TR sections that specifically address the major symptoms—for example, inhalant-induced psychotic disorders (see Section 11.4).

Inhalant Dependence and Inhalant Abuse

Most persons probably use inhalants for a short time without developing a pattern of long-term use resulting in dependence and abuse. Nonetheless, dependence and abuse of inhalants occur and are diagnosed according to the standard DSM-IV-TR criteria for those syndromes (see Tables 9.1–3 and 9.1–4 in Section 9.1).

Inhalant Intoxication

The DSM-IV-TR diagnostic criteria for inhalant intoxication (Table 9.8–2) specify the presence of maladaptive behavioral changes and at least two physical symptoms. The intoxicated state is often characterized by apathy, diminished social and occupational functioning, impaired judgment, and impulsive or aggressive behavior, and it can be accompanied by nausea,

Table 9.8–3
DSM-IV-TR Diagnostic Criteria for Inhalant-Related Disorder Not Otherwise Specified

The inhalant-related disorder not otherwise specified category is for disorders associated with the use of inhalants that are not classifiable as inhalant dependence, inhalant abuse, inhalant intoxication, inhalant intoxication delirium, inhalant-induced persisting dementia, inhalant-induced psychotic disorder, inhalant-induced mood disorder, or inhalant-induced anxiety disorder.

From American Psychiatric Association. *Diagnostic and Statistical Manual of Mental Disorders.* 4th ed. Text rev. Washington, DC: American Psychiatric Association; copyright 2000, with permission.

anorexia, nystagmus, depressed reflexes, and diplopia. With high doses and long exposures, a user's neurological status can progress to stupor and unconsciousness, and a person may later be amnestic for the period of intoxication. Clinicians can sometimes identify a recent user of inhalants by rashes around the patient's nose and mouth; unusual breath odors; the residue of the inhalant substances on the patient's face, hands or clothing; and irritation of the patient's eyes, throat, lungs, and nose.

Inhalant Intoxication Delirium

Delirium can be induced by the effects of the inhalants themselves, by pharmacodynamic interactions with other substances, and by the hypoxia that may be associated with either the inhalant or its method of inhalation. If the delirium results in severe behavioral disturbances, short-term treatment with a dopamine receptor antagonist, such as haloperidol (Haldol), may be necessary. Benzodiazepines should be avoided because of the possibility of increasing the patient's respiratory depression.

Inhalant-Induced Persisting Dementia

Inhalant-induced persisting dementia, like delirium, may be due to the neurotoxic effects of the inhalants themselves, the neurotoxic effects of the metals (e.g., lead) commonly used in inhalants, or the effects of frequent and prolonged periods of hypoxia. The dementia caused by inhalants is likely to be irreversible in all but the mildest cases.

Inhalant-Induced Psychotic Disorder

Inhalant-induced psychotic disorder is a DSM-IV-TR diagnosis. Clinicians can specify hallucinations or delusions as the predominant symptoms. Paranoid states are probably the most common psychotic syndromes during inhalant intoxication.

Inhalant-Induced Mood Disorder and Inhalant-Induced Anxiety Disorder

Inhalant-induced mood disorder and inhalant-induced anxiety disorder are DSM-IV-TR diagnoses that allow the classification of inhalant-related disorders characterized by prominent mood and anxiety symptoms. Depressive disorders are the most common mood disorders associated with inhalant use, and panic disorders and generalized anxiety disorder are the most common anxiety disorders.

Inhalant-Related Disorder Not Otherwise Specified

Inhalant-related disorder not otherwise specified is the recommended DSM-IV-TR diagnosis for inhalant-related disorders that do not fit into one of the diagnostic categories discussed above (Table 9.8–3).

CLINICAL FEATURES

In small initial doses, inhalants may be disinhibiting and may produce feelings of euphoria and excitement and pleasant floating sensations, the effects for which persons presumably use the drugs. High doses of inhalants can cause psychological symptoms of fearfulness, sensory illusions, auditory and visual hallucinations, and distortions of body size. The neurological symptoms can include slurred speech, decreased speed of talking, and ataxia. Long-term use can be associated with irritability, emotional lability, and impaired memory.

Tolerance for the inhalants does develop; although not recognized by DSM-IV-TR, a withdrawal syndrome can accompany the cessation of inhalant use. The withdrawal syndrome does not occur frequently; when it does, it can be characterized by sleep disturbances, irritability, jitteriness, sweating, nausea, vomiting, tachycardia, and (sometimes) delusions and hallucinations.

Adverse Effects

Inhalants are associated with many potentially serious adverse effects. Death can result from respiratory depression, cardiac arrhythmias, asphyxiation, aspiration of vomitus, or accident or injury (e.g., driving while intoxicated with inhalants). Other serious adverse effects of long-term inhalant use include irreversible hepatic or renal damage and permanent muscle damage associated with rhabdomyolysis. The combination of organic solvents and high concentrations of copper, zinc, and heavy metals has been associated with the development of brain atrophy, temporal lobe epilepsy, decreased IQ, and electroencephalogram changes. Several studies of house painters and factory workers who have been exposed to solvents for long periods have shown evidence of brain atrophy on computed tomography scans and of decreases in cerebral blood flow. Additional adverse effects include cardiovascular and pulmonary symptoms (e.g., chest pain and bronchospasm), gastrointestinal symptoms (e.g., pain, nausea, vomiting, and hematemesis), and other neurological signs and symptoms (e.g., peripheral neuritis, headache, paresthesia, cerebellar signs, and lead encephalopathy). There are reports of brain atrophy, renal tubular acidosis, and long-term motor impairment in toluene users. Several reports concern serious adverse effects on fetal development when a pregnant woman uses or is exposed to inhalant substances.

TREATMENT

Inhalant intoxication, like alcohol intoxication, usually requires no medical attention and resolves spontaneously. However, effects of the intoxication, such as coma, bronchospasm, laryngospasm, cardiac arrhythmias, trauma, or burns, need treatment. Otherwise, care primarily involves reassurance, quiet support, and attention to vital signs and level of consciousness.

No established treatment exists for the cognitive and memory problems of inhalant-induced persisting dementia. Street outreach and extensive social service support have been offered to severely deteriorated, inhalant-dependent, homeless adults. Patients may require extensive support within their families or in foster or domiciliary care.

The course and treatment of inhalant-induced psychotic disorder are like those of inhalant intoxication. The disorder is brief, lasting a few hours to (at most) a very few weeks beyond the intoxication. Vigorous treatment of such life-threatening complications as respiratory or cardiac arrest, together with conservative management of the intoxication itself, is appropriate. Confusion, panic, and psychosis mandate special attention to patient safety. Severe agitation may require cautious control with haloperidol (5 mg intramuscularly per 70 kg body weight). Sedative drugs should be avoided, as they may aggravate the psychosis. Inhalant-induced anxiety and mood disorders may precipitate suicidal ideation, and patients should be carefully evaluated for that possibility. Antianxiety and antidepressants are not useful in the acute phase of the disorder; they may be of use if there is a coexisting anxiety or depressive illness.

▲ 9.9 Nicotine-Related Disorders

The landmark 1988 publication called *The Surgeon General's Report on the Health Consequences of Smoking: Nicotine Addiction* increased the awareness of the hazards of smoking to the American public. But the fact that approximately 30 percent continue to smoke despite the mountain of data showing how dangerous the habit is to their health is testament to the powerfully addictive properties of nicotine. The ill effects of cigarette and cigar smoking are reflected in the estimate that 60 percent of the direct health care costs in the United States go to treat tobacco-related illnesses and amount to an estimated $1 billion a day.

EPIDEMIOLOGY

The World Health Organization (WHO) estimates there are 1 billion smokers worldwide, and they smoke 6 trillion cigarettes a year. The WHO also estimates that tobacco kills more than 3 million persons each year. Although the number of persons in the United States who smoke is decreasing, the number of persons smoking in developing countries is increasing. The rate of quitting smoking has been highest among well-educated white men and lower among women, blacks, teenagers, and those with low levels of education.

Tobacco is the most common form of nicotine. It is smoked in cigarettes, cigars, and pipes and used as snuff and chewing tobacco (also called *smokeless tobacco*), both of which are increasingly popular in the United States. Approximately 32 percent of all persons in the United States currently use snuff or chewing tobacco, but approximately 6 percent of young adults ages 19 to 25 use those forms of tobacco.

Currently, approximately 25 percent of Americans smoke, 25 percent are former smokers, and 50 percent have never smoked cigarettes. The prevalence of pipe, cigar, and smokeless tobacco use is less than 2 percent. The prevalence of smoking in the United States was decreasing approximately 1 percent a year, but it has not changed in the last 4 years. The mean age of onset of smoking is 16, and few persons start after 20. Dependence features appear to develop quickly. Classroom and other programs to prevent initiation are only mildly effective, but increased taxation does decrease initiation.

More than 75 percent of smokers have tried to quit, and approximately 40 percent try to quit each year. On a given attempt, only 30 percent remain abstinent for even 2 days, and only 5 to 10 percent stop permanently. However, most smokers make five to ten attempts, so eventually 50 percent of "ever smokers" quit. In the past, 90 percent of successful attempts to quit involved no treatment. However, with the advent of over-the-counter (OTC) and nonnicotine medications in 1998, approximately one-third of all attempts involved the use of medication. According to the text revision of the fourth edition of the *Diagnostic and Statistical Manual of Mental Disorders* (DSM-IV-TR), approximately 85 percent of current daily smokers are nicotine dependent. Nicotine withdrawal occurs in approximately 50 percent of smokers who try to quit.

Education

Level of education attainment is correlated with tobacco usage. Thirty-seven percent of adults who had not completed high school smoked cigarettes, whereas only 17 percent of college graduates smoked.

Psychiatric Patients

Psychiatrists must be particularly concerned and knowledgeable about nicotine dependence because of the high proportion of psychiatric patients who smoke. Approximately 50 percent of all psychiatric outpatients, 70 percent of outpatients with bipolar I disorder, almost 90 percent of outpatients with schizophrenia, and 70 percent of substance use disorder patients smoke. Moreover, data indicate that patients with depressive disorders or anxiety disorders are less successful in their attempts to quit smoking than other persons; thus, a holistic health approach for these patients probably includes helping them address their smoking habits in addition to the primary mental disorder. The high percentage of schizophrenic patients who smoke has been attributed to the ability of nicotine to reduce their extraordinary sensitivity to outside sensory stimuli and to increase their concentration.

Death

Death is the primary adverse effect of cigarette smoking. Tobacco use is associated with approximately 400,000 premature deaths each year in the United States—25 percent of all deaths. The causes of death include chronic bronchitis and emphysema (51,000 deaths), bronchogenic cancer (106,000 deaths), 35 percent of fatal myocardial infarctions (115,000 deaths), cerebrovascular disease, cardiovascular disease, and almost all cases of chronic obstructive pulmonary disease and lung cancer. The increased use of chewing tobacco and snuff (smokeless tobacco) has been associated with the development of oropharyngeal cancer, and the resurgence of cigar smoking is likely to lead to an increase in the occurrence of this type of cancer.

Researchers have found that 30 percent of U.S. cancer deaths are caused by tobacco smoke, the single most lethal carcinogen in the United States. Smoking (mainly cigarette smoking) causes cancer of the lung, upper respiratory tract, esophagus, bladder, and pancreas and probably of the stomach, liver, and kidney. Smokers are eight times more likely than nonsmokers to develop lung cancer, and lung cancer has surpassed breast cancer as the leading cause of cancer-related deaths in women. Even secondhand smoke (discussed below) causes a few thousand cancer deaths each year in the United States, about the same number as are caused by radon exposure. Despite these staggering statistics, smokers can dramatically lower their chances of developing smoke-related cancers simply by quitting.

NEUROPHARMACOLOGY

The psychoactive component of tobacco is nicotine, which affects the central nervous system (CNS) by acting as an agonist at the nicotinic subtype of acetylcholine receptors. Approximately 25 percent of the nicotine inhaled during smoking reaches the bloodstream, through which nicotine reaches the brain within 15 seconds. The half-life of nicotine is approximately 2 hours. Nicotine is believed to produce its positive reinforcing and addictive properties by activating the dopaminergic pathway projecting from the ventral tegmental area to the cerebral cortex and the limbic system. In addition to activating this dopamine reward system, nicotine causes an increase in the concentrations of circulating norepinephrine and epinephrine and an increase in the release of vasopressin, β-endorphin, adrenocorticotropic hormone, and cortisol. These hormones are thought to contribute to the basic stimulatory effects of nicotine on the CNS.

DIAGNOSIS

DSM-IV-TR lists three nicotine-related disorders (Table 9.9–1) but contains specific diagnostic criteria for only nicotine withdrawal (Table 9.9–2) in the nicotine-related disorders section. The other nicotine-related disorders recognized by DSM-IV-TR are nicotine dependence and nicotine-related disorder not otherwise specified.

Nicotine Dependence

DSM-IV-TR allows for the diagnosis of nicotine dependence (see Table 9.1–4 in Section 9.1 of this chapter) but not nicotine abuse. Dependence on nicotine develops quickly, probably

Table 9.9–1
DSM-IV-TR Nicotine-Related Disorders

Nicotine use disorder
Nicotine dependence
Nicotine-induced disorder
Nicotine withdrawal
Nicotine-related disorder not otherwise specified

From American Psychiatric Association. *Diagnostic and Statistical Manual of Mental Disorders.* 4th ed. Text rev. Washington, DC: American Psychiatric Association; copyright 2000, with permission.

Table 9.9–2
DSM-IV-TR Diagnostic Criteria for Nicotine Withdrawal

A. Daily use of nicotine for at least several weeks.
B. Abrupt cessation of nicotine use, or reduction in the amount of nicotine used, followed within 24 hours by four (or more) of the following signs:
  (1) dysphoric or depressed mood
  (2) insomnia
  (3) irritability, frustration, or anger
  (4) anxiety
  (5) difficulty concentrating
  (6) restlessness
  (7) decreased heart rate
  (8) increased appetite or weight gain
C. The symptoms in Criterion B cause clinically significant distress or impairment in social, occupational, or other important areas of functioning.
D. The symptoms are not due to a general medical condition and are not better accounted for by another mental disorder.

From American Psychiatric Association. *Diagnostic and Statistical Manual of Mental Disorders.* 4th ed. Text rev. Washington, DC: American Psychiatric Association; copyright 2000, with permission.

because nicotine activates the ventral tegmental area dopaminergic system, the same system affected by cocaine and amphetamine. The development of dependence is enhanced by strong social factors that encourage smoking in some settings and by the powerful effects of tobacco company advertising. Persons are likely to smoke if their parents or siblings smoke and serve as role models. Several recent studies have also suggested a genetic diathesis toward nicotine dependence. Most persons who smoke want to quit and have tried many times to quit but have been unsuccessful.

Nicotine Withdrawal

DSM-IV-TR does not have a diagnostic category for nicotine intoxication but does have a diagnostic category for nicotine withdrawal (Table 9.9–2). Withdrawal symptoms can develop within 2 hours of smoking the last cigarette, generally peak in the first 24 to 48 hours, and can last for weeks or months. The common symptoms include an intense craving for nicotine, tension, irritability, difficulty concentrating, drowsiness and paradoxical trouble sleeping, decreased heart rate and blood pressure, increased appetite and weight gain, decreased motor performance, and increased muscle tension. A mild syndrome of nicotine withdrawal can appear when a smoker switches from regular to low-nicotine cigarettes.

Nicotine-Related Disorder Not Otherwise Specified

Nicotine-related disorder not otherwise specified is a diagnostic category for nicotine-related disorders that do not fit into one of the categories discussed above (Table 9.9–3). Such diagnoses may include nicotine intoxication, nicotine abuse, and mood disorders and anxiety disorders associated with nicotine use.

Table 9.9–3
DSM-IV-TR Diagnostic Criteria for Nicotine-Related Disorder Not Otherwise Specified

The nicotine-related disorder not otherwise specified category is for disorders associated with the use of nicotine that are not classifiable as nicotine dependence or nicotine withdrawal.

From American Psychiatric Association. *Diagnostic and Statistical Manual of Mental Disorders.* 4th ed. Text rev. Washington, DC: American Psychiatric Association; copyright 2000, with permission.

Table 9.9–4
Typical Quit Rates of Common Therapies

Therapy	Rate (%)
Self-quit	5
Self-help books	10
Physician advice	10
Over-the-counter patch or gum	15
Medication plus advice	20
Behavior therapy alone	20
Medication plus group therapy	30

CLINICAL FEATURES

Behaviorally, the stimulatory effects of nicotine produce improved attention, learning, reaction time, and problem-solving ability. Tobacco users also report that cigarette smoking lifts their mood, decreases tension, and lessens depressive feelings. Results of studies of the effects of nicotine on cerebral blood flow suggest that short-term nicotine exposure increased cerebral blood flow without changing cerebral oxygen metabolism, but long-term nicotine exposure decreases cerebral blood flow. In contrast to its stimulatory CNS effects, nicotine acts as a skeletal muscle relaxant.

Adverse Effects

Nicotine is a highly toxic alkaloid. Doses of 60 mg in an adult are fatal secondary to respiratory paralysis; doses of 0.5 mg are delivered by smoking an average cigarette. In low doses, the signs and symptoms of nicotine toxicity include nausea, vomiting, salivation, pallor (caused by increased peristalsis), diarrhea, dizziness, headache, increased blood pressure, tachycardia, tremor, and cold sweats. Toxicity is also associated with an inability to concentrate, confusion, and sensory disturbances. Nicotine is further associated with a decrease in the user's amount of rapid eye movement sleep. Tobacco use during pregnancy has been associated with an increased incidence of low-birth-weight babies and an increased incidence of newborns with persistent pulmonary hypertension.

Health Benefits of Smoking Cessation

Smoking cessation has major and immediate health benefits for persons of all ages and provides benefits for persons with and without smoking-related diseases. Former smokers live longer than those who continue to smoke. Smoking cessation decreases the risk for lung cancer and other cancers, myocardial infarction, cerebrovascular diseases, and chronic lung diseases. Women who stop smoking before pregnancy or during the first 3 to 4 months of pregnancy reduce their risk for having low-birth-weight infants to that of women who never smoked. The health benefits of smoking cessation substantially exceed any risks from the average 5-pound (2.3 kg) weight gain or any adverse psychological effects after quitting.

TREATMENT

Psychiatrists should advise all patients who are not in crisis to quit smoking. For patients who are ready to stop smoking, it is best to set a "quit date." Most clinicians and smokers prefer abrupt cessation, but because there are no good data to indicate that abrupt cessation is better than gradual cessation, patient preference for gradual cessation should be respected. Brief advice should focus on the need for medication or group therapy, weight gain concerns, high-risk situations, making cigarettes unavailable, and so forth. Because relapse is often rapid, the first follow-up phone call or visit should be 2 to 3 days after the quit date. These strategies have been shown to double self-initiated quit rates (Table 9.9–4).

Psychosocial Therapies

Behavior therapy is the most widely accepted and well-proved psychological therapy for smoking. Behavior therapy consists of several techniques, three of which are supported by good evidence. Skills training and relapse prevention identify high-risk situations and plan and practice behavioral or cognitive coping skills for these situations. Stimulus control involves eliminating cues for smoking in the environment. Rapid smoking has smokers smoke repeatedly to the point of nausea in sessions to associate smoking with unpleasant, rather than pleasant, sensations. This last therapy appears to be effective but requires a good therapeutic alliance and patient compliance.

Psychopharmacological Therapies

Nicotine Replacement Therapies.   All nicotine replacement therapies double cessation rates, presumably because they reduce nicotine withdrawal. These therapies can also be used to reduce withdrawal in patients on smoke-free wards. Replacement therapies use a short period of maintenance (6 to 12 weeks) often followed by a gradual reduction period (6 to 12 weeks).

Nicotine gum (Nicorette) is an OTC product that releases nicotine via chewing and buccal absorption. A 2-mg variety for those who smoke less than 25 cigarettes a day and a 4-mg variety for those who smoke more than 25 cigarettes a day are available. Smokers are to use one to two pieces of gum per hour after abrupt cessation. Venous blood concentrations from the gum are one-third to one-half the between-cigarette levels. Acidic beverages (coffee, tea, soda, and juice) should not be used before, during, or after gum use because they decrease absorption. Compliance with the gum has often been a problem. Adverse effects are minor and include bad taste and sore jaws. Approximately 20 percent of those who quit use the gum for long periods, but 2 percent use gum for longer than a year; long-term use does not appear to be harmful. The major advantage of nicotine gum is its ability to provide relief in high-risk situations.

Nicotine patches, also sold OTC, are available in a 16-hour no-taper preparation (Habitrol) and a 24- or 16-hour tapering preparation (Nicoderm CQ). Patches are administered each morning and produce blood concentrations about half those of smoking. Compliance is high, and the only major adverse effects are rashes and, with 24-hour wear, insomnia. Long-term use does not occur. Using gum and patches in high-risk situations increases quit rates by another 5 to 10 percent. No studies have been done to determine the relative efficacies of 24- or 16-hour patches or of taper and no-taper patches.

Nicotine nasal spray (Nicotrol), available only by prescription, produces nicotine concentrations in the blood that are more similar to those from smoking a cigarette, and it appears to be especially helpful for heavily dependent smokers. However, the spray causes rhinitis, watering eyes, and coughing in more than 70 percent of patients. Although initial data suggested abuse liability, further trials have not found this.

The nicotine inhaler, a prescription product, was designed to deliver nicotine to the lungs, but the nicotine is actually absorbed in the upper throat. Resultant nicotine levels are low. The major asset of the inhaler is that it provides a behavioral substitute for smoking. The inhaler also doubles quit rates. These devices require frequent puffing, which can cause minor adverse effects.

Nonnicotine Medications. Nonnicotine therapy may help smokers who object philosophically to the notion of replacement therapy and smokers who fail replacement therapy. Bupropion (Zyban) (marketed as Wellbutrin for depression) is an antidepressant medication that has both dopaminergic and adrenergic actions. Daily dosages of 300 mg reliably double quit rates in smokers with and without a history of depression. In one study, combined bupropion and nicotine patch had higher quit rates than either alone. Adverse effects include insomnia and nausea, but these are rarely significant. Seizures have not occurred in smoking trials. Interestingly, nortriptyline (Pamelor) appears to be effective for smoking cessation.

Clonidine (Catapres) decreases sympathetic activity from the locus ceruleus and thus is thought to abate withdrawal symptoms. Whether given as a patch or orally, 0.2 to 0.4 mg a day of clonidine appears to double quit rates; however, the scientific database for the efficacy of clonidine is neither as extensive nor as reliable as that for nicotine replacement; also, clonidine can cause drowsiness and hypotension. Some patients benefit from benzodiazepine therapy (10 to 30 mg per day) for the first 2 to 3 weeks of abstinence.

A nicotine vaccine that produces nicotine-specific antibodies in the brain is under investigation at the National Institute on Drug Abuse.

Smoke-Free Environment

Secondhand smoke may contribute to lung cancer death and coronary heart disease in adult nonsmokers. Each year, an estimated 3,000 lung cancer deaths and 62,000 deaths from coronary heart disease in adult nonsmokers are attributed to secondhand smoke. Among children, secondhand smoke is implicated in sudden infant death syndrome, low birth weight, chronic middle ear infections, and respiratory illnesses (e.g., asthma, bronchitis, and pneumonia). Two national health objectives for 2010 are to reduce cigarette smoking among adults to 12 per-

cent and the proportion of nonsmokers exposed to environment tobacco smoke to 45 percent.

Involuntary exposure to secondhand smoke remains a common public health hazard that is preventable by appropriate regulatory policies. Bans on smoking in public places reduce exposure to secondhand smoke and the number of cigarettes smoked by smokers. There is nearly universal support for bans in schools and day-care centers and strong support for bans in indoor work areas and restaurants. Clean indoor air policies are one way to change social norms about smoking and reduce tobacco consumption.

▲ 9.10 Opioid-Related Disorders

Opioids have been used for at least 3,500 years, mostly in the form of crude opium or in alcoholic solutions of opium. Morphine was first isolated in 1806 and codeine in 1832. Over the next century, pure morphine and codeine gradually replaced crude opium for medicinal purposes, although nonmedical use of opium (as for smoking) still persists in some parts of the world. The words *opiate* and *opioid* come from the word *opium*, the juice of the opium poppy, *Papaver somniferum*, which contains approximately 20 opium alkaloids, including morphine.

Opioid dependence is a cluster of physiological, behavioral, and cognitive symptoms, which, taken together, indicates repeated and continuing use of opioid drugs despite significant problems related to such use. Drug dependence in general has also been defined by the World Health Organization as a syndrome in which the use of a drug or class of drugs takes on a much higher priority for a given person than other behaviors that once had a higher value. These brief definitions each have as their central features an emphasis on the drug-using behavior itself, its maladaptive nature, and how the choice to engage in that behavior shifts and becomes constrained as a result of interaction with the drug over time.

Opioid abuse is a term used to designate a pattern of maladaptive use of an opioid drug leading to clinically significant impairment or distress and occurring within a 12-month period, but one in which the symptoms have never met the criteria for opioid dependence.

The *opioid-induced disorders* as defined by the text revision of the fourth edition of the *Diagnostic and Statistical Manual of Mental Disorders* (DSM-IV-TR) include opioid intoxication, opioid withdrawal, opioid-induced sleep disorder, opioid-induced sexual dysfunction, opioid intoxication delirium, opioid-induced psychotic disorder, opioid-induced mood disorder, and opioid-induced anxiety disorder. DSM-IV-TR also includes *opioid-related disorder not otherwise specified* for situations that do not meet the criteria for any of the other opioid-related disorders.

EPIDEMIOLOGY

Persons with opioid dependence use heroin (see below) most widely. According to DSM-IV-TR, the lifetime prevalence for heroin use is approximately 1 percent, with 0.2 percent having taken the drug during the prior year. The number of current heroin users has been questionably estimated to be between 600,000 and 800,000. The number of persons estimated to have used heroin at any time in their lives ("lifetime users") is approximately 2 million. The male-to-female ratio of persons with heroin dependence is approximately 3 to 1. Users of opioids typically started to use substances in their teens and early 20s; currently, most persons with opioid dependence are in their 30s and 40s. According to DSM-IV-TR, the tendency for dependence to remit generally begins after age 40 years and has been called "maturing out." However, many persons have remained opioid dependent for 50 years or longer.

NEUROPHARMACOLOGY

The primary effects of the opioids are mediated through the opioid receptors, which were discovered in the second half of the 1970s. The μ-opioid receptors are involved in the regulation and mediation of analgesia, respiratory depression, constipation, and dependence; the κ-opioid receptors, with analgesia, diuresis, and sedation; and the δ-opioid receptors, possibly with analgesia.

In 1974, enkephalin, an endogenous pentapeptide with opioid-like actions, was identified. This discovery led to the identification of three classes of endogenous opioids within the brain, including the endorphins and the enkephalins. Endorphins are involved in neural transmission and pain suppression. They are released naturally in the body when a person is physically hurt and account in part for the absence of pain during acute injuries.

The opioids also have significant effects on the dopaminergic and noradrenergic neurotransmitter systems. Several types of data indicate that the addictive rewarding properties of opioids are mediated through activation of the ventral tegmental area dopaminergic neurons that project to the cerebral cortex and the limbic system.

Heroin is the most commonly abused opioid and is more potent and lipid soluble than morphine. Because of those properties, heroin crosses the blood–brain barrier faster and has a more rapid onset than morphine. Heroin was first introduced as a treatment for morphine addiction, but heroin, in fact, is more dependence producing than morphine. Codeine, which occurs naturally as about 0.5 percent of the opiate alkaloids in opium, is absorbed easily through the gastrointestinal tract and is subsequently transformed into morphine in the body. Results of at least one study using positron emission tomography have suggested that one effect of all opioids is decreased cerebral blood flow in selected brain regions in persons with opioid dependence.

Tolerance and Dependence

Tolerance does not develop uniformly to all actions of opioid drugs. Tolerance to some actions of opioids can be so high that a hundredfold increase in dose is required to produce the original effect. For example, terminally ill cancer patients may need 200 to 300 mg a day of morphine, whereas a dose of 60 mg can easily be fatal to an opioid-naïve person. The symptoms of opioid withdrawal do not appear unless a person has been using opioids for a long time or when cessation is particularly abrupt, as occurs functionally when an opioid antagonist is given. The long-term use of opioids results in changes in the number and sensitivity of opioid receptors, which mediate at least some of the effects of tolerance and withdrawal. Although long-term use is associated with increased sensitivity of the dopaminergic, cholinergic, and serotonergic neurons, the effect of opioids on the norad-

renergic neurons is probably the primary mediator of the symptoms of opioid withdrawal. Short-term use of opioids apparently decreases the activity of the noradrenergic neurons in the locus ceruleus, long-term use activates a compensatory homeostatic mechanism within the neurons, and opioid withdrawal results in a rebound hyperactivity. This hypothesis also provides an explanation for why clonidine (Catapres), an α_2-adrenergic receptor agonist that decreases the release of norepinephrine, is useful in the treatment of opioid withdrawal symptoms.

COMORBIDITY

Approximately 90 percent of persons with opioid dependence have an additional psychiatric disorder. The most common comorbid psychiatric diagnoses are major depressive disorder, alcohol use disorders, antisocial personality disorder, and anxiety disorders. Approximately 15 percent of persons with opioid dependence attempt to commit suicide at least once. The high prevalence of comorbidity with other psychiatric diagnoses highlights the need to develop a broad-based treatment program that also addresses patients' associated psychiatric disorders.

ETIOLOGY

Psychosocial Factors

Opioid dependence is not limited to low socioeconomic classes, although the incidence of opioid dependence is greater in these groups than in higher socioeconomic classes. Social factors associated with urban poverty probably contribute to opioid dependence. Approximately 50 percent of urban heroin users are children of single parents or divorced parents and are from families in which at least one other member has a substance-related disorder. Children from such settings are at high risk for opioid dependence, especially if they also evidence behavioral problems in school or other signs of conduct disorder.

Some consistent behavior patterns seem to be especially pronounced in adolescents with opioid dependence. These patterns have been called the *heroin behavior syndrome*: underlying depression, often of an agitated type and frequently accompanied by anxiety symptoms; impulsiveness expressed by a passive-aggressive orientation; fear of failure; use of heroin as an antianxiety agent to mask feelings of low self-esteem, hopelessness, and aggression; limited coping strategies and low frustration tolerance, accompanied by the need for immediate gratification; sensitivity to drug contingencies, with a keen awareness of the relation between good feelings and the act of drug taking; feelings of behavioral impotence counteracted by momentary control over the life situation by means of substances; and disturbances in social and interpersonal relationships with peers maintained by mutual substance experiences.

Biological and Genetic Factors

There is evidence for genetically transmitted vulnerability factors that increase the likelihood of developing drug dependence. Monozygotic twins are more likely than dizygotic twins to be concordant for opioid dependence.

A person with an opioid-related disorder may have had genetically determined hypoactivity of the opiate system. Researchers are investigating the possibility that such hypoactivity may be

Table 9.10–1
DSM-IV-TR Opioid-Related Disorders

Opioid use disorders
Opioid dependence
Opioid abuse
Opioid-induced disorders
Opioid intoxication
    Specify if:
        With perceptual disturbances
Opioid withdrawal
Opioid intoxication delirium
Opioid-induced psychotic disorder, with delusions
    Specify if:
        With onset during intoxication
Opioid-induced psychotic disorder, with hallucinations
    Specify if:
        With onset during intoxication
Opioid-induced mood disorder
    Specify if:
        With onset during intoxication
Opioid-induced sexual dysfunction
    Specify if:
        With onset during intoxication
Opioid-induced sleep disorder
    Specify if:
        With onset during intoxication
        With onset during withdrawal
Opioid-related disorder not otherwise specified

From American Psychiatric Association. *Diagnostic and Statistical Manual of Mental Disorders.* 4th ed. Text rev. Washington, DC: American Psychiatric Association; copyright 2000, with permission.

Table 9.10–2
DSM-IV-TR Diagnostic Criteria for Opioid Intoxication

A. Recent use of an opioid.
B. Clinically significant maladaptive behavioral or psychological changes (e.g., initial euphoria followed by apathy, dysphoria, psychomotor agitation or retardation, impaired judgment, or impaired social or occupational functioning) that developed during, or shortly after, opioid use.
C. Pupillary constriction (or pupillary dilation due to anoxia from severe overdose) and one (or more) of the following signs, developing during, or shortly after, opioid use:
    (1) drowsiness or coma
    (2) slurred speech
    (3) impairment in attention or memory
D. The symptoms are not due to a general medical condition and are not better accounted for by another mental disorder.
Specify if:
    With perceptual disturbances

From American Psychiatric Association. *Diagnostic and Statistical Manual of Mental Disorders.* 4th ed. Text rev. Washington, DC: American Psychiatric Association; copyright 2000, with permission.

9.10–3) within the section on opioid-related disorders. The diagnostic criteria for the other opioid-related disorders are contained within the DSM-IV-TR sections that deal specifically with the predominant symptom—for example, opioid-induced mood disorder.

caused by too few or less sensitive opioid receptors by release of too little endogenous opioid, or by overly high concentrations of a hypothesized endogenous opioid antagonist. A biological predisposition to an opioid-related disorder may also be associated with abnormal functioning in either the dopaminergic or the noradrenergic neurotransmitter system.

Psychodynamic Theory

In psychoanalytic literature, the behavior of persons addicted to narcotics has been described in terms of libidinal fixation, with regression to pregenital, oral, or even more archaic levels of psychosexual development. The need to explain the relation of drug abuse, defense mechanisms, impulse control, affective disturbances, and adaptive mechanisms led to the shift from psychosexual formulations to formulations emphasizing ego psychology. Serious ego pathology is often thought to be associated with substance abuse and is considered to indicate profound developmental disturbances. Problems of the relation between the ego and affects emerge as a key area of difficulty.

DIAGNOSIS

DSM-IV-TR lists several opioid-related disorders (Table 9.10–1) but contains specific diagnostic criteria only for opioid intoxication (Table 9.10–2) and opioid withdrawal (Table

Table 9.10–3
DSM-IV-TR Diagnostic Criteria for Opioid Withdrawal

A. Either of the following:
    (1) cessation of (or reduction in) opioid use that has been heavy and prolonged (several weeks or longer)
    (2) administration of an opioid antagonist after a period of opioid use
B. Three (or more) of the following, developing within minutes to several days after Criterion A:
    (1) dysphoric mood
    (2) nausea or vomiting
    (3) muscle aches
    (4) lacrimation or rhinorrhea
    (5) pupillary dilation, piloerection, or sweating
    (6) diarrhea
    (7) yawning
    (8) fever
    (9) insomnia
C. The symptoms in Criterion B cause clinically significant distress or impairment in social, occupational, or other important areas of functioning.
D. The symptoms are not due to a general medical condition and are not better accounted for by another mental disorder.

From American Psychiatric Association. *Diagnostic and Statistical Manual of Mental Disorders.* 4th ed. Text rev. Washington, DC: American Psychiatric Association; copyright 2000, with permission.

Opioid Dependence and Opioid Abuse

Opioid dependence and opioid abuse are defined in DSM-IV-TR according to the general criteria for these disorders (see Table 9.1–4).

Opioid Intoxication

DSM-IV-TR defines opioid intoxication as including maladaptive behavioral changes and some specific physical symptoms of opioid use (Table 9.10–2). In general, altered mood, psychomotor retardation, drowsiness, slurred speech, and impaired memory and attention in the presence of other indicators of recent opioid use strongly suggest a diagnosis of opioid intoxication. DSM-IV-TR allows for the specification of "with perceptual disturbances."

Opioid Withdrawal

The general rule about the onset and duration of withdrawal symptoms is that substances with short durations of action tend to produce short, intense withdrawal syndromes, and substances with long durations of action produce prolonged but mild withdrawal syndromes. An exception to the rule, narcotic antagonist-precipitated withdrawal after long-acting opioid dependence can be severe.

An abstinence syndrome can be precipitated by administration of an opioid antagonist. The symptoms may begin within seconds of such an intravenous injection and may peak in approximately 1 hour. Opioid craving rarely occurs in the context of analgesic administration for pain from physical disorders or surgery. The full withdrawal syndrome, including intense craving for opioids, usually occurs only secondary to abrupt cessation of use in persons with opioid dependence.

Morphine and Heroin.   The morphine and heroin withdrawal syndrome begins 6 to 8 hours after the last dose, usually after a 1- to 2-week period of continuous use or after the administration of a narcotic antagonist. The withdrawal syndrome reaches its peak intensity during the second or third day and subsides during the next 7 to 10 days, but some symptoms may persist for 6 months or longer.

Meperidine.   The withdrawal syndrome from meperidine begins quickly, reaches a peak in 8 to 12 hours, and ends in 4 to 5 days.

Methadone.   Methadone withdrawal usually begins 1 to 3 days after the last dose and ends in 10 to 14 days.

Symptoms.   Opioid withdrawal (Table 9.10–3) consists of severe muscle cramps and bone aches, profuse diarrhea, abdominal cramps, rhinorrhea, lacrimation, piloerection or gooseflesh (from which comes the term *cold turkey* for the abstinence syndrome), yawning, fever, papillary dilation, hypertension, tachycardia, and temperature dysregulation, including hypothermia and hyperthermia. Persons with opioid dependence seldom die from opioid withdrawal, unless they have a severe preexisting physical illness such as cardiac disease. Residual symptoms—such as insomnia, bradycardia, temperature dysregulation, and a craving for opioids—may persist for months after withdrawal. Associated features of opioid withdrawal include restlessness, irritability, depression, tremor,

weakness, nausea, and vomiting. At any time during the abstinence syndrome, a single injection of morphine or heroin eliminates all the symptoms.

Opioid Intoxication Delirium

Opioid intoxication delirium is most likely to happen when opioids are used in high doses, are mixed with other psychoactive compounds, or are used by a person with preexisting brain damage or a central nervous system disorder (e.g., epilepsy).

Opioid-Induced Psychotic Disorder

Opioid-induced psychotic disorder can begin during opioid intoxication. The DSM-IV-TR diagnostic criteria are contained in the section on schizophrenia and other psychotic disorders. Clinicians can specify whether hallucinations or delusions are the predominant symptoms.

Opioid-Induced Mood Disorder

Opioid-induced mood disorder can begin during opioid intoxication. Opioid-induced mood disorder symptoms may have a manic, depressed, or mixed nature, depending on a person's response to opioids. A person coming to psychiatric attention with opioid-induced mood disorder usually has mixed symptoms, combining irritability, expansiveness, and depression.

Opioid-Induced Sleep Disorder and Opioid-Induced Sexual Dysfunction

Opioid-induced sleep disorder and opioid-induced sexual dysfunction are diagnostic categories in DSM-IV-TR. Hypersomnia is likely to be more common with opioids than insomnia. The most common sexual dysfunction is likely to be impotence.

Opioid-Related Disorder Not Otherwise Specified

DSM-IV-TR includes diagnoses for opioid-related disorders with symptoms of delirium, abnormal mood, psychosis, abnormal sleep, and sexual dysfunction. Clinical situations that do not fit into these categories exemplify appropriate cases for the use of the DSM-IV-TR diagnosis of opioid-related disorder not otherwise specified (Table 9.10–4).

Table 9.10–4
DSM-IV-TR Diagnostic Criteria for Opioid-Related Disorder Not Otherwise Specified

The opioid-related disorder not otherwise specified category is for disorders associated with the use of opioids that are not classifiable as opioid dependence, opioid abuse, opioid intoxication, opioid withdrawal, opioid intoxication delirium, opioid-induced psychotic disorder, opioid-induced mood disorder, opioid-induced sexual dysfunction, or opioid-induced sleep disorder.

From American Psychiatric Association. *Diagnostic and Statistical Manual of Mental Disorders.* 4th ed. Text rev. Washington, DC: American Psychiatric Association; copyright 2000, with permission.

CLINICAL FEATURES

Opioids can be taken orally, snorted intranasally, and injected intravenously (IV) or subcutaneously. Opioids are subjectively addictive because of the euphoric high (the rush) that users experience, especially those who take the substances IV. The associated symptoms include a feeling of warmth, heaviness of the extremities, dry mouth, itchy face (especially the nose), and facial flushing. The initial euphoria is followed by a period of sedation, known in street parlance as "nodding off." Opioid use can induce dysphoria, nausea, and vomiting in opioid-naïve persons.

The physical effects of opioids include respiratory depression, papillary constriction, smooth muscle contraction (including the ureters and the bile ducts), constipation, and changes in blood pressure, heart rate, and body temperature. The respiratory depressant effects are mediated at the level of the brainstem.

Adverse Effects

The most common and most serious adverse effect associated with the opioid-related disorders is the potential transmission of hepatitis and HIV through the use of contaminated needles by more than one person. Persons can experience idiosyncratic allergic reactions to opioids, which result in anaphylactic shock, pulmonary edema, and death if they do not receive prompt and adequate treatment. Another serious adverse effect is an idiosyncratic drug interaction between meperidine and monoamine oxidase inhibitors, which can produce gross autonomic instability, severe behavioral agitation, coma, seizures, and death. Opioids and monoamine oxidase inhibitors should not be given together for this reason.

Opioid Overdose

Death from an overdose of an opioid is usually attributable to respiratory arrest from the respiratory depressant effect of the drug. The symptoms of overdose include marked unresponsiveness, coma, slow respiration, hypothermia, hypotension, and bradycardia. When presented with the clinical triad of coma, pinpoint pupils, and respiratory depression, clinicians should consider opioid overdose as a primary diagnosis. They can also inspect the patient's body for needle tracks in the arms, legs, ankles, groin, and even the dorsal vein of the penis.

MPTP-Induced Parkinsonism

In 1976, after ingesting an opioid contaminated with *N*-methyl-4-phenyl-1,2,3,6-tetrahydropyridine (MPTP), several persons developed a syndrome of irreversible parkinsonism. The mechanism for the neurotoxic effect is as follows: MPTP is converted into 1-methyl-4-phenylpyridinium (MPP+) by the enzyme monoamine oxidase and is then taken up by dopaminergic neurons. Because MPP+ binds to melanin in substantia nigra neurons, MPP+ is concentrated in these neurons and eventually kills the cells. Positron emission tomography studies of persons who ingested MPTP but remained asymptomatic have shown a decreased number of dopamine-binding sites in the substantia nigra. This decrease reflects a loss in the number of dopaminergic neurons in that region.

TREATMENT AND REHABILITATION

Overdose Treatment

The first task is to ensure an adequate airway. Tracheopharyngeal secretions should be aspirated; an airway may be inserted. The patient should be ventilated mechanically until naloxone, a specific opioid antagonist, can be given. Naloxone is administered IV at a slow rate—initially approximately 0.8 mg per 70 mg per 70 kg of body weight. Signs of improvement (increased respiratory rate and papillary dilation) should occur promptly. In opioid-dependent patients, too much naloxone may produce signs of withdrawal as well as reversal of overdosage. If there is no response to the initial dosage, naloxone administration may be repeated after intervals of a few minutes. In the past, it was thought that if no response was observed after 4 to 5 mg, the central nervous system depression was probably not due solely to opioids. The duration of action of naloxone is short compared with that of many opioids, such as methadone and levomethadyl acetate, and repeated administration may be required to prevent recurrence of opioid toxicity.

Withdrawal and Detoxification

Methadone.   Methadone is a synthetic narcotic (an opioid) that substitutes for heroin and can be taken orally. When given to addicts to replace their usual substance of abuse, the drug suppresses withdrawal symptoms. A daily dose of 20 to 80 mg suffices to stabilize a patient, although daily doses of up to 120 mg have been used. Methadone has a duration of action exceeding 24 hours; thus, once-daily dosing is adequate. Methadone maintenance is continued until the patient can be withdrawn from methadone, which itself causes dependence. An abstinence syndrome occurs with methadone withdrawal, but patients are detoxified from methadone more easily than from heroin. Clonidine (0.1 to 0.3 mg three to four times a day) is usually given during the detoxification period.

Methadone maintenance has several advantages. First, it frees persons with opioid dependence from using injectable heroin and thus reduces the chance of spreading the human immunodeficiency virus (HIV) through contaminated needles. Second, methadone produces minimal euphoria and rarely causes drowsiness or depression when taken for a long time. Third, methadone allows patients to engage in gainful employment instead of criminal activity. The major disadvantage of methadone use is that patients remain dependent on a narcotic.

Other Opioid Substitutes.   Levomethadyl (ORLAAM), also called L-α-acetylmethadol (LAMM), a longer-acting opioid than methadone, is also used to treat persons with opioid dependence. In contrast to the daily methadone treatment, LAMM can be administered in dosages of 30 to 80 mg three times a week; because of this less frequent dosing regimen, an increasing number of programs are using LAMM.

Buprenorphine is an opioid partial agonist and is an analgesic with opioid antagonist activity approved only for treatment of moderate-to-severe pain. Buprenorphine in a daily dose of 8 to 10 mg appears to reduce heroin use. Buprenorphine also is effective in thrice-weekly dosing because of its slow dissociation from opioid receptors.

Opioid Antagonists.   Opioid antagonists block or antagonize the effects of opioids. Unlike methadone, they do not exert narcotic effects and do not cause dependence. Opioid antagonists include naloxone, which is used in the treatment of opioid overdose because it reverses the effects of narcotics, and naltrexone, the longest-acting (72 hours) antagonist. The theory for using an antagonist for opioid-related disorders is that blocking opioid agonist effects, particularly euphoria, discourages persons with opioid dependence from substance-seeking behavior and thus deconditions this behavior. The major weakness of the antagonist treatment model is the lack of any mechanism that compels a person to continue to take the antagonist.

Pregnant Women with Opioid Dependence

Neonatal addiction is a significant problem. Approximately three-fourths of all infants born to addicted mothers experience the withdrawal syndrome.

Neonatal Withdrawal.   Although opioid withdrawal rarely is fatal for the otherwise healthy adult, it is hazardous to the fetus and can lead to miscarriage or fetal death. Maintaining a pregnant woman with opioid dependence on a low dosage of methadone (10 to 40 mg daily) may be the least hazardous course to follow. At this dosage, neonatal withdrawal is usually mild and can be managed with low doses of paregoric. If pregnancy begins while a woman is taking high doses of methadone, the dosage should be reduced slowly (e.g., 1 mg every 3 days), and fetal movements should be monitored. If withdrawal is necessary or desired, it is least hazardous during the second trimester.

Fetal Acquired Immune Deficiency Syndrome Transmission.   Acquired immune deficiency syndrome (AIDS) is the other major risk to the fetus of a woman with opioid dependence. Pregnant women can pass HIV, the causative agent of AIDS, to the fetus through the placental circulation. An HIV-infected mother can also pass HIV to the infant through breast-feeding. The use of zidovudine (Retrovir) alone or in combination with other anti-HIV medication in infected women can decrease the incidence of HIV in newborns.

Psychotherapy

The entire range of psychotherapeutic modalities is appropriate for treating opioid-related disorders. Individual psychotherapy, behavioral therapy, cognitive-behavioral therapy, family therapy, support groups (e.g., Narcotics Anonymous), and social skills training may all prove effective for specific patients. Social skills training should be particularly emphasized for patients with few social skills. Family therapy is usually indicated when the patient lives with family members.

Therapeutic Communities

Therapeutic communities are residences in which all members have a problem of substance abuse. Abstinence is the rule; to be admitted to such a community, a person must show a high level of motivation. The goals are to effect a complete change of lifestyle, including abstinence from substances; to develop personal honesty, responsibility, and useful social skills; and to eliminate antisocial attitudes and criminal behavior.

Self-Help

Narcotics Anonymous is a self-help group of abstinent drug addicts modeled on the 12-step principles of Alcoholics Anonymous. Such groups now exist in most large cities and can provide useful group support. The outcome of patients treated in 12-step programs is generally good, but the anonymity that is at the core of the 12-step model has made detailed evaluation of its efficacy in treating opioid dependence difficult.

Education and Needle Exchange

Although the essential treatment of opioid use disorder is encouraging persons to abstain from opioids, education about the transmission of HIV must receive equal attention. Persons with opioid dependence who use IV or subcutaneous routes of administration must be taught available safe-sex practices. Free needle-exchange programs are often subject to intense political and societal pressures but, where allowed, should be made available to persons with opioid dependence.

▲ 9.11 Phencyclidine (or Phencyclidine-like)-Related Disorders

Phencyclidine (1,1[phenylcyclohexyl]piperidine; PCP), also known as "angel dust," was developed and is classified as a dissociative anesthetic. Its use as an anesthetic in humans, however, was associated with disorientation, agitation, delirium, and unpleasant hallucinations on awakening. Therefore, PCP is no longer used as an anesthetic in humans, although it is used in some countries as an anesthetic in veterinary medicine. Although PCP has a long duration of action and is very potent by any route of administration, PCP use carries a high risk of behavioral, physiological, and neurological toxicity, and it is highly reinforcing. A related compound, ketamine (Ketalar), also referred to as "special K," is still used as a human anesthetic in the Untied States; it has not been associated with the same adverse effects and is also subject to abuse. PCP was first used illicitly in San Francisco in the late 1960s. Since then, approximately 30 chemical analogues have been produced and are intermittently available on the streets of major U.S. cities.

EPIDEMIOLOGY

PCP and some related substances are relatively easy to synthesize in illegal laboratories and relatively inexpensive to buy on the streets. The variable quality of the laboratories, however, results in a range of potency and purity. PCP use varies most markedly with geography. Some areas of some cities have a tenfold higher usage rate of PCP than other areas. The highest PCP use in the United States is in Washington, D.C., where PCP accounts for 18 percent of all substance-related deaths. In Los Angeles, Chicago, and Baltimore, the comparable figure is 6 percent. Most users of PCP also use other substances, particularly alcohol, but also opiates, opioids, marijuana, amphetamines, and cocaine. PCP is frequently added to marijuana, with severe untoward effects on users. PCP is associated with 3 percent of substance abuse deaths and 32 percent of substance-related emergency room visits nationally.

NEUROPHARMACOLOGY

PCP and its related compounds are variously sold as a crystalline powder, paste, liquid, or drug-soaked paper (blotter). PCP is most commonly used as an additive to a cannabis- or parsley-containing cigarette. Experienced users report that the effects of 2 to 3 mg of smoked PCP occur in approximately 5 minutes and plateau in 30 minutes. The bioavailability of PCP is approximately 75 percent when taken by intravenous administration and approximately 30 percent when smoked. The half-life of PCP in humans is approximately 20 hours, and the half-life of ketamine in humans is approximately 2 hours.

The primary pharmacodynamic effect of PCP and ketamine is as an antagonist at N-methyl-D-aspartate (NMDA) subtype of glutamate receptors. PCP binds to a site within the NMDA-associated calcium channel and prevents the influx of calcium ions. PCP also activates the dopaminergic neurons of the ventral tegmental area, which project to the cerebral cortex and the limbic system. Activation of these neurons is usually involved in mediating the reinforcing qualities of PCP.

Tolerance for the effects of PCP occurs in humans, although physical dependence generally does not occur. In animals that are administered more PCP per pound for longer times than virtually any humans, however, PCP does induce physical dependence, with marked withdrawal symptoms of lethargy, depression, and craving. Physical symptoms of withdrawal in humans are rare, probably as a function of dose and duration of use. Although physical dependence on PCP is rare in humans, psychological dependence on PCP, as well as ketamine, is common, and some users become psychologically dependent on the PCP-induced psychological state.

The fact that PCP is made in illicit laboratories contributes to the increased likelihood of impurities in the final product. One such contaminant is 1-piperidenocyclohexane carbonitrite, which releases hydrogen cyanide in small quantities when ingested. Another contaminant is piperidine, which can be recognized by its strong, fishy odor.

DIAGNOSIS

DSM-IV-TR lists a number of PCP (or PCP-like)-related disorders (Table 9.11–1) but outlines the specific diagnostic criteria for only PCP intoxication (Table 9.11–2) within the PCP (or PCP-like)-related disorder section.

PCP Dependence and PCP Abuse

DSM-IV-TR uses the general criteria for PCP dependence and PCP abuse (See Tables 9.1–3 and 9.1–4 in Section 9.1 of this chapter). Some long-term users of PCP are said to be "crystallized," a syndrome characterized by dulled thinking, decreased reflexes, loss of memory, loss of impulse control, depression, lethargy, and impaired concentration.

PCP Intoxication

Short-term PCP intoxication can have potentially severe complications and must often be considered a psychiatric emergency. DSM-IV-TR gives specific criteria for PCP intoxication (Table 9.11–2). Clinicians can specify the presence of perceptual disturbances.

Table 9.11–1
DSM-IV-TR Phencyclidine-Related Disorders

Phencyclidine use disorders
Phencyclidine dependence
Phencyclidine abuse
Phencyclidine-induced disorders
Phencyclidine intoxication
   Specify if:
      With perceptual disturbances
Phencyclidine intoxication delirium
Phencyclidine-induced psychotic disorder, with delusions
   Specify if:
      With onset during intoxication
Phencyclidine-induced psychotic disorder, with hallucination
   Specify if:
      With onset during intoxication
Phencyclidine-induced mood disorder
   Specify if:
      With onset during intoxication
Phencyclidine-induced anxiety disorder
   Specify if:
      With onset during intoxication
Phencyclidine-related disorder not otherwise specified

From American Psychiatric Association. *Diagnostic and Statistical Manual of Mental Disorders*. 4th ed. Text rev. Washington, DC: American Psychiatric Association; copyright 2000, with permission.

Table 9.11–2
DSM-IV-TR Diagnostic Criteria for Phencyclidine Intoxication

A. Recent use of phencyclidine (or a related substance).
B. Clinically significant maladaptive behavioral changes (e.g., belligerence, assaultiveness, impulsiveness, unpredictability, psychomotor agitation, impaired judgment, or impaired social or occupational functioning) that developed during, or shortly after, phencyclidine use.
C. Within an hour (less when smoked, "snorted," or used intravenously), two (or more) of the following signs:
   (1) vertical or horizontal nystagmus
   (2) hypertension or tachycardia
   (3) numbness or diminished responsiveness to pain
   (4) ataxia
   (5) dysarthria
   (6) muscle rigidity
   (7) seizures or coma
   (8) hyperacusis
D. The symptoms are not due to a general medical condition and are not better accounted for by another mental disorder.
Specify if:
   With perceptual disturbances

From American Psychiatric Association. *Diagnostic and Statistical Manual of Mental Disorders*. 4th ed. Text rev. Washington, DC: American Psychiatric Association; copyright 2000, with permission.

Some patients may be brought to psychiatric attention within hours of ingesting PCP, but often 2 to 3 days elapse before psychiatric help is sought. The long interval between drug ingestion and the appearance of the patient in a clinic usually reflects the attempts of friends to deal with the psychosis by "talking down." Persons who lose consciousness are brought for help earlier than those who remain conscious. Most patients recover completely within a day or two, but some remain psychotic for as long as 2 weeks. Patients who are first seen in a coma often exhibit disorientation, hallucinations, confusion, and difficulty communicating on regaining consciousness. These symptoms may also be seen in noncomatose patients, but their symptoms appear to be less severe than those of comatose patients. Behavioral disturbances sometimes are severe; they may include public masturbation, stripping off clothes, violence, urinary incontinence, crying, and inappropriate laughing. Patients frequently have amnesia for the entire period of the psychosis.

A 17-year-old male was brought to the emergency room by the police, after being found, disoriented, on the street. As the police attempted to question him, he became increasingly agitated; when they attempted to restrain him, he became assaultive. Attempts to question or examine him in the emergency room evoked increased agitation. Initially it was impossible to determine vital signs or to draw blood. Based upon the observation of horizontal, vertical, and rotatory nystagmus, a diagnosis of PCP intoxication was entertained. Within a few minutes of being placed in a darkened examination room, his agitation decreased markedly.

His blood pressure was 170/100; other vital signs were within normal limits. Blood was drawn for toxicological examination. The patient agreed to take 20 mg of diazepam (Valium) orally. Thirty minutes later, he was less agitated and could be interviewed, although he responded to questions in a fragmented fashion and was slightly dysarthric. He stated that he must have inadvertently taken a larger-than-usual dose of "dust," which he reported having used once or twice a week for several years. He denied use of any other substance and any history of mental disorder. He was disoriented to time and place. The qualitative toxicology screen revealed PCP and no other drugs. Results of neurological examination were within normal limits but very brisk deep tendon reflexes were noted.

Some 90 minutes after arrival his temperature, initially normal, was 38°C, his blood pressure had increased to 182/110, and he responded poorly to stimulation. He was admitted to a medical bed. His blood pressure and level of consciousness continued to fluctuate over the ensuing 18 hours. Results of hematological and biochemical analyses of blood, as well as urinalyses, remained within normal limits. A history obtained from his family revealed that he had had multiple emergency room visits for complications from PCP use during the previous several years. He had completed a 30-day residential treatment program and had participated in several outpatient programs but had consistently relapsed. The patient was discharged after vital signs and level of consciousness had been within normal limits for 8 hours. At discharge, nystagmus and dysarthria were no longer present. A referral to an outpatient treatment program was made. (Courtesy of Steven R. Zukin, M.D.)

Table 9.11–3
DSM-IV-TR Diagnostic Criteria for Phencyclidine-Related Disorder Not Otherwise Specified

The phencyclidine-related disorder not otherwise specified category is for disorders associated with the use of phencyclidine that are not classifiable as phencyclidine dependence, phencyclidine abuse, phencyclidine intoxication, phencyclidine intoxication delirium, phencyclidine-induced psychotic disorder, phencyclidine-induced mood disorder, or phencyclidine-induced anxiety disorder.

From American Psychiatric Association. *Diagnostic and Statistical Manual of Mental Disorders.* 4th ed. Text rev. Washington, DC: American Psychiatric Association; copyright 2000, with permission.

PCP Intoxication Delirium

PCP intoxication delirium is included as a diagnostic category in the text revision of the fourth edition of the *Diagnostic and Statistical Manual of Mental Disorders* (DSM-IV-TR). An estimated 25 percent of all PCP-related emergency room patients may meet the criteria for the disorder, which can be characterized by agitated, violent, and bizarre behavior.

PCP-Induced Psychotic Disorder

PCP-induced psychotic disorder is included as a diagnostic category in DSM-IV-TR. Clinicians can further specify whether the predominant symptoms are delusions or hallucinations. An estimated 6 percent of PCP-related emergency room patients may meet the criteria for the disorder. Approximately 40 percent of these patients have physical signs of hypertension and nystagmus, and 10 percent have been injured accidentally during the psychosis. The psychosis can last from 1 to 30 days, with an average of 4 to 5 days.

PCP-Induced Mood Disorder

PCP-induced mood disorder is included as a diagnostic category in DSM-IV-TR. An estimated 3 percent of PCP-related emergency room patients meet the criteria for the disorder, with most fitting the criteria for a manic-like episode. Approximately 40 to 50 percent have been accidentally injured during the course of their manic symptoms.

PCP-Induced Anxiety Disorder

PCP-induced anxiety disorder is included as a diagnostic category in DSM-IV-TR. Anxiety is probably the most common symptom causing a PCP-intoxicated person to seek help in an emergency room.

PCP-Related Disorder Not Otherwise Specified

The diagnosis of PCP-related disorder not otherwise specified is the appropriate diagnosis for a patient who does not fit into any of the previously described diagnoses (Table 9.11–3).

CLINICAL FEATURES

The amount of PCP varies greatly from PCP-laced cigarette to cigarette; 1 g may be used to make as few as four or as many as several dozen cigarettes. Less than 4 mg of PCP is considered a low dose, and doses above 10 mg are considered high. The variability of dose makes it difficult to predict the effect, although smoking PCP is the easiest and most reliable way for users to titrate the dose.

Persons who have just taken PCP are frequently uncommunicative, appear to be oblivious, and report active fantasy production. They experience speedy feelings, euphoria, bodily warmth, tingling, peaceful floating sensations, and, occasionally, feelings of depersonalization, isolation, and estrangement. Sometimes, they have auditory and visual hallucinations. They often have striking alterations of body image, distortions of space and time perception, and delusions. They may experience intensified dependence feelings, confusion, and disorganization of thought. Users may be sympathetic, sociable, and talkative at one moment but hostile and negative at another. Anxiety is sometimes reported; it is often the most prominent presenting symptom during an adverse reaction. Nystagmus, hypertension, and hyperthermia are common effects of PCP. Head-rolling movements, stroking, grimacing, muscle rigidity on stimulation, repeated episodes of vomiting, and repetitive chanting speech are sometimes observed.

The short-term effects last 3 to 6 hours and sometimes give way to a mild depression in which the user becomes irritable, somewhat paranoid, and occasionally belligerent, irrationally assaultive, suicidal, or homicidal. The effects can last for several days. Users sometimes find that it takes 1 to 2 days to recover completely; laboratory tests show that PCP may remain in the patient's blood and urine for more than a week.

DIFFERENTIAL DIAGNOSIS

Depending on a patient's status at the time of admission, the differential diagnosis may include sedative or narcotic overdose, psychotic disorder as a consequence of the use of psychedelic drugs, and brief psychotic disorder. Laboratory analysis may help to establish the diagnosis, particularly in the many cases in which the substance history is unreliable or unattainable.

TREATMENT AND REHABILITATION

The treatment for each of the PCP (or PCP-like)-related disorders is symptomatic. Talking down, which may work after hallucinogen use, is generally not useful for PCP intoxication. Benzodiazepines and dopamine receptor antagonists are the drugs of choice for controlling behavior pharmacologically. Physicians must monitor the patient's level of consciousness, blood pressure, temperature, and muscle activity and must be ready to treat severe medical abnormalities as necessary.

Clinicians must carefully monitor unconscious patients, particularly those who have toxic reactions to PCP; excessive secretions may interfere with already compromised respiration. In an alert patient who has recently taken PCP, gastric lavage presents a risk of inducing laryngeal spasm and aspiration of emesis. Muscle spasms and seizures are best treated with diazepam. The environment should afford minimal sensory stimulation. Ideally, one person stays with the patient in a quiet, dark room. Four-point restraint is dangerous because it may lead to rhabdomyolysis; total body immobilization may occasionally be necessary. A benzodiazepine is often effective in reducing

agitation, but a patient with severe behavioral disturbances may require short-term treatment with a dopamine receptor antagonist—for example, haloperidol (Haldol). For patients with severe hypertension, a hypotensive-inducing drug such as phentolamine (Regitine) may be needed. Ammonium chloride in the early stage and ascorbic acid or cranberry juice later on are used to acidify the patient's urine and to promote the elimination of the substance, although the efficacy of the procedure is controversial.

If the symptoms are not severe and if the clinician can be certain that enough time has elapsed for all the PCP to be absorbed, the patient may be monitored in the outpatient department and, if the symptoms improve, released to family or friends. Even at low doses, however, symptoms may worsen, and the person should be hospitalized to prevent violence and suicide.

In most cases, once any acute medical complications are successfully treated, both peripheral and central nervous system complications, including psychosis, resolve completely within 24 to 72 hours. In the case of prolonged PCP-induced psychotic disorder, the rule is complete recovery within 4 to 6 weeks, regardless of whether antipsychotics have been administered. However, the rate of subsequent relapse to PCP use is very high. Persistence of a psychotic disorder beyond 8 weeks indicates the possible presence of an underlying psychotic disorder exacerbated, but not caused, by PCP.

Ketamine

Ketamine is a dissociative anesthetic agent, originally derived from PCP, that is available for use in human and veterinary medicine. It has become a drug of abuse, with sources exclusively from stolen supplies, and is available as a powder or in solution for intranasal, oral, inhalational, or (rarely) intravenous use. Ketamine functions by working at the NMDA receptor and, like PCP, can cause hallucinations and a dissociated state in which the patient has an altered sense of the body and reality and little concern for the environment.

Ketamine causes cardiovascular stimulation and no respiratory depression. On physical examination the patient may be hypertensive and tachycardic, have increased salivation, and have bidirectional and/or rotary nystagmus. The onset of action is within seconds when used intravenously, and analgesia lasting 40 minutes and dissociative effects lasting for hours have been described. Cardiovascular status should be monitored and supportive care administered. A dystonic reaction has been described, as have flashbacks, but a more common complication is related to a lack of concern for the environment or personal safety.

▲ 9.12 Sedative-, Hypnotic-, or Anxiolytic-Related Disorders

The drugs associated with this class of substance-related disorders are the benzodiazepines (e.g., diazepam [Valium], flunitrazepam [Rohypnol]), barbiturates (e.g., secobarbital [Seconal]), and the barbiturate-like substances, which include methaqualone (formerly known as Quaalude) and meprobamate (Equanil). The major non-psychiatric indications for these drugs are as antiepileptics, muscle relaxants, anesthetics, and anesthetic adjuvants. Alcohol and all drugs of this class are cross-tolerant, and their effects are additive. Physical and psychological dependence develop to all the drugs, and all are associated with withdrawal symptoms.

Sedatives are drugs that reduce subjective tension and induce mental calmness. The term *sedative* is virtually synonymous with the term *anxiolytic*, a drug that reduces anxiety. Hypnotics are drugs used to induce sleep. The differentiation between anxiolytics and sedatives as daytime drugs and hypnotics as nighttime drugs is not accurate. When sedatives and anxiolytics are given in high doses, they can induce sleep just as the hypnotics do. Conversely, when hypnotics are given in low doses, they can induce daytime sedation much as the sedatives and anxiolytics do. In some literature, especially older literature, the sedatives, anxiolytics, and hypnotics are grouped together as *the minor tranquilizers*. This term is poorly defined and subject to ambiguous meanings and, therefore, is best avoided.

SUBSTANCES

Benzodiazepines

Many benzodiazepines, differing primarily in their half-lives, are available in the United States. Examples of benzodiazepines are diazepam, flurazepam (Dalmane), oxazepam (Serax), and chlordiazepoxide (Librium). Benzodiazepines are used primarily as anxiolytics, hypnotics, antiepileptics, and anesthetics, as well as for alcohol withdrawal. After their introduction in the United States in the 1960s, benzodiazepines rapidly became the most prescribed drugs; approximately 15 percent of all persons in this country have had a benzodiazepine prescribed by a physician. Increasing awareness of the risks for dependence on benzodiazepines and increased regulatory requirements, however, have decreased the number of benzodiazepine prescriptions. The Drug Enforcement Agency classifies all benzodiazepines as Schedule IV controlled substances.

Flunitrazepam, a benzodiazepine used in Mexico, South America, and Europe, but not available in the United States, has become a drug of abuse. When taken with alcohol, it has been associated with promiscuous sexual behavior and rape. It is illegal to bring flunitrazepam into the United States. Although misused in the United States, it remains a standard anxiolytic in many countries.

Barbiturates

Before the introduction of benzodiazepines, barbiturates were frequently prescribed, but because of their high abuse potential, their use is much rarer today than in the past. Pentobarbital, secobarbital, and amobarbital (Amytal) are now under the same federal legal controls as morphine.

The first barbiturate, barbital (Veronal), was introduced in the United States in 1903. Barbital and phenobarbital (Solfoton, Luminal), which was introduced shortly thereafter, are long-acting drugs with half-lives of 12 to 24 hours. Amobarbital is an intermediate-acting barbiturate with a half-life of 6 to 12 hours. Amobarbital is an intermediate-acting barbiturate with a half-life of 6 to 12 hours. Pentobarbital and secobarbital are short-acting barbiturates with half-lives of 3 to 6 hours.

Barbiturate-like Substances

The most commonly abused barbiturate-like substance is methaqualone, which is no longer manufactured in the United States. It is often used by young persons who believe that the substance heightens the pleasure of sexual activity. Abusers of methaqualone commonly take one or two standard tablets (usually 300 mg per tablet) to obtain the desired effects. The street names for methaqualone include "mandrakes" (from the U.K. preparation Mandrax) and "soapers" (from the brand name Sopor). "Luding out" (from the brand name Quaalude) means getting high on methaqualone, which is often combined with excessive alcohol intake.

EPIDEMIOLOGY

According to DSM-IV-TR, approximately 6 percent of individuals have used either sedatives or tranquilizers illicitly, including 0.3 percent who reported illicit use of sedatives in the prior year and 0.1 percent who reported use of sedatives in the prior month. The age group with the highest lifetime prevalence of sedative (3 percent) or tranquilizer (6 percent) use was 26- to 34-year-olds, while those ages 18 to 25 were most likely to have used them in the prior year. About one-fourth to one-third of all substance-related emergency room visits involve substances of this class. The patients have a female-to-male ratio of 3 to 1 and a white-to-black ratio of 2 to 1. Some persons use benzodiazepines alone, but persons who use cocaine often use benzodiazepines to reduce withdrawal symptoms, and opioid abusers use them to enhance the euphoric effects of opioids. Because they are easily obtained, benzodiazepines are also used by abusers of stimulants, hallucinogens, and phencyclidine to help reduce the anxiety that can be caused by those substances.

Whereas barbiturate abuse is common among mature adults who have long histories of abuse of these substances, benzodiazepines are abused by a younger age group, usually under 40 years of age. This group may have a slight male predominance and has a white-to-black ratio of approximately 2 to 1. Benzodiazepines are probably not abused as frequently as other substances for the purpose of getting "high," or inducing a euphoric feeling. Rather, they are used when a person wishes to experience a general relaxed feeling.

NEUROPHARMACOLOGY

The benzodiazepines, barbiturates, and barbiturate-like substances all have their primary effects on the γ-aminobutyric acid (GABA) type A (GABA$_A$) receptor complex, which contains a chloride ion channel, a binding site for GABA, and a well-defined binding site for benzodiazepines. The barbiturates and barbiturate-like substances are also believed to bind somewhere on the GABA$_A$ receptor complex. When a benzodiazepine, barbiturate, or barbiturate-like substance does bind to the complex, the effect is to increase the affinity of the receptor for its endogenous neurotransmitter, GABA, and to increase the flow of chloride ions through the channel into the neuron. The influx of negatively charged chloride ions into the neuron is inhibitory, and hyperpolarizes the neuron relative to the extracellular space.

Although all the substances in this class induce tolerance and physical dependence, the mechanisms behind these effects are best understood for the benzodiazepine. After long-term benzodiazepine use, the receptor effects caused by the agonist are attenuated. Specifically, GABA stimulation of the GABA$_A$ receptors results in less chloride influx than was caused by

Table 9.12–1
DSM-IV-TR Sedative-, Hypnotic-, or Anxiolytic-Related Disorders

Sedative, hypnotic, or anxiolytic use disorders
Sedative, hypnotic, or anxiolytic dependence
Sedative, hypnotic, or anxiolytic abuse
Sedative-, hypnotic-, or anxiolytic-induced disorders
Sedative, hypnotic, or anxiolytic intoxication
Sedative, hypnotic, or anxiolytic withdrawal
   Specify if:
      With perceptual disturbances
Sedative, hypnotic, or anxiolytic intoxication delirium
Sedative, hypnotic, or anxiolytic withdrawal delirium
Sedative-, hypnotic-, or anxiolytic-induced persisting dementia
Sedative-, hypnotic-, or anxiolytic-induced psychotic disorder, with delusions
   Specify if:
      With onset during intoxication
      With onset during withdrawal
Sedative-, hypnotic-, or anxiolytic-induced psychotic disorder, with hallucinations
   Specify if:
      With onset during intoxication
      With onset during withdrawal
Sedative-, hypnotic-, or anxiolytic-induced mood disorder
   Specify if:
      With onset during intoxication
      With onset during withdrawal
Sedative-, hypnotic-, or anxiolytic-induced anxiety disorder
   Specify if:
      With onset during withdrawal
Sedative-, hypnotic-, or anxiolytic-induced sexual dysfunction
   Specify if:
      With onset during intoxication
Sedative-, hypnotic-, or anxiolytic-induced sleep disorder
   Specify if:
      With onset during intoxication
      With onset during withdrawal
Sedative-, hypnotic-, or anxiolytic-related disorder not otherwise specified

From American Psychiatric Association. *Diagnostic and Statistical Manual of Mental Disorders.* 4th ed. Text rev. Washington, DC: American Psychiatric Association; copyright 2000, with permission.

Table 9.12–2
DSM-IV-TR Diagnostic Criteria for Sedative, Hypnotic, or Anxiolytic Intoxication

A. Recent use of a sedative, hypnotic, or anxiolytic.
B. Clinically significant maladaptive behavioral or psychological changes (e.g., inappropriate sexual or aggressive behavior, mood lability, impaired judgment, impaired social or occupational functioning) that developed during, or shortly after, sedative, hypnotic, or anxiolytic use.
C. One (or more) of the following signs, developing during, or shortly after, sedative, hypnotic, or anxiolytic use:
   (1) slurred speech
   (2) incoordination
   (3) unsteady gait
   (4) nystagmus
   (5) impairment in attention or memory
   (6) stupor or coma
D. The symptoms are not due to a general medical condition and are not better accounted for by another mental disorder.

From American Psychiatric Association. *Diagnostic and Statistical Manual of Mental Disorders.* 4th ed. Text rev. Washington, DC: American Psychiatric Association; copyright 2000, with permission.

9.12–1) but includes specific diagnostic criteria only for sedative, hypnotic, or anxiolytic intoxication (Table 9.12–2) and sedative, hypnotic or anxiolytic withdrawal (Table 9.12–3). The diagnostic criteria for other sedative-, hypnotic-, or anxiolytic-related disorders are outlined in the DSM-IV-TR sections that are specific for the major symptom—for example, sedative-, hypnotic-, or anxiolytic-induced psychotic disorder.

Table 9.12–3
DSM-IV-TR Diagnostic Criteria for Sedative, Hypnotic, or Anxiolytic Withdrawal

A. Cessation of (or reduction in) sedative, hypnotic, or anxiolytic use that has been heavy and prolonged.
B. Two (or more) of the following, developing within several hours to a few days after Criterion A:
   (1) autonomic hyperactivity (e.g., sweating or pulse rate greater than 100)
   (2) increased hand tremor
   (3) insomnia
   (4) nausea or vomiting
   (5) transient visual, tactile, or auditory hallucinations or illusions
   (6) psychomotor agitation
   (7) anxiety
   (8) grand mal seizures
C. The symptoms in Criterion B cause clinically significant distress or impairment in social, occupational, or other important areas of functioning.
D. The symptoms are not due to a general medical condition and are not better accounted for by another mental disorder.
Specify if:
   With perceptual disturbances

From American Psychiatric Association. *Diagnostic and Statistical Manual of Mental Disorders.* 4th ed. Text rev. Washington, DC: American Psychiatric Association; copyright 2000, with permission.

GABA stimulation before the benzodiazepine administration. This downregulation of receptor response is not due to a decrease in receptor number or to decreased affinity of the receptor for GABA. The basis for the downregulation seems to be in the coupling between the GABA binding site and the activation of the chloride ion channel. This decreased efficiency in coupling may be regulated within the $GABA_A$ receptor complex itself or by other neuronal mechanisms.

DIAGNOSIS

The text revision of the fourth edition of *Diagnostic and Statistical Manual of Mental Disorders* (DSM-IV-TR) lists a number of sedative-, hypnotic-, or anxiolytic-related disorders (Table

Dependence and Abuse

Sedative, hypnotic, or anxiolytic dependence and sedative, hypnotic, or anxiolytic abuse are diagnosed according to the general criteria in DSM-IV-TR for substance dependence and substance abuse (see Tables 9.1–3 and 9.1–4 in Section 9.1).

Intoxication

DSM-IV-TR contains a single set of diagnostic criteria for intoxication by any sedative, hypnotic, or anxiolytic substance (Table 9.12–2). Although the intoxication syndromes induced by all these drugs are similar, subtle clinical differences are observable, especially with intoxications that involve low doses. The diagnosis of intoxication by one of this class of substances is best confirmed by obtaining a blood sample for substance screening.

Benzodiazepines. Benzodiazepine intoxication can be associated with behavioral disinhibition, potentially resulting in hostile or aggressive behavior in some persons. The effect is perhaps most common when benzodiazepines are taken in combination with alcohol. Benzodiazepine intoxication is associated with less euphoria than is intoxication by other drugs in this class. This characteristic is the basis for the lower abuse and dependence potential of benzodiazepines than of barbiturates.

Barbiturates and Barbiturate-like Substances. When barbiturates and barbiturate-like substances are taken in relatively low doses, the clinical syndrome of intoxication is indistinguishable from that associated with alcohol intoxication. The symptoms include sluggishness, incoordination, difficulty thinking, poor memory, slow speech and comprehension, faulty judgment, disinhibited sexual aggressive impulses, narrowed range of attention, emotional lability, and exaggerated basic personality traits. The sluggishness usually resolves after a few hours, but depending primarily on the half-life of the abused substance, impaired judgment, distorted mood, and impaired motor skills may remain for 12 to 24 hours. Other potential symptoms are hostility, argumentativeness, moroseness, and, occasionally, paranoid and suicidal ideation. The neurological effects include nystagmus, diplopia, strabismus, ataxic gait, positive Romberg's sign, hypotonia, and decreased superficial reflexes.

Withdrawal

DSM-IV-TR contains a single set of diagnostic criteria for withdrawal from any sedative, hypnotic, or anxiolytic substance (Table 9.12–3). Clinicians can specify "with perceptual disturbances" if illusions, altered perceptions, or hallucinations are present but accompanied by intact reality testing. Remember that benzodiazepines are associated with a withdrawal syndrome and that withdrawal from benzodiazepines can also result in serious medical complications, such as seizures.

Benzodiazepines. The severity of the withdrawal syndrome associated with the benzodiazepines varies significantly depending on the average dose and the duration of use, but a mild withdrawal syndrome can follow even short-term use of relatively low doses of benzodiazepines. A significant withdrawal syndrome is likely to occur at cessation of dosages in the 40-mg-a-day range for diazepam, for example, although 10 to 20 mg a day, taken for a month, can also result in a withdrawal syndrome when drug administration is stopped. The onset of withdrawal symptoms usually occurs 2 to 3 days after the cessation of use, but with long-acting drugs, such as diazepam, the latency before onset may be 5 or 6 days. The symptoms include anxiety, dysphoria, intolerance for bright lights and loud noises, nausea, sweating, muscle twitching, and sometimes seizures (generally at dosages of 50 mg a day or more of diazepam).

Barbiturates and Barbiturate-like Substances. The withdrawal syndrome for barbiturate and barbiturate-like substances ranges from mild symptoms (e.g., anxiety, weakness, sweating, and insomnia) to severe symptoms (e.g., seizures, delirium, cardiovascular collapse, and death). Persons who have been abusing phenobarbital in the range of 400 mg a day may experience mild withdrawal symptoms; those who have been abusing the substance in the range of 800 mg a day experience orthostatic hypotension, weakness, tremor, and severe anxiety. Approximately 75 percent of these persons have withdrawal-related seizures. Users of dosages higher than 800 mg a day may experience anorexia, delirium, hallucinations, and repeated seizures.

Most symptoms appear in the first 3 days of abstinence, and seizures generally occur on the second or third day, when the symptoms are worst. If seizures do occur, they always precede the development of delirium. The symptoms rarely occur more than a week after stopping the substance. A psychotic disorder, if it develops, starts on the third to eighth day. The various associated symptoms generally run their course within 2 to 3 days but may last as long as 2 weeks. The first episode of the syndrome usually occurs after 5 to 15 years of heavy substance use.

Delirium

DSM-IV-TR allows for the diagnosis of sedative, hypnotic, or anxiolytic intoxication delirium and sedative, hypnotic, or anxiolytic withdrawal delirium. Delirium that is indistinguishable from delirium tremens associated with alcohol withdrawal is seen more commonly with barbiturate withdrawal than with benzodiazepine withdrawal. Delirium associated with intoxication can be seen with either barbiturates or benzodiazepines if the dosages are high enough.

Persisting Dementia

DSM-IV-TR allows for the diagnosis of sedative-, hypnotic-, or anxiolytic-induced persisting dementia. The existence of the disorder is controversial, since there is uncertainty whether a persisting dementia is due to the substance use itself or to associated features of the substance use. One must evaluate the diagnosis further by using DSM-IV-TR criteria to ascertain validity.

Persisting Amnestic Disorder

DSM-IV-TR allows for the diagnosis of sedative-, hypnotic-, or anxiolytic-induced persisting amnestic disorder. Amnestic disorders associated with sedatives, hypnotics, and anxiolytics may be underdiagnosed. One exception is the increased number of reports of amnestic episodes associated with short-term use of benzodiazepines with short half-lives (e.g., triazolam [Halcion]).

Table 9.12–4
DSM-IV-TR Diagnostic Criteria for Sedative-, Hypnotic-, or Anxiolytic-Related Disorder Not Otherwise Specified

The sedative-, hypnotic-, or anxiolytic-related disorder not otherwise specified category is for disorders associated with the use of sedatives, hypnotics, or anxiolytics that are not classifiable as sedative, hypnotic, or anxiolytic dependence; sedative, hypnotic, or anxiolytic abuse; sedative, hypnotic, or anxiolytic intoxication; sedative, hypnotic, or anxiolytic withdrawal; sedative, hypnotic, or anxiolytic intoxication delirium; sedative, hypnotic, or anxiolytic withdrawal delirium; sedative-, hypnotic-, or anxiolytic-induced persisting dementia; sedative-, hypnotic-, or anxiolytic-induced persisting amnestic disorder; sedative-, hypnotic-, or anxiolytic-induced psychotic disorder; sedative-, hypnotic-, or anxiolytic-induced mood disorder; sedative-, hypnotic-, or anxiolytic-induced anxiety disorder; sedative-, hypnotic-, or anxiolytic-induced sexual dysfunction; or sedative-, hypnotic-, or anxiolytic-induced sleep disorder.

From American Psychiatric Association. *Diagnostic and Statistical Manual of Mental Disorders.* 4th ed. Text rev. Washington, DC: American Psychiatric Association; copyright 2000, with permission.

Psychotic Disorders

The psychotic symptoms of barbiturate withdrawal can be indistinguishable from those of alcohol-associated delirium tremens. Agitation, delusions, and hallucinations are usually visual, but sometimes tactile or auditory features develop after approximately 1 week of abstinence. Psychotic symptoms associated with intoxication or withdrawal are more common with barbiturates than with benzodiazepines and are diagnosed as sedative-, hypnotic-, or anxiolytic-induced psychotic disorders. Clinicians can further specify whether delusions or hallucinations are the predominant symptoms.

Other Disorders

Sedative, hypnotic, and anxiolytic use has also been associated with mood disorders, anxiety disorders, sleep disorders, and sexual dysfunctions. When none of the previously discussed diagnostic categories is appropriate for a person with a sedative, hypnotic, or anxiolytic use disorder, the appropriate diagnosis is sedative-, hypnotic-, or anxiolytic-related disorder not otherwise specified (Table 9.12–4).

CLINICAL FEATURES

Patterns of Abuse

Oral Use. Sedatives, hypnotics, and anxiolytics can all be taken orally, either occasionally to achieve a time-limited specific effect or regularly to obtain a constant, usually mild, intoxication state. The occasional use pattern is associated with young persons who take the substance to achieve specific effects—relaxation for an evening, intensification of sexual activities, and a short-lived period of mild euphoria. The user's personality and expectations about the substance's effects and the setting in which the substance is taken also affect the substance-induced experience. The regular use pattern is associated with middle-aged, middle-class persons who usually obtain the substance from a family physician as a prescription for insomnia or anxiety. Abusers of this type may have prescriptions from several physicians, and the pattern of abuse may go undetected until obvious signs of abuse or dependence are noticed by the person's family, coworkers, or physicians.

Intravenous Use. A severe form of abuse involves the intravenous (IV) use of this class of substances. The users are mainly young adults intimately involved with illegal substances. Intravenous barbiturate use is associated with a pleasant, warm, drowsy feeling, and users may be inclined to use barbiturates more than opioids because barbiturates are less costly. The physical dangers of injection include transmission of the human immunodeficiency virus, cellulites, vascular complications from accidental injection into an artery, infections, and allergic reactions to contaminants. Intravenous use is associated with rapid and profound tolerance and dependence and a severe withdrawal syndrome.

Overdose

Benzodiazepines. In contrast to the barbiturates and the barbiturate-like substances, the benzodiazepines have a large margin of safety when taken in overdoses, a feature that contributed significantly to their rapid acceptance. The ratio of lethal dose to effective dose is approximately 200 to 1 or higher, because of the minimal degree of respiratory depression associated with the benzodiazepines. Even when grossly excessive amounts (more than 2 g) are taken in suicide attempts, the symptoms include only drowsiness, lethargy, ataxia, some confusion, and mild depression of the user's vital signs. A much more serious condition prevails when benzodiazepines are taken in overdose in combination with other sedative-hypnotic substances, such as alcohol. In such cases, small doses of benzodiazepines can cause death. The availability of flumazenil (Romazicon), a specific benzodiazepine antagonist, has reduced the lethality of the benzodiazepines. Flumazenil can be used in emergency rooms to reverse the effects of the benzodiazepines.

Barbiturates. Barbiturates are lethal when taken in overdose because they induce respiratory depression. In addition to intentional suicide attempts, accidental or unintentional overdoses are common. Barbiturates in home medicine cabinets are a common cause of fatal drug overdoses in children. As with benzodiazepines, the lethal effects of the barbiturates are additive to those of other sedatives or hypnotics, including alcohol and benzodiazepines. Barbiturate overdose is characterized by the induction of coma, respiratory arrest, cardiovascular failure, and death.

The lethal dose varies with the route of administration and the degree of tolerance for the substance after a history of long-term abuse. For the most commonly abused barbiturates, the ratio of lethal dose to effective dose ranges between 3 to 1 and 30 to 1. Dependent users often take an average daily dose of 1.5 g of a short-acting barbiturate, and some have been reported to take as much as 2.5 g a day for months.

The lethal dose is not much greater for the long-term abuser than for the neophyte. Tolerance develops quickly to the point at which withdrawal in a hospital becomes necessary to prevent accidental death from overdose.

Barbiturate-like Substances.   The barbiturate-like substances vary in their lethality and are usually intermediate between the relative safety of the benzodiazepines and the high lethality of the barbiturates. An overdose of methaqualone, for example, may result in restlessness, delirium, hypertonia, muscle spasms, and convulsions and, in very high doses, death. Unlike barbiturates, methaqualone rarely causes severe cardiovascular or respiratory depression, and most fatalities result from combining methaqualone with alcohol.

TREATMENT AND REHABILITATION

Withdrawal

Benzodiazepines.   Because some benzodiazepines are eliminated from the body slowly, symptoms of withdrawal may continue to develop for several weeks. To prevent seizures and other withdrawal symptoms, clinicians should gradually reduce the dosage. Several reports indicate that carbamazepine (Tegretol) may be useful in the treatment of benzodiazepine withdrawal. Table 9.12–5 lists guidelines for treating benzodiazepine withdrawal.

Barbiturates.   To avoid sudden death during barbiturate withdrawal, clinicians must follow conservative clinical guidelines. Clinicians should not give barbiturates to a comatose or grossly intoxicated patient. A clinician should attempt to determine a patient's usual daily dose of barbiturates and then verify the dosage clinically. For example, a clinician can give a test dose of 200 mg of pentobarbital every hour until a mild intoxication occurs but withdrawal symptoms are absent. The clinician can then taper the total daily dose at a rate of approximately 10 percent of the total daily dose. Once the correct dosage is determined, a long-acting barbiturate can be used for the detoxification period. During this process, the patient may begin to experience withdrawal symptoms, in which case the clinician should halve the daily decrement.

In the withdrawal procedure, phenobarbital may be substituted for the more commonly abused short-acting barbiturates. The effects of phenobarbital last longer, and because there is less fluctuation of barbiturate blood levels, phenobarbital does not cause observable toxic signs or a serious overdose. An adequate dose is 30 mg of phenobarbital for every 100 mg of the short-acting substance. The user should be maintained for at least 2 days at that level before the dosage is reduced further. The regimen is analogous to the substitution of methadone for heroin.

After withdrawal is complete, the patient must overcome the desire to start taking the substance again. Although substitution of nonbarbiturate sedatives or hypnotics for barbiturates has been suggested as a preventive therapeutic measure, this often results in replacing one substance dependence with another. If a user is to remain substance free, follow-up treatment, usually with psychiatric help and community support, is vital. Otherwise, a patient will almost certainly return to barbiturates of a substance with similar hazards.

Overdose

The treatment of overdose of this class of substances involves gastric lavage, activated charcoal, and careful monitoring of vital signs and central nervous system activity. Overdose patients who

Table 9.12–5
Guidelines for Treatment of Benzodiazepine Withdrawal

1. Evaluate and treat concomitant medical and psychiatric conditions
2. Obtain drug history and urine and blood sample for drug and ethanol assay
3. Determine required dose of benzodiazepine or barbiturate for stabilization, guided by history, clinical presentation, drug-ethanol assay, and (in some cases) challenge dose
4. Detoxification from supratherapeutic dosages:
   a. Hospitalize if there are medical or psychiatric indications, poor social supports, or polysubstance dependence or the patient is unreliable
   b. Some clinicians recommend switching to longer-acting benzodiazepine for withdrawal (e.g., diazepam, clonazepam); others recommend stabilizing on the drug that patient was taking or on phenobarbital
   c. After stabilization reduce dosage by 30 percent on the second or third day and evaluate the response, keeping in mind that symptoms that occur after decreases in benzodiazepines with short elimination half-lives (e.g., lorazepam) appear sooner than with those with longer elimination half-lives (e.g., diazepam)
   d. Reduce dosage further by 10 to 25 percent every few days if tolerated
   e. Use adjunctive medications if necessary—carbamazepine, β-adrenergic receptor antagonists, valproate, clonidine, and sedative antidepressants have been used but their efficacy in the treatment of the benzodiazepine abstinence syndrome has not been established
5. Detoxification from therapeutic dosages:
   a. Initiate 10 to 25 percent dose reduction and evaluate response
   b. Dose, duration of therapy, and severity of anxiety influence the rate of taper and need for adjunctive medications
   c. Most patients taking therapeutic doses have uncomplicated discontinuation
6. Psychological interventions may assist patients in detoxification from benzodiazepines and in the long-term management of anxiety

Courtesy of Domenic A. Ciraulo, M.D., and Ofra Sarid-Segal, M.D.

come to medical attention while awake should be kept from slipping into unconsciousness. Vomiting should be induced, and activated charcoal should be administered to delay gastric absorption. If a patient is comatose, the clinician must establish an intravenous fluid line, monitor the patient's vital signs, insert an endotracheal tube to maintain a patent airway, and provide mechanical ventilation if necessary. Hospitalization of a comatose patient in an intensive care unit is usually required during the early stages of recovery from such overdoses.

LEGAL ISSUES

State and federal agencies have attempted to restrict the distribution of benzodiazepines by requiring special reporting forms. For example, through the use of New York State official prescription forms (formerly called *triplicate forms*), the names of doctors and patients are kept on file in a data bank. Governments have taken such measures to stem the tide of abuse. But most abuse results from the illicit manufacture, sale, and diversion of substances, particularly to cocaine and opioid addicts, not from physicians' prescriptions or legitimate pharmaceutical companies. The attempt to curtail the use of substances with unquestionable, invaluable therapeutic benefits exemplifies increasing government interference in the practice of medicine and in the confidential relationship between doctor and patient. Such restrictions do little to curb cocaine, opioid, or benzodiazepine abuse.

Recent surveys of psychiatric patients (except those diagnosed as substance abusers) have demonstrated high rates of benzodiazepine prescription use but almost uniformly low abuse; thus, physicians should not withhold benzodiazepines from their patients with emotional problems for fear of abuse.

▲ 9.13 Anabolic Steroid Abuse

Anabolic steroids are a family of drugs that includes the natural male hormone testosterone and a group of many synthetic analogues of testosterone synthesized since the 1940s (Table 9.13–1). All these drugs possess various degrees of anabolic (muscle-building) and *androgenic* (masculinizing) effects.

EPIDEMIOLOGY

An estimated 1 million persons in the United States have used steroids illegally at least once. Users are primarily middle class and white. Male users of anabolic steroids greatly outnumber female users by approximately 6 to 1; approximately half the users started before the age of 16. In one survey, 1.5 percent of persons surveyed reported a lifetime nonmedical use of these drugs. The highest use was among 18- to 25-year-olds, and 26- to 34-year-olds had the next highest rate of use. Estimates for the rate of use in body builders have ranged up to 50 to 80 percent.

NEUROPHARMACOLOGY

After oral administration of testosterone, only small amounts of the drug reach systemic circulation unchanged. The low bioavailability of orally administered testosterone results from metabolism of the drug in the gastrointestinal mucosa during first pass through the liver. The synthetic androgens (e.g., fluoxymesterone and methyltestosterone) are also less extensively metabolized after oral administration. In plasma, testosterone is 98 percent bound to a specific testosterone-estradiol-binding globulin. The plasma half-life of testosterone reportedly ranges from 10 to 100 minutes. Testosterone is metabolized principally in the liver to various 17-ketosteroids.

ETIOLOGY

Persons who use these drugs are usually involved in activities that require strength and endurance. Psychodynamic vulnerability to anabolic steroid misuse includes low self-esteem and disturbances in the image and appearance of the body. Adolescent users—both heterosexual and homosexual—equate an Adonis-like body with the ability to attract sexual partners.

DIAGNOSIS AND CLINICAL FEATURES

Steroids may initially induce euphoria and hyperactivity. After relatively short periods, however, their use can become associated with increased anger, arousal, irritability, hostility, anxiety, somatization, and depression (especially during times when steroids are not used). Several studies have demonstrated that 2 to 15 percent of anabolic steroid abusers experience hypomanic or manic episodes, and a smaller percentage may have clearly psychotic symptoms. Also disturbing is a correlation between steroid abuse and violence ("roid rage" in the parlance of users). Steroid abusers with no record of antisocial behavior or violence have committed murders and other violent crimes.

Adverse Effects

Anabolic Steroids.   Anabolic steroid use has obvious physical effects. Steroid use causes rapid development and enhancement of muscle bulk, definition, and power. Men who abuse steroids may have acne, premature balding, yellowing of the skin and the eyes, gynecomastia, and decreased size of the testicles and the prostate. Young boys abusing steroids can have painful enlargement of the genitalia. The use of steroids in young adolescents can also lead to stunted growth by causing premature closure of the bone plates. In women who abuse steroids, the voice may deepen, the breasts shrink, the clitoris enlarges, and the menstrual cycle becomes irregular.

Anabolic steroid use can also produce abnormal liver function test results, decrease high-density lipoprotein blood levels,

Table 9.13–1
Examples of Commonly Used Anabolic Steroids[a]

Compounds usually administered orally
Fluoxymesterone (Halotestin, Android-F, Ultandren)
Methandienone (formerly called methandrostenolone) (Dianabol)
Methyltestosterone (Android, Testred, Virilon)
Mibolerone (Cheque Drops[b])
Oxandrolone (Anavar)
Oxymetholone (Anadrol, Hemogenin)
Mesterolone (Mestoranum, Proviron)
Stanozolol (Winstrol)
Compounds usually administered intramuscularly
Nandrolone decanoate (Deca-Durabolin)
Nandrolone phenpropionate (Durabolin)
Methenolone enanthate (Primobolan depot)
Boldenone undecylenate (Equipoise[b])
Stanozolol (Winstrol-V[b])
Testosterone esters blends (Sustanon, Sten)
Testosterone cypionate
Testosterone enanthate (Delatestryl)
Testosterone propionate (Testoviron, Androlan)
Testosterone undecanoate (Andriol, Restandol)
Trenbolone acetate (Finajet, Finaplix[b])
Trenbolone hexahydrobencylcarbonate (Parabolan)

[a]Many of the brand names listed above are foreign, but are included because of the widespread illicit use of foreign steroid preparations in the United States.
[b]Veterinary compound.

and increase low-density lipoprotein blood levels. Decreased spermatogenesis has been reported, as has an association between anabolic steroid abuse and myocardial infarction and cerebrovascular disease.

Dehydroepiandrosterone and Androstenedione.

Dehydroepiandrosterone (DHEA) and androstenedione are adrenal androgens marketed as food supplements and sold over the counter in health food stores. They are not approved or regulated by the Food and Drug Administration (FDA). They are steroid precursors of both androgens and estrogens; persons taking these substances report increased physical and psychological well-being. The adverse effects of the drugs in high doses are similar to those of anabolic steroids and include voice change, acne, hirsutism, and prostatic cancer. Because DHEA is available in U.S. health food stores and may have addictive potential, increased reports of misuse and adverse effects should be expected.

Mr. A is a 26-year-old single white man. He is 69 inches tall and presently weighs 204 pounds with a body fat of 11 percent. He reports that he began lifting weights at age 17, at which time he weighed 155 pounds. Within a year of beginning his weightlifting he began taking anabolic steroids after obtaining them through a friend at his gymnasium. His first cycle of steroids, lasting for 9 weeks, involved methandienone, 30 mg orally a day, and testosterone cypionate, 600 mg intramuscularly a week. During these 9 weeks he gained 20 pounds of muscle mass. He was so pleased with these results that he took five further cycles of anabolic steroids over the next 6 years. During his most ambitious cycle, approximately 1 year ago, he used testosterone cypionate, 600 mg per week; nandrolone decanoate (Deca-Durabolin), 400 mg a week; stanozolol (Winstrol), 12 mg a day; and oxandrolone (Anavar), 10 mg a day.

During each of the cycles Mr. A has noted euphoria, irritability, and grandiose feelings. These symptoms were most prominent during his most recent cycle, when he felt invincible. During this cycle he also noted a decreased need for sleep, racing thoughts, and a tendency to spend excessive amounts of money. For example, he impulsively purchased a $2,700 stereo system when he realistically could not afford to spend more than $500. He also became uncharacteristically irritable with his girlfriend, and on one occasion put his fist through the side window of her car during an argument—an act inconsistent with his normally mild-mannered personality. After this cycle of steroids ended, he became moderately depressed for about 2 months, with hypersomnia, anorexia, markedly decreased libido, and occasional suicidal ideation.

Mr. A smoked marijuana almost daily during his last 2 years of high school and continues to smoke at least twice a week. He has experimented briefly with hallucinogens, cocaine, opiates, and stimulants, but has rarely used them in the last 5 years. However, he has used a number of drugs to lose weight in preparation for bodybuilding contests. These include ephedrine, amphetamine, triiodothyronine, and thyroxin. Recently, he has also begun to use the opioid agonist-antagonist nalbuphine (Nubain) intravenously to treat muscle aches from weightlifting. He reports that intravenous nalbuphine use is widespread among other anabolic steroid users of his acquaintance.

Mr. A exhibits characteristic features of muscle dysmorphia. He checks his appearance dozens of times a day in mirrors, or when he sees his reflection in a store window or even in the back of a spoon. He becomes anxious if he misses even one day of working out at the gym, and acknowledges that his preoccupation with weightlifting has cost him both social and occupational opportunities. Although he has a 48-inch chest and 19-inch biceps, he has frequently declined invitations to go to the beach or a swimming pool for fear that he would look too small when seen in a bathing suit. He is anxious because he has lost some weight since the end of his previous cycle of steroids and is eager to resume another cycle of anabolic steroids in the near future. (Courtesy of Harrison G. Pope, Jr., M.D., and Kirk J. Brower, M.D.)

▲ 9.14 Other Substance-Related Disorders

Substances that can be categorized according to some schema are described in the previous sections. This section deals with a diverse group of drugs not covered previously that cannot be easily grouped together. The text revision of the fourth edition of *Diagnostic and Statistical Manual of Mental Disorders* (DSM-IV-TR) includes a diagnostic category for these substances called other (or unknown) substance-related disorders. Some of these substances are discussed below.

GAMMA HYDROXYBUTYRATE

Gamma hydroxybutyrate (GHB) is a naturally occurring transmitter in the brain that is related to sleep regulation. GHB increases dopamine levels in the brain. In general, GHB is a central nervous system depressant with effects through the endogenous opioid system. It is used to induce anesthesia and long-term sedation, but its unpredictable duration of action limits its use. It has recently been studied for the treatment of alcohol and opioid withdrawal and narcolepsy.

GHB is abused for its intoxicating effects and consciousness-altering properties. It is variously referred to as "GBH" and "liquid ecstasy" and is sold illicitly in various forms (e.g., powder and liquid). Similar chemicals, which the body converts to GHB, include gamma butyrolactone (GBL) and 1,4-butanediol. Adverse effects include nausea, vomiting, respiratory problems, seizures, comas, and death. In some reports, GHB abuse has been linked to Wernicke-Korsakoff–like syndrome.

NITRITE INHALANTS

The nitrite inhalants include amyl, butyl, and isobutyl nitrites, all of which are called "poppers" in popular jargon. Nitrite

9.14. Other Substance-Related Disorders

Table 9.14–1
DSM-IV-TR Criteria for
Polysubstance Dependence

This diagnosis is reserved for behavior during the same 12-month period in which the person was repeatedly using at least three groups of substances (not including caffeine and nicotine), but no single substance has predominated. Further, during this period, the dependence criteria were met for substances as a group but not for any specific substance.

From American Psychiatric Association. *Diagnostic and Statistical Manual of Mental Disorders.* 4th ed. Text rev. Washington, DC: American Psychiatric Association; copyright 2000, with permission.

inhalants are used by persons seeking the associated mild euphoria, altered sense of time, feeling of fullness in the head, and possibly, increased sexual feelings. The nitrite compounds are used by some persons to heighten sexual stimulation during orgasm and, in some cases, to relax the anal sphincter for penile penetration. Under such circumstances, a person may use the substance for a few or a dozen times within several hours.

Adverse reactions include a toxic syndrome characterized by nausea, vomiting, headache, hypotension, drowsiness, and irritation of the respiratory tract. Some evidence indicates that nitrite inhalants may adversely affect immune function. Because sildenafil (Viagra) is lethal when combined with nitrite compounds, persons at risk should be cautioned never to use the two together.

NITROUS OXIDE

Nitrous oxide, commonly known as "laughing gas," is a widely available anesthetic agent that is subject to abuse because of its ability to produce feelings of lightheadedness and of floating, sometimes experienced as pleasurable or specifically as sexual. With long-term abuse patterns, nitrous oxide use has been associated with delirium and paranoia. Female dental assistants exposed to high levels of nitrous oxide have reportedly experienced reduced fertility.

OTHER SUBSTANCES

The spice *nutmeg* can be ingested in a number of preparations. When nutmeg is taken in sufficiently high doses, it can induce depersonalization, derealization, and a feeling of heaviness in the limbs. In high-enough doses, *morning glory seeds* can produce a syndrome resembling that seen with lysergic acid diethylamide (LSD), characterized by altered sensory perceptions and mild visual hallucinations. *Catnip* can produce

cannabis-like intoxication in low doses and LSD-like intoxication in high doses. *Betel nuts*, when chewed, can produce a mild euphoria and a feeling of floating in space. *Kava*, derived from a pepper plant native to the South Pacific, produces sedation and incoordination and is associated with hepatitis, lung abnormalities, and weight loss. Some persons abuse over-the-counter and prescription medications such as cortisol, antiparkinsonian agents, and antihistamines. *Ephedra*, a natural substance found in herbal tea, acts like epinephrine and, when abused, produces cardiac arrhythmia and fatalities.

A controversial possible substance of abuse is *chocolate* derived from the cacao bean. Anandamide, an ingredient in chocolate, stimulates the same receptors as marijuana. Other compounds in chocolate include tryptophan, the precursor of serotonin, and phenylalanine, an amphetamine-like substance, both of which improve mood. So called chocoholics may be self-medicating themselves because of a depressive diathesis.

POLYSUBSTANCE-RELATED DISORDER

Substance users often abuse more than one substance. In DSM-IV-TR, a diagnosis of polysubstance dependence is appropriate if, for a period of at least 12 months, a person has repeatedly used substances from at least three categories (not including nicotine and caffeine), even if the diagnostic criteria for a substance-related disorder are not met for any single substance, as long as, during this period, the criteria for substance dependence have been met for the substances considered as a group (Table 9.14–1).

TREATMENT AND REHABILITATION

Treatment approaches for the substances covered in this section vary according to substances, patterns of abuse, availability of psychosocial support systems, and patients' individual features. Two major treatment goals for substance abuse have been determined: the first is abstinence from the substance, and the second is the physical, psychiatric, and psychosocial well-being of the patient. In some cases, it may be necessary to initiate treatment on an inpatient unit. Although an outpatient setting is more desirable than an inpatient setting, the temptations available to an outpatient for repeated use may present too high a hurdle for the initiation of treatment. Inpatient treatment is also indicated in the case of severe medical or psychiatric symptoms, a history of failed outpatient treatments, a lack of psychosocial supports, or a particularly severe or long-term history of substance abuse. After an initial period of detoxification, patients need a sustained period of rehabilitation. Throughout treatment, individual, family, and group therapies can be effective. Education about substance abuse and support for patients' efforts are essential factors in treatment.

Schizophrenia, which afflicts approximately 1 percent of the population, usually begins before age 25, persists throughout life, and affects people of all social classes. Both patients and their families often suffer from poor care and social ostracism because of widespread ignorance about the disorder. Although schizophrenia is discussed as if it were a single disease, it probably comprises a group of disorders with heterogeneous etiologies, and it includes patients whose clinical presentations, treatment response, and courses of illness are varied. Clinicians should appreciate that the diagnosis of schizophrenia is based entirely on the psychiatric history and mental status examination. There is no laboratory test for schizophrenia.

HISTORY

The magnitude of the clinical problem of schizophrenia has consistently attracted the attention of major figures in psychiatry and neurology throughout the history of the disorder. Two of these people were Emil Kraepelin (1856–1926) and Eugen Bleuler (1857–1939). Earlier, Benedict Morel (1809–1873), a French psychiatrist, had used the term *démence précoce* for deteriorated patients whose illness began in adolescence; Karl Ludwig Kahlbaum (1828–1899) had described the symptoms of catatonia; Ewold Hacker (1843–1909) had written about the bizarre behavior of patients with hebephrenia.

Emil Kraepelin

Kraepelin translated Morel's *démence précoce* to *dementia precox,* a term that emphasized the distinct cognitive process (dementia) and early onset (precox) of the disorder. Patients with dementia precox were described as having a long-term deteriorating course and the common clinical symptoms of hallucinations and delusions. Kraepelin distinguished these patients from those classified as having manic-depressive psychosis who underwent distinct episodes of illness alternating with periods of normal functioning. The major symptoms of patients with paranoia were persistent persecutory delusions, and these patients were described as lacking the deteriorating course of dementia precox and the intermittent symptoms of manic-depressive psychosis. Although Kraepelin had acknowledged that approximately 4 percent of his patients recovered completely and 13 percent had significant remissions, later researchers sometimes mistakenly stated that he had considered dementia precox to have an inevitable deteriorating course.

Eugen Bleuler

Bleuler coined the term *schizophrenia,* which replaced *dementia precox* in the literature. He chose the term to express the presence of schisms between thought, emotion, and behavior in patients with the disorder. Bleuler stressed that, unlike Kraepelin's concept of dementia precox, schizophrenia need not have a deteriorating course. Before the publication of the third edition of the *Diagnostic and Statistical Manual of Mental Disorders* (DSM-III), the incidence of schizophrenia increased in the United States (where psychiatrists followed Bleuler's principles) to perhaps as much as twice the incidence in Europe (where psychiatrists followed Kraepelin's principles). After the publication of DSM-III, the diagnosis of schizophrenia in the United States moved toward Kraepelin's concept. Bleuler's term *schizophrenia,* however, has become the internationally accepted label for the disorder. This term is often misconstrued, especially by lay people, to mean split personality. Split personality, now called *dissociative identity disorder,* is categorized in DSM-IV-TR as a dissociative disorder and thus differs completely from schizophrenia.

The Four As. Bleuler identified specific *fundamental* (or *primary*) *symptoms* of schizophrenia to develop his theory about the internal mental schisms of patients. These symptoms included associational disturbances, especially looseness; affective disturbances, autism, and ambivalence, summarized as the four As: *a*ssociations, *a*ffect, *a*utism, and *a*mbivalence. Bleuler also identified *accessory* (*secondary*) *symptoms,* adding much to the understanding of schizophrenia.

EPIDEMIOLOGY

In the United States, the lifetime prevalence of schizophrenia is approximately 1 percent, which means that approximately 1 person in 100 will develop schizophrenia during his or her lifetime. The Epidemiologic Catchment Area (ECA) study sponsored by the National Institute of Mental Health (NIMH) reported a lifetime prevalence of 0.6 to 1.9 percent. According to DSM-IV-TR, the annual incidence of schizophrenia ranges from 0.5 to 5.0 per 10,000, with some geographic variation (e.g., the incidence is higher for people born in urban areas of industrialized nations). Schizophrenia is found in all societies and geographical areas and incidence and prevalence rates are roughly equal worldwide. In the U.S., approximately 0.05 percent of the total population is treated for schizophrenia in any single year and only approximately half of all patients with schizophrenia obtain treatment, in spite of the severity of the disorder (Table 10–1).

Gender and Age

Schizophrenia is equally prevalent in men and women. The two sexes differ, however, in the onset and course of illness. Onset is earlier in men than in women. More than half of all male schizophrenic patients but only one-third of all female schizophrenic patients are first admitted

**Table 10–1
Prevalence of Schizophrenia in
Specific Populations**

Population	Prevalence (%)
General population	1.0
Nontwin sibling of a schizophrenia patient	8.0
Child with one parent with schizophrenia	12.0
Dizygotic twin of a schizophrenia patient	12.0
Child of two parents with schizophrenia	40.0
Monozygotic twin of a schizophrenia patient	47.0

to a psychiatric hospital before age 25. The peak ages of onset are 8 to 25 years for men and 25 to 35 years for women. Unlike men, women display a bimodal age distribution with a second peak occurring in middle age. Approximately 3 percent to 10 percent of women present with disease onset after age 40. Approximately 90 percent of the patients in treatment for schizophrenia are between 15 and 55 years old. Onset of schizophrenia before age 10 or after age 60 is extremely rare. Some studies have indicated that men are more likely to be impaired by negative symptoms than are women and that women are more likely to have better social functioning than are men prior to disease onset. In general, the outcome for female schizophrenic patients is better than the outcome for male schizophrenic patients. When onset occurs after age 45, the disorder is characterized as late-onset schizophrenia.

Infection and Birth Season

A robust finding in schizophrenia research is that people who develop schizophrenia are more likely to have been born in the winter and early spring and less likely to have been born in late spring and summer. In the Northern Hemisphere, including the United States, people with schizophrenia are more often born in the months from January to April. In the Southern Hemisphere, people with schizophrenia are more often born in the months from July to September. One hypothesis is that a season-specific risk factor, such as a virus or a seasonal change in diet, may be operative. Viral hypotheses include slow viruses, retroviruses, and virally activated autoimmune reactions. Some studies show that the frequency of schizophrenia is increased after exposure to influenza—which occurs in the winter—during the second trimester of pregnancy. Another hypothesis is that people with a genetic predisposition for schizophrenia have a decreased biological advantage to survive season-specific insults.

Geographical Distribution

Schizophrenia is not evenly distributed throughout the United States or the world. Historically, the prevalence of schizophrenia in the northeastern and western United States was greater than in other areas, although this unequal distribution has eroded. Some geographical regions of the world, such as Ireland, have an unusually high prevalence of schizophrenia, and researchers have interpreted these geographical pockets of schizophrenia as possible support for an infective (for example, viral) cause of schizophrenia.

Reproductive Factors

The use of psychotherapeutic drugs, the open-door policies in hospitals, the deinstitutionalization in state hospitals, the emphasis on reha-

bilitation, and the community-based care for patients with schizophrenia have all led to an increase in the marriage and fertility rates among persons with schizophrenia. Because of these factors, the number of children born to schizophrenic parents is continually increasing. The fertility rate for schizophrenic people is close to that for the general population. There is a relation between fertility rates and genetic transmission. First-degree biological relatives of schizophrenic persons have a ten times greater risk for developing the disease than the general population.

Medical Illness

People with schizophrenia have a higher mortality rate from accidents and natural causes than does the general population. Institution-related or treatment-related variables do not explain the increased mortality rate, but the higher rate may be related to the fact that the diagnosis and treatment of medical and surgical conditions in schizophrenic patients can be clinical challenges. Several studies have shown that up to 80 percent of all schizophrenic patients have significant concurrent medical illnesses and that up to 50 percent of these conditions may be undiagnosed.

Suicide Risk

Suicide is a leading cause of mortality in people suffering from schizophrenia. Estimates vary, but as many as 10 percent of people with schizophrenia may die because of a suicide attempt. Although the risk for suicide is greater in people with schizophrenia than in the general population, some risk factor—such as being male, white, and socially isolated—are similar in both groups. Factors such as depressive illness, a history of suicide attempts, unemployment, and recent rejection also increase the risk for suicide in both populations. Previous studies have revealed other risk factors that are unique to this disorder. Among these are being young and male and having a chronic illness with numerous exacerbations. A postdischarge course involving high levels of psychopathology and functional impairment increases the risk for suicide. In addition, people who have a realistic awareness of the deteriorative effects of the illness and a nondelusional assessment of their future mental deterioration, hopelessness, excessive dependence on treatment, or loss of faith in treatment increase the risk of suicide in people with schizophrenia. The risk of mortality is especially high in the young, during the early postdischarge period, and early in the course of illness, although the risk persists across the person's life span. Risk factors identified in previous studies may be helpful in assessing acute suicidal risk in a specific individual. Further research is needed to better understand what risk factors are most predictive of future suicide in people with schizophrenia and what interventions are most helpful in preventing suicide.

Substance Use

Cigarette Smoking. Most surveys have reported that more than three-fourths of all schizophrenic patients smoke cigarettes, compared with less than half of psychiatric patients as a whole. In addition to the well-known health risks associated with smoking, cigarette smoking affects other aspects of a schizophrenic patient's care. Several studies have reported that cigarette smoking is associated with the use of high dosages of antipsychotic drugs, possibly because cigarette smoking increases the metabolism rate of these drugs. On the other hand, cigarette smoking is associated with a decrease in antipsychotic drug-related parkinsonism, possibly because of nicotine-dependent activation of dopamine neurons. Recent studies have demonstrated that nicotine may decrease positive symptoms, such as hallucinations, in schizophrenic patients by its effect on nicotine receptors in the brain that reduce the perception of outside stimuli, especially noise.

Other Substances.   Comorbidity of schizophrenia and other substance-related disorders is common, although the implications of substance abuse in schizophrenic patients are unclear. Approximately 30 to 50 percent of patients with schizophrenia may meet the diagnostic criteria for alcohol abuse or alcohol dependence; the two most commonly used other substances are cannabis (approximately 15 to 25 percent) and cocaine (approximately 5 to 10 percent). Patients report that they use these substances to obtain pleasure and to reduce their depression and anxiety. Most studies have associated the comorbidity of substance-related disorders in patients who have schizophrenia with poor prognosis.

Population Factors

The prevalence of schizophrenia has been correlated with local population density in cities with populations of more than 1 million people. The correlation is weaker in cities of 100,000 to 500,000 people and is absent in cities with fewer than 10,000 people. The effect of population density is consistent with the observation that the incidence of schizophrenia in children of either one or two schizophrenic parents is twice as high in cities as in rural communities. These observations suggest that social stressors in urban settings affect the development of schizophrenia in people at risk.

Socioeconomic and Cultural Factors

Schizophrenia has been described in all cultures and socioeconomic status groups. In industrialized nations, a disproportionate number of schizophrenic patients are in the low socioeconomic groups, an observation explained by two alternative hypotheses. The *downward drift hypothesis* suggests that affected people move into, or fail to rise out of, a low socioeconomic group because of this illness. The *social causation hypothesis* proposes that stresses experienced by members of low socioeconomic groups contribute to the development of schizophrenia.

Some investigators have presented data indicating that, in addition to the stress of industrialization as a cause of schizophrenia, the stress of immigration can lead to a schizophrenia-like condition. Some studies report a high prevalence of schizophrenia among recent immigrants, a finding implicating abrupt cultural change as a stressor involved in the cause of schizophrenia. Perhaps consistent with both hypotheses is the observation that the prevalence of schizophrenia increases among Third World populations as contact with technologically advanced cultures increases.

Theorists advocating a social cause for schizophrenia argue that cultures may be more or less schizophrenogenic, depending on the perceptions of mental illness in the culture, the nature of the patient's role, the system of social and family supports, and the complexity of social communication. Schizophrenia has been reported to be prognostically more benign in developing countries where patients are reintegrated into their communities and families more completely than they are in highly developed Western societies.

Economics.   The financial cost of the illness in the United States is estimated to exceed that of all cancers combined; it begins early in life; it causes significant and long-lasting impairments; it makes heavy demands for hospital care; and requires ongoing clinical care, rehabilitation, and support services; approximately 1 percent of the national income goes toward the treatment of mental illness (excluding substance-related disorders). Schizophrenia accounts for 2.5 percent of all health care expenditures. Costs of treatment and indirect costs to society (for example, lost production and mortality) amount to almost $50 billion annually. Approximately 75 percent of people with severe schizophrenia are unable to work and are unemployed.

Hospitalization.   The development of effective antipsychotic drugs and changes in political and popular attitudes toward the treatment and the rights of people who are mentally ill have resulted in a dramatic change in the patterns of hospitalization for schizophrenic patients over the past 50 years. The probability of readmission within 2 years after discharge from the first hospitalization is approximately 40 to 60 percent. Patients with schizophrenia occupy approximately 50 percent of all mental hospital beds and account for approximately 16 percent of all psychiatric patients who receive any treatment. The problem of people who are homeless in large cities seems related to the deinstitutionalization of schizophrenic patients who were not adequately followed up. Although the exact percentage of homeless persons who are schizophrenic is difficult to obtain, an estimated one-third to two-thirds of homeless people are probably afflicted with schizophrenia.

ETIOLOGY

Schizophrenia is discussed as if it were a single disease, but the diagnostic category includes a group of disorders, probably with heterogeneous causes, but with somewhat similar behavioral symptoms. Patients with schizophrenia show differing clinical presentations, treatment responses, and courses of illness.

Stress–Diathesis Model

According to the stress–diathesis model for the integration of biological, psychosocial, and environmental factors, a person may have a specific vulnerability (diathesis) that, when acted on by a stressful influence, allows the symptoms of schizophrenia to develop. In the most general stress–diathesis model, the diathesis or the stress can be biological, environmental, or both. The environmental component can be either biological (for example, an infection) or psychological (for example, a stressful family situation or the death of a close relative). The biological basis of a diathesis can be further shaped by epigenetic influences, such as substance abuse, psychosocial stress, and trauma.

Neurobiology

The cause of schizophrenia is unknown. In the past decade, however, an increasing amount of research has indicated a pathophysiological role for certain areas of the brain, including the limbic system, the frontal cortex, cerebellum, and the basal ganglia. These four areas are interconnected, so that dysfunction in one area may involve a primary pathological process in another. Brain imaging of living people and neuropathological examination of postmortem brain tissue have implicated the limbic system as a potential site for the primary pathological process in at least some, perhaps even most, schizophrenic patients.

Two areas of active research are the time that a neuropathological lesion appears in the brain and the interaction of the lesion with environmental and social stressors. The basis for the appearance of the brain abnormality may lie in abnormal development (for example, abnormal migration of neurons along the radial glial cells during development) or in degeneration of neurons after development (for example, abnormally early preprogrammed cell death, as appears to occur in Huntington's disease). The fact that monozygotic twins have a 50 percent discordance rate, however, implies a little-understood interaction between the environment and the development of schizophrenia. On the other hand, the factors regulating gene expression are just beginning to be understood. Although monozygotic twins have the same genetic information, differential gene regulation during their lives perhaps allows one monozygotic twin to have schizophrenia, whereas the other does not.

Dopamine Hypothesis.   The simplest formulation of the *dopamine hypothesis of schizophrenia* posits that schizophrenia results from too much dopaminergic activity. The theory evolved from two observations. First, the efficacy and the potency of most antipsychotic drugs, (that is, the dopamine receptor antagonists) are correlated with their abilities to act as antagonists of the dopamine D_2 receptor. Second, drugs that increase dopaminergic activity, notably amphetamine, are psychotomimetic. The basic theory does not elaborate on whether the dopaminergic hyperactivity is due to too much release of dopamine, too many dopamine receptors, hypersensitivity of the dopamine receptors to dopamine, or a combination of these mechanisms. Which dopamine tracts in the brain are involved is also not specified in the theory, although the mesocortical and mesolimbic tracts are most often implicated. The dopaminergic neurons in these tracts project from their cell bodies in the midbrain to dopaminoceptive neurons in the limbic system and the cerebral cortex.

A significant role for dopamine in the pathophysiology of schizophrenia is consistent with studies that have measured plasma concentrations of the major dopamine metabolite, homovanillic acid. Several preliminary studies have indicated that under carefully controlled experimental conditions, plasma homovanillic acid concentrations can reflect central nervous system concentrations of homovanillic acid. These studies have reported a positive correlation between high pretreatment concentrations of homovanillic acid and two factors: the severity of the psychotic symptoms and the treatment response to antipsychotic drugs. Studies of plasma homovanillic acid have also reported that after a transient increase, plasma homovanillic acid concentrations decline steadily. This decline is correlated with symptom improvement in at least some patients. The dopamine hypothesis of schizophrenia continues to be refined and expanded, and new dopamine receptors continue to be identified. One study has reported an increase in D_4 receptors in postmortem brain samples from schizophrenia patients.

Other Neurotransmitters.   Although the neurotransmitter dopamine has received the most attention in schizophrenia research, increasing attention is being paid to other neurotransmitters for at least two reasons. First, because schizophrenia is likely to be a heterogeneous disorder, it is possible that abnormalities in different neurotransmitters lead to the same behavioral syndrome. For instance, hallucinogenic substances that affect serotonin, such as lysergic acid diethylamide, and high doses of substances that affect dopamine, such as amphetamine, can cause psychotic symptoms that are difficult to distinguish from schizophrenia. Second, neuroscience research has shown that a single neuron may contain more than one neurotransmitter and may have neurotransmitter receptors for a half dozen more neurotransmitters. Thus, the various neurotransmitters in the brain are involved in complex interactional relations, and abnormal functioning may result from changes in any single neurotransmitter.

SEROTONIN.   Serotonin has received much attention in schizophrenia research since the observation was made that the serotonin-dopamine antagonist (SDA) drugs (for example, clozapine, risperidone, sertindole) have potent serotonin-related activities. Specifically, antagonism at the serotonin 5-HT$_2$ receptor has been emphasized as important in reducing psychotic symptoms and in mitigating against the development of D_2-antagonism-related movement disorders. Examination of the receptor affinity profiles for each of the serotonin-dopamine antagonists reveals no uniform pattern or ratio of activities other than their relatively higher affinity for serotonin 5-HT$_2$ receptors than for D_2 receptors. Clozapine has its greatest affinity for histamine receptors, whereas quetiapine binds most tightly to α-adrenergic receptors, and ziprasidone is the only member of the group to interact strongly with 5-HT$_1$ receptors. The affinity for 5-HT$_2$ and D_2 receptors varies over more than a 100-fold range within this class of drugs. Yet each is a more effective antipsychotic agent than hundreds of related compounds that differ only slightly in their affinities. It appears, therefore, that multiple neurotransmitter systems interact in a particular balance of activity levels to regulate the signs and symptoms of schizophrenia and, moreover, that antipsychotic drugs can modulate these circuits by subtly perturbing any of several neurotransmitter systems. As suggested in the research on mood disorders, serotonin activity has been implicated in suicidal and impulsive behavior that can also be seen in schizophrenic patients.

NOREPINEPHRINE.   Several investigators have reported that long-term antipsychotic drug administration decreases the activity of noradrenergic neurons in the locus ceruleus and that the therapeutic effects of some antipsychotic drugs may involve their activities at α-adrenergic and α_2-adrenergic receptors. Although the relation between dopaminergic and noradrenergic activity remains unclear, an increasing amount of data suggest that the noradrenergic system modulates the dopaminergic system in such a way that abnormalities of the noradrenergic system predispose a patient to relapse frequently.

GABA.   The inhibitory amino acid neurotransmitter γ-aminobutyric acid (GABA) has also been implicated in the pathophysiology of schizophrenia. The available data are consistent with the hypothesis that some patients with schizophrenia have a loss of GABAergic neurons in the hippocampus. The loss of inhibitory GABAergic neurons could theoretically lead to the hyperactivity of dopaminergic and noradrenergic neurons.

GLUTAMATE. The hypotheses proposed about glutamate include those of hyperactivity, hypoactivity, and glutamate-induced neurotoxicity. Glutamate has been implicated because the acute ingestion of phencyclidine, a glutamate antagonist, produces a syndrome similar to schizophrenia.

NEUROPEPTIDES. Two neuropeptides, cholecystokinin and neurotensin, are found in a number of brain regions implicated in schizophrenia. Their concentrations are altered in psychotic states.

Neuropathology.

In the 19th century, neuropathologists failed to find a neuropathological basis for schizophrenia, and thus they classified schizophrenia as a functional disorder. By the end of the 20th century, however, researchers made significant strides in revealing a potential neuropathological basis for schizophrenia, primarily in the limbic system and the basal ganglia, including neuropathological or neurochemical abnormalities in the cerebral cortex, the thalamus, and the brainstem. The loss of brain volume widely reported in schizophrenic brains appears to result from a reduced density of the axons, dendrites, and synapses that mediate associative functions of the brain. Synaptic density is highest at age 1, then is pared down to adult values in early adolescence. One theory, based in part on the observation that patients often develop schizophrenic symptoms during adolescence, holds that schizophrenia results from an excessive pruning of synapses during this phase of development.

LIMBIC SYSTEM. Because of its role in controlling emotions, the limbic system has been hypothesized to be involved in the pathophysiological basis of schizophrenia. In fact, this area of the brain has proved to be the most fertile for neuropathological studies of schizophrenia. Many well-controlled studies of postmortem schizophrenic brain samples have shown a decrease in the size of the region including the amygdala, the hippocampus, and the parahippocampal gyrus. This neuropathological finding agrees with the observations made by magnetic resonance imaging (MRI) study of patients with schizophrenia. A disorganization of the neurons within the hippocampus of schizophrenic patients has also been reported.

BASAL GANGLIA. The basal ganglia have been of theoretical interest in schizophrenia for at least two reasons. First, many patients with schizophrenia show odd movements, even in the absence of medication-induced movement disorders (for example, tardive dyskinesia). The odd movements can include an awkward gait, facial grimacing, and stereotypies. Inasmuch as the basal ganglia are involved in the control of movement, disease in the basal ganglia is thereby implicated in the pathophysiology of schizophrenia. Second, of all the neurological disorders that can have psychosis as an associated symptom, the movement disorders involving the basal ganglia (for example, Huntington's disease) are the ones most commonly associated with psychosis in affected patients. Furthermore, the basal ganglia are reciprocally connected to the frontal lobes, and the abnormalities in frontal lobe function seen in some brain-imaging studies may be due to disease in the basal ganglia rather than in the frontal lobes themselves.

Neuropathological studies of the basal ganglia have produced variable and inconclusive reports about cell loss or the reduction of volume of the globus pallidus and the substantia nigra. In contrast, many studies have shown an increase in the number of D_2 receptors in the caudate, the putamen, and the nucleus accumbens. The question remains, however, whether the increase is secondary to the patients' having received antipsychotic medications. Some investigators have begun to study the serotonergic system in the basal ganglia; a role for serotonin in psychotic disorders is suggested by the clinical usefulness of antipsychotic drugs with serotonergic activity (for example, clozapine, risperidone).

Neuroimaging.

Brain-imaging techniques now allow researchers to make specific measurements of neurochemicals or brain function in living patients. Calculations of the data derived from the brain-imaging machines are constructed from many assumptions, however, and differences in these mathematical models between two research groups can potentially lead to different conclusions about the same data.

COMPUTED TOMOGRAPHY. Studies using computed tomography (CT) have consistently shown that the brains of patients with schizophrenia have lateral and third ventricular enlargement and some degree of reduction in cortical volume. These findings can be interpreted as consistent with a decrease in the usual amount of brain tissue in affected patients; whether this decrease is due to abnormal development or to degeneration is unknown.

Other CT studies have reported abnormal cerebral asymmetry, reduced cerebellar volume, and brain density changes in patients with schizophrenia. Many CT studies have correlated the presence of CT scan abnormalities with the presence of negative or deficit symptoms, neuropsychiatric impairment, increased neurological signs, frequent extrapyramidal symptoms from antipsychotic drugs, and poor premorbid adjustment.

MAGNETIC RESONANCE IMAGING. One of the most important MRI studies examined monozygotic twins who were discordant for schizophrenia. The study found that virtually all the affected twins had larger cerebral ventricles than did the nonaffected twins, although the cerebral ventricles of most affected twins fell within a normal range.

Several reports have shown that the volumes of the hippocampal-amygdala complex and the parahippocampal gyrus are reduced in patients with schizophrenia. One recent study found a reduction of these brain areas in the left hemisphere and not in the right, although other studies have found bilateral reductions in volume. Some studies have correlated the reduction in limbic system volume with the degree of psychopathology or other measures of severity of illness. There have also been reports of differential T1 and T2 relaxation times in schizophrenic patients, particularly as measured in the frontal and temporal regions.

FUNCTIONAL MRI. Several studies involving patients with schizophrenia have shown differences in sensorimotor cortex activation compared to normals and decreased blood flow to the occipital lobes.

MAGNETIC RESONANCE SPECTROSCOPY. One study that used magnetic resonance spectroscopy (MRS) found hypoactivity in the dorsolateral prefrontal cortex. These data about the hypoactivity of that brain region supported the findings of other brain-imaging studies—for example, those of positron emission tomography (PET). Another finding is that of decreased concentrations of N-acetyl aspartate in the hippocampus and frontal lobes of patients with schizophrenia and in the temporal lobes of persons with a first episode of psychosis. N-acetyl aspartate is a marker of neurons.

POSITRON EMISSION TOMOGRAPHY. One PET study found that a sample of patients with schizophrenia had reduced metabolic activity in the anterior left portion of the thalamus as measured by [^{18}F]luorodeoxyglucose PET and also had reduced volume in the same area as measured by MRI scan. Altered thalamic architecture and activity may play a role in schizophrenia.

A second type of PET study has used radioactive ligands to estimate the quantity of D_2 receptors present. The two most discussed studies disagree. One group reported an increased number of D_2 receptors in the basal ganglia, and the other group reported no change in the number of D_2 receptors in the basal ganglia. The controversy remains unresolved.

Applied Electrophysiology.   Electroencephalographic studies indicate that many schizophrenic patients have abnormal records, increased sensitivity to activation procedures (for example, frequent spike activity after sleep deprivation), decreased alpha activity, increased theta and delta activity, possibly more than usual epileptiform activity, and possibly more than usual left-sided abnormalities. There is also an inability for schizophrenic patients to filter out irrelevant sounds and to be extremely sensitive to background noise. The flooding of sound that results makes concentration difficult and may be a factor in the production of auditory hallucinations. This sound sensitivity may be associated with a genetic defect.

COMPLEX PARTIAL EPILEPSY.   Schizophrenia-like psychoses have been reported to occur more frequently than expected in patients with complex partial seizures, especially seizures involving the temporal lobes. Factors associated with the development of psychosis in these patients include a left-sided seizure focus, medial temporal location of the lesion, and early onset of seizures. The first-rank symptoms described by Schneider may be similar to symptoms of patients with complex partial epilepsy and may reflect the presence of a temporal lobe disorder when seen in patients with schizophrenia.

EVOKED POTENTIALS.   A large number of abnormalities in evoked potential among patients with schizophrenia have been described. The P300 has been most studied and is defined as a large, positive evoked-potential wave that occurs approximately 300 ms after a sensory stimulus is detected. In patients with schizophrenia, the P300 has been reported to be statistically smaller and later than in comparison groups. Abnormalities in the P300 wave have also been reported to be more common in children who, because they have affected parents, are at high risk for schizophrenia. The evoked-potential data have been interpreted as indicating that although patients with schizophrenia are unusually sensitive to a sensory stimulus (larger early-evoked potentials), they compensate for the increased sensitivity by blunting the processing of information at higher cortical levels indicated by smaller late-evoked potentials).

Eye Movement Dysfunction.   The inability to accurately follow a moving visual target is the defining basis for the disorders of smooth visual pursuit and disinhibition of saccadic eye movements seen in patients with schizophrenia. Eye movement dysfunction may be a trait marker for schizophrenia; it is independent of drug treatment and clinical state and is also seen in first-degree relatives of schizophrenic probands. Various studies have reported abnormal eye movements in 50 to 85 percent of patients with schizophrenia, compared with approximately 25 percent in nonschizophrenic psychiatric patients and less than 10 percent in nonpsychiatrically ill control subjects. Because eye movement is partly controlled by centers in the frontal lobes, a disorder in eye movement is consistent with theories that implicate a frontal lobe pathological process in schizophrenia.

Psychoneuroimmunology.   Several immunological abnormalities have been associated with patients who have schizophrenia. The abnormalities include decreased T-cell interleukin-2 production, reduced number and responsiveness of peripheral lymphocytes, abnormal cellular and humoral reactivity to neurons, and the presence of brain-directed (antibrain) antibodies. The data can be interpreted variously as representing the effects of a neurotoxic virus or of an endogenous autoimmune disorder. Most carefully conducted investigations that have searched for evidence of neurotoxic viral infections in schizophrenia have had negative results, although epidemiological data show a high incidence of schizophrenia after prenatal exposure to influenza during several epidemics of the disease. Other data supporting a viral hypothesis are an increased number of physical anomalies at birth, an increased rate of pregnancy and birth complications, seasonality of birth consistent with viral infection, geographical clusters of adult cases, and seasonality of hospitalizations. Nonetheless, the inability to detect genetic evidence of viral infection reduces the significance of all circumstantial data. The possibility of autoimmune brain antibodies has some data to support it; the pathophysiological process, if it exists, however, probably explains only a subset of the population with schizophrenia.

Psychoneuroendocrinology.   Many reports describe neuroendocrine differences between groups of patients with schizophrenia and groups of control subjects. For example, the dexamethasone-suppression test has been reported to be abnormal in various subgroups of patients with schizophrenia, although the practical or predictive value of the test in schizophrenia has been questioned. One carefully done report, however, has correlated persistent nonsuppression on the dexamethasone-suppression test in schizophrenia with a poor long-term outcome. Some data suggest decreased concentrations of luteinizing hormone–follicle stimulating hormone, perhaps correlated with age of onset and length of illness. Two additional reported abnormalities may be correlated with the presence of negative symptoms: a blunted release of prolactin and growth hormone to gonadotropin-releasing hormone or thyrotropin-releasing hormone stimulation and a blunted release of growth hormone to apomorphine stimulation.

Genetic Factors

A wide range of genetic studies strongly suggests a genetic component to the inheritance of schizophrenia. In the 1930s, classic studies of the genetics of schizophrenia showed that a person is likely to have schizophrenia when other members of the family have the disorder and that the likelihood of the person's having schizophrenia is correlated with the closeness of the relationship (for example, first-degree or second-degree relative; Table 10–1). Monozygotic twins have the highest concordance rate. In studies of adopted monozygotic twins, twins reared by adoptive parents are seen to have schizophrenia at the same rate as their twin siblings brought up by their biological parents. This finding suggests that the genetic influence outweighs the environmental influence, a finding corroborated by the observation that the more severe the schizophrenia, the more likely the twins are to be concordant for the disorder. One study supports the stress-diathesis model and shows that adopted monozygotic twins who later had schizophrenia were likely to have been adopted by psychologically disordered families.

Many associations between chromosomal sites and schizophrenia have been reported since the application of the techniques of molecular biology became widespread. More than half of all chromosomes have been associated with schizophrenia in various reports, but the long arms of chromosomes 5, 11, and 18, the short arm of chromosome 19, and the X chromosome have most commonly been implicated. Loci on chromosomes 6, 8, and 22 have also been implicated. The literature is best summarized as indicating a potentially heterogeneous genetic basis for schizophrenia.

Psychosocial Factors

If schizophrenia is a disease of the brain, it is likely to parallel diseases of other organs (for example, myocardial infarctions and diabetes) whose courses are affected by psychosocial stress. Also like other chronic diseases (for example, chronic congestive pulmonary disease), drug therapy alone is rarely sufficient to obtain maximal clinical improvement. Thus, clinicians should consider the psychosocial factors affecting schizophrenia. Although, historically, theorists have attributed the development of schizophrenia to psychosocial factors, contemporary clinicians can benefit from using the relevant theories and guidelines of these past observations and hypotheses.

Psychoanalytic Theories.

Sigmund Freud postulated that schizophrenia resulted from severe developmental fixations that occurred early in life. He postulated that an ego defect contributed to the symptoms of schizophrenia. Ego defects occur when the ego is not yet, or is just beginning to be, established. Intrapsychic conflicts arising from the early fixations of the ego and ego defects, which may have resulted from poor early object relations, cause the psychotic symptoms. Central to Freud's theories of schizophrenia were a decathexis of objects and a regression in response to frustration and conflict with others. Many of Freud's ideas about schizophrenia, however, were colored by his lack of intensive involvement with schizophrenic patients.

In the classic psychoanalytic view of schizophrenia, the ego defect affects the interpretation of reality and the control of inner drives, such as sex and aggression. The disturbances occur as a consequence of distortions in the reciprocal relationship between the infant and the mother. As described by Margaret Mahler, the child is unable to separate from and to progress beyond the closeness and complete dependence that characterize the mother–child relationship in the oral phase of development. A person with schizophrenia never achieves object constancy, which is characterized by a sense of secure identity and which results from a close attachment to the mother during infancy. Paul Federn concluded that the fundamental disturbance in schizophrenia is the patient's early inability to achieve differentiation from others. Some psychoanalysts hypothesize that the defect in ego functions permits intense hostility and aggression to distort the mother–infant relationship and leads to a personality organization vulnerable to stress. The onset of symptoms during adolescence occurs when teenagers need a strong ego to function independently, to separate from the parents, to identify tasks, to control increased internal drives, and to cope with intense external simulation.

Harry Stack Sullivan viewed schizophrenia as a disturbance in interpersonal relatedness. The patient's massive anxiety creates a sense of unrelatedness that is transformed into distortions called *parataxic distortion* that are persecutory. To Sullivan, schizophrenia is an adaptive method to avoid panic, terror, and disintegration of the sense of self. The source of pathologic anxiety is external to the infant, the result of cumulative experimental traumas during development.

Psychoanalytic theory also postulates that the various symptoms of schizophrenia have symbolic meaning for individual patients. For example, fantasies of the world coming to an end may indicate a perception that a person's internal world has broken down. Feelings of grandeur may reflect reactivated narcissism, in which people believe that they are omnipotent. Hallucinations may be substitutes for patients' inability to deal with objective reality and may represent their inner wishes or fears. Delusions, similar to hallucinations, are regressive, restitutive attempts to create a new reality or to express hidden fears or impulses.

Regardless of theoretical model, all psychodynamic approaches are founded on the premise that psychotic symptoms have meaning in schizophrenia. Patients, for example, may become grandiose after an injury to their self-esteem. Similarly, all theories recognize that human relatedness may be terrifying for people with schizophrenia. Although the research on the efficacy of psychotherapy with schizophrenia shows mixed results, concerned people who offer compassion and a sanctuary in a confusing world must be a cornerstone of any overall treatment plan. Long-term follow-up studies show that some patients who bury psychotic episodes probably do not benefit from exploratory psychotherapy, but those who are able to integrate the psychotic experience into their lives may benefit from some insight-oriented approaches.

Learning Theories.

According to learning theorists, children who later have schizophrenia learn irrational reactions and ways of thinking by imitating parents who have their own significant emotional problems. In learning theory, the poor interpersonal relationships of people with schizophrenia develop because of poor models for learning during childhood.

Family Dynamics.

No well-controlled evidence indicates that a specific family pattern plays a causative role in the development of schizophrenia. Clinicians must understand this important point: Many parents of schizophrenic children harbor anger against the psychiatric community for formerly correlating dysfunctional families with the development of schizophrenia. Advocacy organizations such as the National Alliance for the Mentally Ill (NAMI) have done much to educate parents that they should not blame themselves if schizophrenia develops in a child of theirs. Some patients with schizophrenia do come from dysfunctional families, just as many nonpsychiatrically ill people do. It is also clinically relevant, however, not to overlook pathological family behavior that can significantly increase the emotional stress with which a vulnerable patient with schizophrenia must cope.

DOUBLE BIND.

The double bind concept was formulated by Gregory Bateson and Donald Jackson to describe a hypothetical family in which children receive conflicting parental messages about their behavior, attitudes, and feelings. In Bateson's hypothesis, children withdraw into a psychotic state to escape the unsolvable confusion of the double bind. Unfortunately, the family studies that were conducted to validate the theory were seriously flawed methodologically. The theory has value only as a descriptive pattern, not as an etiological explanation of schizophrenia.

SCHISMS AND SKEWED FAMILIES.

Theodore Lidz described two abnormal patterns of family behavior. In one family type, with a prominent schism between the parents, one parent is overly close to a child of the opposite sex. In the other family type, a skewed relationship between a child and one parent involves a power struggle between the parents and the resulting dominance of one parent.

Pseudomutual and Pseudohostile Families. As described by Lyman Wynne, some families suppress emotional expression by consistently using a pseudomutual or pseudohostile verbal communication. In such families, a unique verbal communication develops, and when a child leaves home and must relate to other people, problems may arise. The child's verbal communication may be incomprehensible to outsiders.

Expressed Emotion. Parents or other caretakers may behave with criticism, hostility, and overinvolvement toward a person with schizophrenia. Many studies have indicated that in families with high levels of expressed emotion (often abbreviated EE), the relapse rate for schizophrenia is high. The assessment of expressed emotion involves analyzing both what is said and the manner in which it is said.

Social Theories. Some theories have suggested that industrialization and urbanization are involved in the causes of schizophrenia. Although some data support such theories, these stresses are now thought to have their major effects on the timing of the onset and severity of the illness.

DIAGNOSIS

The DSM-IV-TR diagnostic criteria are listed in Table 10–2. The presence of hallucinations or delusions is not necessary for the diagnosis of schizophrenia; a patient's disorder is diagnosed as schizophrenia when the patient exhibits two of the symptoms listed as symptoms 3 through 5 in Criterion A. Criterion B requires that impaired functioning, although not deteriorations, be present during the active phase of the illness. Symptoms must persist for at least 6 months and a diagnosis of schizoaffective disorder or mood disorder must be absent. At least one of the following must be present: (1) thought echo, thought insertion or withdrawal, or thought broadcasting; or (2) delusions of control, influence or passivity; (3) hallucinatory voices giving a running commentary on the patient's behavior or discussing the patient between themselves, or other types of hallucinatory voices coming from some part of the body; and (4) persistent delusions of other kinds that are culturally inappropriate and completely impossible (e.g., being able to control the weather or being in communication with aliens from another world).

The diagnosis can also be made if at least two of the following are present: (1) persistent hallucinations in any modality, when occurring every day for at least 1 month, or when accompanied by delusions (which may be fleeting or half-formed); (2) neologisms, breaks or interpolations in the train of thought resulting in incoherence or irrelevant speech; (3) catatonic behavior, such as excitement, posturing or waxy flexibility, negativism, mutism, and stupor; and (4) negative symptoms, such as marked apathy, paucity of speech, and blunting and incongruity of emotional responses (it must be clear that these are not due to depression or to antipsychotic medication).

Subtypes

DSM-IV-TR classifies the subtypes of schizophrenia as paranoid, disorganized, catatonic, undifferentiated, and residual (Table 10–3), based predominantly on clinical presentation. These subtypes are not closely correlated with different prognoses; for such differentiation, specific predictors of prognosis are best consulted

Table 10–2
DSM-IV-TR Diagnostic Criteria for Schizophrenia

A. *Characteristic symptoms:* Two (or more) of the following, each present for a significant portion of time during a 1-month period (or less if successfully treated):

  (1) delusions

  (2) hallucinations

  (3) disorganized speech (e.g., frequent derailment or incoherence)

  (4) grossly disorganized or catatonic behavior

  (5) negative symptoms, i.e., affective flattening, alogia, or avolition

Note: Only one Criterion A symptom is required if delusions are bizarre or hallucinations consist of a voice keeping up a running commentary on the person's behavior or thoughts, or two or more voices conversing with each other.

B. *Social/occupational dysfunction:* For a significant portion of the time since the onset of the disturbance, one or more major areas of functioning such as work, interpersonal relations, or self-care are markedly below the level achieved prior to the onset (or when the onset is in childhood or adolescence, failure to achieve expected level of interpersonal, academic, or occupational achievement).

C. *Duration:* Continuous signs of the disturbance persist for at least 6 months. This 6-month period must include at least 1 month of symptoms (or less if successfully treated) that meet Criterion A (i.e., active-phase symptoms) and may include periods of prodromal or residual symptoms. During these prodromal or residual periods, the signs of the disturbance may be manifested by only negative symptoms or two or more symptoms listed in Criterion A present in an attenuated form (e.g., odd beliefs, unusual perceptual experiences).

D. *Schizoaffective and mood disorder exclusion:* Schizoaffective disorder and mood disorder with psychotic features have been ruled out because either (1) no major depressive, manic, or mixed episodes have occurred concurrently with the active-phase symptoms; or (2) if mood episodes have occurred during active-phase symptoms, their total duration has been brief relative to the duration of the active and residual periods.

E. *Substance/general medical condition exclusion:* The disturbance is not due to the direct physiological effects of a substance (e.g., a drug of abuse, a medication) or a general medical condition.

F. *Relationship to a pervasive developmental disorder:* If there is a history of autistic disorder or another pervasive developmental disorder, the additional diagnosis of schizophrenia is made only if prominent delusions or hallucinations are also present for at least a month (or less if successfully treated).

Classification of longitudinal course (can be applied only after at least 1 year has elapsed since the initial onset of active-phase symptoms):

Episodic with interepisode residual symptoms (episodes are defined by the reemergence of prominent psychotic symptoms); also *specify* if: **with prominent negative symptoms**

Episodic with no interepisode residual symptoms

Continuous (prominent psychotic symptoms are present throughout the period of observation); also *specify* if: **with prominent negative symptoms**

Single episode in partial remission: also *specify* if: **with prominent negative symptoms**

Single episode in full remission

Other or unspecified pattern

Table 10–3
DSM-IV-TR Diagnostic Criteria for Schizophrenia Subtypes

Paranoid type

A type of schizophrenia in which the following criteria are met:

A. Preoccupation with one or more delusions or frequent auditory hallucinations.

B. None of the following is prominent: disorganized speech, disorganized or catatonic behavior, or flat or inappropriate affect.

Disorganized type

A type of schizophrenia in which the following criteria are met:

A. All of the following are prominent:

(1) disorganized speech

(2) disorganized behavior

(3) flat or inappropriate affect

B. The criteria are not met for catatonic type.

Catatonic type

A type of schizophrenia in which the clinical picture is dominated by at least two of the following:

(1) motoric immobility as evidenced by catalepsy (including waxy flexibility) or stupor

(2) excessive motor activity (that is apparently purposeless and not influenced by external stimuli)

(3) extreme negativism (an apparently motiveless resistance to all instructions or maintenance of a rigid posture against attempts to be moved) or mutism

(4) peculiarities of voluntary movement as evidenced by posturing (voluntary assumption of inappropriate or bizarre postures), stereotyped movements, prominent mannerisms, or prominent grimacing

(5) echolalia or echopraxia

Undifferentiated type

A type of schizophrenia in which symptoms that meet Criterion A are present, but the criteria are not met for the paranoid, disorganized, or catatonic type.

Residual type

A type of schizophrenia in which the following criteria are met:

A. Absence of prominent delusions, hallucinations, disorganized speech, and grossly disorganized or catatonic behavior.

B. There is continuing evidence of the disturbance, as indicated by the presence of negative symptoms or two or more symptoms listed in Criterion A for schizophrenia, present in an attenuated form (e.g., odd beliefs, unusual perceptual experiences).

From American Psychiatric Association. *Diagnostic and Statistical Manual of Mental Disorders.* 4th ed. Text rev. Washington, DC: American Psychiatric Association; copyright 2000, with permission.

Table 10–4
Features Weighting toward Good to Poor Prognosis in Schizophrenia

Good Prognosis	Poor Prognosis
Late onset	Young onset
Obvious precipitating factors	No precipitating factors
Acute onset	Insidious onset
Good premorbid social, sexual, and work histories	Poor premorbid social, sexual, and work histories
Mood disorder symptoms (especially depressive disorders)	Withdrawn, autistic behavior
Married	Single, divorced, or widowed
Family history of mood disorders	Family history of schizophrenia
Good support systems	Poor support systems
Positive symptoms	Negative symptoms
	Neurological signs and symptoms
	History of perinatal trauma
	No remissions in 3 years
	Many relapses
	History of assaultiveness

disorganized or catatonic type are absent. Classically, the paranoid type of schizophrenia is characterized mainly by the presence of delusions of persecution or grandeur. Patients with paranoid schizophrenia usually have their first episode of illness at an older age than do patients with catatonic or disorganized schizophrenia. Patients in whom schizophrenia occurs in the late 20s or 30s have usually established a social life that may help them through their illness, and the ego resources of paranoid patients tend to be greater than those of patients with catatonic and disorganized schizophrenia. Patients with paranoid type of schizophrenia show less regression of their mental faculties, emotional responses, and behavior than do patients with other types of schizophrenia.

Patients with paranoid schizophrenia are typically tense, suspicious, guarded, reserved, and sometimes hostile or aggressive, but they can occasionally conduct themselves adequately in social situations. Their intelligence in areas not invaded by their psychosis tends to remain intact.

(Table 10–4). The tenth revision of *International Statistical Classification of Diseases and Related Health Problems* (ICD-10), by contrast, uses nine subtypes: paranoid schizophrenia, hebephrenia, catatonic schizophrenia, undifferentiated schizophrenia, postschizophrenic depression, residual schizophrenia, simple schizophrenia, other schizophrenia, and schizophrenia, unspecified, with eight possibilities for classifying the course of the disorder, ranging from continuous to complete remission.

Paranoid Type.

The paranoid type of schizophrenia is characterized by preoccupation with one or more delusions of frequent auditory hallucinations and that specific behaviors suggestive of the

A 44-year-old single, unemployed man was brought into an emergency room by the police for striking an elderly woman in his apartment building. He complained that the woman he struck was a bitch and that she and "the others" deserved more than that for what they put him through.

The patient had been continually ill since the age of 22. During his first year of law school, he gradually became more and more convinced that his classmates were making fun of him. He noticed that they would snort and sneeze whenever he entered the classroom. When a girl he was dating broke off the relationship with him, he believed that she had been replaced by a look-alike. He called the police and asked for their help in solving the "kidnapping." His academic performance in school declined dramatically, and he was asked to leave and seek psychiatric care.

The patient got a job as an investment counselor at a bank, which he held for 7 months. However, he was getting an increasing number of distracting "signals" from coworkers, and he became more and more suspicious and withdrawn. At that time he first reported hearing voices. He was eventually fired and soon thereafter was hospitalized for the first time, at age 24. He has not worked since.

The patient has been hospitalized 12 times; the longest stay was for 8 months. However, in the past 5 years he was hospitalized only once, for 3 weeks. During the hospitalizations he received various antipsychotic drugs. Although outpatient medication had been prescribed, he usually stopped taking it shortly after leaving the hospital. Aside from twice-yearly lunch meetings with his uncle and his contact with mental health workers, he was totally isolated socially. He lived on his own and managed his own financial affairs, including a modest inheritance. He read the Wall Street Journal daily. He cooked and cleaned for himself.

The patient maintained that his apartment was the center of a large communication system that involved all three major television networks, his neighborhood, and apparently hundreds of "actors" in his neighborhood. There were secret cameras in his apartment that carefully monitored all his activities. When he was watching television, many of his minor actions (e.g., getting up to go to the bathroom) were soon directly commented on by the announcer. Whenever he went outside, the "actors" had all been warned to keep him under surveillance; everyone on the street watched him. His neighbors operated two "machines"; one was responsible for all his voices except the "joker." He was not certain who controlled that voice, which visited him only occasionally and was very funny. The other voices, which he heard many times each day, were generated by that machine, which he sometimes thought was directly run by the neighbor whom he attacked. For example, when he was going over his investments, those "harassing" voices constantly told him which stocks to buy. The other machine he called "the dream machine." That machine put erotic dreams into his head, usually of black women.

The patient described other unusual experiences. For example, he recently went to a shoe store 30 miles from his home in the hope of getting some shoes that would not be "altered." However, he soon found out that like the rest of the shoes he bought, special nails had been put into the bottoms of the shoe to annoy him. He was amazed that his decision about which shoe store to go to must have been known to his "harasser" before he himself knew it, so that they had time to get the altered shoes made up especially for him. He realized that great effort and "millions of dollars'" were involved in keeping him under surveillance. He sometimes thought that was all part of a large experiment to discover the secret of his superior intelligence.

At the interview, the patient was well groomed, and his speech was coherent and goal directed. His affect was, at most, only mildly blunted. He was initially angry at police. After several weeks of treatment with an antipsychotic that failed to control his psychotic symptoms, he was transferred to a long-stay facility with the plan to arrange a structured living situation for him.

DISCUSSION

The patient's long illness apparently began with delusions of reference (his classmates making fun of him by snorting and sneezing when he entered the classroom). Over the years his delusions had become increasingly complex and bizarre (his neighbors were actually actors; his thoughts were monitored; a machine put erotic dreams into his head). In addition, he had prominent hallucinations of voices that harassed him.

Bizarre delusions and prominent hallucinations are the characteristic psychotic symptoms of schizophrenia. The diagnosis was confirmed by the marked disturbance in his work and social functioning and the absence of a sustained mood disturbance and of any known organic factor that could account for the disturbance.

All the patient's delusions and hallucinations seemed to involve the single theme of a conspiracy to harass him. That systematized persecutory delusion—the absence of incoherence, marked loosening of associations, flat or grossly inappropriate affect or catatonic or grossly disorganized behavior—indicates the paranoid type. Schizophrenia, paranoid type, is further specified as continuous if, as in this case, all past and present active phases of the illness have been of the paranoid type. The prognosis for the continuous paranoid type is better than the prognosis for the disorganized and undifferentiated types. The patient did, in fact, do remarkably well in spite of a chronic psychotic illness; over the past 5 years he had been able to take care of himself.

Disorganized Type.   The disorganized (formerly called *hebephrenic*) type of schizophrenia is characterized by a marked regression to primitive, disinhibited, and unorganized behavior and by the absence of symptoms that meet the criteria for the catatonic type. The onset of this subtype is generally early, before age 25. Disorganized patients are usually active but in an aimless, nonconstructive manner. Their thought disorder is pronounced, and their contact with reality is poor. Their personal appearance and their social behavior are dilapidated, their emotional responses are inappropriate, and they often burst into laughter without any apparent reason. Incongruous grinning and grimacing are common in these patients, whose behavior is best described as silly or fatuous.

Catatonic Type.   The catatonic type of schizophrenia, which was common several decades ago, has become rare in Europe and North America. The classic feature of the catatonic type is a marked disturbance in motor function; this disturbance may involve stupor, negativism, rigidity, excitement, or posturing (Fig. 10–1). Sometimes, the patient shows a rapid alteration between extremes of excitement and stupor. Associated features include stereotypies, mannerisms, and waxy flexibility. Mutism is particularly common. During catatonic stupor or excitement, patients need careful supervision to prevent them from hurting themselves or others. Medical care may be needed because of malnutrition, exhaustion, hyperpyrexia, or self-inflicted injury.

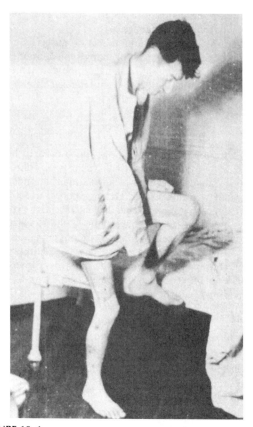

FIGURE 10–1
A chronic schizophrenic patient stands in a cataleptic position. He maintained this uncomfortable position for hours. (Courtesy of New York Academy of Medicine, New York, NY.)

A young, unmarried woman, age 20, was admitted to a psychiatric hospital because she had become violent toward her parents, had been observed gazing into space with a rapt expression, and had been talking to invisible persons. She had been seen to strike odd postures. Her speech had become incoherent.

She had been a good student in high school, then went to business school and, a year before admission to the hospital, started to work in an office as a stenographer. She had always been shy, and although she was quite attractive, she had not been dating much. Another girl, who worked in the same office, told the patient about boys and petting and began to exert a great deal of influence over her. The second girl would communicate with her from across the room. Even when they went home at night, the patient would get voice messages telling her to do certain things. Then pictures began to appear on the wall, most of them ugly and sneering. Those pictures had names—one was named shyness, another distress, another envy. Her office friend sent her messages to knock on the wall, to hit the pictures.

The patient was agitated, noisy, and uncooperative in the hospital for several weeks after she arrived, and required sedation. She was given a course of insulin coma therapy, with no significant or sustained improvement. Later she received several courses of electroconvulsive treatment, which also failed to influence the schizophrenic process to any significant degree. Ten years later, when antipsychotic drugs became available, she received pharmacotherapy.

Despite all those therapeutic efforts, her condition throughout her many years of stay in a mental hospital has remained one of chronic catatonic stupor. She is mute and practically devoid of any spontaneity, but she responds to simple requests. She stays in the same position for hours or sits curled up in a chair. Her facial expression is fixed and stony. (Courtesy of Robert Cancro, M.D., Med.D.Sc., and Heinz E. Lehmann, M.D.)

Undifferentiated Type.   Frequently, patients who are clearly schizophrenic cannot be easily fitted into one or another type. DSM-IV-TR classifies these patients as having schizophrenia of the undifferentiated type.

Residual Type.   According to DSM-IV-TR, the residual type of schizophrenia is characterized by the presence of continuing evidence of the schizophrenic disturbance in the absence of a complete set of active symptoms or of sufficient symptoms to meet the diagnosis of another type of schizophrenia. Emotional blunting, social withdrawal, eccentric behavior, illogical thinking, and mild loosening of associations commonly appear in the residual type. When delusions or hallucinations occur, they are neither prominent nor accompanied by strong affect.

Other Subtypes

The subtyping of schizophrenia has had a long history; other subtyping schemes appear in the literature, especially literature from countries other than the United States.

Bouffée Délirante (Acute Delusional Psychosis).
This French diagnostic concept differs from a diagnosis of schizophrenia primarily on the basis of a symptom duration of less than 3 months. The diagnosis is similar to the DSM-IV-TR diagnosis of schizophreniform disorder. French clinicians report that approximately 40 percent of patients with a diagnosis of *bouffée délirante* progress in their illness and are eventually classified as having schizophrenia.

Latent.   The concept of latent schizophrenia was developed during a time when theorists conceived of the disorder in broad diagnostic terms. Currently, patients must be very mentally ill to warrant a diagnosis of schizophrenia, but with a broad diagnostic concept of schizophrenia, the condition of patients who would not currently be thought of as severely ill could have received a diagnosis of schizophrenia. Latent schizophrenia, for example, was often the diagnosis used for patients with what are now called *schizoid* and *schizotypal personality disorders*. These patients may occasionally show peculiar behaviors or thought disorders but do not consistently manifest psychotic symptoms. In the past, the syndrome was also termed *borderline schizophrenia*.

Oneiroid.   The *oneiroid state* refers to a dream-like state in which patients may be deeply perplexed and not fully oriented in time and place. The term *oneiroid schizophrenic* has been used for patients who are deeply engaged in their hallucinatory experiences to the exclusion of involvement in the real world. When an oneiroid state is present, clinicians should be particularly careful to examine patients for medical or neurological causes of the symptoms.

Paraphrenia.　This term is sometimes used as a synonym for *paranoid schizophrenia* or for either a progressively deteriorating course of illness or the presence of a well-systemized delusional system. The multiple meanings of the term render it ineffective in communicating information.

Pseudoneurotic Schizophrenia.　Occasionally, patients who initially have such symptoms as anxiety, phobias, obsessions, and compulsions later reveal symptoms of thought disorder and psychosis. These patients are characterized by symptoms of pananxiety, panphobia, panambivalence, and sometimes a chaotic sexuality. Unlike people with anxiety disorders, pseudoneurotic patients have free-floating anxiety that rarely subsides. In clinical descriptions, the patients seldom become overtly and severely psychotic. These patients are currently diagnosed in DSM-IV-TR as having borderline personality disorder.

Simple Deteriorative Disorder (Simple Schizophrenia).　Simple deteriorative disorder is characterized by a gradual, insidious loss of drive and ambition. Patients with the disorder are usually not overtly psychotic and do not experience persistent hallucinations or delusions. Their primary symptom is withdrawal from social and work-related situations. The syndrome must be differentiated from depression, a phobia, a dementia, or an exacerbation of personality traits. Clinicians should be sure that patients truly meet the diagnostic criteria for schizophrenia before making the diagnosis. Simple deteriorative disorder appears as a diagnostic category in an appendix of DSM-IV-TR (Table 10–5) indicating the need for further study.

Postpsychotic Depressive Disorder of Schizophrenia.　After an acute schizophrenia episode, some patients become depressed. The symptoms of postpsychotic depressive disorder of schizophrenia can closely resemble the symptoms of the residual phase of schizophrenia as well as the side effects of commonly used antipsychotic medications. The diagnoses should not be made if they are substance induced or part of a mood disorder due to a general medical condition. These depressive states occur in up to 25 percent of patients with schizophrenia and are associated with an increased risk of suicide.

Table 10–5
DSM-IV-TR Research Criteria for Simple Deteriorative Disorder (Simple Schizophrenia)

A. Progressive development over a period of at least a year of all of the following:
  (1) marked decline in occupational or academic functioning
  (2) gradual appearance and deepening of negative symptoms such as affective flattening, alogia, and avolition
  (3) poor interpersonal rapport, social isolation, or social withdrawal
B. Criterion A for schizophrenia has never been met.
C. The symptoms are not better accounted for by schizotypal or schizoid personality disorder, a psychotic disorder, a mood disorder, an anxiety disorder, a dementia, or mental retardation and are not due to the direct physiological effects of a substance or a general medical condition.

From American Psychiatric Association. *Diagnostic and Statistical Manual of Mental Disorders.* 4th ed. Text rev. Washington, DC: American Psychiatric Association; copyright 2000, with permission.

Early-Onset Schizophrenia.　A small minority of patients manifest schizophrenia in childhood. Such children may at first present diagnostic problems, particularly with differentiation from mental retardation and autistic disorder. Recent studies have established that the diagnosis of childhood schizophrenia may be based on the same symptoms used for adult schizophrenia. Its onset is usually insidious, its course tends to be chronic, and the prognosis is mostly unfavorable.

Late-Onset Schizophrenia.　Late-onset schizophrenia is clinically indistinguishable from schizophrenia but has an onset after age 45. This condition tends to appear more frequently in women and also tends to be characterized by a predominance of paranoid symptoms. The prognosis is favorable, and these patients usually do well on antipsychotic medication.

Other Diagnostic Criteria

A variety of research clinicians, some of whom have already been mentioned (for example, Langfeldt, Schneider, and Jaspers), constructed their own criteria to describe the essential features of schizophrenia. The DSM-IV-TR are most extensively used by researchers.

Psychological Testing

In general, patients with schizophrenia perform similarly to patients with neurologically caused mental disorders. The data are consistent with the idea that schizophrenia is a brain disease that disrupts the normal functioning of many cognitive abilities. Patients with schizophrenia generally perform poorly on a wide range of neuropsychological tests. Vigilance, memory, and concept formation are most affected and consistent with pathological involvement in the frontotemporal cortex.

Objective measures of neuropsychological performance, such as the Halstead-Reitan battery and the Luria-Nebraska battery, often give abnormal findings, such as bilateral frontal and temporal lobe dysfunction, including impairments in attention, retention time, and problem-solving ability. Motor ability is also impaired, possibly related to brain asymmetry.

Intelligence Tests.　When groups of patients with schizophrenia are compared with groups of nonschizophrenic psychiatric patients or with the general population, the schizophrenic patients tend to score lower on intelligence tests. Statistically, the evidence suggests that low intelligence is often present at the onset, and intelligence may continue to deteriorate with the progression of the disorder. Other findings are impairments in learning and memory, especially in the ability for sustained attention on visual or motor tasks.

Projective and Personality Tests.　Projective tests, such as the Rorschach test and the Thematic Apperception Test (TAT), may indicate bizarre ideation. Personality inventories, such as the Minnesota Multiphasic Personality Inventory (MMPI), often give abnormal results in schizophrenia, but the contribution to diagnosis and treatment planning is minimal.

CLINICAL FEATURES

A discussion of the clinical signs and symptoms of schizophrenia raises three key issues. First, no clinical sign or symptom is pathognomonic for schizophrenia; every sign or symptom seen in schizophrenia occurs in other psychiatric and neurological disorders. This observation is contrary to the often-heard clinical opinion that certain signs and symptoms are diagnostic of schizophrenia. Therefore, a patient's history is essential for the diagnosis of schizophrenia; clinicians cannot diagnose schizophrenia simply by a mental status examination, which may vary. Second, a patient's symptoms change with time. For example, a patient may have intermittent hallucinations and a varying ability to perform adequately in social situations, or significant symptoms of a mood disorder may come and go during the course of schizophrenia. Third, clinicians must take into account the patient's educational level, intellectual ability, and cultural and subcultural membership. An impaired ability to understand abstract concepts, for example, may reflect either the patient's education or his or her intelligence. Religious organizations and cults may have customs that seem strange to outsiders but that are normal to those within the cultural setting.

Premorbid Signs and Symptoms

In theoretical formulations of the course of schizophrenia, premorbid signs and symptoms appear before the prodromal phase of the illness. The differentiation implies that premorbid signs and symptoms exist before the disease process evidences itself and that the prodromal signs and symptoms are parts of the evolving disorder. In the typical but not invariable premorbid history of schizophrenia, patients have had schizoid or schizotypal personalities characterized as quiet, passive, and introverted; as children they had few friends. Preschizophrenic adolescents may have no close friends and no dates and may avoid team sports. They may enjoy watching movies and television or listening to music to the exclusion of social activities. Some adolescent patients may show an acute onset of obsessive-compulsive behavior as part of the prodromal picture.

The validity of the prodromal signs and symptoms, almost invariably recognized after the diagnosis of schizophrenia has been made, is uncertain; once schizophrenia is diagnosed, the retrospective remembrance of early signs and symptoms is affected. Nevertheless, although the first hospitalization is often thought to mark the beginning of the disorder, signs and symptoms have often been present for months or even years. The signs may have started with complaints about somatic symptoms, such as headache, back and muscle pain, weakness, and digestive problems. The initial diagnosis may be malingering or somatization disorder. Family and friends may eventually notice that the person has changed and is no longer functioning well in occupational, social, and personal activities. During this stage, a patient may begin to develop an interest in abstract ideas, philosophy, the occult, or religious questions. Additional prodromal signs and symptoms can include markedly peculiar behavior, abnormal affects, unusual speech, bizarre ideas, and strange perceptual experiences.

Positive and Negative Symptoms

In 1980, T. J. Crow proposed a classification of schizophrenic patients into types I and II, based on the presence or the absence of positive (or productive) and negative (or deficit) symptoms. Although the system was not accepted as part of the DSM-IV-TR classification, the clinical distinction of the two types has significantly influenced psychiatric research. The *positive symptoms* include delusions and hallucinations. The *negative symptoms* include affective flattening or blunting, poverty of speech (alogia) or speech content, blocking, poor grooming, lack of motivation, anhedonia, and social withdrawal. Type I patients tend to have mostly positive symptoms, normal brain structures on CT scans, and relatively good responses to treatment. Type II patients tend to have mostly negative symptoms, structural brain abnormalities on CT scans, and poor responses to treatments. A third category, disorganized, includes disorganized speech (thought disorder), disorganized behavior, cognitive defects, and attention deficits. Nancy Anderson has studied positive and negative symptoms extensively.

Mental Status Examination

General Description.
The appearance of a patient with schizophrenia can range from that of a completely disheveled, screaming, agitated person to an obsessively groomed, completely silent, and immobile person. Between these two poles, patients may be talkative and may exhibit bizarre postures (Fig. 10–1). Their behavior may become agitated or violent, apparently in an unprovoked manner but usually in response to hallucinations. By contrast, in catatonic stupor, often referred to as *catatonia,* patients seem completely lifeless and may exhibit such signs as muteness, negativism, and automatic obedience. Waxy flexibility, once a common sign in catatonia, has become rare. A person with a less extreme subtype of catatonia may show marked social withdrawal and egocentricity, lack of spontaneous speech or movement, and an absence of goal-directed behavior. Patients with catatonia may sit immobile and speechless in their chairs, respond only with short answers to questions, and move only when directed to. Other obvious behavior may include an odd clumsiness or stiffness in body movements, signs now seen as possibly indicating a disease process in the basal ganglia. Patients with schizophrenia often are poorly groomed, fail to bathe, and dress much too warmly for the prevailing temperatures. Other odd behaviors include tics, stereotypies, mannerisms, and, occasionally, *echopraxia,* in which patients imitate the posture or the behaviors of the examiner.

PRECOX FEELING.   Some experienced clinicians report a precox feeling, an intuitive experience of their inability to establish an emotional rapport with a patient. Although the experience is common, no data indicate that it is a valid or reliable criterion in the diagnosis of schizophrenia.

Mood, Feelings, and Affect.
Two common affective symptoms in schizophrenia are reduced emotional responsiveness, sometimes severe enough to warrant the label of anhedonia, and overly active and inappropriate emotions such as extremes of rage, happiness, and anxiety. A flat or blunted affect can be a symptom of the illness itself, of the parkinsonian side effects of antipsychotic medications, or of depression, and differentiating these symptoms can be a clinical challenge. Overly emotional patients may describe exultant feelings of omnipotence, religious ecstasy, terror at the disintegration of their souls, or paralyzing anxiety about the destruction of the universe. Other feeling tones include perplexity, terror, a sense

of isolation overwhelming ambivalence, and depression. (Postpsychotic depressive disorder of schizophrenia is further discussed in Section 14.4.)

Perceptual Disturbances.   Any of the five senses may be affected by hallucinatory experiences in patients with schizophrenia. The most common hallucinations, however, are auditory, with voices that are often threatening, obscene, accusatory, or insulting. Two or more voices may converse among themselves, or a voice may comment on the patient's life or behavior. Visual hallucinations are common, but tactile, olfactory, and gustatory hallucinations are unusual; their presence should prompt the clinician to consider the possibility of an underlying medical or neurological disorder that is causing the entire syndrome.

CENESTHETIC HALLUCINATIONS.   Cenesthetic hallucinations are unfounded sensations of altered states in bodily organs. Examples of cenesthetic hallucinations include a burning sensation in the brain, a pushing sensation in the blood vessels, and a cutting sensation in the bone marrow.

ILLUSIONS.   As differentiated from hallucinations, *illusions* are distortions of real images or sensations, whereas *hallucinations* are *not* based on real images or sensations. Illusions can occur in schizophrenic patients during active phases, but they can also occur during the prodromal phases and during periods of remission. Whenever illusions or hallucinations occur, clinicians should consider the possibility of a substance-related cause for the symptoms, even when patients have already received diagnoses of schizophrenia.

Thought.   Disorders of thought are the most difficult symptoms for many clinicians and students to understand but may be the core symptoms of schizophrenia. Dividing the disorders of thought into disorders of thought content, form of thought, and thought process is one way to clarify them.

THOUGHT CONTENT.   Disorders of thought content reflect the patient's ideas, beliefs, and interpretations of stimuli. Delusions, the most obvious example of a disorder of thought content, are varied in schizophrenia and may assume persecutory, grandiose, religious, or somatic forms.

Patients may believe that an outside entity controls their thoughts or behavior or conversely, that they control outside events in an extraordinary fashion (for example, by causing the sun to rise and set or by preventing earthquakes). Patients may have an intense and consuming preoccupation with esoteric, abstract, symbolic, psychological, or philosophical ideas. Patients may also worry about allegedly life-threatening but bizarre and implausible somatic conditions, such as the presence of aliens inside the patient's testicles, affecting his ability to father children.

The phrase *loss of ego boundaries* describes the lack of a clear sense of where the patient's own body, mind, and influence end and where those of other animate and inanimate objects begin. For example, patients may think that other people, the television, or the newspapers are making reference to them (*ideas of reference*). Other symptoms of the loss of ego boundaries include the sense that the patient has physically fused with an outside object (for example, a tree or another person) or that the patient has disintegrated and fused with the entire universe. With such a state of mind, some patients with schizophrenia doubt their sex or their sexual orientation. These symptoms should not be confused with transvestism, transsexuality, or homosexuality.

FORM OF THOUGHT.   Disorders of the form of thought are objectively observable in patients' spoken and written language. The disorders include looseness of associations, derailment, incoherence, tangentiality, circumstantiality, neologisms, echolalia, verbigeration, word salad, and mutism. Although looseness of associations was once described as pathognomonic for schizophrenia, the symptom is frequently seen in mania. Distinguishing between looseness of associations and tangentiality can be difficult for even the most experienced clinicians.

THOUGHT PROCESS.   Disorders in thought process concern the way ideas and language are formulated. The examiner infers a disorder from what and how the patient speaks, writes, or draws. The examiner may also assess the patient's thought process by observing his or her behavior, especially in carrying out discrete tasks, for example, in occupational therapy. Disorders of thought process include flight of ideas, thought blocking, impaired attention, poverty of thought content, poor abstraction abilities, perseveration, idiosyncratic associations (for example, identical predicates and clang associations), overinclusion, and circumstantiality.

Impulsiveness, Violence, Suicide, and Homicide.   Patients with schizophrenia may be agitated and have little impulse control when ill. They may also have decreased social sensitivity and appear to be impulsive when, for example, they grab another patient's cigarettes, change television channels abruptly, or throw food on the floor. Some apparently impulsive behavior, including suicide and homicide attempts, may be in response to hallucinations commanding the patient to act.

VIOLENCE.   Violent behavior (excluding homicide) is common among untreated schizophrenic patients. Delusions of a persecutory nature, previous episodes of violence, and neurological deficits are risk factors for violent or impulsive behavior. Management includes appropriate antipsychotic medication. Emergency treatment consists of restraints and seclusion. Acute sedation with lorazepam (Ativan), 1 to 2 mg intramuscularly, repeated every hour as needed, may be necessary to prevent the patient from doing harm to others. If a clinician finds himself being fearful in the presence of a schizophrenic patient, that should be taken as an internal clue that the patient may be on the verge of acting out violently. In such cases, the interview should be terminated or conducted with an attendant at the ready.

SUICIDE.   Approximately 50 percent of all schizophrenic patients attempt suicide, and 10 to 15 percent of patients with schizophrenia die by suicide. Perhaps the most underappreciated factor involved in the suicide of these patients is depression that has been misdiagnosed as flat affect or as a medication side effect. Other precipitants of suicide include feelings of absolute emptiness, a need to escape from mental torture, or auditory hallucinations that command patients to kill themselves. The risk factors for suicide are the patient's awareness of the illness, male sex, college education, young age, a change in the course of the disease, an improvement after a relapse, dependence on the hospital, overly high ambitions, previous suicide attempts early in the course of the illness, and living alone. In the hospital, patients should be monitored closely if they are suicidal.

HOMICIDE.   In spite of the sensational attention that the news media provide when a patient with schizophrenia murders someone, the available data indicate that these patients are no more likely to commit homicide than is a member of the general population. When a patient with schizophrenia does commit homicide, it may be for unpredictable or bizarre reasons based on hallucinations or delusions. Possible predictors of homicidal activity are a history of previous violence, dangerous behavior while hospitalized, and hallucinations or delusions involving such violence.

Sensorium and Cognition

Orientation.   Patients with schizophrenia are usually oriented to person, time, and place. The lack of such orientation should prompt clinicians to investigate the possibility of a medical or neurological brain disorder. Some patients with schizophrenia may give incorrect or bizarre answers to questions about orientation, for example, "I am Christ; this is heaven; and it is A.D. 35."

Memory.   Memory, as tested in the mental status examination, is usually intact. It may be impossible, however, to get a patient to attend closely enough to the memory tests for the ability to be assessed adequately.

Judgment and Insight.   Classically, patients with schizophrenia are described as having poor insight into the nature and the severity of their disorder. The so-called lack of insight is associated with poor compliance with treatment. When examining schizophrenic patients, clinicians should carefully define various aspects of insight, such as awareness of symptoms, trouble in getting along with people, and the reasons for these problems. Such information can be clinically useful in tailoring a treatment strategy and theoretically useful in postulating what areas of the brain contribute to the observed lack of insight (for example, the parietal lobes).

Reliability.   A patient with schizophrenia is no less reliable than is any other psychiatric patient. The nature of the disorder, however, requires the examiner to verify important information through additional sources.

Neurological Findings

Localizing and nonlocalizing neurological signs (also known as *hard* and *soft signs*, respectively) have been reported to be present more commonly in patients with schizophrenia than in other psychiatric patients. Nonlocalizing signs include dysdiadochokinesia, astereognosis, primitive reflexes, and diminished dexterity. The presence of neurological signs and symptoms correlates with increased severity of illness, affective blunting, and a poor prognosis. Other abnormal neurological signs include tics, stereotypies, grimacing, impaired fine motor skills,

abnormal motor tone, and abnormal movements. One study has found that only approximately 25 percent of patients with schizophrenia are aware of their own abnormal involuntary movements and that the lack of awareness is correlated with lack of insight about the primary psychiatric disorder and the duration of illness.

Eye Examination.   In addition to the disorder of smooth ocular pursuit, (saccadic movement) patients with schizophrenia have an elevated blink rate. The elevated blink rate is thought to reflect hyperdopaminergic activity. In primates, blinking can be increased by dopamine agonists and reduced by dopamine antagonists.

Speech.   Although the disorders of speech in schizophrenia (for example, looseness of associations) are classically thought of as indicating a thought disorder, they may also indicate a *forme fruste* of an aphasia, perhaps implicating the dominant parietal lobe. The inability of schizophrenic patients to perceive the prosody of speech or to inflect their own speech can be seen as a neurological symptom of a disorder in the nondominant parietal lobe. Other parietal lobe-like symptoms in schizophrenia include the inability to carry out tasks (that is, *apraxia*), right–left disorientation, and lack of concern about the disorder.

Other Physical Findings

An increased incidence of minor physical anomalies is associated with the diagnosis of schizophrenia. Such anomalies, most likely associated with early stages of embryonic and fetal growth, usually during the first trimester, have been reported in 30 to 75 percent of patients with schizophrenia, compared with 0 to 13 percent of the general population. Some current studies suggest that the anomalies are more common in men than in women and are probably associated with genetic factors, although obstetric complications cannot be ruled out as causative factors. Compulsive water drinking may occur in some patients who can consume up to 10 L a day and develop hyponatremia.

DIFFERENTIAL DIAGNOSIS
Secondary Psychotic Disorders

A wide range of nonpsychiatric medical conditions and a variety of substances can induce symptoms of psychosis and catatonia. The most appropriate diagnosis for such psychosis or catatonia is *psychotic disorder due to a general medical condition, catatonic disorder due to a general medical condition*, or *substance-induced psychotic disorder*. The psychiatric manifestations of many nonpsychiatric medical conditions can come early in the course of the illness, often before the development of other symptoms. Therefore, clinicians must consider a wide range of nonpsychiatric medical conditions in the differential diagnosis of psychosis, even in the absence of obvious physical symptoms. Patients with neurological disorders generally have more insight into their illnesses and more distress from their psychiatric symptoms than do patients with schizophrenia. This fact can help clinicians distinguish the two groups of patients.

When evaluating a patient with psychotic symptoms, clinicians should follow the general guidelines for assessing nonpsychiatric conditions. First, clinicians should aggressively pursue an undiagnosed nonpsychiatric medical condition when a patient exhibits any unusual or rare symptoms or any variation in the level of consciousness. Second, clinicians should attempt to obtain a complete family history, including a history of medical, neurological, and psychiatric disorders. Third, clinicians should consider the possibility of a nonpsychiatric medical condition, even in patients with previous diagnoses of schizophrenia. A patient with schizophrenia is just as likely to have a brain tumor that produces psychotic symptoms as is a nonschizophrenic patient.

Malingering and Factitious Disorders

In a patient who imitates the symptoms of schizophrenia but does not actually have the disorder, either malingering or a factitious disorder may be an appropriate diagnosis. People have faked schizophrenic symptoms and have been admitted into and treated at psychiatric hospitals. The condition of patients who are completely in control of their symptom production may qualify for a diagnosis of malingering; such patients usually have some obvious financial or legal reason to be considered mentally ill. The condition of patients who are less in control of their falsification of psychotic symptoms may qualify for a diagnosis of a factitious disorder. Some patients with schizophrenia, however, may falsely complain of an exacerbation of psychotic symptoms to obtain increased assistance benefits or to gain admission to a hospital. (Factitious disorders are the subject of Chapter 16.)

Other Psychotic Disorders

The psychotic symptoms of schizophrenia can be identical to those of schizophreniform disorder, brief psychotic disorder, schizoaffective disorder, and delusional disorders. *Schizophreniform disorder* differs from schizophrenia in that the symptoms have a duration of at least 1 month but less than 6 months. *Brief psychotic disorder* is the appropriate diagnosis when the symptoms have lasted at least 1 day but less than 1 month and when the patient has not returned to the premorbid state of functioning within that time. When a manic or depressive syndrome develops concurrently with the major symptoms of schizophrenia, *schizoaffective disorder* is the appropriate diagnosis. Nonbizarre delusions present for at least 1 month without other symptoms of schizophrenia or a mood disorder warrant the diagnosis of *delusional disorder.*

Mood Disorders

The differential diagnosis of schizophrenia and mood disorders can be difficult but must be made because of the availability of specific and effective treatments for mania and depression. Compared with the duration of the primary symptoms, affective or mood symptoms in schizophrenia should be brief. Before making a premature diagnosis of schizophrenia, and without more information than that gleaned from a single mental status examination, clinicians should delay a final diagnosis or should assume the presence of mood disorder. After remission of a schizophrenic episode, some patients experience a postpsychotic or secondary depression. Treatment with a selective serotonin reuptake inhibitor (SSRI) or a tricyclic antidepressant is indicated in that situation.

Personality Disorders

Various personality disorders may have some features of schizophrenia. Schizotypal, schizoid, and borderline personality disorders are the personality disorders with the most similar symptoms. Severe obsessive-compulsive personality disorder may mask an underlying schizophrenic process.

Personality disorders, unlike schizophrenia, have mild symptoms and a history of occurring throughout a patient's life; they also lack an identifiable date of onset.

COURSE AND PROGNOSIS

Course

A premorbid pattern of symptoms may be the first evidence of illness, although the import of the symptoms is usually recognized only retrospectively. Characteristically, the symptoms begin in adolescence and are followed by the development of prodromal symptoms in days to a few months. Social or environmental changes, such as going away to college, using a substance, or a relative's death, may precipitate the disturbing symptoms, and the prodromal syndrome may last a year or more before the onset of overt psychotic symptoms.

The classic course of schizophrenia is one of exacerbations and remissions. After the first psychotic episode, a patient gradually recovers and may then function relatively normally for a long time. Patients usually relapse, however, and the pattern of illness during the first 5 years after the diagnosis generally indicates the patient's course. A further deterioration in the patient's baseline functioning follows each relapse of the psychosis. This failure to return to baseline functioning after each relapse is the major distinction between schizophrenia and the mood disorders. Sometimes, a clinically observable postpsychotic depression follows a psychotic episode, and the schizophrenic patient's vulnerability to stress is usually lifelong. Positive symptoms tend to become less severe with time, but the socially debilitating negative or deficit symptoms may increase in severity.

Although approximately one-third of all schizophrenic patients have some marginal or integrated social existence, most have lives characterized by aimlessness, inactivity, frequent hospitalizations, and, in urban settings, homelessness and poverty.

Prognosis

Several studies have shown that over the 5- to 10-year period after the first psychiatric hospitalization for schizophrenia, only approximately 10 to 20 percent of patients can be described as having a good outcome. More than 50 percent of patients can be described as having a poor outcome, with repeated hospitalizations, exacerbations of symptoms, episodes of major mood disorders, and suicide attempts. In spite of these glum figures, schizophrenia does not always run a deteriorating course, and several factors have been associated with a good prognosis (Table 10–4).

Reported recovery rates range from 10 to 60 percent, and a reasonable estimate is that 20 to 30 percent of all schizophrenic patients are able to lead somewhat normal lives. Approximately 20 to 30 percent of patients continue to experience moderate symptoms, and 40 to 60 percent of patients remain significantly impaired by their disorder for their entire lives. Patients with schizophrenia do poorer than do patients with mood disorders, although 20 to 25 percent of mood disorder patients are also severely disturbed at long-term follow-up.

TREATMENT

Three observations about schizophrenia warrant attention when clinicians consider the treatment of the disorder. First, regardless of cause, schizophrenia occurs in a person with a unique individual, familial, and social psychological profile. Two factors—how the patient has been affected by the disorder and how the patient will be helped by the treatment—must shape the treatment approach. Second, many investigators consider that a 50 percent concordance rate for schizophrenia among monozygotic twins suggests that unknown but probably specific environmental and psychological factors have contributed to the development of the disorder. Thus, just as pharmacological agents are used to treat presumed chemical imbalances, nonpharmacological strategies must treat nonbiological issues. Third, the complexity of schizophrenia usually renders any single therapeutic approach insufficient to deal with the multifaceted disorder.

Although antipsychotic medications are the mainstay of the treatment for schizophrenia, research has found that psychosocial interventions, including psychotherapy, can augment the clinical improvement. Psychosocial modalities should be carefully integrated into the drug treatment regimen and should support it. Most patients with schizophrenia benefit more from the combined use of antipsychotic drugs and psychosocial treatment than from either treatment used alone.

Hospitalization

Hospitalization is indicated primarily for diagnostic purposes, for stabilization of medications, for patients' safety because of suicidal or homicidal ideation, and for grossly disorganized or inappropriate behavior, including the inability to take care of basic needs such as food, clothing, and shelter. Establishing an effective association between patients and community support systems is a primary goal of hospitalization. Other aspects of clinical management flow logically from medical models of the disorder. Because physicians are concerned with patients' rehabilitation and adjustment, they must consider their specific disabilities when planning treatment strategies. Physicians must also educate patients and their families and caretakers about schizophrenia.

Hospitalization decreases patients' stress and helps them structure their daily activities. The severity of a patient's illness and the availability of outpatient treatment facilities determine the length of the hospital stay. Research has shown that short stays of 4 to 6 weeks are just as effective as long-term hospitalizations and that hospital settings with active behavioral approaches produce better results than do custodial institutions.

Hospital treatment plans should be oriented toward practical issues of self-care, quality of life, employment, and social rela-

tionships. During hospitalization, patients should be coordinated with aftercare facilities including their family homes, foster families, board-and-care homes, and halfway houses. Day care centers and home visits by counselors can sometimes help patients to remain out of the hospital for long periods and can improve the quality of their daily lives.

Biological Therapies

Pharmacotherapy. Antipsychotic medications, introduced in the early 1950s, have revolutionized the treatment of schizophrenia. Approximately two to four times as many patients relapse when treated with a placebo as do those treated with antipsychotic drugs. These medications, however, treat the symptoms of the disorder and do not cure schizophrenia.

The antipsychotic drugs include two major classes: dopamine receptor antagonists (e.g., chlorpromazine [Thorazine], haloperidol [Haldol]) and SDAs (e.g., risperidone [Risperdal] and clozapine). These drugs are discussed in detail in Chapter 32.

DOPAMINE RECEPTOR ANTAGONISTS. The dopamine receptor antagonists are effective in the treatment of schizophrenia, particularly of the positive symptoms (for example, delusions). The drugs have two major shortcomings. First, only a small percentage of patients (perhaps 25 percent) are helped enough to recover a reasonable amount of normal mental functioning. As noted earlier, even with treatment, approximately 50 percent of patients with schizophrenia lead severely debilitated lives. Second, the dopamine receptor antagonists are associated with both annoying and serious adverse effects. The most common annoying effects are akathisia and parkinsonian-like symptoms of rigidity and tremor. The potential serious effects include tardive dyskinesia and neuroleptic malignant syndrome.

SEROTONIN-DOPAMINE ANTAGONISTS. The SDAs produce minimal or no extrapyramidal symptoms, interact with different subtypes of dopamine receptors than do the standard antipsychotics, and affect both serotonin and glutamate receptors. They also produce fewer neurological and endocrinological side effects and are effective in treating negative symptoms of schizophrenia, for example, withdrawal. Also called *atypical antipsychotic drugs*, they appear to be effective for a broader range of patients with schizophrenia than are the typical dopamine receptor antagonist antipsychotic agents. They are at least as effective as haloperidol for positive symptoms of schizophrenia, are uniquely effective for the negative symptoms, and cause few, if any, extrapyramidal symptoms. Some approved SDAs include clozapine, risperidone, olanzapine (Zyprexa), sertindole, quetiapine, and ziprasidone. These drugs are likely to replace the dopamine receptor antagonists as the drugs of first choice for treatment of schizophrenia.

THERAPEUTIC PRINCIPLES. The use of antipsychotic medications in schizophrenia should follow five major principles.

1. Clinicians should carefully define the target symptoms to be treated.
2. An antipsychotic that has worked well in the past for a patient should be used again. In the absence of such information, the choice of an antipsychotic is usually based on the side effect profile. Currently available data indicate that SDAs may offer a superior side effect profile and the possibility of superior efficacy.

3. The minimum length of an antipsychotic trial is 4 to 6 weeks at adequate dosages. If the trial is unsuccessful, a different antipsychotic drug, usually from a different class, can be tried. An unpleasant reaction by the patient to the first dose of an antipsychotic drug, however, correlates strongly with future poor response and noncompliance. Negative experiences can include a peculiar subjective negative feeling, oversedation, or an acute dystonic reaction. When a severe and negative initial reaction is observed, clinicians may consider switching to a different antipsychotic drug in less than 4 weeks.

4. In general, the use of more than one antipsychotic medication at a time is rarely, if ever, indicated. In especially treatment-resistant patients, however, combinations of antipsychotics with other drugs—for example, carbamazepine (Tegretol)—may be indicated.

5. Patients should be maintained on the lowest possible effective dosage of medication. The maintenance dosage is often lower than that used to achieve symptom control during the psychotic episode.

INITIAL WORKUP. In spite of the annoyance of the neurological effects and the looming possibility of tardive dyskinesia, antipsychotic drugs are remarkably safe, especially when given during a relatively short period. Thus, in emergency situations, clinicians can administer the drugs, with the exception of clozapine, without conducting a physical or laboratory examination of the patient. In the usual assessment, however, clinicians should obtain a complete blood count with white blood cell indexes, liver function tests, and an electrocardiogram, especially in women older than 40 and men older than 30. The major contraindications to antipsychotic drugs are (1) a history of serious allergic response, (2) the possibility that a patient has ingested a substance that will interact with the antipsychotic to induce central nervous system depression (for example, alcohol, opioids, opiates, barbiturates, or benzodiazepines) or anticholinergic delirium (for example, drugs containing atropine, scopolamine, and possibly phencyclidine), (3) the presence of a severe cardiac abnormality, (4) a high risk for seizures from organic or idiopathic causes, and (5) the presence of narrow-angle glaucoma if an antipsychotic drug with significant anticholinergic activity is to be used.

TREATMENT OF REFRACTORY ILLNESS. In the acute state, virtually all patients eventually respond to repeated doses of an antipsychotic drug—every 1 to 2 hours by intramuscular administration or every 2 to 3 hours by mouth. A benzodiazepine is sometimes needed to sedate the patient further. The failure of a patient to respond in the acute state should cause clinicians to consider the possibility of an organic lesion.

Noncompliance with antipsychotic drugs is a major reason for relapse and for failure of a drug trial. Another major reason for a failed drug trial is insufficient time for the trial. It is generally a mistake to increase the dosage or to change antipsychotic medications in the first 2 weeks of treatment. If a patient is improving on the current regimen at the end of 2 weeks, continued treatment with the same regimen will probably result in steady clinical improvement. If, however, a patient has shown little or no improvement in 2 weeks, the possible reasons for a drug failure, including noncompliance, should be considered. In a noncompliant patient, the use of a liquid preparation or depot forms of fluphenazine (Prolixin) or haloperidol (Haldol) may be indicated. Because of the diversity in the metabolism of drugs, clinicians should obtain plasma levels when the laboratory capability is available. Plasma levels of antipsychotic drugs provide only a gross measure of compliance, absorption, and metabolism. There are no clearly defined therapeutic blood level ranges for antipsychotic drugs similar to those for some antidepressants. Because neurological side effects are a common reason for noncompliance in patients with schizophrenia and a major cause of relapse, the more favorable side effect profiles of atypical agents may lead to improved compliance and better outcome.

Having eliminated other possible reasons for the therapeutic failure of an antipsychotic drug, clinicians may try a second antipsychotic drug with a chemical structure different from that of the first one. Additional strategies include supplementing the antipsychotic drug with lithium (Eskalith), an anticonvulsant such as carbamazepine or valproate (Depakene), or a benzodiazepine. The use of so-called megadose antipsychotic therapy (for example, 100 to 200 mg of haloperidol) is rarely indicated because almost no data support the practice.

Other Biological Therapies. Although much less effective than antipsychotic drugs, electroconvulsive therapy may be indicated for catatonic patients and for patients who for some reason cannot take antipsychotic drugs. Patients who have been ill for less than 1 year are most likely to respond. Maintenance electroconvulsive therapy may be of value in patients nonresponsive to pharmacological therapies.

In the past, psychosurgery, particularly frontal lobotomy, was used for the treatment of schizophrenia with variable outcomes. Although sophisticated approaches to psychosurgery for schizophrenia may eventually be developed, psychosurgery is no longer considered an appropriate treatment. It is, however, practiced on a limited experimental basis, for severe intractable cases.

Psychosocial Therapies

Psychosocial therapies include a variety of methods to increase social abilities, self-sufficiency, practical skills, and interpersonal communication in schizophrenic patients. The goal is to enable persons who are severely ill to develop social and vocational skills for independent living. Such treatment is carried out at many sites: hospitals, outpatient clinics, mental health centers, day hospitals, and home or social clubs.

Social Skills Training. Social skills training is sometimes referred to as *behavioral skills therapy*. The therapy can be directly supportive and useful to the patient along with pharmacological therapy. In addition to the symptoms seen in patients with schizophrenia, some of the most noticeable symptoms involve the person's relationships with others, including poor eye contact, unusual delays in response, odd facial expressions, lack of spontaneity in social situations, and inaccurate perceptions or lack of perception of emotions in other people. Behavioral skills training addresses these behaviors through the use of videotapes of others and of the patient, role playing in therapy, and homework assignments for the specific skills being practiced. Social skills training has been shown to reduce relapse rates as measured by the need for hospitalization.

Family-Oriented Therapies. Because patients with schizophrenia are often discharged in an only partially remitted state, a family to which a patient returns can often benefit from a brief but intensive (as often as daily) course of family therapy. The therapy should focus on the immediate situation and should include identifying and avoiding potentially troublesome situations. When problems do emerge with the patient in the family, the aim of the therapy should be to resolve the problem quickly.

In wanting to help, family members too often encourage a relative with schizophrenia to resume regular activities too quickly, both from ignorance about the disorder and from denial of its severity. Without being overly discouraging, therapists must help the family and the patient understand and learn about schizophrenia and must encourage the discussion of the psychotic episode and the events leading up to it. Ignoring the psychotic episode, a common occurrence, often increases the shame associated with the event and does not exploit the freshness of the episode to understand it better. Psychotic symptoms often frighten family members, and talking openly with the psychiatrist and with the relative with schizophrenia often eases all parties. Therapists can direct later family therapy toward long-range application of stress-reducing and coping strategies and toward the patient's gradual reintegration into everyday life.

Therapists must control the emotional intensity of family sessions with patients with schizophrenia. The excessive expression of emotion during a session can damage a patient's recovery process and can undermine potentially successful future family therapy. Several studies have shown that family therapy is especially effective in reducing relapses. Each study, however, used a different type of family therapy. And the commonality among therapies remains unclear. In controlled studies, family therapy dramatically reduced the annual relapse rate, which is 25 to 50 percent for patients not undergoing family therapy, compared with 5 to 10 percent for those who undergo the therapy.

National Alliance for the Mentally Ill. NAMI and similar organizations are support groups for family members and friends of patients who are mentally ill and for patients themselves. Useful sources to which to refer family members, these organizations offer emotional and practical advice about obtaining care in the sometimes complex health care delivery system. NAMI has also waged a campaign to destigmatize mental illness and to increase government awareness of the needs and rights of people who are mentally ill and of their families.

Case Management. Because a variety of professionals with specialized skills, such as psychiatrists, social workers, and occupational therapists, among others, are involved in a treatment program, it is helpful to have one person aware of all the forces acting on the patient. The case manager ensures that their efforts are coordinated and that the patient keeps appointments and complies with treatment plans; the case manager may make home visits and even accompany the patient to work. The success of the program depends on the educational background, training, and competence of the case manager, which is variable. Case managers often have too many cases to manage effectively. The ultimate benefits of the program have yet to be demonstrated.

Assertive Community Treatment. The Assertive Community Treatment (ACT) program was originally developed by researchers in Madison, Wisconsin, in the 1970s, for the delivery of services for persons with chronic mental illness. Patients are assigned to one multidisciplinary team (case manager, psychiatrist, nurse, general physicians, etc.). The team has a fixed caseload of patients and delivers all services when and where needed by the patient, 24 hours a day, 7 days a week. This is mobile and intensive intervention that provides treatment, rehabilitation, and support activities. These include home delivery of medications, monitoring of mental and physical health, in vivo social skills, and frequent contact with family members. There is a high staff-to-patient ratio (1:12). ACT programs can effectively decrease the risk of rehospitalization for persons with schizophrenia, but are labor-intensive and expensive programs to administer.

Group Therapy. Group therapy for people with schizophrenia generally focuses on real-life plans, problems, and relationships. Groups may be behaviorally oriented, psychodynamically or insight oriented, or supportive. Some investigators doubt that dynamic interpretation and insight therapy are valuable for typical patients with schizophrenia. But group therapy is effective in reducing social isolation, increasing the sense of cohesiveness, and improving reality testing for patients with schizophrenia. Groups led in a supportive manner, rather than in an interpretative way, appear to be most helpful for schizophrenic patients.

Cognitive Behavioral Therapy. Cognitive behavioral therapy has been used in schizophrenic patients to improve cognitive distortions, reduce distractibility, and correct errors in judgment. There are reports of ameliorating delusions and hallucinations in some patients using this method. Patients who might benefit generally have some insight into their illness.

Individual Psychotherapy. Studies of the effects of individual psychotherapy in the treatment of schizophrenia have provided data that the therapy is helpful and is additive to the effects of pharmacological treatment. In psychotherapy with a schizophrenic patient, developing a therapeutic relationship that the patient experiences as safe is critical. The therapist's reliability, the emotional distance between the therapist and the patient, and the genuineness of the therapist as interpreted by the patient all affect the therapeutic experience. The psychotherapy for a schizophrenic patient should be thought of in terms of decades, rather than sessions, months, or even years.

Some clinicians and researchers have emphasized that the ability of a patient with schizophrenia to form a therapeutic alliance with a therapist can predict the outcome. Schizophrenic patients who are able to form a good therapeutic alliance are likely to remain in psychotherapy, to remain compliant with their medications, and to have good outcomes at 2-year follow-up evaluations.

The relationship between clinicians and patients differs from that encountered in the treatment of nonpsychotic patients. Establishing a relationship is often difficult. People with schizophrenia are desperately lonely, yet defend against closeness and trust; they are likely to become suspicious, anxious, or hostile or to regress when someone attempts to draw close. Therapists should scrupulously observe a patient's distance and privacy and should demonstrate simple directness, patience, sincerity, and sensitivity to social conventions in preference to premature informality and the condescending use of first names. The patient is likely to perceive exaggerated warmth or professions of friendship as attempts at bribery, manipulation, or exploitation.

In the context of a professional relationship, however, flexibility is essential in establishing a working alliance with the patient. A therapist may have meals with the patient, sit on the floor, go for a walk, eat at a restaurant, accept and give gifts, play table tennis, remember the patient's birthday, or just sit silently with the patient. The major aim is to convey the idea that the therapist is trustworthy, wants to understand the patient and tries to do so, and has faith in the patient's potential as a human being, no matter how disturbed, hostile, or bizarre the patient may be at the moment.

A flexible type of psychotherapy called *personal therapy* is a recently developed form of individual treatment for schizophrenia patients. Its objective is to enhance personal and social adjustment and to forestall relapse. It is a select method using social skills and relaxation exercises, psychoeducation, self reflection, self aware-ness, and exploration of individual vulnerability to stress. The therapist provides a setting that stresses acceptance and empathy. Patients receiving personal therapy show improvement in social adjustment (a composite measure that includes work performance, leisure, and interpersonal relationships) and have a lower relapse rate after 3 years than patients not receiving personal therapy.

Vocational Therapy

A variety of methods and settings are used to help patients regain old skills or develop new ones. These include sheltered workshops, job clubs, and part-time or transitional employment programs. Enabling patients to become gainfully employed is both a means toward and a sign of recovery. Many schizophrenic patients are capable of performing high-quality work in spite of their illness. Others may exhibit exceptional skill or even brilliance in a limited field as a result of some idiosyncratic aspect of their disorder.

11 ▲

Other Psychotic Disorders

▲ 11.1 Schizophreniform Disorder

Schizophreniform disorder is similar to schizophrenia except that its symptoms last at least 1 month but less than 6 months. Patients with schizophreniform disorder return to their baseline level of functioning once the disorder has resolved. In contrast, for a patient to meet the diagnostic criteria for schizophrenia, the symptoms must have been present for at least 6 months. Gabriel Langfeldt first used the term *schizophreniform* in 1939, at the University Psychiatric Clinic in Oslo, Norway, to describe a disorder characterized by a brief and self-contained psychotic episode.

EPIDEMIOLOGY

Little is known about the incidence, prevalence, and sex ratio of schizophreniform disorder. The disorder is most common in adolescents and young adults and is less than half as common as schizophrenia. A lifetime prevalence rate of 0.2 percent and a 1-year prevalence rate of 0.1 percent have been reported.

ETIOLOGY

The cause of schizophreniform disorder is not known. In general, some patients have a disorder similar to schizophrenia, whereas others have a disorder similar to a mood disorder. Because of the generally good outcome, the disorder probably has similarities to the episodic nature of mood disorders.

Brain Imaging

Although some data indicate that patients with schizophreniform disorder may have enlarged cerebral ventricles, as determined by computed tomography (CT) and magnetic resonance imaging (MRI), other data indicate that, unlike the enlargement seen in schizophrenia, the ventricular enlargement in schizophreniform disorder is not correlated with outcome measures or other biological measures.

Other Biological Measures

Although brain imaging studies point to a similarity between schizophreniform disorder and schizophrenia, at least one study of electrodermal activity has indicated a difference. Patients with schizophrenia born during the winter and spring months (a period of high risk for the

birth of these patients) had hyporesponsive skin conductances, but this association was absent in patients with schizophreniform disorder. The significance and the meaning of this single study are difficult to interpret, but the results do suggest caution in assuming similarity between patients with schizophrenia and those with schizophreniform disorder. Data from at least one study of eye tracking in the two groups also indicate that they may differ in some biological measures.

DIAGNOSTIC AND CLINICAL FEATURES

The DSM-IV-TR criteria for schizophreniform are listed in Table 11.1–1. Schizophreniform disorder in its typical presentation is a rapid-onset psychotic disorder without a significant prodrome. Hallucinations, delusions, or both will be present; negative symptoms of alogia and avolition may be present. Affect may be flattened, which is seen as a poor prognostic sign. Speech may be grossly disorganized and confused, and behavior may be disorganized or catatonic. The symptoms of psychosis, the negative symptoms, and those affecting speech and behavior will last at least 1 month but may last longer. The patient's degree of perplexity about what is happening should be assessed, as this is a differentiating prognostic sign.

Although the above is the typical presentation, a picture exactly resembling that of schizophrenia may also occur. In that case, the onset may be insidious, premorbid functioning may have been poor, and affect is quite blunted. The only differentiation from schizophrenia for this type of presentation will be duration of the total episode of illness. When it has lasted 6 months, the diagnosis becomes schizophrenia. In making the diagnosis in the case with insidious onset, the "attenuated symptoms" of the acute episode may have lasted for some time. If they have been present for at least 5 months and then the acute episode lasts 1 month, the diagnosis of schizophrenia is appropriate, without a prior diagnosis of schizophreniform disorder.

In the typical form of the disorder, the patient returns to baseline functioning by the end of 6 months. Theoretically, repeated episodes of schizophreniform illness are possible, each lasting less than 6 months, but rarely is functioning not lost with repeated episodes of this severe illness, and schizophrenia is a more likely consideration.

DIFFERENTIAL DIAGNOSIS

Although the major differential diagnoses are with brief psychotic disorder and schizophrenia, the rapid onset of acute psychosis may be the most important diagnostic point in a patient's course of illness. The clinician should focus on the prior 6

Table 11.1–1
DSM-IV-TR Diagnostic Criteria for
Schizophreniform Disorder

A. Criteria A, D, and E of schizophrenia are met.

B. An episode of the disorder (including prodromal, active, and residual phases) lasts at least 1 month but less than 6 months. (When the diagnosis must be made without waiting for recovery, it should be qualified as "provisional.")

Specify if:

Without good prognostic features

With good prognostic features: as evidenced by two (or more) of the following:

(1) onset of prominent psychotic symptoms within 4 weeks of the first noticeable change in usual behavior or functioning

(2) confusion or perplexity at the height of the psychotic episode

(3) good premorbid social and occupational functioning

(4) absence of blunted or flat affect

From American Psychiatric Association. *Diagnostic and Statistical Manual of Mental Disorders.* 4th ed. Text rev. Washington, DC: American Psychiatric Association; copyright 2000, with permission.

months, taking a detailed history of occupational and social functioning, the pattern of onset, the presence or absence of mood changes, alcohol and substance abuse, and other illness and prescriptive medication. Of special interest will be any family history of psychiatric illness, mood disorders, or schizophrenia-like illnesses in particular. A recent study showed a high prevalence of personality disorders after recovery from the psychosis. One could hypothesize that the personality disorder predisposes one to psychosis, especially when under stress.

The separation of mood disorders with psychotic features from a rapid-onset schizophreniform disorder may be difficult and tests the clinician's skills. Negative symptoms such as alogia, avolition, and blunted affect may be difficult to distinguish from the loss of interest and pleasure seen with major depressive episodes. Appetite, sleep, and other neurovegetative symptoms may also occur with both. The presence of the psychotic features of the illness, in the absence of these mood features, will assist the clinician in making the diagnosis of schizophreniform disorder, but this may take time to evolve.

To differentiate from brief psychotic disorder, a time cutoff has been established, more than 1 day but less than 1 month. During this period, the diagnosis must be brief psychotic disorder. In diagnostic systems prior to DSM-IV-TR, the presence or absence of a stressor was used to differentiate these two conditions further, but it is no longer used in the nosology, except as a descriptor or modifier. Differentiation is based solely on the time line.

COURSE AND PROGNOSIS

The course of schizophreniform disorder is for the most part defined in the criteria. It is a psychotic illness lasting more than 1 month and less than 6 months. The real issue is what happens to persons with this illness over time. Most estimates of progression to schizophrenia range between 60 and 80 percent. What happens to the other 20 to 40 percent is currently not known. Some will have a second or third episode during which they will deteriorate into a more chronic condition of schizophrenia. A few, however,

may have only this single episode and then are able to continue on with their lives. While this is clearly the outcome desired by all clinicians and family members, it is probably a rare occurrence and should not be held out as likely.

TREATMENT

Hospitalization is often necessary in treating patients with schizophreniform disorder and allows for an effective assessment, treatment, and supervision of a patient's behavior. The psychotic symptoms can usually be treated by a 3- to 6-month course of antipsychotic drugs (for example, risperidone [Risperdal]). Several studies have shown that patients with schizophreniform disorder respond much more rapidly to antipsychotic treatment than do patients with schizophrenia. One study found that approximately 75 percent of patients with schizophreniform disorder, compared with only 20 percent of the patients with schizophrenia, responded to antipsychotic medications within 8 days. Electroconvulsive therapy (ECT) may be indicated for some patients, especially those with marked catatonic or depressed features. A trial of lithium (Eskalith), carbamazepine (Tegretol), or valproate (Depakene) may be warranted for treatment and prophylaxis if a patient has a recurrent episode. Psychotherapy is usually necessary to help patients integrate the psychotic experience into their understanding of their minds, brains, and lives.

Finally, a majority of patients with schizophreniform disorder progress to full-blown schizophrenia in spite of treatment. In those cases, a new course of management consistent with a chronic illness must be formulated.

▲ 11.2 Schizoaffective Disorder

As the term implies, *schizoaffective disorder* has features of both schizophrenia and affective disorders (now called *mood disorders*). The diagnostic criteria for schizoaffective disorder have changed over time, mostly as a reflection of changes in the diagnostic criteria for schizophrenia and the mood disorders; however, it remains the best diagnosis for those patients who present with mixtures of both.

EPIDEMIOLOGY

The lifetime prevalence of schizoaffective disorder is less than 1 percent, possibly in the range of 0.5 to 0.8 percent. These figures, however, are estimates; various studies of schizoaffective disorder have used varying diagnostic criteria. In clinical practice, a preliminary diagnosis of schizoaffective disorder is frequently used when a clinician is uncertain of the diagnosis.

Gender and Age Differences

The depressive type of schizoaffective disorder may be more common in older people than in younger people, and the bipolar type may be more common in young adults than in older adults. The prevalence of the disorder has been reported to be lower in men than in women, particularly married women; the age of onset for women is later than the age for men, as in schizophrenia. Men with schizoaffective disorder are likely to exhibit antisocial behavior and to have marked flatness or inappropriateness of affect.

ETIOLOGY

The cause of schizoaffective disorder is unknown, but four conceptual models have been advanced. Schizoaffective disorder may be either a type of schizophrenia or a type of mood disorder. Schizoaffective disorder may be the simultaneous expression of schizophrenia and a mood disorder. Schizoaffective disorder may be a distinct third type of psychosis, one that is not related to either schizophrenia or a mood disorder. Fourth, and most likely, is that schizoaffective disorder is a heterogeneous group of disorders encompassing all the first three possibilities.

Although much of the family and genetic research in schizoaffective disorder is based on the premise that schizophrenia and the mood disorders are completely separate entities, some data indicate that they may be genetically related. Some confusion arising in the family studies of schizoaffective disorder patients may reflect the nonabsolute distinction between the two primary disorders. Not surprisingly, therefore, studies of the relatives of patients with schizoaffective disorder have reported inconsistent results. An increased prevalence of schizophrenia is not found among the relatives of probands with schizoaffective disorder, bipolar type; the relatives of patients with schizoaffective disorder, depressive type, however, may be at higher risk for schizophrenia than for a mood disorder.

Depending on the type of schizoaffective disorder studied, an increased prevalence of schizophrenia or mood disorders may be found in the relatives of schizoaffective disorder probands. The possibility that schizoaffective disorder is distinct from schizophrenia and mood disorders is not supported by the observation that only a small percentage of the relatives of schizoaffective disorder probands have schizoaffective disorder.

As a group, patients with schizoaffective disorder have a better prognosis than do patients with schizophrenia and a worse prognosis than do patients with mood disorders. As a group, patients with schizoaffective disorder respond to lithium and tend to have a nondeteriorating course.

DIAGNOSIS AND CLINICAL FEATURES

DSM-IV-TR diagnostic criteria are provided in Table 11.2–1. These criteria are a product of several revisions that have sought to clarify several diagnoses including schizophrenia, bipolar disorder, and major depressive disorder. The diagnostician must accurately diagnose the affective illness, making sure it meets the criteria of either a manic or depressive episode but also determining the exact length of each episode (not always an easy or possible task). The length of each episode is critical for two reasons. First, to meet Criterion B (psychotic symptoms in the absence of the mood syndrome), one has to know when the affective episode ends and the psychosis continues. Second, to meet Criterion C, the length of all mood episodes must be combined and compared with the total length of the illness. If

**Table 11.2–1
DSM-IV-TR Diagnostic Criteria for
Schizoaffective Disorder**

A. An uninterrupted period of illness during which, at some time, there is either a major depressive episode, a manic episode, or a mixed episode concurrent with symptoms that meet Criterion A for schizophrenia.

   Note: The major depressive episode must include Criterion A1: depressed mood.

B. During the same period of illness, there have been delusions or hallucinations for at least 2 weeks in the absence of prominent mood symptoms.

C. Symptoms that meet criteria for a mood episode are present for a substantial portion of the total duration of the active and residual periods of the illness.

D. The disturbance is not due to the direct physiological effects of a substance (e.g., a drug of abuse, a medication) or a general medical condition.

Specify type:

   Bipolar type: if the disturbance includes a manic or a mixed episode (or a manic or a mixed episode and major depressive episodes)

   Depressive type: if the disturbance only includes major depressive episodes

From American Psychiatric Association. *Diagnostic and Statistical Manual of Mental Disorders.* 4th ed. Text rev. Washington, DC: American Psychiatric Association; copyright 2000, with permission.

the mood component is present for a substantial portion of the total illness, then that criterion is met. Calculating the total length of the episodes can be difficult, and it does not help that the term "substantial portion" is not defined. In practice, most clinicians look for the mood component to be 15 to 20 percent of the total illness. Patients who have one full manic episode lasting 2 months but who have suffered from symptoms of schizophrenia for 10 years do not meet the criteria for schizoaffective disorder. Instead, the diagnosis would be a mood episode superimposed on schizophrenia. It is unclear whether the bipolar or depressive type specifiers are helpful, although they may direct treatment options. These subtypes are often confused with earlier subtypes (schizophrenic versus affective type) thought to have implications in course and prognosis. As with most psychiatric diagnoses, schizoaffective disorder should not be used if the symptoms are caused by substance abuse or a secondary medical condition.

Ms. AD was a 29-year-old unmarried white woman, with a 10-year history of schizoaffective disorder bipolar type. She was first hospitalized after child protection took her son away for alleged child abuse. When the patient was interviewed at that time, she was described as "dressed like a gypsy," with heavy makeup and pressured speech. She told the treatment team that her son had been abused by his father, a well-known rock star. During this time she was stabilized on lithium and haloperidol (Haldol). Ms. AD's manic symptoms resolved, but her belief that she was a rock star's girlfriend remained. Since that first hospitalization she has lost custody of her son. She remains delusional about the child's famous father, and, in addition, she believes that people are out to get her. She has had three distinct episodes of mania during which she needs little sleep and has racing thoughts and pressured speech. She has been intermittently compliant with medications and is currently receiving haloperidol in a long-acting form. In the 10 years of her illness she has never been free of her delusions. She has not been able to work and receives federal disability assistance. (Courtesy of John Lauriello, M.D., Brenda R. Erickson, M.D., and Samuel J. Keith, M.D.)

DIFFERENTIAL DIAGNOSIS

The psychiatric differential diagnosis includes all the possibilities usually considered for mood disorders and for schizophrenia. In any differential diagnosis of psychotic disorders, a complete medical workup should be performed to rule out organic causes of the symptoms. A history of substance use with or without a positive toxicology screening test may indicate a substance-induced disorder. Preexisting medical conditions, their treatment, or both may cause psychotic and mood disorders. Any suspicion of a neurological abnormality warrants consideration of a brain scan to rule out anatomical pathology and an electroencephalogram to determine any possible seizure disorders (e.g., temporal lobe epilepsy). Psychotic disorder due to seizure disorder is more common than that seen in the general population. It tends to be characterized by paranoia, hallucinations, and ideas of reference. Epileptic patients with psychosis are believed to have a better level of function than patients with schizophrenic spectrum disorders. Better control of the seizures can reduce the psychosis.

COURSE AND PROGNOSIS

Considering the uncertainty and evolving diagnosis of schizoaffective disorder, determining the long-term course and prognosis is difficult. Given the definition of the diagnosis, one might expect patients with schizoaffective disorder to have either a course similar to an episodic mood disorder, a chronic schizophrenic course, or some intermediate outcome. It has been presumed that an increasing presence of schizophrenic symptoms predicted worse prognosis. After 1 year, patients with schizoaffective disorder had different outcomes depending on whether their predominant symptoms were affective (better prognosis) or schizophrenic (worse prognosis). One study that followed patients diagnosed with schizoaffective disorder for 8 years found that the outcomes of these patients more closely resembled schizophrenia than a mood disorder with psychotic features.

TREATMENT

Mood stabilizers are a mainstay of treatment for bipolar disorders and would be expected to be important in the treatment of patients with schizoaffective disorder. One study that compared lithium with carbamazepine showed superiority for carbamazepine for schizoaffective disorder, depressive type, but no difference in the two agents for the bipolar type. In practice, however, these medications are used extensively alone, in combination with each other, or with an antipsychotic agent. In manic episodes, schizoaffective patients should be treated aggressively with dosages of a mood stabilizer in the middle to high therapeutic blood concentration range. As the patient enters a maintenance phase, the dosage can be reduced to low to middle range to avoid adverse effects and potential effects on organ systems (e.g., thyroid and kidney) and to improve ease of use and compliance. Laboratory monitoring of plasma drug concentrations and periodic screening of thyroid, kidney, and hematological functioning should be performed. As in all cases of intractable mania, the use of electroconvulsive therapy (ECT) should be considered.

By definition, many schizoaffective patients suffer from major depressive episodes. Treatment with antidepressants mirrors treatment of bipolar depression. Care should be taken not to precipitate a cycle of rapid switches from depression to mania with the antidepressant. The choice of antidepressant should take into account previous antidepressant successes or failures. Selective serotonin reuptake inhibitors (SSRIs) (e.g., fluoxetine [Prozac] and sertraline [Zoloft]) are often used as first-line agents. However, agitated or insomniac patients may benefit from a tricyclic antidepressant. As in all cases of depression, use of ECT should be considered. As mentioned above, antipsychotic agents are important in the treatment of the psychotic symptoms of schizoaffective disorder.

Psychosocial Treatment

Patients benefit from a combination of family therapy, social skills training, and cognitive rehabilitation. Because the psychiatric field has had difficulty deciding the exact diagnosis and prognosis of schizoaffective disorder, this uncertainty must be explained to the patient. The range of symptoms can be quite large, as patients contend with both ongoing psychosis and varying mood states. It can be very difficult for family members to keep up with the changing nature and needs of these patients. Medication regimens can be more complicated, with multiple medications frequent, and psychopharmacological education is important.

▲ 11.3 Delusional Disorder and Shared Psychotic Disorder

According to the text revision of the fourth edition of the *Diagnostic and Statistical Manual of Mental Disorders* (DSM-IV-TR), the diagnosis of delusional disorder is made when a person exhibits nonbizarre delusions of at least 1 month's duration that cannot be attributed to other psychiatric disorders. Definitions of the term *delusion* and types relevant to delusional disorders are presented in Table 11.3–1. *Nonbizarre* means that the delusions must be about situations that can occur in real life, such as being followed, infected, loved at a distance, and so on; that is, they usually have to do with phenomena that, although not real, are nonetheless possible. There are several types of delusions, and the predominant type is specified when the diagnosis is made.

Table 11.3–1
DSM-IV-TR Definition of Delusion and Certain Common Types Associated with Delusional Disorders

Delusion A false belief based on incorrect inference about external reality that is firmly sustained despite what almost everyone else believes and despite what constitutes incontrovertible and obvious proof of evidence to the contrary. The belief is not one ordinarily accepted by other members of the person's culture or subculture (e.g., it is not an article of religious faith). When a false belief involves a value judgment, it is regarded as a delusion only when the judgment is so extreme as to defy credibility. Delusional conviction occurs on a continuum and can sometimes be inferred from an individual's behavior. It is often difficult to distinguish between a delusion and an overvalued idea (in which case the individual has an unreasonable belief or idea but does not hold it as firmly as is the case with a delusion). Delusions are subdivided according to their content. Some of the more common types are listed below:

Bizarre—A delusion that involves a phenomenon that the person's culture would regard as totally implausible.

Delusional jealousy—The delusion that one's sexual partner is unfaithful.

Erotomanic—A delusion that another person, usually of higher status, is in love with the individual.

Grandiose—A delusion of inflated worth, power, knowledge, identity, or special relationship to a deity or famous person.

Mood-congruent—See mood-congruent psychotic features.

Mood-incongruent—See mood-incongruent psychotic features.

Of being controlled—A delusion in which feelings, impulses, thoughts, or actions are experienced as being under the control of some external force rather than being under one's own control.

Of reference—A delusion whose theme is that events, objects, or other persons in one's immediate environment have a particular and unusual significance. These delusions are usually of a negative or pejorative nature, but also may be grandiose in content. This differs from an idea of reference, in which the false belief is not as firmly held nor as fully organized into a true belief.

Persecutory—A delusion in which the central theme is that one (or someone to whom one is close) is being attacked, harassed, cheated, persecuted, or conspired against.

Somatic—A delusion whose main content pertains to the appearance or functioning of one's body.

Thought broadcasting—The delusion that one's thoughts are being broadcast out loud so that they can be perceived by others.

Thought insertion—The delusion that certain of one's thoughts are not one's own, but rather are inserted into one's mind.

Mood-congruent psychotic features—Delusions or hallucinations whose content is entirely consistent with the typical themes of a depressed or manic mood. If the mood is depressed, the content of the delusions or hallucinations would involve themes of personal inadequacy, guilt, disease, death, nihilism, or deserved punishment. The content of the delusion may include themes of persecution if these are based on self-derogatory concepts such as deserved punishment. If the mood is manic, the content of the delusions or hallucinations would involve themes of inflated worth, power, knowledge, or identity, or a special relationship to a deity or a famous person. The content of the delusion may include themes of persecution if these are based on concepts such as inflated worth or deserved punishment.

Mood-incongruent psychotic features—Delusions or hallucinations whose content is not consistent with the typical themes of a depressed or manic mood. In the case of depression, the delusions or hallucinations would not involve themes of personal inadequacy, guilt, disease, death, nihilism, or deserved punishment. In the case of mania, the delusions or hallucinations would not involve themes of inflated worth, power, knowledge, or identity, or a special relationship to a deity or a famous person. Examples of mood-incongruent psychotic features include persecutory delusions (without self-derogatory or grandiose content), thought insertion, thought broadcasting, and delusions of being controlled whose content has no apparent relationship to any of the themes listed above.

From American Psychiatric Association. *Diagnostic and Statistical Manual of Mental Disorders.* 4th ed. Text rev. Washington, DC: American Psychiatric Association; copyright 2000, with permission.

EPIDEMIOLOGY

The prevalence of delusional disorder in the United States is currently estimated to be 0.025 to 0.03 percent. Thus, delusional disorder is much rarer than schizophrenia, which has a prevalence of approximately 1 percent, and the mood disorders, which have a prevalence of approximately 5 percent. The annual incidence of delusional disorder is 1 to 3 new cases per 100,000 people. According to DSM-IV-TR, delusional disorders account for only 1 to 2 percent of all admissions for inpatient mental health facilities. The mean age of onset is approximately 40 years, but the range for the age of onset runs from 18 to the 90s. There is a slight preponderance of female patients. Men are more likely to develop paranoid delusions than women, who are more likely to develop delusions of erotomania. Many patients are married and employed, but there may be some association with recent immigration and low socioeconomic status.

The onset of the disorder ranges from adolescence to old age (18 to 80), but most cases are diagnosed in middle-aged persons (40 to 45).

ETIOLOGY

The cause of delusional disorder is unknown. Patients currently classified as having delusional disorder probably have a heterogeneous group of conditions with delusions as the predominant symptom. The central concept about the cause of delusional disorder is its distinctness from schizophrenia and the mood disorders. Delusional disorder is much more rare than either schizophrenia or mood disorders, with a later onset than schizophrenia and a much less pronounced female predominance than that in the mood disorders. The most convincing data come from family studies that report an increased prevalence of delusional disorder and related personality traits (for example, suspiciousness, jealousy, and secretiveness) in the relatives of delusional disorder probands. Family studies have reported neither an increased incidence of schizophrenia and mood disorders in the families of delusional disorder probands nor an increased incidence of delusional disorder in the families of schizophrenic probands. Long-term follow-up of patients with delusional disorder indicates that the diagnosis of delusional disorder is relatively stable, with less than one-fourth of the patients eventually being reclassified as having schizophrenia and less than 10 percent of patients eventually being reclassified as having a mood disorder. These data indicate that delusional disorder is not simply an early stage in the development of one or both of these two more common disorders.

Biological Factors

A wide range of nonpsychiatric medical conditions and substances, including clear-cut biological factors, can cause delusions, but not everyone with a brain tumor, for example, has delusions. Unique and as-yet not understood factors in a patient's brain and personality are likely to be relevant to the specific pathophysiology of delusional disorder.

The neurological conditions most commonly associated with delusions are conditions that affect the limbic system and the basal ganglia. Patients whose delusions are caused by neurological diseases and who show no intellectual impairment tend to have complex delusions similar to those in patients with delusional disorder. Conversely, patients with neurological disorder with intellectual impairments often have simple delusions unlike those in patients with delusional disorder. Thus, delusional disorder may involve the limbic system or basal ganglia in patients who have intact cerebral cortical functioning.

Delusional disorder may arise as a normal response to abnormal experiences in the environment, the peripheral nervous system, or the central nervous system. Thus, if patients have erroneous sensory experiences of being followed (for example, hearing footsteps), they may come to believe that they are actually being followed. This hypothesis hinges on the presence of hallucinatory-like experiences that need to be explained. The presence of such hallucinatory experiences in delusional disorder has not been proved.

Psychodynamic Factors

Practitioners have a strong clinical impression that many patients with delusional disorder are socially isolated and have attained less-than-expected levels of achievement. Specific psychodynamic theories about the cause and the evolution of delusional symptoms involve suppositions regarding hypersensitive people and specific ego mechanisms: reaction formation, projection, and denial.

Freud's Contributions.   Freud believed that delusions, rather than being symptoms of the disorder, are part of a healing process. In 1896, he described projection as the main defense mechanism in paranoia. Later, Freud read *Memories of My Nervous Illness*, an autobiographical account by Daniel Paul Schreber. Although he never met Schreber, Freud theorized from his review of the autobiography that unconscious homosexual tendencies are defended against by denial and projection. According to classic psychodynamic theory, the dynamics underlying the formation of delusions for a female patient are the same as for a male patient. Careful studies of patients with delusions have been unable to corroborate Freud's theories, although they may be relevant to individual cases. Overall, there is no higher incidence of homosexual ideation or activity in patients with delusions than in other groups. Freud's major contribution, however, was to demonstrate the role of projection in the formation of delusional thought.

Paranoid Pseudocommunity.   Norman Cameron described seven situations that favor the development of delusional disorders: an increased expectation of receiving sadistic treatment, situations that increase distrust and suspicion, social isolation, situations that increase envy and jealousy, situations that lower self-esteem, situations that cause people to see their own defects in others, and situations that increase the potential for rumination over probable meanings and motivations. When frustration from any combination of these conditions exceeds the limit that people can tolerate, they become withdrawn and anxious; they realize that something is wrong, seek an explanation for the problem, and crystallize a delusional system as a solution. Elaboration of the delusion to include imagined people and attribution of malevolent motivations to both real and imagined people result in the organization of the pseudocommunity—a perceived community of plotters. This delusional entity hypothetically binds together projected fears and wishes to justify the patient's aggression and to provide a tangible target for the patient's hostilities.

Other Psychodynamic Factors.   Clinical observations indicate that many, if not all, paranoid patients experience a lack of trust in relationships. This distrust has been hypothesized to be related to a consistently hostile family environment, often with an overcontrolling mother and a distant or sadistic father.

Erik Erikson's concept of trust versus mistrust in early development is a useful model to explain the suspiciousness of the paranoid who never went through the healthy experience of having his or her needs satisfied by what Erikson termed the "outer-providers." Thus, they feel a general distrust of their environment.

Defense Mechanisms.   Patients with delusional disorder use primarily the defense mechanisms of reaction formation, denial, and projection. They use reaction formation as a defense against aggression, dependence needs, and feelings of affection and transform the need for dependence into staunch independence. Patients use denial to avoid awareness of painful reality. Consumed with anger and hostility and unable to face responsibility for the rage, they project their resentment and anger onto others and use projection to protect themselves from recognizing unacceptable impulses in themselves.

Other Relevant Factors.   Delusions have been linked to a variety of additional factors such as social and sensory isolation, socioeconomic deprivation, and personality disturbance. The deaf, the visually impaired, and possibly immigrants with limited ability in a new language may be more vulnerable to delusion formation than the normal population. Vulnerability is heightened with advanced age. Delusional disturbance and other paranoid features are common in the elderly. In short, multiple factors are associated with the formation of delusions, and the source and pathogenesis of delusional disorders per se have yet to be specified.

DIAGNOSIS AND CLINICAL FEATURES

The DSM-IV-TR diagnostic criteria are listed in Table 11.3–2.

Mental Status

General Description.   Patients are usually well groomed and well dressed, without evidence of gross disintegration of personality or of daily activities, yet they may seem eccentric, odd, suspicious, or hostile. They are sometimes litigious and may make this inclination clear to the examiner. What is usually most

**Table 11.3–2
DSM-IV-TR Diagnostic Criteria for
Delusional Disorder**

A. Nonbizarre delusions (i.e., involving situations that occur in real life, such as being followed, poisoned, infected, loved at a distance, or deceived by spouse or lover, or having a disease) of at least 1 month's duration.

B. Criterion A for schizophrenia has never been met. **Note:** Tactile and olfactory hallucinations may be present in delusional disorder if they are related to the delusional theme.

C. Apart from the impact of the delusion(s) or its ramifications, functioning is not markedly impaired and behavior is not obviously odd or bizarre.

D. If mood episodes have occurred concurrently with delusions, their total duration has been brief relative to the duration of the delusional periods.

E. The disturbance is not due to the direct physiological effects of a substance (e.g., a drug of abuse, a medication) or a general medical condition.

Specify type (the following types are assigned based on the predominant delusional theme):

Erotomanic type: delusions that another person, usually of higher status, is in love with the individual

Grandiose type: delusions of inflated worth, power, knowledge, identity, or special relationship to a deity or famous person

Jealous type: delusions that the individual's sexual partner is unfaithful

Persecutory type: delusions that the person (or someone to whom the person is close) is being malevolently treated in some way

Somatic type: delusions that the person has some physical defect or general medical condition

Mixed type: delusions characteristic of more than one of the above types but no one theme predominates

Unspecified type

From American Psychiatric Association. *Diagnostic and Statistical Manual of Mental Disorders.* 4th ed. Text rev. Washington, DC: American Psychiatric Association; copyright 2000, with permission.

remarkable about patients with delusional disorder is that the mental status examination shows them to be remarkably normal except for the presence of a markedly abnormal delusional system. Patients may attempt to engage clinicians as allies in their delusions, but a clinician should not pretend to accept the delusion; this collusion further confounds reality and sets the stage for eventual distrust between the patient and the therapist.

By definition, patients with delusional disorder do not have prominent or sustained hallucinations. According to DSM-IV-TR, tactile or olfactory hallucinations may be present if they are consistent with the delusion (for example, somatic delusion of body odor). A few delusional patients have other hallucinatory experiences—virtually always auditory rather than visual.

Types

Persecutory Type.

The delusion of persecution is a classic symptom of delusional disorder; persecutory type and jealousy type delusions are probably the forms seen most frequently by psychiatrists. In contrast to persecutory delusions in schizophrenia, the clarity, logic, and systematic elaboration of the persecutory theme

in delusional disorder leave a remarkable stamp on this condition. The absence of other psychopathology, of deterioration in personality, or of deterioration in most areas of functioning also contrasts with the typical manifestations of schizophrenia.

Jealous Type.

Delusional disorder with delusions of infidelity has also been called *conjugal paranoia* (e.g., the delusion that a spouse is or has been unfaithful). The eponym *Othello syndrome* has been used to describe morbid jealousy that can arise from multiple concerns. The delusion usually afflicts men, often those with no prior psychiatric illness. It may appear suddenly and serve to explain a host of present and past events involving the spouse's behavior. The condition is difficult to treat and may diminish only on separation, divorce, or death of the spouse.

Marked jealousy (usually termed *pathological* or *morbid jealousy*) is thus a symptom of many disorders including schizophrenia (where female patients more commonly display this feature), epilepsy, mood disorders, drug abuse, and alcoholism—for which treatment is directed at the primary disorder. Jealousy is a powerful emotion; when it occurs in delusional disorder or as part of another condition it can be potentially dangerous and has been associated with violence, notably both suicide and homicide. The forensic aspects of the symptom have been noted repeatedly, especially its role as a motive for murder. However, physical and verbal abuse occur more frequently than extreme actions among individuals with this symptom. Caution and care in deciding how to deal with such presentations are essential not only for diagnosis, but also from the point of view of safety.

Erotomanic Type.

Patients with erotomania have delusions of secret lovers. Most frequently the patient is a woman, but men are also susceptible to the delusion. The patient believes that a suitor, usually more socially prominent than herself, is in love with her. The delusion becomes the central focus of the patient's existence, and the onset can be sudden.

Erotomania, the *psychose passionelle*, is also referred to as *de Clérambault's syndrome* to emphasize its occurrence in different disorders. Besides being the key symptom in some cases of delusional disorder, it is known to occur in schizophrenia, mood disorder, and other organic disorders.

Patients with erotomania frequently show certain characteristics: they are generally but not exclusively women, unattractive in appearance, in low-level jobs, and they lead withdrawn, lonely lives being single and having few sexual contacts. They select secret lovers who are substantially different from themselves. They exhibit what has been called *paradoxical conduct*, the delusional phenomenon of interpreting all denials of love, no matter how clear, as secret affirmations of love. The course may be chronic, recurrent, or brief. Separation from the love object may be the only satisfactory means of intervention. Although men are less commonly afflicted by this condition than women, they may be more aggressive and possibly violent in their pursuit of love. Hence, in forensic populations, men with this condition predominate. The object of aggression may not be the loved individual but companions or protectors of the love object who are viewed as trying to come between the lovers. The tendency toward violence among men with erotomania may lead initially to police rather than psychiatric contact. In certain cases, resentment and rage in response to an absence of reaction from all forms of love communication may escalate to a point that the love object is in danger. So-called stalkers, who continually follow their perceived lovers, frequently have delusions. Although most stalkers are men, women also stalk, and both groups have a high potential for violence.

Somatic Type.   Delusional disorder with somatic delusions has been called *monosymptomatic hypochondriacal psychosis.* The condition differs from other conditions with hypochondriacal symptoms in degree of reality impairment. In delusional disorder the delusion is fixed, unarguable, and presented intensely, because the patient is totally convinced of the physical nature of the disorder. In contrast, persons with hypochondriasis often admit that their fear of illness is largely groundless. The content of the somatic delusion may vary widely from case to case. There are three main types: (1) delusions of infestation (including parasitosis); (2) delusions of dysmorphophobia, such as of misshapenness, personal ugliness, or exaggerated size of body parts (this category seems closest to that of body dysmorphic disorder); and (3) delusions of foul body odors or halitosis. This latter category, sometimes referred to as *olfactory reference syndrome*, appears somewhat different from the category of delusions of infestation in that patients with the former have an earlier age of onset (mean, 25 years), male predominance, single status, and absence of past psychiatric treatment. Otherwise the three groups, although individually low in prevalence, appear to overlap.

The frequency of these conditions is low, but they may be underdiagnosed because patients present to dermatologists, plastic surgeons, and infectious disease specialists more often than to psychiatrists in the unremitting search for curative treatment.

Patients with this condition have a poor prognosis without treatment. It affects both sexes roughly equally. A previous history or family history of psychotic disorder is uncommon. In younger patients, a history of substance abuse or head injury is frequent. Although anger and hostility are commonplace, shame, depression, and avoidant behavior are even more characteristic. Suicide, apparently motivated by anguish, is not uncommon.

Grandiose Type.   Delusions of grandeur (megalomania) have been noted for years. They were described in Kraepelin's paranoia and have been associated with conditions fitting the description of delusional disorder. Whether this subtype occurs in clinical practice sufficiently enough to warrant a classification is debatable.

A 51-year-old man was arrested for disturbing the peace. Police had been called to a local park to stop him from carving his initials and those of a recently formed religious cult into various trees surrounding a pond in the park. When confronted, he had scornfully argued that, having been chosen to begin a new townwide religious revival, it was necessary for him to publicize his intent in a permanent fashion. The police were unsuccessful at preventing the man from cutting another tree and made the arrest. Psychiatric examination was ordered at the state hospital, and the patient was observed there for several weeks. He denied any emotional

difficulty and had never received psychiatric treatment. There was no history of euphoria or mood swings. The patient was angry about being hospitalized and only gradually permitted the doctor to interview him. In a few days, however, he was busy preaching to his fellow patients and letting them know that he had been given a special mandate from God to bring in new converts through his ability to heal. Eventually, his preoccupation with special powers diminished and no other evidence of psychopathology was observed. The patient was discharged, having received no medication at all. Two months later he was arrested at a local theater, this time for disrupting the showing of a film that depicted subjects he believed to be satanic.

Mixed Type.   The category of mixed type applies to patients with two or more delusional themes. However, this diagnosis should be reserved for cases in which no single delusional type predominates.

Unspecified Type.   The category of unspecified type is reserved for cases in which the predominant delusion cannot be subtyped within the previous categories. A possible example is certain delusions of misidentification, for example, Capgras' syndrome, named after the French psychiatrist who described the *illusion des sosies* or the illusion of doubles. The delusion in Capgras' syndrome is the belief that a familiar person has been replaced by an impostor. Others have described variants of the Capgras' syndrome, namely the delusion that persecutors or familiar persons can assume the guise of strangers (*Frégoli's phenomenon*) and the very rare delusion that familiar persons could change themselves into other persons at will (*intermetamorphosis*). Each disorder is not only rare but may be associated with schizophrenia, dementia, epilepsy, and other organic disorders. Reported cases have been predominantly in women, have had associated paranoid features, and have included feelings of depersonalization or derealization. The delusion may be short-lived, recurrent, or persistent. It is unclear whether delusional disorder can appear with such a delusion. Certainly, the Frégoli and intermetamorphosis delusions have bizarre content and are unlikely, but the delusion in Capgras' syndrome is a possible candidate for delusional disorder. The role of hallucination or perceptual disturbance in this condition needs to be explicated. Cases have appeared after sudden brain damage.

In the 19th century, the French psychiatrist Jules Cotard described several patients who suffered from a syndrome called *délire de négation,* sometimes referred to as *nihilistic delusional disorder* or *Cotard syndrome*. Patients with the syndrome complain of having lost not only possessions, status, and strength but also their heart, blood, and intestines. The world beyond them is reduced to nothingness. This relatively rare syndrome is usually considered a precursor to a schizophrenic or depressive episode. With the common use today of antipsychotic drugs, the syndrome is seen even less frequently than in the past.

Shared Psychotic Disorder

Shared psychotic disorder (also referred to over the years as *shared paranoid disorder, induced psychotic disorder, folie à deux, folie impose,* and *double insanity*) was first described by Lasegue and Falret in 1877. It is probably rare, but incidence and prevalence figures are lacking and the literature consists

Table 11.3–3
DSM-IV-TR Diagnostic Criteria for Shared Psychotic Disorder

A. A delusion develops in an individual in the context of a close relationship with another person(s), who has an already-established delusion.

B. The delusion is similar in content to that of the person who already has the established delusion.

C. The disturbance is not better accounted for by another psychotic disorder (e.g., schizophrenia) or a mood disorder with psychotic features and is not due to the direct physiological effects of a substance (e.g., a drug of abuse, a medication) or a general medical condition.

From American Psychiatric Association. *Diagnostic and Statistical Manual of Mental Disorders.* 4th ed. Text rev. Washington, DC: American Psychiatric Association; copyright 2000, with permission.

almost entirely of case reports. The disorder is characterized by the transfer of delusions from one person to another. Both persons are closely associated for a long time and typically live together in relative social isolation. In its most common form, (which is covered by the DSM-IV-TR criteria in Table 11.3–3), the individual who first has the delusion (the primary case) is often chronically ill and typically is the influential member of a close relationship with a more suggestible person (the secondary case) who also develops the delusion. The secondary case is frequently less intelligent, more gullible, more passive, or more lacking in self-esteem than the primary case. If the pair separates, the secondary case may abandon the delusion, but this outcome is not uniformly seen. The occurrence of the delusion is attributed to the strong influence of the more dominant member. Old age, low intelligence, sensory impairment, cerebrovascular disease, and alcohol abuse are among the factors associated with this peculiar form of psychotic disorder. A genetic predisposition to idiopathic psychoses has also been suggested as a possible risk factor.

Other special forms have been reported, such as *folie simultanée,* where two people become psychotic simultaneously and share the same delusion. Occasionally, more than two individuals are involved (e.g., *folie à trois, quatre, cinq*; also *folie à famille*), but such cases are especially rare. The most common relationships in *folie à deux* are sister–sister, husband–wife, and mother–child, but other combinations have also been described. Almost all cases involve members of a single family.

DIFFERENTIAL DIAGNOSIS

Delirium, Dementia, and Substance-Related Disorders

Delirium and dementia should be considered in the differential diagnosis of a patient with delusions. Delirium can be differentiated by the presence of a fluctuating level of consciousness or impaired cognitive abilities. Delusions early in the course of a dementing illness, as in dementia of the Alzheimer's type, may give the appearance of a delusional disorder; neuropsychological testing, however, usually detects cognitive impairment. Although alcohol abuse is an associated feature for patients with delusional disorder, delusional disorder should be distinguished from alcohol-induced psychotic disorder with hallucinations. Intoxication with sympathomimetics (including amphetamine), marijuana, or L-dopa is likely to result in delusional symptoms.

Other Disorders

The psychiatric differential diagnosis for delusional disorder includes malingering and factitious disorder with predominantly psychological signs and symptoms. The nonfactitious disorders in the differential diagnosis are schizophrenia, mood disorders, obsessive-compulsive disorder, somatoform disorders, and paranoid personality disorder. Delusional disorder is distinguished from schizophrenia by the absence of other schizophrenic symptoms and by the nonbizarre quality of the delusions; patients with delusional disorder also lack the impaired functioning seen in schizophrenia. The somatic type of delusional disorder may resemble a depressive disorder or a somatoform disorder. The somatic type of delusional disorder is differentiated from depressive disorders by the absence of other signs of depression and by the lack of a pervasive quality to the depression. Delusional disorder can be differentiated from somatoform disorders by the degree to which the somatic belief is held by the patient. Patients with somatoform disorders allow for the possibility that their disorder does not exist, whereas patients with delusional disorder have no doubt of its reality. Separating paranoid personality disorder from delusional disorder requires the sometimes difficult clinical distinction between extreme suspiciousness and a frank delusion. In general, if clinicians doubt that a symptom is a delusion, the diagnosis of delusional disorder should not be made.

COURSE AND PROGNOSIS

Some clinicians and some research data indicate that an identifiable psychosocial stressor often accompanies the onset of the disorder. The nature of the stressor may be such that a degree of suspicion or concern on the part of the person is warranted. Examples of such stressors are recent immigration, social conflict with family members or friends, and social isolation. A sudden onset is generally thought to be more common than an insidious onset. Some clinicians believe that a person with delusional disorder is likely to be below average in intelligence and that the premorbid personality of such a person is likely to be extroverted, dominant, and hypersensitive. The person's initial suspicions or concerns gradually become elaborate, consume much of the person's attention, and finally become delusional. People may begin quarreling with coworkers, may seek protection from the FBI or the police, or may begin visiting many medical or surgical physicians to seek consultations, lawyers about suits, or police about delusional suspicions.

Delusional disorder is thought to be a fairly stable diagnosis. Less than 25 percent of all cases of delusional disorder are later diagnosed as schizophrenia, and less than 10 percent of such patients have a mood disorder. Approximately 50 percent of patients have recovered at long-term follow-up, 20 percent show a decrease in symptoms, and 30 percent have no change in symptoms. The following factors correlate with a good prognosis: high levels of occupational, social, and functional adjustments; female sex; onset before age 30; sudden onset; short duration of illness; and the presence of precipitating factors.

Although reliable data are limited, patients with persecutory, somatic, and erotic delusions are thought to have a better prognosis than patients with grandiose and jealous delusions.

TREATMENT

Delusional Disorder

Delusional disorder has generally been regarded as resistant to treatment, and interventions have often focused on managing the morbidity of the disorder by reducing the impact of the delusion on the patient's (and family's) life. However, in recent years the outlook has become less pessimistic or restricted in planning effective treatment for these conditions. The goals of treatment are to establish the diagnosis, to decide on appropriate interventions, and to manage complications. Fundamental to the success of these goals is an effective and therapeutic doctor–patient relationship, which is far from easy to establish. The patients do not complain about psychiatric symptoms and often enter treatment against their will; even the psychiatrist may be drawn into their delusional nets.

In shared psychiatric disorder, it is essential that the patients be separated. If hospitalization is indicated, they should be placed on different units and have no contact. In general, the healthier of the two will give up the delusional belief (sometimes without any other therapeutic intervention). The sicker of the two will maintain the false fixed belief.

Psychotherapy

The essential element in effective psychotherapy is to establish a relationship in which patients begin to trust a therapist. Individual therapy seems to be more effective than group therapy; insight-oriented supportive, cognitive, and behavioral therapies are often effective. A therapist should initially neither agree with nor challenge a patient's delusions. Although therapists must ask about a delusion to establish its extent, persistent questioning about it should probably be avoided. Physicians may stimulate the motivation to receive help by emphasizing a willingness to help patients with their anxiety or irritability, without suggesting that the delusions be treated, but therapists should not actively support the notion that the delusions are real.

The unwavering reliability of therapists is essential in psychotherapy. Therapists should be on time and make appointments as regularly as possible, with the goal of developing a solid and trusting relationship with a patient. Overgratification may actually increase patients' hostility and suspiciousness because ultimately they must realize that not all demands can be met. Therapists can avoid overgratification by not extending the designated appointment period, by not giving extra appointments unless absolutely necessary, and by not being lenient about the fee.

A useful approach in building a therapeutic alliance is to empathize with the patient's internal experience of being overwhelmed by persecution. It may be helpful to make such comments as, "You must be exhausted, considering what you've been through." Without agreeing with every delusional misperception, a therapist can acknowledge that, from the patient's perspective, such perceptions create much distress. The ultimate goal is to help patients entertain the possibility of a doubt about their perceptions. As they become less rigid, feelings of weakness and inferiority, associated with some depression, may

surface. When a patient allows feelings of vulnerability to enter into the therapy, a positive therapeutic alliance has been established, and constructive therapy becomes possible.

When family members are available, clinicians may decide to involve them in the treatment plan. Without being delusionally seen as siding with the enemy, a clinician should attempt to enlist the family as allies in the treatment process. Consequently, both the patient and the family members need to understand that the therapist maintains physician–patient confidentiality and that communications from relatives are discussed with the patient. The family may benefit from the therapist's support and may thus be supportive of the patient.

A good therapeutic outcome depends on a psychiatrist's ability to respond to the patient's mistrust of others and the resulting interpersonal conflicts, frustrations, and failures. The mark of successful treatment may be a satisfactory social adjustment rather than an abatement of the patient's delusions.

Hospitalization

Patients with delusional disorder can generally undergo treatment as outpatients, but clinicians should consider hospitalization for several reasons. First, patients may need a complete medical and neurological evaluation to determine whether a nonpsychiatric medical condition is causing the delusional symptoms. Second, patients need an assessment of their ability to control violent impulses, such as to commit suicide and homicide, that may be related to the delusional material. Third, patients' behavior about the delusions may have significantly affected their ability to function within their family or occupational settings; they may require professional intervention to stabilize social or occupational relationships.

If a physician is convinced that a patient would receive the best treatment in a hospital, then the physician should attempt to persuade the patient to accept hospitalization; failing that, legal commitment may be indicated. If a physician convinces a patient that hospitalization is inevitable, the patient often voluntarily enters a hospital to avoid legal commitment.

Pharmacotherapy

In an emergency, severely agitated patients should be given an antipsychotic drug intramuscularly. Although adequately conducted clinical trials with large numbers of patients have not been conducted, most clinicians think that antipsychotic drugs are the treatment of choice for delusional disorder. Patients are likely to refuse medication because they can easily incorporate the administration of drugs into their delusional systems; physicians should not insist on medication immediately after hospitalization but, rather, should spend a few days establishing rapport with patients. Physicians should explain potential side effects to patients, so that patients do not later suspect that the physician lied.

A patient's history of medication response is the best guide to choose a drug. A physician should often start with low doses (for example, 2 mg of haloperidol [Haldol]) and increase the dose slowly. If a patient fails to respond to the drug at a reasonable dosage in a 6-week trial, antipsychotic drugs from other classes should be given clinical trials. Some investigators have indicated that pimozide (Orap) may be particularly effective in delusional disorder, especially in patients with somatic delusions. A common cause of drug failure is noncompliance, which should also be evaluated. Compliance with drug treatment is facilitated if the patient is receiving concurrent psychotherapy.

If the patient receives no benefit from antipsychotic medication, the drug should be discontinued. In patients who do respond to antipsychotic drugs, some data indicate that maintenance doses can be low. Although essentially no studies have evaluated the use of antidepressants, lithium (Eskalith), or anticonvulsants (such as carbamazepine [Tegretol] and valproate [Depakene]) in the treatment of delusional disorder, trials with these drugs may be warranted in patients who are unresponsive to antipsychotic drugs. Trials of these drugs should also be considered when a patient has either the features of a mood disorder or a family history of mood disorders.

▲ 11.4 Brief Psychotic Disorder, Psychotic Disorder Not Otherwise Specified, and Secondary Psychotic Disorders

BRIEF PSYCHOTIC DISORDER

Brief psychotic disorder is an acute and transient psychotic syndrome. According to the text revision of the fourth revised edition of *Diagnostic and Statistical Manual of Mental Disorders* (DSM-IV-TR), the disorder lasts from 1 day to 1 month, and the symptoms may resemble those for schizophrenia (e.g., delusions and hallucinations). In addition, the disorder may develop in response to a severe psychosocial stressor or group of stressors. Because of the variable and unstable nature of the disorder, it is sometimes a difficult diagnosis to make in clinical practice.

Epidemiology

The disorder is uncommon and occurs more often among younger patients (20s and 30s) than older patients. Reliable data on sex and sociocultural determinants are limited, although some findings suggest a higher incidence in women and persons in developing countries. Such epidemiological patterns are sharply distinct from those of schizophrenia.

Some clinicians indicate that the disorder may be seen most frequently in patients from low socioeconomic classes and in those who have experienced disasters or major cultural changes (such as immigrants). Persons who have gone through major psychosocial stressors may be at greater risk for subsequent brief psychotic disorder.

Comorbidity

The disorder is often seen in patients with personality disorders (most commonly, histrionic, paranoid, schizoid, schizotypal, and borderline personality disorders).

Etiology

The cause of brief psychotic disorder is unknown. Patients who have a personality disorder may have a biological or psychological vulnerability toward the development of psychotic symptoms, particularly those with borderline, schizoid, schizotypal, or paranoid qualities. Some patients with brief psychotic disorder have a history of schizophrenia or mood disorders in their families, but this is inconclusive. Psychodynamic formulations have emphasized the presence of inadequate coping mechanisms and the possibility of secondary gain for those patients with psychotic symptoms. Additional psychodynamic theories suggest that the psychotic symptoms are a defense against a prohibited fantasy, the fulfillment of an unattained wish, or an escape from a stressful psychosocial situation.

Diagnosis

DSM-IV-TR describes a continuum of diagnoses for psychotic disorders, based primarily on the duration of the symptoms. For psychotic symptoms that last at least 1 day but less than 1 month and that are not associated with a mood disorder, a substance-related disorder, or a psychotic disorder due to a general medical condition, a diagnosis of brief psychotic disorder is likely to be appropriate (Table 11.4–1). DSM-IV-TR describes three subtypes: (1) the presence of stressors, (2) the absence of stressors, and (3) a postpartum onset discussed below.

Clinical Features

The symptoms of brief psychotic disorder always include at least one major symptom of psychosis, usually with an abrupt onset, but do not always include the entire symptom pattern seen in schizophrenia. Some clinicians have observed that labile mood, confusion, and impaired attention may be more common at the onset of brief psychotic disorder than at the onset of eventual chronic psychotic disorders. Characteristic symptoms in brief psychotic disorder include emotional volatility, strange or bizarre behavior, screaming or muteness, and impaired memory for recent events. Some of the symptoms suggest a diagnosis of delirium and warrant a medical workup, especially to rule out adverse reactions to drugs.

Precipitating Stressors.   The clearest examples of precipitating stressors are major life events that would cause any person significant emotional upset. Such events include the loss of a close family member or a severe automobile accident. Some clinicians argue that the severity of the event must be considered in relation to the patient's life. This view, although reasonable, may broaden the definition of precipitating stressor to include events unrelated to the psychotic episode. Others have argued that the stressor may be a series of modestly stressful events rather than a single markedly stressful event, but evaluating the amount of stress caused by a sequence of events calls for an almost impossibly high degree of clinical judgment.

Differential Diagnosis

Clinicians must not assume that the correct diagnosis for a briefly psychotic patient is brief psychotic disorder, even when a clear pre-

Table 11.4–1
DSM-IV-TR Diagnostic Criteria for Brief Psychotic Disorder

A. Presence of one (or more) of the following symptoms:
  (1) delusions
  (2) hallucinations
  (3) disorganized speech (e.g., frequent derailment or incoherence)
  (4) grossly disorganized or catatonic behavior
  Note: Do not include a symptom if it is a culturally sanctioned response pattern.
B. Duration of an episode of the disturbance is at least 1 day but less than 1 month, with eventual full return to premorbid level of functioning.
C. The disturbance is not better accounted for by a mood disorder with psychotic features, schizoaffective disorder, or schizophrenia and is not due to the direct physiological effects of a substance (e.g., a drug of abuse, a medication) or a general medical condition.

Specify if:

  With marked stressor(s) (brief reactive psychosis): if symptoms occur shortly after and apparently in response to events that, singly or together, would be markedly stressful to almost anyone in similar circumstances in the person's culture

  Without marked stressor(s): if psychotic symptoms do *not* occur shortly after, or are not apparently in response to events that, singly or together, would be markedly stressful to almost anyone in similar circumstances in the person's culture

  With postpartum onset: if onset within 4 weeks postpartum

From American Psychiatric Association. *Diagnostic and Statistical Manual of Mental Disorders.* 4th ed. Text rev. Washington, DC: American Psychiatric Association; copyright 2000, with permission.

Table 11.4–2
Good Prognostic Features for Brief Psychotic Disorder

Good premorbid adjustment
Few premorbid schizoid traits
Severe precipitating stressor
Sudden onset of symptoms
Affective symptoms
Confusion and perplexity during psychosis
Little affective blunting
Short duration of symptoms
Absence of schizophrenic relatives

Course and Prognosis

By definition, the course of brief psychotic disorder is less than 1 month. Nonetheless, the development of such a significant psychiatric disorder may signify a patient's mental vulnerability. Approximately one-half of patients who are first classified as having brief psychotic disorder later display chronic psychiatric syndromes such as schizophrenia and mood disorders. Patients with brief psychotic disorder, however, generally have good prognoses, and European studies have indicated that 50 to 80 percent of all patients have no further major psychiatric problems. The length of the acute and residual symptoms is often just a few days. Occasionally, depressive symptoms follow the resolution of the psychotic symptoms, and suicide is a concern during both the psychotic phase and the postpsychotic depressive phase.

Several indicators have been associated with a good prognosis (Table 11.4–2). Patients with these features are unlikely to have subsequent episodes, and schizophrenia or a mood disorder is unlikely to develop later.

Treatment

Hospitalization. An acutely psychotic patient may need a brief hospitalization for both evaluation and protection. Evaluation requires close monitoring of symptoms and assessment of the patient's level of danger to self and others. In addition, the quiet and structured setting of a hospital may help patients regain their sense of reality. While clinicians wait for the setting or the drugs to have their effects, seclusion, physical restraints, or one-to-one monitoring of the patient may be necessary.

Pharmacotherapy. The two major classes of drugs to be considered in the treatment of brief psychotic disorder are the antipsychotic drugs and the anxiolytics. When an antipsychotic drug is chosen, a high-potency or atypical antipsychotic drug such as haloperidol (Haldol) or risperidone (Risperdal) may be used. Alternatively, anxiolytics such as benzodiazepines can be used in the short-term treatment of psychosis. They can be effective for a short time and are associated with fewer side effects than are the antipsychotic drugs. In rare cases, the benzodiazepines are associated with increased agitation and, more rarely still, with withdrawal seizures, which usually occur only with the sustained use of high dosages. Clinicians should avoid long-term use of any medication in the treatment of the disorder. If maintenance medication is necessary, a clinician may have to reconsider the diagnosis.

cipitating psychosocial factor is identified. Such a factor may be merely coincidental. If psychotic symptoms are present longer than 1 month, the diagnoses of schizophreniform disorder, schizoaffective disorder, schizophrenia, mood disorders with psychotic features, delusional disorder, and psychotic disorder not otherwise specified need to be entertained. However, if psychotic symptoms of sudden onset are present for less than a month in response to an obvious stressor, the diagnosis of brief psychotic disorder is strongly suggested. Other diagnoses to consider in the differential diagnosis include factitious disorder with predominantly psychological signs and symptoms, malingering, psychotic disorder caused by a general medical condition, and substance-induced psychotic disorder. In factitious disorder, symptoms are intentionally produced; in malingering there is a specific goal involved in appearing psychotic (e.g., to gain admission to the hospital), and when associated with a medical condition or drugs, the cause becomes apparent with proper medical or drug workups. If the patient admits to using illicit substances, the clinician can make the assessment of substance intoxication or substance withdrawal without the use of laboratory testing. Patients with epilepsy or delirium can also show psychotic symptoms that resemble those seen in brief psychotic disorder. Additional psychiatric disorders to be considered in the differential diagnosis include dissociative identity disorder and psychotic episodes associated with borderline and schizotypal personality disorders.

Psychotherapy. Although hospitalization and pharmaco-therapy are likely to control short-term situations, the difficult part of treatment is the psychological integration of the experience (and possibly the precipitating trauma, if one was present) into the lives of the patients and their families. Psychotherapy is of use in providing an opportunity to discuss the stressors and the psychotic episode. Exploration and development of coping strategies are the major topics in psychotherapy. Associated issues include helping patients deal with the loss of self-esteem and to regain self-confidence. An individualized treatment strategy based on increasing problem-solving skills while strengthening the ego structure through psychotherapy appears to be the most efficacious. Involvement of the family in the treatment process may be crucial to a successful outcome.

PSYCHOTIC DISORDER NOT OTHERWISE SPECIFIED

The psychotic disorder not otherwise specified category is used for patients who have psychotic symptoms (e.g., delusions, hallucinations, and disorganized speech and behavior) but who do not meet the diagnostic criteria for other specifically defined psychotic disorders. In some cases, the diagnosis of psychotic disorder not otherwise specified may be used when not enough information is available to make a specific diagnosis. DSM-IV-TR criteria are given in Table 11.4–3. Two disorders are described below.

Autoscopic Psychosis

The characteristic symptom of autoscopic psychosis is a visual hallucination of all or part of the person's own body. The hallucinatory perception, which is called a *phantom*, is usually colorless and transparent, and because the phantom imitates the person's movements, it is perceived as though it appears in a mirror. The phantom tends to appear suddenly and without warning.

Epidemiology. Autoscopy is a rare phenomenon. Some people have an autoscopic experience only once or a few times; others have the experience more often. Although the data are limited, sex, age, heredity, and intelligence do not seem to be related to the occurrence of the syndrome.

Etiology. The cause of the autoscopic phenomenon is unknown. A biological hypothesis is that abnormal, episodic activity in areas of the temporoparietal lobes is involved with the sense of self, perhaps combined with abnormal activity in parts of the visual cortex. Psychological theories have associated the syndrome with personalities characterized by imagination, visual sensitivity, and, possibly, narcissistic personality disorder traits. Such people may be likely to experience autoscopic phenomena during periods of stress.

Course and Prognosis. The classic descriptions of the phenomenon indicate that, in most cases, the syndrome is neither progressive nor incapacitating. Affected people usually maintain some emotional distance from the phenomenon, an observation that suggests a specific neuroanatomical lesion. Rarely do the symptoms reflect the onset of schizophrenia or other psychotic disorders.

Table 11.4–3
DSM-IV-TR Diagnostic Criteria for Psychotic Disorder Not Otherwise Specified

This category includes psychotic symptomatology (i.e., delusions, hallucinations, disorganized speech, grossly disorganized or catatonic behavior) about which there is inadequate information to make a specific diagnosis or about which there is contradictory information, or disorders with psychotic symptoms that do not meet the criteria for any specific psychotic disorder.

Examples include

1. Postpartum psychosis that does not meet criteria for mood disorder with psychotic features, brief psychotic disorder, psychotic disorder due to a general medical condition, or substance-induced psychotic disorder
2. Psychotic symptoms that have lasted for less than 1 month but that have not yet remitted, so that the criteria for brief psychotic disorder are not met
3. Persistent auditory hallucinations in the absence of any other features
4. Persistent nonbizarre delusions with periods of overlapping mood episodes that have been present for a substantial portion of the delusional disturbance
5. Situations in which the clinician has concluded that a psychotic disorder is present, but is unable to determine whether it is primary, due to a general medical condition, or substance induced

From American Psychiatric Association. *Diagnostic and Statistical Manual of Mental Disorders.* 4th ed. Text rev. Washington, DC: American Psychiatric Association; copyright 2000, with permission.

Postpartum Psychosis

Postpartum psychosis (sometimes called *puerperal psychosis*) is an example of psychotic disorder not otherwise specified that occurs in women who have recently delivered a baby. The syndrome is most often characterized by the mother's depression, delusions, and thoughts of harming either her infant or herself. Such ideation of suicide or infanticide must be carefully monitored; some mothers have acted on these ideas. Most available data suggest a close relation between postpartum psychosis and the mood disorders, particularly bipolar disorders and major depressive disorder.

Epidemiology. The incidence of postpartum psychosis is approximately 1 per 1,000 childbirths, although some reports have indicated that the incidence may be as high as 2 per 1,000. Approximately 50 to 60 percent of affected women have just had their first child, and approximately 50 percent of cases involve deliveries associated with nonpsychiatric perinatal complications. Approximately 50 percent of the affected women have a family history of mood disorders. Although postpartum psychosis is fundamentally a disorder of women, some rare cases affect fathers. In these instances, a husband may feel displaced by the child and may compete for the mother's love and attention. Such men, however, probably have a coexisting major mental disorder that has been exacerbated by the stress of fatherhood.

Etiology. The most robust data indicate that an episode of postpartum psychosis is essentially an episode of a mood disorder, usually a bipolar disorder but possibly a depressive disorder. Relatives of those with postpartum psychosis have an incidence of mood disorders that is similar to the incidence in relatives of people with mood disorders. Schizoaffective disorder and delusional disorder are rarely appropriate diagnoses. The validity of diagnoses of mood disorders is usually verified in the year after the birth, when as many as two-thirds of the patients have a second episode of the underlying disorder. The delivery process may best be seen as a nonspecific stress that causes the development of an episode of a major mood disorder, perhaps through a major hormonal mechanism.

A few instances of postpartum psychosis result from a general medical condition associated with perinatal events, such as infection, drug intoxication from, for example, scopolamine (Donnagel) and meperidine (Demerol), toxemia, and blood loss. The sudden decrease in estrogen and progesterone concentrations immediately after delivery may also contribute to the disorder, but treatment with these hormones has not been effective.

Some investigators have claimed that a purely psychosocial causal mechanism is suggested by the preponderance of primiparous mothers and by the association between postpartum psychosis and recent stressful events. Psychodynamic studies of postpartum mental illness have also suggested the presence of conflicted feelings in the mother about her mothering experience. Some women may not have wanted to become pregnant; others may feel trapped in unhappy marriages by motherhood. Marital discord during pregnancy has been associated with an increased incidence of illness, although the discord may be related to the slow development of mood disorder symptoms in the mother.

Diagnosis.   Specific diagnostic criteria are not included in DSM-IV-TR. The diagnosis can be made when psychosis occurs in close temporal association with childbirth, although a DSM-IV-TR diagnosis of a mood disorder should be considered in the differential diagnosis. Characteristic symptoms include delusions, cognitive deficits, motility disturbances, mood abnormalities, and occasional hallucinations. The content of the psychotic material revolves around mothering and pregnancy. DSM-IV-TR also allows for the diagnoses of brief psychotic disorder and mood disorders with postpartum onset (see Table 12.1–21).

Clinical Features.   The symptoms of postpartum psychosis can often begin within days of the delivery, although the mean time to onset is 2 to 3 weeks and almost always within 8 weeks of delivery. Characteristically, patients begin to complain of fatigue, insomnia, and restlessness and may have episodes of tearfulness and emotional lability. Later, suspiciousness, confusion, incoherence, irrational statements, and obsessive concerns about the baby's health and welfare may be present. Delusions may be present in 50 percent of all patients and hallucinations in approximately 25 percent. Complaints regarding the inability to move, stand, or walk are also common.

Patients may have feelings of not wanting to care for the baby, of not loving the baby, and, in some cases, of wanting to do harm to the baby or to themselves or both. Delusional material may involve the idea that the baby is dead or defective. Patients may deny the birth and express thoughts of being unmarried, virginal, persecuted, influenced, or perverse. Hallucinations with similar content may involve voices telling the patient to kill the baby.

Differential Diagnosis.   As with any psychotic disorder, clinicians should consider the possibility of either a psychotic disorder due to a general medical condition or a substance-induced psychotic disorder. Potential general medical conditions include hypothyroidism and Cushing's syndrome. Substance-induced psychotic disorder may be associated with the use of pain medications such as pentazocine (Talwin) or of antihypertensive drugs during pregnancy. Other potential medical causes include infections, toxemia, and neoplasms.

Women with a history of a mood disorder should be classified as having a recurrence of the disorder. Postpartum psychosis should not be confused with the so-called postpartum blues, a normal condition that occurs in up to 50 percent of women after childbirth. Postpartum blues is self-limited, lasts only a few days, and is characterized by tearfulness, fatigue, anxiety, and irritability that begin shortly after childbirth and lessen in severity over the course of a week. Postpartum nonpsychotic depression lacks delusional or hallucinatory activity. It is more severe than transient postpartum blues, occurs in 10 to 20 percent of women, and is characterized by despondent mood, feelings of inadequacy as a parent, and sleep disturbances. There may be ruminative or obsessional thoughts of harming their babies, but they lack delusional conviction. These patients should be carefully observed because it is sometimes difficult to differentiate between delusions and obsession and especially difficult to predict whether the patient will act on her fear of or wish to harm her baby.

Course and Prognosis.   The onset of florid psychotic symptoms is usually preceded by prodromal signs such as insomnia, restlessness, agitation, lability of mood, and mild cognitive deficits. Once the psychosis occurs, the patient may be a danger to herself or to her newborn, depending on the content of her delusional system and her degree of agitation. In one study, 5 percent of the patients committed suicide and 4 percent committed infanticide. A favorable outcome is associated with a good premorbid adjustment and a supportive family network.

The course of postpartum psychosis may be similar to that seen in patients with mood disorders. Specifically, mood disorders are usually episodic disorders, and patients with postpartum psychosis often experience another episode of symptoms within a year or two of the birth. Subsequent pregnancies are associated with an increased risk of another episode, sometimes as high as 50 percent.

Treatment.   Postpartum psychosis is a psychiatric emergency. Antidepressants and lithium (Eskalith), sometimes in combination with an antipsychotic, are the treatments of choice. Breast-feeding may have to be interrupted. Suicidal patients may require transfer to a psychiatric unit to help prevent a suicide attempt.

The mother is usually helped by contact with her baby if she so desires, but the visits must be closely supervised, especially if the mother is preoccupied with harming the infant. Psychotherapy is indicated after the period of acute psychosis, and therapy is usually directed at the conflictual areas that have become evident during the evaluation. Therapy may involve helping the patient accept and be at ease with the mothering role. Changes in environmental factors may also be indicated. Increased support from the husband and others in the environment may help reduce the woman's stress. Most studies report high rates of recovery from the acute illness.

PSYCHOTIC DISORDER DUE TO A GENERAL MEDICAL CONDITION AND SUBSTANCE-INDUCED PSYCHOTIC DISORDER

The evaluation of a psychotic patient requires consideration of the possibility that the psychotic symptoms result from a general medical condition such as a brain tumor or the ingestion of a substance such as phencyclidine (PCP).

Epidemiology

Relevant epidemiological data about psychotic disorder due to a general medical condition and substance-induced psychotic disorder are lacking. The disorders are most often encountered in patients who abuse alcohol or other substances on a long-term basis.

Etiology

Physical conditions such as cerebral neoplasms, particularly of the occipital or temporal areas, can cause hallucinations. Sensory deprivation, as in people who are blind or deaf, can also result in hallucinatory or delusional experiences. Lesions involving the temporal lobe and other cerebral regions, especially the right hemisphere and the parietal lobe, are associated with delusions.

Psychoactive substances are common causes of psychotic syndromes. The most commonly involved substances are alcohol, indole hallucinogens such as lysergic acid diethylamide (LSD), amphetamine, cocaine, mescaline, PCP, and ketamine. Many other substances, including steroids and thyroxine, can produce hallucinations.

Diagnosis

Psychotic Disorder Due to a General Medical Condition.
The DSM-IV-TR diagnosis of psychotic disorder due to a general medical condition (Table 11.4–4) is defined in DSM-IV-TR by specifying the predominant symptoms. When the diagnosis is used, the medical condition, along with the predominant symptoms pattern, should be included in the diagnosis—for example, psychotic disorder due to a brain tumor, with delusions. The DSM-IV-TR criteria further specify that the disorder does not occur exclusively while a patient is delirious or demented and that the symptoms are not better accounted for by another mental disorder.

Substance-Induced Psychotic Disorder.
The diagnostic category of substance-induced psychotic disorder in DSM-IV-TR (Table 11.4–5) is reserved for those with substance-induced psychotic symptoms and impaired reality testing. People with substance-induced psychotic symptoms (for example, hallucinations) but with intact reality testing should be classified as having a substance-related disorder (for example, PCP intoxication with perceptual disturbances). The full diagnosis of substance-induced psychotic disorder should include the type of substance involved, the stage of substance use when the disorder began (for example, during intoxication or withdrawal), and the clinical phenomena (for example, hallucinations or delusions).

Table 11.4–4
DSM-IV-TR Diagnostic Criteria for Psychotic Disorder Due to a General Medical Condition

A. Prominent hallucinations or delusions.
B. There is evidence from the history, physical examination, or laboratory findings that the disturbance is the direct physiological consequence of a general medical condition.
C. The disturbance is not better accounted for by another mental disorder.
D. The disturbance does not occur exclusively during the course of a delirium.

Code based on predominant symptom:
With delusions: if delusions are the predominant symptom
With hallucinations: if hallucinations are the predominant symptom
Coding note: Include the name of the general medical condition on Axis I, e.g., psychotic disorder due to malignant lung neoplasm, with delusions; also code the general medical condition on Axis III.
Coding note: If delusions are part of vascular dementia, indicate the delusions by coding the appropriate subtype, e.g., vascular dementia, with delusions.

From American Psychiatric Association. *Diagnostic and Statistical Manual of Mental Disorders*. 4th ed. Text rev. Washington, DC: American Psychiatric Association; copyright 2000, with permission.

Clinical Features

Hallucinations. Hallucinations may occur in one or more sensory modalities. Tactile hallucinations (such as the sensation of bugs crawling on the skin) are characteristic of cocaine use. Auditory hallucinations are usually associated with psychoactive substance abuse; auditory hallucinations may also occur in people who are deaf. Olfactory hallucinations can result from temporal lobe epilepsy; visual hallucinations may occur in people who are blind because of cataracts. Hallucinations are either recurrent or persistent and are experienced in a state of full wakefulness and alertness; a hallucinating patient shows no significant changes in cognitive functions. Visual hallucinations often take the form of scenes involving diminutive (Lilliputian) human figures or small animals. Rare musical hallucinations typically feature religious songs. Patients with psychotic disorder due to a general medical condition and substance-induced psychotic disorder may act on their hallucinations. In alcohol-related hallucinations, threatening, critical, or insulting third-person voices speak about the patients and may tell them to harm either themselves or others. Such patients are dangerous and are at significant risk for suicide or homicide.

Delusions. Secondary and substance-induced delusions are usually present in a state of full wakefulness. Patients experience no change in the level of consciousness, although mild cognitive impairment may be observed. Patients may appear confused, disheveled, or eccentric, with tangential or even incoherent speech. Hyperactivity and apathy may be present, and an associated dysphoric mood is thought to be common. The delusions may be systematized or fragmentary, with varying content, but persecutory delusions are the most common.

Table 11.4–5
DSM-IV-TR Diagnostic Criteria for Substance-Induced Psychotic Disorder

A. Prominent hallucinations or delusions. **Note:** Do not include hallucinations if the person has insight that they are substance induced.

B. There is evidence from the history, physical examination, or laboratory findings of either (1) or (2):

    (1) the symptoms in Criterion A developed during, or within a month of, substance intoxication or withdrawal

    (2) medication use is etiologically related to the disturbance

C. The disturbance is not better accounted for by a psychotic disorder that is not substance induced. Evidence that the symptoms are better accounted for by a psychotic disorder that is not substance induced might include the following: the symptoms precede the onset of the substance use (or medication use); the symptoms persist for a substantial period of time (e.g., about a month) after the cessation of acute withdrawal or severe intoxication, or are substantially in excess of what would be expected given the type or amount of the substance used or the duration of use; or there is other evidence that suggests the existence of an independent non-substance-induced psychotic disorder (e.g., a history of recurrent non-substance-related episodes).

D. The disturbance does not occur exclusively during the course of a delirium.

Note: This diagnosis should be made instead of a diagnosis of substance intoxication or substance withdrawal only when the symptoms are in excess of those usually associated with the intoxication or withdrawal syndrome and when the symptoms are sufficiently severe to warrant independent clinical attention.

Code [Specific substance]-induced psychotic disorder:

(Alcohol, with delusions; alcohol, with hallucinations; amphetamine [or amphetamine-like substance], with delusions; amphetamine [or amphetamine-like substance], with hallucinations; cannabis, with delusions; cannabis, with hallucinations; cocaine, with delusions; cocaine, with hallucinations; hallucinogen, with delusions; hallucinogen, with hallucinations; inhalant, with delusions; inhalant, with hallucinations; opioid, with delusions; opioid, with hallucinations; phencyclidine [or phencyclidine-like substance], with delusions; phencyclidine [or phencyclidine-like substance], with hallucinations; sedative, hypnotic, or anxiolytic, with delusions; sedative, hypnotic, or anxiolytic, with hallucinations; other [or unknown] substance, with delusions; other [or unknown] substance, with hallucinations)

Specify if:

With onset during intoxication: if criteria are met for intoxication with the substance and the symptoms develop during the intoxication syndrome

With onset during withdrawal: if criteria are met for withdrawal from the substance and the symptoms develop during, or shortly after, a withdrawal syndrome

From American Psychiatric Association. *Diagnostic and Statistical Manual of Mental Disorders.* 4th ed. Text rev. Washington, DC: American Psychiatric Association; copyright 2000, with permission.

Differential Diagnosis

Psychotic disorder due to a general medical condition and substance-induced psychotic disorder must be distinguished from delirium, in which patients have a clouded sensorium, from dementia, in which patients have major intellectual deficits, and from schizophrenia, in which patients have other symptoms of thought disorder and impaired functioning. Psychotic disorder due to a general medical condition and substance-induced psychotic disorder must also be differentiated from psychotic mood disorders, in which other affective symptoms are pronounced.

Treatment

Treatment involves identifying the general medical condition or the particular substance involved. At this point, treatment is directed toward the underlying condition and the patient's immediate behavioral control. Hospitalization may be necessary to evaluate patients completely and to ensure their safety. Antipsychotic agents (for example, olanzapine [Zyprexa] and haloperidol [Haldol]) may be necessary for immediate and short-term control of psychotic or aggressive behavior, although benzodiazepines may also be useful for controlling agitation and anxiety.

▲ 11.5 Culture-Bound Syndromes

Although all psychiatric diagnoses are influenced by their cultural context, the most dramatic example of the difficulty in applying Western-based nosological concepts can be found in the so-called culture-bound syndromes. The term evolved to denote recurrent, locality-specific patterns of aberrant behavior and troubling experiences that appear to fall outside conventional Western psychiatric categories. The descriptive phrases formerly used to refer to such phenomena include "cultural and ethnic psychoses and neuroses" and "atypical and exotic psychotic syndromes." The *culture-bound syndrome* is now generally accepted to refer to culturally based signs and symptoms of mental distress or maladaptive behavior that are prominent in folk belief and practice. Such patterns are informed by native cultural assumptions, sorcery, breaches of taboo, intrusions of a disease object, intrusions of a disease-causing spirit, or loss of soul.

REPRESENTATIVE SYNDROMES

Representative culture-bound syndromes from around the world with some of their clinical features are described below. The descriptions are adapted from the fourth revised edition of the *Diagnostic and Statistical Manual of Mental Disorders* (DSM-IV-TR).

Amok. A dissociative episode characterized by a period of brooding followed by an outburst of violent, aggressive, or homicidal behavior directed at persons and objects. The episode tends to be precipitated by a perceived slight or insult and seems to be prevalent only among men. The episode is often accompanied by persecutory ideas, automatisms, amnesia, exhaustion, and a return to premorbid state following the episode. Some instances of *amok* may occur during a brief psychotic episode or constitute onset or an exacerbation of a chronic psychotic process. The original reports that used this term were from Malaysia. A similar behavior patter is found in Laos, Philippines, Polynesia (*cafard* or *cathard*), Papua New Guinea, and Puerto Rico (*mal de pelea*) and among the Navajo (*iich'aa*).

Ataque de nervios. An idiom of distress principally reported among Latinos from the Caribbean, but recognized among many Latin American and Latin Mediterranean groups. Commonly reported symptoms include uncontrollable shouting, attacks of crying, trembling, heat in the chest rising into the head, and verbal or physical aggression. Dissociative experiences, seizure-like or fainting episodes, and suicidal gestures are prominent in some attacks but absent in others. A general feature of an *ataque de nervios* is a sense of being out of control. *Ataque de nervios* frequently occurs as a direct result of a stressful event relating to the family (e.g., death of a close relative, separation or divorce from a spouse, conflicts with a spouse or children, or witnessing an accident involving a family member). Persons may experience amnesia for what occurred during the *ataque de nervios*, but they otherwise return rapidly to their usual level of functioning. Although descriptions of some *ataque de nervios* most closely fit the DSM-IV-TR description of panic attacks, the association of most *ataques* with a precipitating event and the frequent absence of the hallmark symptoms of acute fear or apprehension distinguish them from panic disorder. *Ataques* span the range from normal expressions of distress not associated with a mental disorder to symptom presentations associated with anxiety, mood, dissociative, or somatoform disorders.

Bilis and colera (also referred to as *muina*). The underlying cause is thought to be strongly experienced anger or rage. Anger is viewed among Latino groups as a particularly powerful emotion that can have direct effects on the body and exacerbate existing symptoms. The major effect of anger is to disturb core body balances (which are understood as a balance between hot and cold valences in the body). Symptoms can include acute nervous tension, headache, trembling, screaming, stomach disturbances, and, in more severe cases, loss of consciousness. Chronic fatigue may result from an acute episode.

Brain fag. A term initially used in West Africa to refer to a condition experienced by high school or university students in response to the challenges of schooling. Symptoms include difficulties in concentrating, remembering, and thinking. Students often state that their brains are "fatigued." Additional somatic symptoms are usually centered around the head and neck and include pain, pressure or tightness, blurring of vision, heat, or burning. "Brain tiredness" or fatigue from "too much thinking" is an idiom of distress in many cultures, and resulting syndromes can resemble certain anxiety, depressive, and somatoform disorders.

Dhat. A folk diagnostic term used in India to refer to severe anxiety and hypochondriacal concerns associated with the discharge of semen, whitish discoloration of urine, and feelings of weakness and exhaustion. Similar to *jiryan* (India), *sukra prameha* (Sri Lanka), and *shen-k'uei* (China).

Falling-out or black-out. Episodes that occur primarily in southern United States and Caribbean groups. They are characterized by a sudden collapse, which sometimes occurs without warning but is sometimes preceded by feelings of dizziness or "swimming" in the head. The person's eyes are usually open, but the person claims an inability to see. Those affected usually hear and understand what is occurring around them but feel powerless to move. This may correspond to a diagnosis of conversion disorder or a dissociative disorder.

Ghost sickness. A preoccupation with death and the deceased (sometimes associated with witchcraft), frequently observed among members of many American Indian tribes. Various symptoms can be attributed to ghost sickness, including bad dreams, weakness, feeling of danger, loss of appetite, fainting, dizziness, fear, anxiety, hallucinations, loss of consciousness, confusion, feeling of futility, and a sense of suffocation.

Hwa-byung (also known as *wool-hwa-byung*). A Korean folk syndrome literally translated into English as "anger syndrome" and attributed to the suppression of anger. The symptoms include insomnia, fatigue, panic, fear of impending death, dysphoric affect, indigestion, anorexia, dyspnea, palpitations, generalized aches and pains, and a feeling of a mass in the epigastrium.

Koro. A term, probably of Malaysian origin, that refers to an episode of sudden and intense anxiety that the penis (or, in women, the vulva and nipples) will recede into the body and possibly cause death. The syndrome is reported in South and East Asia, where it is known by a variety of local terms, such as *shuk yang* and *suo yang* (Chinese), *jinjinia bemar* (Assam), or *rok-joo* (Thailand). It is occasionally found in the West. *Koro* at times occurs in localized epidemic form in East Asian areas. The diagnosis is included in the second edition of *Chinese Classification of Mental Disorders* (CCMD-2).

Latah. Hypersensitivity to sudden fright, often with echopraxia, echolalia, command obedience, and dissociative or trance-like behavior. The term *latah* is of Malaysian or Indonesian origin, but the syndrome has been found in many parts of the world. Other terms for the condition are *amurakh, irkunik, ikota, olan, myriachit,* and *menkeiti* (Siberian groups); *bah tschi, bah-tsi, baah-ji* (Thailand); *imu* (Ainu, Sakhalin, Japan); and *mali-mali* and *siok* (Philippines). In Malaysia it is more frequent in middle-aged women.

Locura. A term used by Latinos in the United States and Latin America to refer to a severe form of chronic psychosis. The condition is attributed to an inherited vulnerability, to the effect to multiple life difficulties, or to a combination of both factors. Symptoms exhibited by persons with *locura* include incoherence, agitation, auditory and visual hallucinations, inability to follow rules of social interaction, unpredictability, and possibly violence.

Mal de ojo. A concept widely found in Mediterranean cultures and elsewhere in the world. *Mal de ojo* is a Spanish phrase translated into English as "evil eye." Children are especially at risk. Symptoms include fitful sleep, crying without apparent cause, diarrhea, vomiting, and fever in a child or infant. Sometimes adults (especially women) have the condition.

Nervios. A common idiom of distress among Latinos in the United States and Latin America. A number of other ethnic groups have related, although often somewhat distinctive, ideas of nerves (such as *nerva* among Greeks in North America). *Nervios* refers both to a general state of vulnerability to stressful life experiences and to a syndrome brought on by difficult life circumstances. The term *nervios* includes a wide range of symptoms of emotional distress, somatic disturbance, and inability to function. Common symptoms include headaches and brain aches, irritability, stomach disturbances, sleep difficulties, nervousness, easy tearfulness, inability to concentrate, trembling, tingling sensations, and *mareos* (dizziness with occasional vertigo-like exacerbations). *Nervios* tends to be an ongoing problem, although variable in the degree of disability that is manifested. *Nervios* is a very broad syndrome that spans the range from patients free of a mental disorder to presentations resembling depressive, dissociative, somatoform, or psychotic disorders. Differential diagnosis depends on the constellation of symptoms experienced, the kinds of social events that are associated with the onset and progress of *nervios*, and the level of disability experienced.

Piblokto. An abrupt dissociative episode accompanied by extreme excitement of up to 30 minutes duration and frequency followed by convulsive seizure and coma lasting up to 12 hours. It is observed primarily in circumpolar natives and sub-Arctic Inuit communities, although regional variations in name exist. The person may be withdrawn or mildly irritable for a period of hours or days before the attack and typically reports complete amnesia for the attack. During the attack, persons may tear off clothing, break furniture, shout obscenities, eat feces, flee from protective shelters, or perform irrational or dangerous acts.

Qi-gong psychotic reactions. Acute, time-limited episodes characterized by dissociative, paranoid, or other psychotic or nonpsychotic symptoms that may occur after participation in the Chinese folk health-enhancing practice of *qi-gong* (exercise of vital energy). Especially vulnerable are persons who become overly involved in the practice. This diagnosis is included in CCMD-2.

Rootwork. A set of cultural interpretations that ascribe illness to hexing, witchcraft, sorcery, or evil influence of another person. Symptoms may include generalized anxiety and gastrointestinal complaints (e.g., nausea, vomiting, diarrhea), weakness, dizziness, the fear of being poisoned, and sometimes fear of being killed (voodoo death). Roots, spells, or hexes can be put or placed on another person, causing a variety of emotional and psychological problems. The hexed person may even fear death until the root has been taken off (eliminated), usually through the work of a root doctor (a healer in this tradition), who can also be called on to bewitch an enemy. Rootwork is found in the southern United States among both African-American and European-American populations and in Caribbean societies. It is also known as *mal puesto* or *brujeria* in Latino societies.

Sangue dormido ("sleeping blood"). A syndrome found among Portuguese Cape Verde Islanders (and immigrants from there to the United States). It includes pain, numbness, tremor, paralysis, convulsions, stroke, blindness, heart attack, infection, and miscarriages.

Shejing shuariu ("neurasthenia"). In China, a condition characterized by physical and mental fatigue, dizziness, headaches, other pains, concentration difficulties, sleep disturbance, and memory loss. Other symptoms include gastrointestinal problems, sexual dysfunction, irritability, excitability, and various signs suggesting disturbance of the autonomic nervous system. In many cases, the symptoms would meet the criteria for the DSM-IV-TR mood or anxiety disorder. The diagnosis is included in CCMD-2.

Shen-k'uei (Taiwan), *shenkui* (China). A Chinese folk label describing marked anxiety or panic syndromes with accompanying somatic complaints for which no physical cause can be demonstrated. Symptoms include dizziness, backache, fatigability, general weakness, insomnia, frequent dreams, and complaints of sexual dysfunctions, such as premature ejaculation and impotence. Symptoms are attributed to excessive semen loss from frequent intercourse, masturbation, nocturnal emission, or passing of white turbid urine believed to contain semen. Excessive semen loss is feared because of the belief that it represents the loss of one's vital essence and can therefore be life threatening.

Shin-byung. A Korean folk label for a syndrome in which initial phases are characterized by anxiety and somatic complaints (general weakness, dizziness, fear, anorexia, insomnia, gastrointestinal problems), with subsequent dissociation and possession by ancestral spirits.

Spell. A trance state in which persons "communicate" with deceased relatives or spirits. At times the state is associated with brief periods of personality change. The culture-specific syndrome is seen among African-Americans and European-Americans from the southern United States. Spells are not considered to be medical events in the folk tradition but may be misconstrued as psychotic episodes in clinical settings.

Susto (fright or "soul loss"). A folk illness prevalent among some Latinos in the United States and among people in Mexico, Central America, and South America. *Susto* is also referred to as *espanto, pasmo, tripa ida, perdida del alma,* or *chibih. Susto* is an illness attributed to a frightening event that causes the soul to leave the body and results in unhappiness and sickness. Persons with *susto* also experience significant strains in key social roles. Symptoms may appear any time from days to years after fright is experienced. It is believed that in extreme cases, *susto* may result in death. Typical symptoms include appetite disturbances, inadequate or excessive sleep, troubled sleep or dreams, feelings of sadness, lack of motivation to do anything, and feelings of low self-worth or dirtiness. Somatic symptoms accompanying *susto* include muscle aches and pains, headache, stomachache, and diarrhea. Ritual healings are focused on calling the soul back to the body and cleansing the person to restore bodily and spiritual balance. Different experiences of *susto* may be related to major depressive disorder, posttraumatic stress disorders, and somatoform disorders. Similar etiological beliefs and symptom configurations are found in many parts of the world.

Taijin kyofu sho. A culturally distinctive phobia in Japan, in some ways resembling social phobia in DSM-IV-TR. The syndrome refers to an intense fear that one's body, its parts, or its functions displease, embarrass, or are offensive to other people in appearance, odor, facial expressions, or movements. The syndrome is included in the official Japanese diagnostic system of mental disorders.

Zar. A general term applied in Ethiopia, Somalia, Egypt, Sudan, Iran, and other North African and Middle Eastern societies to the experience of spirits possessing a person. Persons possessed by a spirit may experience dissociative episodes that may include shouting, laughing, hitting the head against the wall, singing, or weeping. They may show apathy and withdrawal, refusing to eat or carry out daily tasks or may develop a long-term relationship with the possessing spirit. Such behavior is not considered pathological locally.

CULTURE AND PSYCHOPHARMACOLOGY

Pharmacogenetics

The field of pharmacogenetics grew out of observations of significant ethnic differences in response to drugs, in differential development, and in side effects profiles, leading to the discovery of defects or deficiencies in the genetically controlled activity of enzyme systems responsible for the metabolism of psychotropic medications and toxins such as alcohol.

Acetylation Status

Observations of ethnic differences in the side-effects profile of the antituberculosis drug isoniazid (Nydrazid, Rifamate) led to the classification of people as slow or rapid acetylators, which, among other biological effects, determines their metabolism of psychotropic medications such as clonazepam (Klonopin) and phenelzine (Nardil).

Alcohol Metabolism

P. H. Wolf, while studying racial differences in alcohol sensitivity, observed that approximately 80 percent of Asians and 50 percent of Native Americans exhibited the flushing response to alcohol (compared with 10 percent of whites) and concluded that these differences had a genetic basis. They have been proved to be related to genetic polymorphism of isoenzymes of alcohol dehydrogenase (ADH) and aldehyde dehydrogenase (ALDH), enzymes critical for complete metabolism of alcohol and other neurotransmitters and that play a role in development of alcoholism or its avoidance. For example, Asians who are either homozygous or heterozygous for the atypical Asian-type ALDH2 gene are alcohol sensitive and have a low risk for alcoholism and alcohol liver disease.

Native Americans have a high frequency of both alcohol flushing and alcohol-related problems. Akira Yoshida's research team reported in 1993 that they had practically no detectable Asian-type ADH2 and ALDH2 genes, a major alcohol-rejecting genetic factor.

Cytochrome P450 Isoenzymes

The cytochrome P450 enzyme system is key in the metabolism of psychotropic and nonpsychotropic drugs as well as a great variety of environmental toxins that find their way into the diets of animals and humans. The genetic defects that render these enzymes less effective and make humans poor metabolizers are unequally distributed among ethnic populations. This is particularly the case for two cytochrome P450 (CYP) isoenzymes: CYP 2D6 (debrisoquin hydroxylase) and CYP 2Cmp (mephenytoin hydroxylase). The percentage of CYP 2D6 poor metabolizers is lower for Asians (0.5 to 2.4 percent) and higher for whites (2.9 to 10 percent). Similar interethnic variance exists in the frequency of poor metabolizers of CYP 2Cmp, low among whites (3 percent), intermediate for African-Americans (18 percent), and higher (up to 20 percent) in Asian and Japanese populations.

These interethnic differences in the P450 isoenzymes are of great importance in psychiatry and psychopharmacology because of their role in the metabolism of antipsychotics, antidepressants, sedatives such as barbiturates and benzodiazepines, and β-adrenergic receptor antagonists (β-blockers) such as propranolol (Inderal).

12 ▲

Mood Disorders

▲ 12.1 Major Depression and Bipolar Disorder

Mood disorders encompass a large group of disorders in which pathological mood and related disturbances dominate the clinical picture. Known in previous editions of the *Diagnostic and Statistical Manual of Mental Disorders* (DSM) as affective disorders, the term *mood disorders* is preferred because it refers to sustained emotional states, not merely to the external (affective) expression of a transitory emotional state. Mood disorders are best considered as syndromes (rather than discrete diseases) consisting of a cluster of signs and symptoms sustained over a period of weeks to months that represent a marked departure from a person's habitual functioning and tend to recur, often in periodic or cyclical fashion. Mood may be normal, elevated, or depressed. Normal persons experience a wide range of moods and have an equally large repertoire of affective expressions; they feel more or less in control of their moods and affects. In mood disorders, the sense of control is lost and there is a subjective experience of great distress.

Patients with an elevated mood demonstrate expansiveness, flight of ideas, decreased sleep, heightened self-esteem, and grandiose ideas. Patients with depressed mood show loss of energy and interest, guilt feelings, difficulty in concentrating, loss of appetite, and thoughts of death or suicide. Other signs and symptoms include changes in activity level, cognitive abilities, speech, and vegetative functions (e.g., sleep, appetite, sexual activity, and other biological rhythms). These disorders virtually always result in impaired interpersonal, social, and occupational functioning.

Patients who are afflicted only with major depressive episodes are said to have major depressive disorder or unipolar depression. Patients with both manic and depressive episodes or patients with manic episodes alone are said to have bipolar disorder. The terms *unipolar mania, pure mania,* or *euphoric mania* are sometimes used for bipolar patients who do not have depressive episodes. Hypomania is an episode of manic symptoms that does not meet the full text revision of the fourth edition of DSM (DSM-IV-TR) criteria for a manic episode.

The field of psychiatry has considered major depression and bipolar disorder to be to separate disorders, particularly in the last 20 years. However, reconsideration has been given more recently to the possibility that bipolar disorder is actually a more severe expression of major depression. Many patients diagnosed as having major depressive disorder reveal, on careful examination, past episodes of manic or hypomanic behavior that have gone undetected. In addition, depression usually causes a greater sense of distress for the patient than does mania, thus, patients are more likely to seek help. For this reason it has been suggested that there is a relative overdiagnosis of unipolar major depressive disorder.

DSM-IV-TR CLASSIFICATION OF MOOD DISORDERS

According to DSM-IV-TR, a major depressive disorder (also known as *unipolar depression*) occurs without a history of a manic, mixed, or hypomanic episode. A major depressive episode must last at least 2 weeks, and, typically, a person diagnosed with major depressive episode must also experience at least four symptoms from a list that includes changes in appetite and weight, changes in sleep and activity, lack of energy, feelings of guilt, problems in thinking and making decisions, and recurring thoughts of death or suicide.

A manic episode is a distinct period of an abnormally and persistently elevated, expansive, or irritable mood for at least 1 week, less if a patient must be hospitalized. A hypomanic episode has a duration of at least 4 days and is similar to a manic episode except that it is not severe enough to cause impairment in social or occupational functioning, and no psychotic features are present. Both mania and hypomania are associated with inflated self-esteem, decreased need for sleep, distractibility, great physical and mental activity, and overinvolvement in pleasurable behavior. According to DSM-IV-TR, bipolar I disorder is defined as having a clinical course of one or more manic episodes and sometimes of major depressive episodes. A mixed episode is a period of at least 1 week in which both a manic episode and a major depressive episode occur almost daily. A variant of bipolar disorder characterized by episodes of hypomania rather than mania is known as *bipolar II disorder.*

Two additional mood disorders, dysthymic disorder and cyclothymic disorder (see Section 12.2) have also been appreciated clinically for some time. Dysthymic disorder and cyclothymic disorder are characterized by the presence of symptoms that are less severe than the symptoms of major depressive disorder and of bipolar I disorder, respectively. DSM-IV-TR defines dysthymic disorder as characterized by at least 2 years of depressed mood that is not severe enough to fit the diagnosis of major depressive episode. Cyclothymic disorder is characterized by at least 2 years of frequently occurring hypomanic

173

symptoms that cannot fit the diagnosis of manic episode and of depressive symptoms that cannot fit the diagnosis of major depressive episode.

DSM-IV-TR includes three mood disorder research categories (minor depressive disorder, recurrent brief depressive disorder, and premenstrual dysphoric disorder). Other DSM-IV-TR diagnoses are mood disorder due to a general medical condition and substance-induced mood disorder. These categories are designed to broaden the recognition of mood disorder diagnoses, to describe mood disorder symptoms more specifically than in the past, and to facilitate the differential diagnosis of mood disorders. Finally, DSM-IV-TR includes three residual disorders—bipolar disorder not otherwise specified, depressive disorder not otherwise specified, and mood disorder not otherwise specified.

EPIDEMIOLOGY

Incidence and Prevalence

Major depressive disorder is a common disorder with a lifetime prevalence of approximately 15 percent, perhaps as high as 25 percent for women. The incidence of major depressive disorder is 10 percent in primary care patients and 15 percent in medical inpatients. Bipolar I disorder is less common than is major depressive disorder, with a lifetime prevalence of approximately 1 percent, similar to the figure for schizophrenia. Table 12.1–1 lists the lifetime prevalence of mood disorders.

Sex

An almost universal observation, independent of country or culture, is the twofold greater prevalence of major depressive disorder in women than in men. The reasons for the difference have been hypothesized to involve hormonal differences, the effects of childbirth, differing psy-

Table 12.1–1
Lifetime Prevalence of Some DSM-IV-TR Mood Disorders

Mood Disorder	Lifetime Prevalence
Depressive disorders	
Major depressive disorder (MDD)	10–25% for women; 5–12% for men
Recurrent, with full interepisode recovery, superimposed on dysthymic disorder	Approximately 3% of persons with MDD
Recurrent, without full interepisode recovery, superimposed on dysthymic disorder (double depression)	Approximately 20–25% of persons with MDD
Dysthymic disorder	Approximately 6%
Bipolar disorders	
Bipolar I disorder	0.4–1.6%
Bipolar II disorder	Approximately 0.5%
Bipolar I disorder or bipolar II disorder, with rapid cycling	5–15% of persons with bipolar disorder
Cyclothymic disorder	0.4–1.0%

Data are from American Psychiatric Association. *Diagnostic and Statistical Manual of Mental Disorders.* 4th ed. Text rev. Washington, DC: American Psychiatric Association; copyright 2000, with permission.

chosocial stressors for women and for men, and behavioral models of learned helplessness. In contrast to major depressive disorder, bipolar I disorder has an equal prevalence among men and women. Manic episodes are more common in men and depressive episodes are more common in women. When mania episodes occur in women, they are more likely than men to present a mixed picture—for example, mania and depression. Women also have a higher rate of being rapid cyclers, defined as having four or more manic episodes in a 1-year period.

Age

The onset of bipolar I disorder is earlier than that for major depressive disorder. The age of onset for bipolar I disorder ranges from childhood (as early as age 5 or 6) to 50 years or even older in rare cases, with a mean age of 30. The mean age of onset for major depressive disorder is approximately 40 years, with 50 percent of all patients having an onset between the ages of 20 and 50. Major depressive disorder can also begin in childhood or in old age. Recent epidemiological data suggest that the incidence of major depressive disorder may be increasing among people younger than 20. This may be related to the increased use of alcohol and drugs of abuse in this age group.

Marital Status

Major depressive disorder occurs most often in people without close interpersonal relationships or in those who are divorced or separated. Bipolar I disorder is more common in divorced and single people than among married people, but this difference may reflect the early onset and the resulting marital discord characteristic of the disorder.

Socioeconomic and Cultural Factors

No correlation has been found between socioeconomic status and major depressive disorder. A higher-than-average incidence of bipolar I disorder is found is among the upper socioeconomic groups, but this may be because of biased diagnostic practices in which bipolar disorder is overdiagnosed. Depression is more common in rural areas than in urban areas. Bipolar I disorder is more common in people who did not graduate from college than in college graduates, a fact that may also reflect the relatively early age of onset for the disorder. The prevalence of mood disorder does not differ among races. There is a tendency, however, for examiners to underdiagnose mood disorder and overdiagnose schizophrenia in patients who have a different racial or cultural background than themselves.

ETIOLOGY

Biological Factors

Many studies have reported abnormalities in biogenic amine metabolites—such as 5-hydroxyindoleacetic acid (5-HIAA), homovanillic acid (HVA), and 3-methoxy-4-hydroxyphenylglycol (MHPG)—in blood, urine, and cerebrospinal fluid (CSF) of patients with mood disorders. The data reported are most consistent with the hypothesis that mood disorders are associated with heterogeneous dysregulations of the biogenic amines.

Biogenic Amines.   Of the biogenic amines, norepinephrine and serotonin are the two neurotransmitters most implicated in the pathophysiology of mood disorders.

NOREPINEPHRINE. The correlation suggested by basic science studies between the downregulation of β-adrenergic receptors and clinical antidepressant responses is probably the single most compelling piece of data indicating a direct role for the noradrenergic system in depression. Other evidence has also implicated the presynaptic $β_2$-adrenergic receptors in depression, as activation of these receptors results in a decrease in the amount of norepinephrine released. Presynaptic $β_2$-adrenergic receptors are also located on serotonergic neurons and regulate the amount of serotonin released. Clinically effective antidepressant drugs with noradrenergic effects—for example, sertraline (Effexor)—are further support of a role for norepinephrine in the pathophysiology of at least some of the symptoms of depression.

SEROTONIN. With the huge effect that the selective serotonin reuptake inhibitors (SSRIs)—for example, fluoxetine (Prozac)—have made on the treatment of depression, serotonin has become the biogenic amine neurotransmitter most commonly associated with depression. The identification of multiple serotonin receptor subtypes has also increased the excitement within the research community about the development of even more specific treatments for depression. Besides the fact that SSRIs and other serotonergic antidepressants are effective in the treatment of depression, other data indicate that serotonin is involved in the pathophysiology of depression. Depletion of serotonin may precipitate depression, and some patients with suicidal impulses have low cerebrospinal fluid concentrations of serotonin metabolites and low concentrations of serotonin uptake sites on platelets.

DOPAMINE. Although norepinephrine and serotonin are the biogenic amines most often associated with the pathophysiology of depression, dopamine has also been theorized to play a role. The data suggest that dopamine activity may be reduced in depression and increased in mania. The discovery of new subtypes of the dopamine receptors and increasing understanding of the presynaptic and postsynaptic regulation of dopamine function have further enriched the research into the relation between dopamine and mood disorders. Drugs that reduce dopamine concentrations—for example, reserpine (Serpasil)—and diseases that reduce dopamine concentrations (such as Parkinson's disease) are associated with depressive symptoms. In contrast, drugs that increase dopamine concentrations, such as tyrosine, amphetamine, and bupropion (Wellbutrin), reduce the symptoms of depression. Two recent theories about dopamine and depression are that the mesolimbic dopamine pathway may be dysfunctional in depression and that the dopamine D_1 receptor may be hypoactive in depression.

Other Neurochemical Factors. Although the data are not yet conclusive, amino acid neurotransmitters (particularly γ-aminobutyric acid) and neuroactive peptides (particularly vasopressin and the endogenous opiates) have been implicated in the pathophysiology of mood disorders. Some investigators have suggested that second-messenger systems—such as adenylate cyclase, phosphatidylinositol, and calcium regulation—may also be of causal relevance. The amino acids glutamate and glycine appear to be the major excitatory neurotransmitters in the central nervous system. Glutamate and glycine bind to sites associated with the *N*-methyl-D-aspartate (NMDA) receptor and, in excess, can have neurotoxic effects. The hippocampus has a high concentration of NMDA receptors; it is thus possible that glutamate in conjunction with hypercortisolemia mediates the neurocognitive effects of chronic stress. There is emerging evidence that drugs that antagonize NMDA receptors have antidepressants effects.

Neuroendocrine Regulation. The hypothalamus is central to the regulation of the neuroendocrine axes and itself receives many neuronal inputs that use biogenic amine neurotransmitters. Various neuroendocrine dysregulations have been reported in patients with mood disorders, and thus the abnormal regulation of neuroendocrine axes may be a result of abnormal functioning of biogenic amine-containing neurons. Although it is theoretically possible for a particular dysregulation of a neuroendocrine axis (such as the thyroid or adrenal axis) to be involved in the cause of a mood disorder, the dysregulations are more likely reflections of a fundamental underlying brain disorder. The major neuroendocrine axes of interest in mood disorders are the adrenal, thyroid, and growth hormone axes. Other neuroendocrine abnormalities that have been described in patients with mood disorders include decreased nocturnal secretion of melatonin, decreased prolactin release to tryptophan administration, decreased basal levels of follicle-stimulating hormone (FSH) and luteinizing hormone (LH), and decreased testosterone levels in men.

ADRENAL AXIS
Role of Cortisol. A correlation between the hypersecretion of cortisol and depression is one of the oldest observations in biological psychiatry. Basic and clinical research of this relation has produced an understanding of how cortisol release is regulated in people with and without depression. Approximately 50 percent of depressed patients have elevated cortical levels. Neurons in the paraventricular nucleus release corticotropin-releasing hormone (CRH), which stimulates the release of adrenocorticotropic hormone (ACTH) from the anterior pituitary. ACTH is coreleased with β-endorphin and β-lipotropin, two peptides synthesized from the same precursor protein from which ACTH is synthesized. ACTH, in turn, stimulates the release of cortisol from the adrenal cortex. The cortisol feedback on the loop works through at least two mechanisms. A fast feedback mechanism, sensitive to the rate of cortisol concentration increase, operates through cortisol receptors on the hippocampus and results in a decreased release of ACTH. A slow feedback mechanism sensitive to the steady-state cortisol concentration is thought to operate through pituitary and adrenal receptors.

Dexamethasone-Suppression Test. Dexamethasone (Decadron) is a synthetic analogue of cortisol. Many researchers have noted that a significant proportion, perhaps 50 percent, of depressed patients do not have the normal cortisol suppression response to a single dose of dexamethasone. Although the dexamethasone-suppression test (DST) was initially thought to be of diagnostic usefulness, many patients with other psychiatric disorders also show a positive result (nonsuppression of cortisol); thus, the test is not entirely valid for indicating mood disorders. New data indicate that the DST may, however, correlate with the likelihood of a relapse: Depressed patients whose DSTs do not normalize with clinical responses to treatment are more likely to relapse than are those whose DSTs do normalize.

THYROID AXIS. In approximately 5 to 10 percent of persons with depression, thyroid disorders are often found. One direct clinical implication of the association is the critical importance of testing all affectively ill patients to determine their thyroid status. Approximately one-third of all patients with major depressive disorder who have an otherwise normal thyroid axis have been found to have a blunted release of thyrotropin, the thyroid-stimulating hormone (TSH), to an infusion of the thyrotropin-releasing hormone (TRH) protirelin. This same abnormality has been reported in a wide range of other psychiatric diagnoses, however, so the diagnostic usefulness of the test is limited. Moreover, attempts to subtype depressed patients on the basis of their TRH test results have been contradictory.

GROWTH HORMONE.   Several studies have shown a statistical difference between depressed patients and others in the regulation of growth hormone release. Depressed patients have a blunted sleep-induced stimulation of growth hormone release. Inasmuch as sleep abnormalities are common symptoms of depression, a neuroendocrine marker related to sleep is an avenue for research. Studies have also found that depressed patients have a blunted response to clonidine (Catapres)-induced increases in growth hormone secretion.

Somatostatin.   In addition to inhibition of growth hormone and release of CRH, somatostatin inhibits γ-aminobutyric acid, ACTH, and TSH. Somatostatin levels are lower in the cerebrospinal fluid of people with depression as compared to those with schizophrenia or normals, and increased levels have been observed in mania.

Prolactin.   Prolactin release from the pituitary is stimulated by serotonin and inhibited by dopamine. Most studies have not found significant abnormalities of basal or circadian prolactin secretion in depression.

Sleep Abnormalities.

Problems with sleeping—initial and terminal insomnia, multiple awakenings, hypersomnia—are common and classic symptoms of depression, and perceived decreased need for sleep is a classic symptom of mania. Researchers have long recognized that the sleep electroencephalograms (EEGs) of many depressed people show abnormalities. Common abnormalities are delayed sleep onset, shortened rapid eye movement (REM) latency (the time between falling asleep and the first REM period), an increased length of the first REM period, and abnormal delta sleep. Some investigators have attempted to use the sleep EEG in the diagnostic assessment of patients with mood disorders.

Circadian Rhythms.

The abnormalities of sleep architecture in depression and the transient clinical improvement associated with sleep deprivation have led to theories that depression reflects an abnormal regulation of circadian rhythms. Some experimental studies with animals indicate that many of the standard antidepressant treatments are effective in changing the setting of internal biological clocks (endogenous *zeitgebers*).

Kindling.

Kindling is the electrophysiological process in which repeated subthreshold stimulation of a neuron eventually generates an action potential. At the organ level, repeated subthreshold stimulation of an area of the brain results in a seizure. The clinical observation that anticonvulsants—for example, carbamazepine (Tegretol) and valproic acid (Depakene)—are useful in the treatment of mood disorders, particularly bipolar I disorder, has given rise to the theory that the pathophysiology of mood disorders may involve kindling in the temporal lobes. Although kindling has been found in laboratory animals, it never has been convincingly demonstrated in humans, and the salutary effects of anticonvulsants in bipolar disorder may also be due to electrochemical alterations unrelated to epilepsy.

Neuroimmune Regulation.

Researchers have reported immunological abnormalities in depressed people and in those grieving the loss of a relative, spouse, or close friend. The dysregulation of the cortisol axis may affect the immune status; there may be abnormal hypothalamic regulation of the immune system. A less likely possibility is that, in some patients, a primary pathophysiological process involving the immune system leads to the psychiatric symptoms of mood disorders.

Brain Imaging.

Structural brain imaging studies with computed tomography (CT) and magnetic resonance imaging (MRI) have produced interesting data. Although the studies have not reported consistent findings, the data indicate the following: A significant set of bipolar I disorder patients, predominantly men, have enlarged cerebral ventricles; ventricular enlargement is less common in patients with major depressive disorder than in those with bipolar I disorder, except that patients with major depressive disorder with psychotic features do tend to have enlarged cerebral ventricles. MRI studies have also indicated that patients with major depressive disorder have smaller caudate nuclei and smaller frontal lobes than do control subjects, and the depressed patients also have abnormal hippocampal T1 relaxation times compared with control subjects. At least one MRI study reported that patients with bipolar I disorder have a significantly increased number of deep white matter lesions when compared with control subjects.

Many reports in the literature concern cerebral blood flow in mood disorders, usually measured by using single photon emission computed tomography (SPECT) or positron emission tomography (PET). A slight majority of the studies have shown decreased blood flow affecting the cerebral cortex in general and the frontal cortical areas in particular. In contrast, investigators in one study found increases in cerebral blood flow in patients with major depressive disorder. They found state-dependent increases in the cortex, the basal ganglia, and the medial thalamus, with the suggestion of a trait-dependent increase in the amygdala. Further studies are needed.

Another brain imaging technique that is being applied to a broad range of mental disorders is magnetic resonance spectroscopy (MRS). MRS studies of patients with bipolar I disorder have produced data consistent with the hypothesis that the pathophysiology of the disorder may involve an abnormal regulation of membrane phospholipid metabolism. ^{7}Li MRS is also used to study brain and plasma concentrations of lithium in patients with bipolar I disorder.

Neuroanatomical Considerations.

Both the symptoms of mood disorders and biological research findings support the hypothesis that mood disorders involve pathology of the limbic system, the basal ganglia, and the hypothalamus. People with neurological disorders of the basal ganglia and the limbic system (especially excitatory lesions of the nondominant hemisphere) are likely to show depressive symptoms. The limbic system and the basal ganglia are intimately connected, and the limbic system may well play a major role in the production of emotions. Depressed patients' alterations in sleep, appetite, and sexual behavior and biological changes in endocrine, immunological, and chronobiological measures suggest dysfunction of the hypothalamus. Depressed patients' stooped posture, motor slowness, and minor cognitive impairment are similar to the signs of disorders of the basal ganglia, such as Parkinson's disease and other subcortical dementias.

Genetic Factors

Genetic data strongly indicate that a significant genetic factor is involved in the development of a mood disorder, but the pattern of genetic inheritance occurs by means of complex mechanisms. Not only is it impossible to exclude psychosocial effects, but nongenetic factors probably have causative roles in the development of mood disorders in at least some people. A genetic component plays a more significant role in transmitting bipolar I disorder than in major depressive disorder.

Family Studies.   Family studies have repeatedly found that first-degree relatives of bipolar I disorder probands (the first ill subject identified in a family) are 8 to 18 times more likely than are the first-degree relatives of control subjects to have bipolar I disorder and two to ten times more likely to have major depressive disorder. Family studies have also found that the first-degree relatives of major depressive disorder probands are 1.5 to 2.5 times more likely to have bipolar I disorder than are the first-degree relatives of normal control subjects and two to three times more likely to have major depressive disorder. The likelihood of having a mood disorder decreases as the degree of relationship widens. For example, a second-degree relative, such as a cousin, is less likely to be affected than is a first-degree relative, like a brother. The inheritability of bipolar I disorder is also apparent in the fact that approximately 50 percent of all bipolar I disorder patients have at least one parent with a mood disorder, most often major depressive disorder. If one parent has bipolar I disorder, there is a 25 percent chance that any child has a mood disorder; if both parents have bipolar I disorder, there is a 50 to 75 percent chance that their child has a mood disorder.

Adoption Studies.   Two of three adoption studies have found a strong genetic component for the inheritance of major depressive disorder; the only adoption study for bipolar I disorder also indicated a genetic basis. These adoption studies have shown that the biological children of affected parents remain at increased risk of a mood disorder, even if they are reared in nonaffected adoptive families. Such studies have also shown that the biological parents of adopted mood-disordered children have a prevalence of mood disorder similar to that of the parents of nonadopted mood-disordered children. The prevalence of mood disorders in the adoptive parents is similar to the baseline prevalence in the general population.

Twin Studies.   Twin studies have shown that the concordance rate for bipolar I disorder in monozygotic twins is 33 to 90 percent, depending on the particular study; for major depressive disorder, the concordance rate in monozygotic twins is approximately 50 percent. By contrast, the concordance rates in dizygotic twins are approximately 5 to 25 percent for bipolar I disorder and 10 to 25 percent for major depressive disorder.

Linkage Studies.   The availability of modern techniques of molecular biology, including restriction fragment length polymorphisms, has led to many studies, most of which are inconclusive. Associations between the mood disorders, particularly bipolar I disorder, and genetic markers have been reported for chromosomes 5, 11, 18, and X. The D_2 receptor gene is located on chromosome 5. The gene for tyrosine hydroxylase, the rate-limiting enzyme for catecholamine synthesis, is located on chromosome 11. In one study, markers on chromosome 18 have been found in 28 nuclear families with bipolar disorder.

CHROMOSOME ELEVEN AND BIPOLAR I DISORDER.   In 1987, a study reported an association between bipolar I disorder among members of an Old Order Amish family and genetic markers on the short arm of chromosome 11. With subsequent extension of the pedigree and the development of bipolar I disorder in previously unaffected family members, the statistical association ceased to apply. That turn of events effectively illustrated the degree of caution that must be used in carrying out and interpreting genetic linkage studies in mental disorders.

X CHROMOSOME AND BIPOLAR I DISORDER.   Linkage has long been suggested between bipolar I disorder and a region on the X chromosome that contains genes for color blindness and glucose-6-phosphate dehydrogenase deficiency. As with most linkage studies in psychiatry, the application of molecular genetic techniques has produced contradictory results; some studies find a linkage and others do not. The most conservative interpretation is the possibility that an X-linked gene is a factor in the development of bipolar I disorder in some patients and families.

Psychosocial Factors

Life Events and Environmental Stress.   There is a long-standing clinical observation that stressful life events more often precede first rather than subsequent episodes of mood disorders. This association has been reported for both patients with major depressive disorder and bipolar I disorder. One theory proposed to explain this observation is that the stress accompanying the first episode results in long-lasting changes in the brain's biology. These long-lasting changes may produce changes in the functional states of various neurotransmitter and intraneuronal signaling systems, changes that may even include the loss of neurons and an excessive reduction in synaptic contacts. As a result, a person has a high risk of undergoing subsequent episodes of a mood disorder, even without an external stressor.

Some clinicians believe that life events play the primary or principal role in depression; others suggest that life events have only a limited role in the onset and timing of depression. The most compelling data indicate that the life event most often associated with a person's later developing of depression is losing a parent before age 11. The environmental stressor most often associated with the onset of an episode of depression is the loss of a spouse. Another risk factor is unemployment—persons out of work are three times more likely to report symptoms of an episode of major depression than those who are employed.

Personality Factors.   No single personality trait or type uniquely predisposes a person to depression; all humans, of whatever personality pattern, can and do become depressed under appropriate circumstances. People with certain personality disorders—obsessive-compulsive, historic, and borderline—may be at greater risk for depression than are people with antisocial or paranoid personality disorders. The latter can use projection and other externalizing defense mechanisms to protect themselves from their inner rage. No evidence indicates that any particular personality disorder is associated with a later development of bipolar I disorder; however, patients with dysthymic disorder and cyclothymic disorder are at risk of later developing major depression or bipolar I disorder.

Psychodynamic Factors in Depression.   The psychodynamic understanding of depression defined by Sigmund Freud and expanded by Karl Abraham is known as the *classic view of depression*. That theory involves four key points: (1) Disturbances in the infant–mother relationship during the oral phase (the first 10 to 18 months of life) predispose to subsequent vulnerability to depression; (2) depression can be linked to real or imagined object loss; (3) introjection of the departed objects is a defense mechanism invoked to deal with the distress connected with the object's loss; and (4) because the lost object is regarded with a mixture of love and hate, feelings of anger are directed inward at the self.

Melanie Klein understood depression as involving the expression of aggression toward loved ones, much as Freud did. Edward Bibring regarded depression as a phenomenon that sets in when a person becomes aware of the discrepancy between extraordinarily high ideals and the inability to meet those goals. Edith Jacobson saw the state of depression as similar to a powerless, helpless child victimized by a tormented parent. The self is experienced as identified with the negative aspects of the tormenting parent, while the sadistic qualities of that parent are transformed into cruel superego. Silvano Arieti observed that many depressed people have lived their lives for someone else rather than for themselves. He referred to this person for whom depressed patients live as the *dominant other*, which may be a principle, an ideal, or an institution, as well as an individual. Depression sets in when patients realize that the person or ideal for whom they have been living is never going to respond in a manner that will meet their expectations. Heinz Kohut's conceptualization of depression, derived from his self-psychological theory, rests on the assumption that the developing self has specific needs that must be met by parents to give the child a positive sense of self-esteem and self-cohesion. When others do not meet these needs, there is a massive loss of self-esteem that presents as depression. John Bowlby believed that damaged early attachments and traumatic separation in childhood predispose to depression. Adult losses are said to revive the traumatic childhood loss and so precipitate adult depressive episodes.

Psychodynamic Factors in Mania.   Most theories of mania view manic episodes as a defense against underlying depression. Karl Abraham, for example, believed that manic episodes may reflect an inability to tolerate a developmental tragedy, such as the loss of a parent. The manic state may also result from a tyrannical superego, which produces intolerable self-criticism that is then replaced by euphoric self-satisfaction. Bertram Lewin regarded the manic patient's ego as overwhelmed by pleasurable impulses such as sex or by feared impulses such as aggression. Klein also viewed mania as a defensive reaction to depression using manic defenses such as omnipotence, in which the person develops delusions of grandeur.

Other Formulations of Depression

Cognitive Theory.
According to cognitive theory, depression results from specific cognitive distortions present in persons prone to depression. Those distortions, referred to as *depressogenic schemata*, are cognitive templates that perceive both internal and external data in ways that are altered by early experiences. Beck postulated a cognitive triad of depression that consists of (1) views about the self—a negative self-precept, (2) about the environment—a tendency to experience the world as hostile and demanding, and (3) about the future—the expectation of suffering and failure. Therapy consists of modifying these distortions.

Table 12.1–2
DSM-IV-TR Criteria for Major Depressive Episode

A. Five (or more) of the following symptoms have been present during the same 2-week period and represent a change from previous functioning; at least one of the symptoms is either (1) depressed mood or (2) loss of interest or pleasure.
Note: Do not include symptoms that are clearly due to a general medical condition, or mood-incongruent delusions or hallucinations.

(1) depressed mood most of the day, nearly every day, as indicated by either subjective report (e.g., feels sad or empty) or observation made by others (e.g., appears tearful). **Note:** In children and adolescents, can be irritable mood

(2) markedly diminished interest or pleasure in all, or almost all, activities most of the day, nearly every day (as indicated by either subjective account or observation made by others)

(3) significant weight loss when not dieting or weight gain (e.g., a change of more than 5% of body weight in a month), or decrease or increase in appetite nearly every day. **Note:** In children, consider failure to make expected weight gains.

(4) insomnia or hypersomnia nearly every day

(5) psychomotor agitation or retardation nearly every day (observable by others, not merely subjective feelings of restlessness or being slowed down)

(6) fatigue or loss of energy nearly every day

(7) feelings of worthlessness or excessive or inappropriate guilt (which may be delusional) nearly every day (not merely self-reproach or guilt about being sick)

(8) diminished ability to think or concentrate, or indecisiveness, nearly every day (either by subjective account or as observed by others)

(9) recurrent thoughts of death (not just fear of dying), recurrent suicidal ideation without a specific plan, or a suicide attempt or a specific plan for committing suicide

B. The symptoms do not meet criteria for a mixed episode.

C. The symptoms cause clinically significant distress or impairment in social, occupational, or other important areas of functioning.

D. The symptoms are not due to the direct physiological effects of a substance (e.g., a drug of abuse, a medication) or a general medical condition (e.g., hypothyroidism).

E. The symptoms are not better accounted for by bereavement, i.e., after the loss of a loved one, the symptoms persist for longer than 2 months or are characterized by marked functional impairment, morbid preoccupation with worthlessness, suicidal ideation, psychotic symptoms, or psychomotor retardation.

From American Psychiatric Association. *Diagnostic and Statistical Manual of Mental Disorders.* 4th ed. Text rev. Washington, DC: American Psychiatric Association; copyright 2000, with permission.

Learned Helplessness.   The learned helplessness theory of depression connects depressive phenomena to the experience of uncontrollable events. For example, when dogs in a laboratory were exposed to electrical shocks from which they could not escape, they showed behaviors that differentiated them from dogs who had not been exposed to such uncontrollable events. After exposure to the shocks, they would not cross a barrier to stop the flow of electric shock when put in a new learning situation. According to the learned helplessness theory, the dogs learned that outcomes were independent of responses, so they had both cognitive motivational deficit (i.e., they would not attempt to escape the shock) and emotional deficit (indicating a decreased reactivity to

Table 12.1–3
DSM-IV-TR Criteria for Manic Episode

A. A distinct period of abnormally and persistently elevated, expansive, or irritable mood, lasting at least 1 week (or any duration if hospitalization is necessary).

B. During the period of mood disturbance, three (or more) of the following symptoms have persisted (four if the mood is only irritable) and have been present to a significant degree:

(1) inflated self-esteem or grandiosity

(2) decreased need for sleep (e.g., feels rested after only 3 hours of sleep)

(3) more talkative than usual or pressure to keep talking

(4) flight of ideas or subjective experience that thoughts are racing

(5) distractibility (i.e., attention too easily drawn to unimportant or irrelevant external stimuli)

(6) increase in goal-directed activity (either socially, at work or school, or sexually) or psychomotor agitation

(7) excessive involvement in pleasurable activities that have a high potential for painful consequences (e.g., engaging in unrestrained buying sprees, sexual indiscretions, or foolish business investments)

C. The symptoms do not meet criteria for a mixed episode.

D. The mood disturbance is sufficiently severe to cause marked impairment in occupational functioning or in usual social activities or relationships with others, or to necessitate hospitalization to prevent harm to self or others, or there are psychotic features.

E. The symptoms are not due to the direct physiological effects of a substance (e.g., a drug of abuse, a medication, or other treatment) or a general medical condition (e.g., hyperthyroidism).

Note: Manic-like episodes that are clearly caused by somatic antidepressant treatment (e.g., medication, electroconvulsive therapy, light therapy) should not count toward a diagnosis of bipolar I disorder.

From American Psychiatric Association. *Diagnostic and Statistical Manual of Mental Disorders.* 4th ed. Text rev. Washington, DC: American Psychiatric Association; copyright 2000, with permission.

Table 12.1–4
DSM-IV-TR Criteria for Hypomanic Episode

A. A distinct period of persistently elevated, expansive, or irritable mood, lasting throughout at least 4 days, that is clearly different from the usual nondepressed mood.

B. During the period of mood disturbance, three (or more) of the following symptoms have persisted (four if the mood is only irritable) and have been present to a significant degree:

(1) inflated self-esteem or grandiosity

(2) decreased need for sleep (e.g., feels rested after only 3 hours of sleep)

(3) more talkative than usual or pressure to keep talking

(4) flight of ideas or subjective experience that thoughts are racing

(5) distractibility (i.e., attention too easily drawn to unimportant or irrelevant external stimuli)

(6) increase in goal-directed activity (either socially, at work or school, or sexually) or psychomotor agitation

(7) excessive involvement in pleasurable activities that have a high potential for painful consequences (e.g., the person engages in unrestrained buying sprees, sexual indiscretions, or foolish business investments)

C. The episode is associated with an unequivocal change in functioning that is uncharacteristic of the person when not symptomatic.

D. The disturbance in mood and the change in functioning are observable by others.

E. The episode is not severe enough to cause marked impairment in social or occupational functioning, or to necessitate hospitalization, and there are no psychotic features.

F. The symptoms are not due to the direct physiological effects of a substance (e.g., a drug of abuse, a medication, or other treatment) or a general medical condition (e.g., hyperthyroidism).

Note: Hypomanic-like episodes that are clearly caused by somatic antidepressant treatment (e.g., medication, electroconvulsive therapy, light therapy) should not count toward a diagnosis of bipolar II disorder.

From American Psychiatric Association. *Diagnostic and Statistical Manual of Mental Disorders.* 4th ed. Text rev. Washington, DC: American Psychiatric Association; copyright 2000, with permission.

the shock). In the reformulated view of learned helplessness as applied to human depression, internal causal explanations are thought to produce a loss of self-esteem after adverse external events. Behaviorists who subscribe to the theory stress that improvement of depression is contingent on the patient's learning a sense of control and mastery of the environment.

DIAGNOSIS

In addition to the diagnostic criteria for major depressive disorder and bipolar disorders, DSM-IV-TR includes specific criteria for mood episodes (Tables 12.1–2 through 12.1–5) and criteria such as severity (Tables 12.1–6 through 12.1–8) to qualify the most recent episode.

Major Depressive Disorder

DSM-IV-TR lists the criteria for a major depressive episode separately from the diagnostic criteria for depression-related diagnoses (Table 12.1–2) and also lists severity descriptors for a major depressive episode (Table 12.1–6).

Major Depressive Disorder, Single Episode.   DSM-IV-TR specifies the diagnostic criteria for the first episode of major depressive disorder (Table 12.1–9). The differentiation between these patients and those who have two or more episodes of major depressive disorder is justified because of the uncertain course of the former patients' disorder. Several studies have reported data consistent with the notion that major depression covers a heterogeneous population of disorders. One type of study assessed the stability of a diagnosis of major depression in a patient over time. The studies found that 25 to 50 percent of the patients were later reclassified as having a different psychiatric condition or a nonpsychiatric medical condition with psychiatric symptoms. A second type of study evaluated first-degree relatives of affectively ill patients to determine the presence and types of psychiatric diagnoses present in these relatives over time. Both types of studies found that depressed patients with more depressive symptoms are more likely to have stable diagnoses over time and are more likely to have affectively ill relatives than are depressed patients with fewer depressive

Table 12.1–5
DSM-IV-TR Criteria for Mixed Episode

A. The criteria are met both for a manic episode and for a major depressive episode (except for duration) nearly every day during at least a 1-week period.

B. The mood disturbance is sufficiently severe to cause marked impairment in occupational functioning or in usual social activities or relationships with others, or to necessitate hospitalization to prevent harm to self or others, or there are psychotic features.

C. The symptoms are not due to the direct physiological effects of a substance (e.g., a drug of abuse, a medication, or other treatment) or a general medical condition (e.g., hyperthyroidism).

Note: Mixed-like episodes that are clearly caused by somatic antidepressant treatment (e.g., medication, electroconvulsive therapy, light therapy) should not count toward a diagnosis of bipolar I disorder.

From American Psychiatric Association. *Diagnostic and Statistical Manual of Mental Disorders.* 4th ed. Text rev. Washington, DC: American Psychiatric Association; copyright 2000, with permission.

Table 12.1–6
DSM-IV-TR Criteria for Severity/Psychotic/Remission Specifiers for Current (or Most Recent) Major Depressive Episode

Note: Code in fifth digit. Mild, moderate, severe without psychotic features, and severe with psychotic features can be applied only if the criteria are currently met for a major depressive episode. In partial remission and in full remission can be applied to the most recent major depressive episode in major depressive disorder and to a major depressive episode in bipolar I or II disorder only if it is the most recent type of mood episode.

Mild: Few, if any, symptoms in excess of those required to make the diagnosis and symptoms result in only minor impairment in occupational functioning or in usual social activities or relationships with others.

Moderate: Symptoms or functional impairment between "mild" and "severe."

Severe without psychotic features: Several symptoms in excess of those required to make the diagnosis, **and** symptoms markedly interfere with occupational functioning or with usual social activities or relationships with others.

Severe with psychotic features: Delusions or hallucinations. If possible, specify whether the psychotic features are mood-congruent or mood-incongruent:

    Mood-congruent psychotic features: Delusions or hallucinations whose content is entirely consistent with the typical depressive themes of personal inadequacy, guilt, disease, death, nihilism, or deserved punishment.

    Mood-incongruent psychotic features: Delusions or hallucinations whose content does not involve typical depressive themes of personal inadequacy, guilt, disease, death, nihilism, or deserved punishment. Included are such symptoms as persecutory delusions (not directly related to depressive themes), thought insertion, thought broadcasting, and delusions of control.

In partial remission: Symptoms of a major depressive episode are present but full criteria are not met, or there is a period without any significant symptoms of a major depressive episode lasting less than 2 months following the end of the major depressive episode. (If the major depressive episode was superimposed on dysthymic disorder, the diagnosis of dysthymic disorder alone is given once the full criteria for a major depressive episode are no longer met.)

In full remission: During the past 2 months, no significant signs or symptoms of the disturbance were present.

Unspecified.

From American Psychiatric Association. *Diagnostic and Statistical Manual of Mental Disorders.* 4th ed. Text rev. Washington, DC: American Psychiatric Association; copyright 2000, with permission.

Table 12.1–7
DSM-IV-TR Criteria for Severity/Psychotic/Remission Specifiers for Current (or Most Recent) Manic Episode

Note: Code in fifth digit. Mild, moderate, severe without psychotic features, and severe with psychotic features can be applied only if the criteria are currently met for a manic episode. In partial remission and in full remission can be applied to a manic episode in bipolar I disorder only if it is the most recent type of mood episode.

Mild: Minimum symptom criteria are met for a manic episode.

Moderate: Extreme increase in activity or impairment in judgment.

Severe without psychotic features: Almost continual supervision required to prevent physical harm to self or others.

Severe with psychotic features: Delusions or hallucinations. If possible, specify whether the psychotic features are mood-congruent or mood-incongruent:

    Mood-congruent psychotic features: Delusions or hallucinations whose content is entirely consistent with the typical manic themes of inflated worth, power, knowledge, identity, or special relationship to a deity or famous person.

    Mood-incongruent psychotic features: Delusions or hallucinations whose content does not involve typical manic themes of inflated worth, power, knowledge, identity, or special relationship to a deity or famous person. Included are such symptoms as persecutory delusions (not directly related to grandiose ideas or themes), thought insertion, and delusions of being controlled.

In partial remission: Symptoms of a manic episode are present but full criteria are not met, or there is a period without any significant symptoms of a manic episode lasting less than 2 months following the end of the manic episode.

In full remission: During the past 2 months, no significant signs or symptoms of the disturbance were present.

Unspecified.

From American Psychiatric Association. *Diagnostic and Statistical Manual of Mental Disorders.* 4th ed. Text rev. Washington, DC: American Psychiatric Association; copyright 2000, with permission.

symptoms. Also, patients with bipolar I disorder and bipolar II disorder (recurrent major depressive episodes with hypomania) are likely to have stable diagnoses over time.

Major Depressive Disorder, Recurrent. Patients who are experiencing at least a second episode of depression are classified in DSM-IV-TR as having major depressive disorder, recurrent (Table 12.1–10). The major problem with diagnosing recurrent episodes of major depressive disorder is choosing the criteria to designate the resolution of each period. Two variables are the degree of resolution of the symptoms and the length of the resolution. DSM-IV-TR requires that distinct episodes of depression be separated by at least 2 months, during which time a patient has no significant symptoms of depression.

Bipolar I Disorder

DSM-IV-TR contains a separate list of criteria for a manic episode (Table 12.1–3). DSM-IV-TR requires the presence of a distinct period of abnormal mood lasting at least 1 week and includes separate bipolar I disorder diagnoses for a single manic episode and a specific type of recurrent episode, based on the symptoms of the most recent episode.

Table 12.1–8
DSM-IV-TR Criteria for Severity/Psychotic/Remission Specifiers for Current (or Most Recent) Mixed Episode

Note: Code in fifth digit. Mild, moderate, severe without psychotic features, and severe with psychotic features can be applied only if the criteria are currently met for a mixed episode. In partial remission and in full remission can be applied to a mixed episode in bipolar I disorder only if it is the most recent type of mood episode.

Mild: No more than minimum symptom criteria are met for both a manic episode and a major depressive episode.

Moderate: Symptoms or functional impairment between "mild" and "severe."

Severe without psychotic features: Almost continual supervision required to prevent physical harm to self or others.

Severe with psychotic features: Delusions or hallucinations. If possible, specify whether the psychotic features are mood-congruent or mood-incongruent:

Mood-congruent psychotic features: Delusions or hallucinations whose content is entirely consistent with the typical manic or depressive themes.

Mood-incongruent psychotic features: Delusions or hallucinations whose content does not involve typical manic or depressive themes. Included are such symptoms as persecutory delusions (not directly related to grandiose or depressive themes), thought insertion, and delusions of being controlled.

In partial remission: Symptoms of a mixed episode are present but full criteria are not met, or there is a period without any significant symptoms of a mixed episode lasting less than 2 months following the end of the mixed episode.

In full remission: During the past 2 months, no significant signs or symptoms of the disturbance were present.

Unspecified.

From American Psychiatric Association. *Diagnostic and Statistical Manual of Mental Disorders.* 4th ed. Text rev. Washington, DC: American Psychiatric Association; copyright 2000, with permission.

Table 12.1–9
DSM-IV-TR Diagnostic Criteria for Major Depressive Disorder, Single Episode

A. Presence of a single major depressive episode.

B. The major depressive episode is not better accounted for by schizoaffective disorder and is not superimposed on schizophrenia, schizophreniform disorder, delusional disorder, or psychotic disorder not otherwise specified.

C. There has never been a manic episode, a mixed episode, or a hypomanic episode. **Note:** This exclusion does not apply if all of the manic-like, mixed-like, or hypomanic-like episodes are substance or treatment induced or are due to the direct physiological effects of a general medical condition.

If the full criteria are currently met for a major depressive episode, *specify* its current clinical status and/or features:

Mild, moderate, severe without psychotic features/severe with psychotic features

Chronic

With catatonic features

With melancholic features

With atypical features

With postpartum onset

If the full criteria are not currently met for a major depressive episode, *specify* the current clinical status of the major depressive disorder or features of the most recent episode:

In partial remission, in full remission

Chronic

With catatonic features

With melancholic features

With atypical features

With postpartum onset

From American Psychiatric Association. *Diagnostic and Statistical Manual of Mental Disorders.* 4th ed. Text rev. Washington, DC: American Psychiatric Association; copyright 2000, with permission.

The designation bipolar I disorder is synonymous with what was known as bipolar disorder—a syndrome in which a complete set of mania symptoms occurs during the course of the disorder. DSM-IV-TR has formalized the diagnostic criteria for bipolar II disorder; it is characterized by depressive episodes and hypomanic episodes (Table 12.1–4) during the course of the disorder, but the episodes of manic-like symptoms do not quite meet the diagnostic criteria for a full manic syndrome.

DSM-IV-TR specifically states that manic episodes clearly precipitated by antidepressant treatment (for example, pharmacotherapy, electroconvulsive therapy [ECT]) are not indicative of bipolar I disorder.

Bipolar I Disorder, Single Manic Episode. According to DSM-IV-TR, patients must be experiencing their first manic episode to meet the diagnostic criteria for bipolar I disorder, single manic episode (Table 12.1–11). This requirement rests on the fact that patients who are having their first episode of bipolar I disorder depression cannot be distinguished from patients with major depressive disorder.

Bipolar I Disorder, Recurrent. The issues about defining the end of an episode of depression also apply to defining the end of an episode of mania. In DSM-IV-TR, episodes are considered distinct when they are separated by at least 2

months without significant symptoms of mania or hypomania. DSM-IV-TR specifies diagnostic criteria for recurrent bipolar I disorder based on the symptoms of the most recent episode: bipolar I disorder, most recent episode manic (Table 12.1–12); bipolar I disorder, most recent episode hypomanic (Table 12.1–13); bipolar I disorder, most recent episode depressed (Table 12.1–14); bipolar I disorder, most recent episode mixed (Table 12.1–15); bipolar I disorder, most recent episode unspecified (Table 12.1–16).

Bipolar II Disorder

The diagnostic criteria for bipolar II disorder specify a particular severity, frequency, and duration of the hypomanic symptoms. The diagnostic criteria for a hypomanic episode (Table 12.1–4) are listed separately from the criteria for bipolar II disorder (Table 12.1–17). The criteria have been established to decrease the overdiagnosis of hypomanic episodes and the incorrect classification of patients with major depressive disorder as patients with bipolar II disorder. Clinically, psychiatrists may find it difficult to distinguish euthymia from hypomania in a patient who has been chronically depressed for many months or years. As with bipolar I disorder, antidepressant-induced hypomanic episodes are not diagnostic of bipolar II disorder.

Table 12.1–10
DSM-IV-TR Diagnostic Criteria for Major Depressive Disorder, Recurrent

A. Presence of two or more major depressive episodes.
   Note: To be considered separate episodes, there must be an interval of at least 2 consecutive months in which criteria are not met for a major depressive episode.

B. The major depressive episodes are not better accounted for by schizoaffective disorder and are not superimposed on schizophrenia, schizophreniform disorder, delusional disorder, or psychotic disorder not otherwise specified.

C. There has never been a manic episode, a mixed episode, or a hypomanic episode. **Note:** This exclusion does not apply if all of the manic-like, mixed-like, or hypomanic-like episodes are substance or treatment induced or are due to the direct physiological effects of a general medical condition.

If the full criteria are currently met for a major depressive episode, *specify* its current clinical status and/or features:

   Mild, moderate, severe without psychotic features/severe with psychotic features
   Chronic
   With catatonic features
   With melancholic features
   With atypical features
   With postpartum onset

If the full criteria are not currently met for a major depressive episode, *specify* the current clinical status of the major depressive disorder or features of the most recent episode:

   In partial remission, in full remission
   Chronic
   With catatonic features
   With melancholic features
   With atypical features
   With postpartum onset

Specify:
   Longitudinal course specifiers (with and without interepisode recovery)
   With seasonal pattern

From American Psychiatric Association. *Diagnostic and Statistical Manual of Mental Disorders*. 4th ed. Text rev. Washington, DC: American Psychiatric Association; copyright 2000, with permission.

Specifiers Describing Most Recent Episode

In addition to the severity/psychotic/remission specifiers, DSM-IV-TR defines additional symptom features that can be used to describe patients with various mood disorders. Two of the cross-sectional features (melancholic and atypical) are limited to describing depressive episodes. Two others (catatonic features and with postpartum onset) can be applied to describing depressive and manic episodes.

With Psychotic Features.

The presence of psychotic features (Table 12.1–6) in major depressive disorder reflects severe disease and is a poor prognostic indicator. Clinicians and researchers had dichotomized depressive illness along a psychotic–neurotic continuum. A review of the literature comparing psychotic with nonpsychotic major depressive disorder indicates that the two conditions may be distinct in their pathogenesis. One difference is that bipolar I disorder is more common in the families of probands with psychotic depression than in the families of probands with nonpsychotic depression.

Table 12.1–11
DSM-IV-TR Diagnostic Criteria for Bipolar I Disorder, Single Manic Episode

A. Presence of only one manic episode and no past major depressive episodes.
   Note: Recurrence is defined as either a change in polarity from depression or an interval of at least 2 months without manic symptoms.

B. The manic episode is not better accounted for by schizoaffective disorder and is not superimposed on schizophrenia, schizophreniform disorder, delusional disorder, or psychotic disorder not otherwise specified.

Specify if:
   Mixed: if symptoms meet criteria for a mixed episode

If the full criteria are currently met for a manic, mixed, or major depressive episode, *specify* its current clinical status and/or features:

   Mild, moderate, severe without psychotic features/severe with psychotic features
   With catatonic features
   With postpartum onset

If the full criteria are not currently met for a manic, mixed, or major depressive episode, *specify* the current clinical status of the bipolar I disorder or features of the most recent episode:

   In partial remission, in full remission
   With catatonic features
   With postpartum onset

From American Psychiatric Association. *Diagnostic and Statistical Manual of Mental Disorders*. 4th ed. Text rev. Washington, DC: American Psychiatric Association; copyright 2000, with permission.

Table 12.1–12
DSM-IV-TR Diagnostic Criteria for Bipolar I Disorder, Most Recent Episode Manic

A. Currently (or most recently) in a manic episode.

B. There has previously been at least one major depressive episode, manic episode, or mixed episode.

C. The mood episodes in Criteria A and B are not better accounted for by schizoaffective disorder and are not superimposed on schizophrenia, schizophreniform disorder, delusional disorder, or psychotic disorder not otherwise specified.

If the full criteria are currently met for a manic episode, *specify* its current clinical status and/or features:

   Mild, moderate, severe without psychotic features/severe with psychotic features
   With catatonic features
   With postpartum onset

If the full criteria are not currently met for a manic episode, *specify* the current clinical status of the bipolar I disorder and/or features of the most recent manic episode:

   In partial remission, in full remission
   With catatonic features
   With postpartum onset

Specify:
   Longitudinal course specifiers (with and without interepisode recovery)
   With seasonal pattern (applies only to the pattern of major depressive episodes)
   With rapid cycling

From American Psychiatric Association. *Diagnostic and Statistical Manual of Mental Disorders*. 4th ed. Text rev. Washington, DC: American Psychiatric Association; copyright 2000, with permission.

Table 12.1–19
DSM-IV-TR Criteria for Atypical Features Specifier

Specify if:

With atypical features (can be applied when these features predominate during the most recent 2 weeks of a current major depressive episode in major depressive disorder or in bipolar I or bipolar II disorder when a current major depressive episode is the most recent type of mood episode, or when these features predominate during the most recent 2 years of dysthymic disorder; if the major depressive episode is not current, it applies if the feature predominates during any 2-week period)

A. Mood reactivity (i.e., mood brightens in response to actual or potential positive events)

B. Two (or more) of the following features:
   (1) significant weight gain or increase in appetite
   (2) hypersomnia
   (3) leaden paralysis (i.e., heavy, leaden feelings in arms or legs)
   (4) long-standing pattern of interpersonal rejection sensitivity (not limited to episodes of mood disturbance) that results in significant social or occupational impairment

C. Criteria are not met for with melancholic features or with catatonic features during the same episode.

From American Psychiatric Association. *Diagnostic and Statistical Manual of Mental Disorders.* 4th ed. Text rev. Washington, DC: American Psychiatric Association; copyright 2000, with permission.

with these features are compared with those patients without the features, the patients with atypical features are found to have a younger age of onset, a more severe degree of psychomotor slowing, and more frequent coexisting diagnoses of panic disorder, substance abuse or dependence, and somatization disorder. The high incidence and severity of anxiety symptoms in patients with atypical features has been correlated in some research with the likelihood of their being misclassified as having an anxiety disorder rather than a mood disorder. Patients with atypical features may also be likely to have a long-term course, a diagnosis of bipolar I disorder, or a seasonal pattern to their disorder. The major treatment implication of patients with atypical features is that they are more likely to respond to monoamine oxidase inhibitors (MAOIs) than to tricyclic drugs.

Yet the significance of atypical features remains controversial, as does the preferential treatment response to MAOIs. Moreover, the absence of specific diagnostic criteria has limited researchers' ability to assess the criteria's validity and the disorder's prevalence and to ascertain the existence of any other biological or psychological factors that may differentiate it from other symptom patterns.

The DSM-IV-TR atypical features can be applied to the most recent major depressive episode in major depressive disorder, bipolar I disorder, bipolar II disorder, or dysthymic disorder (Table 12.1–19).

Ms. G is a 17-year-old high school senior who is referred for evaluation after she attempted suicide with an overdose of pills. Earlier on the night of the suicide attempt, she had a fight with her mother over a request to order pizza. The patient remembers her mother saying that she was a "spoiled brat" and asking whether she would be happier living elsewhere. The patient, feeling rejected and despondent,

went to her room and wrote a note saying that she was having a mental breakdown and that she loved her parents but could not communicate with them. She added a request that her favorite glass animals be given to a particular friend. The parents, who had gone out to a movie, returned home later that evening to find their daughter comatose and immediately rushed her to the hospital emergency room.

During the last couple of months, Ms. G has been crying frequently and has lost interest in her friends, school, and social activities. She has been eating more and more and has recently begun to gain weight, which her mother is very unhappy about. Ms. G says that her mother is always harping about "taking care of herself," and in fact, the argument on the night of her suicide attempt was about Ms. G's desire to order a pizza that her mother did not think she needed. Ms. G's mother reports that all her daughter seems to want to do is sleep and that she never wants to go out with her friends or help around the house. When questioned about changes in her sleep habits, Ms. G admits that she has been feeling very tired lately and that she often feels as if there is nothing to make it worth getting out of bed. She does mention that she is excited about an upcoming visit from her boyfriend, who attends a college a considerable distance away and has not been home for several months.

Upon evaluation, it is apparent that this teenager, the third of three children of upper-middle-class and very intelligent parents, is struggling with a view of herself as less bright, clever, and attractive than her two siblings. She feels ignored and essentially rejected by her seemingly omnipresent mother. The daughter is having difficulty developing a sense of separation from her mother and an image of her individual identity. She experienced her mother's directives as interference with her efforts to express autonomy and independence. (From *DSM-IV Case Studies.*)

With Catatonic Features.

The decision to include a specific classification for catatonic features (Table 12.1–20) in the mood disorders category was motivated by two factors. First, because the authors intended DSM-IV-TR to serve as a guide in the differential diagnosis of mental disorders, the inclusion of a specifically catatonic type of mood disorder helps balance the presence of a catatonic type of schizophrenia. As a symptom, catatonia can be present in several mental disorders, most commonly schizophrenia and the mood disorders. Second, although as yet incompletely studied, the presence of catatonic features in patients with mood disorders will probably be shown to have prognostic and treatment significance.

The hallmark symptoms of catatonia—stuporousness, blunted affect, extreme withdrawal, negativism, and marked psychomotor retardation—can be seen in both catatonic and noncatatonic schizophrenia, major depressive disorder (often with psychotic features), and medical and neurological disorders, but catatonic symptoms are probably most commonly associated with bipolar I disorder. Clinicians often do not associate catatonic symptoms with this disorder because of the marked contrast between the symptoms of stuporous catatonia and the classic symptoms of mania. Because catatonic symptoms are a behavioral syndrome appearing in several medical and psychiatric conditions, catatonic symptoms do not imply a single diagnosis. In DSM-IV-TR, catatonic features can be applied to the most recent manic episode or

Table 12.1–20
DSM-IV-TR Criteria for Catatonic Features Specifier

Specify if:

With catatonic features (can be applied to the current or most recent major depressive episode, manic episode, or mixed episode in major depressive disorder, bipolar I disorder, or bipolar II disorder)

The clinical picture is dominated by at least two of the following:

(1) motoric immobility as evidenced by catalepsy (including waxy flexibility) or stupor

(2) excessive motor activity (that is apparently purposeless and not influenced by external stimuli)

(3) extreme negativism (an apparently motiveless resistance to all instructions or maintenance of a rigid posture against attempts to be moved) or mutism

(4) peculiarities of voluntary movement as evidenced by posturing (voluntary assumption of inappropriate or bizarre postures), stereotyped movements, prominent mannerisms, or prominent grimacing

(5) echolalia or echopraxia

From American Psychiatric Association. *Diagnostic and Statistical Manual of Mental Disorders.* 4th ed. Text rev. Washington, DC: American Psychiatric Association; copyright 2000, with permission.

major depressive episode in major depressive disorder, bipolar I disorder, or bipolar II disorder.

Postpartum Onset.   DSM-IV-TR allows for the specification of a postpartum mood disturbance if the onset of symptoms is within 4 weeks postpartum (Table 12.1–21). Postpartum mental disorders commonly include psychotic symptoms such as hallucinations and delusions. See page 166 for a more complete discussion of these disorders.

Chronic.   DSM-IV-TR allows for the specification of *chronic* to describe major depressive episodes that occur as a part of major depressive disorder, bipolar I disorder, and bipolar II disorder (Table 12.2–22).

Describing Course of Recurrent Episodes

DSM-IV-TR includes criteria for three distinct course specifiers for mood disorders. One of the course specifiers, with rapid

Table 12.1–21
DSM-IV-TR Criteria for Postpartum Onset Specifier

Specify if:

With postpartum onset (can be applied to the current or most recent major depressive, manic, or mixed episode in major depressive disorder, bipolar I disorder, or bipolar II disorder; or to brief psychotic disorder)

Onset of episode within 4 weeks postpartum

From American Psychiatric Association. *Diagnostic and Statistical Manual of Mental Disorders.* 4th ed. Text rev. Washington, DC: American Psychiatric Association; copyright 2000, with permission.

Table 12.1–22
DSM-IV-TR Criteria for Chronic Specifier

Specify if:

Chronic (can be applied to the current or most recent major depressive episode in major depressive disorder and to a major depressive episode in bipolar I or II disorder only if it is the most recent type of mood episode)

Full criteria for a major depressive episode have been met continuously for at least the past 2 years.

From American Psychiatric Association. *Diagnostic and Statistical Manual of Mental Disorders.* 4th ed. Text rev. Washington, DC: American Psychiatric Association; copyright 2000, with permission.

cycling (Table 12.1–23), is restricted to bipolar I disorder and bipolar II disorder. Two other course specifiers, with seasonal pattern (Table 12.1–24) and with or without full interepisode recovery (Table 12.1–25), can be applied to bipolar I disorder, bipolar II disorder, and major depressive disorder, recurrent. The course specifier *with postpartum onset* can be applied to major depressive or manic episodes in bipolar I disorder, bipolar II disorder, major depressive disorder, and brief psychotic disorder.

Rapid Cycling.   Patients with rapid cycling bipolar I disorder are likely to be female and to have had depressive and hypomanic episodes. No data indicate that rapid cycling has a familial pattern of inheritance, and thus an external factor such as stress or drug treatment may be involved in the pathogenesis of rapid cycling. The DSM-IV-TR criteria specify that the patient must have at least four episodes within a 12-month period (Table 12.1–23).

Seasonal Pattern.   Patients with a seasonal pattern to their mood disorders tend to experience depressive episodes during a particular season, most commonly winter. The pattern has become known as seasonal affective disorder, although this term is not used in DSM-IV-TR (Table 12.1–24). Two types of evidence indicate that the seasonal pattern may represent a separate diagnostic entity. First, the patients are likely to respond to treatment with light therapy, although adequate studies to evaluate

Table 12.1–23
DSM-IV-TR Criteria for Rapid-Cycling Specifier

Specify if:

With rapid cycling (can be applied to bipolar I disorder or bipolar II disorder)

At least four episodes of a mood disturbance in the previous 12 months that meet criteria for a major depressive, manic, mixed, or hypomanic episode.

Note: Episodes are demarcated either by partial or full remission for at least 2 months or a switch to an episode of opposite polarity (e.g., major depressive episode to manic episode).

From American Psychiatric Association. *Diagnostic and Statistical Manual of Mental Disorders.* 4th ed. Text rev. Washington, DC: American Psychiatric Association; copyright 2000, with permission.

Table 12.1–24
DSM-IV-TR Criteria for Seasonal Pattern Specifier

Specify if:

With seasonal pattern (can be applied to the pattern of major depressive episodes in bipolar I disorder, bipolar II disorder, or major depressive disorder, recurrent)

A. There has been a regular temporal relationship between the onset of major depressive episodes in bipolar I or bipolar II disorder or major depressive disorder, recurrent, and a particular time of the year (e.g., regular appearance of the major depressive episode in the fall or winter).

Note: Do not include cases in which there is an obvious effect of seasonal-related psychosocial stressors (e.g., regularly being unemployed every winter).

B. Full remissions (or a change from depression to mania or hypomania) also occur at a characteristic time of the year (e.g., depression disappears in the spring).

C. In the last 2 years, two major depressive episodes have occurred that demonstrate the temporal seasonal relationships defined in Criteria A and B, and no nonseasonal major depressive episodes have occurred during that same period.

D. Seasonal major depressive episodes (as described above) substantially outnumber the nonseasonal major depressive episodes that may have occurred over the individual's lifetime.

light therapy in nonseasonally depressed patients have not been conducted. Second, one positron emission tomography study showed that patients show decreased metabolic activity in the orbital frontal cortex and in the left inferior parietal lobule. Future studies will probably focus on differentiating depressed people with seasonal pattern from other depressed people.

Longitudinal Course Specifiers. DSM-IV-TR includes specific descriptions of longitudinal courses for major depressive disorder, bipolar I disorder, and bipolar II disorder (Table 12.1–25). These longitudinal course specifiers allow clinicians and researchers to prospectively identify any treatment or prognostic significance in various longitudinal courses. Although preliminary studies of the DSM-IV-TR longitudinal course specifiers indicate that clinicians can assess the longitudinal course, more and larger studies are needed to develop a solid appreciation of the assessment and implications of variations in the longitudinal course.

Table 12.1–25
DSM-IV-TR Criteria for Longitudinal Course Specifiers

Specify if (can be applied to recurrent major depressive disorder or bipolar I or II disorder):

With full interepisode recovery: if full remission is attained between the two most recent mood episodes

Without full interepisode recovery: if full remission is not attained between the two most recent mood episodes

CLINICAL FEATURES

The two basic symptom patterns in mood disorders are those of depression and mania. Depressive episodes can occur in both major depressive disorder and bipolar I disorder. In many studies, researchers have attempted to find reliable differences between bipolar I disorder depressive episodes and episodes of major depressive disorder, but the differences are elusive. In a clinical situation, only the patient's history, family history, and future course can help differentiate the two conditions. Some patients with bipolar I disorder have mixed states with both manic and depressive features, and some seem to experience brief—minutes to a few hours—episodes of depression during manic episodes.

Depressive Episodes

A depressed mood and a loss of interest or pleasure are the key symptoms of depression. Patients may say that they feel blue, hopeless, in the dumps, or worthless. For a patient, the depressed mood often has a distinct quality that differentiates it from the normal emotion of sadness or grief. Patients often describe the symptom of depression as one of agonizing emotional pain and sometimes complain about being unable to cry, a symptom that resolves as they improve.

Approximately two-thirds of all depressed patients contemplate suicide, and 10 to 15 percent commit suicide. Those recently hospitalized with a suicide attempt or suicidal ideation had a higher lifetime risk of successful suicide than those never hospitalized. Some depressed patients sometimes seem unaware of their depression and do not complain of a mood disturbance, even though they exhibit withdrawal from family, friends, and activities that previously interested them. Almost all depressed patients (97 percent) complain about reduced energy; they find difficulty in finishing tasks, are impaired at school and work, and have decreased motivation to undertake new projects. Approximately 80 percent of patients complain of trouble in sleeping, especially early-morning awakening (that is, terminal insomnia) and multiple awakenings at night, during which they ruminate about their problems. Many patients have decreased appetite and weight loss, but others experience increased appetite and weight gain and sleep longer than usual. These patients are classified in DSM-IV-TR as having atypical features.

Anxiety is a common symptom of depression and affects as many as 90 percent of all depressed patients. The various changes in food intake and rest can aggravate coexisting medical illnesses, such as diabetes, hypertension, chronic obstructive lung disease, and heart disease. Other vegetative symptoms include abnormal menses and decreased interest and performance in sexual activities. Sexual problems can sometimes lead to inappropriate referrals, such as to marital counseling and sex therapy, when clinicians fail to recognize the underlying depressive disorder. Anxiety (including panic attacks), alcohol abuse, and somatic complaints (such as constipation and headaches) often complicate the treatment of depression. Approximately 50 percent of all patients describe a diurnal variation in their symptoms, with an increased severity in the morning and a lessening of symptoms by evening. Cognitive symptoms include subjective reports of an inability to concentrate (84 percent of patients in one study) and impairments in thinking (67 percent of patients in another study).

Depression in Children and Adolescents. School phobia and excessive clinging to parents may be symptoms of depression in children. Poor academic performance, substance abuse, antisocial behavior, sexual promiscuity, truancy, and running away may be symptoms of depression in adolescents. (This subject is further discussed in Chapter 45.)

Depression in Older People. Depression is more common in older people than it is in the general population. Various studies have reported prevalence rates ranging from 25 to almost 50 percent, although the percentage of these cases that are caused by major depressive disorder is uncertain. Several studies have reported data indicating that depression in older people may be correlated with low socioeconomic status, the loss of a spouse, a concurrent physical illness, and social isolation. Other studies have indicated that depression in older people is underdiagnosed and undertreated, perhaps particularly by general practitioners. The underrecognition of depression in older people may occur because the disorder more often appears with somatic complaints in older than in younger age groups. Further, ageism may influence and cause them to accept more depressive symptoms as normal in older patients.

Manic Episodes

An elevated, expansive, or irritable mood is the hallmark of a manic episode. The elevated mood is euphoric and often infectious and can even cause a countertransferential denial of illness by an inexperienced clinician. Although uninvolved people may not recognize the unusual nature of a patient's mood, those who know the patient recognize it as abnormal. Alternatively, the mood may be irritable, especially when a patient's overtly ambitious plans are thwarted. Patients often exhibit a change of predominant mood from euphoria early in the course of the illness to later irritability.

The treatment of manic patients in an inpatient ward can be complicated by their testing of the limits of ward rules, their tendency to shift responsibility for their acts onto others, their exploitation of the weaknesses of others, and their propensity to dividing staff. Outside the hospital, manic patients often drink alcohol excessively, perhaps in an attempt to self-medicate. The patient's disinhibited nature is reflected in an excessive use of the telephone, especially in the making of long-distance calls during the early-morning hours.

Pathological gambling, a tendency to disrobe in public places, wearing clothing and jewelry of bright colors in unusual or outlandish combinations, and an inattention to small details (such as forgetting to hang up the telephone) are also symptomatic of the disorder. Patients act impulsively and at the same time with a sense of conviction and purpose. Manic patients are often preoccupied by religious, political, financial, sexual, or persecutory ideas that can evolve into complex delusional systems. Occasionally, manic patients become regressed and play with their urine and feces.

Mania in Adolescents. Mania in adolescents is often misdiagnosed as antisocial personality disorder or schizophrenia. Symptoms of mania in adolescents may include psychosis, alcohol or other substance abuse, suicide attempts, academic problems, philosophical brooding, obsessive-compulsive disorder symptoms, multiple somatic complaints, marked irritability resulting in fights, and other antisocial behaviors. Although many of these symptoms are seen in normal adolescence, severe or persistent symptoms should cause clinicians to consider bipolar I disorder in the differential diagnosis.

Bipolar II Disorder

The clinical features of bipolar II disorder are those of major depressive disorder combined with those of a hypomanic episode. Although the data are limited, a few studies indicate that bipolar II disorder is associated with more marital disruption and with onset at an earlier age than is bipolar I disorder. Evidence also indicates that patients with bipolar II disorder are at greater risk of both attempting and completing suicide than are patients with bipolar I disorder and major depressive disorder.

Coexisting Disorders

Anxiety. In the anxiety disorders, DSM-IV-TR notes the existence of mixed anxiety-depressive disorder. Significant symptoms of anxiety can and often do coexist with significant symptoms of depression. Whether patients who exhibit significant symptoms of both anxiety and depression are affected by two distinct disease processes or by a single disease process that produces both sets of symptoms is not yet resolved. Patients of both types may constitute the group of patients with mixed anxiety-depressive disorder.

Alcohol Dependence. Alcohol dependence frequently coexists with mood disorders. Both patients with major depressive disorder and those with bipolar I disorder are likely to meet the diagnostic criteria for an alcohol use disorder. The available data indicate that alcohol dependence in women is more strongly associated with a coexisting diagnosis of depression than is alcohol dependence in men. In contrast, the genetic and family data about men who have both a mood disorder and alcohol dependence indicate that they are likely to be suffering from two genetically distinct disease processes.

Other Substance-Related Disorders. Substance-related disorders other than alcohol dependence are also commonly associated with mood disorders. The abuse of substances may be involved in precipitating an episode of illness or, conversely, may represent patients' attempts to treat their own illnesses. Although manic patients seldom use sedatives to dampen their euphoria, depressed patients often use stimulants, such as cocaine and amphetamines, to relieve their depression.

Medical Conditions. Depression commonly coexists with medical conditions, especially in older people. When depression and medical conditions coexist, clinicians must try to determine whether the underlying medical condition is pathophysiologically related to the depression or whether any drugs that the patient is taking for the medical condition are causing the depression. Many studies indicate that treatment of a coexisting major depressive disorder can improve the course of the underlying medical disorder, including cancer.

MENTAL STATUS EXAMINATION
Depressive Episodes

General Description. Generalized psychomotor retardation is the most common symptom, although psychomotor agitation is also seen, especially in older patients. Hand wringing and hair pulling are the most common symptoms of agitation. Classically, a depressed patient has a stooped posture, no spontaneous movements, and a downcast, averted gaze. On clinical examination, depressed patients exhibiting gross symptoms of psychomotor retardation may appear identical to patients with catatonic schizophrenia. This fact is recognized in DSM-IV-TR by the inclusion of the symptom qualifier "with catatonic features" for some mood disorders.

Mood, Affect, and Feelings. Depression is the key symptom, although approximately 50 percent of patients deny depressive feelings and do not appear to be particularly depressed. Family members or employers often bring or send these patients for treatment because of social withdrawal and generally decreased activity.

Speech. Many depressed patients evidence a decreased rate and volume of speech; they respond to questions with single words and exhibit delayed responses to questions. The examiner may literally have to wait 2 or 3 minutes for a response to a question.

Perceptual Disturbances. Depressed patients with delusions or hallucinations are said to have a major depressive episode with psychotic features. Even in the absence of delusions or hallucinations, some clinicians use the term *psychotic depression* for grossly regressed depressed patients—mute, not bathing, soiling. Such patients are probably better described as having catatonic features.

Delusions and hallucinations that are consistent with a depressed mood are said to be mood congruent. Mood-congruent delusions in a depressed person include those of guilt, sinfulness, worthlessness, poverty, failure, persecution, and terminal somatic illnesses (such as cancer and "rotting" brain). The content of mood-incongruent delusions or hallucinations is not consistent with a depressed mood. Mood-incongruent delusions in a depressed person involve grandiose themes of exaggerated power, knowledge, and worth—for example, the belief that a person is being persecuted because he or she is the Messiah. Although relatively rare, hallucinations can also occur in major depressive episodes with psychotic features.

Thought. Depressed patients customarily have a negative view of the world and of themselves. Their thought content often includes nondelusional ruminations about loss, guilt, suicide, and death. Approximately 10 percent of all depressed patients have marked symptoms of a thought disorder, usually thought blocking and profound poverty of content.

Sensorium and Cognition
ORIENTATION. Most depressed patients are oriented to person, place, and time, although some may not have enough energy or interest to answer questions about these subjects during an interview.

MEMORY. Approximately 50 to 75 percent of all depressed patients have a cognitive impairment, sometimes referred to as *depressive pseudodementia*. Such patients commonly complain of impaired concentration and forgetfulness.

Impulse Control. Approximately 10 to 15 percent of all depressed patients commit suicide, and approximately two-thirds have suicidal ideation. Depressed patients with psychotic features occasionally consider killing a person involved with their delusional systems, but the most severely depressed patients often lack the motivation or the energy to act in an impulsive or violent way. Patients with depressive disorders are at increased risk of suicide as they begin to improve and to regain the energy needed to plan and carry out a suicide (paradoxical suicide). It is usually clinically unwise to give a depressed patient a large prescription for antidepressants, especially tricyclic drugs, at the time of discharge from the hospital.

Judgment and Insight. The patient's judgment is best assessed by reviewing his or her actions in the recent past and their behavior during the interview. Depressed patients' insight into their disorder is often excessive; patients overemphasize their symptoms, their disorder, and their life problems. It is difficult to convince such patients that improvement is possible.

Reliability. In interviews and conversations, depressed patients overemphasize the bad and minimize the good. A common clinical mistake is to unquestioningly believe a depressed patient who states that a previous trial of antidepressant medications did not work. Such statements may be false, and they require confirmation from another source. Psychiatrists should not view patients' misinformation as an intentional fabrication; the admission of any hopeful information may be impossible for a person in a depressed state of mind.

Objective Rating Scales for Depression. Objective rating scales for depression can be useful in clinical practice for documenting the depressed patient's clinical state.

ZUNG. The Zung Self-Rating Depression Scale is a 20-item report scale. A normal score is 34 or less; a depressed score is 50 or more. The scale provides a global index of the intensity of a patient's depressive symptoms, including the affective expression of depression.

RASKIN. The Raskin Depression Scale is a clinician-rated scale that measures the severity of a patient's depression, as reported by the patient and as observed by the physician, on a five-point scale of three dimensions: verbal report, displayed behavior, and secondary symptoms. The scale has a range of 3 to 13; a normal score is 3, and a depressed score is 7 or more.

HAMILTON. The Hamilton Rating Scale for Depression (HAM-D) is a widely used depression scale with up to 24 items, each of which is rated 0 to 4 or 0 to 2, with a total score of 0 to 76. The clinician evaluates the patient's answers to questions about feelings of guilt, thoughts of suicide, sleep habits, and other symptoms of depression, and the ratings are derived from the clinical interview.

Manic Episodes
GENERAL DESCRIPTION. Manic patients are excited, talkative, sometimes amusing, and frequently hyperactive. At times, they are grossly psychotic and disorganized and require physical restraints and the intramuscular injection of sedating drugs.

MOOD, AFFECT, AND FEELINGS. Manic patients classically are euphoric, but they can also be irritable, especially when mania has been present for some time. These patients also have a low frustration tolerance, which may lead to feelings of anger and hostility. Manic patients may be emotionally labile, switching from laughter to irritability to depression in minutes or hours.

SPEECH.   Manic patients cannot be interrupted while they are speaking, and they are often intrusive nuisances to those around them. Their speech is often disturbed. As the mania gets more intense, speech becomes louder, more rapid, and difficult to interpret, then filled with puns, jokes, rhymes, plays on words, and irrelevancies as the activated state increases. At a still greater activity level, associations become loosened, the ability to concentrate fades, and flight of ideas, word salad, and neologisms appear. In acute manic excitement, speech may be totally incoherent and indistinguishable from that of a person with schizophrenia.

PERCEPTUAL DISTURBANCES.   Delusions occur in 75 percent of all manic patients. Mood-congruent manic delusions are often concerned with great wealth, extraordinary abilities, or power. Bizarre and mood-incongruent delusions and hallucinations also appear in mania.

THOUGHT.   Manic patients' thought content includes themes of self-confidence and self-aggrandizement. Manic patients are often easily distracted, and cognitive functioning in the manic state is characterized by an unrestrained and accelerated flow of ideas.

SENSORIUM AND COGNITION.   Although the cognitive deficits of patients with schizophrenia have been much discussed, less has been written about similar deficits in patients with bipolar I disorder, who may have similar minor cognitive deficits. The reported cognitive deficits can be interpreted as reflecting diffuse cortical dysfunction; subsequent work may localize the abnormal areas. Grossly, orientation and memory are intact, although some manic patients may be so euphoric that they answer incorrectly. Emil Kraepelin called the symptom "delirious mania."

IMPULSE CONTROL.   Approximately 75 percent of all manic patients are assaultive or threatening. Manic patients do attempt suicide and homicide, but the incidence of these behaviors is unknown. Patients who threaten important people (such as the President of the United States) more often have bipolar I disorder than schizophrenia.

JUDGMENT AND INSIGHT.   Impaired judgment is a hallmark of manic patients. They may break laws about credit cards, sexual activities, and finances and sometimes involve their families in financial ruin. Manic patients also have little insight into their disorder.

RELIABILITY.   Manic patients are notoriously unreliable in their information. Because lying and deceit are common in mania, inexperienced clinicians may treat manic patients with inappropriate disdain.

DIFFERENTIAL DIAGNOSIS

Major Depressive Disorder

Medical Disorders.   The DSM-IV-TR diagnosis of mood disorder due to a general medical condition describes a mood disorder caused by a nonpsychiatric medical condition. The DSM-IV-TR diagnosis of substance-induced mood disorder describes a mood disorder caused by a substance. Both these diagnostic categories are discussed in Section 12.3.

Failure to obtain a good clinical history or to consider the context of a patient's current life situation may lead to diagnostic errors. Clinicians should have depressed adolescents tested for mononucleosis, and patients who are markedly overweight or underweight should be tested for adrenal and thyroid dysfunctions. Homosexuals, bisexual men, and people who abuse an intravenous substance should be tested for acquired immune deficiency syndrome (AIDS). Older patients should be evaluated for viral pneumonia and other medical conditions.

Many neurological and medical disorders and pharmacological agents can produce symptoms of depression (see Table 12.3–8 in Section 12.3). Patients with depressive disorders often first visit their general practitioners with somatic complaints. Most medical causes of depressive disorders can be detected with a comprehensive medical history, a complete physical and neurological examination, and routine blood and urine tests. The workup should include tests for thyroid and adrenal functions, because disorders of both these endocrine systems can appear as depressive disorders. In substance-induced mood disorder, a reasonable rule of thumb is that any drug a depressed patient is taking should be considered a potential factor in the mood disorder. Cardiac drugs, antihypertensives, sedatives, hypnotics, antipsychotics, antiepileptics, antiparkinsonian drugs, analgesics, antibacterials, and antineoplastics are all commonly associated with depressive symptoms.

NEUROLOGICAL CONDITIONS.   The most common neurological problems that manifest depressive symptoms are Parkinson's disease, dementing illnesses (including dementia of the Alzheimer's type), epilepsy, cerebrovascular diseases, and tumors. Approximately 50 to 75 percent of all patients with Parkinson's disease have marked symptoms of depressive disorder that do not correlate with the patient's degree of physical disability, age, or duration of illness but do correlate with the presence of abnormalities found on neuropsychological tests. The symptoms of depressive disorder may be masked by the almost identical motor symptoms of Parkinson's disease. Depressive symptoms often respond to antidepressant drugs or ECT. The interictal changes associated with temporal lobe epilepsy can mimic a depressive disorder, especially if the epileptic focus is on the right side. Depression is a common complicating feature of cerebrovascular diseases, particularly in the 2 years after the episode. Depression is more common in anterior brain lesions than in posterior brain lesions and in both cases often respond to antidepressant medications. Tumors of the diencephalic and temporal regions are particularly likely to be associated with depressive disorder symptoms.

PSEUDODEMENTIA.   Clinicians can usually differentiate the pseudodementia of major depressive disorder from the dementia of a disease, such as dementia of the Alzheimer's type, on clinical grounds. The cognitive symptoms in major depressive disorder have a sudden onset, and other symptoms of the disorder, such as self-reproach, are also present. A diurnal variation in the cognitive problems, which is not seen in primary dementias, may occur. Depressed patients with cognitive difficulties often do not try to answer questions ("I don't know"), whereas patients with dementia may confabulate. In depressed patients, recent memory is more affected than is remote memory. And, during an interview, depressed patients can sometimes be coached and encouraged into remembering, an ability that demented patients lack.

OTHER MOOD DISORDERS. Clinicians must consider the range of DSM-IV-TR diagnosis categories available before arriving at a final diagnosis. First, they must rule out mood disorder caused by a general medical condition and substance-induced mood disorder. Next, clinicians must determine whether a patient has had episodes of mania-like symptoms, indicating bipolar I disorder (complete manic and depressive syndromes), bipolar II disorder (recurrent major depressive episodes with hypomania), or cyclothymic disorder (incomplete depressive and manic syndromes). If a patient's symptoms are limited to those of depression, clinicians must assess the severity and duration of the symptoms to differentiate among major depressive disorder (complete depressive syndrome for 2 weeks), minor depressive disorder (incomplete but episodic depressive syndrome), recurrent brief depressive disorder (complete depressive syndrome but for less than 2 weeks per episode), and dysthymic disorder (incomplete depressive syndrome without clear episodes).

OTHER MENTAL DISORDERS. Substance-related disorders, psychotic disorders, eating disorders, adjustment disorders, somatoform disorders, and anxiety disorders are all commonly associated with depressive symptoms and must be considered in the differential diagnosis of a patient with depressive symptoms. Perhaps the most difficult differential is that between anxiety disorders with depression and depressive disorders with marked anxiety. The difficulty of making this differentiation is reflected in the inclusion of the diagnosis of mixed anxiety-depressive disorder in DSM-IV-TR. An abnormal result on the DST, the presence of shortened REM latency on a sleep EEG, and a negative lactate infusion test result support a diagnosis of major depressive disorder in particularly troublesome cases.

UNCOMPLICATED BEREAVEMENT. Uncomplicated bereavement is not considered a mental disorder, even though approximately one-third of all bereaved spouses for a time meet the diagnostic criteria for major depressive disorder. Some patients with uncomplicated bereavement do develop major depressive disorder, but the diagnosis is not made unless a resolution of the grief does not occur; the differentiation is based on the symptoms' severity and length. In major depressive disorder, common symptoms that evolve from unresolved bereavement are a morbid preoccupation with worthlessness, suicidal ideation, feelings that the person has committed an act (not just an omission) that caused the spouse's death, mummification (keeping the deceased's belongings exactly as they were), and a particularly severe anniversary reaction, which sometimes includes a suicide attempt.

Bipolar I Disorder

When a patient with bipolar I disorder has a depressive episode, the differential diagnosis is the same as that for a patient being considered for a diagnosis of major depressive disorder. When a patient is manic, however, the differential diagnosis includes bipolar I disorder, bipolar II disorder, cyclothymic disorder, mood disorder caused by a general medical condition, and substance-induced mood disorder. For manic symptoms, borderline, narcissistic, histrionic, and antisocial personality disorders need special consideration.

Schizophrenia. A great deal has been published about the clinical difficulty of distinguishing a manic episode from schizophrenia. Although difficult, a differential diagnosis is possible with a few clinical guidelines. Merriment, elation, and an infectiousness of mood are much more common in manic episodes than in schizophrenia. The combination of a manic mood, rapid or pressured speech, and hyperactivity weighs heavily toward a diagnosis of a manic episode. The onset in a manic episode is often rapid and is perceived as a marked change from a patient's previous behavior. Half of all patients with bipolar I disorder have a family history of mood disorder. Catatonic features may be a depressive phase of bipolar I disorder. When evaluating patients with catatonia, clinicians should carefully look for a history of manic or depressive episodes and for a family history of mood disorders. Manic symptoms in people from minority groups (particularly blacks and Hispanics) are often misdiagnosed as schizophrenic symptoms.

Medical Conditions. In contrast to depressive symptoms, which are present in almost all psychiatric disorders, manic symptoms are more distinctive, although they can be caused by a wide range of medical and neurological conditions and substances (Table 12.1–5). Antidepressant treatment can also be associated with the precipitation of mania in some patients.

Bipolar II Disorder

The differential diagnosis of patients being evaluated for a mood disorder should include the other mood disorders, psychotic disorders, and borderline disorder. The differentiation between major depressive disorder and bipolar I disorder on one hand and bipolar II disorder on the other hand rests on the clinical evaluation of the mania-like episodes. Clinicians should not mistake euthymia in a chronically depressed patient as a hypomanic or manic episode. Patients with borderline personality disorder often have a severely disrupted life, similar to that of patients with bipolar II disorder, because of the multiple episodes of significant mood disorder symptoms.

COURSE AND PROGNOSIS

The many studies of the course and prognosis of mood disorder have generally concluded that mood disorders tend to have long courses and that patients tend to have relapses. Although mood disorders are often considered benign in contrast to schizophrenia, they exact a profound toll on affected patients. Another common conclusion from studies is that life stressors more frequently precede the first episode of mood disorders than subsequent episodes. This finding has been interpreted to indicate that psychosocial stress may play a role in the initial cause of mood disorders and that, even though the initial episode may resolve, a long-lasting change in the biology of the brain puts a patient at great risk for subsequent episodes.

Major Depressive Disorder

Course

ONSET. Approximately 50 percent of patients undergoing their first episode of major depressive disorder had significant depressive symptoms before the first identified episode. One implication of this observation is that early identification and treatment of early symptoms may prevent the development of a full depressive episode. Although symptoms may have been present, patients with major depressive disorder usually have not had a premorbid personality disorder. The first depressive episode occurs before age 40 in approximately 50 percent of patients. A later onset is associated with the absence of a family history of mood disorders, antisocial personality disorder, and alcohol abuse.

DURATION. An untreated depressive episode lasts 6 to 13 months; most treated episodes last approximately 3 months. The withdrawal of antidepressants before 3 months has elapsed almost always results in the return of the symptoms. As the course of the disorder progresses, patients tend to have more frequent episodes that last longer. Over a 20-year period, the mean number of episodes is five or six.

DEVELOPMENT OF MANIC EPISODES. Approximately 5 to 10 percent of patients with an initial diagnosis of major depressive disorder have a manic episode 6 to 10 years after the first depressive episode. The mean age for this switch is 32 years, and it often occurs after two to four depressive episodes. Although the data are inconsistent and controversial, some clinicians report that the depression of patients who are later classified as having bipolar I disorder is often characterized by hypersomnia, psychomotor retardation, psychotic symptoms, a history of postpartum episodes, a family history of bipolar I disorder, and a history of antidepressant-induced hypomania.

Prognosis.   Major depressive disorder is not a benign disorder. It tends to be chronic, and patients tend to relapse. Patients who have been hospitalized for a first episode of major depressive disorder have approximately a 50 percent chance of recovering in the first year. The percentage of patients recovering after hospitalization decreases with time. Many unrecovered patients remain affected with dysthymic disorder. Recurrences of major depressive episodes are also common. Approximately 25 percent of patients experience a recurrence in the first 6 months after release from a hospital, approximately 30 to 50 percent in the first 2 years, and approximately 50 to 75 percent in 5 years. The incidence of relapse is lower than these figures in patients who continue prophylactic psychopharmacological treatment and in patients who have had only one or two depressive episodes. Generally, as a patient experiences more and more depressive episodes, the time between the episodes decreases, and the severity of each episode increases.

PROGNOSTIC INDICATORS.   Many studies have focused on identifying both good and bad prognostic indicators in the course of major depressive disorder. Mild episodes, the absence of psychotic symptoms, and a short hospital stay are good prognostic indicators. Psychosocial indicators of a good course include a history of solid friendships during adolescence, stable family functioning, and a generally sound social functioning for the 5 years preceding the illness. Additional good prognostic signs are the absence of a comorbid psychiatric disorder and of a personality disorder, no more than one previous hospitalization for major depressive disorder, and an advanced age of onset. The possibility of a poor prognosis is increased by coexisting dysthymic disorder, abuse of alcohol and other sub-

stances, anxiety disorder symptoms, and a history of more than one previous depressive episode. Men are more likely than women to experience a chronically impaired course.

Bipolar I Disorder

Course.   The natural history of bipolar I disorder is such that it is often useful to make a graph of a patient's disorder and to keep it up-to-date as treatment progresses (Fig. 12.1–1). Although cyclothymic disorder is sometimes diagnosed retrospectively in patients with bipolar I disorder, no identified personality traits are specifically associated with bipolar I disorder.

Bipolar I disorder most often starts with depression (75 percent of the time in women, 67 percent in men) and is a recurring disorder. Most patients experience both depressive and manic episodes, although 10 to 20 percent experience only manic episodes. The manic episodes typically have a rapid onset (hours or days) but may evolve over a few weeks. An untreated manic episode lasts approximately 3 months; therefore, clinicians should not discontinue drugs before that time. Ninety percent of persons who have a single manic episode are likely to have another. As the disorder progresses, the time between episodes often decreases. After approximately five episodes, however, the interepisode interval often stabilizes at 6 to 9 months. Five to 15 percent of persons with bipolar disorder have four or more episodes per year and can be classified as rapid cyclers.

BIPOLAR I DISORDER IN CHILDREN AND OLDER PEOPLE. Bipolar I disorder can affect both the very young and older people. The incidence of bipolar I disorder in children and adolescents is approximately 1 percent, and the onset can be as early as age 8. Common misdiagnoses are schizophrenia and oppositional defiant disorder.

Bipolar I disorder with such an early onset is associated with a poor prognosis. Manic symptoms are common in older people, although the range of causes is broad and includes nonpsychiatric medical conditions, dementia, delirium, and bipolar I disorder. Currently available data indicate that the onset of true bipolar I disorder in older people is relatively uncommon.

Prognosis.   Patients with bipolar I disorder have a poorer prognosis than do patients with major depressive disorder. Approximately 40 to 50 percent of bipolar I disorder patients may have a second manic episode within 2 years of the first episode. Although lithium (Eskalith) prophylaxis improves the course and prognosis of bipolar I disorder, probably only 50 to 60 percent of patients achieve significant control of their symptoms with lithium. One 4-year follow-up study of patients with bipolar I disorder found that a premorbid poor occupational status, alcohol dependence, psychotic features, depressive features, interepisode depressive features, and male gender were all factors that weighed toward a poor prognosis. Short duration of manic episodes, advanced age of onset, few suicidal thoughts, and few coexisting psychiatric or medical problems weigh toward a good prognosis.

Approximately 7 percent of all patients with bipolar I disorder do not have a recurrence of symptoms; 45 percent have more than one episode, and 40 percent have a chronic disorder. Patients may have from 2 to 30 manic episodes, although the mean number is approximately nine. Approximately 40 percent of all patients have more than ten episodes. On long-term fol-

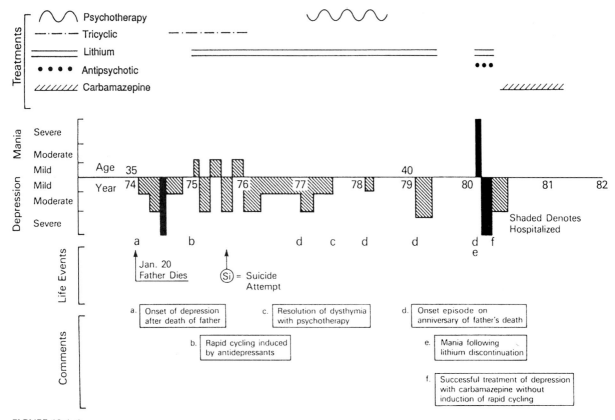

FIGURE 12.1–1
Graphing the course of a mood disorder. Prototype of a life chart. (Courtesy of Robert M. Post, M.D.)

low-up, 15 percent of all patients with bipolar I disorder are well, 45 percent are well but have multiple relapses, 30 percent are in partial remission, and 10 percent are chronically ill. One-third of all patients with bipolar I disorder have chronic symptoms and evidence of significant social decline.

Bipolar II Disorder

The course and prognosis of bipolar II disorder have just begun to be studied. Preliminary data indicate, however, that the diagnosis is stable, as shown by the high likelihood that patients with bipolar II disorder will have the same diagnosis up to 5 years later. The data thus show that bipolar II disorder is a chronic disease that warrants long-term treatment strategies.

TREATMENT

The treatment of patients with mood disorders must be directed toward several goals. First, the patient's safety must be guaranteed. Second, a complete diagnostic evaluation of the patient must be carried out. Third, a treatment plan that addresses not only the immediate symptoms but also the patient's prospective well-being must be initiated. Although current treatment emphasizes pharmacotherapy and psychotherapy addressed to the individual patient, stressful life events are also associated with increases in relapse rates among patients with mood disorders. Thus, treatment must reduce the number and severity of the stressors in patients' lives.

Overall, the treatment of mood disorders is rewarding for psychiatrists. Specific treatments are now available for both manic and depressive episodes, and available data indicate that prophylactic treatment is also effective. Because the prognosis for each episode is good, optimism is always warranted and is welcomed by both the patient and the patient's family, even if initial treatment results are not promising. Mood disorders are chronic, however, and the psychiatrist must advise the patient and the family about future treatment strategies.

Hospitalization

The first and most critical decision a physician must make is whether to hospitalize a patient or to attempt outpatient treatment. Clear indications for hospitalization are the need for diagnostic procedures, the risk of suicide or homicide, and a patient's grossly reduced ability to get food and shelter. A history of rapidly progressing symptoms and the rupture of a patient's usual support systems are also indications for hospitalization.

A physician may safely treat mild depression or hypomania in the office if he or she evaluates the patient frequently. Clinical signs of impaired judgment, weight loss, or insomnia should be minimal. The patient's support system should be strong, neither overinvolved nor withdrawing from the patient. Any adverse changes in the patient's symptoms or behavior or the attitude of the patient's support system may be sufficient to warrant hospitalization.

Patients with mood disorders are often unwilling to enter a hospital voluntarily and may have to be involuntarily committed. These patients are often incapable of making decisions because of their slowed thinking, negative *Weltanschauung* (world view), and hopelessness. Manic patients often have such a complete lack of insight into their disorder that hospitalization seems absolutely absurd to them.

Psychosocial Therapy

Although most studies indicate—and most clinicians and researchers believe—that a combination of psychotherapy and pharmacotherapy is the most effective treatment for major depressive disorder, some data suggest another view: Either pharmacotherapy or psychotherapy alone is effective, at least in patients with mild major depressive episodes, and the regular use of combined therapy adds to the cost of treatment and exposes patients to unnecessary side effects.

Three types of short-term psychotherapies—cognitive therapy, interpersonal therapy, and behavior therapy—have been studied to determine their efficacy in the treatment of major depressive disorder. Although its efficacy in treating major depressive disorder is not as well researched as these three therapies, psychoanalytically oriented psychotherapy has long been used for depressive disorders, and many clinicians use the technique as their primary method. What differentiates the three short-term psychotherapy methods from the psychoanalytically oriented approach are the active and directive roles of the therapist, the directly recognizable goals, and the end points for short-term therapy.

Although less research has been conducted on psychodynamic theory of depression than on some other forms of psychotherapy, the accumulating evidence is encouraging regarding the efficacy of dynamic therapy. In a randomized controlled trial comparing psychodynamic therapy with cognitive-behavior therapy, the outcomes of the depressed patients in the study showed no differences between the two treatments.

Cognitive Therapy. Cognitive therapy, developed originally by Aaron Beck, focuses on the cognitive distortions postulated to be present in major depressive disorder. Such distortions include selective attention to the negative aspects of circumstances and unrealistically morbid inferences about consequences. For example, apathy and low energy are results of a patient's expectation of failure in all areas. The goal of cognitive therapy is to alleviate depressive episodes and to prevent their recurrence by helping patients identify and test negative cognitions; develop alternative, flexible, and positive ways of thinking; and rehearse new cognitive and behavioral responses.

Studies have shown that cognitive therapy is effective in the treatment of major depressive disorder. Most of the studies found that cognitive therapy is equal in efficacy to pharmacotherapy and associated with fewer side effects and with better follow-up than is pharmacotherapy. Some of the best-controlled studies have indicated that the combination of cognitive therapy and pharmacotherapy is more efficacious than either therapy alone, although other studies have not found that additive effect. At least one study, the National Institute of Mental Health's Treatment of Depression Collaborative Research Program, found that pharmacotherapy, either alone or with psychotherapy, may be the treatment of choice for patients with severe major depressive episodes.

Interpersonal Therapy. Interpersonal therapy, developed by Gerald Klerman, focuses on one or two of a patient's current interpersonal problems. This therapy is based on two assumptions. First, current interpersonal problems are likely to have their roots in early dysfunctional relationships. Second, current interpersonal problems are likely to be involved in precipitating or perpetuating the current depressive symptoms. Several controlled trials have compared interpersonal therapy, cognitive therapy, pharmacotherapy, and the combination of pharmacotherapy with psychotherapy. These trials indicated that interpersonal therapy is effective in the treatment of major depressive disorder and, not surprisingly, may be specifically helpful in addressing interpersonal problems. The data about the efficacy of interpersonal therapy in the treatment of severe major depressive episodes are less reliable, although some information indicates that interpersonal therapy may be the most effective method for severe major depressive episodes when the treatment choice is psychotherapy alone.

The interpersonal therapy program usually consists of 12 to 16 weekly sessions and is characterized by an active therapeutic approach. Intrapsychic phenomena, such as defense mechanisms and internal conflicts, are not addressed. Discrete behaviors—such as lack of assertiveness, impaired social skills, and distorted thinking—may be addressed but only in the context of their meaning in or their effect on interpersonal relationships.

Behavior Therapy. Behavior therapy is based on the hypothesis that maladaptive behavioral patterns result in a person's receiving little positive feedback, and perhaps outright rejection, from society. By addressing maladaptive behaviors in therapy, patients learn to function in the world in such a way that they receive positive reinforcement. Although individual and group therapies have been studied, behavior therapy for major depressive disorder has not yet been the subject of many controlled studies. The data to date indicate that behavior therapy is an effective treatment for major depressive disorder.

Psychoanalytically Oriented Therapy. The psychoanalytic approach to mood disorders is based on psychoanalytic theories about depression and mania. The goal of psychoanalytic psychotherapy is to effect a change in a patient's personality structure or character, not simply to alleviate symptoms. Improvements in interpersonal trust, intimacy, coping mechanisms, the capacity to grieve, and the ability to experience a wide range of emotions are some of the aims of psychoanalytic therapy. Treatment often requires the patient to experience periods of heightened anxiety and distress during the course of therapy, which may continue for several years.

Family Therapy. Family therapy is not generally viewed as a primary therapy for the treatment of major depressive disorder, but increasing evidence indicates that helping a patient with a mood disorder to reduce and cope with stress can lessen the chance of a relapse. Family therapy is indicated if the disorder jeopardizes a patient's marriage or family functioning or if the mood disorder is promoted or maintained by the family situation. Family therapy examines the role of the mood-disordered member in the overall psychological well-being of the whole family; it also examines the role of the entire family in the maintenance of the patient's symptoms. Patients with mood disorders have a high rate of divorce, and approximately 50 percent of all spouses report that they would not have married or had children if they had known that the patient was going to develop a mood disorder.

Pharmacotherapy

Although the specific, short-term psychotherapies such as interpersonal therapy and cognitive therapy have influenced the treatment approaches to major depressive disorder, the pharmacotherapeutic approach to mood disorders has revolutionized their treatment and has dramatically affected the courses of mood disorders and reduced their inherent costs to society. Physicians must integrate pharmacotherapy with psychotherapeutic interventions. If physicians view mood disorders as fundamentally evolving from psychodynamic issues, their ambivalence about the use of drugs may result in a poor response, noncompliance, and probably inadequate dosages for too short a treatment period. Alternatively, if physicians ignore the psychosocial needs of a patient, the outcome of pharmacotherapy may be compromised.

Major Depressive Disorder.

Effective and specific treatments, such as tricyclic drugs, for major depressive disorder have been available for 40 years. The use of specific pharmacotherapy approximately doubles the chance that a depressed patient will recover in 1 month. Nevertheless, problems remain in the treatment of major depressive disorder: Some patients do not respond to the first treatment; all currently available antidepressants may take up to 3 to 4 weeks to exert significant therapeutic effects, although they may begin to show their effects earlier; and, until relatively recently, all available antidepressants have been toxic in overdoses and have had adverse effects. The introduction of the SSRIs, such as fluoxetine, paroxetine (Paxil), and sertraline (Zoloft), as well as bupropion, venlafaxine (Effexor), nefazodone, and mirtazapine (Remeron), offers clinicians drugs that are equally effective but safer and better tolerated than previous drugs. Recent indications for antidepressant medications (for example, eating disorders and anxiety disorders) make the grouping of these drugs under the single label of antidepressants somewhat confusing.

The principal indication for antidepressants is a major depressive episode. The first symptoms to improve are often poor sleep and appetite patterns. Agitation, anxiety, depressive episodes, and hopelessness are the next symptoms to improve. Other target symptoms include low energy, poor concentration, helplessness, and decreased libido.

PATIENT EDUCATION.

Adequate patient education about the use of antidepressants is as critical to treatment success as is choosing the most appropriate drug and dosage. When introducing the topic of a drug trial to a patient, physicians should emphasize that major depressive disorder is a combination of biological and psychological factors, all of which benefit from drug therapy. Physicians should also stress that the patient will not become addicted to antidepressants, because these drugs do not provide immediate gratification. Further, it will probably take 3 to 4 weeks for the effects of the antidepressant to be felt, and even if the patient shows no improvement by that time, other medications are available. Some clinicians say that the appearance of side effects shows that the drug is working, but the expected side effects should be explained in detail. For example, some patients taking SSRIs may experience agitation, gastrointestinal upset, or nausea before any reduction in depres-

sion. The adverse effects pass with time. With tricyclic drugs and MAOIs, physicians may find it useful to tell the patient that sleep and appetite will improve first, followed by a sense of returned energy, and that the feeling of depression, unfortunately, will be the last symptom to change.

Physicians must always consider the risk of suicide in patients with mood disorder. Most antidepressants are lethal if taken in large amounts. It is unwise to give large prescriptions to most patients with mood disorder when they are discharged from the hospital unless another person monitors the drug's administration.

ALTERNATIVES TO DRUG TREATMENT.

Two organic therapies that are alternatives to pharmacotherapy are ECT and phototherapy. ECT is generally used when a patient is unresponsive to pharmacotherapy or cannot tolerate pharmacotherapy, or the clinical situation is so severe that the rapid improvement seen with ECT is needed. Although the use of ECT is often limited to these three situations, it is an effective antidepressant treatment and can be reasonably considered as the treatment of choice in some patients, such as older depressed people. Phototherapy is a novel treatment that has been used with patients with a seasonal pattern to their mood disorder. It can be used alone in mild cases of mood disorder with a seasonal pattern. For severely affected patients, it can be used in combination with pharmacotherapy, although studies of the efficacy of this combination have not yet produced definitive results.

AVAILABLE DRUGS.

The SSRIs are the most widely used antidepressant drugs in the United States. They are the agents of choice because of their effectiveness, ease of use, and relative lack of adverse effects, even at high dosages. Because they are well tolerated, they have been prescribed by clinicians in a wide range of specialties. Of the other newer agents, citalopram (Celexa), escitalopram (Lexapro), bupropion, venlafaxine (Effexor), fluvoxamine (Luvox), and nefazodone have gained widespread use among psychiatrists. Each of these agents is safer than the tricyclic and tetracyclic drugs and MAOIs, and each has been shown to be as effective for depression in clinical trials. The tricyclic and tetracyclic drugs, trazodone (Desyrel), alprazolam (Xanax), and mirtazapine, may cause sedation. The MAOIs require dietary restrictions. These drugs are less widely used because of their adverse effects. Sympathomimetic drugs, such as dextroamphetamine (Dexedrine) and methylphenidate (Ritalin), may produce a rapid improvement of mood (within 1 week) and are indicated in closely monitored situations. (See Chapter 32 for an extensive discussion of drugs used in depression and mania.)

PHARMACOLOGICAL ACTIONS.

In patients who tolerate full therapeutic dosages of the various available antidepressants, no one agent has shown an obvious superiority. There are marked differences, however, in adverse effect profiles, and individual patients may respond to one antidepressant and not to another. Most antidepressants interact with either serotonergic or noradrenergic neurotransmission or with both. Moreover, potentiation of either of these neurotransmitter systems has been shown to stimulate the other system, such that the details of the pharmacodynamics of each drug are difficult to translate into a prediction of efficacy.

The MAOIs are less frequently chosen because they may cause a hypertensive crisis if patients ingest foods with a high content of tyramine, which requires strict adherence to a simple set of dietary guidelines. Alprazolam, a benzodiazepine, is U.S.

Food and Drug Administration (FDA)–approved for treatment of depression, but it is rarely used because of concerns about sedation and because it may be addictive and may be very difficult to discontinue. Sympathomimetics, although among the most effective antidepressants, are rarely used because of concerns for abuse, even though this is unlikely at the low dosages usually necessary for treatment of depression.

ADVERSE EFFECTS. One of the most serious concerns about antidepressants is their lethality when taken in overdoses. Tricyclic and tetracyclic drugs are, by far, the most lethal of the antidepressants; the SSRIs, bupropion, trazodone, nefazodone, mirtazapine, venlafaxine, and the MAOIs are safer, although even these drugs can be lethal when taken in overdose in combination with alcohol or other drugs. Another concern about antidepressants is their cardiac safety. Again, tricyclic and tetracyclic drugs are generally the least safe. Hypotension is a potentially serious adverse effect of many antidepressants, particularly in older people. Among the conventional antidepressants, amoxapine (Asendin), maprotiline (Ludiomil), nortriptyline, and trazodone are associated with little hypotension, and bupropion and the SSRIs are associated with the least hypotension. One set of adverse effects that many clinicians inappropriately ignore are the sexual adverse effects of antidepressants. Almost all the antidepressants, except nefazodone and mirtazapine, have been associated with decreased libido, erectile dysfunction, or anorgasmia. The serotonergic drugs are probably more closely associated with sexual adverse effects than are the noradrenergic compounds.

DRUG–DRUG INTERACTIONS. Another increasing concern among clinicians prescribing drugs for depressive disorders and conditions are possible drug–drug interactions, especially in regard to the hepatic cytochrome P450 (CYP) enzyme. The CYP isoenzyme system is involved in the metabolism of most drugs, but some people are genetically at risk for developing high blood concentrations of drugs that are metabolized by one of the CYP enzymes, such as CYP 2D6.

TYPE-SPECIFIC TREATMENTS. Some clinical types of major depressive episodes may have varying responses to particular antidepressants. For example, patients with major depressive disorder with atypical features (sometimes called *hysteroid dysphoria*) may preferentially respond to treatment with MAOIs. Two other specific groups are patients with depressed bipolar I disorder and with major depressive episodes with psychotic features.

Lithium is a potential first-line pharmacological agent in treating depression in patients with bipolar I disorder and in some patients with major depressive disorder with a marked periodicity to their disorder. Patients with bipolar I disorder who are being treated with conventional antidepressants must be observed carefully for the emergence of manic symptoms.

Antidepressants alone are not likely to be effective in the treatment of major depressive episodes with psychotic features. One exception may be amoxapine, an antidepressant closely related to loxapine (Loxitane), an antipsychotic; however, clinicians usually use a combination of an antidepressant and an antipsychotic. Several studies have also shown that ECT is effective for this indication—perhaps more effective than pharmacotherapy.

GENERAL CLINICAL GUIDELINES. The most common clinical mistake leading to an unsuccessful trial of an antidepressant drug is the use of too low a dosage for too short a time. Unless adverse events prevent it, the dosage of an antidepressant should be raised to the maximum recommended level and maintained at that level for at least 4 or 5 weeks before a drug trial can be considered unsuccessful. Alternatively, if a patient is improving clinically on a low dosage of the drug, this dosage should not be raised unless clinical improvement stops before the maximal benefit is obtained. When a patient does not begin to respond to appropriate dosages of a drug after 2 or 3 weeks, clinicians may decide to obtain a plasma concentration of the drug if the test is available for the particular drug being used. The test may indicate either noncompliance or particularly unusual pharmacokinetic disposition of the drug and may thereby suggest an alternative dosage.

DURATION AND PROPHYLAXIS. Antidepressant treatment should be maintained for at least 6 months or the length of a previous episode, whichever is greater. Several studies show that prophylactic treatment with antidepressants is effective in reducing the number and severity of recurrences. Conclusions drawn from one study were that, when episodes are less than 2 1/2 years apart, prophylactic treatment for 5 years is probably indicated. Another factor suggesting prophylactic treatment is the seriousness of previous depressive episodes. Episodes that have involved significant suicidal ideation or impairment of psychosocial functioning may indicate that clinicians should consider prophylactic treatment. When antidepressants are stopped, they should be tapered gradually over 1 to 2 weeks, depending on the half-life of the particular compound. Several studies indicate that maintenance antidepressant medication appears to be safe and effective for the treatment of chronic depression.

FAILURE OF DRUG TRIAL. When the first antidepressant drug has been used for an adequate trial and, if appropriate, clinicians are sure that adequate plasma concentrations were obtained, there are two options if symptoms have not satisfactorily improved: to augment the drug with lithium, liothyronine (the levorotatory isomer of triiodothyronine [T_3]), or L-tryptophan, or to switch to an alternative primary agent. A now rarely used strategy is to combine a tricyclic or tetracyclic drug with an MAOI. When switching agents, clinicians should switch a patient who has been taking a tricyclic or tetracyclic drug to an SSRI (or possibly an MAOI) and should switch a patient who has been taking an SSRI to bupropion, venlafaxine, nefazodone, a tricyclic or tetracyclic drug, mirtazapine, trazodone, or possibly an MAOI. At least 2 weeks should elapse between the use of an SSRI and the use of an MAOI, and the two drugs should never be used concurrently, because a serotonin syndrome might develop.

Lithium. Lithium (900 to 1,200 mg a day, serum level between 0.6 and 0.8 mEq/L) can be added to the antidepressant dosage for 7 to 14 days. This approach converts a significant number of antidepressant nonresponders to responders. The mechanism of action is unknown, although the lithium may potentiate the serotonergic neuronal system. Some data indicate that pretreatment with the antidepressant alone is necessary for this effect and that beginning treatment with the two drugs simultaneously is not as effective as starting with an antidepressant and then adding lithium.

Liothyronine. The addition of 25 to 50 mg a day of liothyronine to an antidepressant regimen for 7 to 14 days may convert antidepressant nonresponders to responders. The adverse effects of liothyronine are minor but may include headaches and feelings of warmth. The mechanism of action for liothyronine augmentation is not known, although the modulation of β-adrenergic receptors and the presence of undetectable thyroid axis abnormalities in major depressive disorder have been suggested. If liothyronine augmentation is successful, the liothyronine should be continued for 2 months and then tapered at the rate of 12.5 mg a day every 3 to 7 days.

L-Tryptophan. L-Tryptophan, the amino acid precursor to serotonin, has been used as an adjuvant both to antidepressant drugs in major depressive disorder and to lithium in bipolar I disorder. L-Tryptophan has also been used alone as an antidepressant and a hypnotic. L-Tryptophan–containing products have been recalled in the United States because of an outbreak of eosinophilia-myalgia syndrome associated with the use of L-tryptophan. The symptoms of the syndrome include fatigue, myalgia, shortness of breath, rashes, and swelling of the extremities. Congestive heart failure and death can also occur. Although several studies have shown that L-tryptophan is an effective adjuvant in the treatment of mood disorders, the drug should not be used for any purpose until the problem with the syndrome is completely resolved. The syndrome is probably related to a contaminant in a single manufacturing plant, but this hypothesis has yet to be tested.

Tricyclic or Tetracyclic Drug and MAOI Combinations. The combination of a tricyclic or tetracyclic drug and an MAOI is sometimes used for patients who have not responded to several other pharmacological treatments. With the availability of a broad range of antidepressants, however, this combination therapy is rarely used. Because of the high incidence of adverse effects, it is not a treatment of first, second, or even third choice. When this combination is used, clinicians should initiate treatment with the two drugs simultaneously at low dosages for each and should then raise the dosages slowly. Imipramine or trimipramine (Surmontil) and an MAOI should not be used in combination because of their high incidence of toxic effects, including restlessness, dizziness, tremulousness, muscle twitching, sweating, convulsions, hyperpyrexia, and sometimes death.

When a patient has been taking a tricyclic or tetracyclic drug, physicians should quarter the dosage of the drug for 5 to 7 days and then slowly add the MAOI to the regimen. When the patient has been taking an MAOI, physicians should stop the drug for 2 weeks and then start the two drugs simultaneously. The reasons for this strategy are that MAOIs irreversibly inhibit monoamine oxidase and that it takes approximately 2 weeks for normal MAO activity levels to be achieved after the use of MAOIs. Figure 12.1–2 provides a useful treatment algorithm.

Bipolar I Disorder. Lithium, divalproex (Depakote), and olanzapine (Zyprexa) are the only FDA–approved treatments for the manic phase of bipolar disorder, but carbamazepine (Tegretol) is also a well-established treatment. Gabapentin (Neurontin) and lamotrigine (Lamictal) are promising treatments for refractory or treatment-intolerant patients. The efficacy of the latter two agents is not well established, but their clinical use is expanding. Topiramate (Topamax) is another anticonvulsant showing benefit in bipolar patients. ECT is highly effective in all phases of bipolar disorder. Carbamazepine, divalproex, and valproic acid (Depakene) appear more effective than lithium in the treatment of mixed or dysphoric mania, rapid cycling, and psychotic mania, and in the treatment of patients with a history of multiple manic episodes or comorbid substances abuse.

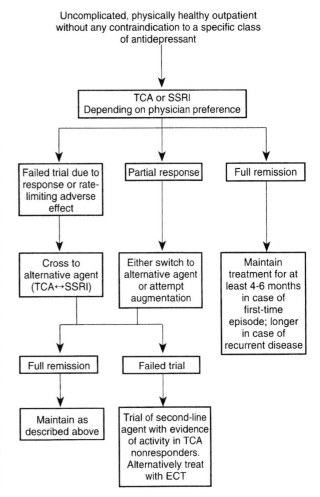

FIGURE 12.1–2

Algorithm for treating patient with major depressive disorder. ECT, electroconvulsive therapy; SSRI, selective serotonin reuptake inhibitor; TCA, tricyclic antidepressant. (Reprinted with permission from Preskorn SH, Burke M. Somatic therapy for major depressive disorder: selection of an antidepressant. *J Clin Psychiatry* 1992;53 [9 Suppl]:10.)

Treatment of acute manic episodes often requires adjunctive use of potent sedative drugs. Drugs commonly used at the start of treatment include clonazepam (1 mg every 4 to 6 hours) and lorazepam (Ativan) (2 mg every 4 to 6 hours). Haloperidol (Haldol) (2 to 10 mg/day), olanzapine (2.6 to 10 mg/day), and risperidone (Risperdal) (0.5 to 6 mg/day) are also of use. Bipolar patients may be particularly sensitive to the side effects of typical antipsychotics. The atypical antipsychotics (e.g., olanzapine [Zyprexa] [10 to 15 mg/day]) are often used as monotherapy for acute control and may have intrinsic antimanic properties. Physicians should attempt to taper these adjunctive agents when the patient stabilizes.

Patients who do not respond adequately to one mood stabilizer may do well with combination treatment. Lithium and valproic acid are commonly used together. Increased neurotoxicity is a risk, but the combination is safe. Other combinations include lithium plus carbamazepine plus valproic acid (requires increasing laboratory monitoring for drug interactions and hepatic toxicity) and combinations with the newer anticonvulsants.

LITHIUM. Lithium is still a standard treatment for bipolar I disorder. The adverse effects that may limit the use of lithium and cause clinicians to consider using either carbamazepine or valproate include renal effects (thirst, polyuria), nervous system effects (tremor, memory loss), metabolic effects (weight gain), gastrointestinal effects (diarrhea), dermatological effects (acne, psoriasis), and thyroid effects (goiter, myxedema). Of potentially serious concern with lithium treatment are its effects on the kidneys, which can include moderate and occasionally severe impairment of tubular function; uncommon, moderate, and unspecific morphological changes; and, rarely, a nephrotic syndrome. These many adverse effects require careful monitoring of patients' renal and thyroid status.

Compliance with lithium treatment is increased with the early initiation of treatment, adequate treatment of concomitant illness, treatment of coexisting substance abuse, early detection and prevention of side effects, and the patient's participation in individual and group psychotherapy. Responsiveness to lithium treatment is improved when adequate lithium levels are maintained, adjunctive medication is used as indicated, and laboratory and clinical monitoring is carried out. Nonresponsiveness to lithium treatment is most likely with severe illness, the presence of schizoaffective disorder symptoms, mixed manic and depressive symptoms, somatic symptoms, alcohol and other substance abuse, rapid cycling, and the absence of a family history of bipolar I disorder. A blood level of 0.8 to 1.2 mEq/L is the effective range.

VALPROATE. The efficacy data for valproate are now sufficient to warrant its use as a first-line drug. A significant number of patients seem to tolerate valproate better than they tolerate lithium and carbamazepine. Valproic acid and divalproex have a broad therapeutic index and appear effective at levels of 50 to 125 g/mL. Pretreatment workup includes a complete blood cell count and liver function tests. A pregnancy test is needed because this drug can cause neural tube defects in developing fetuses. It can cause thrombocytopenia and increased transaminase levels, both of which are usually benign and self-limited but require increased blood monitoring. Fatal hepatic toxicity has been reported only in children younger than 10 years of age who received multiple anticonvulsants. Typical side effects include hair loss (which can be treated with zinc and selenium), tremor, weight gain, and sedation. Gastrointestinal upset is common but can be minimized by using enteric-coated tablets (Depakote) and titrating gradually. Valproic acid can be loaded for acute symptom control by administering at 20 mg/kg in divided doses. This strategy also produces a therapeutic level and may improve symptoms within 7 days. For outpatients, more physically brittle patients, or less severely ill patients, medication can be started at 250 to 750 mg/day and gradually titrated to a therapeutic level. Blood level can be checked after 3 days at a particular dosage.

Carbamazepine. Carbamazepine is usually titrated to response rather than blood level, although many clinicians titrate to reach levels of 4 to 12 µg/mL. Pretreatment evaluation should include liver function tests and a complete blood cell count as well as electrocardiogram, electrolytes, reticulocytes, and pregnancy test. Side effects include nausea, sedation, and ataxia. Hepatic toxicity, hyponatremia, or bone marrow suppression may occur. Rash occurs in 10 percent of patients. Exfoliative rashes

(Stevens-Johnson syndrome) are rare but potentially fatal. The drug can be started at 200 to 600 mg/day, with adjustments every 5 days based on clinical response. Improvement may be seen 7 to 14 days after a therapeutic dose has been achieved. Drug interactions complicate carbamazepine use and probably relegate it to second-line status. It is a potent enzyme inducer and can lower levels of other psychotropics, such as haloperidol. Carbamazepine induces its own metabolism (autoinduction), and the dosage often needs to be increased during the first few months of treatment to maintain a therapeutic level and clinical response.

OTHER ANTICONVULSANTS. Lamotrigine and gabapentin are anticonvulsants that may have antidepressant, antimanic, and mood-stabilizing properties. They do not require blood monitoring. Gabapentin is excreted exclusively by the kidneys. It has a benign side effect profile that can include sedation or activation, dizziness, and fatigue. It does not interact with other drugs. Dose reduction in patients with renal insufficiency is required. Gabapentin can be titrated aggressively, and therapeutic response has been reported at dosages of 300 to 3,600 mg/day. It has a short half-life, and dosing to three times a day is required. Lamotrigine requires gradual titration to decrease the risk for rash, which occurs in 10 percent of patients. Stevens-Johnson syndrome occurs in 0.1 percent of patients treated with lamotrigine. Other side effects include nausea, sedation, ataxia, and insomnia. Dosage can be initiated at 25 to 50 mg/day for 2 weeks and then increased slowly to 150 to 250 mg twice daily. Valproate raises lamotrigine levels. In the presence of valproate, lamotrigine titration should be slower and dosages lower (e.g., 25 mg orally four times daily for 2 weeks, with 25-mg increases every 2 weeks to a maximum of 150 mg/day).

Topiramate has shown preliminary efficacy in bipolar disorders. Its side effects include fatigue and cognitive dulling. This drug has the unique property of causing weight loss. One series of overweight patients with bipolar disorder lost an average of 5 percent of their body weight while taking topiramate as an adjunct to other medications. The starting dosage is usually 25 to 50 mg/day to a maximum of 400 mg/day.

Other Agents.

Other agents used in bipolar disorder include verapamil (Isoptin, Calan), nimodipine (Nimotop), clonidine (Catapres), clonazepam, and levothyroxine (Levoxyl, Levothroid, Synthroid). Clozapine (Clozaril) has been shown to have potent antimanic and mood-stabilizing properties in treatment-refractory patients. ECT may be considered in particularly severe or drug-resistant cases as another alternative treatment of bipolar I disorder.

RAPID CYCLING. The development of rapid cycling in patients with bipolar I disorder has been associated with the use of conventional antidepressants, especially tricyclic drugs, and with the presence of hypothyroidism. In addition to the use of thyroid treatments—that is, levothyroxine (T4) (Levothroid) 0.3 to 0.5 mg a day—some researchers and clinicians have reported preliminary positive results with the use of other psychopharmacological agents, including bupropion and nimodipine.

MAINTENANCE. The decision to maintain a patient on lithium (or other drug) prophylaxis is based on the severity of the patient's disorder, the risk of adverse effects from the particular drug, and the quality of the patient's support systems. Maintenance treatment is generally indicated for the prophylaxis of bipolar I disorder in any patient who has had more than one episode. The rationale for this practice is the relative safety of the available drugs, their demonstrated efficacy, and the significant potential for psychosocial problems if another bipolar I disorder episode occurs. During long-term treatment, laboratory monitoring is required for lithium, valproic acid, and carbamazepine.

Bipolar II Disorder. The treatment of bipolar II disorder must be approached cautiously; treatment for depressive episodes with antidepressants can frequently precipitate a manic episode. Whether typical bipolar I disorder medication strategies (for example, lithium and anticonvulsants) are effective in the treatment of patients with bipolar II disorder is still under investigation. A trial of such agents seems warranted, especially when treatment with antidepressants alone has not been successful.

▲ 12.2 Dysthymia and Cyclothymia

DYSTHYMIC DISORDER

According to the text revision of the fourth edition of *Diagnostic and Statistical Manual of Mental Disorders* (DSM-IV-TR), the most typical features of dysthymic disorder are feelings of inadequacy, guilt, irritability, and anger; withdrawal from society; loss of interest; and inactivity and lack of productivity. The term *dysthymia*, which means "ill humored," was introduced in 1980. Before that time, most patients now classified as having dysthymic disorder were classified as having depressive neurosis (also called *neurotic depression*).

Dysthymic disorder is distinguished from major depressive disorder by the fact that patients complain that they have always been depressed. Thus, most cases are of early onset, beginning in childhood or adolescence and certainly by the time patients reach their 20s. A late-onset subtype, much less prevalent and not well characterized clinically, has been identified among middle-aged and geriatric populations, largely through epidemiological studies in the community. The family history of patients with dysthymia is typically replete with both depressive and bipolar disorders, which is one of the more robust findings supporting its link to primary mood disorder.

Epidemiology

Dysthymic disorder is common among the general population and affects 5 to 6 percent of all people. It is seen among patients in general psychiatric clinics, where it affects between one-half and one-third of all clinic patients. The reported prevalence of dysthymic disorder among young adolescents is approximately 8 percent in boys and 5 percent in girls; however, there are no gender differences for incidence rates. The disorder is more common in women younger than 64 years of age than in men of any age and is more common among unmarried and young people and in those with low incomes. Dysthymic disorder frequently coexists with other mental disorders, particularly major depressive disorder, and in persons with major depressive disor-

der there is a lessened likelihood of full remission between episodes. The patients may also have coexisting anxiety disorders (especially panic disorder), substance abuse, and borderline personality disorder. Dysthymic disorder is more common among those with first-degree relatives with major depressive disorder. Patients with dysthymic disorder are likely to be taking a wide range of psychiatric medications, including antidepressants, antimanic agents such as lithium (Eskalith) and carbamazepine (Tegretol), and sedative-hypnotics.

Etiology

Biological Factors. Some studies of biological measures in dysthymic disorder support its classification with the mood disorders; other studies question this association. One hypothesis drawn from the data is that the biological basis for the symptoms of dysthymic disorder and major depressive disorder are similar, but the biological bases for the underlying pathophysiology in the two disorders differs.

SLEEP STUDIES. Decreased rapid eye movement (REM) latency and increased REM density are two state markers of depression in major depressive disorder that also occur in a significant proportion of patients with dysthymic disorder. Some investigators have reported preliminary data indicating that the presence of these sleep abnormalities in patients with dysthymic disorder predicts a response to antidepressant drugs.

NEUROENDOCRINE STUDIES. The two most studied neuroendocrine axes in major depressive disorder and dysthymic disorder are the adrenal axis and the thyroid axis, which have been tested by using the dexamethasone-suppression test (DST) and the thyrotropin-releasing hormone (TRH)-stimulation test, respectively. Although the results of studies are not absolutely consistent, most studies indicate that patients with dysthymic disorder are less likely to have abnormal results on a DST than are patients with major depressive disorder. Fewer studies of the TRH-stimulation test have been conducted, but they have produced preliminary data indicating that abnormalities in the thyroid axis may be a trait variably associated with chronic illness. A higher percentage of patients with dysthymic disorder have thyroid axis abnormalities than do normal control subjects.

Psychosocial Factors. Psychodynamic theories about the development of dysthymic disorder posit that the disorder results from personality and ego development and culminates in difficulty in adapting to adolescence and young adulthood. Karl Abraham, for example, thought that the conflicts of depression center on oral- and anal-sadistic traits. Anal traits include excessive orderliness, guilt, and concern for others; they are postulated to be a defense against preoccupation with anal matter and with disorganization, hostility, and self-preoccupation. A major defense mechanism used is reaction formation. Low self-esteem, anhedonia, and introversion are often associated with the depressive character.

FREUD. In "Mourning and Melancholia," Sigmund Freud asserted that an interpersonal disappointment early in life can cause a vulnerability to depression that leads to ambivalent love relationships as an adult; real or threatened losses in adult life then trigger depression. People prone to depression are orally dependent and require constant narcissistic gratification. When deprived

Table 12.2–1
DSM-IV-TR Diagnostic Criteria for Dysthymic Disorder

A. Depressed mood for most of the day, for more days than not, as indicated either by subjective account or observation by others, for at least 2 years. **Note:** In children and adolescents, mood can be irritable and duration must be at least 1 year.

B. Presence, while depressed, of two (or more) of the following:

(1) poor appetite or overeating

(2) insomnia or hypersomnia

(3) low energy or fatigue

(4) low self-esteem

(5) poor concentration or difficulty making decisions

(6) feelings of hopelessness

C. During the 2-year period (1 year for children or adolescents) of the disturbance, the person has never been without the symptoms in Criteria A and B for more than 2 months at a time.

D. No major depressive episode has been present during the first 2 years of the disturbance (1 year for children and adolescents); i.e., the disturbance is not better accounted for by chronic major depressive disorder, or major depressive disorder, in partial remission.

Note: There may have been a previous major depressive episode provided there was a full remission (no significant signs or symptoms for 2 months) before development of the dysthymic disorder. In addition, after the initial 2 years (1 year in children or adolescents) of dysthymic disorder, there may be superimposed episodes of major depressive disorder, in which case both diagnoses may be given when the criteria are met for a major depressive episode.

E. There has never been a manic episode, a mixed episode, or a hypomanic episode, and criteria have never been met for cyclothymic disorder.

F. The disturbance does not occur exclusively during the course of a chronic psychotic disorder, such as schizophrenia or delusional disorder.

G. The symptoms are not due to the direct physiological effects of a substance (e.g., a drug of abuse, a medication) or a general medical condition (e.g., hypothyroidism).

H. The symptoms cause clinically significant distress or impairment in social, occupational, or other important areas of functioning.

Specify if:

Early onset: if onset is before age 21 years

Late onset: if onset is age 21 years or older

Specify (for most recent 2 years of dysthymic disorder):

With atypical features

From American Psychiatric Association. *Diagnostic and Statistical Manual of Mental Disorders.* 4th ed. Text rev. Washington, DC: American Psychiatric Association; copyright 2000, with permission.

of love, affection, and care, they become clinically depressed; when they experience a real loss, they internalize or introject the lost object and turn their anger on it and, thus, on themselves.

COGNITIVE THEORY. The cognitive theory of depression also applies to dysthymic disorder. It holds that a disparity between actual and fantasized situations leads to diminished self-esteem and a sense of helplessness. The success of cognitive therapy in

the treatment of some patients with dysthymic disorder may provide some support for the theoretical model.

Diagnosis and Clinical Features

The DSM-IV-TR diagnosis criteria for dysthymic disorder (Table 12.2–1) stipulate the presence of a depressed mood most of the time for at least 2 years (or 1 year for children and adolescents). To meet the diagnostic criteria, a patient should not have symptoms that are better accounted for as major depressive disorder and should never have had a manic or hypomanic episode. DSM-IV-TR allows clinicians to specify whether the onset was early (before age 21) or late (age 21 or older). DSM-IV-TR also allows for the specification of atypical features in dysthymic disorder (Table 12.1–1).

The profile of dysthymic disorder overlaps with that of major depressive disorder but differs from it in that symptoms tend to outnumber signs (more subjective than objective depression). This means that disturbances in appetite and libido are uncharacteristic, and psychomotor agitation or retardation is not observed. This all translates into a depression with attenuated symptomatology. However, subtle endogenous features are observed: inertia, lethargy, and anhedonia that are characteristically worse in the morning. Because patients presenting clinically often fluctuate in and out of a major depression, the core DSM-IV-TR criteria for dysthymic disorder tend to emphasize vegetative dysfunction, whereas the alternative Criterion B for dysthymic disorder (Table 12.2–2) in a DSM-IV-TR appendix lists cognitive symptoms.

A 27-year-old male grade-school teacher presented with the chief complaint that life was a painful duty that had always lacked luster for him. He said he felt enveloped by a sense of gloom that was nearly always with him. Although he was respected by his peers, he felt "like a grotesque failure, a self-concept I have had since childhood." He stated that he merely performed his responsibilities as a teacher and that he had never derived any pleasure from anything he had done in life. He said he had never had any romantic feelings; sexual activity, in which he had engaged with two different women, had involved pleasureless orgasm. He said he felt empty, going through life without any sense of direction, ambition, or passion, a realization that itself was tormenting. (Courtesy of Hagop S. Akiskal, M.D.)

Dysthymic Variants. Dysthymia is not uncommon in patients with chronically disabling physical disorders, particularly among elderly adults. Dysthymia-like clinically significant subthreshold depression lasting 6 or more months has also been described in neurological conditions, including stroke. According to a recent World Health Organization (WHO) conference, this condition aggravates the prognosis of the underlying neurological disease and, therefore, deserves pharmacotherapy.

Differential Diagnosis

The differential diagnosis for dysthymic disorder is essentially identical to that for major depressive disorder. Many substances and medical illnesses can cause chronic depressive symptoms.

Table 12.2–2
DSM-IV-TR Alternative Research Criterion B for Dysthymic Disorder

B. Presence, while depressed, of three (or more) of the following:

(1) low self-esteem or self-confidence, or feelings of inadequacy

(2) feelings of pessimism, despair, or hopelessness

(3) generalized loss of interest or pleasure

(4) social withdrawal

(5) chronic fatigue or tiredness

(6) feelings of guilt, brooding about the past

(7) subjective feelings of irritability or excessive anger

(8) decreased activity, effectiveness, or productivity

(9) difficulty in thinking, reflected by poor concentration, poor memory, or indecisiveness

From American Psychiatric Association. *Diagnostic and Statistical Manual of Mental Disorders.* 4th ed. Text rev. Washington, DC: American Psychiatric Association; copyright 2000, with permission.

Two disorders are particularly important to consider in the differential diagnosis of dysthymic disorder—minor depressive disorder and recurrent brief depressive disorder.

Minor Depressive Disorder. Minor depressive disorder (discussed in Section 12.3) is characterized by episodes of depressive symptoms that are less severe than those seen in major depressive disorder. The difference between dysthymic disorder and minor depressive disorder is primarily the episodic nature of the symptoms in the latter. Between episodes, patients with minor depressive disorder have a euthymic mood, whereas patients with dysthymic disorder have virtually no euthymic periods.

Recurrent Brief Depressive Disorder. Recurrent brief depressive disorder (discussed in Section 12.3) is characterized by brief periods (less than 2 weeks) during which depressive episodes are present. Patients with the disorder would meet the diagnostic criteria for major depressive disorder if their episodes lasted longer. Patients with recurrent brief depressive disorder differ from patients with dysthymic disorder on two counts: They have an episodic disorder, and the severity of their symptoms is greater.

Double Depression. An estimated 40 percent of patients with major depressive disorder also meet the criteria for dysthymic disorder, a combination often referred to as *double depression*. Available data support the conclusion that patients with double depression have a poorer prognosis than do patients with only major depressive disorder. The treatment of patients with double depression should be directed toward both disorders, as the resolution of the symptoms of major depressive episode still leaves these patients with significant psychiatric impairment.

Alcohol and Substance Abuse. Patients with dysthymic disorder commonly meet the diagnostic criteria for a substance-related disorder. This comorbidity can be logical: Patients with dysthymic disorder tend to develop coping methods for their chronically depressed state. Therefore, they are likely to use alcohol, or stimulants such as cocaine, or marijuana, the choice perhaps depending primarily on a patient's social context. The presence of a comorbid diagnosis of substance abuse presents a diagnostic dilemma for clinicians; the long-term use of many substances can result in a symptom picture indistinguishable from that of dysthymic disorder.

Course and Prognosis

Approximately 50 percent of patients with dysthymic disorder experience an insidious onset of symptoms before age 25. Despite the early onset, patients often suffer with the symptoms for a decade before seeking psychiatric help and may consider early-onset dysthymic disorder simply as part of life. Patients with an early onset of symptoms are at risk for either major depressive disorder or bipolar I disorder in the course of their disorder. Studies of patients with the diagnosis of dysthymic disorder indicated that approximately 20 percent progressed to major depressive disorder, 15 percent to bipolar II disorder, and less than 5 percent to bipolar I disorder.

The prognosis for patients with dysthymic disorder is variable. Antidepressive agents (for example, fluoxetine [Prozac] and bupropion [Wellbutrin]) and specific types of psychotherapies (for example, cognitive and behavior therapies) have positive effects on the course and prognosis of dysthymic disorder. The available data about previously available treatments indicate that only 10 to 15 percent of patients are in remission 1 year after the initial diagnosis. Approximately 25 percent of all patients with dysthymic disorder never attain a complete recovery. Overall, however, the prognosis is good with treatment.

Treatment

Historically, patients with dysthymic disorder either received no treatment or were seen as candidates for long-term, insight-oriented psychotherapy. Contemporary data offer the most objective support for cognitive therapy, behavior therapy, and pharmacotherapy. The combination of pharmacotherapy and either cognitive or behavior therapy may be the most effective treatment for the disorder.

Cognitive Therapy. Cognitive therapy is a technique in which patients are taught new ways of thinking and behaving to replace faulty negative attitudes about themselves, the world, and the future. It is a short-term therapy program oriented toward current problems and their resolution.

Behavior Therapy. Behavior therapy for depressive disorders is based on the theory that depression is caused by a loss of positive reinforcement as a result of separation, death, or sudden environmental change. The various treatment methods focus on specific goals to increase activity, to provide pleasant experiences, and to teach patients how to relax. Altering personal behavior in depressed patients is believed to be the most effective way to change the associated depressed thoughts and feelings. Behavior therapy is often used to treat the learned helplessness of some patients who seem to meet every life challenge with a sense of impotence.

Insight-Oriented Psychoanalytic Psychotherapy. Individual insight-oriented psychotherapy is the most common treatment method for dysthymic disorder, and many clinicians believe it to be the treatment of choice. The psychotherapeutic approach attempts to relate the development and the maintenance of depressive symptoms and maladaptive personality features to unresolved conflicts from early childhood. Insight into depressive equivalents (such as substance abuse) or into childhood disappointments as antecedents to adult depression can be gained through treatment. Ambivalent current relationships with parents, friends, and others in the patient's current life are examined. Patients' understanding of how they try to gratify an excessive need for outside approval to counter low self-esteem and a harsh superego is an important goal in the therapy.

Dysthymic disorder involves a chronic state of depression that for certain people becomes a way of life. These people consciously experience themselves to be at the mercy of a tormenting internal object that is unrelenting in its persecution. Usually conceptualized as a harsh superego, the internal agency criticizes them, punishes them for not measuring up to expectations, and generally contributes to their feelings of misery and unhappiness. This pattern may be associated with self-defeating tendencies because patients do not feel that they deserve to be successful. They may also have a long-standing sense of despair about ever getting their emotional needs met by important people in their lives. The patients' bleak outlook on life and their pessimism about relationships result in a self-fulfilling prophecy—many people avoid them because their company is unpleasant.

Interpersonal Therapy. In interpersonal therapy for depressive disorders, a patient's current interpersonal experiences and ways of coping with stress are examined to reduce depressive symptoms and to improve self-esteem. Interpersonal therapy lasts for approximately 12 to 16 weekly sessions and can be combined with antidepressant medication.

Family and Group Therapies. Family therapy may help both the patient and the patient's family deal with the symptoms of the disorder, especially when a biologically based subaffective syndrome seems to be present. Group therapy may help withdrawn patients learn new ways to overcome their interpersonal problems in social situations.

Pharmacotherapy. Because of long-standing and commonly held theoretical beliefs that dysthymic disorder is primarily a psychologically determined disorder, many clinicians avoid prescribing antidepressants for patients, but many studies have shown therapeutic success with antidepressants. The data generally indicate that selective serotonin reuptake inhibitors (SSRIs) are of use for patients with dysthymic disorder. Reports indicate that the SSRIs may be the drugs of choice. Similarly, bupropion may also be an effective treatment for patients with dysthymic disorder. Monoamine oxidase inhibitors (MAOIs) are effective in a subgroup of dysthymic patients, a group who may also respond to the judicious use of amphetamines.

FAILURE OF THERAPEUTIC TRIAL. A therapeutic trial of an antidepressant in the treatment of dysthymic disorder should include maximal tolerated dosages for a minimum of 8 weeks before clinicians conclude that the trial was not effective. When a drug trial is unsuccessful, clinicians should reconsider the diagnosis, especially the possibility of an underlying medical disorder (especially a thyroid disorder) or adult attention-deficit disorder. When a reconsideration of the differential diagnosis still suggests that dysthymic disorder is the most likely diagnosis, clinicians may follow the same therapeutic strategy as for major depressive disorder and may attempt to augment the first antidepressant by adding lithium or liothyronine (Cytomel), although augmentation strategies for dysthymic disorder have not been studied. As an alternative, clinicians may decide to switch to an antidepressant from a completely different class of drugs. For example, if a trial with an SSRI is unsuccessful, a clinician may switch to bupropion, a MAOI, or tricyclics. There are some reports of augmentation with testosterone in men who are treatment resistant.

Hospitalization. Hospitalization is usually not indicated for patients with dysthymic disorder, but particularly severe symptoms, marked social or professional incapacitation, the need for extensive diagnostic procedures, and suicidal ideation are all indications for hospitalization.

CYCLOTHYMIC DISORDER

Cyclothymic disorder is symptomatically a mild form of bipolar II disorder, characterized by episodes of hypomania and mild depression. In DSM-IV-TR, cyclothymic disorder is defined as a "chronic, fluctuating disturbance" with many periods of hypomania and of depression. The disorder is differentiated from bipolar II disorder, which is characterized by the presence of major, not minor, depressive and hypomanic episodes. As with dysthymic disorder, the inclusion of cyclothymic disorder with the mood disorders implies a relation, probably biological, to bipolar I disorder. Some psychiatrists, however, consider cyclothymic disorder to have no biological component, to be distinct from bipolar I disorder, and to result from chaotic object relations early in life.

Contemporary understanding of cyclothymic disorder is based to some extent on the observations of Emil Kraepelin and Kurt Schneider that one-third to two-thirds of patients with mood disorders exhibit personality disorders. Kraepelin described four types of personality disorders: depressive (gloomy), manic (cheerful and uninhibited), irritable (labile and explosive), and cyclothymic. He described the irritable personality as simultaneously depressive and manic and the cyclothymic personality as the alternation of the depressive and manic personalities.

Epidemiology

Patients with cyclothymic disorder may constitute from 3 to 5 percent of all psychiatric outpatients, perhaps particularly those with significant complaints about marital and interpersonal difficulties. In the general population, the lifetime prevalence of cyclothymic disorder is estimated to be approximately 1 percent. This figure is probably lower than the actual prevalence, because, as with patients with bipolar I disorder, the patients may not be aware that they have a psychiatric problem. Cyclothymic disorder, like dysthymic disorder, frequently coexists with borderline personality disorder. An estimated 10 percent of outpatients and 20 percent of inpatients with borderline personality disorder have a coexisting diagnosis of cyclothymic disorder. The female-to-male ratio in cyclothymic disorder is approximately 3 to 2, and 50 to 75 percent of all patients have an onset between ages 15 and 25. Families of persons with cyclothymic disorder often contain members with substance-related disorder.

Etiology

As with dysthymic disorder, there is controversy about whether cyclothymic disorder is related to the mood disorders, either biologically or psychologically. Some researchers have postulated that cyclothymic disorder has a closer relation to borderline personality disorder than to the mood disorders. In spite of these controversies, the preponderance of biological and genetic data favors the ideas of cyclothymic disorder as a bona fide mood disorder.

Biological Factors.   The strongest evidence for the hypothesis that cyclothymic disorder is a mood disorder is the genetic data. Approximately 30 percent of all patients with cyclothymic disorder have positive family histories for bipolar I disorder; this rate is similar to the rate for patients with bipolar I disorder. Moreover, the pedigrees of families with bipolar I disorder often contain generations of patients with bipolar I disorder linked by a generation with cyclothymic disorder. Conversely, the prevalence of cyclothymic disorder in the relatives of patients with bipolar I disorder is much higher than is the prevalence of cyclothymic disorder, either in the relatives of patients with other mental disorders or in people who are mentally healthy. The observations that approximately one-third of patients with cyclothymic disorder subsequently have major mood disorders, that they are particularly sensitive to antidepressant-induced hypomania, and that approximately 60 percent respond to lithium add further support to the idea of cyclothymic disorder as a mild or attenuated form of bipolar II disorder.

Psychosocial Factors.   Most psychodynamic theories postulate that the development of cyclothymic disorder lies in traumas and fixations during the oral stage of infant development. Freud hypothesized that the cyclothymic state is the ego's attempt to overcome a harsh and punitive superego. Hypomania is explained psychodynamically as the lack of self-criticism and an absence of inhibitions occurring when a depressed person throws off the burden of an overly harsh superego. The major defense mechanism in hypomania is denial, by which the patient avoids external problems and internal feelings of depression.

Patients with cyclothymic disorder are characterized by periods of depression alternating with periods of hypomania. Psychoanalytic exploration reveals that such patients defend themselves against underlying depressive themes with their euphoric or hypomanic periods. Hypomania is frequently triggered by a profound interpersonal loss. The false euphoria generated in such instances is a patient's way to deny dependence on love objects while simultaneously disavowing any aggression or destructiveness that may have contributed to the loss of the loved person. Hypomania may also be associated with an unconscious fantasy that the lost object has been restored. This denial is generally short-lived, and the patient soon resumes the preoccupation with suffering and misery characteristic of dysthymic disorder.

Diagnosis and Clinical Features

Although many patients seek psychiatric help for depression, their problems are often related to the chaos that their manic episodes have caused. Clinicians must consider a diagnosis of cyclothymic disorder when a patient appears with what may seem to be sociopathic behavioral problems. Marital difficulties and instability in relationships are common complaints because patients with cyclothymic disorder are often promiscuous and irritable while in manic and mixed states. Although there are anecdotal reports of increased productivity and creativity when

Table 12.2–3
DSM-IV-TR Diagnostic Criteria for Cyclothymic Disorder

A. For at least 2 years, the presence of numerous periods with hypomanic symptoms and numerous periods with depressive symptoms that do not meet criteria for a major depressive episode. **Note:** In children and adolescents, the duration must be at least 1 year.

B. During the above 2-year period (1 year in children and adolescents), the person has not been without the symptoms in Criterion A for more than 2 months at a time.

C. No major depressive episode, manic episode, or mixed episode has been present during the first 2 years of the disturbance.

   Note: After the initial 2 years (1 year in children and adolescents) of cyclothymic disorder, there may be superimposed manic or mixed episodes (in which case both bipolar I disorder and cyclothymic disorder may be diagnosed) or major depressive episodes (in which case both bipolar II disorder and cyclothymic disorder may be diagnosed).

D. The symptoms in Criterion A are not better accounted for by schizoaffective disorder and are not superimposed on schizophrenia, schizophreniform disorder, delusional disorder, or psychotic disorder not otherwise specified.

E. The symptoms are not due to the direct physiological effects of a substance (e.g., a drug of abuse, a medication) or a general medical condition (e.g., hyperthyroidism).

F. The symptoms cause clinically significant distress or impairment in social, occupational, or other important areas of functioning.

From American Psychiatric Association. *Diagnostic and Statistical Manual of Mental Disorders.* 4th ed. Text rev. Washington, DC: American Psychiatric Association; copyright 2000, with permission.

patients are hypomanic, most clinicians report that their patients become disorganized and ineffective in work and school during these periods.

The DSM-IV-TR diagnostic criteria for cyclothymic disorder (Table 12.2–3) stipulate that a patient has never met the criteria for a major depressive episode and did not meet the criteria for a manic episode during the first 2 years of the disturbance. The criteria also require the more or less constant presence of symptoms for 2 years (or 1 year for children and adolescents).

Signs and Symptoms.   The symptoms of cyclothymic disorder are identical to the symptoms of bipolar II disorder, except that they are generally less severe. On occasion, however, the symptoms may be equal in severity but of shorter duration than those seen in bipolar II disorder. Approximately half of all patients with cyclothymic disorder have depression as their major symptom, and these patients are most likely to seek psychiatric help while depressed. Some patients with cyclothymic disorder have primarily hypomanic symptoms and are less likely to consult a psychiatrist than are primarily depressed patients. Almost all patients with cyclothymic disorder have periods of mixed symptoms with marked irritability.

Most patients with cyclothymic disorder seen by psychiatrists have not succeeded in their professional and social lives as a result of their disorder, but a few have become high achievers who have worked especially long hours and have required little sleep. Some people's ability to successfully control the symptoms of the disorder depends on multiple individual, social, and cultural attributes.

The lives of most patients with cyclothymic disorder are difficult. The cycles of the disorder tend to be much shorter than those in bipolar I disorder. In cyclothymic disorder, the changes in mood are irregular and abrupt and sometimes occur within hours. Occasional periods of normal mood and the unpredictable nature of the mood changes produce great stress. Patients often feel that their moods are out of control. In irritable, mixed periods, they may become involved in unprovoked disagreements with friends, family, and coworkers.

Substance Abuse. Alcohol and other substance abuse are common in cyclothymic disorder patients, who use substances either to self-medicate (with alcohol, benzodiazepines, and marijuana) or to achieve even further stimulation (with cocaine, amphetamines, and hallucinogens) when they are manic. Approximately 5 to 10 percent of all patients with cyclothymic disorder have substance dependence. People with this disorder often have a history of multiple geographical moves, involvements in religious cults, and dilettantism.

Differential Diagnosis

When a diagnosis of cyclothymic disorder is under consideration, all the possible medical and substance-related causes of depression and mania such as seizures and particular substances (cocaine, amphetamine, and steroids) must be considered. Borderline, antisocial, histrionic, and narcissistic personality disorders should also be considered in the differential diagnosis. Attention-deficit/hyperactivity disorder (ADHD) can be difficult to differentiate from cyclothymic disorder in children and adolescents. A trial of stimulants helps most patients with attention-deficit/hyperactivity disorder and exacerbates the symptoms of most patients with cyclothymic disorder. The diagnostic category of bipolar II disorder (discussed in Section 12.1) is characterized by the combination of major depressive and hypomanic episodes.

Course and Prognosis

Some patients with cyclothymic disorder are characterized as having been sensitive, hyperactive, or moody as young children. The onset of frank symptoms of cyclothymic disorder often occurs insidiously in the teens or early 20s. The emergence of symptoms at that time hinders a person's performance in school and the ability to establish friendships with peers. The reactions of patients to such a disorder vary; patients with adaptive coping strategies or ego defenses have better outcomes than do patients with poor coping strategies. Approximately one-third of all patients with cyclothymic disorder develop a major mood disorder, most often bipolar II disorder.

Treatment

Biological Therapy. The mood stabilizers and antimanic drugs are the first line of treatment for patients with cyclothymic disorder. Although the experimental data are limited to studies with lithium, other antimanic agents—for example, car-

bamazepine and valproate (Depakene)—are reported to be effective. Dosages and plasma concentrations of these agents should be the same as those in bipolar I disorder. Antidepressant treatment of depressed patients with cyclothymic disorder should be done with caution, because these patients have increased susceptibility to antidepressant-induced hypomanic or manic episodes. Approximately 40 to 50 percent of all patients with cyclothymic disorder who are treated with antidepressants experience such episodes. Anticonvulsants such as gabapentin have been of use in some patients. Clonazepam has been useful to control cyclothymic patients who are agitated periodically.

Psychosocial Therapy. Psychotherapy for patients with cyclothymic disorder is best directed toward increasing patients' awareness of their condition and helping them develop coping mechanisms for their mood swings. Therapists usually need to help patients repair any damage, both work and family related, done during episodes of hypomania. Because of the long-term nature of cyclothymic disorder, patients often require lifelong treatment. Family and group therapies may be supportive, educational, and therapeutic for patients and for those involved in their lives. The psychiatrist conducting psychotherapy is able to evaluate the degree of cyclothymia and so provide an early-warning system to prevent full-blown manic attacks before they occur.

▲ 12.3 Other Mood Disorders

DEPRESSIVE DISORDER NOT OTHERWISE SPECIFIED

If a patient exhibits depressive symptoms as the major feature and does not meet the diagnostic criteria for any other mood disorder, the most appropriate diagnosis is a depressive disorder not otherwise specified (Table 12.3–1). There are three types: (1) minor depressive disorder, (2) recurrent brief disorder, and (3) premenstrual dysphoric disorder.

Minor Depressive Disorder

The literature in the United States on minor depressive disorder is limited, in part by the fact that the term *minor depression* is used to describe a wide range of disorders, including what is called dysthymic disorder in fourth revised edition of the *Diagnostic and Statistical Manual of Mental Disorders* (DSM-IV-TR). The information about this disorder is supplemented considerably in an appendix of DSM-IV-TR by the introduction of specific diagnostic guidelines that allow researchers to use a single definition of the disorder.

Epidemiology. The epidemiology of minor depressive disorder is unknown, but preliminary data indicate that it may be as common as major depressive disorder—that is, approximately 5 percent prevalence in the general population. Preliminary data also indicate that the

Table 12.3–1
DSM-IV-TR Diagnostic Criteria for Depressive Disorder Not Otherwise Specified

The depressive disorder not otherwise specified category includes disorders with depressive features that do not meet the criteria for major depressive disorder, dysthymic disorder, adjustment disorder with depressed mood, or adjustment disorder with mixed anxiety and depressed mood. Sometimes depressive symptoms can present as part of an anxiety disorder not otherwise specified. Examples of depressive disorder not otherwise specified include

1. Premenstrual dysphoric disorder: in most menstrual cycles during the past year, symptoms (e.g., markedly depressed mood, marked anxiety, marked affective lability, decreased interest in activities) regularly occurred during the last week of the luteal phase (and remitted within a few days of the onset of menses). These symptoms must be severe enough to markedly interfere with work, school, or usual activities and be entirely absent for at least 1 week postmenses.
2. Minor depressive disorder: episodes of at least 2 weeks of depressive symptoms but with fewer than the five items required for major depressive disorder.
3. Recurrent brief depressive disorder: depressive episodes lasting from 2 days up to 2 weeks, occurring at least once a month for 12 months (not associated with the menstrual cycle).
4. Postpsychotic depressive disorder of schizophrenia: a major depressive episode that occurs during the residual phase of schizophrenia.
5. A major depressive episode superimposed on delusional disorder, psychotic disorder not otherwise specified, or the active phase of schizophrenia.
6. Situations in which the clinician has concluded that a depressive disorder is present but is unable to determine whether it is primary, due to a general medical condition, or substance induced.

disorder is more common in women than in men. Minor depressive disorder probably affects people of virtually any age, from childhood onward.

Etiology.   The cause of minor depressive disorder is unknown. The same causative considerations given major depressive disorder should be considered. Specifically, the biological theories involve the activities of noradrenergic and serotonergic biogenic amine systems and the thyroid and adrenal neuroendocrine axes. The psychological theories center on issues of loss, guilt, and punitive superegos.

Diagnosis and Clinical Features.   Except that they are of lesser severity, the clinical features of minor depressive disorder are virtually identical to those of major depressive disorder (Table 12.3–2). The central symptom of both disorders is the same—a depressed mood. Periods of sadness as part of the vicissitudes of living should not be confused with minor depressive disorder.

Differential Diagnosis.   The differential diagnosis for minor depressive disorder is the same as that for major depressive disorder. Of special importance for the differential diagnosis of minor depressive disorder are dysthymic disorder and recurrent brief depressive disorder. Dysthymic disorder is characterized by the presence of chronic depres-

Table 12.3–2
DSM-IV-TR Research Criteria for Minor Depressive Disorder

A. A mood disturbance, defined as follows:
   (1) at least two (but less than five) of the following symptoms have been present during the same 2-week period and represent a change from previous functioning; at least one of the symptoms is either (a) or (b):
      (a) depressed mood most of the day, nearly every day, as indicated by either subjective report (e.g., feels sad or empty) or observation made by others (e.g., appears tearful). **Note:** In children and adolescents, can be irritable mood.
      (b) markedly diminished interest or pleasure in all, or almost all, activities most of the day, nearly every day (as indicated by either subjective account or observation made by others)
      (c) significant weight loss when not dieting or weight gain (e.g., a change of more than 5% of body weight in a month), or decrease or increase in appetite nearly every day. **Note:** In children, consider failure to make expected weight gains.
      (d) insomnia or hypersomnia nearly every day
      (e) psychomotor agitation or retardation nearly every day (observable by others, not merely subjective feelings of restlessness or being slowed down)
      (f) fatigue or loss of energy nearly every day
      (g) feelings of worthlessness or excessive or inappropriate guilt (which may be delusional) nearly every day (not merely self-reproach or guilt about being sick)
      (h) diminished ability to think or concentrate, or indecisiveness, nearly every day (either by subjective account or as observed by others)
      (i) recurrent thoughts of death (not just fear of dying), recurrent suicidal ideation without a specific plan, or a suicide attempt or a specific plan for committing suicide
   (2) the symptoms cause clinically significant distress or impairment in social, occupational, or other important areas of functioning
   (3) the symptoms are not due to the direct physiological effects of a substance (e.g., a drug of abuse, a medication) or a general medical condition (e.g., hypothyroidism)
   (4) the symptoms are not better accounted for by bereavement (i.e., a normal reaction to the death of a loved one)
B. There has never been a major depressive episode, and criteria are not met for dysthymic disorder.
C. There has never been a manic episode, a mixed episode, or a hypomanic episode, and criteria are not met for cyclothymic disorder. **Note:** This exclusion does not apply if all of the manic-, mixed-, or hypomanic-like episodes are substance or treatment induced.
D. The mood disturbance does not occur exclusively during schizophrenia, schizophreniform disorder, schizoaffective disorder, delusional disorder, or psychotic disorder not otherwise specified.

sive symptoms, whereas recurrent brief depressive disorder is characterized by multiple brief episodes of severe depressive symptoms.

Course and Prognosis.   No definitive data on the course and the prognosis of minor depressive disorder are available, but minor depressive disorder, probably like major depressive disorder, has a long-term course that may require long-term treatment. A significant proportion of patients with minor depressive disorder are probably at risk for other mood disorders, including dysthymic disorder, bipolar I disorder, bipolar II disorder, and major depressive disorder.

Treatment.   The treatment of minor depressive disorder can include psychotherapy, pharmacotherapy, or both. Some psychotherapists advocate using multiple psychotherapeutic approaches, but using the psychotherapy data for major depressive disorder is a more conservative approach. Insight-oriented psychotherapy, cognitive therapy, interpersonal therapy, and behavior therapy are the psychotherapeutic treatments for major depressive disorder and, by implication, for minor depressive disorder. Patients with minor depressive disorder are probably responsive to pharmacotherapy, particularly selective serotonin reuptake inhibitors (SSRIs) and bupropion (Wellbutrin).

Recurrent Brief Depressive Disorder

Recurrent brief depressive disorder is characterized by multiple, relatively brief episodes (of less than 2 weeks) of depressive symptoms that, except for their brief duration, meet the diagnostic criteria for major depressive disorder. Recurrent brief depressive disorder has been written about mostly in the European literature, but with its introduction as a research category in the appendix of DSM-IV-TR, the diagnosis is likely to gain rapid acceptance in the United States. This acceptance will likely be further facilitated by clinicians' increasing awareness that recurrent brief depressive disorder is relatively common and associated with significant morbidity.

Epidemiology.   Extensive studies of the epidemiology of recurrent brief depressive disorder have not been conducted in the United States. Available data indicate that the 10-year prevalence rate for the disorder is estimated to be 10 percent for people in their 20s; the 1-year prevalence rate for the general population is estimated to be 5 percent. These numbers indicate that recurrent brief depressive disorder is most common among young adults, but many more studies must be conducted to refine the data.

Etiology.   One study showed that patients with recurrent brief depressive disorder share several biological abnormalities with patients with major depressive disorder as compared with control subjects who are mentally healthy. The variables include nonsuppression on the dexamethasone-suppression test (DST), a blunt response to thyrotropin-releasing hormone (TRH), and a shortening of rapid eye movement (REM) sleep latency. The data are consistent with the idea that recurrent brief depressive disorder is closely related to major depressive disorder in its cause and pathophysiology. The available data also suggest a close relation between the two disorders and indicate that family histories of mood disorders are similar for recurrent brief depressive disorder and major depressive disorder.

Diagnosis and Clinical Features.   The clinical features of recurrent brief depressive disorder are almost identical to those of major depressive disorder (Table 12.3–3). One subtle difference is that the lives of patients with recurrent brief depressive disorder may seem more disrupted or chaotic because of the frequent changes in their moods than the lives of patients with major depressive disorder, whose depressive episodes occur at a measured pace. In one study, the mean length of time between depressive disorder episodes in recurrent brief

Table 12.3–3
DSM-IV-TR Research Criteria for Recurrent Brief Depressive Disorder

A. Criteria, except for duration, are met for a major depressive episode.

B. The depressive periods in Criterion A last at least 2 days but less than 2 weeks.

C. The depressive periods occur at least once a month for 12 consecutive months and are not associated with the menstrual cycle.

D. The periods of depressed mood cause clinically significant distress or impairment in social, occupational, or other important areas of functioning.

E. The symptoms are not due to the direct physiological effects of a substance (e.g., a drug of abuse, a medication) or a general medical condition (e.g., hypothyroidism).

F. There has never been a major depressive episode, and criteria are not met for dysthymic disorder.

G. There has never been a manic episode, a mixed episode, or a hypomanic episode, and criteria are not met for cyclothymic disorder. **Note:** This exclusion does not apply if all of the manic-, mixed-, or hypomanic-like episodes are substance or treatment induced.

H. The mood disturbance does not occur exclusively during schizophrenia, schizophreniform disorder, schizoaffective disorder, delusional disorder, or psychotic disorder not otherwise specified.

From American Psychiatric Association. *Diagnostic and Statistical Manual of Mental Disorders.* 4th ed. Text rev. Washington, DC: American Psychiatric Association; copyright 2000, with permission.

depressive disorder was calculated to be 18 days. Results of another study showed that episodes of sleep disturbances closely coincide with the episodes of depression and thus help clinicians establish the periodicity of the depressive episodes.

Differential Diagnosis.   The differential diagnosis for recurrent brief depressive disorder is the same as that for major depressive disorder. Clinicians should consider bipolar disorders and major depressive disorder with seasonal pattern in the differential diagnosis. Research into recurrent brief depressive disorder may find an association with the rapid cycling type of bipolar disorder. Clinicians should also assess whether there is a seasonal pattern to the recurrence of depressive episodes in a patient being evaluated for a diagnosis of recurrent brief depressive disorder. At least one researcher has proposed that patients with recurrent brief depressive disorder be subtyped according to the relative frequencies of their depressive episodes. This differentiation is not included in DSM-IV-TR, although it may yet prove to have prognostic or treatment implications.

Course and Prognosis.   The course and the prognosis for patients with recurrent brief depressive disorder are not well known. On the basis of available data, their course, including age of onset, and their prognosis are similar to those of patients with major depressive disorder.

Treatment.   The treatment of patients with recurrent brief depressive disorder should be similar to the treatment of patients with major depressive disorder. The main treatments are psychotherapy (insight-oriented psychotherapy, cognitive therapy, interpersonal therapy, or behavioral therapy) and pharmacotherapy with the standard antidepressant drugs. Some of the treatments for bipolar I disorder—lithium (Eskalith) and anticonvulsants—may be of therapeutic value. There is controversy about whether these patients should be on life-long medication based on the belief that each recurrence may be worse than the one before.

Premenstrual Dysphoric Disorder

In an appendix, DSM-IV-TR includes suggested diagnostic criteria for premenstrual dysphoric disorder to help researchers and clinicians evaluate the validity of the diagnosis. Premenstrual dysphoric disorder has also been referred to as *late luteal phase dysphoric disorder*. The generally recognized syndrome involves mood symptoms (for example, lability), behavior symptoms (for example, changes in eating patterns), and physical symptoms (for example, breast tenderness, edema, and headaches). This pattern of symptoms occurs at a specific time during the menstrual cycle, and the symptoms resolve for some period of time between menstrual cycles.

Epidemiology. Because of the absence of generally agreed-on diagnostic criteria, the epidemiology of premenstrual dysphoric disorder is not known with certainty. One study reported that approximately 40 percent of women have at least mild premenstrual symptoms and that from 2 to 10 percent meet the full diagnostic criteria for the disorder.

Etiology. The cause of premenstrual dysphoric disorder is unknown. However, because the symptoms are timed to the menstrual cycle, the hormonal changes occurring during the menstrual cycle are probably involved in producing symptoms. A common theory characterizes the disorder as the result of an abnormally high estrogen-to-progesterone ratio in affected women. Other hypotheses suggest that the biogenic amine neurons of affected women are abnormally affected by changes in the hormones, that the disorder is an example of a chronobiological phase disorder, and that it is the result of abnormal prostaglandin activity. In addition to the biological theories, societal and personal issues about menstruation and womanhood may affect the symptoms of individual patients.

Diagnosis and Clinical Features. The most common mood and cognitive symptoms are lability of mood, irritability, anxiety, decreased interest in activities, increased fatigability, and difficulty in concentrating (Table 12.3–4). Behavioral symptoms often include changes in appetite and sleep patterns. The most common somatic complaints are headache, breast tenderness, and edema. In affected women, the symptoms appear during most (if not all) menstrual cycles, although they usually remit before the end of the blood flow. Affected women are symptom free for at least 1 week during each menstrual cycle.

Differential Diagnosis. If symptoms are present throughout the menstrual cycle, with no intercycle symptom relief, clinicians should consider one of the nonmenstrual cycle-related mood disorders and anxiety disorders. The presence of especially severe symptoms, even if cyclical, should prompt clinicians to consider other mood disorders and anxiety disorder.

Course and Prognosis. The course and the prognosis of premenstrual dysphoric disorder have not been studied enough to reach

Table 12.3–4
DSM-IV-TR Research Criteria for Premenstrual Dysphoric Disorder

A. In most menstrual cycles during the past year, five (or more) of the following symptoms were present for most of the time during the last week of the luteal phase, began to remit within a few days after the onset of the follicular phase, and were absent in the week postmenses, with at least one of the symptoms being either (1), (2), (3), or (4):

  (1) markedly depressed mood, feelings of hopelessness, or self-deprecating thoughts

  (2) marked anxiety, tension, feelings of being "keyed up," or "on edge"

  (3) marked affective lability (e.g., feeling suddenly sad or tearful or increased sensitivity to rejection)

  (4) persistent and marked anger or irritability or increased interpersonal conflicts

  (5) decreased interest in usual activities (e.g., work, school, friends, hobbies)

  (6) subjective sense of difficulty in concentrating

  (7) lethargy, easy fatigability, or marked lack of energy

  (8) marked change in appetite, overeating, or specific food cravings

  (9) hypersomnia or insomnia

  (10) a subjective sense of being overwhelmed or out of control

  (11) other physical symptoms, such as breast tenderness or swelling, headaches, joint or muscle pain, a sensation of "bloating," weight gain

Note: In menstruating females, the luteal phase corresponds to the period between ovulation and the onset of menses, and the follicular phase begins with menses. In nonmenstruating females (e.g., those who have had a hysterectomy), the timing of luteal and follicular phases may require measurement of circulating reproductive hormones.

B. The disturbance markedly interferes with work or school or with usual social activities and relationships with others (e.g., avoidance of social activities, decreased productivity and efficiency at work or school).

C. The disturbance is not merely an exacerbation of the symptoms of another disorder, such as major depressive disorder, panic disorder, dysthymic disorder, or a personality disorder (although it may be superimposed on any of these disorders).

D. Criteria A, B, and C must be confirmed by prospective daily ratings during at least two consecutive symptomatic cycles. (The diagnosis may be made provisionally prior to this confirmation.)

any reasonable conclusions. Anecdotally, the symptoms tend to be chronic unless effective treatment is initiated.

Treatment. Treatment of premenstrual dysphoric disorder includes support for the patient about the presence and recognition of the symptoms. Progesterone supplementation, fluoxetine (Sarafem), and alprazolam (Xanax) have all been reported to be effective, although no treatment has been conclusively demonstrated to be effective in multiple, well-controlled trials. Some clinicians have found that small doses of amphetamine (5 to 15 mg/day) during the menses help avoid and reduce pain.

Table 12.3–5
DSM-IV-TR Research Criteria for Postpsychotic Depressive Disorder of Schizophrenia

A. Criteria are met for a major depressive episode.

Note: The major depressive episode must include Criterion A1: depressed mood. Do not include symptoms that are better accounted for as medication side effects or negative symptoms of schizophrenia.

B. The major depressive episode is superimposed on and occurs only during the residual phase of schizophrenia.

C. The major depressive episode is not due to the direct physiological effects of a substance or a general medical condition.

From American Psychiatric Association. *Diagnostic and Statistical Manual of Mental Disorders.* 4th ed. Text rev. Washington, DC: American Psychiatric Association; copyright 2000, with permission.

Postpsychotic Depressive Disorder of Schizophrenia

Postpsychotic depressive disorder in schizophrenic patients is categorized in an appendix in DSM-IV-TR.

Epidemiology. In the absence of specific diagnostic criteria, the reported incidence of postpsychotic depression of schizophrenia varies widely from less than 10 percent to more than 70 percent. A reasonable estimate based on large studies is approximately 25 percent, although a definitive incidence figure must wait for controlled studies using the DSM-IV-TR criteria.

Prognostic Significance. Patients with postpsychotic depressive disorder of schizophrenia are likely to have had poor premorbid adjustment, marked schizoid personality disorder traits, and an insidi-

Table 12.3–6
DSM-IV-TR Diagnostic Criteria for Bipolar Disorder Not Otherwise Specified

The bipolar disorder not otherwise specified category includes disorders with bipolar features that do not meet criteria for any specific bipolar disorder. Examples include

1. Very rapid alternation (over days) between manic symptoms and depressive symptoms that meet symptom threshold criteria but not minimal duration criteria for manic, hypomanic, or major depressive episodes
2. Recurrent hypomanic episodes without intercurrent depressive symptoms
3. A manic or mixed episode superimposed on delusional disorder, residual schizophrenia, or psychotic disorder not otherwise specified
4. Hypomanic episodes, along with chronic depressive symptoms, that are too infrequent to qualify for a diagnosis of cyclothymic disorder
5. Situations in which the clinician has concluded that a bipolar disorder is present but is unable to determine whether it is primary, due to a general medical condition, or substance induced

From American Psychiatric Association. *Diagnostic and Statistical Manual of Mental Disorders.* 4th ed. Text rev. Washington, DC: American Psychiatric Association; copyright 2000, with permission.

Table 12.3–7
DSM-IV-TR Diagnostic Criteria for Mood Disorder Due to a General Medical Condition

A. A prominent and persistent disturbance in mood predominates in the clinical picture and is characterized by either (or both) of the following:
(1) depressed mood or markedly diminished interest or pleasure in all, or almost all, activities
(2) elevated, expansive, or irritable mood

B. There is evidence from the history, physical examination, or laboratory findings that the disturbance is the direct physiological consequence of a general medical condition.

C. The disturbance is not better accounted for by another mental disorder (e.g., adjustment disorder with depressed mood in response to the stress of having a general medical condition).

D. The disturbance does not occur exclusively during the course of a delirium.

E. The symptoms cause clinically significant distress or impairment in social, occupational, or other important areas of functioning.

Specify type:

With depressive features: if the predominant mood is depressed but the full criteria are not met for a major depressive episode

With major depressive-like episode: if the full criteria are met (except Criterion D) for a major depressive episode

With manic features: if the predominant mood is elevated, euphoric, or irritable

With mixed features: if the symptoms of both mania and depression are present but neither predominates

Coding note: Include the name of the general medical condition on Axis I, e.g., mood disorder due to hypothyroidism, with depressive features; also code the general medical condition on Axis III.

Coding note: If depressive symptoms occur as part of a preexisting vascular dementia, indicate the depressive symptoms by coding the appropriate subtype, i.e., vascular dementia, with depressed mood.

From American Psychiatric Association. *Diagnostic and Statistical Manual of Mental Disorders.* 4th ed. Text rev. Washington, DC: American Psychiatric Association; copyright 2000, with permission.

ous onset of their psychotic symptoms. They are also likely to have first-degree relatives with mood disorders. Although the findings have not been consistent, postpsychotic depressive disorder of schizophrenia has been associated with a less favorable prognosis, a higher likelihood of relapse, and an increased incidence of suicide than is seen in schizophrenic patients without postpsychotic depressive disorder.

Diagnosis and Differential Diagnosis. The clinical boundaries of the diagnosis are hard to define operationally. The symptoms of postpsychotic depressive disorder of schizophrenia can closely resemble the symptoms of the residual phase of schizophrenia as well as the side effects of commonly used antipsychotic medications. Distinguishing the diagnosis from schizoaffective disorder, depressive type, is also difficult. The DSM-IV-TR criteria for a major depressive episode must be met and the symptoms must occur only during the residual phase of schizophrenia (Table 12.3–5). The symptoms cannot be substance induced or part of a mood disorder due to a general medical condition.

Table 12.3–8
DSM-IV-TR Diagnostic Criteria for Substance-Induced Mood Disorder

A. A prominent and persistent disturbance in mood predominates in the clinical picture and is characterized by either (or both) of the following:

    (1) depressed mood or markedly diminished interest or pleasure in all, or almost all, activities

    (2) elevated, expansive, or irritable mood

B. There is evidence from the history, physical examination, or laboratory findings of either (1) or (2):

    (1) the symptoms in Criterion A developed during, or within a month of, substance intoxication or withdrawal

    (2) medication use is etiologically related to the disturbance

C. The disturbance is not better accounted for by a mood disorder that is not substance induced. Evidence that the symptoms are better accounted for by a mood disorder that is not substance induced might include the following: the symptoms precede the onset of the substance use (or medication use); the symptoms persist for a substantial period of time (e.g., about a month) after the cessation of acute withdrawal or severe intoxication or are substantially in excess of what would be expected given the type or amount of the substance used or the duration of use; or there is other evidence that suggests the existence of an independent non-substance-induced mood disorder (e.g., a history of recurrent major depressive episodes).

D. The disturbance does not occur exclusively during the course of a delirium.

E. The symptoms cause clinically significant distress or impairment in social, occupational, or other important areas of functioning.

Note: This diagnosis should be made instead of a diagnosis of substance intoxication or substance withdrawal only when the mood symptoms are in excess of those usually associated with the intoxication or withdrawal syndrome and when the symptoms are sufficiently severe to warrant independent clinical attention.

Code [Specific substance]-induced mood disorder: Alcohol; amphetamine [or amphetamine-like substance]; cocaine; hallucinogen; inhalant; opioid; phencyclidine [or phencyclidine-like substance]; sedative, hypnotic, or anxiolytic; other [or unknown] substance

Specify type:

    With depressive features: if the predominant mood is depressed

    With manic features: if the predominant mood is elevated, euphoric, or irritable

    With mixed features: if symptoms of both mania and depression are present and neither predominates

Specify if:

    With onset during intoxication: if the criteria are met for intoxication with the substance and the symptoms develop during the intoxication syndrome

    With onset during withdrawal: if criteria are met for withdrawal from the substance and the symptoms develop during, or shortly after, a withdrawal syndrome

From American Psychiatric Association. *Diagnostic and Statistical Manual of Mental Disorders.* 4th ed. Text rev. Washington, DC: American Psychiatric Association; copyright 2000, with permission.

Treatment. The use of antidepressants (for example, fluoxetine [Prozac]) in the treatment of postpsychotic depressive disorder of schizophrenia has been reported in several studies. Approximately half the studies have reported positive effects, and the other half have reported no effects in the relief of the depressive symptoms. Antidepressant medications probably relieve depressive symptoms in some patients, but the mixed results of the studies reflect the current inability to distinguish patients who will respond from those who will not.

BIPOLAR DISORDER NOT OTHERWISE SPECIFIED

If patients exhibit depressive and manic symptoms as the major features of their disorder and do not meet the diagnostic criteria for any other mood disorder or other DSM-IV-TR mental disorder, the most appropriate diagnosis is bipolar disorder not otherwise specified (Table 12.3–6).

ATYPICAL DEPRESSION

Atypical depression refers to fatigue superimposed on a history of somatic anxiety and phobias, together with reverse vegetative signs (mood worse in the evening, insomnia, tendency to oversleep and overeat), so that weight gain rather than weight loss occurs. Sleep is disturbed in the first half of the night in many persons with atypical depressive disorder, so irritability, hypersomnolence, and daytime fatigue would be expected. The temperaments of these patients are characterized by inhibited-sensitive traits. Selective serotonin reuptake inhibitors (SSRIs) may be of help; however, the MAOIs seem to show some specificity for such patients. Others are helped by psychostimulants such as amphetamine.

SECONDARY MOOD DISORDERS

Secondary mood disorders consist of two broad categories that must be considered in the differential diagnosis of any patient with mood disorder symptoms. They are (1) mood disorder due to a general medical condition and (2) substance-induced mood disorder.

Mood Disorders Due to a General Medical Condition

When depressive or manic symptoms are present in a patient with a general medical condition, attributing the depressive symptoms either to the general medical condition or to a mood disorder can be difficult. Many general medical conditions present depressive symptoms, such as poor sleep, decreased appetite, and fatigue. This category is discussed extensively in Section 7.5. Table 12.3–7 lists the DSM-IV-TR criteria for the disorder.

Substance-Induced Mood Disorder

Substance-induced mood disorder must always be considered in the differential diagnosis of mood disorder symptoms. Clini-

Table 12.3–9
DSM-IV-TR Diagnostic Criteria for Mood Disorder Not Otherwise Specified

This category includes disorders with mood symptoms that do not meet the criteria for any specific mood disorder and in which it is difficult to choose between depressive disorder not otherwise specified and bipolar disorder not otherwise specified (e.g., acute agitation).

From American Psychiatric Association. *Diagnostic and Statistical Manual of Mental Disorders.* 4th ed. Text rev. Washington, DC: American Psychiatric Association; copyright 2000, with permission.

cians should consider three possibilities. First, a patient may be taking drugs for the treatment of nonpsychiatric medical problems. Second, a patient may have been accidentally and perhaps unknowingly exposed to neurotoxic chemicals. Third, the patient may have taken a substance for recreational purposes or may be dependent on such a substance.

Epidemiology.   The epidemiology of substance-induced mood disorder is unknown. The prevalence is probably high, however, given the widespread use of so-called recreational drugs, the fact that many prescription drugs can cause depression and mania, and the fact that toxic chemicals abound in the environment and the workplace.

Etiology.   Medications, especially antihypertensives, are probably the most frequent cause of substance-induced mood disorder, although a wide range of drugs can produce depression and mania. Drugs such as reserpine (Serpasil) and methyldopa (Aldomet), both antihypertensive agents, can precipitate a depressive disorder, presumably by depleting serotonin, as happens in more than 10 percent of all persons who take the drugs.

Diagnosis and Clinical Features.   The DSM-IV-TR diagnostic criteria for substance-induced mood disorder allow the specification of the substance involved, the time of onset (during intoxication or withdrawal), and the nature of the symptoms (for example, manic or

depressed) (Table 12.3–8). A maximum of 1 month between the use of the substance and the appearance of the symptoms is allowed in DSM-IV-TR, although the usual time frame is probably shorter. In some cases, the diagnosis may be warranted after more than 1 month.

Substance-induced manic and depressive features can be identical to those of bipolar I disorder and major depressive disorder. Substance-induced mood disorder, however, may show more waxing and waning of symptoms and a fluctuation in patients' level of consciousness.

Differential Diagnosis.   The presence of a history of mood disorders in the patient or a patient's family weighs toward the diagnosis of a primary mood disorder, although such a history does not rule out the possibility of substance-induced mood disorder. Substances may also trigger an underlying mood disorder in a patient who is biologically vulnerable to mood disorders.

Course and Prognosis.   The course and prognosis of substance-induced mood disorder are variable. Shortly after the substance has been cleared from the body, a normal mood usually returns. Sometimes, however, the substance exposure seems to precipitate a long-lasting mood disorder that may take weeks or months to resolve completely.

Treatment.   The primary treatment of substance-induced mood disorder is the identification of the causally involved substance. Stopping the intake of the substance is usually sufficient to cause the mood disorder symptoms to abate. If the symptoms linger, treatment with appropriate psychiatric drugs may be necessary.

Mood Disorder Not Otherwise Specified

If patients exhibit mood symptoms that are difficult to distinguish between depression and mania and do not meet the diagnostic criteria for any other mood disorder or other DSM-IV-TR mental disorder, the most appropriate diagnosis is mood disorder not otherwise specified (Table 12.3–9). In view of the many types of mood disorders, this diagnosis should rarely be used. Clinicians are urged to attempt to use a more specific diagnosis if at all possible.

13 ▲

Anxiety Disorders

▲ 13.1 Overview

Anxiety disorders are among the most prevalent psychiatric conditions in the United States and around the world. Studies have shown that they increase morbidity, utilization of health care services, and functional impairment. Understanding the neuroanatomy and molecular biology of anxiety promises new insights into etiology and more specific (and thus more effective) treatments in the future.

SYMPTOMS OF ANXIETY

The experience of anxiety has two components: the awareness of the physiological sensations (such as palpitations and sweating) and the awareness of being nervous or frightened. In addition to motor and visceral effects (Table 13.1–1), anxiety affects thinking, perception, and learning. It tends to produce confusion and distortions of perception, not only of time and space but also of people and the meanings of events. These distortions can interfere with learning by lowering concentration, reducing recall, and impairing the ability to relate one item to another—that is, to make associations.

An important aspect of emotions is their effect on the selectivity of attention. Anxious people are apt to select certain things in their environment and overlook others in their effort to prove that they are justified in considering the situation frightening. If they falsely justify their fear, they augment their anxieties by the selective response and set up a vicious circle of anxiety, distorted perception, and increased anxiety. If, alternatively, they falsely reassure themselves by selective thinking, appropriate anxiety may be reduced, and they may fail to take necessary precautions.

PATHOLOGICAL ANXIETY

Epidemiology

The anxiety disorders make up one of the most common groups of psychiatric disorders. The National Comorbidity Study reported that one in four people has met the diagnostic criteria for at least one anxiety disorder and that there is a 12-month prevalence rate of 17.7 percent. Women (30.5 percent lifetime prevalence) are more likely to have an anxiety disorder than are men (19.2 percent lifetime prevalence). Finally, the prevalence of anxiety disorders decreases with higher socioeconomic status.

Contributions of Psychological Sciences

Three major schools of psychological theory—psychoanalytic, behavioral, and existential—have contributed theories about the causes of anxiety. Each theory has both conceptual and practical usefulness in treating anxiety disorders.

Psychoanalytic Theories. Although Sigmund Freud originally believed that anxiety stemmed from a physiological buildup of libido, he ultimately redefined anxiety as a signal of the presence of danger in the unconscious. Anxiety was viewed as the result of psychic conflict between unconscious sexual or aggressive wishes and corresponding threats from the superego or external reality. In response to this signal, the ego mobilized defense mechanisms to prevent unacceptable thoughts and feelings from emerging into conscious awareness. Today, many neurobiologists continue to substantiate many of Freud's original ideas and theories. One example is the role of the amygdala, which subserves the fear response without any reference to conscious memory and substantiates Freud's concept of an unconscious memory system for anxiety responses. From a psychodynamic perspective, the goal of therapy is not necessarily to eliminate all anxiety but to increase anxiety tolerance—that is, the capacity to experience anxiety and use it as a signal to investigate the underlying conflict that has created it. Anxiety appears in response to various situations during the life cycle, and an attempt to eradicate it by psychopharmacological means may do nothing to address the life situation or its internal correlates that have induced the state of anxiety.

Cognitive-Behavioral Theories. The behavioral or learning theories of anxiety have spawned some of the most effective treatments for anxiety disorders. According to these theories, anxiety is a conditioned response to specific environmental stimuli. In a model of classic conditioning, people without food allergies may become sick after eating contaminated shellfish in a restaurant. Subsequent exposures to shellfish may cause these people to feel sick. Through generalization, they may come to distrust all food prepared by others. As an alternative causal possibility, they may learn to have an internal response of anxiety by imitating the anxiety responses of their parents (social learning theory). In either case, treatment is usually a form of desensitization by repeated exposure to the anxiogenic stimulus, coupled with cognitive psychotherapeutic approaches.

In recent years, proponents of behavioral theories have shown increasing interest in cognitive approaches to conceptualizing and treating anxiety disorders, and cognitive theorists

Table 13.1–1
Peripheral Manifestations of Anxiety

Diarrhea
Dizziness, light-headedness
Hyperhidrosis
Hyperreflexia
Hypertension
Palpitations
Pupillary mydriasis
Restlessness (e.g., pacing)
Syncope
Tachycardia
Tingling in the extremities
Tremors
Upset stomach ("butterflies")
Urinary frequency, hesitancy, urgency

have proposed alternatives to traditional learning theory causal models of anxiety. According to conceptualizations of nonphobic anxiety states, faulty, distorted, or counterproductive thinking patterns accompany or precede maladaptive behaviors and emotional disorders. According to one model, patients with anxiety disorders tend to overestimate the degree of danger and the probability of harm in a given situation and tend to underestimate their abilities to cope with perceived threats to their physical or psychological well-being. This model asserts that patients with panic disorder often have thoughts of loss of control and fears of dying that follow inexplicable physiological sensations (such as palpitations, tachycardia, and light-headedness) but that precede and then accompany panic attacks.

Existential Theories.   Existential theories of anxiety provide models for generalized anxiety disorder, in which there is no specifically identifiable stimulus for a chronically anxious feeling. The central concept of existential theory is that people become aware of feelings of profound nothingness in their lives, feelings that may be even more discomforting than an acceptance of their inevitable death. Anxiety is their response to the vast void in existence and meaning. Such existential concerns may have increased since the development of weapons of mass destruction.

Contributions of Biological Sciences

Biological theories of anxiety have developed from preclinical studies with animal models of anxiety, the study of patients in whom biological factors were ascertained, the growing knowledge about basic neuroscience, and the actions of psychotherapeutic drugs. One pole of thought posits that measurable biological changes in patients with anxiety disorders reflect the results of psychological conflicts; the opposite pole posits that the biological events precede the psychological conflicts. Both situations may exist in specific persons, and a range of biologically based sensitivities may exist among persons with the symptoms of anxiety disorders.

Autonomic Nervous System.   Stimulation of the autonomic nervous system causes certain symptoms—cardiovascular (e.g., tachycardia), muscular (e.g., headache), gastrointestinal

(e.g., diarrhea), and respiratory (e.g., tachypnea). These peripheral manifestations of anxiety are neither peculiar to anxiety disorders nor necessarily correlated with the subjective experience of anxiety. In the first third of the 20th century, Walter Cannon demonstrated that cats exposed to barking dogs exhibit behavioral and physiological signs of fear that are associated with the adrenal release of epinephrine. The James-Lange theory states that subjective anxiety is a response to peripheral phenomena. It is currently generally thought that central nervous system anxiety precedes the peripheral manifestations of anxiety, except when a specific peripheral cause is present, such as when a patient has a pheochromocytoma. The autonomic nervous systems of some patients with anxiety disorder, especially those with panic disorder, exhibit increased sympathetic tone, adapt slowly to repeated stimuli, and respond excessively to moderate stimuli.

Neurotransmitters.   The three major neurotransmitters associated with anxiety on the bases of animal studies and responses to drug treatment are norepinephrine, serotonin, and γ-aminobutyric acid (GABA). Much of the basic neuroscience information about anxiety comes from animal experiments involving behavioral paradigms and psychoactive agents. One such animal model of anxiety is the conflict test, in which the animal is simultaneously presented with stimuli that are positive (for example, food) and negative (for example, electric shock). Anxiolytic drugs (for example, benzodiazepines) tend to facilitate the adaptation of the animal to this situation, whereas other drugs (for example, amphetamines) further disrupt the animal's behavioral responses.

NOREPINEPHRINE.   The general theory about the role of norepinephrine in anxiety disorders is that affected patients may have a poorly regulated noradrenergic system with occasional bursts of activity. The cell bodies of the noradrenergic system are primarily localized to the locus ceruleus in the rostral pons, and they project their axons to the cerebral cortex, the limbic system, the brainstem, and the spinal cord. Experiments in primates have demonstrated that stimulation of the locus ceruleus produces a fear response in the animals and that ablation of the same area inhibits or completely blocks the ability of the animals to form a fear response.

Human studies have found that, in patients with panic disorder, β-adrenergic agonists (for example, isoproterenol [Isuprel]) and $α_2$-adrenergic antagonists (for example, yohimbine [Yocon]) can provoke frequent and severe panic attacks. Conversely, clonidine (Catapres), an $α_2$-adrenergic agonist, reduces anxiety symptoms in some experimental and therapeutic situations. A less consistent finding is that patients with anxiety disorders, particularly panic disorder, have elevated cerebrospinal fluid or urinary levels of the noradrenergic metabolite 3-methoxy-4-hydroxyphenylglycol.

SEROTONIN.   The identification of many serotonin receptor types has stimulated the search for the role of serotonin in the pathogenesis of anxiety disorders. The interest in this relation was initially motivated by the observation that serotonergic antidepressants have therapeutic effects in some anxiety disorders—for example, clomipramine (Anafranil) in obsessive-compulsive disorder. The effectiveness of buspirone (BuSpar), a serotonin 5-HT$_{1A}$ receptor agonist, in the treatment of anxiety disorders also suggests the possibility of an association between serotonin and anxiety. The cell bodies of most serotonergic neurons are located in the raphe nuclei in the rostral brainstem and project to the cerebral cortex, the limbic system (especially the amygdala and the hippocampus), and the hypothalamus. Although the administration of serotonergic agents to animals results in behavior suggestive of anxiety, the data on similar effects in humans are less robust. Several reports indicate that m-chlorophenylpiperazine (mCPP), a drug with multiple serotonergic and nonserotonergic effects, and fenfluramine (Pondimin), which causes the release of serotonin, do cause increased anxiety in patients with anxiety disorders; and many anecdotal reports indicate that serotonergic hallucinogens and stimulants—for example, lysergic acid diethylamide (LSD) and 3,4-methylenedioxymethamphetamine (MDMA)—are associated with the development of both acute and chronic anxiety disorders in people who use these drugs.

GABA. A role of GABA in anxiety disorders is most strongly supported by the undisputed efficacy of benzodiazepines, which enhance the activity of GABA at the $GABA_A$ receptor, in the treatment of some types of anxiety disorders. Although low-potency benzodiazepines are most effective for the symptoms of generalized anxiety disorder, high-potency benzodiazepines, such as alprazolam (Xanax), are effective in the treatment of panic disorder. Studies in primates have found that autonomic nervous system symptoms of anxiety disorders are induced when a benzodiazepine inverse agonist, β-carboline-3-carboxylic acid (BCCE), is administered. BCCE also causes anxiety in normal control volunteers. A benzodiazepine antagonist, flumazenil, causes frequent severe panic attacks in patients with panic disorder. These data have led researchers to hypothesize that some patients with anxiety disorders have abnormal functioning of their $GABA_A$ receptors, although this connection has not been shown directly.

APLYSIA. A neurotransmitter model for anxiety disorders is based on the study of *Aplysia california,* by Nobel prize winner Eric Kandel, M.D. *Aplysia* is a sea snail that reacts to danger by moving away, withdrawing into its shell, and decreasing its feeding behavior. These behaviors can be classically conditioned, so that the snail responds to a neutral stimulus as if it were a dangerous stimulus. The snail can also be sensitized by random shocks, so that it exhibits a flight response in the absence of real danger. Parallels have previously been drawn between classic conditioning and human phobic anxiety. The classically conditioned *Aplysia* shows measurable changes in presynaptic facilitation, resulting in the release of increased amounts of neurotransmitter. Although the sea snail is a simple animal, this work shows an experimental approach to complex neurochemical processes potentially involved in anxiety disorders in humans.

Brain-Imaging Studies. A range of brain-imaging studies, almost always conducted with a specific anxiety disorder, have produced several possible leads in the understanding of anxiety disorders. Structural studies—for example, computed tomography (CT) and magnetic resonance imaging (MRI)—occasionally show some increase in the size of cerebral ventricles. In one study, the increase was correlated with the length of time patients had been taking benzodiazepines. In one MRI study, a specific defect in the right temporal lobe was noted in patients with panic disorder. Several other brain-imaging studies have reported abnormal findings in the right hemisphere but not the left hemisphere; this finding suggests that some types of cerebral asymmetries may be important in the development of anxiety disorder symptoms in specific patients. Functional brain-imaging studies—for example, positron emission tomography (PET), single photon emission computed tomography (SPECT), and electroencephalography (EEG)—of patients with anxiety disorder have variously reported abnormalities in the frontal cortex, the occipital and temporal areas, and, in a study of panic disorder, the parahippocampal gyrus. Several functional neuroimaging studies have implicated the caudate nucleus in the pathophysiology of obsessive-compulsive disorder. A conservative interpretation of these data is that some patients with anxiety disorders have a demonstrable functional cerebral pathological condition and that the condition may be causally relevant to their anxiety disorder symptoms.

Genetic Studies. Genetic studies have produced solid data that at least some genetic component contributes to the development of anxiety disorders. Almost half of all patients with panic disorder have at least one affected relative. The figures for other anxiety disorders, although not as high, also indicate a higher frequency of the illness in first-degree relatives of affected patients than occurs in the relatives of nonaffected persons. Although adoption studies with anxiety disorders have not been reported, data from twin registers also support the hypothesis that anxiety disorders are at least partially genetically determined. It becomes clear that a linkage exists between genetics and anxiety disorders but that no anxiety disorder is likely to be the result of a simple Mendelian abnormality. A recent report has attributed about 4 percent of the intrinsic variability of anxiety within the general population to a polymorphic variant of the gene for the serotonin transporter, which is the site of action of many serotonergic drugs. People with the variant produce less transporter and have higher levels of anxiety.

Neuroanatomical Considerations. The locus ceruleus and the raphe nuclei project primarily to the limbic system and the cerebral cortex. In combination with the data from brain-imaging studies, these areas have become the focus of much hypothesis-building about the neuroanatomical substrates of anxiety disorders.

LIMBIC SYSTEM. In addition to receiving noradrenergic and serotonergic innervation, the limbic system also contains a high concentration of $GABA_A$ receptors. Ablation and stimulation studies in nonhuman primates have also implicated the limbic system in the generation of anxiety and fear responses. Two areas of the limbic system have received special attention in the literature: increased activity in the septohippocampal pathway, which may lead to anxiety, and the cingulate gyrus, which has been implicated particularly in the pathophysiology of obsessive-compulsive disorder.

CEREBRAL CORTEX. The frontal cerebral cortex is connected with the parahippocampal region, the cingulate gyrus, and the hypothalamus and therefore may be involved in the production of anxiety disorders. The temporal cortex has also been implicated as a pathophysiological site in anxiety disorders. This association is based in part on the similarity in clinical presentation and electrophysiology between some patients with temporal lobe epilepsy and patients with obsessive-compulsive disorder.

DSM-IV-TR

The fourth revised edition of the *Diagnostic and Statistical Manual of Mental Disorders* (DSM-IV-TR) lists the following anxiety disorders: panic disorder with and without agoraphobia, agoraphobia without history of panic disorder, specific and social phobias, obsessive-compulsive disorder, posttraumatic stress disorder, acute stress disorder, generalized anxiety disorder, anxiety disorder due to a general medical condition, substance-induced anxiety disorder, and anxiety disorder not otherwise specified. These are discussed in the sections that follow.

▲ 13.2 Panic Disorder and Agoraphobia

Panic disorder is characterized by the spontaneous, unexpected occurrence of panic attacks that consist of discreet periods of intense fear varying from several attacks during the day to only a few attacks during a year. Panic disorder is often accompanied by agoraphobia, the fear of being alone in public places (such as supermarkets), particularly places from which a rapid exit would be difficult in the course of a panic attack.

EPIDEMIOLOGY

Epidemiological studies have reported lifetime prevalence rates of 1.5 to 5 percent for panic disorder and 3 to 5.6 percent for panic attacks. Women are two to three times more likely to be affected than are men, although underdiagnosis of panic disorder in men may contribute to the skewed distribution. There are few if any differences among Hispanics, whites, and blacks. The only social factor identified as contributing to the development of panic disorder is a recent history of divorce or separation. Panic disorder most commonly develops in young adulthood (the mean age of presentation is approximately 25 years), but both panic disorder and agoraphobia can develop at any age. Panic disorder has been reported to occur in children and adolescents, and it is probably underdiagnosed in these age groups.

The lifetime prevalence of agoraphobia has been reported as ranging from as low as 0.6 percent to as high as 6 percent. The major factor leading to this wide range of estimates is the use of varying diagnostic criteria and assessment methods. In many cases, the onset of agoraphobia follows a traumatic event.

COMORBIDITY

Ninety-one percent of patients with panic disorder and 84 percent of those with agoraphobia have at least one other psychiatric disorder. According to the fourth revised edition of the *Diagnostic and Statistical Manual of Mental Disorders*, (DSM-IV-TR), 10 to 15 percent of persons with panic disorder have comorbid major depressive disorder. Approximately one-third of persons with both disorders have major depressive disorders

before the onset of panic disorder; approximately two-thirds first experience panic disorder during or after the onset of major depression.

Anxiety disorders also commonly occur in persons with panic disorder and agoraphobia. Fifteen to 30 percent of persons with panic disorder also have social phobia, 2 to 20 percent have specific phobia, 15 to 30 percent have generalized anxiety disorder, 2 to 10 percent have posttraumatic stress disorder, and up to 30 percent have obsessive-compulsive disorder. Other common comorbidity conditions are hypochondriasis, personality disorders, and substance-related disorders.

ETIOLOGY

Biological Factors

Research on the biological basis of panic disorder has produced a range of findings; one interpretation is that the symptoms of panic disorder are related to a range of biological abnormalities in brain structure and function. Most work has taken place in the area of using biological stimulants to induce panic attacks in patients with panic disorder. These and other studies have produced hypotheses implicating both peripheral and central nervous system dysregulation in the pathophysiology of panic disorder. The autonomic nervous systems of some patients with panic disorder have been reported to exhibit increased sympathetic tone, to adapt slowly to repeated stimuli, and to respond excessively to moderate stimuli. Studies of the neuroendocrine status of these patients have shown several abnormalities, although the studies have been inconsistent in their findings.

The major neurotransmitter systems that have been implicated are those for norepinephrine, serotonin, and γ-aminobutyric acid (GABA). Serotonergic dysfunction is quite evident in panic disorder and various studies with mixed serotonin agonist-antagonist drugs have demonstrated increased rates of anxiety. Such responses may be due to postsynaptic serotonin hypersensitivity in panic disorder. There is preclinical evidence that attenuation of local inhibitory GABAergic transmission in the basolateral amygdala, midbrain, and hypothalamus can elicit anxietylike physiological responses. The totality of the biological data has led to a focus on the brainstem (particularly the noradrenergic neurons of the locus ceruleus and the serotonergic neurons of the median raphe nucleus), the limbic system (possibly responsible for the generation of anticipatory anxiety), and the prefrontal cortex (possibly responsible for the generation of phobic avoidance). Among the various neurotransmitters involved, the noradrenergic system has also attracted much attention, particularly the presynaptic α_2-receptors playing a significant role. They have been identified by pharmacological challenges with α_2-receptor agonist clonidine (Catapres) and the α_2-receptor antagonist yohimbine, which stimulates firing of the locus ceruleus and elicits high rates of panic-like activity in panic disorder patients.

Panic-Inducing Substances. Panic-inducing substances (sometimes called *panicogens*) induce panic attacks in a majority of patients with panic disorder and in a much smaller proportion of people without panic disorder or a history of panic attacks. (The use of panic-inducing substances is strictly limited to research settings; there are no clinically indicated reasons to stimulate panic attacks in patients.) So-called respiratory panic-inducing substances cause respiratory stimulation and a shift in the acid-base balance. These substances include carbon dioxide (5 to 35 percent mixtures), sodium lactate, and bicarbonate. Neurochemical panic-inducing substances, which act through specific neurotransmitter systems, include yohimbine (Yocon), an α_2-adrenergic receptor antagonist; fenfluramine (Pondimin), a serotonin-releasing agent; m-chlorophenylpiperazine (mCPP), an agent with multiple serotonergic effects; μ-carboline drugs; GABA$_B$ receptor inverse agonists; flumazenil, a GABA$_B$ receptor antagonist; cholecystokinin; and caffeine. Isoproterenol (Isuprel) is also a panic-inducing substance, although its mechanism of action in inducing panic attacks is poorly understood. The respiratory panic-inducing substances may act initially at the peripheral cardiovascular baroreceptors and relay their signal by vagal afferents to the nucleus tractus solitarii and then on to the nucleus paragigantocellularis of the medulla. The hyperventilation in panic disorder patients may be due to a hypersensitive suffocation alarm system whereby increasing P$_{CO_2}$ and brain lactate concentrations prematurely activate a physiological asphyxic monitor. The neurochemical panic-inducing substances are presumed to primarily affect the noradrenergic, serotonergic, and GABA receptors of the central nervous system directly.

Brain Imaging.   Structural brain-imaging studies, for example, magnetic resonance imaging (MRI), in patients with panic disorder have implicated pathological involvement in the temporal lobes, particularly the hippocampus. One MRI study reported abnormalities, especially cortical atrophy, in the right temporal lobe of these patients. Functional brain-imaging studies, for example, positron emission tomography (PET), have implicated a dysregulation of cerebral blood flow. Specifically, anxiety disorders and panic attacks are associated with cerebral vasoconstriction, which may result in central nervous system symptoms such as dizziness and in peripheral nervous system symptoms that may be induced by hyperventilation and hypocapnia. Most functional brain-imaging studies have used a specific panic-inducing substance (for example, lactate, caffeine, or yohimbine) in combination with PET or single photon emission computed tomography (SPECT) to assess the effects of the panic-inducing substance and the induced panic attack on cerebral blood flow.

Mitral Valve Prolapse.   Although great interest was formerly expressed in an association between mitral valve prolapse and panic disorder, research has almost completely erased any clinical significance or relevance to the association. Mitral valve prolapse is a heterogeneous syndrome consisting of the prolapse of one of the mitral valve leaflets, resulting in a midsystolic click on cardiac auscultation. Research studies have found that the prevalence of panic disorder in patients with mitral valve prolapse is the same as the prevalence of panic disorder in patients without mitral valve prolapse.

Genetic Factors

Although the number of well-controlled studies of the genetic basis of panic disorder and agoraphobia is small, the data to date support the conclusion that the disorders have a distinct genetic component. In addition, some data indicate that panic disorder with agoraphobia is a severe form of panic disorder and is thus more likely to be inherited. Various studies have found a fourfold to eightfold increase in the risk for panic disorder among the first-degree relatives of panic disorder patients

compared with first-degree relatives of other psychiatric patients. The twin studies conducted to date have generally reported that monozygotic twins are more likely to be concordant for panic disorder than are dizygotic twins. At this point, there are no data indicating association between a specific chromosomal location or mode of transmission and this disorder.

Psychosocial Factors

Both cognitive-behavioral and psychoanalytic theories have been developed to explain the pathogenesis of panic disorder and agoraphobia. The success of cognitive-behavioral approaches to the treatment of these disorders may add credence to the cognitive-behavioral theories.

Cognitive-Behavioral Theories.   Behavioral theories posit that anxiety is a response learned either from modeling parental behavior or through the process of classic conditioning. In a classic conditioning approach to panic disorder and agoraphobia, a noxious stimulus (such as a panic attack) that occurs with a neutral stimulus (such as a bus ride) can result in the avoidance of the neutral stimulus. Other behavioral theories posit a linkage between the sensation of minor somatic symptoms (such as palpitations) and the generation of a panic attack. Although cognitive-behavioral theories can help explain the development of agoraphobia or an increase in the number or severity of panic attacks, they do not explain the occurrence of the first unprovoked and unexpected panic attack that an affected patient experiences.

Psychoanalytic Theories.   Psychoanalytic theories conceptualize panic attacks as arising from an unsuccessful defense against anxiety-provoking impulses. What was previously a mild signal anxiety becomes an overwhelming feeling of apprehension, complete with somatic symptoms. To explain agoraphobia, psychoanalytic theories emphasize the loss of a parent in childhood and a history of separation anxiety. Being alone in public places revives the childhood anxiety about being abandoned. The defense mechanisms used include repression, displacement, avoidance, and symbolization. Traumatic separations during childhood may affect children's developing nervous systems in such a manner that they become susceptible to anxieties in adulthood. There may be a predisposing neurophysiological vulnerability that may interact with certain kinds of environmental stressors to produce the end result of a panic attack.

Many patients describe panic attacks as coming out of the blue, as though no psychological factors were involved, but psychodynamic exploration frequently reveals a clear psychological trigger for the panic attack. Although panic attacks are correlated neurophysiologically with the locus ceruleus, the onset of panic is generally related to environmental or psychological factors. Patients with panic disorder have a higher incidence of stressful life events, particularly loss, compared with control subjects in the months before the onset of panic disorder. Moreover, the patients typically experience greater distress about life events than do control subjects.

The hypothesis that stressful psychological events produce neurophysiological changes in panic disorder is supported by a study of female twins. The research findings revealed that panic disorder was strongly associated with both parental separation and parental death before children had reached the age of 17. Separa-

Table 13.2–1
Psychodynamic Themes in Panic Disorder

1. Difficulty tolerating anger
2. Physical or emotional separation from significant person both in childhood and in adult life
3. May be triggered by situations of increased work responsibilities
4. Perception of parents as controlling, frightening, critical, and demanding
5. Internal representations of relationships involving sexual or physical abuse
6. A chronic sense of feeling trapped
7. Vicious cycle of anger at parental rejecting behavior followed by anxiety that the fantasy will destroy the tie to parents
8. Failure of signal anxiety function in ego related to self fragmentation and self–other boundary confusion
9. Typical defense mechanisms: reaction formation, undoing, somatization, and externalization.

tion from the mother early in life was clearly more likely to result in panic disorder than was paternal separation in the cohort of 1,018 pairs of female twins. Another etiological factor in women patients appears to be childhood physical and sexual abuse. Approximately 60 percent of women with panic disorder have a history of childhood sexual abuse compared to 31 percent of women with other anxiety disorders. Further support for psychological mechanisms in panic disorder can be inferred from a study of panic disorder in which patients received successful treatment with cognitive therapy. Before the therapy, the patients responded to panic attack induction with lactate. After successful cognitive therapy, lactate infusion no longer resulted in a panic attack.

The research indicates that the cause of panic attacks is likely to involve the unconscious meaning of stressful events and that the pathogenesis of the panic attacks may be related to neurophysiological factors triggered by the psychological reactions. Psychodynamic clinicians should always do a thorough investigation of possible triggers whenever assessing a patient with panic disorder. The psychodynamics of panic disorder are summarized in Table 13.2–1.

DIAGNOSIS

Panic Attacks

In DSM-IV-TR, the criteria for a panic attack are listed as a separate set of criteria (Table 13.2–2). Panic attacks can occur in mental disorders other than panic disorder, particularly in specific phobia, social phobia, and posttraumatic stress disorder. Unexpected panic attacks occur at any time and are not associated with any identifiable situational stimulus, but panic attacks need not be unexpected. Attacks in patients with social and specific phobias are usually expected or cued to a recognized or specific stimulus. Some panic attacks do not fit easily into the distinction between unexpected and expected, and these attacks are referred to as *situationally predisposed panic attacks*; they may or may not occur when a patient is exposed to a specific trigger, or they may occur either immediately after exposure or after a considerable delay.

Panic Disorder

DSM-IV-TR contains two diagnostic criteria for panic disorder, one without agoraphobia (Table 13.2–3) and the other

Table 13.2–2
DSM-IV-TR Criteria for Panic Attack

Note: A panic attack is not a codable disorder. Code the specific diagnosis in which the panic attack occurs (e.g., panic disorder with agoraphobia).

A discrete period of intense fear or discomfort, in which four (or more) of the following symptoms developed abruptly and reached a peak within 10 minutes:

(1) palpitations, pounding heart, or accelerated heart rate
(2) sweating
(3) trembling or shaking
(4) sensations of shortness of breath or smothering
(5) feeling of choking
(6) chest pain or discomfort
(7) nausea or abdominal distress
(8) feeling dizzy, unsteady, lightheaded, or faint
(9) derealization (feelings of unreality) or depersonalization (being detached from oneself)
(10) fear of losing control or going crazy
(11) fear of dying
(12) paresthesias (numbness or tingling sensations)
(13) chills or hot flushes

From American Psychiatric Association. *Diagnostic and Statistical Manual of Mental Disorders.* 4th ed. Text rev. Washington, DC: American Psychiatric Association; copyright 2000, with permission.

Table 13.2–3
DSM-IV-TR Diagnostic Criteria for Panic Disorder without Agoraphobia

A. Both (1) and (2):
  (1) recurrent unexpected panic attacks
  (2) at least one of the attacks has been followed by 1 month (or more) of one (or more) of the following:
    (a) persistent concern about having additional attacks
    (b) worry about the implications of the attack or its consequences (e.g., losing control, having a heart attack, "going crazy")
    (c) a significant change in behavior related to the attacks
B. Absence of agoraphobia
C. The panic attacks are not due to the direct physiological effects of a substance (e.g., a drug of abuse, a medication) or a general medical condition (e.g., hyperthyroidism).
D. The panic attacks are not better accounted for by another mental disorder, such as social phobia (e.g., occurring on exposure to feared social situations), specific phobia (e.g., on exposure to a specific phobic situation), obsessive-compulsive disorder (e.g., on exposure to dirt in someone with an obsession about contamination), posttraumatic stress disorder (e.g., in response to stimuli associated with a severe stressor), or separation anxiety disorder (e.g., in response to being away from home or close relatives).

From American Psychiatric Association. *Diagnostic and Statistical Manual of Mental Disorders.* 4th ed. Text rev. Washington, DC: American Psychiatric Association; copyright 2000, with permission.

Table 13.2–4
DSM-IV-TR Diagnostic Criteria for Panic Disorder with Agoraphobia

A. Both (1) and (2):
  (1) recurrent unexpected panic attacks
  (2) at least one of the attacks has been followed by 1 month (or more) of one (or more) of the following:
    (a) persistent concern about having additional attacks
    (b) worry about the implications of the attack or its consequences (e.g., losing control, having a heart attack, "going crazy")
    (c) a significant change in behavior related to the attacks
B. The presence of agoraphobia
C. The panic attacks are not due to the direct physiological effects of a substance (e.g., a drug of abuse, a medication) or a general medical condition (e.g., hyperthyroidism).
D. The panic attacks are not better accounted for by another mental disorder, such as social phobia (e.g., occurring on exposure to feared social situations), specific phobia (e.g., on exposure to a specific phobic situation), obsessive-compulsive disorder (e.g., on exposure to dirt in someone with an obsession about contamination), posttraumatic stress disorder (e.g., in response to stimuli associated with a severe stressor), or separation anxiety disorder (e.g., in response to being away from home or close relatives).

From American Psychiatric Association. *Diagnostic and Statistical Manual of Mental Disorders.* 4th ed. Text rev. Washington, DC: American Psychiatric Association; copyright 2000, with permission.

Table 13.2–5
DSM-IV-TR Criteria for Agoraphobia

Note: Agoraphobia is not a codable disorder. Code the specific disorder in which the agoraphobia occurs (e.g., panic disorder with agoraphobia or agoraphobia without history of panic disorder).

A. Anxiety about being in places or situations from which escape might be difficult (or embarrassing) or in which help may not be available in the event of having an unexpected or situationally predisposed panic attack or panic-like symptoms. Agoraphobic fears typically involve characteristic clusters of situations that include being outside the home alone; being in a crowd or standing in a line; being on a bridge; and traveling in a bus, train, or automobile.

Note: Consider the diagnosis of specific phobia if the avoidance is limited to one or only a few specific situations, or social phobia if the avoidance is limited to social situations.

B. The situations are avoided (e.g., travel is restricted) or else are endured with marked distress or with anxiety about having a panic attack or panic-like symptoms, or require the presence of a companion.
C. The anxiety or phobic avoidance is not better accounted for by another mental disorder, such as social phobia (e.g., avoidance limited to social situations because of fear of embarrassment), specific phobia (e.g., avoidance limited to a single situation like elevators), obsessive-compulsive disorder (e.g., avoidance of dirt in someone with an obsession about contamination), posttraumatic stress disorder (e.g., avoidance of stimuli associated with a severe stressor), or separation anxiety disorder (e.g., avoidance of leaving home or relatives).

From American Psychiatric Association. *Diagnostic and Statistical Manual of Mental Disorders.* 4th ed. Text rev. Washington, DC: American Psychiatric Association; copyright 2000, with permission.

with agoraphobia (Table 13.2–4), but both require the presence of panic attacks as described in Table 13.2–2. Some community surveys have indicated that panic attacks are common, and a major issue in developing diagnostic criteria for panic disorder was the determination of a threshold number or frequency of panic attacks required to meet the diagnosis. Setting the threshold too low results in the diagnosis of panic disorder in patients who do not have an impairment from an occasional panic attack; setting the threshold too high results in a situation in which patients who are impaired by their panic attacks do not meet the diagnostic criteria. DSM-IV-TR does not specify a minimum number of panic attacks or a time frame but does require that at least one attack be followed by at least a month-long period of concern about having another panic attack (also known as *anticipatory anxiety*) or about the implications of the attack or a significant change in behavior. DSM-IV-TR also requires that the panic attacks generally be unexpected but allows for expected or situationally predisposed attacks.

Agoraphobia without History of Panic Disorder

Table 13.2–5 lists criteria for agoraphobia. The DSM-IV-TR diagnostic criteria for agoraphobia without history of panic disorder (Table 13.2–6) are based on the fear of a sudden incapacitating or embarrassing symptom. In contrast, the ICD-10 criteria require the presence of interrelated or overlapping phobias but do not require that fear of incapacitating or embarrassing symptoms be present.

The DSM-IV-TR criteria also address the avoidance of situations that are based on a concern related to a medical disorder

(for example, fear of a myocardial infarction in a patient with severe heart disease).

CLINICAL FEATURES

Panic Disorder

The first panic attack is often completely spontaneous, although panic attacks occasionally follow excitement, physical exertion,

Table 13.2–6
DSM-IV-TR Diagnostic Criteria for Agoraphobia without History of Panic Disorder

A. The presence of agoraphobia related to fear of developing panic-like symptoms (e.g., dizziness or diarrhea).
B. Criteria have never been met for panic disorder.
C. The disturbance is not due to the direct physiological effects of a substance (e.g., a drug of abuse, a medication) or a general medical condition.
D. If an associated general medical condition is present, the fear described in Criterion A is clearly in excess of that usually associated with the condition.

From American Psychiatric Association. *Diagnostic and Statistical Manual of Mental Disorders.* 4th ed. Text rev. Washington, DC: American Psychiatric Association; copyright 2000, with permission.

sexual activity, or moderate emotional trauma. DSM-IV-TR emphasizes that at least the first attacks must be unexpected (uncued) to meet the diagnostic criteria for panic disorder. Clinicians should attempt to ascertain any habit or situation that commonly precedes a patient's panic attacks. Such activities may include the use of caffeine, alcohol, nicotine, or other substances; unusual patterns of sleeping or eating; and specific environmental settings, such as harsh lighting at work.

The attack often begins with a 10-minute period of rapidly increasing symptoms. The major mental symptoms are extreme fear and a sense of impending death and doom. Patients are usually unable to name the source of their fear; they may feel confused and have trouble in concentrating. The physical signs often include tachycardia, palpitations, dyspnea, and sweating. Patients often try to leave whatever situation they are in to seek help. The attack generally lasts 20 to 30 minutes and rarely more than an hour. A formal mental status examination during a panic attack may reveal rumination, difficulty in speaking (for example, stammering), and an impaired memory. Patients may experience depression or depersonalization during an attack. The symptoms may disappear quickly or gradually. Between attacks, patients may have anticipatory anxiety about having another attack. The differentiation between anticipatory anxiety and generalized anxiety disorder can be difficult, although pain disorder patients with anticipatory anxiety are able to name the focus of their anxiety.

Somatic concerns of death from a cardiac or respiratory problem may be the major focus of patients' attention during panic attacks. Patients may believe that the palpitations and chest pain indicate that they are about to die. As many as 20 percent of such patients actually have syncopal episodes during a panic attack. The patients may be seen in emergency rooms as young (20s), physically healthy persons who nevertheless insist that they are about to die from a heart attack. Rather than immediately diagnosing hypochondriasis, the emergency room physician should consider a diagnosis of panic disorder. Hyperventilation may produce respiratory alkalosis and other symptoms. The age-old treatment of breathing into a paper bag sometimes helps.

Agoraphobia

Patients with agoraphobia rigidly avoid situations in which it would be difficult to obtain help. They prefer to be accompanied by a friend or a family member in busy streets, crowded stores, closed-in spaces (such as tunnels, bridges, and elevators), and closed-in vehicles (such as subways, buses, and airplanes). The patients may insist that they be accompanied every time they leave the house. The behavior may result in marital discord, which may be misdiagnosed as the primary problem. Severely affected patients may simply refuse to leave the house. Particularly before a correct diagnosis is made, patients may be terrified that they are going crazy.

Associated Symptoms

Depressive symptoms are often present in panic disorder and agoraphobia, and, in some patients, a depressive disorder coexists with the panic disorder. Some studies have found that the lifetime risk of suicide in persons with panic disorder is higher

Table 13.2–7
Organic Differential Diagnosis for Panic Disorder

Cardiovascular diseases	
Anemia	Hypertension
Angina	Mitral valve prolapse
Congestive heart failure	Myocardial infarction
Hyperactive β-adrenergic state	Paradoxical atrial tachycardia
Pulmonary diseases	
Asthma	Pulmonary embolus
Hyperventilation	
Neurological diseases	
Cerebrovascular disease	Migraine
Epilepsy	Multiple sclerosis
Huntington's disease	Transient ischemic attack
Infection	Tumor
Ménière's disease	Wilson's disease
Endocrine diseases	
Addison's disease	Hypoglycemia
Carcinoid syndrome	Hypoparathyroidism
Cushing's syndrome	Menopausal disorders
Diabetes	Pheochromocytoma
Hyperthyroidism	Premenstrual syndrome
Drug intoxications	
Amphetamine	Hallucinogens
Amyl nitrite	Marijuana
Anticholinergics	Nicotine
Cocaine	Theophylline
Drug withdrawal	
Alcohol	Opiates and opioids
Antihypertensives	Sedative-hypnotics
Other conditions	
Anaphylaxis	Systemic infections
B_{12} deficiency	Systemic lupus erythematosus
Electrolyte disturbances	Temporal arteritis
Heavy metal poisoning	Uremia

than it is in persons with no mental disorder. Clinicians should be alert to the risk of suicide. In addition to agoraphobia, other phobias and obsessive-compulsive disorder can coexist with panic disorder. The psychosocial consequences of panic disorder and agoraphobia, in addition to marital discord, can include time lost from work, financial difficulties related to the loss of work, and alcohol and other substance abuse.

DIFFERENTIAL DIAGNOSIS
Panic Disorder

The differential diagnosis for a patient with panic disorder includes a large number of medical disorders (Table 13.2–7), as well as many mental disorders.

Medical Disorders.   Whenever a patient, regardless of age or risk factors, reports to an emergency room with symptoms of a potentially fatal condition (for example, myocardial infarction), a complete medical history must be obtained and a physical examination performed. Standard laboratory procedures include a complete blood count; studies of electrolytes, fasting glucose, calcium concentrations, liver function, urea, creatinine, and thyroid; a urinalysis; a drug screen; and an electrocardiogram. Once the presence of an immediately life-threatening condition is ruled out, the clinical suspicion is panic disorder.

The possibility that additional medical diagnostic procedures will reveal a medical condition must be weighed against the potentially adverse effects of the procedure in helping the patient accept a diagnosis of panic disorder. Nevertheless, the presence of atypical symptoms (such as vertigo, loss of bladder control, and unconsciousness) or the late onset of the first panic attack (older than age 45 years) should cause clinicians to reconsider the presence of an underlying nonpsychiatric medical condition.

The standard workup helps clinicians evaluate patients for the presence of thyroid, parathyroid, adrenal, and substance-related causes of panic attacks. Symptoms of chest pain, especially in patients with cardiac risk factors (for example, obesity and hypertension), may warrant further cardiac tests, including a 24-hour electrocardiogram, a stress test, a chest X-ray, and the measurement of cardiac enzymes. The presence of atypical neurological symptoms may warrant obtaining an electroencephalogram or an MRI to assess the possibility that the patient has temporal lobe epilepsy, multiple sclerosis, or a space-occupying brain lesion. The rare possibility that a patient has carcinoid syndrome or pheochromocytoma can best be checked by measuring a 24-hour urine sample for serotonin metabolites or catecholamines.

Although hypoglycemia was once thought to be associated with panic disorder, especially in the lay literature, available data now indicate that hypoglycemia is rarely a cause of panic attacks in the absence of other symptoms that point to hypoglycemia.

Mental Disorders. The psychiatric differential diagnosis for panic disorder includes malingering, factitious disorders, hypochondriasis, depersonalization disorder, social and specific phobias, posttraumatic stress disorder, depressive disorders, and schizophrenia. In the differential diagnosis, clinicians must determine whether a panic attack was unexpected, situationally bound, or situationally predisposed. Unexpected panic attacks are the hallmark of panic disorder; situationally bound panic attacks generally indicate a different condition, such as social phobia or specific phobia (when exposed to the phobic situation), obsessive-compulsive disorder (when trying to resist a compulsion), or a depressive disorder (when overwhelmed with anxiety). The focus of the anxiety or the fear is also important. Was there no focus (as in panic disorder), or was there a specific focus (for example, a person with social phobia who fears becoming tongue-tied)? Somatoform disorders should also be considered in the differential diagnosis, although a patient may meet the criteria for both somatoform disorder and panic disorder.

SPECIFIC AND SOCIAL PHOBIAS. DSM-IV-TR addresses the sometimes difficult diagnostic task of distinguishing between panic disorder with agoraphobia, on the one hand, and specific and social phobias, on the other hand. Some patients who experience a single panic attack in a specific setting (for example, an elevator) may go on to have a long-lasting avoidance of the specific setting, regardless of whether they ever have another panic attack. These patients meet the diagnostic criteria for a specific phobia, and clinicians must use their judgment about what is the most appropriate diagnosis. In another example, a person who experiences one or more panic attacks may then fear speaking in public. Although the clinical picture is almost identical to the clinical picture in social phobia, a diagnosis of social phobia is excluded because the avoidance of the public situation is based on fear of having a panic attack, rather than on fear of the public speaking itself. Because empirical data on the distinctions are limited, DSM-IV-TR advises clinicians to use their clinical judgment to diagnose difficult cases.

Agoraphobia without History of Panic Disorder

The differential diagnosis for agoraphobia without a history of panic disorder includes all the medical disorders that may cause anxiety or depression. The psychiatric differential diagnosis includes major depressive disorder, schizophrenia, paranoid personality disorder, avoidance personality disorder, and dependent personality disorder.

COURSE AND PROGNOSIS

Panic Disorder

Panic disorder usually has its onset during late adolescence or early adulthood, although onset during childhood, early adolescence, and midlife does occur. Some data implicate increased psychosocial stressors with the onset of panic disorder, although no psychosocial stressor can be definitely identified in most cases.

Panic disorder, in general, is a chronic disorder, although its course is variable both among patients and within a single patient. The available long-term follow-up studies of panic disorder are difficult to interpret because they have not controlled for the effects of treatment. Nevertheless, approximately 30 to 40 percent of patients seem to be symptom free at long-term follow-up; approximately 50 percent have symptoms that are mild enough not to affect their lives significantly; and approximately 10 to 20 percent continue to have significant symptoms.

After the first one or two panic attacks, patients may be relatively unconcerned about their condition; with repeated attacks, however, the symptoms may become a major concern. Patients may attempt to keep the panic attacks secret and thereby cause their families and friends concern about unexplained changes in behavior. The frequency and severity of the attacks may fluctuate. Panic attacks may occur several times in a day or less than once a month. The excessive intake of caffeine or nicotine may exacerbate the symptoms.

Depression may complicate the symptom picture in anywhere from 40 to 80 percent of all patients, as estimated by various studies. Although the patients do not tend to talk about suicidal ideation, they are at increased risk for committing suicide. Alcohol and other substance dependence occurs in approximately 20 to 40 percent of all patients, and obsessive-compulsive disorder may also develop. Family interactions and performance in school and at work commonly suffer. Patients with good premorbid functioning and a brief duration of symptoms tend to have good prognoses.

Agoraphobia

Most cases of agoraphobia are thought to be due to panic disorder. When the panic disorder is treated, the agoraphobia often improves with time. For a rapid and complete reduction of agoraphobia, behavior therapy is sometimes indicated. Agoraphobia without a history of panic disorder is often incapacitating and chronic, and depressive disorders and alcohol dependence often complicate its course.

TREATMENT

With treatment, most patients have a dramatic improvement in the symptoms of panic disorder and agoraphobia. The two most effective treatments are pharmacotherapy and cognitive-behavioral therapy. Family and group therapy may help affected patients and their families adjust to the fact that the patients have the disorder and to the psychosocial difficulties that the disorder may have precipitated.

Pharmacotherapy

Alprazolam (Xanax) and paroxetine (Paxil) are the two drugs approved by the U.S. Food and Drug Administration (FDA) for the treatment of panic disorder. In general, experience is showing superiority of the selective serotonin reuptake inhibitors (SSRIs) and clomipramine (Anafranil) over the benzodiazepines, monoamine oxidase inhibitors (MAOIs), and tricyclic and tetracyclic drugs in terms of effectiveness and tolerance of adverse effects. A few reports have suggested a role for nefazodone (Serzone) and venlafaxine (Effexor), and buspirone (BuSpar) has been suggested as an additive medication in some cases. β-Adrenergic receptor antagonists have not been found to be useful for panic disorder. A conservative approach is to begin with paroxetine, sertraline (Zoloft), or fluvoxamine (Luvox) in isolated panic disorder. If rapid control of severe symptoms is desired, a brief course of alprazolam should be initiated concurrently with the SSRI, followed by slowly tapering off the benzodiazepine. In long-term use, fluoxetine (Prozac) is an effective drug for panic with comorbid depression, although its initial activating properties may mimic panic symptoms for the first several weeks and it may be poorly tolerated on this basis.

Selective Serotonin Reuptake Inhibitors. All SSRIs are effective for panic disorder. Paroxetine has sedative effects and tends to calm patients immediately, which leads to greater compliance and less discontinuation. Fluvoxamine and sertraline are the next best tolerated. Anecdotal reports suggest that patients with panic disorder are particularly sensitive to the activating effects of SSRIs, particularly fluoxetine, which requires that they be started at small doses and titrated up slowly. Once at therapeutic dosages, for example, 20 mg a day of paroxetine, some patients may experience increased sedation. One approach for patients with panic disorder is to begin with 5 or 10 mg a day of paroxetine for 1 to 2 weeks, then increase the dosage by 10 mg a day every 1 to 2 weeks to a maximum of 60 mg. If sedation becomes intolerable, then taper paroxetine down to 10 mg a day and switch to fluoxetine at 10 mg a day and titrate upward slowly. Other strategies can be used based on the experience of the clinician.

Benzodiazepines. Benzodiazepines have the most rapid onset of action against panic, often within the first week, and they can be used for long periods without the development of tolerance to the antipanic effects. Alprazolam has been the most widely used benzodiazepine for panic disorder, but controlled studies have demonstrated equal efficacy for lorazepam (Ativan), and case reports have also indicated that clonazepam (Klonopin) may be effective. Some patients use benzodiazepines as needed when faced with a phobic stimulus. Benzodiazepines can reasonably be used as the first agent for treatment of panic disorder while a serotonergic drug is being slowly titrated to a therapeutic dose. After 4 to 12 weeks, the benzodiazepine can be slowly tapered (over 4 to 10 weeks) while the serotonergic drug is continued. The major reservation among clinicians regarding the use of benzodiazepines for panic disorder is the potential for dependence, cognitive impairment, and abuse, especially after long-term use. Patients should be instructed not to drive or operate dangerous equipment while taking benzodiazepines. Benzodiazepines elicit a sense of well-being, whereas discontinuation of benzodiazepines produces a well-documented and unpleasant withdrawal syndrome. Anecdotal reports and small case series have indicated that addiction to alprazolam is one of the most difficult to overcome, and it may require a comprehensive program of detoxification. Benzodiazepines should be tapered slowly, and all anticipated withdrawal effects should be thoroughly explained to the patient.

Tricyclic and Tetracyclic Drugs.   The most robust data show that among tricyclic drugs, clomipramine and imipramine (Tofranil) are the most effective in the treatment of panic disorder. Clinical experience indicates that the doses must be titrated slowly upward to avoid overstimulation and that the full clinical benefit requires full dosages and may not be achieved for 8 to 12 weeks. Some data support the efficacy of desipramine (Norpramin), and less evidence suggests a role for maprotiline (Ludiomil), trazodone (Desyrel), nortriptyline (Pamelor), amitriptyline (Elavil), and doxepin (Adapin). Tricyclic drugs are less widely used than SSRIs because the tricyclic drugs generally have more severe adverse effects at the higher dosages required for effective treatment of panic disorder.

Monoamine Oxidase Inhibitors.   The most robust data support the effectiveness of phenelzine (Nardil), and some data also support the use of tranylcypromine (Parnate). MAOIs appear less likely to cause overstimulation than either SSRIs or tricyclic drugs, but they may require full dosages for at least 8 to 12 weeks to be effective. The need for dietary restrictions has limited the use of MAOIs, particularly since the appearance of the SSRIs.

Treatment Nonresponse.   If patients fail to respond to one class of drugs, another should be tried. Recent data support the effectiveness of nefazodone and venlafaxine. The combination of an SSRI or a tricyclic drug and a benzodiazepine or of an SSRI and lithium or a tricyclic drug can be tried. Case reports have suggested the effectiveness of carbamazepine (Tegretol), valproate (Depakote), and calcium channel inhibitors. Buspirone may have a role in the augmentation of other medications but has little effectiveness by itself. Clinicians should reassess the patient, particularly to establish the presence of comorbid conditions such as depression, alcohol use, or other substance use.

Duration of Pharmacotherapy.   Once it becomes effective, pharmacological treatment should generally continue for 8 to 12 months. Data indicate that panic disorder is a chronic, perhaps lifelong condition that recurs when treatment is discontinued. Studies have reported that from 30 to 90 percent of panic disorder patients who have received successful treatment have a relapse when their medication is discontinued. Patients may be likely to relapse if they have been given benzodiazepines and the benzodiazepine therapy is terminated in such a way as to cause withdrawal symptoms.

Cognitive and Behavior Therapies

Cognitive and behavior therapies are effective treatments for panic disorder. Various reports have concluded that cognitive and behavior therapies are superior to pharmacotherapy alone; other reports have concluded the opposite. Several studies and reports have found that the combination of cognitive or behavior therapy with pharmacotherapy is more effective than is either therapeutic approach alone. Several studies that included long-term follow-up of patients who received cognitive or behavior therapy have shown that the therapies are effective in producing long-lasting remission of symptoms.

Cognitive Therapy.   The two major foci of cognitive therapy for panic disorder are instruction about a patient's false beliefs and information about panic attacks. The instruction about false beliefs centers on the patient's tendency to misinterpret mild bodily sensations as indicative of impending panic attacks, doom, or death. The information about panic attacks includes explanations that, when panic attacks occur, they are time limited and not life threatening.

José was a 27-year-old laboratory technician who began having full-blown panic attacks 8 months prior to seeking help at our research clinic. While he was unable to identify specific situations that elicited attacks, he was particularly concerned about the possibility of their occurring while he was engaged in laboratory procedures with patients. His attacks typically involved a sudden explosion of autonomic arousal and included palpitations, sweating, dizziness, feelings of unreality, and tingling in his arms and legs. He dreaded the idea that the attacks might recur. In the beginning of his cognitive-behavioral program, he found an educational handout that described the myths of panic attacks (e.g., that they will lead to heart attacks, losing control, or going crazy) particularly reassuring. He began practicing diaphragmatic breathing each evening and, after several weeks, became effective in challenging his negative way of thinking about the consequences of panic attacks. In the latter few weeks of his 12-week program, he practiced exposing himself to physical sensations of panic by doing a variety of interoceptive exercises at home, including hyperventilating for 1 or 2 minutes at a time (designed to help José acclimate to the physical sensations associated with overbreathing), and spinning in a chair repeatedly (designed to help acclimate him to symptoms of dizziness and feelings of unreality). At the conclusion of the treatment program José's panic attacks had disappeared, and at 6-month follow-up he had maintained his treatment gains by attending "booster sessions" with his therapist once every 2 months.

Applied Relaxation.   The goal of applied relaxation (for example, Herbert Benson's relaxation training) is to instill in patients a sense of control about their levels of anxiety and relaxation. Through the use of standardized techniques for muscle relaxation and the imagining of relaxing situations, patients learn techniques that may help them through a panic attack.

Respiratory Training.   Because the hyperventilation associated with panic attacks is probably related to some symptoms such as dizziness and faintness, one direct approach to control panic attacks is to train patients to control the urge to hyperventilate. After such training, patients can use the technique to help control hyperventilation during a panic attack.

In Vivo Exposure.   In vivo exposure used to be a common behavior treatment for panic disorder. The technique involves sequentially greater exposure of a patient to the feared stimulus; over time, the patient becomes desensitized to the experience. Previously, the focus was on external stimuli; recently, the technique has included exposure of the patient to internal feared sensations (for example, tachypnea and fear of having a panic attack).

Other Psychosocial Therapies

Family Therapy.   Families of patients with panic disorder and agoraphobia may also have been affected by the family member's disorder. Family therapy directed toward education and support is often beneficial.

Insight-Oriented Psychotherapy.   Insight-oriented psychotherapy can be of benefit in the treatment of panic disorder and agoraphobia. Treatment focuses on helping patients understand the hypothesized unconscious meaning of the anxiety, the symbolism of the avoided situation, the need to repress impulses, and the secondary gains of the symptoms. A resolution of early infantile and oedipal conflicts is hypothesized to correlate with the resolution of current stresses.

Combined Psychotherapy and Pharmacotherapy.
Even when pharmacotherapy is effective in eliminating the primary symptoms of panic disorder, psychotherapy may be needed to treat secondary symptoms. Psychotherapeutic interventions help patients overcome the fear of going outside. Additionally, some will refuse any medication because they believe that it stigmatizes them as being mentally ill, so psychotherapeutic intervention is required to help them understand and eliminate their resistance to pharmacotherapy.

▲ 13.3 Specific Phobia and Social Phobia

The term *phobia* refers to an excessive fear of a specific object, circumstance, or situation. A specific phobia is a strong, persisting fear of an object or situation, whereas a social phobia is a strong, persisting fear of situations in which embarrassment can occur. People with specific phobias may anticipate harm, such as being bitten by a dog, or may panic at the thought of losing control; for instance, if they fear being in an elevator, they may also worry about fainting after the door closes. People with social phobias (also called *social anxiety disorder*) have excessive fears of humiliation or embarrassment in various social settings, such as in speaking in public, urinating in a public rest room (also called *shy bladder*), and speaking to a date. A generalized social phobia, which is often a chronic and disabling condition characterized by a phobic avoidance of most social situations, can be difficult to distinguish from avoidant personality disorder.

EPIDEMIOLOGY

Epidemiological studies have shown that phobias are among the most common mental disorders in the United States. Approximately 5 to 10 percent of the population is estimated to be afflicted with these troubling and sometimes disabling disorders. Less conservative estimates have ranged as high as 25 percent of the population. The lifetime prevalence of specific phobia is approximately 11 percent, and the lifetime prevalence of social phobia has been reported at 3 to 13 percent.

Specific Phobia

Specific phobia is more common than social phobia. Specific phobia is the most common mental disorder among women and the second most common among men, second only to substance-related disorders. The 6-month prevalence of specific phobia is approximately 5 to 10 per 100 people. The female-to-male ratio is approximately 2 to 1, although the ratio is closer to 1 to 1 for the blood-injection-injury phobia (types of phobia are discussed later in this section). The peak age of onset for the natural environment type and the blood-injection-injury type is in the range of 5 to 9 years, although onset also occurs at older ages. In contrast, the peak age of onset for the situational type (except fear of heights) is higher, in the mid-20s, which is closer to the age of onset for agoraphobia. The feared objects and situations in specific phobias (listed in descending frequency of appearance) are animals, storms, heights, illness, injury, and death.

Social Phobia

Several studies have reported a lifetime prevalence ranging from 3 to 13 percent. The 6-month prevalence for social phobia is approximately 2 to 3 per 100 people. In epidemiological studies, females are affected more often than males, but in clinical samples, the reverse is often true. The reasons for these varying observations are unknown. The peak age of onset for social phobia is in the teens, although onset is common as young as 5 years of age and as old as 35.

COMORBIDITY

Persons with social phobia may have a history of other anxiety disorders, mood disorders, substance-related disorders, and bulimia nervosa. In addition, avoidant personality disorders frequently occur in persons with generalized social phobia.

Reports of comorbidity in specific phobia range from 50 to 80 percent. Common comorbid disorders with specific phobia include anxiety, mood, and substance-related disorders.

ETIOLOGY

Both specific phobia and social phobia have types, and the precise causes of these types are likely to differ. Even within the types, as in all mental disorders, causative heterogeneity is found. The pathogenesis of the phobias, once it is understood, may prove to be a clear model for interactions between biological and genetic factors, on the one hand, and environmental events, on the other hand. In the blood-injection-injury type of specific phobia, affected people may have inherited a particularly strong vasovagal reflex, which becomes associated with phobic emotions.

General Principles

Behavioral Factors. In 1920, John B. Watson wrote an article called "Conditioned Emotional Reactions," in which he recounted his experiences with Little Albert, an infant with a fear of rats and rabbits. Unlike Sigmund Freud's Little Hans, who developed a fear of horses in the natural course of his maturation, Little Albert's difficulties were the direct result of the scientific experiments of psychologists who used conditioning techniques to induce his fear of rats and furry objects.

Watson's hypothesis invoked the traditional pavlovian stimulus-response model of the conditioned reflex to account for the creation of the phobia: Anxiety is aroused by a naturally frightening stimulus (the rat) that occurs in contiguity with a second inherently neutral stimulus (fur or cotton-wool). As a result of the contiguity, especially when the two stimuli are paired on several successive occasions, the originally neutral stimulus takes on the capacity to arouse anxiety by itself. The neutral stimulus, therefore, becomes a conditioned stimulus for anxiety production.

Operant conditioning theory provides another model to explain phobic formations: Anxiety is a drive that motivates the organism to do whatever it can to obviate a painful affect. In the course of its random behavior, the organism learns that certain actions enable it to avoid the anxiety-provoking stimulus. These avoidance patterns remain stable for long periods as a result of the reinforcement they receive from their capacity to diminish activity. This model is readily applicable to phobias in that avoidance of the anxiety-provoking object or situation plays a central part. Such avoidance behavior becomes fixed as a stable symptom because of its effectiveness in protecting the person from the phobic anxiety.

Psychoanalytic Factors. Sigmund Freud's formulation of phobic neurosis is still the analytic explanation of specific phobia and social phobia. Freud hypothesized that the major function of anxiety is to signal the ego that a forbidden unconscious drive is pushing for conscious expression and to alert the ego to strengthen and marshall its defenses against the threatening instinctual force. Freud viewed the phobia—*anxiety hysteria,* as he called it—to be the result of conflicts centered on an unresolved childhood oedipal situation. Because sex drives continue to have a strong incestuous coloring in adults, sexual arousal can kindle an anxiety that is characteristically a fear of castration. In patients with phobias, the sexual conflict is displaced from the person who evokes the conflict to a seemingly unimportant, irrelevant object or situation, which then has the power to arouse the constellation of affects, including signal anxiety. The phobic object or situation may be symbolic of the primary source of the conflict.

Although psychiatrists followed Freud's thought that phobias resulted from castration anxiety, recent psychoanalytic theorists have suggested that other types of anxiety may be involved. In agoraphobia, for example, separation anxiety clearly plays a leading role, and in erythrophobia (a fear of red that can be manifested as a fear of blushing), the element of shame implies the involvement of superego anxiety. Clinical observations have led to the view that anxiety associated with phobias has a variety of sources and colorings.

Phobias illustrate the interaction between a genetic constitutional diathesis and environmental stressors. Longitudinal studies suggest that certain children are constitutionally predisposed to phobias because they are born with a specific temperament known as *behavioral inhibition* to the unfamiliar, but a chronic environmental stress must act on a child's temperamental disposition to create a full-blown phobia. Stressors such as the death of a parent, separation from a parent, criticism or humiliation by an older sibling, and violence in the household may activate the latent diathesis within the child, who then becomes symptomatic.

COUNTERPHOBIC ATTITUDE. Otto Fenichel called attention to the fact that phobic anxiety can be hidden behind attitudes and behavior patterns that represent a denial, either that the dreaded object or situation is dangerous or that the person is afraid of it. Instead of being a passive victim of external circumstances, a person reverses the situation and actively attempts to confront and master whatever is feared. People with counterphobic attitudes seek out situations of danger and rush enthusiastically toward them. Devotees of potentially dangerous sports, such as parachute jumping and rock climbing, may be exhibiting counterphobic behavior. Such patterns may be secondary to phobic anxiety or may be normal means of dealing with a realistically dangerous situation. Children's play may exhibit counterphobic elements, as when children play doctor and give a doll the shot they received earlier that day in the pediatrician's office. This pattern of behavior may involve the related defense mechanism of identifying with the aggressor.

Specific Phobia

The development of specific phobia may result from the pairing of a specific object or situation with the emotions of fear and panic. Various mechanisms for the pairing have been postulated. In general, a nonspecific tendency to experience fear or anxiety forms the backdrop; when a specific event (driving, for example) is paired with an emotional experience (an accident, for example), the person is susceptible to a permanent emotional association between driving or cars and fear or anxiety. The emotional experience itself can be responsive to an external incident, as in a traffic accident, or to an internal incident, most commonly a panic attack. Although a person may never again experience a panic attack and may not meet the diagnostic criteria for panic disorder, he or she may have a generalized fear of driving, not an expressed fear of having a panic attack while driving. Other mechanisms of association between the phobic object and the phobic emotions include modeling, in which a person observes the reaction in another (for example, a parent), and information transfer, in which a person is taught or warned about the dangers of specific objects (for example, venomous snakes).

Genetic Factors. Specific phobia tends to run in families. The blood-injection-injury type has a particularly high familial tendency. Studies have reported that two-thirds to three-fourths of affected probands have at least one first-degree relative with specific phobia of the same type, but the necessary twin and adoption studies have not been conducted to rule out a significant contribution by nongenetic transmission of specific phobia.

Social Phobia

Several studies have reported that some children possibly have a trait characterized by a consistent pattern of behavioral inhibition. This trait may be particularly common in the children of parents who are affected with panic disorder and may develop into severe shyness as the children grow older. At least some people with social phobia may have exhibited behavioral inhibition during childhood. Perhaps associated with this trait, which is thought to be biologically based, are the psychologically based data indicating that the parents of people with social phobia were, as a group, less caring, more rejecting, and more overprotective of their children than were other parents. Some social phobia research has referred to the spectrum from dominance to submission observed in the animal kingdom. For example, dominant humans may tend to walk with their chins in the air and to make eye contact, whereas submissive humans may tend to walk with their chins down and to avoid eye contact.

Neurochemical Factors. The success of pharmacotherapies in treating social phobia has generated two specific neurochemical hypotheses about two types of social phobia. Specifically, the use of β-adrenergic antagonists—for example, propranolol (Inderal)—or performance phobias (such as public speaking) has led to the development of an adrenergic theory for these phobias. Patients with performance phobias may release more norepinephrine or epinephrine, both centrally and peripherally, than do nonphobic people, or such patients may be sensitive to a normal level of adrenergic stimulation. The observation that monoamine oxidase inhibitors (MAOIs) may be more effective than tricyclic drugs in the treatment of generalized social phobia, has led some investigators to hypothesize that dopaminergic activity is related to the pathogenesis of the disorder. Finally, serotonin plays a role in phobias, since selective serotonin uptake inhibitors (SSRIs) have proven effective in treating the disorder.

Genetic Factors. First-degree relatives of people with social phobia are approximately three times more likely to be affected with social phobia than are first-degree relatives of those without mental disorders. And some preliminary data indicate that monozygotic twins are more often concordant than are dizygotic twins, although in social phobia it is particularly important to study twins reared apart to help control for environmental factors.

DIAGNOSIS

Specific Phobia

The text revision of the fourth edition of the *Diagnostic and Statistical Manual of Mental Disorders* (DSM-IV-TR) uses the term *specific phobia*. Table 13.3–1 lists the diagnostic criteria. Criteria A and B have been carefully worded in DSM-IV-TR to allow for the possibility that exposure to a phobic stimulus may result in a panic attack. In contrast to panic disorder, however, in specific phobia, the panic attack is situationally bound to the specific phobic stimulus. Criterion G in DSM-IV-TR includes

Table 13.3–1
DSM-IV-TR Diagnostic Criteria for Specific Phobia

A. Marked and persistent fear that is excessive or unreasonable, cued by the presence or anticipation of a specific object or situation (e.g., flying, heights, animals, receiving an injection, seeing blood).

B. Exposure to the phobic stimulus almost invariably provokes an immediate anxiety response, which may take the form of a situationally bound or situationally predisposed panic attack. **Note:** In children, the anxiety may be expressed by crying, tantrums, freezing, or clinging.

C. The person recognizes that the fear is excessive or unreasonable. **Note:** In children, this feature may be absent.

D. The phobic situation(s) is avoided or else is endured with intense anxiety or distress.

E. The avoidance, anxious anticipation, or distress in the feared situation(s) interferes significantly with the person's normal routine, occupational (or academic) functioning, or social activities or relationships, or there is marked distress about having the phobia.

F. In individuals under age 18 years, the duration is at least 6 months.

G. The anxiety, panic attacks, or phobic avoidance associated with the specific object or situation are not better accounted for by another mental disorder, such as obsessive-compulsive disorder (e.g., fear of dirt in someone with an obsession about contamination), posttraumatic stress disorder (e.g., avoidance of stimuli associated with a severe stressor), separation anxiety disorder (e.g., avoidance of school), social phobia (e.g., avoidance of social situations because of fear of embarrassment), panic disorder with agoraphobia, or agoraphobia without history of panic disorder.

Specify type:

Animal type

Natural environment type (e.g., heights, storms, water)

Blood-injection-injury type

Situational type (e.g., airplanes, elevators, enclosed places)

Other type (e.g., fear of choking, vomiting, or contracting an illness; in children, fear of loud sounds or costumed characters)

From American Psychiatric Association. *Diagnostic and Statistical Manual of Mental Disorders.* 4th ed. Text rev. Washington, DC: American Psychiatric Association; copyright 2000, with permission.

Table 13.3–2
DSM-IV-TR Diagnostic Criteria for Social Phobia

A. A marked and persistent fear of one or more social or performance situations in which the person is exposed to unfamiliar people or to possible scrutiny by others. The individual fears that he or she will act in a way (or show anxiety symptoms) that will be humiliating or embarrassing. **Note:** In children, there must be evidence of the capacity for age-appropriate social relationships with familiar people and the anxiety must occur in peer settings, not just in interactions with adults.

B. Exposure to the feared social situation almost invariably provokes anxiety, which may take the form of a situationally bound or situationally predisposed panic attack. **Note:** In children, the anxiety may be expressed by crying, tantrums, freezing, or shrinking from social situations with unfamiliar people.

C. The person recognizes that the fear is excessive or unreasonable. **Note:** In children, this feature may be absent.

D. The feared social or performance situations are avoided or else are endured with intense anxiety or distress.

E. The avoidance, anxious anticipation, or distress in the feared social or performance situation(s) interferes significantly with the person's normal routine, occupational (academic) functioning, or social activities or relationships, or there is marked distress about having the phobia.

F. In individuals under age 18 years, the duration is at least 6 months.

G. The fear or avoidance is not due to the direct physiological effects of a substance (e.g., a drug of abuse, a medication) or a general medical condition and is not better accounted for by another mental disorder (e.g., panic disorder with or without agoraphobia, separation anxiety disorder, body dysmorphic disorder, a pervasive developmental disorder, or schizoid personality disorder).

H. If a general medical condition or another mental disorder is present, the fear in Criterion A is unrelated to it, e.g., the fear is not of stuttering, trembling in Parkinson's disease, or exhibiting abnormal eating behavior in anorexia nervosa or bulimia nervosa.

Specify if:

Generalized: if the fears include most social situations (also consider the additional diagnosis of avoidant personality disorder)

From American Psychiatric Association. *Diagnostic and Statistical Manual of Mental Disorders.* 4th ed. Text rev. Washington, DC: American Psychiatric Association; copyright 2000, with permission.

the words "not better accounted for" to emphasize the need for clinicians' judgment about diagnosing the symptoms. The specific content of the phobia and the strength of the relation (for example, cued or noncued) between the stimulus and a panic attack also need to be considered.

DSM-IV-TR includes distinctive types of specific phobia: animal type; natural environment type (for example, storms); blood-injection-injury type; situational type (for example, cars); and other type (for specific phobias that do not fit into the previous four types). Preliminary data indicate that the natural environment type is most common in children younger than 10 years old and the situational type most often occurs in people in their early 20s. The blood-injection-injury type is differentiated from the others in that bradycardia and hypotension often follow the initial tachycardia that is common to all phobias. The blood-injection-injury type of specific phobia is particularly likely to affect many members and generations of a family. One type of recently reported specific phobia is space phobia, in which people are afraid of falling when there is no nearby support like a wall or a chair. Some data indicate that affected people may have abnormal right hemisphere function, possibly resulting in a visual-spatial impairment. Balance disorders should also be ruled out in such patients.

Social Phobia

The DSM-IV-TR diagnostic criteria for social phobia (Table 13.3–2) acknowledge that the disorder can be associated with panic attacks. DSM-IV-TR also included a specifier for generalized type, which may be useful in predicting course, prognosis, and treatment response. DSM-IV-TR excluded a diagnosis of social phobia when the symptoms are a result of social avoidance stemming from embarrassment about another psychiatric or nonpsychiatric medical condition.

Mr. M, a 28-year-old computer programmer, seeks treatment because of fears that prevent him from visiting his terminally ill father-in-law in the hospital. He explains that he is afraid of any situation even remotely associated with bodily injury or illness. For example, he cannot bear to have his blood drawn, or to see or even hear about sick people. These fears are the reason he avoids consulting a doctor even when he is sick and avoids visiting sick friends or family members and even listening to descriptions of medical procedures, physical trauma, or illness. He became a vegetarian 5 years ago to avoid thoughts of animals being killed.

The patient dates the onset of these fears to a particular incident when he was 9 and his Sunday school teacher gave a detailed account of a leg operation she had undergone. As he listened, he began to feel anxious and dizzy, he sweated profusely, and finally he fainted. He recalls great difficulty receiving immunizations and being subjected to other routine medical procedures through the rest of his school years, as well as numerous fainting and near-fainting episodes throughout his teenage and adult years whenever he witnessed the slightest physical trauma, heard of an injury or illness, or saw a sick or disfigured person. When he recently saw someone in a store in a wheelchair, he started wondering if the person was in pain and became so distressed that he fainted and fell to the floor. He was greatly embarrassed, when he regained consciousness, by the crowd of people surrounding him.

Mr. M denies any other emotional problems. He enjoys his work, seems to get along well with his wife, and has many friends.

DISCUSSION

Mr. M is afraid of thinking about or being near a situation involving bodily illness or injury. He recognizes that his fear is excessive and unreasonable, but nevertheless he avoids such situations. Although the fear and avoidance behavior apparently does not interfere with his normal routine or school activities, he is quite distressed about having the fear, which is the reason he now seeks treatment.

His fear is unrelated to obsessive-compulsive disorder (e.g., an obsession involving being infected with germs) and to any trauma that might precede posttraumatic stress disorder (e.g., having witnessed mutilation on the battlefield): therefore, neither of these diagnoses is made.

Mr. M has a specific phobia called blood-injection-injury type. He feels faint in the presence of the phobic stimulus, as do many people with this type of phobia. Feeling faint is rarely seen in other specific phobias, such as fear of flying or of animals, or in social phobia or agoraphobia. (From *DSM-IV Casebook*.)

CLINICAL FEATURES

Phobias are characterized by the arousal of severe anxiety when patients are exposed to specific situations or objects or when patients even anticipate exposure to the situations or objects. DSM-IV-TR emphasizes the possibility that panic attacks can and frequently do occur in patients with specific and social pho-bias, but the panic attacks, except perhaps for the first few, are expected. Exposure to the phobic stimulus or anticipation of it almost invariably results in a panic attack in a person who is susceptible to them.

People with phobias, by definition, try to avoid the phobic stimulus; some go to great trouble to avoid anxiety-provoking situations. For example, a phobic patient may take a bus across the United States, rather than fly, to avoid contact with the object of the patient's phobia, an airplane. Perhaps as another way to avoid the stress of the phobic stimulus, many phobic patients have substance-related disorders, particularly alcohol use disorders. Moreover, an estimated one-third of patients with social phobia have major depressive disorder.

The major finding on the mental status examination is the presence of an irrational and ego-dystonic fear of a specific situation, activity, or object; patients are able to describe how they avoid contact with the phobia. Depression is commonly found on the mental status examination and may be present in as many as one-third of all phobic patients.

DIFFERENTIAL DIAGNOSIS

Specific phobia and social phobia need to be differentiated from appropriate fear and normal shyness, respectively. DSM-IV-TR aids in the differentiation by requiring that the symptoms impair the patient's ability to function appropriately. Nonpsychiatric medical conditions that can result in the development of a phobia include the use of substances (particularly hallucinogens and sympathomimetics), central nervous system tumors, and cerebrovascular diseases. Phobic symptoms in these instances are unlikely in the absence of additional suggestive findings on physical, neurological, and mental status examinations. Schizophrenia is also in the differential diagnosis of both specific phobia and social phobia, as schizophrenic patients can have phobic symptoms as part of their psychoses. Unlike patients with schizophrenia, however, phobic patients have insight into the irrationality of their fears and lack the bizarre quality and other psychotic symptoms that accompany schizophrenia.

In the differential diagnosis of both specific phobia and social phobia, clinicians must consider panic disorder, agoraphobia, and avoidant personality disorder. DSM-IV-TR acknowledges that the differentiation among panic disorder, agoraphobia, social phobia, and specific phobia can be difficult in individual cases, and clinicians are advised to use clinical judgment. In general, however, patients with specific phobia or nongeneralized social phobia tend to experience anxiety immediately when presented with the phobic stimulus. Furthermore, the anxiety or panic is limited to the identified situation; patients are not abnormally anxious when they are neither confronted with the phobic stimulus nor caused to anticipate the stimulus.

A patient with agoraphobia is often comforted by the presence of another person in an anxiety-provoking situation, whereas a patient with social phobia is made more anxious than before by the presence of other people. Whereas breathlessness, dizziness, a sense of suffocation, and a fear of dying are common in panic disorder and agoraphobia, the symptoms associated with social phobia usually involve blushing, muscle twitching, and anxiety about scrutiny. The differentiation between social phobia and avoidant personality disorder can be difficult and can require extensive interviews and psychiatric histories.

Specific Phobia

Other diagnoses to consider in the differential diagnosis of specific phobia are hypochondriasis, obsessive-compulsive disorder, and paranoid personality disorder. Hypochondriasis is the fear of having a disease, whereas specific phobia of the illness type is the fear of contracting the disease. Some patients with obsessive-compulsive disorder manifest behavior indistinguishable from that of a patient with specific phobia. For example, patients with obsessive-compulsive disorder may avoid knives because they have compulsive thoughts about killing their children, whereas patients with specific phobia about knives may avoid them for fear of cutting themselves. Patients with paranoid personality disorder have generalized fear that distinguishes them from those with specific phobia.

Social Phobia

Two additional differential diagnostic considerations for social phobia are major depressive disorder and schizoid personality disorder. The avoidance of social situations can often be a symptom in depression, but a psychiatric interview with the patient is likely to elicit a broad constellation of depressive symptoms. In patients with schizoid personality disorder, the lack of interest in socializing, not the fear of socializing, leads to the avoidant social behavior.

COURSE AND PROGNOSIS

Specific phobia exhibits a bimodal age of onset, with a childhood peak for animal phobia, natural environment phobia, and blood-injury-injection phobia and an early adulthood peak for other phobias, such as situational phobia. As with other anxiety disorders, limited prospective epidemiological data exist on the natural course of specific phobia. Because patients with isolated specific phobias rarely present for treatment, research on the course of the disorder in the clinic is limited. The information that is available suggests that most specific phobias that begin in childhood and persist into adulthood continue to persist for many years. The severity of the condition is thought to remain relatively constant, without the waxing and waning course seen with other anxiety disorders.

Social phobia tends to have its onset in late childhood or early adolescence. Social phobia tends to be a chronic disorder, although as with the other anxiety disorders, prospective epidemiological data are limited. Both retrospective epidemiological studies and prospective clinical studies suggest that the disorder can profoundly disrupt the life of an individual over many years. This can include disruption in school or academic achievement, interference with job performance, and social development.

TREATMENT

Behavior Therapy

The most studied and most effective treatment for phobias is probably behavior therapy. The key aspects of successful treatment are (1) the patient's commitment to treatment, (2) clearly identified problems and objectives, and (3) available alternative strategies for coping with the feelings. A variety of behavioral treatment techniques have been employed, the most common being systematic desensitization, a method pioneered by Joseph Wolpe. In this method, the patient is exposed serially to a predetermined list of anxiety-provoking stimuli graded in a hierarchy from the least to the most frightening. Through the use of tranquilizing drugs, hypnosis, and instruction in muscle relaxation, patients are taught how to induce in themselves both mental and physical repose. Once they have mastered the techniques, patients are instructed to employ them to induce relaxation in the face of each anxiety-provoking stimulus. As they become desensitized to each stimulus in the scale, the patients move up to the next stimulus until, ultimately, what previously produced the most anxiety is no longer capable of eliciting the painful affect.

Other behavioral techniques that have more recently been employed involve intensive exposure to the phobic stimulus through either imagery or desensitization in vivo. In imaginal flooding, patients are exposed to the phobic stimulus for as long as they can tolerate the fear until they reach a point at which they can no longer feel it. Flooding (also known as *implosion*) in vivo requires patients to experience similar anxiety through exposure to the actual phobic stimulus.

Insight-Oriented Psychotherapy

Early in the development of psychoanalysis and the dynamically oriented psychotherapies, theorists believed that these methods were the treatments of choice for phobic neurosis, which was then thought to stem from oedipal-genital conflicts. Soon, however, therapists recognized that, despite progress in uncovering and analyzing unconscious conflicts, patients frequently failed to lose their phobic symptoms. Moreover, by continuing to avoid phobic situations, patients excluded a significant degree of anxiety and its related associations from the analytic process. Both Freud and his pupil Sandor Ferenczi recognized that, if progress in analyzing these symptoms was to be made, therapists had to go beyond their analytic roles and actively urge phobic patients to seek the phobic situation and experience the anxiety and resultant insight. Since then, psychiatrists have generally agreed that a measure of activity on the therapist's part is often required to treat phobic anxiety successfully. The decision to apply the techniques of psychodynamic insight-oriented therapy should be based not on the presence of phobic symptoms alone but on positive indications from the patient's ego structure and life patterns for the use of this method of treatment. Insight-oriented therapy enables patients to understand the origin of the phobia, the phenomenon of secondary gain, and the role of resistance and enables them to seek healthy ways of dealing with anxiety-provoking stimuli.

Other Therapeutic Modalities

Hypnosis, supportive therapy, and family therapy may be useful in the treatment of phobic disorders. Hypnosis is used to enhance the therapist's suggestion that the phobic objection is not dangerous, and self-hypnosis can be taught to the patient as a method of relaxation when confronted with the phobic object. Supportive psychotherapy and family therapy are often useful in helping the patient actively confront the phobic object during treatment. Not only can family therapy enlist the aid of the family in treating the patient, but it may help the family understand the nature of the patient's problem.

Specific Phobia

Among the psychotherapies, the most commonly used treatment for specific phobia is exposure therapy. In this method, therapists desensitize patients by using a series of gradual, self-paced exposures to the phobic stimuli, and they teach patients various techniques to deal with anxiety, including relaxation, breathing control, and cognitive approaches. The cognitive approaches include reinforcing the realization that the phobic situation is, in fact, safe. The key aspects of successful behavior therapy are the patient's commitment to treatment, clearly identified problems and objectives, and alternative strategies for coping with the patient's feelings. In the special situation of blood-injection-injury phobia, some therapists recommend that patients tense their bodies and remain seated during the exposure to help avoid the possibility of fainting from a vasovagal reaction to the phobic stimulation. β-Adrenergic antagonists may be useful in the treatment of specific phobia, especially when the phobia is associated with panic attacks. Pharmacotherapy (e.g., benzodiazepines), psychotherapy, or combined therapy directed to the attacks may also be of benefit.

Social Phobia

Both psychotherapy and pharmacotherapy are useful in treating social phobias, and varying approaches are indicated for the generalized type and for performance situations. Some studies indicate that the use of both pharmacotherapy and psychotherapy produces better results than either therapy alone, although the finding may not be applicable to all situations and patients.

Effective drugs for the treatment of social phobia include (1) SSRIs, (2) the benzodiazepines, (3) venlafaxine (Effexor), and (4) buspirone (BuSpar). Most clinicians consider SSRIs the first-line treatment choice for patients with generalized social phobia. The benzodiazepines alprazolam (Xanax) and clonazepam (Klonopin) are also efficacious in both generalized and specific social phobia. Buspirone has shown additive effects when used to augment treatment with SSRIs.

In severe cases, successful treatment of social phobia with both irreversible monoamine oxidase inhibitors (MAOIs), such as phenelzine (Nardil), and reversible inhibitors of monoamine oxidase (RIMAs), such as moclobemide (Aurorix) and brofaromine (Consonar) (which are not available in the United States), have been reported. Therapeutic dosages of phenelzine range from 45 to 90 mg a day, with response rates ranging from 50 to 70 percent, and approximately 5 to 6 weeks are needed to assess the efficacy.

The treatment of social phobia associated with performance situations frequently involves the use of β-adrenergic receptor antagonists shortly before exposure to a phobic stimulus. The two compounds most widely used are atenolol (Tenormin), 50 to 100 mg every morning or 1 hour before the performance, and propranolol (20 to 40 mg). Cognitive, behavioral, and exposure techniques can also be useful in performance situations.

Psychotherapy for the generalized type of social phobia usually involves a combination of behavioral and cognitive methods, including cognitive retraining, desensitization, rehearsal during sessions, and a range of homework assignments.

▲ 13.4 Obsessive-Compulsive Disorder

The essential feature of obsessive-compulsive disorder (OCD) is the symptom of recurrent obsessions or compulsions sufficiently severe to cause marked distress to the person. The obsessions or compulsions are time-consuming and interfere significantly with the person's normal routine, occupational functioning, usual social activities, or relationships. A patient with OCD may have an obsession or a compulsion or both.

An *obsession* is a recurrent and intrusive thought, feeling, idea, or sensation. In contrast to an obsession, which is a mental event, a compulsion is a behavior. Specifically, a *compulsion* is a conscious, standardized, recurrent behavior, such as counting, checking, or avoiding. A patient with OCD realizes the irrationality of the obsession and experiences both the obsession and the compulsion as ego-dystonic.

Although the compulsive act may be carried out in an attempt to reduce the anxiety associated with the obsession, it does not always succeed in doing so. The completion of the compulsive act may not affect the anxiety, and it may even increase the anxiety.

EPIDEMIOLOGY

The lifetime prevalence of OCD in the general population is estimated at 2 to 3 percent. Some researchers have estimated that the disorder is found in as many as 10 percent of outpatients in psychiatric clinics. These figures make OCD the fourth most common psychiatric diagnosis after phobias, substance-related disorders, and major depressive disorder. Epidemiological studies in Europe, Asia, and Africa have confirmed these rates across cultural boundaries.

Among adults, men and women are equally likely to be affected, but among adolescents, boys are more commonly affected than are girls. The mean age of onset is approximately 20 years, although men have a slightly earlier age of onset (mean around 19 years) than do women (mean around 22 years). Overall, the symptoms of approximately two-thirds of affected people have an onset before age 25, and the symptoms of fewer than 15 percent have an onset after age 35. The onset of the disorder can occur in adolescence or childhood, in some cases as early as 2 years of age. Single people are more frequently affected with OCD than are married people, although this finding probably reflects the difficulty that people with the disorder have in maintaining a relationship. OCD occurs less often among blacks than among whites, although access to health care rather than differences in prevalence may explain the variation.

COMORBIDITY

People with OCD are commonly affected by other mental disorders. The lifetime prevalence for major depressive disorder in people with OCD is approximately 67 percent and for social phobia approximately 25 percent. Other common comorbid psychiatric diagnoses in patients with OCD include alcohol use disorders, generalized anxiety disorder, specific phobia, panic disorder, eating disorders, and personality disorders. The incidence of Tourette's disorder in patients with OCD is 5 to 7 percent, and 20 to 30 percent of OCD patients have a history of tics.

ETIOLOGY

Biological Factors

Neurotransmitters

SEROTONERGIC SYSTEM.   The many clinical drug trials that have been conducted support the hypothesis that a dysregulation of serotonin is involved in the symptom formation of obsessions and compulsions in the disorder. Data show that serotonergic drugs are more effective than drugs that affect other neurotransmitter systems, but whether serotonin is involved in the cause of OCD is not clear. Clinical studies have assayed cerebrospinal fluid (CSF) concentrations of serotonin metabolites (for example, 5-hydroxyindoleacetic acid [5-HIAA]) and affinities and numbers of platelet-binding sites of tritiated imipramine (which binds to serotonin reuptake sites) and have reported variable findings of these measures in patients with OCD. In one study, the CSF concentration of 5-HIAA decreased after treatment with clomipramine, focusing attention on the serotonergic system.

NORADRENERGIC SYSTEM.   Currently, less evidence exists for dysfunction in the noradrenergic system in OCD. Anecdotal reports show some improvement in OCD symptoms with oral clonidine.

NEUROIMMUNOLOGY.   There has been a positive link between streptococcal infection and OCD. Group A β-hemolytic streptococcal infection can cause rheumatic fever and approximately 10 to 30 percent of the patients develop Sydenham's chorea and show obsessive-compulsive symptoms. Onset of the infection usually occurs at about 8 years of age to produce those sequelae. The condition is called pediatric autoimmune neuropsychiatric disorder associated with streptococcal infection (PANDAS).

Brain-Imaging Studies.   Various functional brain-imaging studies—for example, positron emission tomography (PET)—have shown increased activity (for example, metabolism and blood flow) in the frontal lobes, the basal ganglia (especially the caudate), and the cingulum of patients with OCD. Pharmacological and behavioral treatments reportedly reverse these abnormalities. Both computed tomographic (CT) and magnetic resonance imaging (MRI) studies have found bilaterally decreased sizes of caudates in patients with OCD. Neurological procedures involving the cingulum are sometimes effective in the treatment of OCD patients.

Genetics.   Available genetic data on OCD support the hypothesis that the disorder has a significant genetic component. The data, however, do not yet distinguish the influence of cultural and behavioral effects on the transmission of the disorder. Studies of concordance for the disorder in twins have consistently found a significantly higher concordance rate for monozygotic twins than for dizygotic twins. Family studies of these patients have shown that 35 percent of the first-degree rel-

atives of OCD patients are also afflicted with the disorder. Family studies of probands with OCD have found increased rates of Tourette's disorder and chronic motor tics only among the relatives of probands with OCD who also have some form of tic disorder. These data suggest that there is a familial and perhaps genetic relationship between Tourette's disorder and chronic motor tics and same cases of OCD.

Behavioral Factors

According to learning theorists, obsessions are conditioned stimuli. A relatively neutral stimulus becomes associated with fear or anxiety through a process of respondent conditioning by being paired with events that are by nature noxious or anxiety-producing. Thus, previously neutral objects and thoughts become conditioned stimuli capable of provoking anxiety or discomfort.

Compulsions are established in a different way. When a person discovers that a certain action reduces anxiety attached to an obsessional thought, he or she develops active avoidance strategies in the form of compulsions or ritualistic behaviors to control the anxiety. Gradually, because of their efficacy in reducing a painful secondary drive (anxiety), the avoidance strategies become fixed as learned patterns of compulsive behaviors. Learning theory provides useful concepts for explaining certain aspects of obsessive-compulsive phenomena—for example, the anxiety-provoking capacity of ideas not necessarily frightening in themselves and the establishment of compulsive patterns of behavior.

Psychosocial Factors

Personality Factors.   OCD differs from obsessive-compulsive personality disorder. Most people with OCD do not have premorbid compulsive symptoms, and such personality traits are neither necessary nor sufficient for the development of OCD. Only approximately 15 to 35 percent of OCD patients have had premorbid obsessional traits.

Psychodynamic Factors.   Sigmund Freud originally conceptualized the condition we now call OCD as *obsessive-compulsive neurosis*. He assumed there was a defensive retreat involved in the face of anxiety-provoking oedipal wishes. He postulated that the patient with an obsessive-compulsive neurosis regressed to the anal phase of psychosexual development.

Although psychoanalytic therapy will not directly change the obsessions or the compulsions associated with the illness, psychodynamic insight may be of great help in understanding problems with treatment compliance, interpersonal difficulties, and personality problems accompanying the Axis I disorder.

Even though the symptoms of OCD may be biologically driven, patients may become invested in maintaining the symptomatology because of secondary gains. For example, a male patient, whose mother stays home to take care of him, may unconsciously wish to hang on to his OCD symptoms because they have the meaning of keeping the attention of his mother.

Another contribution of psychodynamic understanding involves the interpersonal dimensions. Studies have shown that relatives will accommodate the patient through active participation in rituals or significant modifications of their daily routines. This form of family accommodation is correlated with stress in the family, rejecting attitudes toward the patient, and poor family functioning. Often the family members are involved in an effort to reduce the patient's anxiety or to control the patient's expressions of anger. This pattern of relatedness may become internalized and be recreated when the patient enters a treatment setting.

Finally, one other contribution of psychodynamic thinking is to recognize the precipitants that initiate or exacerbate symptoms. Often interpersonal difficulties increase the patient's anxiety and therefore also increase the patient's symptomatology. Research suggests that OCD may be precipitated by a number of environmental stressors, especially those involving pregnancy, childbirth, or parental care of children. An understanding of the stressors may assist the clinician in an overall treatment plan that reduces the stressful events themselves or their meaning to the patient.

OTHER PSYCHODYNAMIC FACTORS.   In classic psychoanalytic theory, OCD was considered a regression from the oedipal phase to the anal psychosexual phase of development. When patients with the disorder feel threatened by anxiety, they regress to a stage associated with the anal phase.

One of the striking features of patients with OCD is the degree to which they are preoccupied with aggression or cleanliness, either overtly in the content of their symptoms or in the associations that lie behind them. Therefore, the psychogenesis of OCD may lie in disturbances in normal growth and development related to the anal-sadistic phase of development.

Ambivalence.   Ambivalence is the direct result of a change in the characteristics of the impulse life. It is an important feature of normal children during the anal-sadistic developmental phase; children feel both love and murderous hate toward the same object, sometimes simultaneously. Patients with OCD often consciously experience both love and hate toward an object. This conflict of opposing emotions is evident in a patient's doing and undoing patterns of behavior and in paralyzing doubt in the face of choices.

Magical Thinking.   In magical thinking, regression uncovers early modes of thought rather than impulses; that is, ego functions, as well as id functions, are affected by regression. Inherent in magical thinking is omnipotence of thought. Many patients with OCD believe that merely by thinking about an event in the external world they can cause the event to occur without intermediate physical actions. This feeling causes them to fear having an aggressive thought.

DIAGNOSIS

As part of the diagnostic criteria for OCD, DSM-IV-TR allows clinicians to specify that patients have the poor insight type of OCD if they generally do not recognize the excessiveness of their obsessions and compulsions (Table 13.4–1).

CLINICAL FEATURES

Obsessions and compulsions have certain features in common: An idea or an impulse intrudes itself insistently and persistently into a person's conscious awareness. A feeling of anxious dread accompanies the central manifestation and frequently leads the person to take countermeasures against the initial idea or

Table 13.4–1
DSM-IV-TR Diagnostic Criteria for Obsessive-Compulsive Disorder

A. Either obsessions or compulsions:
Obsessions as defined by (1), (2), (3), and (4):
(1) recurrent and persistent thoughts, impulses, or images that are experienced, at some time during the disturbance, as intrusive and inappropriate and that cause marked anxiety or distress
(2) the thoughts, impulses, or images are not simply excessive worries about real-life problems
(3) the person attempts to ignore or suppress such thoughts, impulses, or images, or to neutralize them with some other thought or action
(4) the person recognizes that the obsessional thoughts, impulses, or images are a product of his or her own mind (not imposed from without as in thought insertion)
Compulsions as defined by (1) and (2):
(1) repetitive behaviors (e.g., hand washing, ordering, checking) or mental acts (e.g., praying, counting, repeating words silently) that the person feels driven to perform in response to an obsession, or according to rules that must be applied rigidly
(2) the behaviors or mental acts are aimed at preventing or reducing distress or preventing some dreaded event or situation; however, these behaviors or mental acts either are not connected in a realistic way with what they are designed to neutralize or prevent or are clearly excessive

B. At some point during the course of the disorder, the person has recognized that the obsessions or compulsions are excessive or unreasonable. **Note:** This does not apply to children.

C. The obsessions or compulsions cause marked distress, are time consuming (take more than 1 hour a day), or significantly interfere with the person's normal routine, occupational (or academic) functioning, or usual social activities or relationships.

D. If another Axis I disorder is present, the content of the obsessions or compulsions is not restricted to it (e.g., preoccupation with food in the presence of an eating disorder; hair pulling in the presence of trichotillomania; concern with appearance in the presence of body dysmorphic disorder; preoccupation with drugs in the presence of a substance use disorder; preoccupation with having a serious illness in the presence of hypochondriasis; preoccupation with sexual urges or fantasies in the presence of a paraphilia; or guilty ruminations in the presence of major depressive disorder).

E. The disturbance is not due to the direct physiological effects of a substance (e.g., a drug of abuse, a medication) or a general medical condition.

Specify if:
With poor insight: if, for most of the time during the current episode, the person does not recognize that the obsessions and compulsions are excessive or unreasonable

From American Psychiatric Association. *Diagnostic and Statistical Manual of Mental Disorders.* 4th ed. Text rev. Washington, DC: American Psychiatric Association; copyright 2000, with permission.

impulse. The obsession or the compulsion is ego-alien; that is, it is experienced as being foreign to the person's experience of himself or herself as a psychological being. No matter how vivid and compelling the obsession or compulsion, the person usually recognizes it as absurd and irrational. The person suffering from obsessions and compulsions usually feels a strong desire to resist them. Nevertheless, approximately half of all patients offer little resistance to compulsions, although approximately 80 percent of all patients believe that the compulsion is irrational. Sometimes patients overvalue obsessions and compulsions. A patient, for example, may insist that compulsive cleanliness is morally correct, even though he or she may have lost a job because of time spent cleaning.

Symptom Patterns

The presentation of obsessions and compulsions is heterogeneous in adults and in children and adolescents. The symptoms of an individual patient may overlap and change with time, but OCD has four major symptom patterns.

Contamination.   The most common pattern is an obsession of contamination, followed by washing or accompanied by compulsive avoidance of the presumably contaminated object. The feared object is often hard to avoid (for example, feces, urine, dust, or germs). Patients may literally rub the skin off their hands by excessive hand washing or may be unable to leave their homes because of fear of germs. Although anxiety is the most common emotional response to the feared object, obsessive shame and disgust are also common. Patients with contamination obsessions usually believe that the contamination is spread from object to object or person to person by the slightest contact.

Pathological Doubt.   The second most common pattern is an obsession of doubt, followed by a compulsion of checking. The obsession often implies some danger of violence (such as forgetting to turn off the stove or not locking a door). The checking may involve multiple trips back into the house to check the stove, for example. The patients have an obsessional self-doubt and always feel guilty about having forgotten or committed something.

Intrusive Thoughts.   In the third most common pattern, there are intrusive obsessional thoughts without a compulsion. Such obsessions are usually repetitive thoughts of a sexual or aggressive act that is reprehensible to the patient. Patients obsessed with thoughts of aggressive or sexual acts may report themselves to police or confess to a priest.

Symmetry.   The fourth most common pattern is the need for symmetry or precision, which can lead to a compulsion of slowness. Patients can literally take hours to eat a meal or shave their faces.

Other Symptom Patterns.   Religious obsessions and compulsive hoarding are common in patients with OCD. Trichotillomania (compulsive hair pulling) and nail biting may be compulsions related to OCD.

Mental Status Examination

On mental status examinations, patients with OCD may also show symptoms of depressive disorders. Such symptoms are present in approximately 50 percent of all patients. Some OCD patients have character traits suggestive of obsessive-compulsive personality disorder, but most do not. Patients with OCD, especially men, have a higher-than-average celibacy rate. Married patients have a greater-than-usual amount of marital discord.

Ms. B presented for psychiatric admission after being transferred from a medical floor where she had been treated for malnutrition. Ms. B had been found unconscious in her apartment by a neighbor. When brought to the emergency room by ambulance, she was found to be hypotensive and hypokalemic. At psychiatric admission, Ms. B described a long history of recurrent obsessions about cleanliness, particularly related to food items. She reported that it was difficult for her to eat any food unless it had been washed by her three to four times, since she often thought that a food item was dirty. She reported that washing her food decreased the anxiety she felt about the dirtiness of food. Although Ms. B reported that she occasionally tried to eat food that she did not wash (e.g., in a restaurant), she became so worried about contracting an illness from eating such food that she could no longer dine in restaurants. Ms. B reported that her obsessions about the cleanliness of food had become so extreme over the past 3 months that she could eat very few foods, even if she washed them excessively. She recognized the irrational nature of these obsessive concerns, but either could not bring herself to eat or became extremely nervous and nauseous after eating. (Courtesy of Daniel S. Pine, M.D.)

DIFFERENTIAL DIAGNOSIS

Medical Conditions

The DSM-IV-TR diagnostic requirement of personal distress and functional impairment differentiates OCD from ordinary or mildly excessive thoughts and habits. The major neurological disorders to consider in the differential diagnosis are Tourette's disorder, other tic disorders, temporal lobe epilepsy, and, occasionally, trauma and postencephalitic complications.

Tourette's Disorder

The characteristic symptoms of Tourette's disorder are motor and vocal tics that occur frequently and virtually every day. Tourette's disorder and OCD have a similar age of onset and similar symptoms. Approximately 90 percent of people with Tourette's disorder have compulsive symptoms, and as many as two-thirds meet the diagnostic criteria for OCD.

Other Psychiatric Conditions

The major psychiatric considerations in the differential diagnosis of OCD are schizophrenia, obsessive-compulsive personality disorder, phobias, and depressive disorders. OCD can usually be distinguished from schizophrenia by the absence of other schizophrenic symptoms, by the less bizarre nature of the symptoms, and by the patient's insight into the disorder. Obsessive-compulsive personality disorder does not have the degree of functional impairment associated with OCD. Phobias are distinguished by the absence of a relation between the obsessive thoughts and the compulsions. Major depressive disorder can sometimes be associated with obsessive ideas, but patients with only OCD fail to meet the diagnostic criteria for major depressive disorder.

Other psychiatric conditions that may be closely related to OCD are hypochondriasis, body dysmorphic disorder, and possibly other impulse-control disorders, such as kleptomania and pathological gambling. In all these disorders, patients have either a repetitious thought (for example, concern about the body) or a repetitious behavior (for example, stealing). Several research groups are investigating these disorders and other disorders, such as compulsive sexual behavior, their relations to OCD, and their responses to various treatments.

COURSE AND PROGNOSIS

More than half the patients with OCD have a sudden onset of symptoms. The onset of symptoms for approximately 50 to 70 percent of patients occurs after a stressful event, such as a pregnancy, a sexual problem, or the death of a relative. Because many people manage to keep their symptoms secret, there is often a delay of 5 to 10 years before patients come to psychiatric attention, although the delay is probably shortening with increased awareness of the disorder. The course is usually long but variable; some patients experience a fluctuating course, and others experience a constant one.

Approximately 20 to 30 percent of patients have significant improvement in their symptoms, and 40 to 50 percent have moderate improvement. The remaining 20 to 40 percent of patients either remain ill or have a worsening of their symptoms.

Approximately one-third to one-half of patients with OCD have major depressive disorder, and suicide is a risk for all patients with OCD. A poor prognosis is indicated by yielding to (rather than resisting) compulsions, childhood onset, bizarre compulsions, the need for hospitalization, a coexisting major depressive disorder, delusional beliefs, the presence of overvalued ideas (that is, some acceptance of obsessions and compulsions), and the presence of a personality disorder (especially schizotypal personality disorder). A good prognosis is indicated by a good social and occupational adjustment, the presence of a precipitating event, and an episodic nature in the symptoms. The obsessional content does not seem to be related to the prognosis.

TREATMENT

With mounting evidence that OCD is largely determined by biological factors, the classic psychoanalytic theory has fallen out of favor. Moreover, because OCD symptoms appear to be largely refractory to psychodynamic psychotherapy and psychoanalysis, pharmacological and behavioral treatments have become common. But psychodynamic factors may be of considerable benefit in understanding what precipitates exacerbations of the disorder and in treating various forms of resistance to treatment, such as noncompliance with medication.

Many patients with OCD tenaciously resist treatment efforts. They may refuse to take medication and may resist carrying out therapeutic homework assignments and other prescribed activities given by behavior therapists. The obsessive-compulsive symptoms themselves, no matter how biologically based, may have important psychological meanings that make patients reluctant to give them up. A psychodynamic exploration of a patient's resistance to treatment may result in improved compliance.

Well-controlled studies have found that pharmacotherapy, behavior therapy, or a combination of both is effective in significantly reducing the symptoms of patients with OCD. The decision about which therapy to use is based on the clinician's judgment and experience and on the patient's acceptance of the various modalities.

Pharmacotherapy

The efficacy of pharmacotherapy in OCD has been proved in many clinical trials and is enhanced by the observation that the studies find a placebo response rate of approximately 5 percent. This percentage is low, compared with the 30 to 40 percent placebo response rate often seen in studies of antidepressants and anxiolytic drugs.

The drugs, all of which are used to treat depressive disorders or other mental disorders, can be used in their usual dosage ranges. Initial effects are generally seen after 4 to 6 weeks of treatment, although 8 to 16 weeks are usually needed to obtain the maximal therapeutic benefit. Treatment with antidepressant drugs is still controversial, and a significant proportion of patients with OCD who respond to treatment with antidepressant drugs seem to relapse if the drug therapy is discontinued.

The standard approach is to start with a selective serotonin reuptake inhibitor (SSRI) or clomipramine (Anafranil) and then to move to other pharmacological strategies if the serotonin-specific drugs are not effective. The serotonergic drugs have increased the percentage of patients with OCD who are likely to respond to treatment to the range of 50 to 70 percent.

Selective Serotonin Reuptake Inhibitors.
The SSRIs—fluoxetine (Prozac), citalopram (Celexa), escitalopram (Lexapro), fluvoxamine (Luvox), paroxetine (Paxil), sertraline (Zoloft)—have been approved by the U.S. Food and Drug Administration (FDA) for the treatment of OCD. Higher doses have often been necessary for a beneficial effect, such as 80 mg a day of fluoxetine. Although the SSRIs may cause sleep disturbance, nausea and diarrhea, headache, anxiety, and restlessness, these adverse effects are often transient and are generally less troubling than the adverse effects associated with tricyclic drugs, such as clomipramine (Anafranil). The best clinical outcomes occur when SSRIs are used in combination with behavioral therapy.

Clomipramine.
Of all the tricyclic and tetracyclic drugs, clomipramine is the most selective for serotonin reuptake versus norepinephrine reuptake, exceeded in this respect only by the SSRIs. The potency of serotonin reuptake of clomipramine is exceeded only by sertraline and paroxetine. Clomipramine was the first drug to be U.S. FDA approved for the treatment of OCD. Its dosing must be titrated upward over 2 to 3 weeks to avoid gastrointestinal adverse effects and orthostatic hypotension, and, like other tricyclic drugs, it causes significant sedation and anticholinergic effects, including dry mouth and constipation. As with SSRIs, the best outcomes result from a combination of drug and behavioral therapy.

Other Drugs.
If treatment with clomipramine or an SSRI is unsuccessful, many therapists augment the first drug by the addition of valproate (Depakene), lithium (Eskalith), or carbamazepine (Tegretol). Other drugs that can be tried in the treatment of OCD are venlafaxine (Effexor), pindolol (Visken), and the monoamine oxidase inhibitors (MAOIs), especially phenelzine (Nardil). Other pharmacological agents for the treatment of unresponsive patients include buspirone (BuSpar), 5-hydroxytryptamine (5-HT), L-tryptophan, and clonazepam (Klonopin). Antipsychotic agents may be helpful when a tic disorder or Tourette's syndrome is also present.

Behavior Therapy

Although few head-to-head comparisons have been made, behavior therapy is as effective as pharmacotherapies in OCD, and some data indicate that the beneficial effects are longer lasting with behavior therapy. Therefore, many clinicians consider behavior therapy to be the treatment of choice for OCD. Behavior therapy can be conducted in both outpatient and inpatient settings. The principal behavioral approaches in OCD are exposure and response prevention. Desensitization, thought stopping, flooding, implosion therapy, and aversive conditioning have also been used in patients with OCD. In behavior therapy, patients must be truly committed to improvement.

Psychotherapy

In the absence of adequate studies of insight-oriented psychotherapy for OCD, any valid generalizations about its effectiveness are hard to make, although there are anecdotal reports of successes. Individual analysts have seen striking and lasting changes for the better in patients with obsessive-compulsive personality disorder, especially when they are able to come to terms with the aggressive impulses lying behind their character traits. Likewise, analysts and dynamically oriented psychiatrists have observed marked symptomatic improvement in patients with OCD in the course of analysis or prolonged insight psychotherapy.

Supportive psychotherapy undoubtedly has its place, especially for those OCD patients who, despite symptoms of varying degrees of severity, are able to work and make social adjustments. With continuous and regular contact with an interested, sympathetic, and encouraging professional person, patients may be able to function by virtue of this help, without which their symptoms would incapacitate them. Occasionally, when obsessional rituals and anxiety reach an intolerable intensity, it is necessary to hospitalize patients until the shelter of an institution and the removal from external environmental stresses diminish symptoms to a tolerable level.

A patient's family members are often driven to the verge of despair by the patient's behavior. Any psychotherapeutic endeavors must include attention to the family members through the provision of emotional support, reassurance, explanation, and advice on how to manage and respond to the patient.

Other Therapies

Family therapy is often useful in supporting the family, helping reduce marital discord resulting from the disorder, and building a treatment alliance with the family members for the good of the patient. Group therapy is useful as a support system for some patients.

For extreme cases in severely treatment-resistant patients, electroconvulsive therapy (ECT) and psychosurgery may be considered. ECT is not as effective as psychosurgery but should be tried before surgery. The most common psychosurgical procedure for OCD is cingulotomy, which is successful in treating 25 to 30 percent of otherwise treatment-unresponsive patients. The most common complication of psychosurgery is the development of seizures, which are almost always controlled by treatment with phenytoin (Dilantin). Some patients who do not respond to psychosurgery alone and who did not respond to pharmacotherapy or behavior therapy before the operation do respond to pharmacotherapy or behavior therapy after psychosurgery.

▲ 13.5 Posttraumatic Stress Disorder and Acute Stress Disorder

Posttraumatic stress disorder (PTSD) is a syndrome that develops after a person sees, is involved in, or hears of an extreme traumatic stressor. The person reacts to this experience with fear and helplessness, persistently relives the event, and tries to avoid being reminded of it. To make the diagnosis, the symptoms must last for more than a month after the event and must significantly affect important areas of life such as family and work. The revised fourth edition of the *Diagnostic and Statistical Manual of Mental Disorders* (DSM-IV-TR) defines a disorder that is similar to PTSD called *acute stress disorder*, which occurs earlier than PTSD (within 4 weeks of the event) and remits within 2 days to 4 weeks. If symptoms persist after that time, a diagnosis of PTSD is warranted.

EPIDEMIOLOGY

The lifetime prevalence of PTSD is estimated to be approximately 8 percent of the general population, although an additional 5 to 15 percent may experience subclinical forms of the disorder. Among high-risk groups whose members experienced traumatic events, the lifetime prevalence rates range from 5 to 75 percent. Approximately 30 percent of Vietnam veterans experienced PTSD, and an additional 25 percent experienced subclinical forms of the disorder. The lifetime prevalence among women ranges from approximately 10 to 12 percent, and 5 to 6 percent among men. Although PTSD can appear at any age, it is most prevalent in young adults, because they tend be more exposed to precipitating situations. Children can also have the disorder. Men and women differ in the types of traumas to which they are exposed and their liability to develop PTSD. The lifetime prevalence is significantly higher in women, and a higher proportion of women go on to develop the disorder. Historically, men's trauma was usually combat experience, and women's trauma was most commonly assault or rape. The disorder is most likely to occur in those who are single, divorced, widowed, socially withdrawn, or of low socioeconomic level. The most important risk factors, however, for this disorder are the severity, duration, and proximity of a person's exposure to the actual trauma. There seems to be a familial pattern for this disorder, and first-degree biological relatives of persons with a history of depression have an increased risk for developing PTSD after a traumatic event.

COMORBIDITY

Comorbidity rates are high among patients with PTSD, with approximately two-thirds having at least two other disorders.

Common comorbid conditions include depressive disorders, substance-related disorders, other anxiety disorders, and bipolar disorders. Comorbid disorders make persons more vulnerable to develop PTSD.

ETIOLOGY

Stressor

The stressors causing both acute stress and PTSD are overwhelming enough to affect almost anyone. The stressor can arise from experiences in war, torture, natural catastrophes, assault, rape, and serious accidents (for example, in cars and in burning buildings). However, not everyone experiences the disorder after a traumatic event. The stressor alone is not sufficient to cause the disorder. Clinicians must consider individual preexisting biological and psychosocial factors and events that happened before and after the trauma. For example, a member of a group who lived through a disaster can sometimes deal with trauma because others shared the experience. The stressor's subjective meaning to a person is also important. For example, survivors of a catastrophe may experience guilt feelings (*survivor guilt*) that can predispose to or exacerbate PTSD.

Risk Factors

As mentioned above, even when faced with overwhelming trauma, most people do not experience PTSD symptoms. The National Comorbidity Study found that 60 percent of males and 50 percent of females had experienced some significant trauma, but the reported lifetime prevalence of PTSD was only 6.7 percent. Similarly, events that may appear mundane or less than catastrophic to most people may produce PTSD in some.

Psychodynamic Factors

The psychoanalytic model of the disorder hypothesizes that the trauma has reactivated a previously quiescent, yet unresolved psychological conflict. The revival of the childhood trauma results in regression and the use of the defense mechanisms of repression, denial, reaction formation, and undoing. According to Freud, a splitting of consciousness occurs in patients who reported a history of childhood sexual trauma. A preexisting conflict might be symbolically reawakened by the new traumatic event. The ego relives and thereby tries to master and reduce the anxiety. Persons who suffer from alexithymia, the inability to identify or verbalize feeling states, are incapable of soothing themselves when under stress.

Cognitive-Behavioral Factors

The cognitive model of PTSD posits that affected people are unable to process or rationalize the trauma that precipitated the disorder. They continue to experience the stress and attempt to avoid experiencing it by avoidance techniques. Consistent with their partial ability to cope cognitively with the event, people experience alternating periods of acknowledging and blocking the event. The attempt of the brain to process the massive amount of information provoked by the trauma is thought to produce the alternating periods of acknowledging and blocking the event.

The behavioral model of PTSD emphasizes two phases in its development. First, the trauma (the unconditioned stimulus) that produces a fear response is paired, through classic conditioning, with a conditioned stimulus (physical or mental reminders of the trauma, such as sights, smells, or sounds). Second, through instrumental learning, the conditioned stimuli elicit the fear response independent of the original unconditioned stimulus, and people develop a pattern of avoidance of both the conditioned stimulus and the unconditioned stimulus.

Some persons also receive secondary gains from the external world, commonly monetary compensation, increased attention or sympathy, and the satisfaction of dependency needs. These gains reinforce the disorder and its persistence.

Biological Factors

The biological theories of PTSD have developed from both preclinical studies of animal models of stress and from measures of biological variables in clinical populations with the disorder. Many neurotransmitter systems have been implicated by both sets of data. Preclinical models of learned helplessness, kindling, and sensitization in animals have led to theories about norepinephrine, dopamine, endogenous opioids, and benzodiazepine receptors and the hypothalamic-pituitary-adrenal (HPA) axis. In clinical populations, data have supported hypotheses that the noradrenergic and endogenous opiate systems, as well as the HPA axis, are hyperactive in at least some patients with PTSD.

Noradrenergic System.   Soldiers with PTSD-like symptoms exhibited nervousness, increased blood pressure and heart rate, palpitations, sweating, flushing, and tremors—symptoms associated with adrenergic drugs. Studies found increased 24-hour urine epinephrine concentrations in veterans with PTSD and increased urine catecholamine concentrations in sexually abused girls. Further, platelet α_2- and lymphocyte β-adrenergic receptors are downregulated in PTSD, possibly in response to chronically elevated catecholamine concentration. Approximately 30 to 40 percent of PTSD patients report flashbacks after yohimbine (Yocon) administration. Such findings are strong evidence for altered function in the noradrenergic system in PTSD.

Opioid System.   Abnormality in the opioid system is suggested by reduced plasma β-endorphin concentrations in PTSD. Combat veterans with PTSD demonstrate a naloxone-reversible analgesic response to combat-related stimuli, raising the possibility of opioid system hyperregulation similar to that in the HPA axis.

Corticotropin-Releasing Factor and the Hypothalamic-Pituitary-Adrenal Axis.   Several factors point to dysfunction of the HPA axis. Studies have demonstrated low plasma and urinary free cortisol concentrations in PTSD. There are increased glucocorticoid receptors on lymphocytes and challenge with exogenous corticotropin-releasing factor (CRF) shows a blunted adrenocorticotropic hormone (ACTH) response. Further, suppression of cortisol by challenge with low-dose dexamethasone (Decadron) is enhanced in PTSD. This indicates hyperregulation of the HPA axis in PTSD.

Also, some studies have revealed cortisol hypersuppression to occur in trauma-exposed patients who develop PTSD compared to those patients exposed to trauma who do not develop PTSD, indicating that it might be specifically associated with PTSD and not just trauma. Overall, this hyperregulation of the HPA axis differs from the neuroendocrine activity usually seen during stress and in other disorders such as depression.

Recently, the role of the hippocampus in PTSD has received increased attention, although the issue remains controversial. Animal studies have shown that stress is associated with structural changes in the hippocampus, and studies of combat veterans with PTSD have revealed lower average volume in the hippocampal region of the brain. Futhermore, researchers suggest that the hippocampus is not necessarily the only area of the brain to show structural changes in PTSD, since studies on depression have shown similar effects in the amygdala and prefrontal cortex.

DIAGNOSIS

The DSM-IV-TR diagnostic criteria for PTSD (Table 13.5–1) specify that the symptoms of experiencing, avoidance, and hyperarousal have lasted more than 1 month. For patients in whom symptoms have been present less than 1 month, the appropriate diagnosis may be acute stress disorder (Table 13.5–2). The DSM-IV-TR diagnostic criteria for PTSD allow clinicians to specify whether the disorder is acute (if the symptoms have lasted less than 3 months) or chronic (if the symptoms have lasted 3 months or more). DSM-IV-TR also allows clinicians to specify that the disorder was with delayed onset if the onset of the symptoms was 6 months or more after the stressful event.

CLINICAL FEATURES

The principal clinical features of PTSD are the painful reexperiencing of the event, a pattern of avoidance and emotional numbing, and fairly constant hyperarousal. The disorder may not develop until months or even years after the event. The mental status examination often reveals feelings of guilt, rejection, and humiliation. Patients may also describe dissociative states and panic attacks, and illusions and hallucinations may be present. Cognitive testing may reveal that patients have impairments of memory and attention. Associated symptoms can include aggression, violence, poor impulse control, depression, and substance-related disorders. Patients have elevated Sc, D, F, and Ps scores on the Minnesota Multiphasic Personality Inventory, and the Rorschach test findings often include aggressive and violent material.

> Mr. F sought treatment for symptoms that he developed in the wake of an automobile accident that had occurred about 6 weeks prior to his psychiatric evaluation. While driving to work on a mid-January morning, Mr. F lost control of his car on an icy road. His car swerved out of control into oncoming traffic in another lane, collided with another car, and then hit a nearby pedestrian. Mr. F was trapped in his car for 3 hours while rescue workers cut the door of his car. Upon referral, Mr. F reported frequent intrusive thoughts about the accident, including nightmares of the event and recurrent intrusive visions of his car slamming into the pedestrian. He reported that he had altered his driving route to work to avoid the scene of the accident, and he found himself switching the television channel whenever a commercial for snow tires appeared. Mr. F described frequent difficulty falling asleep, poor concentration, and an increased focus on his environment, particularly when he was driving.

Table 13.5–1
DSM-IV-TR Diagnostic Criteria for Posttraumatic Stress Disorder

A. The person has been exposed to a traumatic event in which both of the following were present:
 (1) the person experienced, witnessed, or was confronted with an event or events that involved actual or threatened death or serious injury, or a threat to the physical integrity of self or others
 (2) the person's response involved intense fear, helplessness, or horror. **Note:** In children, this may be expressed instead by disorganized or agitated behavior

B. The traumatic event is persistently reexperienced in one (or more) of the following ways:
 (1) recurrent and intrusive distressing recollections of the event, including images, thoughts, or perceptions. **Note:** In young children, repetitive play may occur in which themes or aspects of the trauma are expressed.
 (2) recurrent distressing dreams of the event. **Note:** In children, there may be frightening dreams without recognizable content.
 (3) acting or feeling as if the traumatic event were recurring (includes a sense of reliving the experience, illusions, hallucinations, and dissociative flashback episodes, including those that occur on awakening or when intoxicated). **Note:** In young children, trauma-specific reenactment may occur.
 (4) intense psychological distress at exposure to internal or external cues that symbolize or resemble an aspect of the traumatic event
 (5) physiological reactivity on exposure to internal or external cues that symbolize or resemble an aspect of the traumatic event

C. Persistent avoidance of stimuli associated with the trauma and numbing of general responsiveness (not present before the trauma), as indicated by three (or more) of the following:
 (1) efforts to avoid thoughts, feelings, or conversations associated with the trauma
 (2) efforts to avoid activities, places, or people that arouse recollections of the trauma
 (3) inability to recall an important aspect of the trauma
 (4) markedly diminished interest or participation in significant activities
 (5) feeling of detachment or estrangement from others
 (6) restricted range of affect (e.g., unable to have loving feelings)
 (7) sense of a foreshortened future (e.g., does not expect to have a career, marriage, children, or a normal life span)

D. Persistent symptoms of increased arousal (not present before the trauma), as indicated by two (or more) of the following:
 (1) difficulty falling or staying asleep
 (2) irritability or outbursts of anger
 (3) difficulty concentrating
 (4) hypervigilance
 (5) exaggerated startle response

E. Duration of the disturbance (symptoms in Criteria B, C, and D) is more than 1 month.

F. The disturbance causes clinically significant distress or impairment in social, occupational, or other important areas of functioning.

Specify if:
 Acute: if duration of symptoms is less than 3 months
 Chronic: if duration of symptoms is 3 months or more
Specify if:
 With delayed onset: if onset of symptoms is at least 6 months after the stressor

From American Psychiatric Association. *Diagnostic and Statistical Manual of Mental Disorders.* 4th ed. Text rev. Washington, DC: American Psychiatric Association; copyright 2000, with permission.

Table 13.5–2
DSM-IV-TR Diagnostic Criteria for Acute Stress Disorder

A. The person has been exposed to a traumatic event in which both of the following were present:

(1) the person experienced, witnessed, or was confronted with an event or events that involved actual or threatened death or serious injury, or a threat to the physical integrity of self or others

(2) the person's response involved intense fear, helplessness, or horror

B. Either while experiencing or after experiencing the distressing event, the individual has three (or more) of the following dissociative symptoms:

(1) a subjective sense of numbing, detachment, or absence of emotional responsiveness

(2) a reduction in awareness of his or her surroundings (e.g., "being in a daze")

(3) derealization

(4) depersonalization

(5) dissociative amnesia (i.e., inability to recall an important aspect of the trauma)

C. The traumatic event is persistently reexperienced in at least one of the following ways: recurrent images, thoughts, dreams, illusions, flashback episodes, or a sense of reliving the experience; or distress on exposure to reminders of the traumatic event.

D. Marked avoidance of stimuli that arouse recollections of the trauma (e.g., thoughts, feelings, conversations, activities, places, people).

E. Marked symptoms of anxiety or increased arousal (e.g., difficulty sleeping, irritability, poor concentration, hypervigilance, exaggerated startle response, motor restlessness).

F. The disturbance causes clinically significant distress or impairment in social, occupational, or other important areas of functioning or impairs the individual's ability to pursue some necessary task, such as obtaining necessary assistance or mobilizing personal resources by telling family members about the traumatic experience.

G. The disturbance lasts for a minimum of 2 days and a maximum of 4 weeks and occurs within 4 weeks of the traumatic event.

H. The disturbance is not due to the direct physiological effects of a substance (e.g., a drug of abuse, a medication) or a general medical condition, is not better accounted for by brief psychotic disorder, and is not merely an exacerbation of a preexisting Axis I or Axis II disorder.

From American Psychiatric Association. *Diagnostic and Statistical Manual of Mental Disorders.* 4th ed. Text rev. Washington, DC: American Psychiatric Association; copyright 2000, with permission.

Posttraumatic Stress Disorders in Children and Adolescents

PTSD occurs in children and adolescents, but most studies of the disorder have focused on adults. DSM-IV-TR has little to say about PTSD as it affects young children, except to describe symptoms such as repetitive dreams of the events, nightmares of monsters, and the development of physical symptoms such as stomachaches and headaches.

High rates of PTSD have been documented in children exposed to such life-threatening events as combat and other war-related trauma, kidnapping, severe illness or burns, bone marrow transplantation, and a number of natural and man-made disasters. Studies on young victims or witnesses to criminal assault, domestic violence, and community violence have revealed high psychiatric morbidity after exposure to violence. As might be expected, the prevalence of PTSD is higher in children than in adults exposed to the same stressor. In certain situations, up to 90 percent of children will develop the disorder. In general, PTSD has been underestimated in children and adolescents.

Child risk factors include demographic factors (e.g., age, sex, socioeconomic status), other life events (positive and negative), social and cultural cognitions, psychiatric comorbidity, and inherent coping strategies. Family factors (e.g., parental psychopathology and functioning, material status, and education) play key roles in determining child symptoms. Parents' responses to traumatic events particularly influence young children who may not completely understand the nature of the trauma or its inherent danger.

Stressor.   Stressors in children may be sudden, single-incident trauma or ongoing or chronic trauma such as physical or sexual abuse. Children also suffer as the result of "indirect" exposure—that is, the unwitnessed death or injury of a loved one, as in situations of disaster, war, or community violence.

Reenactment and Reexperiencing.   Children, like adults, reexperience the traumatic event in the form of distressing intrusive thoughts or memories, flashbacks, and dreams. Children's nightmares may be linked specifically to a trauma theme or may generalize to other fears. Flashbacks occur in children as well as in their adolescent or adult victim counterparts. "Traumatic play," a specific form of reexperiencing seen in young children, consists of repetitive acting out of the trauma or trauma-related themes in play. Older children may incorporate aspects of the trauma into their lives in a process termed *reenactment.* Fantasized actions of interventions or revenge are common; adolescents should be considered at increased risk for impulsive acting out secondary to anger and revenge fantasies. Related behaviors in child and adolescent victims of trauma include sexual acting out, substance use, and delinquency. Children often withdraw and show reduced interest in previously enjoyable activities. Regressive behaviors such as enuresis or fear of sleeping alone may also occur.

Gulf War Syndrome

In the Persian Gulf War against Iraq, which began in 1990 and ended in 1991, approximately 700,000 American soldiers served in the coalition forces. Although morbidity and mortality rates were minimal in comparison to previous wars, on their return, more than 100,000 veterans reported a vast array of health problems, including irritability, chronic fatigue, shortness of breath, muscle and joint pain, migraine headaches, digestive disturbances, skin rash, hair loss, forgetfulness, and difficulty in concentrating. Collectively, these symptoms are called the *Gulf War syndrome,* but no government agency has identified the cause of these symptoms. Many veterans believe that their disorders were caused by exposure to biological and chemical agents such as fumes from burning oil wells and land fills or mustard and other nerve gasses. The U.S. Department of Defense acknowledges that up to 20,000 troops serving in the combat area may have been exposed to chemical weapons but denies that those complaining of the syndrome are suffering from the effects of chemical exposure. The best evidence indicates that the condition is a disorder that in some cases may have been precipitated by exposure to an unidentified toxin. One study of loss of memory found structural change in the right parietal lobe in 18 men with Gulf War syndrome using magnetic resonance spectroscopy (MRS). Such brain abnormalities have been found to correlate with specific clinical symptoms. New data show that damage to the basal ganglia and subsequent neurotransmitter dysfunction in veterans of the Gulf War may provide a neurological basis for this syndrome. The cause has also been attributed to the psychological stress associated with being in a combat area.

Several studies have found higher rates of physical complaints and psychological distress in veterans who had been stationed in the Persian Gulf region versus those who were deployed to Germany or the United States during the war, even after controlling for the demographic effects. This, however, may also be due to toxins in the region and not simply the stress. PTSD (and its related symptoms) is a well-documented condition that occurs in wartime. It was first identified after the Civil War and has been noted in every war thereafter, although by different names. Yet many studies of Gulf War veterans have found lower rates of PTSD than those found among veterans of previous wars, which may lend some support to the notion of a separate syndrome. Likewise, however, some patients may in fact have treatable mood and anxiety disorders but are not diagnosed because their symptoms are primarily somatic.

Torture

The intentional physical and psychological torture of one human by another can have emotionally damaging effects comparable to and possibly worse than those seen with combat and other types of trauma. As defined by the United Nations, *torture* is any deliberate infliction of severe mental pain or suffering, usually through cruel, inhuman, or degrading treatment or punishment. This broad definition includes various forms of interpersonal violence, from chronic domestic abuse to broad-scale genocide. According to Amnesty International, torture is common and widespread in most of the 150 countries worldwide where human rights violations have been documented. Recent figures estimate that between 5 and 35 percent of the world's 14 million refugees have had at least one torture experience; these numbers do not even account for the consequences of the current political, regional, and religious disputes in Eastern Europe, the former Yugoslavia, and the Middle East.

Torture is distinct from most other types of trauma because it is human inflicted and intentional. One individual working for himself or for a higher authority may abuse another in order to punish, exact retribution, or obtain information from the victim. Methods can be physical, for example in the form of beatings, burning of the skin, electric shock, or asphyxiation; or psychological, through threats, humiliation, or being forced to watch others, often loved ones, being tortured. One distinct method of torture that may combine physical and psychological aspects is brainwashing (see section below). While many forms of torture can leave lasting physical scars, which themselves serve as constant reminders of the trauma, it seems that the true purpose is the psychological effect—the torturer invokes fear, helplessness, and, ultimately, physical and mental weakness in the victim. Reported prevalence rates of PTSD among survivors of torture are approximately 36 percent, much higher than the average lifetime prevalence, and researchers concur that the severity and duration of PTSD may be greater when the stres-

sors are of human design. Studies have also revealed substantial comorbidity with depression and other anxiety disorders in victims of torture. Other common psychological complaints include somatization, obsessive-compulsive symptoms, anger-hostility, phobias, paranoid ideation, and psychotic episodes.

Treatment methods for survivors of torture are the same as those for other posttraumatic symptoms and disorders, but clinicians must be especially sensitive to the array of stressful life events that victims of torture have experienced. Many survivors who present for treatment are refugees and face new posttrauma stressors over and above the effects of torture, such as separation from family, difficulty finding work, difficulty obtaining health services, language barriers, loneliness, poverty, and racial discrimination. Religious faith, political education and commitment, strong social support, and mental preparedness for the possibility of torture seem to serve as protective factors against developing PTSD and other psychological consequences after torture. Moreover, cultural and religious factors that influence coping styles may also affect treatment response in survivors of torture.

Brainwashing

First practiced by the Chinese Communists on U.S. prisoners during the Korean War, brainwashing is the deliberate creation of cultural shock. A condition of isolation, alienation, and intimidation is developed for the express purpose of assaulting ego strengths and leaving the person to be brainwashed vulnerable to the imposition of alien ideas and behavior that would usually be rejected. Brainwashing relies on both mental and physical coercion. All people are vulnerable to brainwashing if they are exposed to it for a long enough time, if they are alone and without support, and if they are without hope of escape from the situation. Whether the psychological effects are permanent likely depends on the individual's strength of character and subsequent environment and support system. Help from the mental health care system, in the form of deprogramming, is usually necessary to help brainwashed persons readjust to their usual environments after the brainwashing experience. Supportive therapy is offered, with emphasis on reeducation, restitution of ego strengths that existed before the trauma, and alleviation of the guilt and depression that are remnants of the frightening experience and of the lost confidence and confusion in identity that result from it.

Terrorism

The terrorist activity of September 11, 2001, in which the World Trade Center in New York City and the Pentagon in Washington, DC were destroyed and damaged, resulting in more than 3,500 deaths and injuries, traumatized a nation, many of whose citizens required therapeutic intervention. A survey of more than 500 U.S. adults, taken less than 1 month after the event to assess their reactions and their children's reactions to the terrorist attacks found the following:

Forty-five percent of adults reported one or more substantial symptom of stress, such as distressing recollections of the event, insomnia, nightmares, fearfulness, and irritability, among others. Ninety percent of those interviewed reported minor degrees of symptoms. Susceptibility to symptoms was associated with being female, nonwhite, having previous psychological illness, and being close to the disaster site. Most adults responded to the attack by talking to others about their feelings, by attending religious services, and donating charitable gifts.

More than 80 percent of parents reported that their children had one or more symptoms. An interesting finding was that the level of stress was associated with the extent of television viewing about the disaster.

In a later survey of Manhattan residents conducted 5 to 8 weeks after the World Trade Center collapse published in the *New England Journal of Medicine* in 2002, it was found that 9.8 percent—or an estimated 90,000 people—had PTSD or clinical depression. Another 3.7 percent—or an estimated 34,000 people—met the criteria for both diagnoses. Higher rates for both disorders were found among people who lived close to Ground Zero, who had suffered personal losses as a result of the attacks, who had endured other stressful events during the previous 12 months, or who had experienced extreme panic during or shortly after the attack. The rates of both disorders were higher among Hispanic respondents than among whites, blacks, or Asians, and higher among women than among men. Among people in upper income levels, the incidence was lower for disorders.

Finally, in a study of more than 8,000 children aged 10 through 13 who lived in New York at the time of the terrorist attacks, it was found that 11 percent had symptoms compatible with a diagnosis of PTSD 9 months after the event. An additional 15 percent had signs of agoraphobia (e.g., fear of taking public transportation). Similar to the demographics in adults described above, Hispanic students and girls were disproportionally affected, as were those who were exposed to prior unrelated traumatic events.

DIFFERENTIAL DIAGNOSIS

A major consideration in the diagnosis of PTSD is the possibility that the patient also incurred a head injury during the trauma. Other organic considerations that can both cause and exacerbate the symptoms are epilepsy, alcohol use disorders, and other substance-related disorders. Acute intoxication or withdrawal from some substances may also present a clinical picture that is difficult to distinguish from the disorder until the effects of the substance have worn off.

PTSD is commonly misdiagnosed as another mental disorder and is then inappropriately treated. Clinicians must consider the diagnosis of PTSD in patients who have pain disorder, substance abuse, other anxiety disorders, and mood disorders. In general, PTSD can be distinguished from other mental disorders by interviewing a patient about previous traumatic experiences and by the nature of the current symptoms. Borderline personality disorder, dissociative disorders, factitious disorders, and malingering should also be considered. Borderline personality disorder can be difficult to distinguish from PTSD. The two disorders may coexist or even may be causally related. Patients with dissociative disorders do not usually have the degree of avoidance behavior, the autonomic hyperarousal, or the history of trauma that patients with PTSD report. Partly because of the publicity that PTSD has received, clinicians should also consider the possibility of a factitious disorder and malingering.

COURSE AND PROGNOSIS

PTSD usually develops some time after the trauma. The delay can be as short as 1 week or as long as 30 years. Symptoms can fluctuate over time and may be most intense during periods of stress. Untreated, approximately 30 percent of patients recover completely, 40 percent continue to have mild symptoms, 20 percent continue to have moderate symptoms, and 10 percent remain unchanged or become worse. After 1 year, approximately 50 percent of patients will recover. A good prognosis is predicted by a rapid onset of the symptoms, the short duration of the symptoms (less than 6 months), good premorbid functioning, strong social supports, and the absence of other psychiatric, medical, or substance-related disorders or other risk factors.

In general, the very young and the very old have more difficulty with traumatic events than do those in midlife. For example, approximately 80 percent of young children who sustain a burn injury show symptoms of PTSD 1 or 2 years after the initial injury; only 30 percent of adults who suffer such an injury have a PTSD after 1 year. Presumably, young children do not yet have adequate coping mechanisms to deal with the physical and emotional insults of the trauma. Likewise, older people, when compared with younger adults, are likely to have more rigid coping mechanisms and to be less able to muster a flexible approach to dealing with the effects of trauma. Furthermore, the traumatic effects may be exacerbated by physical disabilities characteristic of late life, particularly disabilities of the nervous system and the cardiovascular system, such as reduced cerebral blood flow, failing vision, palpitations, and arrhythmias. Preexisting psychiatric disability, whether a personality disorder or a more serious condition, also increases the effects of particular stressors. PTSD that is comorbid with other disorders is often more severe, maybe more chronic, and may be difficult to treat. The availability of social supports may also influence the development, severity, and duration of PTSD. In general, patients who have a good network of social support are less likely to have the disorder, are less likely to experience it in its severe forms, and are more likely to recover in less time.

TREATMENT

When a clinician is faced with a patient who has experienced a significant trauma, the major approaches are support, encouragement to discuss the event, and education about a variety of coping mechanisms (for example, relaxation). The use of sedatives and hypnotics can also be helpful. When a patient experienced a traumatic event in the past and now has PTSD, the emphasis should be on education about the disorder and its treatment, both pharmacological and psychotherapeutic. The clinician should also work to destigmatize the notion of mental illness and PTSD.

Pharmacotherapy

Selective serotonin reuptake inhibitors (SSRIs), such as sertraline (Zoloft) and paroxetine (Paxil), are considered first-line treatments for PTSD owing to their efficacy, tolerability, and safety ratings. SSRIs reduce symptoms from all PTSD symptom clusters and are effective in improving symptoms unique to PTSD, not just those similar to those of depression or other anxiety disorders.

The efficacy of imipramine (Tofranil) and amitriptyline (Elavil), two tricyclic drugs, in the treatment of PTSD is supported by a number of well-controlled clinical trials. Although some trials of the two drugs have had negative findings, most of these trials had serious design flaws, including too short a duration. Dosages of imipramine and amitriptyline should be the same as those used to treat depressive disorders, and the minimum length of an adequate trial should be 8 weeks. Patients who respond well should probably continue the pharmacotherapy for at least 1 year before an attempt is made to withdraw the drug. Some studies indicate that pharmacotherapy is more effective in treating the depression, anxiety, and hyperarousal than in treating the avoidance, denial, and emotional numbing.

Other drugs that may be useful in the treatment of PTSD are the monoamine oxidase inhibitors (MAOIs) (e.g., phenelzine [Nardil]), trazodone (Desyrel), and the anticonvulsants (for example, carbamazepine (Tegretol) and valproate [Depakene]). Some studies have also revealed improvement in PTSD in patients treated with reversible monoamine oxidase inhibitors (RIMAs) such as brofaromine. Use of clonidine (Catapres) and propranolol (Inderal), which are antiadrenergic agents, is suggested by the theories about noradrenergic hyperactivity in the disorder. Almost no positive data concern the use of antipsychotic drugs in the disorder, so the use of these drugs—for example, haloperidol (Haldol)—should be reserved for the short-term control of severe aggression and agitation.

Psychotherapy

Psychodynamic psychotherapy may be useful in the treatment of many patients with PTSD. In some cases, reconstruction of the traumatic events with associated abreaction and catharsis may be therapeutic, but psychotherapy must be individualized, because reexperiencing the traumas overwhelms some patients.

Psychotherapeutic interventions for PTSD include behavior therapy, cognitive therapy, and hypnosis. Many clinicians advocate time-limited psychotherapy for the victims of trauma. Such therapy usually takes a cognitive approach and also provides support and security. The short-term nature of the psychotherapy minimizes the risk of dependence and chronicity, but issues of suspicion, paranoia, and trust often adversely affect compliance. Therapists should overcome patients' denial of the traumatic event, encourage them to relax, and remove them from the source of the stress. Patients should be encouraged to sleep, using medication if necessary. Support from people in their environment (such as friends and relatives) should be provided. Patients should be encouraged to review and abreact emotional feelings associated with the traumatic event and to plan for future recovery. Abreaction—experiencing the emotions associated with the event—may be helpful for some patients. The amobarbital (Amytal) interview has been used to facilitate this process.

Psychotherapy after a traumatic event should follow a model of crisis intervention with support, education, and the development of coping mechanisms and acceptance of the event. When PTSD has developed, two major psychotherapeutic approaches can be taken. The first is exposure to the traumatic event through imaging techniques or in vivo exposure. The exposures can be intense, as in implosive therapy, or graded, as in systematic desensitization. The second approach is to teach the patient methods of stress management, including relaxation techniques and cognitive approaches to coping with stress. Some preliminary data indicate that, although stress management techniques are effective more rapidly than are exposure techniques, the results of exposure techniques are more long lasting.

Another psychotherapeutic technique that is relatively novel and somewhat controversial is eye movement desensitization and reprocessing (EMDR), in which the patient focuses on the lateral movement of the clinician's finger while maintaining a mental image of the trauma experience. The general belief is that symptoms can be relieved as patients work through the traumatic event while in a state of deep relaxation. Proponents of this treatment state it is as effective and possibly more effective than other treatments for PTSD and that is preferred by both clinicians and patients who have tried it.

In addition to individual therapy techniques, group therapy and family therapy have been reported to be effective in cases of PTSD. The advantages of group therapy include the sharing of traumatic experiences and support from other group members. Group therapy has been particularly successful with Vietnam veterans and survivors of catastrophic disasters, such as earthquakes. Family therapy often helps sustain a marriage through periods of exacerbated symptoms. Hospitalization may be necessary when symptoms are particularly severe or when there is a risk of suicide or other violence.

▲ 13.6 Generalized Anxiety Disorder

Persons who seem to be pathologically anxious about almost everything are likely to be classified as having generalized anxiety disorder. The text revision of the fourth edition of the *Diagnostic and Statistical Manual of Mental Disorders* (DSM-IV-TR) defines generalized anxiety disorder as excessive anxiety and worry about several events or activities for a majority of days during at least a 6-month period. The worry is difficult to control and is associated with somatic symptoms such as muscle tension, irritability, difficulty sleeping, and restlessness. The anxiety is not focused on features of another Axis I disorder, is not caused by substance use or a general medical condition, and does not occur only during a mood or psychiatric disorder. The anxiety is difficult to control, is subjectively distressing, and produces impairment in important areas of a person's life.

EPIDEMIOLOGY

Generalized anxiety disorder is a common condition; reasonable estimates for its 1-year prevalence range from 3 to 8 percent. The ratio of women to men with the disorder is approximately 2 to 1, but the ratio of women to men who are receiving inpatient treatment for the disorder is approximately 1 to 1. There is a lifetime prevalence of 45 percent.

COMORBIDITY

Generalized anxiety disorder is probably the disorder that most often coexists with another mental disorder, usually social phobia, specific phobia, panic disorder, or a depressive disorder. Perhaps 50 to 90 percent of patients with generalized anxiety disorder have another mental disorder. As many as 25 percent of patients eventually experience panic disorder. An additional high percentage of patients are likely to have major depressive disorder. Other common disorders associated with generalized anxiety disorder are dysthymic disorder, social and specific phobia, and substance-related disorders.

ETIOLOGY

As with most mental disorders, the cause of generalized anxiety disorder is not known. As currently defined, generalized anxiety disorder probably affects a heterogeneous group of people. Perhaps because a certain degree of anxiety is normal and adaptive, differentiating normal anxiety from pathological anxiety and differentiating biological causative factors from psychosocial factors are difficult. Biological and psychological factors probably work together.

Biological Factors

The therapeutic efficacies of benzodiazepines and the azaspirones—for example, buspirone (BuSpar)—have focused biological research efforts on the γ-aminobutyric acid and serotonin neurotransmitter systems. Benzodiazepines (which are benzodiazepine receptor agonists) are known to reduce anxiety, whereas flumazenil (Romazicon) (a benzodiazepine receptor antagonist) and the β-carbolines (benzodiazepine receptor reverse agonists) are known to induce anxiety. Although no convincing data indicate that the benzodiazepine receptors are abnormal in patients with generalized anxiety disorder, some researchers have focused on the occipital lobe, which has the highest concentrations of benzodiazepine receptors in the brain. Other brain areas that have been hypothesized to be involved in generalized anxiety disorder are the basal ganglia, the limbic system, and the frontal cortex. Because buspirone is an agonist at the serotonin 5-HT$_{1A}$ receptor, there is the hypothesis that the regulation of the serotonergic system in generalized anxiety disorder is abnormal. Other neurotransmitter systems that have been the subject of research in generalized anxiety disorder include the norepinephrine, glutamate, and cholecystokinin neurotransmitter systems. Some evidence indicates that patients with generalized anxiety disorder may have a subsensitivity of their α_2-adrenergic receptors, as indicated by a blunted release of growth hormone after clonidine (Catapres) infusion.

Only a limited number of brain-imaging studies of patients with generalized anxiety disorder have been conducted. One positron emission tomography (PET) study reported a lower metabolic rate in basal ganglia and white matter in generalized anxiety disorder patients than in normal control subjects. A few genetic studies have also been conducted in the field. One study found that a genetic relation may exist between generalized anxiety disorder and major depressive disorder in women. Another study showed a distinct but difficult-to-quantitate genetic component in generalized anxiety disorder. Approximately 25 percent of first-degree relatives of patients with generalized anxiety disorder are also affected. Male relatives are likely to have an alcohol use disorder. Some twin studies report a concordance rate of 50 percent in monozygotic twins and 15 percent in dizygotic twins.

A variety of electroencephalogram (EEG) abnormalities have been noted in alpha rhythm and evoked potentials. Sleep EEG studies have reported increased sleep discontinuity, decreased delta sleep, decreased stage 1 sleep, and reduced rapid eye movement (REM) sleep. These changes in sleep architecture are different from the changes seen in depressive disorders.

Psychosocial Factors

The two major schools of thought about psychosocial factors leading to the development of generalized anxiety disorder are the cognitive-behavioral school and the psychoanalytic school. According to the cognitive-behavioral school, patients with generalized anxiety disorder respond to incorrectly and inaccurately perceived dangers. The inaccuracy is generated by selective attention to negative details in the environment, by distortions in information processing, and by an overly negative view of the person's own ability to cope. The psychoanalytic school hypothesizes that anxiety is a symptom of unresolved unconscious conflicts. This psychological theory was first presented by Sigmund Freud in 1909 with his description of Little Hans; before then, Freud had conceptualized anxiety as having a physiological basis.

A hierarchy of anxieties is related to various developmental levels. At the most primitive level, anxiety may relate to the fear of annihilation or of fusion with another person. At a more mature level of development, anxiety is related to separation from a love object. At a still more mature level, anxiety is connected to the loss of love from an important object. Castration anxiety is related to the oedipal phase of development and is considered one of the highest levels of anxiety. Superego anxiety, a person's fear of disappointing his or her own ideals and values (derived from internalized parents), is the most mature form of anxiety.

DIAGNOSIS

The DSM-IV-TR diagnostic criteria (Table 13.6–1) include criteria to help clinicians differentiate among generalized anxiety disorder, normal anxiety, and other mental disorders. The distinction between generalized anxiety disorder and normal anxiety is emphasized by the use of the words "excessive" and "difficult to control" in the criteria and by the specification that the symptoms cause significant impairment or distress.

CLINICAL FEATURES

The primary symptoms of generalized anxiety disorder are anxiety, motor tension, autonomic hyperactivity, and cognitive vigilance. The anxiety is excessive and interferes with other aspects of people's lives. The motor tension is most commonly manifested as shakiness, restlessness, and headaches. The autonomic hyperactivity is commonly manifested by shortness of breath, excessive sweating, palpitations, and various gastrointestinal symptoms. The cognitive vigilance is evidenced by irritability and the ease with which patients are startled.

Patients with generalized anxiety disorder usually seek out a general practitioner or internist for help with a somatic symptom. Alternatively, the patients go to a specialist for a specific symptom—for example, chronic diarrhea. A specific nonpsy-

Table 13.6–1
DSM-IV-TR Diagnostic Criteria for Generalized Anxiety Disorder

A. Excessive anxiety and worry (apprehensive expectation), occurring more days than not for at least 6 months, about a number of events or activities (such as work or school performance).

B. The person finds it difficult to control the worry.

C. The anxiety and worry are associated with three (or more) of the following six symptoms (with at least some symptoms present for more days than not for the past 6 months).
   Note: Only one item is required in children.
   (1) restlessness or feeling keyed up or on edge
   (2) being easily fatigued
   (3) difficulty concentrating or mind going blank
   (4) irritability
   (5) muscle tension
   (6) sleep disturbance (difficulty falling or staying asleep, or restless unsatisfying sleep)

D. The focus of the anxiety and worry is not confined to features of an Axis I disorder, e.g., the anxiety or worry is not about having a panic attack (as in panic disorder), being embarrassed in public (as in social phobia), being contaminated (as in obsessive-compulsive disorder), being away from home or close relatives (as in separation anxiety disorder), gaining weight (as in anorexia nervosa), having multiple physical complaints (as in somatization disorder), or having a serious illness (as in hypochondriasis), and the anxiety and worry do not occur exclusively during posttraumatic stress disorder.

E. The anxiety, worry, or physical symptoms cause clinically significant distress or impairment in social, occupational, or other important areas of functioning.

F. The disturbance is not due to the direct physiological effects of a substance (e.g., a drug of abuse, a medication) or a general medical condition (e.g., hyperthyroidism) and does not occur exclusively during a mood disorder, a psychotic disorder, or a pervasive developmental disorder.

From American Psychiatric Association. *Diagnostic and Statistical Manual of Mental Disorders*. 4th ed. Text rev. Washington, DC: American Psychiatric Association; copyright 2000, with permission.

chiatric medical disorder is rarely found, and patients vary in their doctor-seeking behavior. Some patients accept a diagnosis of generalized anxiety disorder and the appropriate treatment; others seek additional medical consultations for their problems.

Ms. X was a successful, married, 30-year-old attorney who presented for a psychiatric evaluation to treat growing symptoms of worry and anxiety. For the preceding 8 months, Ms. X had noted increased worry about her job performance. For example, while she had always been a superb litigator, she increasingly found herself worrying about her ability to win each new case she was presented. Similarly, while she had always been in outstanding physical condition, she worried increasingly that her health had begun to deteriorate. Ms. X noted frequent somatic symptoms that accompanied her worries. For example, she often felt restless while she worked and while she commuted to her office, thinking about the upcoming challenges of the day. She reported feeling increasingly fatigued, irritable, and tense. She noted that she had increasing difficulty falling asleep at night as she worried about her job performance and impending trials. (Courtesy of Daniel S. Pine, M.D.)

DIFFERENTIAL DIAGNOSIS

The differential diagnosis of generalized anxiety disorder includes all the medical disorders that may cause anxiety. The medical workup should include standard blood chemistry tests, an electrocardiogram, and thyroid function tests. Clinicians must rule out caffeine intoxication, stimulant abuse, alcohol withdrawal, and sedative, hypnotic, or anxiolytic withdrawal. The mental status examination and the history should explore the diagnostic possibilities of panic disorder, phobias, and obsessive-compulsive disorder. In general, patients with panic disorder seek treatment earlier, are more disabled by their disorder, have had a sudden onset of symptoms, and are less troubled by their somatic symptoms than are patients with generalized anxiety disorder. Distinguishing generalized anxiety disorder from major depressive disorder and dysthymic disorder can be difficult; in fact, the disorders frequently coexist. Other diagnostic possibilities are adjustment disorder with anxiety, hypochondriasis, adult attention-deficit/hyperactivity disorder, somatization disorder, and personality disorders.

COURSE AND PROGNOSIS

The age of onset is difficult to specify; most patients with the disorder report that they have been anxious for as long as they can remember. Patients usually come to a clinician's attention in their 20s, although the first contact with a clinician can occur at virtually any age. Only one-third of patients who have generalized anxiety disorder seek psychiatric treatment. Many go to general practitioners, internists, cardiologists, pulmonary specialists, or gastroenterologists, seeking treatment for the somatic component of the disorder. Because of the high incidence of comorbid mental disorders in patients with generalized anxiety disorder, the clinical course and prognosis of the disorder are difficult to predict. Nonetheless, some data indicate that life events are associated with the onset of generalized anxiety disorder: The occurrence of several negative life events greatly increases the likelihood that the disorder will develop. By definition, generalized anxiety disorder is a chronic condition that may well be lifelong.

TREATMENT

The most effective treatment of generalized anxiety disorder is probably one that combines psychotherapeutic, pharmacotherapeutic, and supportive approaches. The treatment may take a significant amount of time for the involved clinician, whether the clinician is a psychiatrist, a family practitioner, or another specialist.

Psychotherapy

The major psychotherapeutic approaches to generalized anxiety disorder are cognitive-behavioral, supportive, and insight-oriented. Data are still limited on the relative merits of those approaches, although the most sophisticated studies have examined cognitive-behavioral techniques, which seem to have both short-term and long-term efficacy. Cognitive approaches directly address patients' hypothesized cognitive distortions, and behavioral approaches address somatic symptoms directly. The major techniques used in behavioral approaches are relaxation and biofeedback. Some preliminary data indicate that the combination of cognitive and behavioral approaches is more effective than either technique used alone. Supportive therapy offers patients reassurance and comfort, although its long-term efficacy is doubtful. Insight-oriented psychotherapy focuses on uncovering unconscious conflicts and identifying ego strengths. The efficacy of insight-oriented psychotherapy for generalized anxiety disorder is reported in many anecdotal case reports, but large controlled studies are lacking.

Most patients experience a marked lessening of anxiety when given the opportunity to discuss their difficulties with concerned and sympathetic physicians. If clinicians discover external situations that are anxiety provoking, they may be able—alone or with the help of the patients or their families—to change the environment and thus reduce the stressful pressures. A reduction in symptoms often allows patients to function effectively in their daily work and relationships and thus to gain new rewards and gratification that are in themselves therapeutic.

In the psychoanalytic perspective, anxiety is sometimes a signal of unconscious turmoil that deserves investigation. The anxiety can be normal, adaptive, maladaptive, too intense, or too mild, depending on the circumstances. Anxiety appears in numerous situations over the course of the life cycle; in many cases, symptom relief is not the most appropriate course of action.

For patients who are psychologically minded and motivated to understand the sources of their anxiety, psychotherapy may be the treatment of choice. Psychodynamic therapy proceeds with the assumption that anxiety may increase with effective treatment. The goal of the dynamic approach may be to increase the patient's anxiety tolerance (a capacity to experience anxiety without having to discharge it), rather than to eliminate anxiety. Empirical research indicates that many patients who have successful psychotherapeutic treatment may continue to experience anxiety after termination of the psychotherapy, but their increased ego mastery allows them to use the anxiety symptoms as a signal to reflect on internal struggles and to expand their insight and understanding. A psychodynamic approach to patients with generalized anxiety disorder involves a search for the patient's underlying fears.

Pharmacotherapy

Because of the long-term nature of the disorder, a treatment plan must be carefully thought out. The three major drugs to be considered for the treatment of generalized anxiety disorder are buspirone, the benzodiazepines, and the selective serotonin reuptake inhibitors (SSRIs). Other drugs that may be useful are the tricyclic drugs (for example, imipramine [Tofranil]), antihistamines, and the β-adrenergic antagonists (for example, propranolol [Inderal]).

Although drug treatment of generalized anxiety disorder is sometimes seen as a 6- to 12-month treatment, some evidence indicates that treatment should be long-term, perhaps lifelong. Approximately 25 percent of patients relapse in the first month after the discontinuation of therapy, and 60 to 80 percent relapse over the course of the next year. Although some patients become dependent on the benzodiazepines, no tolerance develops to the therapeutic effects of either the benzodiazepines, buspirone, or the SSRIs.

Benzodiazepines.   Benzodiazepines have been the drugs of choice for generalized anxiety disorder. They can be prescribed on an as-needed basis, so that patients take a rapidly acting benzodiazepine when they feel particularly anxious. The alternative approach is to prescribe benzodiazepines for a limited period, during which psychosocial therapeutic approaches are implemented.

Several problems are associated with the use of benzodiazepines in generalized anxiety disorder. Approximately 25 to 30 percent of all patients do not respond, and tolerance and dependence may occur. Some patients also experience impaired alertness while taking the drugs and are therefore at risk for accidents involving automobiles and machinery.

The clinical decision to initiate treatment with a benzodiazepine should be a considered and specific one. The patient's diagnosis, the specific target symptoms, and the duration of treatment all should be defined, and the information should be shared with patients. Treatment for most anxiety conditions lasts for 2 to 6 weeks, followed by 1 or 2 weeks of tapering the drug before it is discontinued. The most common clinical mistake with benzodiazepine treatment is to continue treatment indefinitely.

For the treatment of anxiety, it is usual to begin a drug at the low end of its therapeutic range and to increase the dosage to achieve a therapeutic response. The use of a benzodiazepine with an intermediate half-life (8 to 15 hours) is likely to avoid some of the adverse effects associated with the use of benzodiazepines with long half-lives, and the use of divided doses prevents the development of adverse effects associated with high peak plasma levels. The improvement produced by benzodiazepines may go beyond a simple antianxiety effect. For example, the drugs may cause patients to regard various occurrences in a positive light. The drugs may also have a mild disinhibiting action, similar to that observed after ingesting modest amounts of alcohol.

Buspirone.   Buspirone is a 5-HT$_{1A}$ receptor partial agonist and is most likely effective in 60 to 80 percent of patients with generalized anxiety disorder. Data indicate that buspirone is more effective in reducing the cognitive symptoms of generalized anxiety disorder than in reducing the somatic symptoms. Evidence also indicates that patients who have previously undergone treatment with benzodiazepines are not likely to respond to treatment with buspirone. The lack of response may be due to the absence, with buspirone treatment, of some of the nonanxiolytic effects of benzodiazepines (such as muscle relaxation and the additional sense of well-being). The major disadvantage of buspirone is that its effects take 2 to 3 weeks to become evident, in contrast to the almost immediate anxiolytic effects of the benzodiazepines. One approach is to initiate a benzodiazepine and buspirone simultaneously, then taper off the benzodiazepine after 2 to 3 weeks, at which point the buspirone should have reached its maximum effects. Some studies have also reported that long-term combined treatment with benzodiazepine and buspirone may be more effective than either drug alone. Buspirone is not an effective treatment for benzodiazepine withdrawal.

Venlafaxine.   Venlafaxine (Effexor) is effective in treating the insomnia, poor concentration, restlessness, irritability, and excessive muscle tension associated with generalized anxiety disorder.

Selective Serotonin Reuptake Inhibitors.   SSRIs may be effective, especially for patients with comorbid depression. The prominent disadvantage of SSRIs, especially fluoxetine (Prozac), is that they may transiently increase anxiety. For this reason, the SSRIs sertraline (Zoloft) or paroxetine (Paxil) are better choices. It is reasonable to begin treatment with sertraline or paroxetine plus a benzodiazepine, then to taper the benzodiazepine after 2 to 3 weeks. Controlled studies are needed to determine whether SSRIs are as effective for generalized anxiety disorder as they are for panic disorder and obsessive-compulsive disorder.

Other Drugs.   If conventional treatment (e.g., with buspirone or a benzodiazepine) is ineffective or not completely effective, then a clinical reassessment is indicated to rule out comorbid conditions, such as depression, or to better understand the patient's environmental stresses. Other drugs that have proven useful for generalized anxiety disorder include the tricyclic and tetracyclic drugs. The β-adrenergic receptor antagonists may reduce the somatic manifestations of anxiety but not the underlying condition, and their use is usually limited to situational anxieties, such as performance anxiety. Nefazodone (Serzone), also used in depression, has been shown to reduce anxiety and to prevent panic disorder.

▲ 13.7 Anxiety Disorder Due to a General Medical Condition

Many medical disorders are associated with anxiety. Symptoms can include panic attacks, generalized anxiety, obsessions and compulsions, and other signs of distress. In all cases, the signs and symptoms will be due to the direct physiological effects of the medical condition.

EPIDEMIOLOGY

The occurrence of anxiety symptoms related to general medical conditions is common, although the incidence of the disorder varies for each specific general medical condition.

ETIOLOGY

A wide range of medical conditions can cause symptoms similar to those of anxiety disorders. Hyperthyroidism, hypothyroidism, hypoparathyroidism, and vitamin B_{12} deficiency are frequently associated with anxiety symptoms. A pheochromocytoma produces epinephrine, which can cause paroxysmal episodes of anxiety symptoms. Certain lesions of the brain and postencephalitic states reportedly produce symptoms identical to those seen in obsessive-compulsive disorder. Other medical conditions, such as cardiac arrhythmia, can produce physiological symptoms of panic disorder. Hypoglycemia can also mimic the symptoms of an anxiety disorder. The diverse medical conditions that can cause symptoms of anxiety disorder may do so through a common mechanism, the noradrenergic system, although the effects on the serotonergic system are also under study.

DIAGNOSIS

The fourth revised edition of the *Diagnostic and Statistical Manual of Mental Disorders* (DSM-IV-TR) diagnosis of anxiety disorder due to a general medical condition (Table 13.7–1) requires the presence of symptoms of an anxiety disorder. DSM-IV-TR allows clinicians to specify whether the disorder is characterized by symptoms of generalized anxiety, panic attacks, or obsessive-compulsive symptoms.

Table 13.7–1
DSM-IV-TR Diagnostic Criteria for Anxiety Disorder Due to a General Medical Condition

A. Prominent anxiety, panic attacks, or obsessions or compulsions predominate in the clinical picture.
B. There is evidence from the history, physical examination, or laboratory findings that the disturbance is the direct physiological consequence of a general medical condition.
C. The disturbance is not better accounted for by another mental disorder (e.g., adjustment disorder with anxiety in which the stressor is a serious general medical condition).
D. The disturbance does not occur exclusively during the course of a delirium.
E. The disturbance causes clinically significant distress or impairment in social, occupational, or other important areas of functioning.

Specify if:
   With generalized anxiety: if excessive anxiety or worry about a number of events or activities predominates in the clinical presentation
   With panic attacks: if panic attacks predominate in the clinical presentation
   With obsessive-compulsive symptoms: if obsessions or compulsions predominate in the clinical presentation
Coding note: Include the name of the general medical condition on Axis I, e.g., anxiety disorder due to pheochromocytoma, with generalized anxiety; also code the general medical condition on Axis III.

From American Psychiatric Association. *Diagnostic and Statistical Manual of Mental Disorders.* 4th ed. Text rev. Washington, DC: American Psychiatric Association; copyright 2000, with permission.

Clinicians should have an increased level of suspicion for the diagnosis when chronic or paroxysmal anxiety is associated with a physical disease known to cause such symptoms in some patients. Paroxysmal bouts of hypertension in an anxious patient may indicate that a workup for a pheochromocytoma is appropriate. A general medical workup may reveal diabetes, an adrenal tumor, thyroid disease, or a neurological condition. For example, some patients with complex partial epilepsy have extreme episodes of anxiety or fear as their only manifestation of the epileptic activity.

CLINICAL FEATURES

The symptoms of anxiety disorder due to a general medical condition can be identical to those of the primary anxiety disorders. A syndrome similar to panic disorder is the most common clinical picture, and a syndrome similar to a phobia is the least common. Patients who have cardiomyopathy may have the highest incidence of panic disorder secondary to a general medical condition. One study reported that 83 percent of patients with cardiomyopathy awaiting cardiac transplantation had panic disorder. In some studies, approximately 25 percent of patients with Parkinson's disease and chronic obstructive pulmonary disease have symptoms of panic disorder. Other medical disorders associated with panic disorder include chronic pain, primary biliary cirrhosis, and epilepsy, particularly when the focus is in the right parahippocampal gyrus. The highest prevalence of generalized anxiety disorder symptoms in a medical disorder seems to be in Graves' disease, in which as many as two-thirds of all patients meet the criteria for generalized anxiety disorder.

DIFFERENTIAL DIAGNOSIS

Anxiety as a symptom can be associated with many psychiatric disorders, in addition to the anxiety disorders themselves. A mental status examination is necessary to determine the presence of mood symptoms or psychotic symptoms that may suggest another psychiatric diagnosis. For a clinician to conclude that a patient has an anxiety disorder due to a general medical condition, the patient should clearly have anxiety as the predominant symptom and should have a specific causative nonpsychiatric medical disorder. To ascertain the degree to which a general medical condition is causative for the anxiety, the clinician should know whether the medical condition and the anxiety symptoms have been related closely in the literature, the age of onset (primary anxiety disorders usually have their onset before age 35), and the patient's family history of both anxiety disorders and relevant general medical conditions (for example, hyperthyroidism). A diagnosis of adjustment disorder with anxiety must also be considered in the differential diagnosis.

COURSE AND PROGNOSIS

The unremitting experience of anxiety can be disabling and can interfere with every aspect of life, including social, occupational, and psychological functioning. The treatment or the removal of the primary medical cause of the anxiety usually initiates a clear course of improvement in the anxiety disorder symptoms. In some cases, however, the anxiety disorder symptoms continue even after the primary medical condition is treated—for example, after an episode of encephalitis. Some symptoms, particularly obsessive-compulsive disorder symptoms, linger for a longer time than do other anxiety disorder symptoms. When anxiety disorder symptoms are present for a significant period after the medical disorder has been treated, the remaining symptoms should probably be treated as if they were primary—that is, with psychotherapy or pharmacotherapy or both.

TREATMENT

The primary treatment for anxiety disorder due to a general medical condition is the treatment of the underlying medical condition. If a patient also has an alcohol or other substance use disorder, this disorder must also be therapeutically addressed to gain control of the anxiety disorder symptoms. If the removal of the primary medical condition does not reverse the anxiety disorder symptoms, treatment of these symptoms should follow the treatment guidelines for the specific mental disorder. In general, behavioral modification techniques, anxiolytic agents, and serotonergic antidepressants have been the most effective treatment modalities.

SUBSTANCE-INDUCED ANXIETY DISORDER

DSM-IV-TR includes the substance-induced mental disorders in the categories for the relevant mental disorder syndromes. Substance-induced anxiety disorder, therefore, is contained in the category of anxiety disorders.

Epidemiology

Substance-induced anxiety disorder is common, both as the result of the ingestion of so-called recreational drugs and as the result of prescription drug use.

Etiology

A wide range of substances can cause symptoms of anxiety that mimic any of the DSM-IV-TR anxiety disorders. Although sympathomimetics (such as amphetamine, cocaine, and caffeine) have been most associated with the production of anxiety disorder symptoms, many serotonergic drugs (for example, lysergic acid diethylamide [LSD] and methylenedioxymethamphetamine [MDMA]) can also cause both acute and chronic anxiety syndromes in users of these drugs. A wide range of prescription medications is also associated with the production of anxiety disorder symptoms in susceptible persons.

Diagnosis

The DSM-IV-TR diagnostic criteria for substance-induced anxiety disorder require the presence of prominent anxiety, panic attacks, obsessions, or compulsions (Table 13.7–2). The DSM-IV-TR guidelines state that the symptoms should have developed during the use of the substance or within 1 month of the cessation of substance use, but DSM-IV-TR encourages clinicians to use appropriate clinical judgment to assess the relation between substance exposure and anxiety symptoms. The structure of the diagnosis includes specification of the substance (for example, cocaine), specification of the appropriate state during the onset (for example, intoxication), and mention of the specific symptom pattern (for example, panic attacks).

Clinical Features

The associated clinical features of substance-induced anxiety disorder vary with the particular substance involved. Even infrequent use of psychostimulants can result in anxiety disorder symptoms in some persons. Associated with the anxiety disorder symptoms may also be cognitive impairments in comprehension, calculation, and memory. These cognitive deficits are usually reversible when the substance use is stopped.

Differential Diagnosis

The differential diagnosis for substance-induced anxiety disorder includes the primary anxiety disorders, anxiety disorder due to a general medical condition (for which the patient may be receiving an implicated drug), and mood disorders, which are frequently accompanied by symptoms of anxiety disorders. Personality disorders and malingering must be considered in the differential diagnosis, particularly in some urban emergency rooms.

Course and Prognosis

The course and prognosis generally depend on the removal of the causally involved substance and the long-term ability of the affected person to limit the use of the substance. The anxio-

Table 13.7–2
DSM-IV-TR Diagnostic Criteria for Substance-Induced Anxiety Disorder

A. Prominent anxiety, panic attacks, or obsessions or compulsions predominate in the clinical picture.

B. There is evidence from the history, physical examination, or laboratory findings of either (1) or (2):

(1) the symptoms in Criterion A developed during, or within 1 month of, substance intoxication or withdrawal

(2) medication use is etiologically related to the disturbance

C. The disturbance is not better accounted for by an anxiety disorder that is not substance induced. Evidence that the symptoms are better accounted for by an anxiety disorder that is not substance induced might include the following: the symptoms precede the onset of the substance use (or medication use); the symptoms persist for a substantial period of time (e.g., about a month) after the cessation of acute withdrawal or severe intoxication or are substantially in excess of what would be expected given the type or amount of the substance used or the duration of use; or there is other evidence suggesting the existence of an independent non-substance-induced anxiety disorder (e.g., a history of recurrent non-substance-related episodes).

D. The disturbance does not occur exclusively during the course of a delirium.

E. The disturbance causes clinically significant distress or impairment in social, occupational, or other important areas of functioning.

Note: This diagnosis should be made instead of a diagnosis of substance intoxication or substance withdrawal only when the anxiety symptoms are in excess of those usually associated with the intoxication or withdrawal syndrome and when the anxiety symptoms are sufficiently severe to warrant independent clinical attention.

Code [Specific substance]-induced anxiety disorder

Alcohol; amphetamine (or amphetamine-like substance); caffeine; cannabis; cocaine; hallucinogen; inhalant; phencyclidine (or phencyclidine-like substance); sedative, hypnotic, or anxiolytic; other [or unknown] substance

Specify if:

With generalized anxiety: if excessive anxiety or worry about a number of events or activities predominates in the clinical presentation

With panic attacks: if panic attacks predominate in the clinical presentation

With obsessive-compulsive symptoms: if obsessions or compulsions predominate in the clinical presentation

With phobic symptoms: if phobic symptoms predominate in the clinical presentation

Specify if:

With onset during intoxication: if the criteria are met for intoxication with the substance and the symptoms develop during the intoxication syndrome

With onset during withdrawal: if criteria are met for withdrawal from the substance and the symptoms develop during, or shortly after, a withdrawal syndrome

From American Psychiatric Association. *Diagnostic and Statistical Manual of Mental Disorders.* 4th ed. Text rev. Washington, DC: American Psychiatric Association; copyright 2000, with permission.

Table 13.7–3
DSM-IV-TR Diagnostic Criteria for Anxiety Disorder Not Otherwise Specified

This category includes disorders with prominent anxiety or phobic avoidance that do not meet criteria for any specific anxiety disorder, adjustment disorder with anxiety, or adjustment disorder with mixed anxiety and depressed mood. Examples include

1. Mixed anxiety-depressive disorder: clinically significant symptoms of anxiety and depression, but the criteria are not met for either a specific mood disorder or a specific anxiety disorder

2. Clinically significant social phobic symptoms that are related to the social impact of having a general medical condition or mental disorder (e.g., Parkinson's disease, dermatological conditions, stuttering, anorexia nervosa, body dysmorphic disorder)

3. Situations in which the disturbance is severe enough to warrant a diagnosis of an anxiety disorder but the individual fails to report enough symptoms for the full criteria for any specific anxiety disorder to have been met; for example, an individual who reports all of the features of panic disorder without agoraphobia except that the panic attacks are all limited-symptom attacks

4. Situations in which the clinician has concluded that an anxiety disorder is present but is unable to determine whether it is primary, due to a general medical condition, or substance induced

From American Psychiatric Association. *Diagnostic and Statistical Manual of Mental Disorders.* 4th ed. Text rev. Washington, DC: American Psychiatric Association; copyright 2000, with permission.

Treatment

The primary treatment for substance-induced anxiety disorder is the removal of the causally involved substance. Clinicians should then focus on finding an alternative treatment if the substance was a medically indicated drug, on limiting the patient's exposure if the substance was introduced through environmental exposure, or on treating the underlying substance-related disorder. If anxiety disorder symptoms continue even though substance use has stopped, treatment of the anxiety disorder symptoms with appropriate psychotherapeutic or pharmacotherapeutic modalities may be appropriate.

ANXIETY DISORDER NOT OTHERWISE SPECIFIED

Some patients have symptoms of anxiety disorders that do not meet the criteria for any specific DSM-IV-TR anxiety disorder or adjustment disorder with anxiety or mixed anxiety and depressed mood. Such patients are most appropriately classified as having anxiety disorder not otherwise specified. DSM-IV-TR includes four examples of conditions that are appropriate for the diagnosis (Table 13.7–3). One of the examples is mixed anxiety-depressive disorder.

Mixed Anxiety-Depressive Disorder

This disorder describes patients with the condition of both anxiety and depressive symptoms who do not meet the diagnostic criteria for either an anxiety disorder or a mood disorder. The

genic effects of most drugs are reversible. When the anxiety does not reverse with the cessation of the drug, clinicians should reconsider the diagnosis of substance-induced anxiety disorder or consider the possibility that the substance causes irreversible brain damage.

combination of depressive and anxiety symptoms results in a significant functional impairment for the affected person. The condition may be particularly prevalent in primary care practices and outpatient mental health clinics. Opponents have argued that the availability of the diagnosis may discourage clinicians from taking the necessary time to obtain a complete psychiatric history to differentiate true depressive disorders from true anxiety disorders.

Epidemiology.   The coexistence of major depressive disorder and panic disorder is common. As many as two-thirds of all patients with depressive symptoms have prominent anxiety symptoms, and one-third may meet the diagnostic criteria for panic disorder. Researchers have reported that from 20 to 90 percent of all patients with panic disorder have episodes of major depressive disorder. These data suggest that the coexistence of depressive and anxiety symptoms, neither of which meet the diagnostic criteria for other depressive or anxiety disorders, may be common. At this time, however, formal epidemiological data on mixed anxiety-depressive disorder are not available. Nevertheless, some clinicians and researchers have estimated that the prevalence of the disorder in the general population is as high as 10 percent and in primary care clinics as high as 50 percent, although conservative estimates suggest a prevalence of approximately 1 percent in the general population.

Etiology.   Four principal lines of evidence suggest that anxiety symptoms and depressive symptoms are causally linked in some affected patients. First, several investigators have reported similar neuroendocrine findings in depressive disorders and anxiety disorders, particularly panic disorder, including blunted cortisol response to adrenocorticotropic hormone, blunted growth hormone response to clonidine (Catapres), and blunted thyroid-stimulating hormone (TSH) and prolactin responses to thyrotropin-releasing hormone (TRH). Second, several investigators have reported data indicating that hyperactivity of the noradrenergic system is causally relevant to some patients with depressive disorders and with panic disorder. Specifically, these studies have found elevated concentrations of the norepinephrine metabolite 3-methoxy-4-hydroxyphenylglycol (MHPG) in the urine, the plasma, or the cerebrospinal fluid (CSF) of depressed patients and panic disorder patients who were actively experiencing a panic attack. As with other anxiety and depressive disorders, serotonin and γ-aminobutyric acid (GABA) may also be causally involved in mixed anxiety-depressive disorder. Third, many studies have found that serotonergic drugs, such as fluoxetine (Prozac) and clomipramine (Anafranil), are useful in treating both depressive and anxiety disorders. Fourth, a number of family studies have reported data indicating that anxiety and depressive symptoms are genetically linked in at least some families.

Diagnosis.   The DSM-IV-TR criteria (Table 13.7–4) require the presence of subsyndromal symptoms of both anxiety and depression and the presence of some autonomic symptoms, such as tremor, palpitations, dry mouth, and the sensation of a churning stomach. Some preliminary studies have indicated that the sensitivity of general practitioners to a syndrome of mixed anxiety-depressive disorder is low, although this lack of recognition may reflect the lack of an appropriate diagnostic label for the patients.

Table 13.7–4
DSM-IV-TR Research Criteria for Mixed Anxiety-Depressive Disorder

A. Persistent or recurrent dysphoric mood lasting at least 1 month.

B. The dysphoric mood is accompanied by at least 1 month of four (or more) of the following symptoms:
   (1) difficulty concentrating or mind going blank
   (2) sleep disturbance (difficulty falling or staying asleep, or restless, unsatisfying sleep)
   (3) fatigue or low energy
   (4) irritability
   (5) worry
   (6) being easily moved to tears
   (7) hypervigilance
   (8) anticipating the worst
   (9) hopelessness (pervasive pessimism about the future)
   (10) low self-esteem or feelings of worthlessness

C. The symptoms cause clinically significant distress or impairment in social, occupational, or other important areas of functioning.

D. The symptoms are not due to the direct physiological effects of a substance (e.g., a drug of abuse, a medication) or a general medical condition.

E. All of the following:
   (1) criteria have never been met for major depressive disorder, dysthymic disorder, panic disorder, or generalized anxiety disorder
   (2) criteria are not currently met for any other anxiety or mood disorder (including an anxiety or mood disorder, in partial remission)
   (3) the symptoms are not better accounted for by any other mental disorder

From American Psychiatric Association. *Diagnostic and Statistical Manual of Mental Disorders.* 4th ed. Text rev. Washington, DC: American Psychiatric Association; copyright 2000, with permission.

Clinical Features.   The clinical features of mixed anxiety-depressive disorder combine symptoms of anxiety disorders and some symptoms of depressive disorders. In addition, symptoms of autonomic nervous system hyperactivity, such as gastrointestinal complaints, are common and contribute to the high frequency with which the patients are seen in outpatient medical clinics.

Differential Diagnosis.   The differential diagnosis includes other anxiety and depressive disorders and personality disorders. Among the anxiety disorders, generalized anxiety disorder is most likely to overlap with mixed anxiety-depressive disorder. Among the mood disorders, dysthymic disorder and minor depressive disorder are most likely to overlap with mixed anxiety-depressive disorder. Among the personality disorders, avoidant, dependent, and obsessive-compulsive personality disorders may have symptoms that resemble those of mixed anxiety-depressive disorder. A diagnosis of a somatoform disorder should also be considered. Only a psychiatric history, a mental status examination, and a working knowledge of the specific DSM-IV-TR criteria can help clinicians differentiate among these conditions. In Europe and Asia, especially, this condition is commonly diagnosed under the rubric of neurasthenia.

Course and Prognosis.   On the basis of clinical data to date, patients seem to be equally likely to have prominent anxiety symptoms, prominent depressive symptoms, or an equal mixture of the two symptoms at onset. During the course of the illness, anxiety or depressive symptoms may alternate in their predominance. The prognosis is not known.

Treatment.   Because adequate studies comparing treatment modalities for mixed anxiety-depressive disorder are not available, clinicians are probably most likely to provide treatment based on the symptoms present, their severity, and the clinician's own levels of experience with various treatment modalities. Psychotherapeutic approaches may involve time-limited approaches, such as cognitive therapy or behavior modification, although some clinicians use a less structured psychotherapeutic approach, such as insight-oriented psychotherapy. Pharmacotherapy for mixed anxiety-depressive disorder may include antianxiety drugs, antidepressive drugs, or both. Among the anxiolytic drugs, some data indicate that the use of triazolobenzodiazepines (for example, alprazolam [Xanax]) may be indicated because of their effectiveness in treating depression associated with anxiety. A drug that affects the 5-HT_{1A} receptor, such as buspirone, may also be indicated. Among the antidepressants, despite the noradrenergic theories linking anxiety disorders and depressive disorders, the serotonergic antidepressants (for example, fluoxetine) may be most effective in treating mixed anxiety-depressive disorder.

14 ▲

Somatoform and Pain Disorders

The term *somatoform* derives from the Greek *soma* for body, and the somatoform disorders are a broad group of illnesses that have bodily signs and symptoms as a major component. These disorders encompass mind–body interactions in which the brain, in ways still not well understood, sends various signals that impinge on the patient's awareness, indicating a serious problem in the body. Additionally, minor changes in neurochemistry, neurophysiology, and neuroimmunology may result from unknown mental or brain mechanisms that cause illness.

The text revision of the fourth edition of the *Diagnostic and Statistical Manual of Mental Disorders* (DSM-IV-TR) recognizes five specific somatoform disorders: (1) somatization disorder, characterized by many physical complaints affecting many organ systems; (2) conversion disorder, characterized by one or two neurological complaints; (3) hypochondriasis, characterized less by a focus on symptoms than by the patients' beliefs that they have a specific disease; (4) body dysmorphic disorder, characterized by a false belief or exaggerated perception that a body part is defective; and (5) pain disorder, characterized by symptoms of pain that are either solely related to, or significantly exacerbated by, psychological factors. DSM-IV-TR also has two residual diagnostic categories for somatoform disorders: (1) undifferentiated somatoform disorder, which includes somatoform disorders not otherwise described that have been present for 6 months or longer, and (2) somatoform disorder not otherwise specified, which is a category for conditions that do not meet any of the somatoform disorder diagnoses mentioned above.

SOMATIZATION DISORDER

Somatization disorder is characterized by many somatic symptoms that cannot be explained adequately on the basis of physical and laboratory examinations. It usually begins before the age of 30, may continue for years, and is distinguished, according to DSM-IV-TR, by "a combination of pain, gastrointestinal, sexual, and pseudoneurological symptoms." Somatization disorder differs from other somatoform disorders because of the multiplicity of the complaints and the multiple organ systems (for example, gastrointestinal and neurological) that are affected. The disorder is chronic and is associated with significant psychological distress, impairment in social and occupational functioning, and excessive medical-help–seeking behavior.

Somatization disorder has been recognized since the time of ancient Egypt. An early name for somatization disorder was *hysteria*, a condition incorrectly thought to affect only women. (The word *hysteria* is derived from the Greek word for uterus, *hystera*.) In the 17th century, Thomas Sydenham recognized that psychological factors, which he called *antecedent sorrows*, were involved in the pathogenesis of the symptoms. In 1859, Paul Briquet, a French physician, observed the multiplicity of the symptoms and the affected organ systems and commented on the usually chronic course of the disorder. Because of these astute clinical observations, the disorder was called *Briquet's syndrome* for a time, although the term *somatization disorder* became the standard in the United States.

Epidemiology

The lifetime prevalence of somatization disorder in the general population is estimated to be 0.1 or 0.2 percent, although several research groups believe that the actual figure may be closer to 0.5 percent. Women with somatization disorder outnumber men 5 to 20 times, but the highest estimates may be due to the early tendency not to diagnose somatization disorder in male patients. Nevertheless, it is not an uncommon disorder. With a 5-to-1 female-to-male ratio, the lifetime prevalence of somatization disorder among women in the general population may be 1 or 2 percent. Among patients in the offices of general practitioners and family practitioners, as many as 5 to 10 percent may meet the diagnostic criteria for somatization disorder. The disorder is inversely related to social position and occurs most often among patients who have little education and low income levels. Somatization disorder is defined as beginning before age 30; it most often begins during a person's teenage years.

Etiology

Psychosocial Factors. Psychosocial formulations involve interpretation of the symptom as a social communication, the result of which is to avoid obligations (for example, going to a job a person does not like), to express emotions (for example, anger at a spouse), or to symbolize a feeling or a belief (for example, a pain in the gut). Strict psychoanalytic interpretations of symptoms rest on the hypothesis that the symptoms substitute for repressed instinctual impulses.

A behavioral perspective on somatization disorder emphasizes that parental teaching, parental example, and ethnic mores may teach some children to somatize more than do others. In addition, some patients with somatization disorder come from unstable homes and have been physically abused.

Biological and Genetic Factors. Some studies propose that patients have characteristic attention and cognitive impairments that result in the faulty perception and assessment of somatosensory inputs. The impairments include excessive distractibility, inability to habituate to repetitive stimuli, the grouping of cognitive constructs on an impressionistic basis, partial and circumstantial associations, and lack of selectivity, as indicated in some studies of evoked potentials. A limited number of brain-imaging studies have reported decreased metabolism in the frontal lobes and in the nondominant hemisphere.

Genetic data indicate that somatization disorder may have genetic components. Somatization disorder tends to run in families and occurs in 10 to 20 percent of the first-degree female relatives of patients with somatization disorder. Within these families, first-degree male relatives are prone to substance abuse and antisocial personality disorder. One study reported a concordance rate of 29 percent in monozygotic twins and 10 percent in dizygotic twins, an indication of a genetic effect.

Research into cytokines, a new area of basic neuroscience study, may be relevant to somatization disorder and other somatoform disorders. Cytokines are messenger molecules that the immune system uses to communicate within itself and with the nervous system, including the brain. Examples of cytokines are interleukins, tumor necrosis factor, and interferons. Some preliminary experiments indicate that cytokines may help cause some of the nonspecific symptoms of disease, especially of infections, such as hypersomnia, anorexia, fatigue, and depression. Although no data yet support the hypothesis, abnormal regulation of the cytokine system may result in some of the symptoms seen in somatoform disorders.

Diagnosis

For the diagnosis of somatization disorder, DSM-IV-TR requires onset of symptoms before age 30 (Table 14–1). During the course of the disorder, patients must have complained of at least four pain symptoms, two gastrointestinal symptoms, one sexual symptom, and one pseudoneurological symptom, none of which are completely explained by physical or laboratory examinations.

Clinical Features

Patients with somatization disorder have many somatic complaints and long, complicated medical histories. Nausea and vomiting (other than during pregnancy), difficulty in swallowing, pain in the arms and legs, shortness of breath unrelated to exertion, amnesia, and complications of pregnancy and menstruation are among the most common symptoms. Patients frequently believe that they have been sickly most of their lives. Pseudoneurological symptoms suggest, but are not pathognomonic of, a neurological disorder. According to DSM-IV-TR, they include impaired coordination or balance, paralysis or localized weakness, difficulty swallowing or lump in throat, aphonia, urinary retention, hallucinations, loss of touch or pain sensation, double vision, blindness, deafness, seizures, or loss of consciousness other than fainting.

Psychological distress and interpersonal problems are prominent; anxiety and depression are the most prevalent psychiatric conditions. Suicide threats are common, but actual suicide is rare. If suicide does occur, it is often associated with substance abuse. Patients' medical histories are often circumstantial,

Table 14–1
DSM-IV-TR Diagnostic Criteria for Somatization Disorder

A. A history of many physical complaints beginning before age 30 years that occur over a period of several years and result in treatment being sought or significant impairment in social, occupational, or other important areas of functioning.

B. Each of the following criteria must have been met, with individual symptoms occurring at any time during the course of the disturbance:

  (1) *four pain symptoms:* a history of pain related to at least four different sites or functions (e.g., head, abdomen, back, joints, extremities, chest, rectum, during menstruation, during sexual intercourse, or during urination)

  (2) *two gastrointestinal symptoms:* a history of at least two gastrointestinal symptoms other than pain (e.g., nausea, bloating, vomiting other than during pregnancy, diarrhea, or intolerance of several different foods)

  (3) *one sexual symptom:* a history of at least one sexual or reproductive symptom other than pain (e.g., sexual indifference, erectile or ejaculatory dysfunction, irregular menses, excessive menstrual bleeding, vomiting throughout pregnancy)

  (4) *one pseudoneurological symptom:* a history of at least one symptom or deficit suggesting a neurological condition not limited to pain (conversion symptoms such as impaired coordination or balance, paralysis or localized weakness, difficulty swallowing or lump in throat, aphonia, urinary retention, hallucinations, loss of touch or pain sensation, double vision, blindness, deafness, seizures; dissociative symptoms such as amnesia; or loss of consciousness other than fainting)

C. Either (1) or (2):

  (1) after appropriate investigation, each of the symptoms in Criterion B cannot be fully explained by a known general medical condition or the direct effects of a substance (e.g., a drug of abuse, a medication)

  (2) when there is a related general medical condition, the physical complaints or resulting social or occupational impairment are in excess of what would be expected from the history, physical examination, or laboratory findings

D. The symptoms are not intentionally produced or feigned (as in factitious disorder or malingering).

From American Psychiatric Association. *Diagnostic and Statistical Manual of Mental Disorders.* 4th ed. Text rev. Washington, DC: American Psychiatric Association; copyright 2000, with permission.

vague, imprecise, inconsistent, and disorganized. Patients classically but not always describe their complaints in a dramatic, emotional, and exaggerated fashion, with vivid and colorful language; they may confuse temporal sequences and cannot clearly distinguish current from past symptoms. Female patients with somatization disorder may dress in an exhibitionistic manner. Patients may be perceived as dependent, self-centered, hungry for admiration or praise, and manipulative.

Differential Diagnosis

Clinicians must always rule out nonpsychiatric medical conditions that may explain a patient's symptoms. Several medical disorders often show nonspecific, transient abnormalities in the same age group. These medical disorders include multiple sclerosis (MS), myasthenia gravis, systemic lupus erythematosus

(SLE), acquired immune deficiency syndrome (AIDS), acute intermittent porphyria, hyperparathyroidism, hyperthyroidism, and chronic systemic infections. The onset of multiple somatic symptoms in patients older than 40 should be presumed to be caused by a nonpsychiatric medical condition until an exhaustive medical workup has been completed.

Many mental disorders are considered in the differential diagnosis, which is complicated by the observation that at least 50 percent of patients with somatization disorder have a coexisting mental disorder. Patients with major depressive disorder, generalized anxiety disorder, and schizophrenia may all have an initial complaint that focuses on somatic symptoms. In all these disorders, however, the symptoms of depression, anxiety, or psychosis eventually predominate over the somatic complaints. Although patients with panic disorder may complain of many somatic symptoms related to their panic attacks, they are not bothered by somatic symptoms between panic attacks.

Among the other somatoform disorders, hypochondriasis, conversion disorder, and pain somatization disorder, patients with hypochondriasis falsely believe that they have a specific disease, whereas those with somatization disorder are concerned with many symptoms. The symptoms of conversion disorder are limited to one or two neurological symptoms rather than to the wide-ranging symptoms of somatization disorder. Pain disorder is limited to one or two complaints of pain symptoms.

Course and Prognosis

Somatization disorder is chronic and often debilitating. By definition, the symptoms should have begun before age 30 and have been present for several years. Episodes of increased symptom severity and the development of new symptoms are thought to last 6 to 9 months and may be separated by less symptomatic periods lasting 9 to 12 months. Rarely, however, does a patient with somatization disorder go for more than a year without seeking medical attention. There is often an association between periods of increased stress and the exacerbation of somatic symptoms.

Treatment

Somatization disorder is best treated when the patient has a single identified physician as the primary doctor. When more than one clinician is involved, patients have increased opportunities to express somatic complaints. Primary physicians should see patients during regularly scheduled visits, usually at monthly intervals. The visits should be relatively brief, although a partial physical examination should be conducted to respond to each new somatic complaint. Additional laboratory and diagnostic procedures should generally be avoided. Once somatization disorder has been diagnosed, the treating physician should listen to the somatic complaints as emotional expressions rather than as medical complaints. Nevertheless, patients with somatization disorder can also have bona fide physical illnesses; therefore, physicians must always use their judgment about what symptoms to work up and to what extent. A reasonable long-range strategy for a primary care physician who is treating a patient with somatization disorder is to increase the patient's awareness of the possibility that psychological factors are involved in the symptoms until the patient is willing to see a mental health clinician. In complex cases with many medical presentations, a psychiatrist is better able to judge whether to seek medical or surgical consultation because of his or her medical training; however, a nonmedical mental health professional can explore the psychological antecedents of the disorder as well, especially if consulting closely with a physician.

Psychotherapy, both individual and group, decreases these patients' personal health care expenditures by 50 percent, largely by decreasing their rates of hospitalization. In psychotherapy settings, patients are helped to cope with their symptoms, to express underlying emotions, and to develop alternative strategies for expressing their feelings.

Giving psychotropic medications whenever somatization disorder coexists with a mood or anxiety disorder is always a risk, but psychopharmacological treatment, as well as psychotherapeutic treatment, of the coexisting disorder is indicated. Medication must be monitored, because patients with somatization disorder tend to use drugs erratically and unreliably. In patients without coexisting mental disorders, few available data indicate that pharmacological treatment is effective in patients without coexisting mental disorders.

CONVERSION DISORDER

A conversion disorder is a disturbance of bodily functioning that does not conform to current concepts of the anatomy and physiology of the central or the peripheral nervous system. It typically occurs in a setting of stress and produces considerable dysfunction.

DSM-IV-TR defines conversion disorder as characterized by the presence of one or more neurological symptoms (for example, paralysis, blindness, and paresthesias) that cannot be explained by a known neurological or medical disorder. In addition, the diagnosis requires that psychological factors be associated with the initiation or the exacerbation of the symptoms.

Epidemiology

The prevalence of some symptoms of conversion disorder that are not of sufficient severity to warrant the diagnosis may occur in as many as one-third of the general population sometime during their lives. One community reported that the annual incidence of conversion disorder was 22 per 100,000. Among specific populations, the occurrence of conversion disorder may be even higher than that, perhaps making conversion disorder the most common somatoform disorder in some populations. Several studies have reported that 5 to 15 percent of psychiatric consultations in a general hospital and 25 to 30 percent of admissions to a Veterans Administration hospital involve patients with conversion disorder diagnoses. DSM-IV-TR gives a range from a low of 11 to a high of 500 cases per 100,000 population.

The ratio of women to men among adult patients is at least 2 to 1 and as much as 10 to 1; among children there is an even higher predominance in girls. Men with conversion disorder have often been involved in occupational or military accidents. Conversion disorder can have its onset at any time, from childhood to old age, but it is most common in adolescents and young adults. Data indicate that conversion disorder is most common among rural populations, people with little education, those with low intelligence quotients, those in low socioeconomic groups, and military personnel who have been exposed to combat situations. Conversion disorder is commonly associated with comorbid diagnoses of major depressive disorder, anxiety disorders, and schizophrenia.

Comorbidity

Medical and especially neurological disorders occur frequently among patients with conversion disorders. What is typically seen in these comorbid neurological or medical conditions is an elaboration of symptoms stemming from the original organic lesion.

Among the Axis I psychiatric conditions, depressive disorders, anxiety disorders, and somatization disorders are especially noted for their association with conversion disorder. Conversion in schizophrenia is reported but is very uncommon. Studies of patients admitted to a psychiatric hospital for conversion disorder reveal that on further study, one-fourth to one-half have a clinically significant mood disorder or schizophrenia.

Personality disorders also frequently accompany conversion disorder, especially the histrionic type (in 5 to 21 percent of cases) and the passive-dependent type (9 to 40 percent of cases). However, conversion disorders can occur in persons with no predisposing medical, neurological, or psychiatric disorder.

Etiology

Psychoanalytic Factors.   According to psychoanalytic theory, conversion disorder is caused by the repression of unconscious intrapsychic conflict and the conversion of anxiety into a physical symptom. The conflict is between an instinctual impulse (for example, aggression or sexuality) and the prohibitions against its expression. The symptoms allow the partial expression of the forbidden wish or urge but disguise it, so that patients can avoid consciously confronting their unacceptable impulses; that is, the conversion disorder symptom has a symbolic relation to the unconscious conflict. Conversion disorder symptoms also enable patients to communicate that they need special consideration and special treatment. Such symptoms may function as a nonverbal means of controlling or manipulating others.

Learning Theory.   In terms of conditioned learning theory, a conversion symptom can be seen as a piece of classically conditioned learned behavior; symptoms of illness, learned in childhood, are called forth as a means of coping with an otherwise impossible situation.

Biological Factors.   Increasing data implicate biological and neuropsychological factors in the development of conversion disorder symptoms. Preliminary brain-imaging studies have found hypometabolism of the dominant hemisphere and hypermetabolism of the nondominant hemisphere and have implicated impaired hemispheric communication in the cause of conversion disorder. The symptoms may be caused by an excessive cortical arousal that sets off negative feedback loops between the cerebral cortex and the brainstem reticular formation. Elevated levels of corticofugal output, in turn, inhibit the patient's awareness of bodily sensation, which, in some patients with conversion disorder, may explain the observed sensory deficits. Neuropsychological tests sometimes reveal subtle

Table 14–2
DSM-IV-TR Diagnostic Criteria for Conversion Disorder

A. One or more symptoms or deficits affecting voluntary motor or sensory function that suggest a neurological or other general medical condition.

B. Psychological factors are judged to be associated with the symptom or deficit because the initiation or exacerbation of the symptom or deficit is preceded by conflicts or other stressors.

C. The symptom or deficit is not intentionally produced or feigned (as in factitious disorder or malingering).

D. The symptom or deficit cannot, after appropriate investigation, be fully explained by a general medical condition, or by the direct effects of a substance, or as a culturally sanctioned behavior or experience.

E. The symptom or deficit causes clinically significant distress or impairment in social, occupational, or other important areas of functioning or warrants medical evaluation.

F. The symptom or deficit is not limited to pain or sexual dysfunction, does not occur exclusively during the course of somatization disorder, and is not better accounted for by another mental disorder.

Specify type of symptom or deficit:

With motor symptom or deficit
With sensory symptom or deficit
With seizures or convulsions
With mixed presentation

From American Psychiatric Association. *Diagnostic and Statistical Manual of Mental Disorders.* 4th ed. Text rev. Washington, DC: American Psychiatric Association; copyright 2000, with permission.

cerebral impairments in verbal communication, memory, vigilance, affective incongruity, and attention in these patients.

Diagnosis

DSM-IV-TR limits the diagnosis of conversion disorder to those symptoms that affect a voluntary motor or sensory function—that is, neurological symptoms (Table 14–2). Physicians are unable to explain the neurological symptoms solely on the basis of any known neurological condition.

The diagnosis of conversion disorder requires that clinicians find a necessary and critical association between the cause of the neurological symptoms and psychological factors, although the symptoms cannot be the result of malingering or factitious disorder. The diagnosis of conversion disorder also excludes symptoms of pain and sexual dysfunction and symptoms that occur only in somatization disorder. DSM-IV-TR allows the specification of the type of symptom or deficit seen in conversion disorder (Table 14–2).

Clinical Features

Paralysis, blindness, and mutism are the most common conversion disorder symptoms. Conversion disorder may be most commonly associated with passive-aggressive, dependent, antisocial, and histrionic personality disorders. Depressive and anxiety disorder symptoms can often accompany the symptoms of conversion disorder, and affected patients are at risk for suicide.

Mrs. A was a 22-year-old right-handed fundamentalist farmer's wife, homemaker, and mother of three from a sparsely settled Western state. Her past medical history was benign except for a motor vehicle accident 2 years previously that produced a sharp blow to the right temporal area, resulting in several hours' loss of consciousness. She had an unremarkable behavioral history without substance abuse, prolonged depressions, or unexplained somatic symptoms. Her demeanor had always been placid and unassuming. There was no family history of antisocial behavior or substance abuse.

On Thanksgiving Day, while taking her usual solitary afternoon walk along the creek behind the kitchen, she came upon the floating, lifeless bodies of two of her children. She shrieked, swooned, and fell to the ground. Relatives in the house rushed out to assist but could not revive the children. When she was helped up, she asked that her husband guide her back to her room. Later that afternoon she seemed calm, even detached, as others scurried about making arrangements. She admitted to a visitor that she seemed to have lost the gift of sight.

That evening the family physician was called to examine the newly sightless woman. He noted that her pupils were round, equal, and constricted briskly with a bright light; she could not touch the tips of her index fingers together in front of her; she failed to look at her own hands when instructed to do so; and she had no other neurological abnormalities, asymmetries, or complaints. The physician explained to the gathered family and patient that the woman was suffering from nervous shock, needed kind and quiet support, and should refrain from routine household chores for the moment. The physician also suggested that her eyesight would gradually return over the next week or so, perhaps following the funerals of her children. The patient's vision did slowly return over the next days, and she gradually resumed her usual level of care for the home, her surviving child, and other members of the family. (Courtesy of Frederick G. Guggenheim, M.D.)

Sensory Symptoms.

In conversion disorder, anesthesia and paresthesia are common, especially of the extremities. All sensory modalities can be involved, and the distribution of the disturbance is usually inconsistent with that of either central or peripheral neurological disease. Thus, clinicians may see the characteristic stocking-and-glove anesthesia of the hands or feet or the hemianesthesia of the body beginning precisely along the midline.

Conversion disorder symptoms may involve the organs of special sense and can produce deafness, blindness, and tunnel vision. These symptoms may be unilateral or bilateral, but neurological evaluation reveals intact sensory pathways. In conversion disorder blindness, for example, patients walk around without collisions or self-injury, their pupils react to light, and their cortical evoked potentials are normal.

Motor Symptoms.

The motor symptoms include abnormal movements, gait disturbance, weakness, and paralysis. Gross rhythmical tremors, choreiform movements, tics, and jerks may be present. The movements generally worsen when attention is called to them. One gait disturbance seen in conversion disorder is astasia-abasia, which is a wildly ataxic, staggering gait accompanied by gross, irregular, jerky truncal movements and thrashing and waving arm movements. Patients with the symptoms rarely fall; if they do, they are generally not injured.

Other common motor disturbances are paralysis and paresis involving one, two, or all four limbs, although the distribution of the involved muscles does not conform to the neural pathways. Reflexes remain normal; the patients have no fasciculations or muscle atrophy (except after long-standing conversion paralysis); electromyography findings are normal.

Seizure Symptoms.

Pseudoseizures are another symptom in conversion disorder. Clinicians may find it difficult to differentiate a pseudoseizure from an actual seizure by clinical observation alone. Moreover, approximately one-third of the patient's pseudoseizures also have a coexisting epileptic disorder. Tongue biting, urinary incontinence, and injuries after falling can occur in pseudoseizures, although these symptoms are generally not present. Pupillary and gag reflexes are retained after pseudoseizure, and patients have no postseizure increase in prolactin concentrations.

Other Associated Features.

Several psychological symptoms have also been associated with conversion disorder.

PRIMARY GAIN. Patients achieve primary gain by keeping internal conflicts outside their awareness. Symptoms have symbolic value in that they represent an unconscious psychological conflict.

SECONDARY GAIN. Patients accrue tangible advantages and benefits as a result of their being sick, such as being excused from obligations and difficult life situations, receiving support and assistance that might not otherwise be forthcoming, and controlling other persons' behavior.

LA BELLE INDIFFÉRENCE. La belle indifférence is a patient's inappropriately cavalier attitude toward serious symptoms; that is, the patient seems to be unconcerned about what appears to be a major impairment. That bland indifference may be lacking in some patients; it is also seen in some seriously ill medical patients who develop a stoic attitude. The presence or the absence of la belle indifférence is an inaccurate measure of whether a patient has conversion disorder.

IDENTIFICATION. Patients with conversion disorder may unconsciously model their symptoms on those of someone important to them. For example, a parent or a person who has recently died may serve as a model for conversion disorder. During pathological grief reaction, bereaved people commonly have symptoms of the deceased.

Differential Diagnosis

One of the major problems in diagnosing conversion disorder is the difficulty of definitively ruling out a medical disorder. Concomitant nonpsychiatric medical disorders are common in hospitalized patients with conversion disorder, and evidence of a current or previous neurological disorder or of a systemic disease affecting the brain has been reported in 18 to 64 percent of such patients. An estimated 25 to 50 percent of patients classified as having conversion disorder eventually receive diagnoses of neurological or nonpsychiatric medical disorders that could have caused their earlier symptoms. Therefore, a thorough medical and neurological workup is essential in all cases. If the symptoms can be resolved by suggestion, hypnosis, or parenteral amobarbital (Amytal) or lorazepam (Ativan), they are probably the result of conversion disorder.

Neurological disorders (such as dementia and other degenerative diseases), brain tumors, and basal ganglia disease must be considered in the differential diagnosis. For example, weakness may be confused with myasthenia gravis, polymyositis, acquired myopathies, or multiple sclerosis. Optic neuritis may be misdiagnosed as conversion disorder blindness. Other diseases that may cause confusing symptoms are Guillain-Barré syndrome, Creutzfeldt-Jakob disease, and early neurological manifestations of AIDS. Conversion disorder symptoms occur in schizophrenia, depressive disorders, and anxiety disorders, but these other disorders are associated with their own distinct symptoms that eventually make differential diagnosis possible.

Sensorimotor symptoms also occur in somatization disorder. But somatization disorder is a chronic illness that begins early in life and includes symptoms in many other organ systems. In hypochondriasis, patients have no actual loss or distortion of function; the somatic complaints are chronic and are not limited to neurological symptoms, and the characteristic hypochondriacal attitudes and beliefs are present. If the patient's symptoms are limited to pain, pain disorder can be diagnosed. Patients whose complaints are limited to sexual function are classified as having a sexual dysfunction, rather than conversion disorder.

In both malingering and factitious disorder, the symptoms are under conscious, voluntary control. A malingerer's history is usually more inconsistent and contradictory than is that of a patient with conversion disorder, and a malingerer's fraudulent behavior is clearly goal directed.

Course and Prognosis

The initial symptoms of most patients with conversion disorder, perhaps 90 to 100 percent, resolve in a few days or less than a month. A reported 75 percent of patients may not experience another episode, but 25 percent have additional episodes during periods of stress. Associated with a good prognosis are a sudden onset, an easily identifiable stressor, good premorbid adjustment, no comorbid psychiatric or medical disorders, and no ongoing litigation. The longer the conversion disorder symptoms are present, the worse the prognosis. As discussed previously, 25 to 50 percent of patients may later have neurological disorders or nonpsychiatric medical conditions affecting the nervous system. Therefore, patients with conversion disorder must have complete medical and neurological evaluations at the time of the diagnosis.

Treatment

Resolution of the conversion disorder symptom is usually spontaneous, although probably facilitated by insight-oriented supportive or behavior therapy; the most important feature of the therapy is a relationship with a caring and authoritative therapist. With patients who are resistant to the idea of psychotherapy, physicians can suggest that the psychotherapy will focus on issues of stress and coping. Telling such patients that their symptoms are imaginary often makes them worse. Hypnosis, anxiolytics, and behavioral relaxation exercises are effective in some cases. Parenteral amobarbital or lorazepam may be helpful in obtaining additional historic information, especially when a patient has recently experienced a traumatic event. Psychodynamic approaches include psychoanalysis and insight-oriented psychotherapy, in which patients explore intrapsychic conflicts and the symbolism of the conversion disorder symptoms. Brief and direct forms of short-term psychotherapy have also been used to treat conversion disorder. The greater the duration of these patients' sick role and the more they have regressed, the more difficult the treatment.

HYPOCHONDRIASIS

Hypochondriasis is defined as a person's preoccupation with the fear of contracting, or the belief of having, a serious disease. This fear or belief arises when a person misinterprets bodily symptoms or functions. The term *hypochondriasis* is derived from the old medical term *hypochondrium* ("below the ribs") and reflects the common abdominal complaints of many patients with the disorder. Hypochondriasis results from patients' unrealistic or inaccurate interpretations of physical symptoms or sensations, even though no known medical causes can be found. Patients' preoccupations result in significant distress to them and impair their ability to function in their personal, social, and occupational roles.

Epidemiology

One study reported a 6-month prevalence of hypochondriasis of 4 to 6 percent in a general medical clinic population, but it may be as high as 15 percent. Men and women are equally affected by hypochondriasis. Although the onset of symptoms can occur at any age, the disorder most commonly appears in people 20 to 30 years of age. Some evidence indicates that the diagnosis is more common among blacks than among whites, but social position, education level, and marital status do not appear to affect the diagnosis. Hypochondriacal complaints reportedly occur in approximately 3 percent of medical students, usually in the first 2 years, but they are generally transient.

Etiology

In the diagnostic criteria for hypochondriasis, DSM-IV-TR indicates that the symptoms reflect a misinterpretation of bodily symptoms. A reasonable body of data indicates that people with hypochondriasis augment and amplify their somatic sensations; they have lower-than-usual thresholds for and a lower tolerance of physical discomfort. For example, what people normally perceive as abdominal pressure, people with hypochondriasis experience as abdominal pain. They may focus on bodily sensations, misinterpret them, and become alarmed by them because of a faulty cognitive scheme.

A second theory is that hypochondriasis is understandable in terms of a social learning model. The symptoms of hypochondriasis are viewed as a request for admission to the sick role made by a person facing seemingly insurmountable and insolvable problems. The sick role offers an escape that allows a patient to avoid noxious obligations, to postpone unwelcome challenges, and to be excused from usual duties and obligations.

A third theory about hypochondriasis is that it is a variant form of other mental disorders, among which depressive disorders and anxiety disorders are most frequently included. An estimated 80 percent of patients with hypochondriasis may have coexisting depressive or anxiety disorders. Patients who meet the diagnostic criteria for hypochondriasis may be somatizing subtypes of these other disorders.

The psychodynamic school of thought has produced a fourth theory of hypochondriasis. According to this theory, aggressive and hostile wishes toward others are transferred (through repression and displacement) into physical complaints. The anger of patients with hypochondriasis originates in past disappointments, rejections, and losses, but the patients express their anger in the

Table 14–3
DSM-IV-TR Diagnostic Criteria for Hypochondriasis

A. Preoccupation with fears of having, or the idea that one has, a serious disease based on the person's misinterpretation of bodily symptoms.

B. The preoccupation persists despite appropriate medical evaluation and reassurance.

C. The belief in Criterion A is not of delusional intensity (as in delusional disorder, somatic type) and is not restricted to a circumscribed concern about appearance (as in body dysmorphic disorder).

D. The preoccupation causes clinically significant distress or impairment in social, occupational, or other important areas of functioning.

E. The duration of the disturbance is at least 6 months.

F. The preoccupation is not better accounted for by generalized anxiety disorder, obsessive-compulsive disorder, panic disorder, a major depressive episode, separation anxiety, or another somatoform disorder.

Specify if:

With poor insight: if, for most of the time during the current episode, the person does not recognize that the concern about having a serious illness is excessive or unreasonable

From American Psychiatric Association. *Diagnostic and Statistical Manual of Mental Disorders.* 4th ed. Text rev. Washington, DC: American Psychiatric Association; copyright 2000, with permission.

present by soliciting the help and concern of other people and then rejecting them as ineffective. Hypochondriasis is also viewed as a defense against guilt, a sense of innate badness, an expression of low self-esteem, and a sign of excessive self-concern. Pain and somatic suffering thus become means of atonement and expiation (undoing) and can be experienced as deserved punishment for past wrongdoing (either real or imaginary) and for a person's sense of wickedness and sinfulness.

Diagnosis

The DSM-IV-TR diagnostic criteria for hypochondriasis require that patients be preoccupied with the false belief that they have a serious disease and that the false belief be based on a misinterpretation of physical signs or sensations (Table 14–3). The belief must last at least 6 months, despite the absence of pathological findings on medical and neurological examinations. The diagnostic criteria also stipulate that the belief cannot have the intensity of a delusion (more appropriately diagnosed as delusional disorder) and that it not be restricted to distress about appearance (more appropriately diagnosed as body dysmorphic disorder). The symptoms of hypochondriasis must be of an intensity that causes emotional distress or impairs the patient's ability to function in important areas of life. Clinicians may specify the presence of poor insight; patients do not consistently recognize that the concerns about disease are excessive.

Clinical Features

Patients with hypochondriasis believe that they have a serious disease that has not yet been detected, and they cannot be persuaded to the contrary. They may maintain a belief that they have a particular disease; as time progresses, they may transfer their belief to another disease. Their convictions persist despite negative laboratory results, the benign course of the alleged disease over time, and appropriate reassurances from physicians, yet their beliefs are not so fixed as to be delusions. Hypochondriasis is often accompanied by symptoms of depression and anxiety and commonly coexists with a depressive or anxiety disorder.

Although DSM-IV-TR specifies that the symptoms must be present for at least 6 months, transient hypochondriacal states can occur after major stresses, most commonly the death or serious illness of someone important to the patient, or a serious (perhaps life-threatening) illness that has been resolved but that leaves the patient temporarily hypochondriacal in its wake. Such states that last fewer than 6 months should be diagnosed as somatoform disorder not otherwise specified. Transient hypochondriacal responses to external stress generally remit when the stress is resolved, but they can become chronic if reinforced by people in the patient's social system or by health professionals.

Differential Diagnosis

Hypochondriasis must be differentiated from nonpsychiatric medical conditions, especially disorders that show symptoms that are not necessarily easily diagnosed. Such diseases include AIDS, endocrinopathies, myasthenia gravis, multiple sclerosis, degenerative diseases of the nervous system, systemic lupus erythematosus, and occult neoplastic disorders.

Hypochondriasis is differentiated from somatization disorder by the emphasis in hypochondriasis on fear of having a disease and emphasis in somatization disorder on concern about many symptoms. A subtle distinction is that patients with hypochondriasis usually complain about fewer symptoms than do patients with somatization disorder. Somatization disorder usually has an onset before age 30, whereas hypochondriasis has a less specific age of onset. Patients with somatization disorder are more likely to be women than are those with hypochondriasis, which is equally distributed among men and women.

Hypochondriasis must also be differentiated from the other somatoform disorders. Conversion disorder is acute and generally transient and usually involves a symptom rather than a particular disease. The presence or absence of *la belle indifférence* is an unreliable feature with which to differentiate the two conditions. Pain disorder is chronic, as is hypochondriasis, but the symptoms are limited to complaints of pain. Patients with body dysmorphic disorder wish to appear normal but believe that others notice that they are not, whereas those with hypochondriasis seek out attention for their presumed diseases.

Hypochondriacal symptoms can also occur in patients with depressive disorders and anxiety disorders. If a patient meets the full diagnostic criteria for both hypochondriasis and another major mental disorder, such as major depressive disorder or generalized anxiety disorder, the patient should receive both diagnoses, unless the hypochondriacal symptoms occur only during episodes of the other mental disorder. Patients with panic disorder may initially complain that they are affected by a disease (for example, heart trouble), but careful questioning during the medical history usually uncovers the classic symptoms of a panic attack. Delusional hypochondriacal beliefs occur in schizophrenia and other psychotic disorders but can be differentiated from hypochondriasis by their delusional intensity and by the presence of other psychotic symptoms. In addition, schizophrenic patients' somatic delusions tend to be bizarre, idiosyncratic, and out of keeping with their cultural milieus.

Hypochondriasis is distinguished from factitious disorder with physical symptoms and from malingering in that patients with hypochondriasis actually experience and do not simulate the symptoms they report.

Course and Prognosis

The course of hypochondriasis is usually episodic; the episodes last from months to years and are separated by equally long quiescent periods. There may be an obvious association between exacerbations of hypochondriacal symptoms and psychosocial stressors. Although well-conducted large outcome studies have not yet been reported, an estimated one-third to one-half of all patients with hypochondriasis eventually improve significantly. A good prognosis is associated with a high socioeconomic status, treatment-responsive anxiety or depression, the sudden onset of symptoms, the absence of a personality disorder, and the absence of a related nonpsychiatric medical condition. Most children with hypochondriasis recover by late adolescence or early adulthood.

Treatment

Patients with hypochondriasis are usually resistant to psychiatric treatment, although some accept this treatment if it takes place in a medical setting and focuses on stress reduction and education in coping with chronic illness. Group psychotherapy often benefits such patients, in part because it provides the social support and social interaction that seem to reduce their anxiety. Other forms of psychotherapy, such as individual insight-oriented psychotherapy, behavior therapy, cognitive therapy, and hypnosis may be useful.

Frequent, regularly scheduled physical examinations are useful to reassure patients that their physicians are not abandoning them and that their complaints are being taken seriously. Invasive diagnostic and therapeutic procedures should only be undertaken, however, when objective evidence calls for them. When possible, the clinician should refrain from treating equivocal or incidental physical examination findings.

Pharmacotherapy alleviates hypochondriacal symptoms only when a patient has an underlying drug-responsive condition, such as an anxiety disorder or major depressive disorder. When hypochondriasis is secondary to another primary mental disorder, that disorder must be treated in its own right. When hypochondriasis is a transient situational reaction, clinicians must help patients cope with the stress without reinforcing their illness behavior and their use of the sick role as a solution to their problems.

BODY DYSMORPHIC DISORDER

Patients with body dysmorphic disorder have a pervasive subjective feeling of ugliness of some aspect of their appearance despite a normal or nearly normal appearance. The core of the disorder is the person's strong belief or fear that he or she is unattractive or even repulsive. This fear is rarely assuaged by reassurance or compliments, even though the typical patient with this disorder is quite normal in appearance.

The disorder was recognized and named *dysmorphophobia* more than 100 years ago by Emil Kraepelin, who considered it a compulsive neurosis; Pierre Janet called it *obsession de la honte du corps* (obsession with shame of the body). Freud wrote about the condition in his description of the Wolf-Man, who was excessively concerned about his nose.

Epidemiology

Body dysmorphic disorder is a poorly studied condition, partly because patients are more likely to go to dermatologists, internists, or plastic surgeons than to psychiatrists. One study of a group of college students found that more than 50 percent had at least some preoccupation with a particular aspect of their appearance and in approximately 25 percent of the students, the concern had at least some significant effect on their feelings and functioning.

The most common age of onset is between 15 and 30 years, and women are somewhat more often affected than men. Affected patients are likely to be unmarried. Body dysmorphic disorder commonly coexists with other mental disorders. One study found that more than 90 percent of patients with body dysmorphic disorder had experienced a major depressive episode in their lifetimes; approximately 70 percent had experienced an anxiety disorder, and approximately 30 percent had experienced a psychotic disorder.

Etiology

The cause of body dysmorphic disorder is unknown. The high comorbidity with depressive disorders, a higher-than-expected family history of mood disorders and obsessive-compulsive disorder, and the reported responsiveness of the condition to serotonin-specific drugs indicate that in at least some patients the pathophysiology of the disorder may involve serotonin and may be related to other mental disorders. Stereotyped concepts of beauty emphasized in certain families and within the culture at large may significantly affect patients with body dysmorphic disorder. In psychodynamic models, body dysmorphic disorder is seen as reflecting the displacement of a sexual or emotional conflict onto an unrelated body part. Such an association occurs through the defense mechanisms of repression, dissociation, distortion, symbolization, and projection.

Diagnosis

The DSM-IV-TR diagnostic criteria for body dysmorphic disorder stipulate a preoccupation with an imagined defect in appearance or an overemphasis of a slight defect (Table 14–4). The preoccupation causes patients significant emotional distress or markedly impairs their ability to function in important areas.

Clinical Features

The most common concerns involve facial flaws, particularly those involving specific parts (for example, the nose). Sometimes the concern is vague and difficult to understand, such as extreme concern over a "scrunchy" chin. One study found that, on average, patients had concerns about four body regions during the course of the disorder. The specific body part may change during the time a patient is affected with the disorder. Common associated symptoms include ideas or frank delusions of reference (usually about people's noticing the alleged body flaw), either excessive mirror checking or avoidance of reflec-

Table 14–4
DSM-IV-TR Diagnostic Criteria for Body Dysmorphic Disorder

A. Preoccupation with an imagined defect in appearance. If a slight physical anomaly is present, the person's concern is markedly excessive.

B. The preoccupation causes clinically significant distress or impairment in social, occupational, or other important areas of functioning.

C. The preoccupation is not better accounted for by another mental disorder (e.g., dissatisfaction with body shape and size in anorexia nervosa).

From American Psychiatric Association. *Diagnostic and Statistical Manual of Mental Disorders.* 4th ed. Text rev. Washington, DC: American Psychiatric Association; copyright 2000, with permission.

tive surfaces, and attempts to hide the presumed deformity (with makeup or clothing). The effects on a person's life can be significant; almost all affected patients avoid social and occupational exposure. As many as one-third of the patients may be housebound because of worry about being ridiculed for the alleged deformities, and as many as one-fifth attempt suicide. As previously discussed, comorbid diagnoses of depressive disorders and anxiety disorders are common, and patients may also have traits of obsessive-compulsive, schizoid, and narcissistic personality disorders.

Differential Diagnosis

Distortions of body image occur in anorexia nervosa, gender identity disorders, and some specific types of brain damage (for example, neglect syndromes); body dysmorphic disorder should not be diagnosed in these situations. Body dysmorphic disorder must also be distinguished from a person's normal concern about appearance. In body dysmorphic disorder, a person experiences significant emotional distress and functional impairment because of the concern. Although distinguishing between a strongly held idea and a delusion is difficult, if a patient's preoccupation with the perceived body defect is, in fact, of delusional intensity, the appropriate diagnosis is delusional disorder, somatic type. Other diagnostic considerations are narcissistic personality disorder, depressive disorders, obsessive-compulsive disorder, and schizophrenia. In narcissistic personality disorder, concern about a body part is only a minor feature in the general constellation of personality traits. In depressive disorders, schizophrenia, and obsessive-compulsive disorder, the other symptoms of these disorders usually evidence themselves in short order, even when the initial symptom is excessive concern about a body part.

Course and Prognosis

The onset of body dysmorphic disorder is usually gradual. An affected person may experience increasing concern over a particular body part until the person notices that functioning is being affected. Then the person may seek medical or surgical help to address the presumed problem. The level of concern about the problem may wax and wane over time, although the disorder is usually chronic if left untreated.

Treatment

Treatment of patients with body dysmorphic disorder with surgical, dermatological, dental, and other medical procedures to address the alleged defects is almost invariably unsuccessful. Although tricyclic drugs, monoamine oxidase inhibitors (MAOIs), and pimozide (Orap) have been reported to be useful in individual cases, a larger body of data indicate that serotonin-specific drugs—for example, clomipramine (Anafranil) and fluoxetine (Prozac)—are effective in reducing symptoms in at least 50 percent of patients. In any patient with a coexisting mental disorder, such as a depressive disorder or an anxiety disorder, the coexisting disorder should be treated with the appropriate pharmacotherapy and psychotherapy. How long treatment should be continued when the symptoms of body dysmorphic disorder have remitted is unknown.

Relation to Plastic Surgery

Few data exist about the number of patients seeking plastic surgery who have body dysmorphic disorder. One study found that only 2 percent of the patients in a plastic surgery clinic had the diagnosis. The overall percentage may be a much higher, however. Surgical requests are varied: removal of facial sags, jowls, wrinkles, or puffiness; rhinoplasty; breast reduction or enhancement; penile enlargement, among others. Commonly associated with the belief about appearance is an unrealistic expectation of how much surgery will correct the defect. As reality sets in, the person realizes that life's problems are not solved by altering the perceived cosmetic defect. Ideally, such patients will seek out psychotherapy to understand the true nature of their neurotic feelings of inadequacy. Absent that, patients may take out their anger by suing their plastic surgeon—plastic surgeons have one of the highest malpractice-suit rates of any specialty—or by developing a clinical depression.

PAIN DISORDER

DSM-IV-TR defines pain disorder as the presence of pain that is "the predominant focus of clinical attention." Psychological factors play an important role in the disorder. The primary symptom is pain in one or more sites that is not fully accounted for by a nonpsychiatric medical or neurological condition. The symptoms of pain are associated with emotional distress and functional impairment. The disorder has been called *somatoform pain disorder, psychogenic pain disorder, idiopathic pain disorder, and atypical pain disorder.*

Epidemiology

Pain is perhaps the most frequent complaint in medical practice, and intractable pain syndromes are common. Low back pain has disabled an estimated 7 million people in the United States and accounts for more than 8 million physician office visits annually. Pain disorder is diagnosed twice as frequently in women as in men. The peak ages of onset are in the fourth and fifth decades, perhaps because the tolerance for pain declines with age. Pain disorder is most common in people with blue-collar occupations, perhaps because of increased likelihood of job-related injuries. First-degree relatives of patients with pain disorder have an increased likelihood of having the same disorder; thus, genetic inheritance or behavioral mechanisms are possibly involved in its transmission. Depressive disorders, anxiety disorders, and substance abuse are also more common in the families of patients with pain disorder than they are in the general population.

Etiology

Psychodynamic Factors.   Patients who experience bodily aches and pains without identifiable and adequate physical causes may be symbolically expressing an intrapsychic conflict through the body. For patients suffering from alexithymia, in which they are unable to articulate their internal feeling states in words, their bodies express their feelings. Other patients may unconsciously regard emotional pain as weak and somehow lacking in legitimacy. By displacing the problem to the body, they may feel that they have a legitimate claim to the fulfillment of their dependence needs. The symbolic meaning of body disturbances may also relate to atonement for perceived sin, to expiation of guilt, or to suppressed aggression. Many patients have intractable and unresponsive pain because they are convinced that they deserve to suffer.

Pain can function as a method of obtaining love, a punishment for wrongdoing, and a way of expiating guilt and of atoning for an innate sense of badness. Among the defense mechanisms used by patients with pain disorder are displacement, substitution, and repression. Identification plays a part when a patient takes on the role of an ambivalent love object who also has pain, such as a parent.

Behavioral Factors.   Pain behaviors are reinforced when rewarded and are inhibited when ignored or punished. For example, moderate pain symptoms may become intense when followed by the solicitous and attentive behavior of others, by monetary gain, or by the successful avoidance of distasteful activities.

Interpersonal Factors.   Intractable pain has been conceptualized as a means for manipulation and gaining advantage in interpersonal relationships, for example, to ensure the devotion of a family member or to stabilize a fragile marriage. Such secondary gain is most important to patients with pain disorder.

Biological Factors.   The cerebral cortex can inhibit the firing of afferent pain fibers. Serotonin is probably the main neurotransmitter in the descending inhibitory pathways, and endorphins also play a role in the central nervous system modulation of pain. Endorphin deficiency seems to correlate with the augmentation of incoming sensory stimuli. Some patients may have pain disorder, rather than another mental disorder, because of sensory and limbic structural or chemical abnormalities that predispose them to experience pain.

Diagnosis

The DSM-IV-TR diagnostic criteria for pain disorder require the presence of clinically significant complaints of pain (Table 14–5). The complaints of pain must be judged to be significantly affected by psychological factors, and the symptoms must result in a patient's significant emotional distress or functional impairment (e.g., social or occupational). DSM-IV-TR requires that the

Table 14–5
DSM-IV-TR Diagnostic Criteria for Pain Disorder

A. Pain in one or more anatomical sites is the predominant focus of the clinical presentation and is of sufficient severity to warrant clinical attention.

B. The pain causes clinically significant distress or impairment in social, occupational, or other important areas of functioning.

C. Psychological factors are judged to have an important role in the onset, severity, exacerbation, or maintenance of the pain.

D. The symptom or deficit is not intentionally produced or feigned (as in factitious disorder or malingering).

E. The pain is not better accounted for by a mood, anxiety, or psychotic disorder and does not meet criteria for dyspareunia.

Code as follows:

Pain disorder associated with psychological factors: psychological factors are judged to have the major role in the onset, severity, exacerbation, or maintenance of the pain. (If a general medical condition is present, it does not have a major role in the onset, severity, exacerbation, or maintenance of the pain.) This type of pain disorder is not diagnosed if criteria are also met for somatization disorder.

Specify if:

Acute: duration of less than 6 months

Chronic: duration of 6 months or longer

Pain disorder associated with both psychological factors and a general medical condition: both psychological factors and a general medical condition are judged to have important roles in the onset, severity, exacerbation, or maintenance of the pain. The associated general medical condition or anatomical site of the pain (see below) is coded on Axis III.

Specify if:

Acute: duration of less than 6 months

Chronic: duration of 6 months or longer

Note: The following is not considered to be a mental disorder and is included here to facilitate differential diagnosis.

Pain disorder associated with a general medical condition: a general medical condition has a major role in the onset, severity, exacerbation, or maintenance of the pain. (If psychological factors are present, they are not judged to have a major role in the onset, severity, exacerbation, or maintenance of the pain.) The diagnostic code for the pain is selected based on the associated general medical condition if one has been established or on the anatomical location of the pain if the underlying general medical condition is not yet clearly established—for example, low back, sciatic, pelvic, headache, facial, chest, joint, bone, abdominal, breast, renal, ear, eye, throat, tooth, and urinary.

pain disorder be associated primarily with psychological factors or with both psychological factors and a general medical condition. DSM-IV-TR further specifies that pain disorder associated solely with a general medical condition be diagnosed as an Axis III condition and also allows clinicians to specify whether the pain disorder is acute or chronic, depending on whether the duration of symptoms has been 6 months or more.

Clinical Features

Patients with pain disorder do not constitute a uniform group but, instead, are a heterogeneous collection of people with low back pain, headache, atypical facial pain, chronic pelvic pain, and other kinds of pain. A patient's pain may be posttraumatic, neuropathic, neurological, iatrogenic, or musculoskeletal; to meet a diagnosis of pain disorder, however, the disorder must have a psychological factor that is judged to be significantly involved in the pain symptoms and their ramifications.

Patients with pain disorder often have long histories of medical and surgical care. They visit many physicians, request many medications, and may be especially insistent in their desire for surgery. Indeed, they can be completely preoccupied with their pain and cite it as the source of all their misery. Such patients often deny any other sources of emotional dysphoria and insist that their lives are blissful except for their pain. Their clinical picture can be complicated by substance-related disorders, because these patients attempt to reduce the pain through the use of alcohol and other substances.

At least one study has correlated the number of pain symptoms to the likelihood and severity of symptoms of somatization disorder, depressive disorders, and anxiety disorders. Major depressive disorder is present in approximately 25 to 50 percent of all patients with pain disorder, and dysthymic disorder or depressive disorder symptoms are reported in 60 to 100 percent of the patients. Some investigators believe that chronic pain is almost always a variant of a depressive disorder, a masked or somatized form of depression. The most prominent depressive symptoms in patients with pain disorder are anergia, anhedonia, decreased libido, insomnia, and irritability; diurnal variation, weight loss, and psychomotor retardation appear to be less common.

Differential Diagnosis

Purely physical pain can be difficult to distinguish from purely psychogenic pain, especially because the two are not mutually exclusive. Physical pain fluctuates in intensity and is highly sensitive to emotional, cognitive, attentional, and situational influences. Pain that does not vary and is insensitive to any of these factors is likely to be psychogenic. When pain does not wax and wane and is not even temporarily relieved by distraction or analgesics, clinicians can suspect an important psychogenic component.

Pain disorder must be distinguished from other somatoform disorders, although some somatoform disorders can coexist. Patients with hypochondriacal preoccupations may complain of pain, and aspects of the clinical presentation of hypochondriasis, such as bodily preoccupation and disease conviction, can also be present in patients with pain disorder. Patients with hypochondriasis tend to have many more symptoms than do patients with pain disorder, and their symptoms tend to fluctuate more than do the symptoms of patients with pain disorder. Conversion disorder is generally short lived, whereas pain disorder is chronic. In addition, pain is, by definition, not a symptom in conversion disorder. Malingering patients consciously provide false reports, and their complaints are usually connected to clearly recognizable goals.

The differential diagnosis can be difficult because patients with pain disorder often receive disability compensation or a litigation award. Muscle contraction (tension) headaches, for example, have a pathophysiological mechanism to account for the pain and so are not diagnosed as pain disorder. Patients with

pain disorder are not, however, pretending to be in pain. As in all of the somatoform disorders, symptoms are not imaginary.

Course and Prognosis

The pain in pain disorder generally begins abruptly and increases in severity for a few weeks or months. The prognosis varies, although pain disorder can often be chronic, distressful, and completely disabling. When psychological factors predominate in pain disorder, the pain may subside with treatment or after the elimination of external reinforcement. The patients with the poorest prognoses, with or without treatment, have preexisting characterological problems, especially pronounced passivity; are involved in litigation or receive financial compensation; use addictive substances; and have long histories of pain.

Treatment

Because it may not be possible to reduce the pain, the treatment approach must address rehabilitation. Clinicians should discuss the issue of psychological factors early in treatment and should frankly tell patients that such factors are important in the cause and consequences of both physical and psychogenic pain. Therapists should also explain how various brain circuits that are involved with emotions (such as the limbic system) may influence the sensory pain pathways. For example, if a person hits his or her head while happy at a party, the pain can seem to be less than when a person hits his or her head while angry and at work. Nevertheless, therapists must fully understand that the patient's experiences of pain are real.

Pharmacotherapy.   Analgesic medications are not generally helpful for most patients with pain disorder. In addition, substance abuse and dependence are often major problems for patients who receive long-term analgesic treatment. Sedatives and antianxiety agents are not especially beneficial and often become problems in themselves because of their frequent abuse, misuse, and side effects.

Antidepressants, such as tricyclics and selective serotonin reuptake inhibitors (SSRIs), are useful. Whether antidepressants reduce pain through their antidepressant action or exert an independent, direct analgesic effect (possibly by stimulating efferent inhibitory pain pathways) remains controversial. The success of SSRIs supports the hypothesis that serotonin is important in the pathophysiology of the disorder. Amphetamine, which has analgesic effects, may benefit some patients, especially when used as an adjunct to SSRIs, but dosages must be monitored carefully.

Psychotherapy.   Some outcome data indicate that psychodynamic psychotherapy is helpful to patients with pain disorder. The first step in psychotherapy is to develop a solid therapeutic alliance by empathizing with the patient's suffering. Clinicians should not confront somatizing patients with comments such as, "This is all in your head." For the patient, the pain is real, and clinicians must acknowledge the reality of the pain, even though they suspect that it is largely intrapsychic in origin. A useful entry point into the emotional aspects of the pain is to examine its interpersonal ramifications in the patient's life. By exploring marital problems, for example, the psycho-

**Table 14–6
DSM-IV-TR Diagnostic Criteria for
Undifferentiated Somatoform Disorder**

A. One or more physical complaints (e.g., fatigue, loss of appetite, gastrointestinal or urinary complaints).

B. Either (1) or (2):

(1) after appropriate investigation, the symptoms cannot be fully explained by a known general medical condition or the direct effects of a substance (e.g., a drug of abuse, a medication)

(2) when there is a related general medical condition, the physical complaints or resulting social or occupational impairment is in excess of what would be expected from the history, physical examination, or laboratory findings

C. The symptoms cause clinically significant distress or impairment in social, occupational, or other important areas of functioning.

D. The duration of the disturbance is at least 6 months.

E. The disturbance is not better accounted for by another mental disorder (e.g., another somatoform disorder, sexual dysfunction, mood disorder, anxiety disorder, sleep disorder, or psychotic disorder).

F. The symptom is not intentionally produced or feigned (as in factitious disorder or malingering).

From American Psychiatric Association. *Diagnostic and Statistical Manual of Mental Disorders.* 4th ed. Text rev. Washington, DC: American Psychiatric Association; copyright 2000, with permission.

**Table 14–7
DSM-IV-TR Diagnostic Criteria for Somatoform
Disorder Not Otherwise Specified**

This category includes disorders with somatoform symptoms that do not meet the criteria for any specific somatoform disorder. Examples include

1. Pseudocyesis: a false belief of being pregnant that is associated with objective signs of pregnancy, which may include abdominal enlargement (although the umbilicus does not become everted), reduced menstrual flow, amenorrhea, subjective sensation of fetal movement, nausea, breast engorgement and secretions, and labor pains at the expected date of delivery. Endocrine changes may be present, but the syndrome cannot be explained by a general medical condition that causes endocrine changes (e.g., a hormone-secreting tumor).

2. A disorder involving nonpsychotic hypochondriacal symptoms of less than 6 months' duration.

3. A disorder involving unexplained physical complaints (e.g., fatigue or body weakness) of less than 6 months' duration that are not due to another mental disorder.

From American Psychiatric Association. *Diagnostic and Statistical Manual of Mental Disorders.* 4th ed. Text rev. Washington, DC: American Psychiatric Association; copyright 2000, with permission.

therapist may soon get to the source of the patient's psychological pain and the function of the physical complaints in significant relationships. Cognitive therapy has been used to alter negative thoughts and to foster a positive attitude.

Other Therapies.   Biofeedback can be helpful in the treatment of pain disorder, particularly with migraine pain, myofascial pain, and muscle tension states, such as tension headaches. Hypnosis, transcutaneous nerve stimulation, and dorsal column stimulation also have been used. Nerve blocks and surgical ablative procedures are ineffective for most patients with pain disorder; the pain returns after 6 to 18 months.

Pain Control Programs.   It may sometimes be necessary to remove patients from their usual settings and place them in a comprehensive inpatient pain control program. Multidisciplinary pain units use many modalities, such as cognitive, behavior, and group therapies. They provide extensive physical conditioning through physical therapy and exercise and offer vocational evaluation and rehabilitation. Concurrent mental disorders are diagnosed and treated, and patients dependent on analgesics and hypnotics are detoxified. Inpatient multimodal treatment programs generally report encouraging results.

UNDIFFERENTIATED SOMATOFORM DISORDER

According to DSM-IV-TR, undifferentiated somatoform disorder is defined as unexplained physical effects that last for at least 6 months and that are below the threshold for diagnosing somatization disorder. The DSM-IV-TR diagnosis (Table 14–6) is appropriate for patients with one or more physical complaints that

cannot be explained by a known medical condition or that grossly exceed the expected complaints in a medical condition but that do not meet the diagnostic criteria for a specific somatoform disorder. The symptoms must cause patients significant emotional distress or impair their social or occupational functioning.

Two types of symptom patterns may be seen in patients with undifferentiated somatoform disorder: those involving the autonomic nervous system and those involving sensations of fatigue or weakness. In what is sometimes referred to as *autonomic arousal disorder*, some patients are affected with somatoform disorder symptoms that are limited to bodily functions innervated by the autonomic nervous system. Such patients have complaints involving the cardiovascular, respiratory, gastrointestinal, urogenital, and dermatological systems. Other patients complain of mental and physical fatigue, physical weakness and exhaustion, and inability to perform many everyday activities because of their symptoms.

Some clinicians diagnose this syndrome as *neurasthenia*, a description used primarily in Europe and Asia. The syndrome may also overlap chronic fatigue syndrome, which has been hypothesized to involve psychiatric, virological, and immunological factors. Both of these disorders are discussed in the section that follows.

SOMATOFORM DISORDER NOT OTHERWISE SPECIFIED

The DSM-IV-TR diagnostic category of somatoform disorder not otherwise specified (Table 14–7) is a residual category for patients who have symptoms suggestive of a somatoform disorder but who do not meet the specific diagnostic criteria for other somatoform disorders. Such patients may have a symptom not covered in the other somatoform disorders (for example, pseudocyesis) or may not have met the 6-month criterion of the other somatoform disorders.

15 ▲

Chronic Fatigue Syndrome and Neurasthenia

CHRONIC FATIGUE SYNDROME

Chronic fatigue syndrome (referred to as *myalgic encephalomyelitis* in the United Kingdom and Canada) is a multisystem syndrome characterized by 6 months or more of severe, debilitating fatigue, often accompanied by myalgia, headaches, pharyngitis, low-grade fever, cognitive complaint, gastrointestinal symptoms, and tender lymph nodes. The search for an infectious cause of chronic fatigue syndrome has been active because of the high percentage of patients who report abrupt onset after a severe flu-like illness.

In 1988, the U.S. Centers for Disease Control and Prevention (CDC) identified specific diagnostic criteria for chronic fatigue syndrome. Since then, the disorder has captured the attention of both the medical profession and the general public. The problems associated with studying chronic fatigue syndrome are of great interest in the United States today.

Epidemiology

The exact incidence and prevalence of chronic fatigue syndrome are unknown, but the incidence has been estimated at 1 per 1,000. The illness is observed primarily in young adults (ages 20 to 40). Women are at least twice as likely as men to be affected. In the United States, studies show that approximately 25 percent of the general adult population experience fatigue lasting 2 weeks or longer. When the fatigue persists beyond 6 months, it is defined as chronic fatigue. It has been reported that chronic fatigue syndrome has a prevalence of 0.52 percent in women and 0.29 percent in men. A study of patients in primary care clinics found that 24 percent had experienced fatigue lasting longer than 1 year.

Etiology

The cause of the disorder is unknown. The diagnosis can be made only after all other medical and psychiatric causes of chronic fatiguing illness have been excluded. Scientific studies have validated no pathognomonic signs or diagnostic tests for this condition.

Investigators have tried to implicate the Epstein-Barr herpesvirus (EBV) as the etiological agent in chronic fatigue syndrome. Epstein-Barr virus infection, however, is associated with specific antibodies and atypical lymphocytosis, findings that are absent in chronic fatigue syndrome. Results of tests for other viral agents, such as enteroviruses, herpesvirus, and retroviruses, have been negative. Some investigators have found nonspecific markers of immune abnormalities in patients with chronic fatigue syndrome, for example, reduced proliferation responses of peripheral blood lymphocytes, but these responses are similar to those detected in some patients with major depression.

Diagnosis and Clinical Features

Because chronic fatigue syndrome has no pathognomonic features, diagnosis is difficult. Physicians should attempt to delineate as many signs and symptoms as possible to facilitate the process.

The CDC diagnostic criteria for chronic fatigue syndrome are listed in Table 15–1 and include fatigue for at least 6 months, impaired memory or concentration, sore throat, tender or enlarged lymph nodes, muscle pain, arthralgias, headache, sleep disturbance, and postexertional malaise. Fatigue is the most obvious symptom and is characterized by severe mental and physical exhaustion sufficient to cause a 50 percent reduction in patients' activities. For most patients, the onset is gradual; some have an acute onset that resembles a flu-like illness.

Ms. J was a 35-year-old single white librarian with a benign medical past and no psychiatric symptoms prior to developing a flu-like illness. After 10 days the acute episode passed, but she continued to feel lethargic and fatigued readily. Two weeks after the onset of this illness, she returned to work but was unable to complete her usual 8-hour days because of increasing exhaustion and newly developed, gradually evolving, diffuse muscle and joint pain.

Her primary care physician suggested naproxen (Naprosyn) and encouraged her while counseling patience. The physician noted nothing unusual about her mood, and prescribed hypnotic agents to improve her sleep. There was no improvement, however, from 10 mg of zolpidem (Ambien). She then started having squeezing bitemporal headaches. After 3 months, she was referred to a rheumatologist who tried to give her amitriptyline (Elavil) 50 mg at night. She protested vehemently, saying that she was not depressed, just in pain.

Previously, she had been a conscientious employee and had rarely taken leave or missed work because of illness. After 3 months of this illness, however, she was forced to take a leave of absence, returning to live with her mother, since she no longer had any income. She continued to "hurt all over," was lethargic and irritable, and slept poorly because of pain. When she slept, she reported that she no longer awoke refreshed.

259

Table 15–1
CDC Criteria for Chronic Fatigue Syndrome

A. Severe unexplained fatigue for over 6 months that is:
    (1) of a new or definite onset
    (2) not due to continuing exertion
    (3) not resolved by rest
    (4) functionally impairing
B. The presence of four or more of the following new symptoms:
    (1) impaired memory or concentration
    (2) sore throat
    (3) tender lymph nodes
    (4) muscle pain
    (5) pain in several joints
    (6) new pattern of headaches
    (7) unrefreshing sleep
    (8) postexertional malaise lasting more than 24 hours

Differential Diagnosis

Chronic fatigue must be differentiated from endocrine disorders, such as hypothyroidism; neurological disorders, such as multiple sclerosis (MS); infectious disorders, such as acquired immune deficiency syndrome (AIDS) and infectious mononucleosis; and psychiatric disorders, such as depressive disorders. The evaluation process is complex.

Up to 80 percent of patients with chronic fatigue syndrome meet the diagnostic criteria for major depression. The correlation is so high that many psychiatrists believe all cases of the syndrome to be depressive disorders, yet patients with chronic fatigue syndrome rarely report feelings of guilt, suicidal ideation, or anhedonia and show little or no weight loss.

Also, there is usually no family history of depression or other genetic loading for psychiatric disorder and few if any stressful events in patients' lives that might precipitate or account for a depressive illness. In addition, although some patients respond to antidepressant medication, many eventually become refractory to all psychopharmacological agents. Regardless of diagnostic labeling, however, depressive comorbidity requires treatment with either antidepressants or cognitive-behavioral therapy or a combination of both.

Course and Prognosis

Spontaneous recovery is rare in patients with chronic fatigue syndrome, but improvement does occur. Patients with the best prognosis have had no previous or concurrent psychiatric illness, are able to maintain social contacts, and continue to work, even at reduced levels.

Treatment

Treatment of chronic fatigue syndrome is mainly supportive. Physicians must first establish rapport and not dismiss patients' complaints as being without foundation. It is important to encourage patients to continue their daily activities and to resist their fatigue as much as possible. A reduced workload is far better than absence from work.

Psychiatric treatment is desirable, especially when depression is present. In many cases, symptoms improve markedly when patients are in supportive or insight-oriented psychotherapy. Cognitive-behavioral therapy has been reported to be of use. Therapy is geared to help patients overcome and correct mistaken beliefs, such as fear that any activity causing fatigue worsens the disorder. Pharmacological agents, especially antidepressants with nonsedating qualities, such as bupropion (Wellbutrin), may be helpful. Nefazodone (Serzone) was reported to decrease pain and improve sleep and memory in some patients. Analeptics (for instance, amphetamine or methylphenidate [Ritalin]) may help to reduce fatigue.

NEURASTHENIA

The term *neurasthenia* ("nervous exhaustion") was introduced in the 1860s by the American neuropsychiatrist George Miller Beard, who applied it to a condition characterized by chronic fatigue and disability. It remains a diagnostic entity in Europe and Asia. According to current nosology in the United States, the disorder is not considered a distinct diagnosis.

Neurasthenia is characterized by a wide variety of signs and symptoms. The most common findings are chronic weakness and fatigue, aches and pains, and general anxiety or "nervousness." In the fourth revised edition of the *Diagnostic and Statistical Manual of Mental Disorders* (DSM-IV-TR), neurasthenia would be associated with one of the two forms of undifferentiated somatoform disorders—that is, with the group of physical complaints including chronic fatigue and loss of appetite. Because so many signs and symptoms of neurasthenia overlap with and appear in each of these disorders, differential diagnosis may be exceedingly difficult. For example, patients with anxiety disorder do not uncommonly have depressive symptomatology; patients with hypochondriasis often complain of anxiety; and patients with body dysmorphic disorder can have somatic complaints. Clinicians must rigorously apply the diagnostic criteria for anxiety, depressive, and somatoform disorders before making the diagnosis. Hallmarks of chronic fatigue syndrome must also be considered, and differentiating between the two disorders is difficult. Treatment is supportive and similar to that for chronic fatigue syndrome, described above.

16

Factitious Disorders

In factitious disorders, patients intentionally produce signs of medical or mental disorders and misrepresent their histories and symptoms. The only apparent objective of the behavior is to assume the role of a patient without an external incentive. For many people, hospitalization itself is a primary objective and often a way of life. The disorders have a compulsive quality, but the behaviors are considered voluntary in that they are deliberate and purposeful, even if they cannot be controlled. Clinicians can assess whether a symptom is intentional both by direct evidence and by excluding other causes.

In a 1951 article in *Lancet*, Richard Asher coined the term "Münchausen syndrome" to refer to a syndrome in which patients embellish their personal history, chronically fabricate symptoms to gain hospital admission, and move from hospital to hospital. The syndrome was named after Baron Hieronymus Friedrich Freiherr von Münchausen (1720–1791), a German cavalry officer.

EPIDEMIOLOGY

The prevalence of factitious disorders in the general population is unknown, although some clinicians believe that they are more common than acknowledged. They appear to occur more frequently in hospital and health care workers than in the general population. The disorder occurs more frequently in females than in males, and the severe syndromes are more frequent in females. One study reported a 9 percent rate of factitious disorders among all patients admitted to a hospital; another study found factitious fever in 3 percent of all patients. According to the text revision of the fourth edition of *Diagnostic and Statistical Manual of Mental Disorders* (DSM-IV-TR), factitious disorder is diagnosed in approximately 1 percent of patients who are seen in psychiatric consultation in general hospitals. The prevalence appears to be greater in highly specialized treatment settings. Cases of feigned psychological signs and symptoms are reported much less commonly than those of physical signs and symptoms. A databank of people who feign illness has been established to alert hospitals about such patients, many of whom travel from place to place, seek admission under different names, or simulate different illnesses.

In the United States, factitious disorder by proxy (discussed separately below) accounts for fewer than 1,000 of the almost 3 million cases of child abuse reported annually.

COMORBIDITY

A large number of persons diagnosed with factitious disorder have comorbid psychiatric diagnoses (e.g., mood disorders, personality disorders, or substance-related disorders).

ETIOLOGY

Psychosocial Factors

The psychodynamic underpinnings of factitious disorders are poorly understood because engaging the patients in exploratory psychotherapy is difficult. Patients may insist that their symptoms are physical and that psychologically oriented treatment is therefore useless. Anecdotal case reports indicate that many of the patients suffered childhood abuse or deprivation, resulting in frequent hospitalizations during early development. In such circumstances, an inpatient stay may have been regarded as an escape from a traumatic home situation, and the patient may have found a series of caretakers (such as doctors, nurses, and hospital workers) to be loving and caring. In contrast, the patients' families of origin included a rejecting mother or an absent father. The usual history reveals that the patients perceive one or both parents as rejecting figures who are unable to form close relationships. The facsimile of genuine illness, therefore, is used to recreate the desired positive parent–child bond. Hence, the patients transform the physicians and staff members into rejecting parents.

Patients who seek out painful procedures, such as surgical operations and invasive diagnostic tests, may have a masochistic personality makeup in which pain serves as punishment for past sins, imagined or real. Some patients may attempt to master the past and the early trauma of serious medical illness or hospitalization by assuming the role of the patient and reliving the painful and frightening experience over and over again through multiple hospitalizations. Patients who feign psychiatric illness may have had a relative who was hospitalized with the illness they are simulating. Through identification, patients hope to reunite with the relative in a magical way.

Many patients have the poor identity formation and disturbed self-image that is characteristic of someone with borderline personality disorder. Some patients are as-if personalities who have assumed the identities of those around them. If these patients are health professionals, they are often unable to differ-

**Table 16–1
DSM-IV-TR Diagnostic Criteria for
Factitious Disorder**

A. Intentional production or feigning of physical or psychological signs or symptoms.

B. The motivation for the behavior is to assume the sick role.

C. External incentives for the behavior (such as economic gain, avoiding legal responsibility, or improving physical well-being, as in malingering) are absent.

Code based on type:

With predominantly psychological signs and symptoms: if psychological signs and symptoms predominate in the clinical presentation

With predominantly physical signs and symptoms: if physical signs and symptoms predominate in the clinical presentation

With combined psychological and physical signs and symptoms: if both psychological and physical signs and symptoms are present but neither predominates in the clinical presentation

From American Psychiatric Association. *Diagnostic and Statistical Manual of Mental Disorders.* 4th ed. Text rev. Washington, DC: American Psychiatric Association; copyright 2000, with permission.

entiate themselves from the patients with whom they come in contact. The cooperation or encouragement of other people in simulating a factitious illness occurs in a rare variant of the disorder and suggests another possible causative factor. Although most patients act alone, friends or relatives participate in fabricating the illness in some instances.

Significant defense mechanisms are repression, identification, identification with the aggressor, regression, and symbolization.

Biological Factors

Some researchers have proposed than brain dysfunction may be a factor in factitious disorders, especially Münchausen syndrome. It has been hypothesized that impaired information processing contributes to Münchausen patients' pseudologia fantastica and aberrant behavior. No genetic patterns have been established, and electroencephalographic (EEG) studies noted no specific abnormalities in patients with factitious disorders.

DIAGNOSIS AND CLINICAL FEATURES

The diagnostic criteria for factitious disorder in DSM-IV-TR are given in Table 16–1. The psychiatric examination should emphasize securing information from any available friends, relatives, or other informants, because interviews with reliable outside sources often reveal the false nature of the patient's illness. Although time consuming and tedious, verifying all the facts presented by the patient about previous hospitalizations and medical care is essential.

Psychiatric evaluation is requested on a consultation basis in approximately 50 percent of the cases, usually after the presence of a simulated illness is suspected. The psychiatrist is often asked to confirm the diagnosis of factitious disorder. Under these circumstances, it is necessary to avoid pointed or accusatory questioning that may provoke truculence, evasion, or flight from the hospital.

Factitious Disorder with Predominantly Psychological Signs and Symptoms

Some patients show psychiatric symptoms that are judged to be feigned. The feigned symptoms often include depression, hallucinations, dissociative and conversion symptoms, and bizarre behavior. Because the patients do not improve after routine therapeutic measures are administered, they may receive large doses of psychoactive drugs and may undergo electroconvulsive (ECT) therapy.

Factitious psychological symptoms resemble the phenomenon of pseudomalingering, conceptualized as satisfying the need to maintain an intact self-image, which would be marred by admitting psychological problems that are beyond the person's capacity to master through conscious effort. In this case, deception is a transient ego-supporting device.

Psychotic inpatients found to have factitious disorder with predominantly psychological signs and symptoms—that is, exclusively simulated psychotic symptoms—generally have a concurrent diagnosis of borderline personality disorder. In these cases, the outcome appears to be worse than that of bipolar I disorder or schizoaffective disorder.

Patients may appear depressed and may explain their depression by offering a false history of the recent death of a significant friend or relative. Elements of the history that may suggest factitious bereavement include a violent or bloody death, a death under dramatic circumstances, and the dead person's being a child or a young adult. Other patients may describe both recent and remote memory loss or both auditory and visual hallucinations. According to DSM-IV-TR:

> The individual may surreptitiously use psychoactive substances for the purpose of producing symptoms that suggest a mental disorder (e.g., stimulants to produce restlessness or insomnia, hallucinogens to induce altered perceptual states, analgesic to induce euphoria, and hypnotics to induce lethargy). Combinations of psychoactive substances can produce very unusual presentations.

Other symptoms, which also appear in the physical type of factitious disorder, include pseudologia fantastica and impostorship. In pseudologia fantastica, limited factual material is mixed with extensive and colorful fantasies. The listener's interest pleases the patient and thus reinforces the symptom. The history or the symptoms are not the only distortions of truth. Patients often give false and conflicting accounts about other areas of their lives (for example, they may claim the death of a parent, so as to play on the sympathy of others). Imposture is commonly related to lying in these cases. Many patients assume the identity of a prestigious person. Men, for example, report being war heroes and attribute their surgical scars to wounds received during battle or in other dramatic and dangerous exploits.

Factitious Disorder with Predominantly Physical Signs and Symptoms

Factitious disorder with predominantly physical signs and symptoms is the best-known type of Münchausen syndrome. The disorder has also been called *hospital addiction, polysurgical addiction*—producing the so-called washboard abdomen—and *professional patient syndrome*, among other names.

The essential feature of patients with the disorder is their ability to present physical symptoms so well that they are able to gain admission to and stay in a hospital (Table 16–1). To support their history, the patients may feign symptoms suggestive of a disorder that may involve any organ system. They are familiar with the diagnoses of most disorders that usually require hospital admission or medication and can give excellent histories capable of deceiving even experienced clinicians. Clinical presentations are myriad and include hematoma, hemoptysis, abdominal pain, fever, hypoglycemia, lupus-like syndromes, nausea, vomiting, dizziness, and seizures. Urine is contaminated with blood or feces, anticoagulants are taken to simulate bleeding disorders, insulin is used to produce hypoglycemia, and so on. Such patients often insist on surgery and claim adhesions from previous surgical procedures. They may acquire a gridiron- or washboard-like abdomen from multiple procedures. Complaints of pain, especially that simulating renal colic, are common, with the patients wanting narcotics. In approximately half the reported cases, the patients demand treatment with specific medications, usually analgesics. Once in the hospital, they continue to be demanding and difficult. As each test is returned with a negative result, they may accuse doctors of incompetence, threaten litigation, and become generally abusive. Some may abruptly sign out shortly before they believe they are going to be confronted with their factitious behavior.

Factitious Disorder with Combined Psychological and Physical Signs and Symptoms

In combined forms of factitious disorder, both psychological and physical signs and symptoms are present. If neither type predominates in the clinical presentation, a diagnosis of factitious disorder with combined psychological and physical signs and symptoms should be made. In one representative report, a patient alternated between feigned dementia, bereavement, rape, and seizures.

Factitious Disorder Not Otherwise Specified

Some patients with factitious signs and symptoms do not meet the DSM-IV-TR criteria for a specific factitious disorder and should be classified as having factitious disorder not otherwise specified (Table 16–2). The most notable example of the diagnosis is *factitious disorder by proxy*, which is also included in a DSM-IV-TR appendix (Table 16–3). In this diagnosis, a person intentionally produces physical signs or symptoms in another person who is under the first person's care. One apparent purpose of the behavior is for the caretaker to indirectly assume the sick role; another is to be relieved of the caretaking role by having the person hospitalized. The most common case of factitious disorder by proxy involves a mother who deceives medical personnel into believing that her child is ill. The deception may involve a false medical history, the contamination of laboratory samples, the alteration of records, or the induction of injury and illness in the child.

PATHOLOGY AND LABORATORY EXAMINATION

Psychological testing may reveal specific underlying pathology in individual patients. Features that are overrepresented in patients with factitious disorder include normal or above-average

Table 16–2
DSM-IV-TR Diagnostic Criteria for Factitious Disorder Not Otherwise Specified

This category includes disorders with factitious symptoms that do not meet the criteria for factitious disorder. An example is factitious disorder by proxy: the intentional production or feigning of physical or psychological signs or symptoms in another person who is under the individual's care for the purpose of indirectly assuming the sick role (see Table 16–3 for suggested research criteria).

From American Psychiatric Association. *Diagnostic and Statistical Manual of Mental Disorders.* 4th ed. Text rev. Washington, DC: American Psychiatric Association; copyright 2000, with permission.

intelligence quotient (IQ); absence of a formal thought disorder; poor sense of identity, including confusion over sexual identity; poor sexual adjustment; poor frustration tolerance; strong dependence needs; and narcissism. An invalid test profile and elevations of all clinical scales on the Minnesota Multiphasic Personality Inventory-2 (MMPI-2) indicate an attempt to appear more disturbed than is the case ("fake bad").

There are no specific laboratory tests for factitious disorders. However, certain tests (e.g., drug screening) may help confirm the presence of or rule out specific mental or medical disorders.

DIFFERENTIAL DIAGNOSIS

Any disorder in which physical signs and symptoms are prominent should be considered in the differential diagnosis, and the possibility of authentic or concomitant physical illness must always be explored. Additionally, a history of many surgeries in factious disorder patients may predispose patients to complications or actual diseases, necessitating even further surgery. Factitious disorder is on a continuum between somatoform disorders and malingering, the goal being to assume the risk role. On one hand it is unconscious and nonvolitional (somatoform) and on the other hand it is conscious and willful (malingering).

Somatoform Disorders

A factitious disorder is differentiated from somatization disorder (Briquet's syndrome) by the voluntary production of factitious symptoms,

Table 16–3
DSM-IV-TR Research Criteria for Factitious Disorder by Proxy

A. Intentional production or feigning of physical or psychological signs or symptoms in another person who is under the individual's care.

B. The motivation for the perpetrator's behavior is to assume the sick role by proxy.

C. External incentives for the behavior (such as economic gain) are absent.

D. The behavior is not better accounted for by another mental disorder.

From American Psychiatric Association. *Diagnostic and Statistical Manual of Mental Disorders.* 4th ed. Text rev. Washington, DC: American Psychiatric Association; copyright 2000, with permission.

the extreme course of multiple hospitalizations, and the seeming willingness to undergo an extraordinary number of mutilating procedures in patients with the former disorder. Patients with conversion disorder are not usually conversant with medical terminology and hospital routines, and their symptoms have a direct temporal relation or symbolic reference to specific emotional conflicts.

Hypochondriasis differs from factitious disorder in that the hypochondriacal patient, similar to somatoform, does not usually submit to potentially mutilating procedures and hypochondriasis typically has a later age of onset. (Somatoform disorders are discussed in Chapter 14.)

Personality Disorders

Because of their pathological lying, lack of close relationships with others, hostile and manipulative manner, and associated substance abuse and criminal history, factitious disorder patients are often classified as having antisocial personality disorder. Antisocial people, however, do not usually volunteer for invasive procedures or resort to a way of life marked by repeated or long-term hospitalization.

Because of attention seeking and an occasional flair for the dramatic, patients with factitious disorder may be classified as having histrionic personality disorder. Not all factitious disorder patients have a dramatic flair, however; many are withdrawn and bland. Consideration of the person's chaotic lifestyle, history of disturbed interpersonal relationships, identity crisis, substance abuse, self-damaging acts, and manipulative tactics may lead to the diagnosis of borderline personality disorder. People with factitious disorder usually do not have the eccentricities of dress, thought, or communication that characterize schizotypal personality disorder patients. (Personality disorders are discussed in Chapter 24.)

Schizophrenia

The diagnosis of schizophrenia is often based on bizarre lifestyles, but patients with factitious disorder do not usually meet the diagnostic criteria for schizophrenia unless they have the fixed delusion that they are actually ill and act on this belief by seeking hospitalization. Such a practice seems to be the exception; few patients with factitious disorder show evidence of a severe thought disorder or bizarre delusions.

Malingering

Factitious disorders must be distinguished from malingering. Malingerers have an obvious, recognizable environmental goal in producing signs and symptoms, such as hospitalization to secure financial compensation, evade the police, avoid work, or merely obtain free bed and board for the night. Moreover, these patients can usually stop producing their signs and symptoms when they are no longer considered profitable or when the risk becomes too great. (Malingering is discussed in Chapter 29.)

Substance Abuse

Although patients with factitious disorders may have a complicating history of substance abuse, they should not be considered merely as substance abusers but as having coexisting diagnoses.

Ganser's Syndrome

Ganser's syndrome, a controversial condition most typically associated with prison inmates, is characterized by the use of approximate answers. People with the syndrome respond to simple questions with astonishingly incorrect answers. For example, when asked about the color of a blue car, the person answers "red" or answers "2 plus 2 equals 5." Ganser's syndrome may be a variant of malingering in that the patients avoid punishment or responsibility for their actions. Ganser's syndrome is classified in DSM-IV-TR as a dissociative disorder not otherwise specified. However, in factitious disorder with predominantly psychological signs and symptoms, the intentional giving of approximate answers may occur.

COURSE AND PROGNOSIS

Factitious disorders typically begin in early adulthood, although they may appear during childhood or adolescence. The onset of the disorder or of discrete episodes of seeking treatment may follow real illness, loss, rejection, or abandonment. Usually, the patient or a close relative had a hospitalization in childhood or early adolescence for a genuine physical illness. Thereafter, a long pattern of successive hospitalizations begins insidiously and unfolds. As the disorder progresses, the patient becomes knowledgeable about medicine and hospitals. The onset of the disorder in patients who had early hospitalizations for actual illness is earlier than generally reported.

Factitious disorders are incapacitating to the patient and often produce severe traumas or untoward reactions related to treatment. A course of repeated or long-term hospitalization is obviously incompatible with meaningful vocational work and sustained interpersonal relationships. The prognosis in most cases is poor. A few patients occasionally spend time in jail, usually for minor crimes, such as burglary, vagrancy, and disorderly conduct. Patients may also have a history of intermittent psychiatric hospitalization.

Although no adequate data are available about the ultimate outcome for the patients, a few of them probably die as a result of needless medication, instrumentation, or surgery. In view of the patients' often expert simulation and the risks that they take, some may die without the disorder's being suspected. Possible features that indicate a favorable prognosis are (1) the presence of a depressive-masochistic personality; (2) functioning at a borderline, not a continuously psychotic, level; and (3) the attributes of an antisocial personality disorder with minimal symptoms.

TREATMENT

No specific psychiatric therapy has been effective in treating factitious disorders. They deny to themselves and others their true illness and thus avoid possible treatment for it. Ultimately, the patients elude meaningful therapy by abruptly leaving the hospital or failing to keep follow-up appointments.

Treatment is thus best focused on management rather than on cure. Perhaps the single most important factor in successful management is a physician's early recognition of the disorder. In this way, physicians can forestall patients' undergoing a multitude of painful and potentially dangerous diagnostic procedures. Good liaison between psychiatrists and the medical or surgical staff is strongly advised. Although a few cases of individual psychotherapy have been reported in the literature, there is no consensus about the best approach. In general, working in concert with the patient's primary care physician is more effective than working with the patient in isolation.

The personal reactions of physicians and staff members are of great significance in treating and establishing a working alliance with the patients, who invariably evoke feelings of futility, bewilderment, betrayal, hostility, and even contempt. In essence, staff members are forced to abandon a basic element of their relationship with patients: acceptance of the truthfulness of the patients' statements. One appropriate psychiatric intervention is to suggest to the staff ways of remaining aware that even though the patient's illness is factitious, the patient is ill.

Physicians should try not to feel resentment when patients humiliate their diagnostic prowess, and they should avoid any unmasking ceremony that sets up patients as adversaries and precipitates their flight from the hospital. The staff should not perform unnecessary procedures or discharge patients abruptly, both of which are manifestations of anger.

Although the use of confrontation is controversial, at some point in the treatment, patients must be made to face reality. Most patients simply leave treatment when their methods of gaining attention are identified and brought out into the open. In some cases, clinicians should reframe the factitious disorder as a cry for help, so that patients do not view clinicians' responses as punitive.

Education about the disorder and some attempt to understand the patient's motivations may help staff members maintain their professional conduct in the face of extreme frustration. In cases of factitious disorder by proxy, legal intervention has been obtained in several instances, particularly with children. The senselessness of the disorder and the denial of false action by parents are obstacles to successful court action and often make conclusive proof unobtainable. In such cases, the child welfare services should be notified and arrangements made for the ongoing monitoring of the children's health.

Pharmacotherapy of factitious disorders is of limited use. Selective serotonin reuptake inhibitors (SSRIs) may be useful in decreasing impulsive behavior when that is a major component in acting-out factitious behavior.

17 ▲

Dissociative Disorders

Most people see themselves as human beings with one basic personality; they experience a unitary sense of self. People with dissociative disorders, however, have lost the sense of having one consciousness. They feel as though they either have no identity, are confused about who they are, or experience multiple identities. Everything that usually gives people their unique personalities—their integrated thoughts, feelings, and actions—is abnormal in people with dissociative disorders.

In most dissociative states, contradictory representations of the self, which conflict with each other, are kept in separate mental compartments. There are four types: (1) *dissociative amnesia* is characterized by an inability to remember information, usually related to a stressful or traumatic event, that cannot be explained by ordinary forgetfulness, the ingestion of substances, or a general medical condition; (2) *dissociative fugue* is characterized by sudden and unexpected travel away from home or work and is associated with an inability to recall the past and with confusion about a person's personal identity or with the adoption of a new identity; (3) *dissociative identity disorder* (also called *multiple personality disorder*), generally considered the most severe and chronic of the dissociative disorders, is characterized by the presence of two or more distinct personalities within a single person; and (4) *depersonalization disorder* is characterized by recurrent or persistent feelings of detachment from the body or mind. The text revision of the fourth edition of *Diagnostic and Statistical Manual of Mental Disorders* (DSM-IV-TR) includes the diagnostic category of dissociative disorder not otherwise specified for dissociative disorders that do not meet the diagnostic criteria of the other dissociative disorders. DSM-IV-TR also includes in its appendix diagnostic guidelines for dissociative trance disorder, which is currently categorized as a dissociative disorder not otherwise specified. Mental contents coexist in parallel consciousness.

DISSOCIATIVE AMNESIA

The symptom of amnesia is common to dissociative amnesia, dissociative fugue, and dissociative identity disorder. Dissociative amnesia is the appropriate diagnosis when the dissociative phenomena are limited to amnesia. Its key symptom is the inability to recall information, usually about stressful or traumatic events in people's lives. This inability cannot be explained by ordinary forgetfulness, and there is no evidence of an underlying brain disorder. Persons retain the capacity to learn new information.

A common form of dissociative amnesia involves amnesia for personal identity but intact memory of general information.

This clinical picture is exactly the reverse of the one seen in dementia, in which patients may remember their names but forget general information, such as what they had for lunch. Except for their amnesia, patients with dissociative amnesia appear completely intact and function coherently. By contrast, in most amnesias due to a general medical condition (such as postictal and toxic amnesias), patients may be confused and behave in a disorganized manner. Other types of amnesias (e.g., transient global amnesia and postconcussion amnesia) are associated with an ongoing anterograde amnesia, which does not occur in patients with dissociative amnesia.

Epidemiology

Dissociative amnesia is thought to be the most common of the dissociative disorders, although epidemiological data for all the dissociative disorders are limited and uncertain. Dissociative amnesia is thought to occur more often in women than in men and more often in young adults than in older adults, but it can occur at any age. Inasmuch as the disorder is usually associated with stressful and traumatic events, its incidence probably increases during times of war and natural disaster. Cases of dissociative amnesia related to domestic settings—for example, spouse abuse and child abuse—are probably constant in number. Most cases are seen in hospital emergency rooms, where amnesia patients are brought after being found on the street.

Etiology

The newly appreciated complexity of the formation and retrieval of memories may make dissociative amnesia intuitively understandable because of the many potential areas for dysfunction. Most patients with dissociative amnesia are unable to retrieve painful memories of stressful and traumatic events, and thus the emotional content of the memory is clearly related to the pathophysiology and the cause of the disorder.

One relevant observation about people in general is that learning is often state dependent—that is, dependent on the context in which learning occurs. Thus, people can remember where a light switch is located in their car more easily while they are driving than when they are watching television. The theory of state-dependent learning applies to dissociative amnesia in that the memory of a traumatic event is laid down during the event, and the emotional state may be so extraordinary that it is hard for an affected person to remember information learned during that state.

Table 17–1
DSM-IV-TR Diagnostic Criteria for Dissociative Amnesia

A. The predominant disturbance is one or more episodes of inability to recall important personal information, usually of a traumatic or stressful nature, that is too extensive to be explained by ordinary forgetfulness.

B. The disturbance does not occur exclusively during the course of dissociative identity disorder, dissociative fugue, posttraumatic stress disorder, acute stress disorder, or somatization disorder and is not due to the direct physiological effects of a substance (e.g., a drug of abuse, a medication) or a neurological or other general medical condition (e.g., amnestic disorder due to head trauma).

C. The symptoms cause clinically significant distress or impairment in social, occupational, or other important areas of functioning.

From American Psychiatric Association. *Diagnostic and Statistical Manual of Mental Disorders.* 4th ed. Text rev. Washington, DC: American Psychiatric Association; copyright 2000, with permission.

In the psychoanalytic approach to dissociative amnesia, the disorder is considered primarily as a defense mechanism whereby a person alters consciousness as a way of dealing with an emotional conflict or an external stressor. Secondary defenses involved in dissociative amnesia include repression (disturbing impulses are blocked from consciousness) and denial (an aspect of external reality is ignored by the conscious mind).

Diagnosis

The diagnostic criteria for dissociative amnesia in the fourth revised edition of the *Diagnostic and Statistical Manual of Mental Disorders* (DSM-IV-TR) (Table 17–1) emphasize that the forgotten information is usually of a traumatic or stressful nature. Dissociative amnesia can be diagnosed only when the symptoms are not limited to amnesia that occurs in the course of dissociative identity disorder and are not the result of a general medical condition (for example, head trauma) or the ingestion of a substance.

Clinical Features

Although rare episodes of dissociative amnesia occur spontaneously, the history usually reveals a precipitating emotional trauma charged with painful emotions and psychological conflict—for example, a natural disaster in which people witnessed severe injuries or feared for their lives. A fantasized or actual expression of an impulse (sexual or aggressive) with which a person is unable to deal may also act as a precipitant, and amnesia may follow behavior that a person later finds morally reprehensible (for example, violence, an extramarital affair).

Although not necessary for diagnosis, the onset of the amnesia is often abrupt, and patients are usually aware that they have lost their memories. Some patients are upset by the memory loss, but others appear to be unconcerned or indifferent. When patients are not aware of their memory loss but a clinician suspects that they have dissociative amnesia, it is often useful to ask specific questions that may reveal the symptoms. Amnestic patients are usually alert before and after the amnesia

occurs. A few patients, however, report a slight clouding of consciousness during the period immediately surrounding the onset of amnesia. Depression and anxiety are common predisposing factors and frequently appear in a patient's mental status examination. Amnesia may provide a primary or a secondary gain. A woman who is amnestic about the birth of a dead infant achieves a primary gain by protecting herself from painful emotions. A soldier who has a sudden case of amnesia and is then removed from combat as a result exemplifies a secondary gain.

Dissociative amnesia may take one of several forms: Localized amnesia, the most common type, is the loss of memory for the events of a short time (a few hours to a few days); generalized amnesia is the loss of memory for a whole lifetime of experience; selective (also known as *systematized*) amnesia is the failure to recall some but not all events that occurred during a short time.

Confabulation and Self-Monitoring.   Because amnesia can have a disastrous effect on a patient's day-to-day life, many people with chronic amnesia develop adaptive strategies. One such strategy is *confabulation*, the invention of false information to cover up a gap in memory. Other patients will resort to various forms of self-monitoring to protect themselves from memory loss, such as note-taking or the cessation of regular activities.

Differential Diagnosis

The differential diagnosis of dissociative amnesia involves a consideration of both general medical conditions and other mental disorders. Clinicians should conduct a medical history, a physical examination, a laboratory workup, a psychiatric history, and a mental status examination.

Amnesia associated with dementia and delirium is usually associated with many other easily recognized cognitive symptoms. When a patient has amnesia about personal information in these conditions, the dementia or delirium is usually advanced and easily differentiated from dissociative amnesia.

Epilepsy can lead to sudden memory impairment associated with motor and electroencephalogram (EEG) abnormalities. Patients with epilepsy are prone to seizures during periods of stress, and some researchers have hypothesized that an epileptic-like cause may be involved in the dissociative disorders. A history of an aura, head trauma, or incontinence can help clinicians recognize amnesia related to epilepsy.

Transient Global Amnesia.   Transient global amnesia is an acute and transient retrograde amnesia that affects recent more than remote memories. Although patients are usually aware of the amnesia, they may still perform highly complex mental and physical acts during the 6 to 24 hours that transient global amnesia episodes usually last. Recovery from the disorder is usually complete. Transient global amnesia is most often caused by transient ischemic attacks (TIAs) that affect limbic midline brain structures. It can also be associated with migraine headaches, seizures, and intoxication with sedative-hypnotic drugs.

Transient global amnesia can be differentiated from dissociative amnesia in several ways. Dissociative amnesia is not associated with anterograde amnesia during the episode. Patients with transient global amnesia tend to be more upset and concerned about the symptoms than are patients with dissociative amnesia. The personal identity of patients with dissociative amnesia is lost; that of patients with transient global amnesia is retained. The memory loss of patients with dissociative amnesia may be selective for certain areas and usually does not show a temporal gradient; the memory loss of a patient with transient global amnesia is generalized, and remote events are remembered better than recent events. Because of the association of transient global amnesia with vascular problems, the disorder is most common in patients in their 60s and 70s, whereas dissociative amnesia is most common in patients in their 20s to 40s, a period associated with the common psychological stressors seen in these patients. Other vasospastic events in the temporal lobe or thalamus have been reported in which transient amnestic attacks occur, even in young adults.

Other Mental Disorders.   In DSM-IV-TR, sleepwalking disorder is classified as a parasomnia, a type of sleep disorder. Patients suffering from sleepwalking disorder behave in a strange manner that resembles the behavior of someone in a dissociative state. They exhibit an altered state of conscious awareness of their surroundings; they often have vivid hallucinatory recollections of an emotionally traumatic event in the past of which there is no memory during the usual waking state. Such patients are out of contact with the environment, appear preoccupied with a private world, and stare into space if their eyes are open. They may appear emotionally upset, speak excitedly in words and sentences that are frequently hard to understand, or engage in a pattern of seemingly meaningful activities repeated every time an episode occurs. The patients have amnesia for the sleepwalking episode once it has ended.

Although amnesia for a period of immediate past experience is found in patients with sleepwalking disorder and with localized and general amnesia, the state of consciousness during the period for which they are amnestic differs in character. Patients with amnesia, in contrast to sleepwalking disorders, usually give no indication to observers that anything is amiss and seem entirely alert both before and after the amnesia occurs.

Posttraumatic stress disorder, acute stress disorder, and the somatoform disorders (especially somatization disorder and conversion disorder) should be considered in the differential diagnosis and may coexist with dissociative amnesia. The somatoform disorders may be associated with the same traumatic events that are usually seen in dissociative amnesia. Malingering, in this case a deliberate attempt to mimic amnesia, may be difficult to confirm. Any possible secondary gain, especially in regard to escaping punishment for criminal activity, should increase a clinician's suspicion, although such secondary gain does not rule out the diagnosis of dissociative amnesia.

Course and Prognosis

The symptoms of dissociative amnesia usually terminate abruptly, and recovery is generally complete with few recurrences. In some cases, especially if there is secondary gain, the condition may last a long time. Clinicians should try to restore patients' lost memories to consciousness as soon as possible; otherwise, the repressed memory may form a nucleus in the unconscious mind around which future amnestic episodes may develop.

Treatment

Interviewing may give clinicians clues to the psychologically traumatic precipitant. Drug-assisted interviews with short-acting barbiturates, such as thiopental (Pentothal) and sodium amobarbital given intravenously, and benzodiazepines may help

patients recover their forgotten memories. Hypnosis can be used primarily as a means of relaxing patients enough for them to recall what has been forgotten. When patients are placed in a somnolent state, mental inhibitions are diminished and the amnestic material emerges into consciousness and is then recalled. Once the lost memories have been retrieved, psychotherapy is generally recommended to help patients incorporate the memories into their conscious states.

DISSOCIATIVE FUGUE

The behavior of patients with dissociative fugue is unusual and dramatic. The term *fugue* is used to reflect the fact that patients physically travel away from their customary homes or work situations and fail to remember important aspects of their previous identities (name, family, occupation). Such patients often, but not always, take on an entirely new identity and occupation, although the new identity is usually less complete than are the alternate personalities in dissociative identity disorder, and the old and new identities do not alternate, as they do in dissociative identity disorder.

Epidemiology

Dissociative fugue is rare and, like dissociative amnesia, occurs most often during wartime, after natural disasters, and as a result of personal crises with intense internal conflicts. According to DSM-IV-TR, there is a prevalence rate of 0.2 percent in the general population.

Etiology

Although heavy alcohol abuse may predispose people to dissociative fugue, the cause of the disorder is thought to be basically psychological. The essential motivating factor seems to be a desire to withdraw from emotionally painful experiences. Patients with mood disorders and certain personality disorders (e.g., borderline, histrionic, and schizoid personality disorders) are predisposed to develop dissociative fugue.

A variety of stressors and personal factors predispose a person to the development of dissociative fugue. The psychosocial factors include marital, financial, occupational, and war-related stressors. Other associated predisposing features include depression, suicide attempts, organic disorders (especially epilepsy), and a history of substance abuse. A history of head trauma also predisposes a person to dissociative fugue.

Diagnosis and Clinical Features

DSM-IV-TR requires that a person either be confused about his or her identity or assume a new identity (Table 17–2). Unlike dissociative amnesia, the diagnosis of dissociative fugue requires that the onset of the symptoms be sudden. The diagnosis is excluded if the symptoms occur only during the course of dissociative identity disorder or as a result of substance ingestion or a general medical condition (such as temporal lobe epilepsy).

Dissociative fugue has several typical features. Patients wander in a purposeful way, usually far from home and often for days at a time. During this period, they have complete amnesia for their past lives and associations, but, unlike patients with disso-

**Table 17–2
DSM-IV-TR Diagnostic Criteria for
Dissociative Fugue**

A. The predominant disturbance is sudden, unexpected travel away from home or one's customary place of work, with inability to recall one's past.

B. Confusion about personal identity or assumption of a new identity (partial or complete).

C. The disturbance does not occur exclusively during the course of dissociative identity disorder and is not due to the direct physiological effects of a substance (e.g., a drug of abuse, a medication) or a general medical condition (e.g., temporal lobe epilepsy).

D. The symptoms cause clinically significant distress or impairment in social, occupational, or other important areas of functioning.

From American Psychiatric Association. *Diagnostic and Statistical Manual of Mental Disorders.* 4th ed. Text rev. Washington, DC: American Psychiatric Association; copyright 2000, with permission.

ciative amnesia, they are generally unaware that they have forgotten anything. Only when they suddenly return to their former selves do they recall the time antedating the onset of fugue, but then they remain amnestic for the period of the fugue itself. Patients with dissociative fugue do not seem to others to be behaving in extraordinary ways. They lead quiet, prosaic, reclusive existences; work at simple occupations; live modestly; and, in general, do nothing to draw attention to themselves.

Differential Diagnosis

The differential diagnosis for dissociative fugue is similar to that for dissociative amnesia. In dissociative amnesia, a loss of memory results from psychological stress, but there are no episodes of purposeful travel or of a new identity. The wandering that is seen in dementia or delirium is usually distinguished from the traveling of a patient with dissociative fugue by the aimlessness of the former and the absence of complex and socially adaptive behaviors. Complex partial epilepsy may be associated with episodes of travel, but the patients do not usually assume a new identity, and the episodes are generally not precipitated by psychological stress.

Organic fugue states may be caused by a wide variety of medications, including hallucinogenic drugs, steroids, barbiturates, phenothiazines, triazolam (Halcion), and L-asparaginase. The alcohol blackout can be easily confused with dissociative fugue, but this can be differentiated through a good clinical history and alcohol concentrations, if drawn during acute intoxication. The clinician should remember, however, that dissociative fugue and alcohol blackouts can coexist in the same individual. There are reports of triazolam and alcohol together producing episodes of anterograde amnesia.

Course and Prognosis

The fugue is usually brief—hours to days. Less commonly, a fugue lasts many months and involves extensive travel covering thousands of miles. Generally, recovery is spontaneous and rapid. Recurrences are possible.

Treatment

Treatment of dissociative fugue is similar to that of dissociative amnesia. Psychiatric interviewing, drug-assisted interviewing, and hypnosis may help reveal to therapists and patients the psychological stressors that precipitated the fugue episode. Psychotherapy is indicated to help patients incorporate the precipitating stressors into their psyches in a healthy and integrated manner. The treatment of choice for dissociative fugue is expressive-supportive psychodynamic psychotherapy. The most widely accepted technique requires a mixture of abreaction of the past trauma and integration of the trauma into a cohesive self that no longer requires fragmentation to deal with the trauma.

DISSOCIATIVE IDENTITY DISORDER

Dissociative identity disorder is the name that DSM-IV-TR uses for what has been commonly known as *multiple personality disorder*. Dissociative identity disorder is a chronic dissociative disorder, and its cause typically involves a traumatic event, usually childhood physical or sexual abuse. The concept of personality conveys the sense of an integration of the way people think, feel, and behave and the appreciation of themselves as a unitary being. People with dissociative identity disorder have two or more distinct personalities, each of which determines behavior and attitudes during any period that it is the dominant personality. Dissociative identity disorder is usually considered the most serious of the dissociative disorders, although some clinicians who diagnose a variety of patients with the disorder have suggested that there may be a wider range of severities than was previously appreciated.

Epidemiology

Anecdotal and research reports about dissociative identity disorder have varied in their estimates of the prevalence of the disorder. At one extreme, some investigators believe that dissociative identity disorder is extremely rare; at the other extreme, some believe that dissociative identity disorder is vastly underrecognized. Well-controlled studies have reported that from 0.5 to 3.0 percent of general psychiatric hospital admissions meet the diagnostic criteria for dissociative identity disorder, as do perhaps as many as 5 percent of all psychiatric disorders. Patients who receive the diagnosis of dissociative identity disorder are overwhelmingly women—5:1 to 9:1 female to male ratios. Many clinicians and researchers, however, believe that men are underreported in clinical samples because, they believe, most men with the disorder enter the criminal justice system rather than the mental health system.

The disorder is most common in late adolescence and young adult life, with a mean age of diagnosis of 30 years, although patients have usually had symptoms for 5 to 10 years before the diagnosis. Several studies have found that the disorder is more common in first-degree biological relatives of people with the disorder than in the general population.

Dissociative identity disorder frequently coexists with other mental disorders, including anxiety disorders, mood disorders, somatoform disorders, sexual dysfunctions, substance-related disorders, eating disorders, sleeping disorders, and posttraumatic stress disorder. The symptoms of dissociative identity disorder are similar to those seen in borderline personality disorder, and differentiating the two disorders can be difficult. Suicide attempts are common in patients with dissociative identity disorder; some studies have reported that as many as two-thirds of all patients with dissociative identity disorder attempt suicide during the course of their illness.

Etiology

The cause of dissociative identity disorder is unknown, although the histories of the patients invariably (approaching 100 percent) involve a traumatic event, most often in childhood. In general, four types of causative factors have been identified: a traumatic life event, a vulnerability for the disorder to develop, environmental factors, and the absence of external support. The traumatic event is usually childhood physical or sexual abuse, commonly incestuous. Other traumatic events can include the death of a close relative or friend during childhood and the witnessing of a trauma or a death.

The tendency for the disorder to develop may be biologically or psychologically based. The variable ability of people to be hypnotized may be one example of a risk factor for the development of dissociative identity disorder. Epilepsy has been hypothesized to be involved in the cause of dissociative identity disorder, and a high percentage of abnormal EEG activity has been reported in some studies of affected patients. One study of regional cerebral blood flow revealed temporal hyperperfusion in one of the subpersonalities but not in the main personality. Although several studies have found differences in pain sensitivity and other physiological measures among the personalities, the use of these data as proof of the existence of dissociative identity disorder should be approached with great caution.

The environmental factors involved in the pathogenesis of dissociative identity disorder are nonspecific and are likely to involve such factors as role models and the availability of other mechanisms with which to deal with stress. In many cases, a factor in the development of dissociative identity seems to have been the absence of support from significant others, such as parents, siblings, other relatives, and nonrelated people, such as teachers.

Diagnosis and Clinical Features

As a diagnostic criterion (Table 17–3), DSM-IV-TR requires an amnestic component, which research has found to be essential to the complete clinical picture. The diagnosis also requires the presence of at least two distinct personality states. A diagnosis of dissociative personality disorder is excluded if the symptoms are the result of a substance (e.g., alcohol) or of a general medical condition (e.g., complex partial seizures).

In spite of stories in the popular press about patients with more than 20 personalities, the median number of personalities in dissociative identity disorder is in the range of five to ten. Often, only two or three of the personalities are evident at diagnosis; the others are recognized during the course of treatment. DSM-IV-TR reports an average of eight identities for men and 15 for women, which may be somewhat high.

The transition from one personality to another is often sudden and dramatic. During each personality state, patients generally are amnestic about other states and the events that took place when another personality was dominant. Sometimes, however, one per-

Table 17–3
DSM-IV-TR Diagnostic Criteria for Dissociative Identity Disorder

A. The presence of two or more distinct identities or personality states (each with its own relatively enduring pattern of perceiving, relating to, and thinking about the environment and self).

B. At least two of these identities or personality states recurrently take control of the person's behavior.

C. Inability to recall important personal information that is too extensive to be explained by ordinary forgetfulness.

D. The disturbance is not due to the direct physiological effects of a substance (e.g., blackouts or chaotic behavior during alcohol intoxication) or a general medical condition (e.g., complex partial seizures). **Note:** In children, the symptoms are not attributable to imaginary playmates or other fantasy play.

From American Psychiatric Association. *Diagnostic and Statistical Manual of Mental Disorders.* 4th ed. Text rev. Washington, DC: American Psychiatric Association; copyright 2000, with permission.

sonality state is not bound by such amnesia and retains complete awareness of the existence, qualities, and activities of the other personalities. At other times, the personalities are aware of all or some of the others to varying degrees and may experience the others as friends, companions, or adversaries. In classic cases, each personality has a fully integrated, highly complex set of associated memories and characteristic attitudes, personal relationships, and behavior patterns. Most often, the personalities have proper names; occasionally, one or more is given the name of its function—for example, the protector. Although some clinicians have emphasized that one of the personalities tends to be dominant, this is not always the case. In fact, sometimes one personality masquerades as one of the others, but usually a host personality is the one who comes for treatment and carries the patient's legal name. This host personality is likely to be depressed or anxious, may have masochistic personality traits, and may seem overly moral.

The first appearance of the secondary personality or personalities may be spontaneous or may emerge in relation to what seems to be a precipitant (including hypnosis or a drug-assisted interview). The personalities may be of both sexes, of various races and ages, and from families different from the patient's family of origin. The most common subordinate personality is child-like. The personalities are often disparate and may even be opposites.

On examination, patients frequently show nothing unusual in their mental status, other than a possible amnesia for periods of varying durations. Often, only with prolonged interviews or with many contacts can a clinician detect the presence of multiple personalities. Sometimes, by asking a patient to keep a diary, the clinician finds the multiple personalities revealed in the diary entries. An estimated 60 percent of patients switch to alternate personalities only occasionally; another 20 percent of patients not only have rare episodes but also are adept at covering the switches.

Differential Diagnosis

The differential diagnosis includes two other dissociative disorders, dissociative amnesia and dissociative fugue. Both of those disorders, however, lack the shifts in identity and the awareness of the original identity that are seen in dissociative identity disorder. Psychotic disorders, notably schizophrenia, may be confused with dissociative identity disorder only because people with schizophrenia may be delusional and believe that they have separate identities or report hearing other personalities' voices. In schizophrenia, a formal thought disorder, chronic social deterioration, and other distinguishing signs are present. Recently, clinicians have increasingly appreciated rapidly cycling bipolar disorders, whose symptoms appear similar to those of dissociative identity disorder; interviewing, however, reveals the presence of *discrete* personalities in patients with dissociative identity disorder. Borderline personality disorder may coexist with dissociative identity disorder, but the alteration of personalities in dissociative identity disorder may be mistakenly interpreted as nothing more than the irritability of mood and self-image problems characteristic of patients with borderline personality disorder. Malingering presents a difficult diagnostic problem. Clear secondary gain raises suspicion, and drug-assisted interviews may be helpful in making the diagnosis. Among the neurological disorders to consider, complex partial epilepsy is the most likely to imitate the symptoms of dissociative identity disorder.

Course and Prognosis

Dissociative identity disorder can develop in children as young as 3 years of age. In children, the symptoms may appear trance-like and may be accompanied by depressive disorder symptoms, amnestic periods, hallucinatory voices, disavowal of behaviors, changes in abilities, and suicidal or self-injurious behaviors. Although women are more likely to have the disorder than are men, affected children are more likely to be boys than girls; the female predominance develops only in adolescence. Two symptom patterns in affected female adolescents have been observed. One pattern is that of a chaotic life with promiscuity, drug use, somatic symptoms, and suicide attempts. Such patients may be misclassified as having an impulse control disorder, schizophrenia, rapidly cycling bipolar I disorder, or histrionic or borderline personality disorder. A second pattern is characterized by withdrawal and child-like behaviors. Sometimes, these patients are misclassified as having a mood disorder, a somatoform disorder, or generalized anxiety disorder. In male adolescents with dissociative identity disorder, the symptoms may cause them to have trouble with the law or school officials, and they may eventually end up in prison.

The earlier the onset of dissociative identity disorder, the worse the prognosis. One or more of the personalities may function relatively well while others function marginally. The level of impairment ranges from moderate to severe, the determining variables being the number, type, and chronicity of the various personalities. Recovery is generally incomplete. In addition, individual personalities may have their own separate mental disorders; mood disorders, personality disorders, and other dissociative disorders are the most common.

Treatment

The most efficacious approaches to dissociative identity disorder involve insight-oriented psychotherapy, often in association with hypnotherapy or drug-assisted interviewing techniques. Hypnotherapy or drug-assisted interviewing can be useful in obtaining additional history, identifying previously unrecognized personalities, and fostering abreaction. A psychotherapeutic treatment plan should begin by confirming the diagnosis and by identifying and characterizing the various personalities. Therapy usually fosters communication between the personalities to begin reintegration and to help patients control their overall behavior. If any of the personalities are inclined toward self-destructive or otherwise violent behavior, the therapist should engage the patient and the appropriate personalities in treatment contracts about these dangerous behaviors. Hospitalization may be necessary in some cases.

The use of antipsychotic medications in the patients is almost never indicated. Some data indicate that antidepressants and anti-anxiety medications may be useful as adjuvants to psychotherapy. A few uncontrolled studies report that anticonvulsant medications such as carbamazepine (Tegretol) help selected patients.

FORENSIC ISSUES

The intersection between the diagnosis of dissociative identity disorder and the legal system has proven exceedingly controversial. The contentious dispute over its existence, the often sensationalized media attention, and the need to rule out simulation or malingering have made the forensic evaluation of the disorder difficult to perform and to defend. Issues of competency to stand trial and degree of responsibility for the behavior of different alter personality states have received contradictory judicial opinions. The most common defenses are (1) dissociative defendants do not have control over or are not conscious of their alter personalities and therefore cannot be held responsible for their actions; (2) these defendants cannot recall the actions of their alter personalities and therefore cannot participate in their own defense; and (3) a diagnosis of dissociative identity disorder makes it impossible for a defendant to conform to the law or to know right from wrong. Evidentiary questions, such as the admissibility of hypnotic or amobarbital (Amytal) interviews and the independence of testimony by different alter personalities have proven problematic.

In general, most courts have not found dissociation sufficient grounds for a claim of legal incompetence. They have held that the whole human being is responsible for the behavior of any part.

DEPERSONALIZATION DISORDER

DSM-IV-TR characterizes depersonalization disorder as a persistent or recurrent alteration in the perception of the self to the extent that a person's sense of his or her own reality is temporarily lost. Patients with depersonalization disorder may feel that they are mechanical, in a dream, or detached from their bodies. The episodes are ego-dystonic, and the patients realize the unreality of the symptoms.

Some clinicians distinguish between depersonalization and derealization. *Depersonalization* is the feeling that the body or the personal self is strange and unreal; *derealization* is the perception of objects in the external world as being strange and unreal. The distinction provides a more accurate description of each phenomenon than is achieved by grouping them together under the rubric of depersonalization.

Epidemiology

As an occasional isolated experience in the lives of many people, depersonalization is a common phenomenon and is not necessarily pathological. Studies indicate that transient depersonalization may occur in as many as 70 percent of a given population, with no significant difference between men and women. Children fre-

Table 17–4
DSM-IV-TR Diagnostic Criteria for Depersonalization Disorder

A. Persistent or recurrent experiences of feeling detached from, and as if one is an outside observer of, one's mental processes or body (e.g., feeling like one is in a dream).

B. During the depersonalization experience, reality testing remains intact.

C. The depersonalization causes clinically significant distress or impairment in social, occupational, or other important areas of functioning.

D. The depersonalization experience does not occur exclusively during the course of another mental disorder, such as schizophrenia, panic disorder, acute stress disorder, or another dissociative disorder, and is not due to the direct physiological effects of a substance (e.g., a drug of abuse, a medication) or a general medical condition (e.g., temporal lobe epilepsy).

From American Psychiatric Association. *Diagnostic and Statistical Manual of Mental Disorders.* 4th ed. Text rev. Washington, DC: American Psychiatric Association; copyright 2000, with permission.

quently experience depersonalization as they develop the capacity for self-awareness, and adults often undergo a temporary sense of unreality when they travel to new and strange places.

Information about the epidemiology of pathological depersonalization is scanty. In a few recent studies, depersonalization was found to occur in women at least twice as frequently as in men; it is rarely found in people older than 40 years. The mean age of onset is approximately 16 years.

Etiology

Depersonalization may be caused by a psychological, neurological, or systemic disease. Systemic causes include endocrine disorders of the thyroid and the pancreas. Experiences of depersonalization have been associated with epilepsy, brain tumors, sensory deprivation, and emotional trauma, and depersonalization phenomena have been caused by electrical stimulation of the cortex of the temporal lobes during neurosurgery. Depersonalization is associated with an array of substances, including alcohol, barbiturates, benzodiazepines, scopolamine, β-adrenergic antagonists, marijuana, and virtually any phencyclidine (PCP)-like or hallucinogenic substance. Anxiety and depression are predisposing factors, as is severe stress experienced, for example, in combat or in an automobile accident. Depersonalization is a symptom frequently associated with anxiety disorders, depressive disorders, and schizophrenia.

Diagnosis and Clinical Features

The DSM-IV-TR diagnostic criteria for depersonalization disorder (Table 17–4) require persistent or recurrent episodes of depersonalization that result in significant distress to patients or in impairment in their ability to function in social, occupational, or interpersonal relationships. The disorder is largely differentiated from psychotic disorders by the diagnostic requirement that reality testing remains intact in depersonalization disorder. The disorder cannot be diagnosed if the symptoms are better accounted for by another mental disorder, substance ingestion, or general medical condition.

The central characteristic of depersonalization is the quality of unreality and estrangement. Inner mental processes and external events seem to go on exactly as before, but they feel different and no longer appear to have any relation or significance to the person. Parts of the body or the entire physical being may seem foreign, as may mental operations and accustomed behavior. Particularly common is the sensation of a change in the patient's body; for instance, patients may feel that their extremities are bigger or smaller than usual. Hemidepersonalization, the patient's feeling that half of the body is unreal or does not exist, may be related to contralateral parietal lobe disease. Anxiety often accompanies the disorder, and many patients complain of distortions in their senses of time and space.

An occasional phenomenon is doubling; patients feel that the point of consciousness is outside their bodies, often a few feet overhead; from there they observe themselves, as if they were totally separate people. Sometimes, patients believe that they are in two places at the same time, a condition known as *reduplicative paramnesia* or *double orientation*. Most patients are aware of the disturbances in their sense of reality; this awareness is considered one of the salient characteristics of the disorder.

Marlene Steinberg has reported the following examples from interviews with patients with this disorder.

FEELINGS OF UNREALITY

"It's really weird. It's sort of like I'm here, but I'm really not here and that I kind of stepped out of myself, like a ghost . . . I feel really light, you know. I feel kind of empty and light, like I'm going to float away . . . Sometimes I really look at myself that way . . . It's kind of a cold, eerie feeling. I'm just totally numbed by it."

BODILY PERCEPTIONS

"[I]t just doesn't seem real. Everything to me doesn't seem real, my body included . . . I was looking in the mirror and all of a sudden it just felt as if the image in the mirror was looking back out upon myself."

BEHAVIORAL PERCEPTIONS

"You just feel like you're never being yourself, uh, you're not thinking as you normally do. You just feel strange . . . I need to concentrate on things a lot more . . . I feel as if most persons have their brain on automatic. I feel like I have to crank it, like I'm always working at it and always consciously trying to remember things, trying to concentrate . . . It's almost as if I can't visualize things in my mind the way you normally would, when you actually see things . . . I can't do that very well."

EXTERNAL PERCEPTIONS

"[Everything] just feels different, just like it's in a dream, in a daze, things are dulled . . . I remember when this first started and I was in college and I went home and the thing that kept going over in my mind was I want to go home, I want to go home and I was home, but that just kept coming into my mind . . . everything always seems unreal . . . other persons, myself, just everything."

Differential Diagnosis

Depersonalization may occur as a symptom in numerous other disorders. The common occurrence of depersonalization in patients with depressive disorders and schizophrenia should alert clinicians to the possibility that a patient who initially complains of feelings of unreality and estrangement is suffering from one of these more common disorders. A history and the mental status examination should in most cases disclose the characteristic features of depressive disorder and schizophrenia. Because psychotomimetic drugs often induce long-lasting changes in the experience of the reality of the self and the environment, clinicians must inquire about the use of such substances. The presence of other clinical phenomena in patients complaining of a sense of unreality should usually take precedence in determining the diagnosis. In general, the diagnosis of depersonalization disorder is reserved for those conditions in which depersonalization constitutes the predominating symptom.

The fact that depersonalization phenomena may result from gross disturbances in brain function underlies the necessity for a neurological evaluation, especially when the depersonalization is not accompanied by common and obvious psychiatric symptoms. In particular, the possibility of a brain tumor or epilepsy should be considered. The experience of depersonalization may be the earliest presenting symptom of a neurological disorder.

Course and Prognosis

In most patients, the symptoms of depersonalization disorder first appear suddenly; only a few patients report a gradual onset. The disorder starts most often between the ages of 15 and 30 years, but it has been seen in patients as young as 10 years of age; it occurs less frequently after age 30 and almost never in the late decades of life. A few follow-up studies indicate that, in more than 50 percent of cases, depersonalization tends to be a long-lasting condition. In many patients, the symptoms run a steady course without any significant fluctuation of intensity, or the symptoms may occur episodically, interspersed with symptom-free intervals. Little is known about precipitating factors, although the disorder has been observed to begin during a period of relaxation after a person has experienced fatiguing psychological stress. The disorder is sometimes ushered in by an attack of acute anxiety frequently accompanied by hyperventilation.

Treatment

Little attention has been given to the treatment of patients with depersonalization disorder. At this time, data on which a specific pharmacological treatment may be based are insufficient, but the anxiety usually responds to antianxiety agents. An underlying disorder (for example, schizophrenia) can also be treated pharmacologically. Psychotherapeutic approaches are equally untested. As with all patients with neurotic symptoms, the decision to use psychoanalysis or insight-oriented psychotherapy is determined not by the presence of the symptom itself but by a variety of positive indications derived from an assessment of the patient's personality, human relationships, and life situation.

Table 17–5
DSM-IV-TR Diagnostic Criteria for Dissociative Disorder Not Otherwise Specified

This category is included for disorders in which the predominant feature is a dissociative symptom (i.e., a disruption in the usually integrated functions of consciousness, memory, identity, or perception of the environment) that does not meet the criteria for any specific dissociative disorder. Examples include

1. Clinical presentations similar to dissociative identity disorder that fail to meet full criteria for this disorder. Examples include presentations in which (a) there are not two or more distinct personality states, or (b) amnesia for important personal information does not occur.

2. Derealization unaccompanied by depersonalization in adults.

3. States of dissociation that occur in individuals who have been subjected to periods of prolonged and intense coercive persuasion (e.g., brainwashing, thought reform, or indoctrination while captive).

4. Dissociative trance disorder: single or episodic disturbances in the state of consciousness, identity, or memory that are indigenous to particular locations and cultures. Dissociative trance involves narrowing of awareness of immediate surroundings or stereotyped behaviors or movements that are experienced as being beyond one's control. Possession trance involves replacement of the customary sense of personal identity by a new identity, attributed to the influence of a spirit, power, deity, or other person, and associated with stereotyped "involuntary" movements or amnesia and is perhaps the most common dissociative disorder in Asia. Examples include *amok* (Indonesia), *bebainan* (Indonesia), *latah* (Malaysia), *piblokto* (Arctic), *ataque de nervios* (Latin America), and possession (India). The dissociative or trance disorder is not a normal part of a broadly accepted collective cultural or religious practice.

5. Loss of consciousness, stupor, or coma not attributable to a general medical condition.

6. Ganser syndrome: the giving of approximate answers to questions (e.g., "2 plus 2 equals 5") when not associated with dissociative amnesia or dissociative fugue.

From American Psychiatric Association. *Diagnostic and Statistical Manual of Mental Disorders.* 4th ed. Text rev. Washington, DC: American Psychiatric Association; copyright 2000, with permission.

DISSOCIATIVE DISORDER NOT OTHERWISE SPECIFIED

The diagnosis of dissociative disorder not otherwise specified is applied to disorders with dissociative features that do not meet the diagnostic criteria for dissociative amnesia, dissociative fugue, dissociative identity disorder, or depersonalization disorder. The DSM-IV-TR examples of dissociative disorder not otherwise specified (Table 17–5) take into account changes in the diagnostic criteria for the other dissociative disorders. Specifically, example 1 describes patients who do not meet the diagnostic criteria for dissociative identity disorder because the second personality is not sufficiently distinct or because the patient has no amnestic period. According to DSM-IV-TR, derealization in the absence of depersonalization is an example of dissociative disorder not otherwise specified.

Dissociative Trance Disorder

DSM-IV-TR adds, as an example of dissociative disorder not otherwise specified, patients with single or episodic alterations in consciousness

Table 17–6
DSM-IV-TR Research Criteria for Dissociative Trance Disorder

A. Either (1) or (2):

(1) trance, i.e., temporary marked alteration in the state of consciousness or loss of customary sense of personal identity without replacement by an alternate identity, associated with at least one of the following:

   (a) narrowing of awareness of immediate surroundings, or unusually narrow and selective focusing on environmental stimuli

   (b) stereotyped behaviors or movements that are experienced as being beyond one's control

(2) possession trance, a single or episodic alteration in the state of consciousness characterized by the replacement of customary sense of personal identity by a new identity. This is attributed to the influence of a spirit, power, deity, or other person, as evidenced by one (or more) of the following:

   (a) stereotyped and culturally determined behaviors or movements that are experienced as being controlled by the possessing agent

   (b) full or partial amnesia for the event

B. The trance or possession trance state is not accepted as a normal part of a collective cultural or religious practice.

C. The trance or possession trance state causes clinically significant distress or impairment in social, occupational, or other important areas of functioning.

D. The trance or possession trance state does not occur exclusively during the course of a psychotic disorder (including mood disorder with psychotic features and brief psychotic disorder) or dissociative identity disorder and is not due to the direct physiological effects of a substance or a general medical condition.

From American Psychiatric Association. *Diagnostic and Statistical Manual of Mental Disorders.* 4th ed. Text rev. Washington, DC: American Psychiatric Association; copyright 2000, with permission.

that are limited to particular locations or cultures. The example states that the "dissociative or trance disorder is not a normal part of a broadly accepted collective cultural or religious practice." DSM-IV-TR includes in its appendixes a suggested set of diagnostic criteria for dissociative trance disorder (Table 17–6). The DSM-IV-TR diagnostic criteria require that the symptoms cause a patient significant distress or an impairment in the ability to function.

Trance states are altered states of consciousness, and patients exhibit diminished responsivity to environmental stimuli. Children may have repeated amnestic periods or trance-like states after physical abuse or trauma. Possession and trance states are curious and imperfectly understood forms of dissociation. Apparently, trance states commonly appear in mediums who preside over seances. Mediums typically enter a dissociative state, during which a person from the so-called spirit world takes over much of the mediums' conscious awareness and influences their thoughts and speech.

Automatic writing and crystal gazing are less common manifestations of possession or trance states. In automatic writing, the dissociation affects only the arm and the hand that write the message, which often discloses mental contents of which the writer was unaware. Crystal gazing results in a trance state in which visual hallucinations are prominent.

Phenomena related to trance states include highway hypnosis and similar mental states experienced by airplane pilots. The monotony of moving at high speeds through environments that provide little in the way of distractions to the operator of the vehicle leads to a fixation on a single object, for example, a dial on the instrument panel or the never-ending horizon of a road running straight ahead for miles. When trance-like state of consciousness results, visual hallucinations may occur, and the danger of a serious accident is always present. Possibly in the same category are the hallucinations and dissociated mental states of patients who have been confined to respirators for long periods without adequate environmental distractions.

The religions of many cultures recognize that the practice of concentration may lead to a variety of dissociative phenomena, such as hallucinations, paralyses, and other sensory disturbances.

Recovered Memory Syndrome

Under hypnosis or during psychotherapy, the patient may recover a memory of a painful experience or conflict—particularly of sexual or physical abuse—that is etiologically significant. When the repressed material is brought back to consciousness, the person not only may recall the experience but may relive it accompanied by the appropriate affective response (a process called *abreaction*). If the event recalled never really happened but the person believes it to be true and reacts accordingly, it is known as *false memory syndrome*.

The recovered memory syndrome has been surrounded by controversy because victims of past abuse have sued perpetrators, many of whom have been convicted on the recovered memory as the only evidence. Problems arise because memory is subject to distortion, retrospective falsification that may also be influenced by the therapist. In children, the recovery of memories of abuse are often obtained by overzealous prosecuting attorneys or by so-called recovered memory experts, some of whom have no qualifications whatsoever. Such measures are often contaminated by the suggestibility of children and the prejudices of their adult interrogators.

Ganser's Syndrome

Ganser's syndrome is the voluntary production of severe psychiatric symptoms, sometimes described as the giving of approximate answers or talking past the point (for example, when asked to multiply 4 times 5, the patient answers 21). The syndrome may occur in people with other mental disorders, such as schizophrenia, depressive disorders, toxic states, paresis, alcohol use disorders, and factitious disorder. The psychological symptoms generally represent the patient's sense of mental illness rather than any recognized diagnostic category. The syndrome is commonly associated with dissociative phenomena such as amnesia, fugue, perceptual disturbances, and conversion symptoms. Ganser's syndrome is apparently most common in men and in prisoners, although prevalence data and familial patterns are not established. A major predisposing factor is the existence of a severe personality disorder. The differential diagnosis may be extremely difficult. Unless a patient is able to admit the factitious nature of the presenting symptoms or unless conclusive evidence from objective psychological tests indicates that the symptoms are false, clinicians may be unable to determine whether the patient has a true disorder. The syndrome may be recognized by its pansymptomatic nature or by the fact that the symptoms are often worse when patients believe they are being watched. Recovery from the syndrome is sudden; patients claim amnesia for the events. Ganser's syndrome was previously classified as a factitious disorder.

18

Human Sexuality

▲ 18.1 Normal Sexuality

Sexuality depends on four interrelated factors: sexual identity, gender identity, sexual orientation, and sexual behavior. These factors affect personality growth, development, and functioning. Sexuality is something more than physical sex, coital or noncoital, and something less than all behaviors directed toward attaining pleasure.

SEXUAL IDENTITY AND GENDER IDENTITY

Sexual identity is the pattern of a person's biological sexual characteristics: chromosomes, external genitalia, internal genitalia, hormonal composition, gonads, and secondary sex characteristics. In normal development, these characteristics form a cohesive pattern that leaves a person in no doubt about his or her sex. Gender identity is a person's sense of maleness or femaleness.

Sexual Identity

Modern embryological studies have shown that all mammalian embryos, whether genetically male (XY genotype) or genetically female (XX genotype), are anatomically female during the early stages of fetal life. Differentiation of the male from the female results from the action of fetal androgens; the action begins about the sixth week of embryonic life and is completed by the end of the third month. Recent studies have explained the effects of fetal hormones on the masculinization or feminization of the brain. In animals, prenatal hormonal stimulation of the brain is necessary for male and female reproductive and copulatory behavior. The fetus is also vulnerable to exogenously administered androgens during that period. For instance, if a pregnant woman receives sufficient exogenous androgens, her female fetus possessing ovaries can develop external genitalia resembling those of a male.

Gender Identity

By the age of 2 to 3 years, almost everyone has a firm conviction that "I am male" or "I am female." Yet even if maleness and femaleness develop normally, people must still develop a sense of masculinity or femininity.

Gender identity, according to Robert Stoller, "connotes psychological aspects of behavior related to masculinity and femininity." He considers gender social and sex biological: "Most often the two

are relatively congruent, that is, males tend to be manly and females womanly." But sex and gender may develop in conflicting or even opposite ways. Gender identity results from an almost infinite series of cues derived from experiences with family members, teachers, friends, and coworkers and from cultural phenomena. Physical characteristics derived from a person's biological sex—such as physique, body shape, and physical dimensions—interrelate with an intricate system of stimuli, including rewards and punishment and parental gender labels, to establish gender identity.

Thus, formation of gender identity arises from parental and cultural attitudes, the infant's external genitalia, and a genetic influence, which is physiologically active by the sixth week of fetal life. Even though family, cultural, and biological influences may complicate the establishment of a sense of masculinity or femininity, people usually develop a relatively secure sense of identification with their biological sex—a stable gender identity.

Gender Role.   Related to, and in part derived from, gender identity is gender role behavior. John Money and Anke Ehrhardt described gender role behavior as all those things that a person says or does to disclose himself or herself as having the status of boy or man, girl or woman, respectively. A gender role is not established at birth but is built up cumulatively through experiences encountered and transacted through casual and unplanned learning, through explicit instruction and inculcation, and through spontaneously putting two and two together to make sometimes four and sometimes five. The usual outcome is a congruence of gender identity and gender role. Although biological attributes are significant, the major factor in achieving the role appropriate to a person's sex is learning.

Research on sex differences in children's behavior reveals more psychological similarities than differences. However, girls are found to be less prone to tantrums after the age of 18 months than are boys, and boys generally are more physically and verbally aggressive than are girls from age 2 onward. Little girls and little boys are similarly active, but boys are more easily stimulated to sudden bursts of activity when they are in groups. Some researchers speculate that although aggression is a learned behavior, male hormones may have sensitized boys' neural organizations to absorb these lessons more easily than do girls.

People's gender roles can seem to be opposed to their gender identities. People may identify with their own sex and yet adopt the dress, hairstyle, or other characteristics of the opposite sex. Or they may identify with the opposite sex and yet for expediency adopt many behavioral characteristics of their own sex. A further discussion of gender issues appears in Chapter 19.

SEXUAL ORIENTATION

Sexual orientation describes the object of a person's sexual impulses: heterosexual (opposite sex), homosexual (same sex), or bisexual (both sexes).

SEXUAL BEHAVIOR

Physiological Responses

Sexual response is a true psychophysiological experience. Arousal is triggered by both psychological and physical stimuli; levels of tension are experienced both physiologically and emotionally; and with orgasm, there is normally a subjective perception of a peak of physical reaction and release. Psychosexual development, psychological attitudes toward sexuality, and attitudes toward one's sexual partner are directly involved with and affect the physiology of human sexual response. Normal men and women experience a sequence of physiological responses to sexual stimulation. In the first detailed description of these responses, William Masters and Virginia Johnson observed that the physiological process involves increasing levels of vasocongestion and myotonia (tumescence) and the subsequent release of the vascular activity and muscle tone as a result of orgasm (detumescence). The text revision of the fourth edition of *Diagnostic and Statistical Manual of Mental Disorders* (DSM-IV-TR) defines a four-phase response cycle: phase 1, desire; phase 2, excitement; phase 3, orgasm; phase 4, resolution.

Phase 1: Desire.   The classification of the desire (or appetitive) phase, which is distinct from any phase identified solely through physiology, reflects the psychiatric concern with motivations, drives, and personality. The phase is characterized by sexual fantasies and the desire to have sexual activity.

Phase 2: Excitement.   The excitement and arousal phase, brought on by psychological stimulation (fantasy or the presence of a love object) or physiological stimulation (stroking or kissing) or a combination of the two, consists of a subjective sense of pleasure. During this phase, penile tumescence leads to erection in men and vaginal lubrication occurs in women. The nipples of both sexes become erect, although nipple erection is more common in women than in men. A woman's clitoris becomes hard and turgid, and her labia minora become thicker as a result of venous engorgement. Initial excitement may last from several minutes to several hours. With continued stimulation, a man's testes increase 50 percent in size and elevate. A woman's vaginal barrel shows a characteristic constriction along the outer third, known as the *orgasmic platform*. The clitoris elevates and retracts behind the symphysis pubis, and as a result is not easily accessible. Stimulation of the area, however, causes traction on the labia minora and the prepuce and there is intrapreputial movement of the clitoral shaft. Women's breast size increases 25 percent. Continued engorgement of the penis and the vagina produces color changes, particularly in the labia minora, which become bright or deep red. Voluntary contractions of large muscle groups occur, the rates of heartbeat and respiration increase, and blood pressure rises. Heightened excitement lasts from 30 seconds to several minutes.

Phase 3: Orgasm.   The orgasm phase consists of a peaking of sexual pleasure, with the release of sexual tension and the rhythmic contraction of the perineal muscles and the pelvic reproductive organs. A subjective sense of ejaculatory inevitability triggers men's orgasms.

The forceful emission of semen follows. The male orgasm is also associated with four to five rhythmic spasms of the prostate, seminal vesicles, vas, and urethra. In women, orgasm is characterized by 3 to 15 involuntary contractions of the lower third of the vagina and by strong sustained contractions of the uterus, flowing from the fundus downward to the cervix. Both men and women have involuntary contractions of the internal and external anal sphincters. These and the other contractions during orgasm occur at intervals of 0.8 second. Other manifestations include voluntary and involuntary movements of the large muscle groups, including facial grimacing and carpedal spasm. Blood pressure rises 20 to 40 mm (both systolic and diastolic), and the heart rate increases up to 160 beats a minute. Orgasm lasts from 3 to 25 seconds and is associated with a slight clouding of consciousness.

Phase 4: Resolution.   Resolution consists of the disgorgement of blood from the genitalia (detumescence), which brings the body back to its resting state. If orgasm occurs, resolution is rapid and is characterized by a subjective sense of well-being, general relaxation, and muscular relaxation. If orgasm does not occur, resolution may take from 2 to 6 hours and may be associated with irritability and discomfort. After orgasm, men have a refractory period that may last from several minutes to many hours; in that period they cannot be stimulated to further orgasm. Women do not have a refractory period and are capable of multiple and successive orgasms.

HORMONES AND NEUROHORMONES AND SEXUAL BEHAVIOR

In general, substances that increase dopamine levels in the brain increase desire, whereas substances that augment serotonin decrease desire. Testosterone increases libido in both men and women, although estrogen is a key factor in the lubrication involved in female arousal and may increase sensitivity in the woman to stimulation. Progesterone mildly depresses desire in men and women, as do excessive prolactin and cortisol. Oxytocin is involved in pleasurable sensations during sex and is found in increased levels in men and women after orgasm.

Masturbation

Masturbation is usually a normal precursor of object-related sexual behavior. No other form of sexual activity has been more frequently discussed, more roundly condemned, and more universally practiced than masturbation. Research by Alfred Kinsey into the prevalence of masturbation indicated that nearly all men and three-fourths of all women masturbate sometime during their lives.

Longitudinal studies of development show that sexual self-stimulation is common in infancy and childhood. Just as infants learn to explore the functions of their fingers and mouths, so too do they learn to do the same with their genitalia. At approximately 15 to 19 months of age, both sexes begin genital self-stimulation. Pleasurable sensations result from any gentle touch to the genital region. Those sensations, coupled with the ordinary desire for exploration of the body, produce a normal interest in masturbatory pleasure at that time. Children also develop an increased interest in the genitalia of others—parents, children, and even animals. As youngsters acquire playmates, the curiosity about their own and others' genitalia motivates episodes of exhibitionism or genital exploration. Such experiences, unless blocked by guilty fear, contribute to continued pleasure from sexual stimulation.

With the approach of puberty, the upsurge of sex hormones, and the development of secondary sex characteristics, sexual curiosity is intensified, and masturbation increases. Adolescents are physically capable of coitus and orgasm but are usually inhibited by social restraints. The dual and often conflicting pressures of establishing their sexual identities and controlling their sexual impulses produce in teenagers a strong physiological sexual tension that demands release, and masturbation is a normal way to reduce sexual tensions. In general, males learn to masturbate to orgasm earlier than females and masturbate more frequently. An important emotional difference between the adolescent and the youngster of earlier years is the presence of coital fantasies during masturbation in the adolescent. These fantasies are an important adjunct to the development of sexual identity; in the comparative safety of the imagination, the adolescent learns to perform the adult sex role. This autoerotic activity is usually maintained into the young adult years, when it is normally replaced by coitus.

Couples in a sexual relationship do not abandon masturbation entirely. When coitus is unsatisfactory or is unavailable because of illness or the absence of the partner, self-stimulation often serves an adaptive purpose, combining sensual pleasure and tension release. Kinsey reported that when women masturbate, most prefer clitoral stimulation. Masters and Johnson stated that women prefer the shaft of the clitoris to the glans because the glans is hypersensitive to intense stimulation. Most men masturbate by vigorously stroking the penile shaft and glans.

Moral taboos against masturbation have generated myths that masturbation causes mental illness or a decrease in sexual potency. No scientific evidence supports such claims. Masturbation is a psychopathological symptom only when it becomes a compulsion beyond a person's willful control. Then it is a symptom of emotional disturbance, not because it is sexual but because it is compulsive. Masturbation is probably a universal and inevitable aspect of psychosexual development, and in most cases it is adaptive.

HOMOSEXUALITY

In 1973, homosexuality was eliminated as a diagnostic category by the American Psychiatric Association (APA) and in 1980 was removed from DSM. The 10th revision of *International Statistical Classification of Diseases and Related Health Problems* (ICD-10) states: "Sexual orientation alone is not to be regarded as a disorder." This change reflects a change in the understanding of homosexuality, which is now considered to occur with some regularity as a variant of human sexuality, not a pathological disorder. As David Hawkins wrote, "The presence of homosexuality does not appear to be a matter of choice; the expression of it is a matter of choice."

The term *homosexuality* often describes a person's overt behavior, sexual orientation, and sense of personal or social identity. Many people prefer to identify sexual orientation by using terms like *lesbians* and *gay men*, rather than *homosexual*, which may imply pathology and etiology based on its origin as a medical term, and refer to sexual behavior with terms like *same sex* and *male female*. Hawkins wrote that the terms *gay* and *lesbian* refer to a combination of self-perceived identity and social identity; they reflect a person's sense of belonging to a social group that is similarly labeled. Homophobia is a negative attitude toward or fear of homosexuality or homosexuals. Heterosexism is the belief that a heterosexual relationship is preferable to all others; it implies discrimination against those practicing other forms of sexuality.

Coming Out

According to Richelle Klinger and Robert Cabaj, coming out is a "process by which an individual acknowledges his or her sexual orientation in the face of societal stigma and with successful resolution accepts himself or herself." The authors wrote:

Successful coming out involves the individual accepting his or her sexual orientation and integrating it into all spheres (e.g., social, vocational, and familial). Another milestone that individuals and couples must eventually confront is the degree of disclosure of sexual orientation to the external world. Some degree of disclosure is probably necessary for successful coming out.

Difficulty in negotiating coming out and disclosure is a common cause of relationship difficulties. For each individual, problems in resolving the coming out process may contribute to poor self-esteem caused by internalized homophobia and lead to deleterious effects on the individual's ability to function in the relationship. Conflict can also arise within a relationship when there is disagreement on the degree of disclosure between partners.

LOVE AND INTIMACY

Freud postulated that psychological health could be determined by a person's ability to function well in two spheres, work and love. A person able to give and receive love with minimum fear and conflict has the capacity to develop genuinely intimate relationships with others. A desire to maintain closeness to the love object typifies being in love. Mature love is marked by the intimacy that is a special attribute of the relationship between two people. When involved in an intimate relationship, the person actively strives for the growth and happiness of the loved person. Sex frequently acts as a catalyst in the forming and maintenance of intimate relationships. The quality of intimacy in a mature sexual relationship is what Rollo May called "active receiving," in which a person, while loving, permits himself to be loved. May describes the value of sexual love as an expansion of self-awareness, the experience of tenderness, an increase of self-affirmation and pride, and sometimes, at the moment of orgasm, loss of feeling of separateness. In that setting, sex and love are reciprocally enhancing and healthily fused.

Some people suffer from conflicts that prevent them from fusing tender and passionate impulses. This can inhibit the expression of sexuality in a relationship, interfere with feeling of closeness to another person, and diminish a person's sense of adequacy and self-esteem. When these problems are severe, they may prevent the formation of or commitment to an intimate relationship.

▲ 18.2 Abnormal Sexuality and Sexual Dysfunctions

In the fourth revised edition of the *Diagnostic and Statistical Manual of Mental Disorders* (DSM-IV-TR), a *sexual dysfunction* is defined as a disturbance in the sexual response cycle or as pain with sexual intercourse. Seven major categories of sexual dysfunction are listed in DSM-IV-TR: sexual desire disorders, sexual arousal disorders, orgasm disorders, sexual pain disorders, sexual dysfunction caused by a general medical condition, substance-induced sexual dysfunction, and sexual dysfunction not otherwise specified. Each is described in this chapter.

Sexual dysfunctions can be symptomatic of biological (biogenic) problems or intrapsychic or interpersonal (psychogenic) conflicts or a combination of these factors. Sexual function can

Table 18.2–1
DSM-IV-TR Diagnostic Criteria for Hypoactive Sexual Desire Disorder

A. Persistently or recurrently deficient (or absent) sexual fantasies and desire for sexual activity. The judgment of deficiency or absence is made by the clinician, taking into account factors that affect sexual functioning, such as age and the context of the person's life.

B. The disturbance causes marked distress or interpersonal difficulty.

C. The sexual dysfunction is not better accounted for by another Axis I disorder (except another sexual dysfunction) and is not due exclusively to the direct physiological effects of a substance (e.g., a drug of abuse, a medication) or a general medical condition.

Specify type:
   Lifelong type
   Acquired type
Specify type:
   Generalized type
   Situational type
Specify:
   Due to psychological factors
   Due to combined factors

From American Psychiatric Association. *Diagnostic and Statistical Manual of Mental Disorders.* 4th ed. Text rev. Washington, DC: American Psychiatric Association; copyright 2000, with permission.

Table 18.2–2
DSM-IV-TR Diagnostic Criteria for Sexual Aversion Disorder

A. Persistent or recurrent extreme aversion to, and avoidance of, all (or almost all) genital sexual contact with a sexual partner.

B. The disturbance causes marked distress or interpersonal difficulty.

C. The sexual dysfunction is not better accounted for by another Axis I disorder (except another sexual dysfunction).

Specify type:
   Lifelong type
   Acquired type
Specify type:
   Situational type
   Generalized type
Specify:
   Due to psychological factors
   Due to combined factors

From American Psychiatric Association. *Diagnostic and Statistical Manual of Mental Disorders.* 4th ed. Text rev. Washington, DC: American Psychiatric Association; copyright 2000, with permission.

be adversely affected by stress of any kind, by emotional disorders, or by ignorance of sexual function and physiology. The dysfunction may be lifelong or acquired—that is, it can develop after a period of normal functioning. The dysfunction may be generalized or limited to a specific partner or a certain situation.

In considering each of the disorders, clinicians need to rule out an acquired medical condition and the use of a pharmacological substance that could account for or contribute to the dysfunction. If the disorder is biogenic, it is coded on Axis III unless there is substantial evidence of dysfunctional episodes apart from the onset of physiological or pharmacological influences. In some cases, a patient suffers from more than one dysfunction—for example, premature ejaculation and male erectile disorder.

SEXUAL DESIRE DISORDERS

Sexual desire disorders are divided into two classes: hypoactive sexual desire disorder, characterized by a deficiency or absence of sexual fantasies and desire for sexual activity (Table 18.2–1), and sexual aversion disorder, characterized by an aversion to and avoidance of genital sexual contact with a sexual partner or by masturbation (Table 18.2–2). The former condition is more common than the latter and more common among women than among men. An estimated 20 percent of the population have hypoactive sexual desire disorder.

A variety of causative factors are associated with sexual desire disorders. Patients with desire problems often use inhibition of desire in a defensive way to protect against unconscious fears about sex. Sigmund Freud conceptualized low sexual desire as the result of inhibition during the phallic psychosexual phase of development and of unresolved oedipal conflicts. Some men,

fixated at the phallic state of development, are fearful of the vagina and believe that they will be castrated if they approach it. Freud called this concept *vagina dentata*; because men unconsciously believe that the vagina has teeth, they avoid contact with the female genitalia. Equally, women may suffer from unresolved developmental conflicts that inhibit desire. Lack of desire can also be the result of chronic stress, anxiety, or depression.

Abstinence from sex for a prolonged period sometimes results in suppression of sexual impulses. Loss of desire may also be an expression of hostility to a partner or the sign of a deteriorating relationship. In one study of young married couples who ceased having sexual relations for 2 months, marital discord was the reason most frequently given for the cessation or inhibition of sexual activity.

The presence of desire depends on several factors: biological drive, adequate self-esteem, the ability to accept oneself as a sexual person, previous good experiences with sex, the availability of an appropriate partner, and a good relationship in nonsexual areas with a partner. Damage to, or absence of, any of these factors may result in diminished desire.

In making the diagnosis, clinicians must evaluate a patient's age, general health, and life stresses and must attempt to establish a baseline of sexual interest before the disorder began. The need for sexual contact and satisfaction varies among people and over time in any given person. In a group of 100 couples with stable marriages, 8 percent reported having intercourse less than once a month. In another group of couples, one-third reported episodic lack of sexual relations for periods averaging 8 weeks. Married couples have coitus three times a month, on average. The diagnosis should not be made unless the lack of desire is a source of distress to a patient.

SEXUAL AROUSAL DISORDERS

The sexual arousal disorders are divided by DSM-IV-TR into female sexual arousal disorder, characterized by the persistent

Table 18.2–3
DSM-IV-TR Diagnostic Criteria for Female Sexual Arousal Disorder

A. Persistent or recurrent inability to attain, or to maintain until completion of the sexual activity, an adequate lubrication-swelling response of sexual excitement.

B. The disturbance causes marked distress or interpersonal difficulty.

C. The sexual dysfunction is not better accounted for by another Axis I disorder (except another sexual dysfunction) and is not due exclusively to the direct physiological effects of a substance (e.g., a drug of abuse, a medication) or a general medical condition.

Specify type:
   Lifelong type
   Acquired type
Specify type:
   Generalized type
   Situational type
Specify:
   Due to psychological factors
   Due to combined factors

From American Psychiatric Association. *Diagnostic and Statistical Manual of Mental Disorders.* 4th ed. Text rev. Washington, DC: American Psychiatric Association; copyright 2000, with permission.

Table 18.2–4
DSM-IV-TR Diagnostic Criteria for Male Erectile Disorder

A. Persistent or recurrent inability to attain, or to maintain until completion of the sexual activity, an adequate erection.

B. The disturbance causes marked distress or interpersonal difficulty.

C. The erectile dysfunction is not better accounted for by another Axis I disorder (other than a sexual dysfunction) and is not due exclusively to the direct physiological effects of a substance (e.g., a drug of abuse, a medication) or a general medical condition.

Specify type:
   Lifelong type
   Acquired type
Specify type:
   Generalized type
   Situational type
Specify:
   Due to psychological factors
   Due to combined factors

From American Psychiatric Association. *Diagnostic and Statistical Manual of Mental Disorders.* 4th ed. Text rev. Washington, DC: American Psychiatric Association; copyright 2000, with permission.

or recurrent partial or complete failure to attain or maintain the lubrication-swelling response of sexual excitement until the completion of the sexual act, and male erectile disorder, characterized by the recurrent and persistent partial or complete failure to attain or maintain an erection to perform the sex act. The diagnosis takes into account the focus, the intensity, and the duration of the sexual activity in which patients engage (Tables 18.2–3 and 18.2–4). If sexual stimulation is inadequate in focus, intensity, or duration, the diagnosis should not be made.

Female Sexual Arousal Disorder

The prevalence of female sexual arousal disorder is generally underestimated. Women who have excitement-phase dysfunction often have orgasm problems as well. In one study of relatively happy married couples, 33 percent of the women described difficulty in maintaining sexual excitement. Many psychological factors (for example, anxiety, guilt, and fear) are associated with female sexual arousal disorder. In many women, excitement-phase disorders are associated with dyspareunia and with lack of desire.

Physiological studies of sexual dysfunctions indicate that a hormonal pattern may contribute to responsiveness in women who have excitement-phase dysfunction. William Masters and Virginia Johnson found women to be particularly desirous of sex before the onset of the menses. Other women report that they feel the greatest sexual excitement immediately after the menses or at the time of ovulation. Alterations in testosterone, estrogen, prolactin, and thyroxin levels have been implicated in female sexual arousal disorder. Also, medications with antihistaminic or anticholinergic properties cause a decrease in vaginal lubrication. Some evidence indicates that women who are dysfunctional are less aware of the physiological arousal of

their bodies and experience less warmth or less sensation in the genitalia.

Male Erectile Disorder

Male erectile disorder is also called *erectile dysfunction* and *impotence*. A man with lifelong male erectile disorder has never been able to obtain an erection sufficient for vaginal insertion. In acquired male erectile disorder, a man has successfully achieved vaginal penetration at some time in his sexual life but is later unable to do so. In situational male erectile disorder, a man is able to have coitus in certain circumstances but not in others; for example, he may function effectively with a prostitute but be impotent with his wife.

Acquired male erectile disorder has been reported in 10 to 20 percent of all men. Freud declared it common among his patients. Impotence is the chief complaint of more than 50 percent of all men treated for sexual disorders. Lifelong male erectile disorder is rare; it occurs in approximately 1 percent of men younger than 35, but the incidence increases with age. Among young adults, it has been reported in approximately 8 percent of the population. Alfred Kinsey reported that 75 percent of all men were impotent at age 80. All men over 40, Masters and Johnson reported, have a fear of impotence, which the researchers believe reflects the masculine fear of loss of virility with advancing age. Male erectile disorder, however, is not universal in aging men; having an available sex partner is related to continuing potency, as is a history of consistent sexual activity and the absence of vascular disease.

The causes of male erectile disorder may be organic or psychological or a combination of both, but in young and middle-aged men, the cause is usually psychological. A good history is of primary importance in determining the cause of the dysfunction. If a man reports having spontaneous erections at times when he does not plan to have intercourse, having morning erections, or having good erections with masturbation or with partners other than his usual one, the organic causes of his impotence can be considered negligible, and costly diagnostic procedures can be avoided. Male erectile disorder caused by a general medical condition or a pharmacological substance is discussed later in this section.

Freud ascribed one type of impotence to an inability to reconcile feelings of affection toward a woman with feelings of desire for her. Men with such conflicting feelings can function only with women whom they see as degraded. Other factors that have been cited as contributing to impotence include a punitive superego, an inability to trust, and feelings of inadequacy or a sense of being undesirable as a partner. A man may be unable to express a sexual impulse because of fear, anxiety, anger, or moral prohibition. In an ongoing relationship, impotence may reflect difficulties between the partners, particularly when a man cannot communicate his needs or his anger in a direct and constructive way. In addition, episodes of impotence are reinforcing, with the man becoming increasingly anxious before each sexual encounter.

ORGASM DISORDERS

Female Orgasmic Disorder

Female orgasmic disorder, sometimes called *inhibited female orgasm* or *anorgasmia*, is defined as the recurrent or persistent inhibition of female orgasm, as manifested by the recurrent delay in, or absence of, orgasm after a normal sexual excitement phase that a clinician judges to be adequate in focus, intensity, and duration—in short, a woman's inability to achieve orgasm by masturbation or coitus (Table 18.2–5). Women who cannot achieve orgasm by one of these methods are not necessarily categorized as anorgasmic, although some degree of sexual inhibition may be postulated.

Research on the physiology of the female sexual response has shown that orgasms caused by clitoral stimulation and those caused by vaginal stimulation are physiologically identical. Freud's theory that women must give up clitoral sensitivity for vaginal sensitivity to achieve sexual maturity is now considered misleading, but some women report that they gain a special sense of satisfaction from an orgasm precipitated by coitus. Some researchers attribute this satisfaction to the psychological feeling of closeness engendered by the act of coitus, but others maintain that the coital orgasm is a physiologically different experience. Many women achieve orgasm during coitus by a combination of manual clitoral stimulation and penile vaginal stimulation.

A woman with lifelong female orgasmic disorder has never experienced orgasm by any kind of stimulation. A woman with acquired orgasmic disorder has previously experienced at least one orgasm, regardless of the circumstances or means of stimulation, whether by masturbation or while dreaming during sleep. Kinsey found that only 5 percent of married women over 35 years of age had never achieved orgasm by any means. The incidence of orgasm increases with age. According to Kinsey, the first orgasm occurs during adolescence in approximately 50 percent of women as a result of masturbation or genital caressing with a partner; the rest usually experience orgasm as they get older. Lifelong female orgasmic disorder is more common among unmarried than married women. Increased orgasmic potential in women older than 35 has been explained on the basis of less psychological inhibition, greater sexual experience, or both.

Table 18.2–5
DSM-IV-TR Diagnostic Criteria for Female Orgasmic Disorder

A. Persistent or recurrent delay in, or absence of, orgasm following a normal sexual excitement phase. Women exhibit wide variability in the type or intensity of stimulation that triggers orgasm. The diagnosis of female orgasmic disorder should be based on the clinician's judgment that the woman's orgasmic capacity is less than would be reasonable for her age, sexual experience, and the adequacy of sexual stimulation she receives.

B. The disturbance causes marked distress or interpersonal difficulty.

C. The orgasmic dysfunction is not better accounted for by another Axis I disorder (except another sexual dysfunction) and is not due exclusively to the direct physiological effects of a substance (e.g., a drug of abuse, a medication) or a general medical condition.

Specify type:
  Lifelong type
  Acquired type
Specify type:
  Generalized type
  Situational type
Specify:
  Due to psychological factors
  Due to combined factors

From American Psychiatric Association. *Diagnostic and Statistical Manual of Mental Disorders.* 4th ed. Text rev. Washington, DC: American Psychiatric Association; copyright 2000, with permission.

Acquired female orgasmic disorder is a common complaint in clinical populations. One clinical treatment facility reported having approximately four times as many nonorgasmic women in its practice as patients with all other sexual disorders. In another study, 46 percent of women complained of difficulty in reaching orgasm. The true prevalence of problems in maintaining excitement is not known, but inhibition of excitement and orgasmic problems often occur together. The overall prevalence of female orgasmic disorder from all causes is estimated to be 30 percent.

Numerous psychological factors are associated with female orgasmic disorder. They include fears of impregnation, rejection by a sex partner, damage to the vagina, hostility toward men, and feelings of guilt about sexual impulses. For some women, orgasm is equated with loss of control or with aggressive, destructive, or violent impulses; their fear of these impulses may be expressed through inhibition of excitement or orgasm. Cultural expectations and social restrictions on women are also relevant. Many women have grown up to believe that sexual pleasure is not a natural entitlement for so-called decent women. Nonorgasmic women may be otherwise symptom free or may experience frustration in a variety of ways; they may have such pelvic complaints as lower abdominal pain, itching, and vaginal discharge, as well as increased tension, irritability, and fatigue.

Male Orgasmic Disorder

In male orgasmic disorder, sometimes called *inhibited orgasm* or *retarded ejaculation*, a man achieves ejaculation during coitus with great difficulty, if at all (Table 18.2–6). A man with lifelong orgas-

Table 18.2–6
DSM-IV-TR Diagnostic Criteria for Male Orgasmic Disorder

A. Persistent or recurrent delay in, or absence of, orgasm following a normal sexual excitement phase during sexual activity that the clinician, taking into account the person's age, judges to be adequate in focus, intensity, and duration.

B. The disturbance causes marked distress or interpersonal difficulty.

C. The orgasmic dysfunction is not better accounted for by another Axis I disorder (except another sexual dysfunction) and is not due exclusively to the direct physiological effects of a substance (e.g., a drug of abuse, a medication) or a general medical condition.

Specify type:
   Lifelong type
   Acquired type
Specify type:
   Generalized type
   Situational type
Specify:
   Due to psychological factors
   Due to combined factors

From American Psychiatric Association. *Diagnostic and Statistical Manual of Mental Disorders.* 4th ed. Text rev. Washington, DC: American Psychiatric Association; copyright 2000, with permission.

Table 18.2–7
DSM-IV-TR Diagnostic Criteria for Premature Ejaculation

A. Persistent or recurrent ejaculation with minimal sexual stimulation before, on, or shortly after penetration and before the person wishes it. The clinician must take into account factors that affect duration of the excitement phase, such as age, novelty of the sexual partner or situation, and recent frequency of sexual activity.

B. The disturbance causes marked distress or interpersonal difficulty.

C. The premature ejaculation is not due exclusively to the direct effects of a substance (e.g., withdrawal from opioids).

Specify type:
   Lifelong type
   Acquired type
Specify type:
   Generalized type
   Situational type
Specify:
   Due to psychological factors
   Due to combined factors

From American Psychiatric Association. *Diagnostic and Statistical Manual of Mental Disorders.* 4th ed. Text rev. Washington, DC: American Psychiatric Association; copyright 2000, with permission.

mic disorder has never been able to ejaculate during coitus. The disorder is diagnosed as acquired if it develops after previously normal functioning. Some researchers think that orgasm and ejaculation should be differentiated, especially in the case of men who ejaculate but complain of a decreased or absent subjective sense of pleasure during the orgasmic experience (orgasmic anhedonia).

The incidence of male orgasmic disorder is much lower than the incidence of premature ejaculation or impotence. Masters and Johnson reported an incidence of male orgasmic disorder of only 3.8 percent in one group of 447 men with sexual dysfunctions. A general prevalence of 5 percent has been reported.

Lifelong male orgasmic disorder indicates severe psychopathology. A man may come from a rigid, puritanical background; he may perceive sex as sinful and the genitals as dirty; and he may have conscious or unconscious incest wishes and guilt. He usually has difficulties with closeness in areas beyond those of sexual relations. In a few cases, the condition is aggravated by an attention-deficit disorder. A man's distractibility prevents arousal sufficient for climax to occur.

In an ongoing relationship, acquired male orgasmic disorder frequently reflects interpersonal difficulties. The disorder may be a man's way of coping with real or fantasized changes in the relationship, such as plans for pregnancy about which the man is ambivalent, the loss of sexual attraction to the partner, or demands by the partner for greater commitment as expressed by sexual performance. In some men, the inability to ejaculate reflects unexpressed hostility toward a woman. The problem is more common among men with obsessive-compulsive disorder than among others.

Premature Ejaculation

In premature ejaculation, men persistently or recurrently achieve orgasm and ejaculation before they wish to. There is no definite time frame within which to define the dysfunction; the diagnosis is made when a man regularly ejaculates before or immediately after entering the vagina. Clinicians need to consider factors that affect the duration of the excitement phase, such as age, the novelty of the sex partner, and the frequency and duration of coitus (Table 18.2–7). Masters and Johnson conceptualized the disorder in terms of the couple and considered a man a premature ejaculator if he could not control ejaculation for a sufficient time during intravaginal containment to satisfy his partner in at least half their episodes of coitus. This definition assumes that the female partner is capable of an orgasmic response. Like the other dysfunctions, premature ejaculation is not diagnosed when it is caused exclusively by organic factors or when it is not symptomatic of any other clinical psychiatric syndrome.

Premature ejaculation is more commonly reported among college-educated men than among men with less education. The complaint is thought to be related to their concern for partner satisfaction, but the true cause of the increased frequency has not been determined. Premature ejaculation is the chief complaint of approximately 35 to 40 percent of men treated for sexual disorders. Some researchers divide men who experience premature ejaculation into two groups: those who are physiologically predisposed to climax quickly because of shorter nerve latency time and those with a psychogenic or behaviorally conditioned etiology. Difficulty in ejaculatory control may be associated with anxiety regarding the sex act, with unconscious fears about the vagina, or with negative cultural conditioning. Men whose early sexual contacts occurred largely with prostitutes who demanded that the sex act proceed quickly or whose sexual contacts took place in situations in which discovery would be embarrassing (such as in the back seat of a car or in the parental home) might have been conditioned to achieve orgasm rapidly. With young, inexperienced men, who are more likely to have the problem, it may

Table 18.2–8
DSM-IV-TR Diagnostic Criteria for Dyspareunia

A. Recurrent or persistent genital pain associated with sexual intercourse in either a male or a female.

B. The disturbance causes marked distress or interpersonal difficulty.

C. The disturbance is not caused exclusively by vaginismus or lack of lubrication, is not better accounted for by another Axis I disorder (except another sexual dysfunction), and is not due exclusively to the direct physiological effects of a substance (e.g., a drug of abuse, a medication) or a general medical condition.

Specify type:
  Lifelong type
  Acquired type
Specify type:
  Generalized type
  Situational type
Specify:
  Due to psychological factors
  Due to combined factors

From American Psychiatric Association. *Diagnostic and Statistical Manual of Mental Disorders.* 4th ed. Text rev. Washington, DC: American Psychiatric Association; copyright 2000, with permission.

Table 18.2–9
DSM-IV-TR Diagnostic Criteria for Vaginismus

A. Recurrent or persistent involuntary spasm of the musculature of the outer third of the vagina that interferes with sexual intercourse.

B. The disturbance causes marked distress or interpersonal difficulty.

C. The disturbance is not better accounted for by another Axis I disorder (e.g., somatization disorder) and is not due exclusively to the direct physiological effects of a general medical condition.

Specify type:
  Lifelong type
  Acquired type
Specify type:
  Generalized type
  Situational type
Specify:
  Due to psychological factors
  Due to combined factors

From American Psychiatric Association. *Diagnostic and Statistical Manual of Mental Disorders.* 4th ed. Text rev. Washington, DC: American Psychiatric Association; copyright 2000, with permission.

resolve in time. In ongoing relationships, the partner has a great influence on a premature ejaculator, and a stressful marriage exacerbates the disorder. The developmental background and the psychodynamics found in premature ejaculation and in impotence are similar.

SEXUAL PAIN DISORDERS

Dyspareunia

Dyspareunia is recurrent or persistent genital pain occurring in either men or women before, during, or after intercourse. Much more common in women than in men, dyspareunia is related to, and often coincides with, vaginismus. Repeated episodes of vaginismus may lead to dyspareunia and vice versa; in either case, somatic causes must be ruled out. Dyspareunia should not be diagnosed when an organic basis for the pain is found or when, in a woman, it is caused exclusively by vaginismus or by a lack of lubrication (Table 18.2–8). The incidence of dyspareunia is unknown.

In most cases, dynamic factors are considered causative. Chronic pelvic pain is a common complaint in women with a history of rape or childhood sexual abuse. Painful coitus may result from tension and anxiety about the sex act that cause women to involuntarily contract their vaginal muscles. The pain is real and makes intercourse unpleasant or unbearable. Anticipation of further pain may cause women to avoid coitus altogether. If a partner proceeds with intercourse regardless of a woman's state of readiness, the condition is aggravated. Dyspareunia can also occur in men, but it is uncommon and is usually associated with an organic condition, such as herpes, prostatitis, or Peyronie's disease, which consists of sclerotic plaques on the penis that cause penile curvature.

Vaginismus

Vaginismus is an involuntary muscle constriction of the outer third of the vagina that interferes with penile insertion and intercourse.

This response may occur during a gynecological examination when involuntary vaginal constriction prevents the introduction of the speculum into the vagina. The diagnosis is not made when the dysfunction is caused exclusively by organic factors or when it is symptomatic of another Axis I mental disorder (Table 18.2–9).

Vaginismus is less prevalent than is female orgasmic disorder. It most often afflicts highly educated women and those in high socioeconomic groups. Women with vaginismus may consciously wish to have coitus but unconsciously wish to keep a penis from entering their bodies. A sexual trauma such as rape may cause vaginismus; women with psychosexual conflicts may perceive the penis as a weapon. In some cases, pain or the anticipation of pain at the first coital experience causes vaginismus. Clinicians have noted that a strict religious upbringing in which sex is associated with sin is frequent in these patients. Other women have problems in dyadic relationships; if women feel emotionally abused by their partners, they may protest in this nonverbal fashion.

SEXUAL DYSFUNCTION DUE TO A GENERAL MEDICAL CONDITION

The category sexual dysfunction due to a general medical condition covers sexual dysfunction that results in marked distress and interpersonal difficulty; the history, physical examination, or laboratory findings must provide evidence of a general medical condition judged to be causally related to the sexual dysfunction (Table 18.2–10).

Male Erectile Disorder Due to a General Medical Condition

The incidence of psychological, as opposed to organic, male erectile disorder has been the focus of many studies. Statistics indicate that approximately 50 percent of men with erectile disor-

Table 18.2–10
DSM-IV-TR Diagnostic Criteria for Sexual Dysfunction Due to a General Medical Condition

A. Clinically significant sexual dysfunction that results in marked distress or interpersonal difficulty predominates in the clinical picture.

B. There is evidence from the history, physical examination, or laboratory findings that the sexual dysfunction is fully explained by the direct physiological effects of a general medical condition.

C. The disturbance is not better accounted for by another mental disorder (e.g., major depressive disorder).

Select code and term based on the predominant sexual dysfunction:

Female hypoactive sexual desire disorder due to . . . [indicate the general medical condition]: if deficient or absent sexual desire is the predominant feature

Male hypoactive sexual desire disorder due to . . . [indicate the general medical condition]: if deficient or absent sexual desire is the predominant feature

Male erectile disorder due to . . . [indicate the general medical condition]: if male erectile dysfunction is the predominant feature

Female dyspareunia due to . . . [indicate the general medical condition]: if pain associated with intercourse is the predominant feature

Male dyspareunia due to . . . [indicate the general medical condition]: if pain associated with intercourse is the predominant feature

Other female sexual dysfunction due to . . . [indicate the general medical condition]: if some other feature is predominant (e.g., orgasmic disorder) or no feature predominates

Other male sexual dysfunction due to . . . [indicate the general medical condition]: if some other feature is predominant (e.g., orgasmic disorder) or no feature predominates

Coding note: Include the name of the general medical condition on Axis I, e.g., male erectile disorder due to diabetes mellitus; also code the general medical condition on Axis III.

From American Psychiatric Association. *Diagnostic and Statistical Manual of Mental Disorders.* 4th ed. Text rev. Washington, DC: American Psychiatric Association; copyright 2000, with permission.

der have an organic basis for the disorder. The organic causes of male erectile disorder are many, most falling under the categories of cardiovascular, neurological, and endocrine disorders. Side effects of medication may impair male sexual functioning in a variety of ways and are a common cause of erectile disorder. Castration (removal of the testes) does not always lead to sexual dysfunction, as erection may still occur. A reflex arc, fired when the inner thigh is stimulated, passes through the sacral cord erectile center to account for the phenomenon. Other surgical procedures such as prostatectomy are associated with erectile disorder in 25 to 45 percent of cases, depending on the procedure used.

A number of procedures, benign and invasive, are used to help differentiate organically caused impotence from functional impotence. The procedures include monitoring nocturnal penile tumescence (erections that occur during sleep), normally associated with rapid eye movement; monitoring tumescence with a strain gauge; measuring blood pressure in the penis with a penile plethysmograph or an ultrasound (Doppler) flowmeter, both of which assess blood flow in the internal pudendal artery; and mea-

suring pudendal nerve latency time. Other diagnostic tests that delineate organic bases for impotence include glucose tolerance tests, plasma hormone assays, liver and thyroid function tests, prolactin and follicle-stimulating hormone (FSH) determinations, and cystometric examinations. Invasive diagnostic studies include penile arteriography, infusion cavernosonography, and radioactive xenon penography. Invasive procedures require expert interpretation and are used only for patients who are candidates for vascular reconstructive procedures.

Dyspareunia Due to a General Medical Condition

An estimated 30 percent of all surgical procedures on the female genital area result in temporary dyspareunia. In addition, 30 to 40 percent of women with the complaint who are seen in sex therapy clinics have pelvic pathology. Organic abnormalities leading to dyspareunia and vaginismus include irritated or infected hymenal remnants, episiotomy scars, Bartholin's gland infection, various forms of vaginitis and cervicitis, and endometriosis. Postcoital pain has been reported by women with myomata and endometriosis and is attributed to the uterine contractions during orgasm. Postmenopausal women may have dyspareunia resulting from thinning of the vaginal mucosa and reduced lubrication.

Two conditions not readily apparent on physical examination that produce dyspareunia are vulvular vestibulitis and interstitial cystitis. The former may present with chronic vulvar pain, and the latter produces pain most intensely after orgasm. Dyspareunia in men is uncommon. It is usually associated with a medical condition, such as Peyronie's disease that causes penile curvature.

Hypoactive Sexual Desire Disorder Due to a General Medical Condition

Desire commonly decreases after major illness or surgery, particularly when the body image is affected after such procedures as mastectomy, ileostomy, hysterectomy, and prostatectomy. Illnesses that deplete a person's energy, chronic conditions that require physical and psychological adaptation, and serious illnesses that may cause a person to become depressed can all result in a marked lessening of sexual desire in both men and women.

In some cases, biochemical correlates are associated with hypoactive sexual desire disorder. A recent study found markedly lower levels of serum testosterone in men complaining of low desire than in normal controls in a sleep-laboratory situation. Drugs that depress the central nervous system (CNS) or decrease testosterone production can decrease desire.

Other Male Sexual Dysfunction Due to a General Medical Condition

When another dysfunctional feature is predominant (for example, orgasmic disorder) or when no feature predominates, the category other male sexual dysfunction due to a general medical condition is used.

Male orgasmic disorder may have physiological causes and can occur after surgery on the genitourinary tract, such as prostatectomy. It may also be associated with Parkinson's disease and other neurological disorders involving the lumbar or sacral sections of the spinal cord. The anti-

Table 18.2–11
DSM-IV-TR Diagnostic Criteria for Substance-Induced Sexual Dysfunction

A. Clinically significant sexual dysfunction that results in marked distress or interpersonal difficulty predominates in the clinical picture.

B. There is evidence from the history, physical examination, or laboratory findings that the sexual dysfunction is fully explained by substance use as manifested by either (1) or (2):

   (1) the symptoms in Criterion A developed during, or within a month of, substance intoxication

   (2) medication use is etiologically related to the disturbance

C. The disturbance is not better accounted for by a sexual dysfunction that is not substance induced. Evidence that the symptoms are better accounted for by a sexual dysfunction that is not substance induced might include the following: the symptoms precede the onset of the substance use or dependence (or medication use); the symptoms persist for a substantial period of time (e.g., about a month) after the cessation of intoxication, or are substantially in excess of what would be expected given the type or amount of the substance used or the duration of use; or there is other evidence that suggests the existence of an independent non-substance-induced sexual dysfunction (e.g., a history of recurrent non-substance-related episodes).

Note: This diagnosis should be made instead of a diagnosis of substance intoxication only when the sexual dysfunction is in excess of that usually associated with the intoxication syndrome and when the dysfunction is sufficiently severe to warrant independent clinical attention.

Code [Specific substance]-induced sexual dysfunction:

   Alcohol; amphetamine [or amphetamine-like substance]; cocaine; opioid; sedative, hypnotic, or anxiolytic; other [or unknown] substance

Specify if:

   With impaired desire

   With impaired arousal

   With impaired orgasm

   With sexual pain

Specify if:

   With onset during intoxication: if the criteria are met for intoxication with the substance and the symptoms develop during the intoxication syndrome

From American Psychiatric Association. *Diagnostic and Statistical Manual of Mental Disorders.* 4th ed. Text rev. Washington, DC: American Psychiatric Association; copyright 2000, with permission.

can affect a woman's ability to have orgasms. Several drugs also affect some women's capacity to have orgasms. Antihypertensive medications, CNS stimulants, tricyclic drugs, SSRIs, and, frequently, monoamine oxidase inhibitors (MAOIs) have interfered with female orgasmic capacity. One study of women taking MAOIs, however, found that after 16 to 18 weeks of pharmacotherapy, the side effect of the medication disappeared and the women were able to reexperience orgasms, although they continued taking an undiminished dosage of the drug.

SUBSTANCE-INDUCED SEXUAL DYSFUNCTION

The diagnosis of substance-induced sexual dysfunction is used when evidence of substance intoxication or withdrawal is apparent from the history, physical examination, or laboratory findings. Distressing sexual dysfunction occurs within a month of significant substance intoxication or withdrawal (Table 18.2–11). Specified substances include alcohol; amphetamines or related substances; cocaine; opioids; sedatives, hypnotics, or anxiolytics; and other or unknown substances.

Abused recreational substances affect sexual function in various ways. In small doses, many substances enhance sexual performance by decreasing inhibition or anxiety or by causing a temporary elation of mood. With continued use, however, erectile engorgement and orgasmic and ejaculatory capacities become impaired. The abuse of sedatives, anxiolytics, hypnotics, and particularly opiates and opioids nearly always depresses desire. Alcohol may foster the initiation of sexual activity by removing inhibition, but it also impairs performance. Cocaine and amphetamines produce similar effects. Although no direct evidence indicates that sexual drive is enhanced, users initially have feelings of increased energy and may become sexually active. Ultimately, dysfunction occurs. Men usually go through two stages: an experience of prolonged erection without ejaculation, then a gradual loss of erectile capability.

Patients recovering from substance dependency may need therapy to regain sexual function, partly because of psychological readjustment to a nondependent state. Many substance abusers have always had difficulty with intimate interactions. Others who spent their crucial developmental years under the influence of a substance have missed the experiences that would have enabled them to learn social and sexual skills.

PHARMACOLOGICAL AGENTS IMPLICATED IN SEX DYSFUNCTION

Almost every pharmacological agent, particularly those used in psychiatry, has been associated with an effect on sexuality. In men, these effects include decreased sex drive, erectile failure (impotence), decreased volume of ejaculate, and delayed or retrograde ejaculation. In women, decreased sex drive, decreased vaginal lubrication, inhibited or delayed orgasm, and decreased or absent vaginal contractions may occur. Drugs may also enhance the sexual responses and increase the sex drive, but this is less common than are adverse effects.

hypertensive drug guanethidine monosulfate (Ismelin), methyldopa (Aldomet), the phenothiazines, the tricyclic drugs, and the selective serotonin reuptake inhibitors (SSRIs), among others, have been implicated in retarded ejaculation. Male orgasmic disorder must also be differentiated from retrograde ejaculation, in which ejaculation occurs but the seminal fluid passes backward into the bladder. Retrograde ejaculation always has an organic cause. It can develop after genitourinary surgery and is also associated with medications that have anticholinergic side effects, such as the phenothiazines, especially thioridazine (Mellaril).

Other Female Sexual Dysfunction Due to a General Medical Condition

Some medical conditions—specifically, endocrine diseases such as hypothyroidism, diabetes mellitus, and primary hyperprolactinemia—

Psychoactive Drugs

Antipsychotic Drugs. Most antipsychotic drugs are dopamine receptor antagonists that also block adrenergic and cholinergic receptors, thus accounting for adverse sexual effects. Chlorpromazine (Thorazine), thioridazine, and trifluoperazine (Stelazine) are potent anticholinergics that impair erection and cause retrograde ejaculation, in which the seminal fluid backs up into the bladder rather than being propelled through the penile urethra. Patients still have a pleasurable sensation, but the orgasm is dry. When urinating after orgasm, the urine may be milky white because it contains the ejaculate. The condition is startling but harmless and may occur in up to 50 percent of patients taking the drug. Paradoxically, some rare cases of priapism have been reported with antipsychotics.

Antidepressant Drugs.
The tricyclic and tetracyclic antidepressants have anticholinergic effects that interfere with erection and delay ejaculation. Since the anticholinergic effects vary among the cyclic antidepressants, those with the fewest effects (such as desipramine [Norpramin]) produce the fewest sexual side effects. The effects in women of the tricyclics and tetracyclics have not been documented sufficiently; however, few women seem to complain of any effects.

Some men report an increased sensitivity of the glans that is pleasurable and that does not interfere with erection, although it delays ejaculation. In some cases, however, the tricyclic causes a painful ejaculation, perhaps as the result of interference with seminal propulsion caused by interference with, in turn, urethral, prostatic, vas, and epididymal smooth muscle contractions. Clomipramine (Anafranil) has been reported to increase sex drive in some persons. Deprenyl (Selegiline), a selective MAO type B (MAO_B) inhibitor, and bupropion (Wellbutrin) have also been reported to increase sex drive, possibly by dopaminergic activity and increased production of norepinephrine.

Venlafaxine (Effexor) and the SSRIs often have adverse effects because of the rise in serotonin levels. A lowering of the sex drive and a difficulty in reaching orgasm occur in both sexes. Reversal of those negative effects has been achieved with cyproheptadine (Periactin), an antihistamine with antiserotonergic effects, and with methylphenidate (Ritalin), which has adrenergic effects. Trazodone is associated with the rare occurrence of priapism, the symptom of prolonged erection in the absence of sexual stimuli. That symptom appears to result from the α_2-adrenergic antagonism of trazodone.

The MAOIs affect biogenic amines broadly. Accordingly, they produce impaired erection, delayed or retrograde ejaculation, vaginal dryness, and inhibited orgasm. Tranylcypromine (Parnate) has a paradoxical sexually stimulating effect in some persons, possibly as a result of its amphetamine-like properties.

Lithium.
Lithium (Eskalith) regulates mood and in the manic state may reduce hypersexuality, possibly by a dopamine antagonist activity. In some patients, impaired erection has been reported.

Sympathomimetics.
Psychostimulants are sometimes used in the treatment of depression and include amphetamines, methylphenidate, and pemoline (Cylert), which raise the plasma levels of norepinephrine and dopamine. Libido is increased; however, with prolonged use, men may experience a loss of desire and erections.

α-Adrenergic and β-Adrenergic Receptor Antagonists.
α-Adrenergic and β-adrenergic receptor antagonists are used in the treatment of hypertension, angina, and certain cardiac arrhythmias. They diminish tonic sympathetic nerve outflow from vasomotor centers in the brain. As a result, they can cause impotence, decrease the volume of ejaculate, and produce retrograde ejaculation. Changes in libido have been reported in both sexes.

Suggestions have been made to use the side effects of drugs therapeutically. Thus, a drug that delays or interferes with ejaculation (such as fluoxetine [Prozac]) might be used to treat premature ejaculation.

Anticholinergics.
The anticholinergics block cholinergic receptors and include such drugs as amantadine (Symmetrel) and benztropine (Cogentin). They produce dryness of the mucous membranes (including that of the vagina) and impotence.

Antihistamines.
Drugs such as diphenhydramine (Benadryl) have anticholinergic activity and are mildly hypnotic. They may inhibit sexual function as a result. Cyproheptadine, although an antihistamine, also has potent activity as a serotonin antagonist. It is used to block the serotonergic sexual side effects produced by SSRIs, such as delayed orgasm and impotence.

Antianxiety Agents.
The major class of anxiolytics is the benzodiazepines (such as diazepam [Valium]). They act on the γ-aminobutyric acid (GABA) receptors, which are believed to be involved in cognition, memory, and motor control. Because they decrease plasma epinephrine concentrations, they diminish anxiety, and as a result they improve sexual function in people inhibited by anxiety.

Alcohol.
Alcohol suppresses CNS activity generally and can produce erectile disorders in men as a result. Alcohol has a direct gonadal effect that decreases testosterone levels in men; paradoxically, it can produce a slight rise in testosterone levels in women. The latter finding may account for women reporting increased libido after drinking small amounts of alcohol. The long-term use of alcohol reduces the ability of the liver to metabolize estrogenic compounds. In men that produces signs of feminization (such as gynecomastia as a result of testicular atrophy).

Opioids.
Opioids, such as heroin, have adverse sexual effects, such as erectile failure and decreased libido. The alteration of consciousness may enhance the sexual experience in occasional users.

Hallucinogens.
The hallucinogens include lysergic acid diethylamide (LSD), phencyclidine (PCP), psilocybin (from some mushrooms), and mescaline (from peyote cactus). In addition to inducing hallucinations, the drugs cause loss of contact with reality and an expanding and heightening of consciousness. Some users report that the sexual experience is similarly enhanced, but others experience anxiety, delirium, or psychosis, which clearly interferes with sexual function.

Cannabis.
The altered state of consciousness produced by cannabis may enhance sexual pleasure for some persons. Its prolonged use depresses testosterone levels.

Barbiturates and Similarly Acting Drugs.
Barbiturates and similarly acting sedative-hypnotic drugs may enhance sexual responsiveness in people who are sexually unresponsive as a result of anxiety. They have no direct effect on the sex organs; however, they do produce an alteration in consciousness that some people find pleasurable. They are subject to abuse and may be fatal when combined with alcohol or other CNS depressants.

Methaqualone (Quaalude) acquired a reputation as a sexual enhancer, which had no biological basis in fact. It is no longer marketed in the United States.

SEXUAL DYSFUNCTION NOT OTHERWISE SPECIFIED

The category sexual dysfunction not otherwise specified covers sexual dysfunctions that cannot be classified under the categories described above (Table 18.2–12). Examples include people who experience the physiological components of sexual excitement and orgasm but report no erotic sensation or even anesthesia (orgasmic anhedonia). Women with conditions analogous to premature ejaculation in men are classified here. Orgasmic women who desire, but have not experienced, multiple orgasms can be classified under this heading as well. Also, disorders of excessive, rather than inhibited, dysfunction, such as compulsive masturbation or coitus (sex addiction), or those with genital pain occurring during masturbation may be classified here. Other unspecified disorders are found in people who have one or more sexual fantasies about which they feel guilty or otherwise dysphoric, but the range of common sexual fantasies is broad.

Female Premature Orgasm

Data on female premature orgasm are lacking; no separate category of premature orgasm for women is included in DSM-IV-TR. A case of multiple spontaneous orgasms without sexual stimulation has been seen in a woman; the cause was an epileptogenic focus in the temporal lobe. Instances have been reported of women on antidepressants (such as fluoxetine and clomipramine) who experience spontaneous orgasm associated with yawning.

Postcoital Headache

Postcoital headache, characterized by headache immediately after coitus, may last for several hours. It is usually described as throbbing and is localized in the occipital or frontal area. The cause is unknown. There may be vascular, muscle-contraction (tension), or psychogenic causes. Coitus may precipitate migraine or cluster headaches in predisposed people.

Orgasmic Anhedonia

Orgasmic anhedonia is a condition in which a person has no physical sensation of orgasm, even though the physiological component (for example, ejaculation) remains intact. Organic causes, such as sacral and cephalic lesions that interfere with afferent pathways from the genitalia to the cortex, must be ruled out. Psychological causes usually relate to extreme guilt about experiencing sexual pleasure. These feelings produce a dissociative response that isolates the affective component of the orgasmic experience from consciousness.

Masturbatory Pain

People may experience pain during masturbation. Organic causes should always be ruled out; a small vaginal tear or early Peyronie's disease may produce a painful sensation. The condition should be differentiated from compulsive masturbation. People may masturbate to the extent that they do physical damage to their genitals and eventually experience pain during subsequent masturbatory acts. Such cases constitute a separate sexual disorder and should be so classified.

Certain masturbatory practices have resulted in what has been called *autoerotic asphyxiation*. The practices involve masturbating while hanging by the neck to heighten the erotic sensations and the orgasm's intensity through the mechanism of mild hypoxia. Although the people intend to release themselves from the noose after orgasm, an estimated 500 to 1,000 people a year accidentally kill themselves by hanging. Most who indulge in the practice are male; transvestism is often associated with the habit, and most deaths occur among adolescents. Such masochistic practices are usually associated with severe mental disorders, such as schizophrenia and major mood disorders.

TREATMENT

Before 1970, the most common treatment of sexual dysfunctions was individual psychotherapy. Classic psychodynamic theory holds that sexual inadequacy has its roots in early developmental conflicts, and the sexual disorder is treated as part of a pervasive emotional disturbance. Treatment focuses on the exploration of unconscious conflicts, motivation, fantasy, and various interpersonal difficulties. One of the assumptions of therapy is that the removal of the conflicts allows the sexual impulse to become structurally acceptable to the ego and thereby the patient finds appropriate means of satisfaction in the environment. Unfortunately, the symptoms of sexual dysfunctions frequently become secondarily autonomous and continue to persist, even when other problems evolving from the patient's pathology have been resolved. The addition of behavioral techniques is often necessary to cure the sexual problem.

Dual-Sex Therapy

The theoretical basis of dual-sex therapy is the concept of the marital unit or dyad as the object of therapy; the approach represents the major advance in the diagnosis and treatment of sexual disorders in this century. The methodology was originated and developed by Masters and Johnson. In dual-sex therapy, treatment is based on the concept that the couple must be treated when a dysfunctional person is in a relationship. Because both are involved in a sexually distressing situation, both must participate in the therapy program. The sexual problem often reflects other areas of disharmony or misunderstanding in the marriage so that the entire marital relationship is treated, with emphasis on sexual functioning as a part of the relationship. The keystone of the program is the roundtable session in which a male and female therapy team clarifies, dis-

Table 18.2–12
DSM-IV-TR Diagnostic Criteria for Sexual Dysfunction Not Otherwise Specified

This category includes sexual dysfunctions that do not meet criteria for any specific sexual dysfunction. Examples include

1. No (or substantially diminished) subjective erotic feelings despite otherwise normal arousal and orgasm
2. Situations in which the clinician has concluded that a sexual dysfunction is present but is unable to determine whether it is primary, due to a general medical condition, or substance induced

From American Psychiatric Association. *Diagnostic and Statistical Manual of Mental Disorders.* 4th ed. Text rev. Washington, DC: American Psychiatric Association; copyright 2000, with permission.

cusses, and works through problems with the couple. The four-way sessions require active participation by the patients. Therapists and patients discuss the psychological and physiological aspects of sexual functioning, and therapists have an educative attitude. Therapists suggest specific sexual activities, which the couple follows in the privacy of their home. The aim of the therapy is to establish or reestablish communication within the marital unit. Sex is emphasized as a natural function that flourishes in the appropriate domestic climate, and improved communication is encouraged toward that end. In a variation of this therapy that has proved effective, one therapist may treat the couple. Treatment is short-term and behaviorally oriented. The therapists attempt to reflect the situation as they see it, rather than to interpret underlying dynamics. An undistorted picture of the relationship presented by the therapists often corrects the myopic, narrow view held by each marriage partner. This new perspective can interrupt the couple's vicious cycle of relating and can encourage improved, more effective communication. Specific exercises are prescribed for the couple to treat their particular problems. Sexual inadequacy often involves lack of information, misinformation, and performance fear. Therefore, the couple are specifically prohibited from any sexual play other than that prescribed by the therapists. Beginning exercises usually focus on heightening sensory awareness to touch, sight, sound, and smell. Initially, intercourse is interdicted, and the couple learns to give and receive bodily pleasure without the pressure of performance or penetration. At the same time, they learn how to communicate nonverbally in a mutually satisfactory way, and they learn that sexual foreplay is an enjoyable alternative to intercourse and orgasm.

During the sensate focus exercises, the couple receives much reinforcement to reduce their anxiety. They are urged to use fantasies to distract them from obsessive concerns about performance (spectatoring). The needs of both the dysfunctional partner and the nondysfunctional partner are considered. If either partner becomes sexually excited by the exercises, the other is encouraged to bring him or her to orgasm by manual or oral means. Open communication between the partners is urged, and the expression of mutual needs is encouraged. Resistances, such as claims of fatigue or not enough time to complete the exercises, are common and must be dealt with by the therapists. Genital stimulation is eventually added to general body stimulation. The couple are instructed sequentially to try various positions for intercourse, without necessarily completing the act, and to use varieties of stimulating techniques before they are instructed to proceed with intercourse.

Psychotherapy sessions follow each new exercise period, and problems and satisfactions, both sexual and in other areas of the couple's lives, are discussed. Specific instructions and the introduction of new exercises geared to the individual couple's progress are reviewed in each session. Gradually, the couple gains confidence and learns to communicate, verbally and sexually. Dual-sex therapy is most effective when the sexual dysfunction exists apart from other psychopathology.

Specific Techniques and Exercises

Various techniques are used to treat the various dysfunctions. In cases of vaginismus, a woman is advised to dilate her vaginal opening with her fingers or with graduated dilators.

In cases of premature ejaculation, an exercise known as the *squeeze technique* is used to raise the threshold of penile excitability. In this exercise, the man or the woman stimulates the erect penis until the earliest sensations of impending ejaculation are felt. At this point, the woman forcefully squeezes the coronal ridge of the glans, the erection is diminished, and ejaculation is inhibited. The exercise program eventually raises the threshold of the sensation of ejaculatory inevitability and allows the man to become aware of his sexual sensations and confident about his sexual performance. A variant of the exercise is the stop-start technique developed by James H. Semans, in which the woman stops all stimulation of the penis when the man first senses an impending ejaculation. No squeeze is used. Research has shown that the presence or absence of circumcision has no bearing on a man's ejaculatory control; the glans is equally sensitive in the two states. Sex therapy has been most successful in the treatment of premature ejaculation.

A man with a sexual desire disorder or male erectile disorder is sometimes told to masturbate to prove that full erection and ejaculation are possible. Male orgasmic disorder is managed initially by extravaginal ejaculation and then by gradual vaginal entry after stimulation to a point near ejaculation.

In cases of lifelong female orgasmic disorder, the woman is directed to masturbate, sometimes using a vibrator. The shaft of the clitoris is the masturbatory site most preferred by women, and orgasm depends on adequate clitoral stimulation. An area on the anterior wall of the vagina has been identified in some women as a site of sexual excitation known as the *G-spot*; but reports of an ejaculatory phenomenon at orgasm in women after the stimulation of the G-spot have not been satisfactorily verified.

Hypnotherapy

Hypnotherapists focus specifically on the anxiety-producing symptom—that is, the particular sexual dysfunction. The successful use of hypnosis enables patients to gain control over the symptom that has been lowering self-esteem and disrupting psychological homeostasis. The cooperation of the patient is first obtained and encouraged during a series of nonhypnotic sessions with the therapist. Those discussions permit the development of a secure doctor–patient relationship, a sense of physical and psychological comfort on the part of the patient, and the establishment of mutually desired treatment goals. During this time, the therapist assesses the patient's capacity for the trance experience. The nonhypnotic sessions also permit the clinician to take a psychiatric history and perform a mental status examination before beginning hypnotherapy. The focus of treatment is on symptom removal and attitude alteration. The patient is instructed in developing alternative means of dealing with the anxiety-provoking situation, the sexual encounter.

Behavior Therapy

Behavior therapists assume that sexual dysfunction is learned maladaptive behavior, which causes patients to be fearful of sexual interaction. Using traditional techniques, therapists set up a hierarchy of anxiety-provoking situations, ranging from least threatening, for instance, the thought of kissing, to most threatening, the thought of penile penetration. The behavior therapist enables the patient to master the anxiety through a standard program of systematic desensitization, which is designed to inhibit the learned anxious response by encouraging behaviors antithetical to anxiety. The patient first deals with the least anxiety-producing situation in fantasy and progresses by steps to the most anxiety-producing situation. Medication, hypnosis, and special training in deep muscle relaxation are sometimes used to help with the initial mastery of anxiety.

Assertiveness training is helpful in teaching patients to express sexual needs openly and without fear. Exercises in assertiveness are given in conjunction with sex therapy; patients are encouraged to make sexual requests and to refuse to comply with requests perceived as unreasonable. Sexual exercises may be prescribed for patients to perform at home, and a hierarchy may be established, starting with those activities that have proved most pleasurable and successful in the past.

Group Therapy

Group therapy has been used to examine both intrapsychic and interpersonal problems in patients with sexual disorders. A therapy group provides a strong support system for a patient who feels ashamed, anxious, or guilty about a particular sexual problem. It is a useful forum in which to counteract sexual myths, correct misconceptions, and provide accurate information about sexual anatomy, physiology, and varieties of behavior.

Groups for the treatment of sexual disorders can be organized in several ways. Members may all share the same problem, such as premature ejaculation; members may all be of the same sex with different sexual problems; or groups may be composed of both men and women who are experiencing a variety of sexual problems. Group therapy may be an adjunct to other forms of therapy or the prime mode of treatment. Groups organized to treat a particular dysfunction are usually behavioral in approach.

Groups composed of married couples with sexual dysfunctions have also been effective. A group provides the opportunity to gather accurate information, offers consensual validation of individual preferences, and enhances self-esteem and self-acceptance. Techniques such as role playing and psychodrama may be used in treatment. Such groups are not indicated for couples when one partner is uncooperative, when a patient has a severe depressive disorder or psychosis, when a patient finds explicit sexual audiovisual material repugnant, or when a patient fears or dislikes groups.

Analytically Oriented Sex Therapy

One of the most effective treatment modalities is the use of sex therapy integrated with psychodynamic and psychoanalytically oriented psychotherapy. The sex therapy is conducted over a longer period than usual, which allows learning or relearning of sexual satisfaction under the realities of patients' day-to-day lives. The addition of psychodynamic conceptualizations to behavioral techniques used to treat sexual dysfunctions allows the treatment of patients with sexual disorders associated with other psychopathology.

The material and dynamics that emerge in patients in analytically oriented sex therapy are the same as those in psychoanalytic therapy, such as dreams, fear of punishment, aggressive feelings, difficulty trusting a partner, fear of intimacy, oedipal feelings, and fear of genital mutilation. The combined approach of analytically oriented sex therapy is used by the general psy-

chiatrist who carefully judges the optimal timing of sex therapy and the ability of patients to tolerate the directive approach that focuses on their sexual difficulties.

Biological Treatments

Biological treatments, including pharmacotherapy, surgery, and mechanical devices, are used to treat specific cases of sexual disorder. Most of the recent advances involve male sexual dysfunction. Current studies are under way to test biological treatment of sexual dysfunction in women.

Pharmacotherapy.   The major new medications for the treatment of sexual dysfunction are sildenafil (Viagra); oral phentolamine (Vasomax); injectable alprostadil (Impulse, Caverject), an injectable phentolamine; papaverine; and a transurethral alprostadil (MUSE), all used to treat erectile disorder. Congeners of these drugs are in preparation with other routes of administration (e.g., creams, lotions, patches).

Sildenafil is a nitric oxide enhancer that facilitates the inflow of blood to the penis necessary for an erection. The drug takes effect approximately 1 hour after ingestion, and its effect can last up to 4 hours. Sildenafil is not effective in the absence of sexual stimulation. The most common adverse events associated with its use are headaches, flushing, and dyspepsia. The use of sildenafil is contraindicated for people taking organic nitrates. The concomitant action of the two drugs can result in large, sudden, and sometimes fatal drops in systemic blood pressure. Sildenafil is not effective in all cases of erectile dysfunction. It fails to produce an erection rigid enough for penetration in approximately 50 percent of men who have radical prostate surgery or in those with long-standing insulin-dependent diabetes. It is also ineffective in certain cases of nerve damage.

Sildenafil use in women results in vaginal lubrication, but not in increased desire. However, anecdotal reports describe individual women who have experienced intensified excitement with sildenafil.

Oral phentolamine and apomorphine are effective as potency enhancers in some men with minimal erectile dysfunction. Phentolamine reduces sympathetic tone and relaxes corporeal smooth muscle. Adverse events include hypotension, tachycardia, and dizziness. Apomorphine effects are mediated by the autonomic nervous system and result in vasodilatation that facilitates the inflow of blood to the penis. Adverse events include nausea and sweating.

In contrast to the oral medications, injectable and transurethral alprostadil act locally on the penis and can produce erections in the absence of sexual stimulation. Alprostadil contains a naturally occurring form of prostaglandin E, a vasodilating agent. Alprostadil may be administered by direct injection into the corpora cavernosa or by intraurethral insertion or a pellet through a canula. The firm erection produced within 2 to 3 minutes after administration of the drug may last as long as 1 hour. Infrequent and reversible adverse effects of injections include penile bruising and changes in liver function tests. However, possible hazardous sequelae exist, including priapism and sclerosis of the small veins of the penis. Users of transurethral alprostadil sometimes complain of burning sensations in the penis.

Two small trials found different topical agents effective in alleviating erectile dysfunction. One cream consists of three vasoactive substances known to be absorbed through the skin: aminophylline, isosorbide dinitrate, and co-dergocrine mesylate, which is a mixture of ergot alkaloids. The other is a gel containing alprostadil and an additional ingredient, which temporarily makes the outer layer of the skin more permeable.

A cream incorporating alprostadil also has been developed to treat female sexual arousal disorder. The initial results are promising. Also, vaginally applied phentolamine mesylate, an α-adrenergic antagonist, significantly increased vasocongestion and a subjective sense of arousal in a trial of postmenopausal women with arousal problems who were already on hormonal therapy.

Numerous other pharmacological agents have been used to heal the various sexual disorders. Intravenous methohexital sodium (Brevital) has been used in desensitization therapy. Antianxiety agents may have some application in tense patients, although these drugs can also interfere with the sexual response. The side effects of antidepressants, in particular the SSRIs and tricyclic drugs, have been used to prolong the sexual response in patients with premature ejaculation. This approach is particularly useful in patients refractory to behavioral techniques who may fall into the category of physiologically determined premature ejaculation. The use of antidepressants has also been advocated in the treatment of patients who are phobic of sex and in those with a post-traumatic stress disorder following rape. Trazodone is an antidepressant that improves nocturnal erections. The risks of taking such medications must be carefully weighed against their possible benefits. Bromocriptine is used in the treatment of hyperprolactinemia, which is frequently associated with hypogonadism. Such cases are first worked up to rule out pituitary tumors. Bromocriptine (Parlodel), a dopamine agonist, may improve sexual function impaired by hyperprolactinemia. Sometimes the problem requires androgen therapy.

A number of substances have popular standing as aphrodisiacs; for example, ginseng root and yohimbine (Yocon). However, studies have not confirmed any aphrodisiac properties. Yohimbine, an α-adrenergic receptor antagonist, may cause dilation of the penile artery; however, the American Urologic Association does not recommend its use to treat organic erectile dysfunction. Many recreational drugs, including cocaine, amphetamines, alcohol, and cannabis, are considered enhancers of sexual performance. Although they may provide the user with an initial benefit because of their tranquilizing, disinhibiting, or mood-elevating effects, consistent or prolonged use of any of these substances impairs sexual functioning.

Dopaminergic agents have been reported to increase libido and improve sex function. Those drugs include L-dopa, a dopamine precursor, and bromocriptine, a dopamine agonist. The antidepressant bupropion has dopaminergic effects and has increased sex drive in some patients. Selegiline, an MAOI, is selective for MAO_B and is dopaminergic. It improves sexual functioning in older persons.

Hormone Therapy.   Androgens increase the sex drive in women and in men with low testosterone concentrations. Women may experience virilizing effects, some of which are irreversible (e.g., deepening of the voice). In men, prolonged use of androgens produces hypertension and prostatic enlargement. Testosterone is most effective when given parenterally; however, effective oral and transdermal preparations are available.

Women who use estrogens for replacement therapy or for contraception may report decreased libido; in such cases, a combined preparation of estrogen and testosterone has been used effectively. Estrogen, itself, prevents thinning of the vaginal mucous membrane and facilitates lubrication. Two new forms of estrogen, vaginal rings and vaginal tablets, provide alternate administration routes to treat women with arousal problems or genital atrophy. Because tablets and rings do not increase circulating estrogen levels, these devices may be considered for breast cancer patients with arousal problems in view of the mutagenic and cardiovascular complications associated with prolonged estrogen use.

Antiandrogens and Antiestrogens.   Estrogens and progesterone are antiandrogens that have been used to treat compulsive sexual behavior in men, usually in sex offenders. Clomiphene (Clomid) and tamoxifen (Nolvadex) are both antiestrogens and both stimulate gonadotropin-releasing hormone (GnRH) secretion and increase testosterone concentrations, thereby increasing libido. Women being treated for breast cancer with tamoxifen report an increased libido.

Mechanical Treatment Approaches

In male patients with arteriosclerosis (especially of the distal aorta, known as *Leriche's syndrome*), the erection may be lost during active pelvic thrusting. The need for increased blood in the gluteal muscles and others served by the ilial or hypogastric arteries takes blood away (steals) from the pudendal artery and thus interferes with penile blood flow. Relief may be obtained by decreasing pelvic thrusting, which is also aided by the woman-superior coital position.

Vacuum Pump.   Vacuum pumps are mechanical devices that patients without vascular disease can use to obtain erections. The blood drawn into the penis after the creation of the vacuum is kept there by a ring placed around the base of the penis. This device has no adverse effects, but it is cumbersome, and partners must be willing to accept its use. Some women complain that the penis is redder and cooler than when erection is produced by natural circumstances, and they find the process and the result objectionable.

A similar device, called *EROS*, has been developed to create clitoral erections in women. EROS is a small suction cup that fits over the clitoral region and draws blood into the clitoris. There have been studies reporting its success in treating female sexual arousal disorder.

Vibrators used to stimulate the clitoral area have been successful in treating anorgasmic women.

Surgical Treatment

Male Prostheses.   Surgical treatment is infrequently advocated, but penile prosthetic devices are available for men with inadequate erectile responses who are resistant to other treatment methods or who have medically caused deficiencies. There are two main types of prosthesis: a semirigid rod prosthesis that produces a permanent erection that can be positioned close to the body for concealment and an inflatable type that is implanted with its own reservoir and pump for inflation and deflation. The latter type is designed to mimic normal physiological functioning.

Outcome

The results of different treatment methods have varied considerably since Masters and Johnson first reported positive results for their treatment approach in 1970. Masters and Johnson studied the failure rates of their patients (defined as the failure to initiate reversal of the basic symptom of the presenting dysfunction). They compared initial failure rates with 5-year follow-up findings for the same couples. Although some have criticized their definition of the percentage of presumed successes, other studies have confirmed the effectiveness of their approach. Demonstrating the effectiveness of traditional outpatient psychotherapy is just as difficult when therapy is oriented to sexual problems as it is in general. The more severe the psychopathology associated with a problem of long duration, the more adverse the outcome is likely to be.

The more difficult treatment cases involve couples with severe marital discord. Desire disorders are particularly difficult to treat. They require longer, more intensive therapy than some other disorders, and their outcomes are very variable.

When behavioral approaches are used, empirical criteria that predict outcome are more easily isolated. Using these criteria, for instance, couples who regularly practice assigned exercise appear to have a much greater likelihood of success than do more resistant couples or those whose interaction involves sadomasochistic or depressive features or mechanisms of blame and projection. Flexibility of attitude is also a positive prognostic factor. Overall, younger couples tend to complete sex therapy more often than older couples. Couples whose interactional difficulties center on their sex problems, such as inhibition, frustration, or fear of performance failure, are also likely to respond well to therapy.

In general, methods that have proved effective singly or in combination include training in behavioral-sexual skills, systematic desensitization, directive martial counseling, traditional psychodynamic approaches, group therapy, and pharmacotherapy. Although most therapists prefer to treat a couple for sexual dysfunction, treatment of individual persons has also been successful.

▲ 18.3 Sexual Disorder Not Otherwise Specified and Paraphilias

PARAPHILIAS

Paraphilias are abnormal expressions of sexuality. They can range from nearly normal behavior to behavior that is destructive or hurtful only to oneself or to oneself and one's partner, and finally to behavior that is deemed destructive or threatening to the community at large. The fourth revised edition of the *Diagnostic and Statistical Manual of Mental Disorders* (DSM-IV-TR) addresses these differences by designating impulses toward pedophilia, frotteurism, voyeurism, exhibitionism, and sexual sadism clinically significant if the person has acted on these fantasies or if these fantasies cause marked distress or interpersonal difficulty. The remaining paraphilias, such as zoophilia or fetishism, meet the criteria for clinical significance only if they cause marked distress or impairment in social, occupational, or other important areas of functioning even if the urges have been expressed behaviorally. Paraphiliac urges may occur rarely, intermittently, or compulsively. They may be incidental or they may offer the only venue through which sexuality can be expressed.

Epidemiology

Among legally identified cases of paraphilias, pedophilia is most common. Ten to 20 percent of all children have been molested by age 18. Because a child is the object, the act is taken more seriously, and greater effort is spent tracking down the culprit than in other paraphilias. People with exhibitionism who publicly display themselves to young children are also commonly apprehended. Those with voyeurism may be apprehended, but their risk is not great. Twenty percent of adult females have been the targets of people with exhibitionism and voyeurism. Sexual masochism and sexual sadism are underrepresented in any prevalence estimates. Sexual sadism usually comes to attention only in sensational cases of rape, brutality, and lust murder. The excretory paraphilias are scarcely reported, as any activity usually takes place between consenting adults or between prostitute and client. People with fetishism rarely become entangled in the legal system. Those with transvestic fetishism may be arrested occasionally for disturbing the peace or on other misdemeanor charges if they are obviously men dressed in women's clothes, but arrest is more common among those with gender identity disorders. Zoophilia as a true paraphilia is rare.

As usually defined, the paraphilias seem to be largely male conditions. Fetishism almost always occurs in men. More than 50 percent of all paraphilias have their onset before age 18. Patients with paraphilia frequently have three to five paraphilias, either concurrently or at different times in their lives. This pattern of occurrence is especially the case with exhibitionism, fetishism, sexual masochism, sexual sadism, transvestic fetishism, voyeurism, and zoophilia. The occurrence of paraphiliac behavior peaks between ages 15 and 25 and gradually declines; in men over 50, criminal paraphiliac acts are rare. Those that occur are practiced in isolation or with a cooperative partner.

Etiology

Psychosocial Factors.   In the classic psychoanalytic model, people with a paraphilia have failed to complete the normal developmental process toward heterosexual adjustment. Failure to resolve the oedipal crisis by identifying with the father-aggressor (for boys) or mother-aggressor (for girls) results either in improper identification with the opposite-sex parent or in an improper choice of object for libido cathexis. Classic psychoanalytic theory holds that transsexualism and transvestic fetishism are disorders because each involves identification with the opposite-sex parent instead of the same-sex parent; for instance, a man dressing in women's clothes is believed to identify with his mother. Exhibitionism and voyeurism may be an attempt to calm their anxiety about castration. Fetishism is an attempt to avoid anxiety by displacing libidinal impulses to inappropriate objects. People with pedophilia and sexual sadism have a need to dominate and control their victims to compensate for their feelings of powerlessness during the oedipal crisis.

Other theories attribute the development of a paraphilia to early experiences that condition or socialize children into committing a paraphiliac act. Molestation as a child can predispose a person to accept continued abuse as an adult or, conversely, to become an abuser of others. Also, early experiences of abuse that is not specifically sexual, such as spanking, enemas, or verbal humiliation, can be sexualized by a child and can form the basis for a paraphilia. Such experiences can result in the development of an *eroticized child*. The onset of paraphiliac acts can

Table 18.3–1
DSM-IV-TR Diagnostic Criteria for Exhibitionism

A. Over a period of at least 6 months, recurrent, intense sexually arousing fantasies, sexual urges, or behaviors involving the exposure of one's genitals to an unsuspecting stranger.

B. The person has acted on these sexual urges, or the sexual urges or fantasies cause marked distress or interpersonal difficulty.

From American Psychiatric Association. *Diagnostic and Statistical Manual of Mental Disorders.* 4th ed. Text rev. Washington, DC: American Psychiatric Association; copyright 2000, with permission.

Table 18.3–2
DSM-IV-TR Diagnostic Criteria for Fetishism

A. Over a period of at least 6 months, recurrent, intense sexually arousing fantasies, sexual urges, or behaviors involving the use of nonliving objects (e.g., female undergarments).

B. The fantasies, sexual urges, or behaviors cause clinically significant distress or impairment in social, occupational, or other important areas of functioning.

C. The fetish objects are not limited to articles of female clothing used in cross-dressing (as in transvestic fetishism) or devices designed for the purpose of tactile genital stimulation (e.g., a vibrator).

From American Psychiatric Association. *Diagnostic and Statistical Manual of Mental Disorders.* 4th ed. Text rev. Washington, DC: American Psychiatric Association; copyright 2000, with permission.

result from people's modeling their behavior on the behavior of others who have carried out paraphiliac acts, mimicking sexual behavior depicted in the media, or recalling emotionally laden events from the past, such as their own molestation. Learning theory indicates that because the fantasizing of paraphiliac interests begins at an early age and because personal fantasies and thoughts are not shared with others (who could block or discourage them), the use and misuse of paraphiliac fantasies and urges continue uninhibited until late in life.

Biological Factors. Several studies have identified abnormal organic findings in people with paraphilias. Among patients referred to large medical centers, those with positive organic findings included 74 percent with abnormal hormone levels, 27 percent with hard or soft neurological signs, 24 percent with chromosomal abnormalities, 9 percent with seizures, 9 percent with dyslexia, 4 percent with abnormal electroencephalograms (EEGs), 4 percent with major mental disorders, and 4 percent with mental handicaps. The question that remains unanswered is whether these abnormalities are causally related to paraphiliac interests or are incidental findings that bear no relevance to the development of paraphilia.

Diagnosis and Clinical Features

In DSM-IV-TR, the diagnostic criteria for paraphilias include the presence of a pathognomonic fantasy and an intense urge to act out the fantasy or its behavior elaboration. The fantasy, which may distress a patient, contains unusual sexual material that is relatively fixed and shows only minor variations. Arousal and orgasm depend on the mental elaboration or the behavioral playing out of the fantasy. Sexual activity is ritualized or stereotyped and makes use of degraded, reduced, or dehumanized objects.

Exhibitionism. Exhibitionism is the recurrent urge to expose the genitals to a stranger or to an unsuspecting person (Table 18.3–1). Sexual excitement occurs in anticipation of the exposure, and orgasm is brought about by masturbation during or after the event. In almost 100 percent of cases, those with exhibitionism are men exposing themselves to women. The dynamic of men with exhibitionism is to assert their masculinity by showing their penises and by watching the victims' reactions—fright, surprise, and disgust.

Fetishism. In fetishism, the sexual focus is on objects (such as shoes, gloves, pantyhose, and stockings) that are intimately associated with the human body (Table 18.3–2). The particular fetish is linked to

someone closely involved with a patient during childhood and has a quality associated with this loved, needed, or even traumatizing person. Usually, the disorder begins by adolescence, although the fetish may have been established in childhood. Once established, the disorder tends to be chronic.

The disorder is almost exclusively found in men. According to Freud, the fetish serves as a symbol of the phallus to people with unconscious castration fears. Learning theorists believe that the object was associated with sexual stimulation at an early age.

Frotteurism. Frotteurism is usually characterized by a man's rubbing his penis against the buttocks or other body parts of a fully clothed woman to achieve orgasm (Table 18.3–3). The acts usually occur in crowded places, particularly in subways and buses.

Pedophilia. Pedophilia involves recurrent intense sexual urges toward or arousal by children 13 years of age or younger, over a period of at least 6 months. People with pedophilia are at least 16 years of age and at least 5 years older than the victims (Table 18.3–4). When a perpetrator is a late adolescent involved in an ongoing sexual relationship with a 12- or 13-year-old, the diagnosis is not warranted.

Most child molestations involve genital fondling or oral sex. Vaginal or anal penetration of children occurs infrequently except in cases of incest. Although most child victims coming to public attention are girls, this finding appears to be a product of the referral process. Offenders report that when they touch a child, most (60 percent) of the victims are boys. This figure is in sharp contrast to the figure for nontouching victimization of children, such as window peeping and exhibitionism; 99 per-

Table 18.3–3
DSM-IV-TR Diagnostic Criteria for Frotteurism

A. Over a period of at least 6 months, recurrent, intense sexually arousing fantasies, sexual urges, or behaviors involving touching and rubbing against a nonconsenting person.

B. The person has acted on these sexual urges, or the sexual urges or fantasies cause marked distress or interpersonal difficulty.

From American Psychiatric Association. *Diagnostic and Statistical Manual of Mental Disorders.* 4th ed. Text rev. Washington, DC: American Psychiatric Association; copyright 2000, with permission.

Table 18.3–4
DSM-IV-TR Diagnostic Criteria for Pedophilia

A. Over a period of at least 6 months, recurrent, intense sexually arousing fantasies, sexual urges, or behaviors involving sexual activity with a prepubescent child or children (generally age 13 years or younger).

B. The person has acted on these sexual urges, or the sexual urges or fantasies cause marked distress or interpersonal difficulty.

C. The person is at least age 16 years and at least 5 years older than the child or children in Criterion A.

Note: Do not include an individual in late adolescence involved in an ongoing sexual relationship with a 12- or 13-year-old.

Specify if:

Sexually attracted to males
Sexually attracted to females
Sexually attracted to both

Specify if:

Limited to incest

Specify type:

Exclusive type (attracted only to children)
Nonexclusive type

From American Psychiatric Association. *Diagnostic and Statistical Manual of Mental Disorders.* 4th ed. Text rev. Washington, DC: American Psychiatric Association; copyright 2000, with permission.

cent of all such cases are perpetrated against girls. Of those with pedophilia, 95 percent are heterosexual, and 50 percent have consumed alcohol to excess at the time of the incident. In addition to their pedophilia, a significant number of the perpetrators are concomitantly, or have previously been, involved in exhibitionism, voyeurism, or rape.

Incest is related to pedophilia by the frequent selection of an immature child as a sex object, the subtle or overt element of coercion, and occasionally the preferential nature of the adult–child liaison.

Sexual Masochism.
Masochism takes its name from the activities of Leopold von Sacher-Masoch, a 19th-century Austrian novelist whose characters derived sexual pleasure from being abused and dominated by women. According to DSM-IV-TR, people with sexual masochism have a recurrent preoccupation with sexual urges and fantasies involving the act of being humiliated, beaten, bound, or otherwise made to suffer (Table 18.3–5). Sexual masochistic practices are more

Table 18.3–5
DSM-IV-TR Diagnostic Criteria for Sexual Masochism

A. Over a period of at least 6 months, recurrent, intense sexually arousing fantasies, sexual urges, or behaviors involving the act (real, not simulated) of being humiliated, beaten, bound, or otherwise made to suffer.

B. The fantasies, sexual urges, or behaviors cause clinically significant distress or impairment in social, occupational, or other important areas of functioning.

From American Psychiatric Association. *Diagnostic and Statistical Manual of Mental Disorders.* 4th ed. Text rev. Washington, DC: American Psychiatric Association; copyright 2000, with permission.

Table 18.3–6
DSM-IV-TR Diagnostic Criteria for Sexual Sadism

A. Over a period of at least 6 months, recurrent, intense sexually arousing fantasies, sexual urges, or behaviors involving acts (real, not simulated) in which the psychological or physical suffering (including humiliation) of the victim is sexually exciting to the person.

B. The person has acted on these sexual urges with a nonconsenting person, or the sexual urges or fantasies cause marked distress or interpersonal difficulty.

From American Psychiatric Association. *Diagnostic and Statistical Manual of Mental Disorders.* 4th ed. Text rev. Washington, DC: American Psychiatric Association; copyright 2000, with permission.

common among men than among women. Moral masochism involves a need to suffer but is not accompanied by sexual fantasies.

Sexual Sadism.
The DSM-IV-TR diagnostic criteria for sexual sadism are presented in Table 18.3–6. The onset of the disorder is usually before the age of 18 years; most people with sexual sadism are male. According to psychoanalytic theory, sadism is a defense against fears of castration: people with sexual sadism do to others what they fear will happen to them and derive pleasure from expressing their aggressive instincts. The disorder was named after the Marquis de Sade, an 18th-century French author and military officer who was repeatedly imprisoned for his violent sexual acts against women. Sexual sadism is related to rape, although rape is more aptly considered an expression of power. Some sadistic rapists, however, kill their victims after having sex (so-called lust murders).

Voyeurism.
Voyeurism, also known as *scopophilia*, is the recurrent preoccupation with fantasies and acts that involve observing people who are naked or engaged in grooming or sexual activity (Table 18.3–7).

Transvestic Fetishism.
Transvestic fetishism is described as fantasies and sexual urges to dress in opposite-gender clothing as a means of arousal and as an adjunct to masturbation or coitus (Table 18.3–8). Transvestic fetishism typically begins in childhood or early adolescence. As years pass, some men with transvestic fetishism want to dress and live permanently as women. More rarely, women want to dress and live as men. These people are classified in DSM-IV-TR as those with transvestic fetishism and gender dysphoria.

Paraphilia Not Otherwise Specified.
The classification of paraphilia not otherwise specified includes varied paraphilias that do not meet the criteria for any of the aforementioned categories (Table 18.3–9).

Table 18.3–7
DSM-IV-TR Diagnostic Criteria for Voyeurism

A. Over a period of at least 6 months, recurrent, intense sexually arousing fantasies, sexual urges, or behaviors involving the act of observing an unsuspecting person who is naked, in the process of disrobing, or engaging in sexual activity.

B. The person has acted on these sexual urges, or the sexual urges or fantasies cause marked distress or interpersonal difficulty.

From American Psychiatric Association. *Diagnostic and Statistical Manual of Mental Disorders.* 4th ed. Text rev. Washington, DC: American Psychiatric Association; copyright 2000, with permission.

Table 18.3–8
DSM-IV-TR Diagnostic Criteria for Transvestic Fetishism

A. Over a period of at least 6 months, in a heterosexual male, recurrent, intense sexually arousing fantasies, sexual urges, or behaviors involving cross-dressing.

B. The fantasies, sexual urges, or behaviors cause clinically significant distress or impairment in social, occupational, or other important areas of functioning.

Specify if:

   With gender dysphoria: if the person has persistent discomfort with gender role or identity

From American Psychiatric Association. *Diagnostic and Statistical Manual of Mental Disorders.* 4th ed. Text rev. Washington, DC: American Psychiatric Association; copyright 2000, with permission.

TELEPHONE SCATOLOGIA.   Telephone scatologia is characterized by obscene phone calling and involves an unsuspecting partner. Tension and arousal begin in anticipation of phoning; the recipient of the call listens while the telephoner (usually male) verbally exposes his preoccupations or induces her to talk about her sexual activity. The conversation is accompanied by masturbation, which is often completed after the contact is interrupted.

INTERNET SEX.   People also use interactive computer networks, sometimes compulsively, to send obscene messages by electronic mail or to transmit sexually explicit messages and video images. Because of the anonymity of the users in chat rooms who use aliases, on-line sexual activity, also known as *cybersex*, allows some people to engage in all forms of imagined sex acts. Some play the role of the opposite sex ("genderbending"), which represents an alternative method of acting out and expressing homosexual, transvestite, or transsexual fantasies. A danger of on-line sexual activity is that pedophiles may contact children or adolescents who are lured into meeting them and then molested. Some on-line contacts develop into off-line liaisons. Although some people report that the off-line encounters develop into meaningful relationships, most such meetings usually are filled with disappointment and disillusionment, as the fantasized person fails to meet unconscious expectations of perfection. In other situations, when adults meet, rape or even homicide may occur. An estimated 20 percent of Internet users engage in some form of on-line sexual activity, including viewing pornographic images.

NECROPHILIA.   Necrophilia is an obsession with obtaining sexual gratification from cadavers. Most people with this disorder find corpses in morgues, but some have been known to rob graves or even to murder

Table 18.3–9
DSM-IV-TR Diagnostic Criteria for Paraphilia Not Otherwise Specified

This category is included for coding paraphilias that do not meet the criteria for any of the specific categories. Examples include, but are not limited to, telephone scatologia (obscene phone calls), necrophilia (corpses), partialism (exclusive focus on part of body), zoophilia (animals), coprophilia (feces), klismaphilia (enemas), and urophilia (urine).

From American Psychiatric Association. *Diagnostic and Statistical Manual of Mental Disorders.* 4th ed. Text rev. Washington, DC: American Psychiatric Association; copyright 2000, with permission.

to satisfy their sexual urges. According to Richard von Krafft-Ebing, the diagnosis of psychosis is, under all circumstances, justified.

PARTIALISM.   People with the disorder of partialism concentrate their sexual activity on one part of the body to the exclusion of all others. Mouth-genital contact—such as cunnilingus (oral contact with a woman's external genitals), fellatio (oral contact with the penis), and anilingus (oral contact with the anus)—is normally associated with foreplay.

ZOOPHILIA.   In zoophilia, animals—which may be trained to participate—are preferentially incorporated into arousal fantasies or sexual activities, including intercourse, masturbation, and oral-genital contact.

COPROPHILIA AND KLISMAPHILIA.   Coprophilia is attraction to sexual pleasure associated with the desire to defecate on a partner, to be defecated on, or to eat feces (coprophagia). A variant is the compulsive utterance of obscene words (coprolalia). Klismaphilia is the use of enemas as part of sexual stimulation. These paraphilias are associated with fixation at the anal stage of psychosexual development.

UROPHILIA.   Urophilia, a form of urethral eroticism, is interest in sexual pleasure associated with the desire to urinate on a partner or to be urinated on.

MASTURBATION.   Masturbation is a normal activity that is common in all stages of life from infancy to old age, but this viewpoint was not always accepted. Freud believed neurasthenia to be caused by excessive masturbation. In the early 1900s, masturbatory insanity was a common diagnosis in hospitals for the criminally insane in the United States. Masturbation can be defined as a person's achieving sexual pleasure, which usually results in orgasm, by himself or herself (autoeroticism). The frequency of masturbation varies from three to four times a week in adolescence to one to two times a week in adulthood. It is common among married people; Kinsey reported that it occurred on the average of once a month among married couples. Masturbation is abnormal when it is the only type of sexual activity performed in adulthood, when it is done with such frequency as to indicate a compulsion or sexual dysfunction, or when it is consistently preferred to sex with a partner.

HYPOXYPHILIA.   Hypoxyphilia is the desire to achieve an altered state of consciousness secondary to hypoxia while experiencing orgasm. People may use a drug (such as a volatile nitrite or nitrous oxide) to produce hypoxia. Autoerotic asphyxiation is also associated with hypoxic states but should be classified as a form of sexual masochism. (A discussion of autoerotic asphyxiation appears in Chapter 18.2.)

Differential Diagnosis

Clinicians must differentiate a paraphilia from an experimental act that is not recurrent or compulsive and that is done for its novelty. Paraphiliac activity is most likely to occur during adolescence. Some paraphilias (especially the bizarre types) are associated with other mental disorders, such as schizophrenia. Brain diseases may also release perverse impulses.

Course and Prognosis

A poor prognosis for paraphilias is associated with an early age of onset, a high frequency of acts, no guilt or shame about the act, and substance abuse. The course and the prognosis are good when patients have a history of coitus in addition to the paraphilia and when they are self-referred rather than referred by a legal agency.

Treatment

Five types of psychiatric interventions are used to treat people with paraphilias: external control, reduction of sexual drives, treatment of comorbid conditions (such as depression or anxiety), cognitive-behavioral therapy, and dynamic psychotherapy.

Prison is an external control mechanism for sexual crimes that usually does not contain a treatment element. When victimization occurs in a family or work setting, the external control comes from letting supervisors, peers, or other adult family members know of the problem and advising them about eliminating opportunities for the perpetrator to act on his urges.

Drug therapy, including antipsychotic or antidepressant medication, is indicated for the treatment of schizophrenia or depressive disorders if the paraphilia is associated with these disorders. Antiandrogens, such as cyproterone acetate in Europe and medroxyprogesterone acetate (Depo-Provera) in the United States, may reduce the drive to behave sexually by decreasing serum testosterone levels to subnormal concentrations. Serotonergic agents such as fluoxetine (Prozac) have been used in some paraphiliac cases with limited success.

Cognitive-behavioral therapy is used to disrupt learned paraphiliac patterns and modify behavior to make it socially acceptable. The interventions include social skills training, sex education, cognitive restructuring (confronting and destroying the rationalizations used to support victimization of others), and the development of victim empathy. Imaginal desensitization, relaxation technique, and learning what triggers the paraphiliac impulse so that such stimuli can be avoided are also taught. In modified aversive behavior rehearsal, the perpetrator is videotaped acting out his paraphilia with a mannequin. The paraphiliac is then confronted by a therapist and a group of other offenders who ask questions about feelings, thoughts, and motives associated with the act and repeatedly try to correct cognitive distortions and point out lack of victim empathy to the patient.

Insight-oriented psychotherapy is a long-standing treatment approach. Patients have the opportunity to understand their dynamics and the events that caused the paraphilia to develop. In particular, they become aware of the daily events that cause them to act on their impulses (such as a real or fantasized rejection). Treatment helps them deal with life stresses better and enhances their capacity to relate to a life partner. Psychotherapy also allows the patient to regain self-esteem, which in turn allows him or her to approach a partner in a more normal sexual manner. Sex therapy is an appropriate adjunct to the treatment of patients who suffer from specific sexual dysfunctions when they attempt nondeviant sexual activities.

Good prognostic indicators include the presence of only one paraphilia, normal intelligence, the absence of substance abuse, the absence of nonsexual antisocial personality traits, and the presence of a successful adult attachment. However, paraphilias remain significant treatment challenges even under these circumstances.

SEXUAL DISORDER NOT OTHERWISE SPECIFIED

Many sexual disorders are not classifiable as sexual dysfunctions or as paraphilias. These unclassified disorders are rare, poorly documented, not easily classified, or not specifically described in DSM-IV-TR (Table 18.3–10). Some of these are described briefly below.

Table 18.3–10
DSM-IV-TR Diagnostic Criteria for Sexual Disorder Not Otherwise Specified

This category is included for coding a sexual disturbance that does not meet the criteria for any specific sexual disorder and is neither a sexual dysfunction nor a paraphilia. Examples include

1. Marked feelings of inadequacy concerning sexual performance or other traits related to self-imposed standards of masculinity or femininity
2. Distress about a pattern of repeated sexual relationships involving a succession of lovers who are experienced by the individual only as things to be used
3. Persistent and marked distress about sexual orientation

From American Psychiatric Association. *Diagnostic and Statistical Manual of Mental Disorders.* 4th ed. Text rev. Washington, DC: American Psychiatric Association; copyright 2000, with permission.

Postcoital Dysphoria

Postcoital dysphoria occurs during the resolution phase of sexual activity, when people normally experience a sense of general well-being and muscular and psychological relaxation. Some people, instead, become depressed, tense, anxious, and irritable and show psychomotor agitation. The incidence of the disorder is unknown, but it is more common in men than in women. Treatment requires insight-oriented psychotherapy to help patients understand the unconscious antecedents to their behavior and attitudes.

Couple Problems

At times, a complaint arises from the spousal unit or the couple, rather than from an individual dysfunction. For example, one partner may prefer morning sex, but the other functions more readily at night, or the partners have unequal frequencies of desire.

Unconsummated Marriage

A couple involved in an unconsummated marriage have never had coitus and are typically uninformed and inhibited about sexuality. Their feelings of guilt, shame, or inadequacy are increased by their problem, and they experience conflict between their need to seek help and their need to conceal their difficulty. Couples may seek help for the problem after having been married several months or many years.

Body Image Problems

Some people are ashamed of their bodies and experience feelings of inadequacy related to self-imposed standards of masculinity or femininity. They may insist on sex only during total darkness, not allow certain body parts to be seen or touched, or seek unnecessary operative procedures to deal with their imagined inadequacies. Body dysmorphic disorder should be ruled out.

Sex Addiction

The concept of sex addiction developed over the past two decades to refer to persons who compulsively seek out sexual experiences and whose behavior becomes impaired if they are unable to gratify their sexual impulses. The concept of sex addiction derived from the model of addiction to such drugs as heroin or addiction to behavioral patterns, such as gambling. Addiction implies psychological dependence, physical dependence, and the presence of a withdrawal syndrome if the substance (such as the drug) is unavailable or the behavior (such as gambling) is frustrated.

In DSM-IV-TR, the term *sex addiction* is not used, nor is it a disorder that is universally recognized or accepted. Nevertheless, the phenomenon of a person whose entire life revolves around sex-seeking behavior and activities, who spends an excessive amount of time in such behavior, and who often tries to stop such behavior but is unable to do so is well known to clinicians. Such people show repeated and increasingly frequent attempts to have a sexual experience, of which deprivation gives rise to symptoms of distress. Sex addiction is a useful concept heuristically, in that it can alert the clinician to seek an underlying cause for the manifest behavior.

Diagnosis. Sex addicts are unable to control their sexual impulses, which can involve the entire spectrum of sexual fantasy or behavior. Eventually, the need for sexual activity increases, and the person's behavior is motivated solely by the persistent desire to experience the sex act. The history usually reveals a long-standing pattern of such behavior, which the person repeatedly has tried to stop, but without success. Although there may be feelings of guilt and remorse after the act, they are not sufficient to prevent its recurrence. The patient may report that the need to act out is most severe during stressful periods or when angry, depressed, anxious, or otherwise dysphoric. Most acts culminate in a sexual orgasm. Eventually, the sexual activity interferes with the person's social, vocational, or marital life, which begins to deteriorate.

Types of Behavioral Patterns. The paraphilias constitute the behavioral patterns most often found in the sex addict. As defined in DSM-IV-TR, the essential features of a paraphilia are recurrent intense sexual urges of behaviors, including exhibitionism, fetishism, frotteurism, sadomasochism, cross-dressing, voyeurism, and pedophilia. Paraphilias are associated with clinically significant distress and almost invariably interfere with interpersonal relationships, and they often lead to legal complications. In addition to the paraphilias, however, sex addiction can also include behavior that is considered normal, such as coitus and masturbation, except that it is promiscuous and uncontrolled.

Comorbidity. *Comorbidity* (dual diagnosis) refers to the presence of an addiction that coexists with another psychiatric disorder. For example, approximately 50 percent of patients with substance-use disorder also have an additional psychiatric disorder. Similarly, many sex addicts have an associated psychiatric disorder. The diagnosis of comorbidity is often difficult to make because addictive behavior (of all types) can produce extreme anxiety and severe disturbances in mood and affect, especially while the addictive behavior is treated. If, after a period of abstinence, symptoms of a psychiatric disorder remain, the comorbid condition is more easily recognized and diagnosed than during the addictive period. Finally, there is a high correlation between sex addiction and substance-use disorders (up to 80 percent in some studies), which not only complicates the task of diagnosis, but also complicates treatment.

Treatment. Self-help groups based on the 12-step concept used in Alcoholics Anonymous (AA) have been used successfully with many sex addicts. They include such groups as Sexaholics Anonymous (SA), Sex and Love Addicts Anonymous (SLAA), and Sex Addicts Anonymous (SAA). The groups differ in that some are for men or women or for married people or couples. All advocate some degree of abstinence from either the addictive behavior or sex in general. Should a substance-use disorder also be present, the patient often requires referral to AA or Narcotics Anonymous (NA) as well. The patient may enter an inpatient treatment unit when he or she lacks sufficient motivation to control his or her behavior on an outpatient basis or may be a danger to self or others. Additionally, there may be severe medical or psychiatric symptoms that require careful supervision and treatment best carried out in a hospital.

A 42-year-old married businessman with two children was considered a model of virtue in his community. He was active in his church and on the boards of several charitable organizations. He was living a secret life, however, and would lie to his wife, telling her that he was at a board meeting when he was actually visiting massage parlors for paid sex. He eventually was engaging in the behavior four to five times a day, and although he tried to quit many times, he was unable to do so. He knew that he was harming himself by putting his reputation and marriage at risk.

The patient presented himself to the psychiatric emergency room, stating that he would prefer to be dead rather than continue the behavior described. He was admitted with a diagnosis of major depressive disorder and started on a daily dose of 20 mg of fluoxetine. In addition, he received 100 mg of medroxyprogesterone intramuscularly once a day. His need to masturbate diminished markedly and ceased entirely on the third hospital day, as did his mental preoccupation with sex. The medroxyprogesterone was discontinued on the sixth day, when he was discharged. He continued to take fluoxetine, enrolled in a local SA group, and entered individual and couples psychotherapy. His addictive behavior eventually stopped, he was having satisfactory sexual relations with his wife, and he was no longer suicidal or depressed.

Psychotherapy. Insight-oriented psychotherapy may help patients understand the dynamics of their behavioral patterns. Supportive psychotherapy can help repair the interpersonal, social, or occupational damage that occurs. Cognitive-behavioral therapy helps the patient to recognize dysphoric states that precipitate sexual acting out. Marital therapy or couples therapy can aid the patient in regaining self-esteem, which is severely impaired by the time a treatment program is begun. Finally, psychotherapy may be of help in the treatment of any associated psychiatric disorder.

Pharmacotherapy. Most specialists in general addiction avoid the use of pharmacological agents, especially in the early stages of treatment. Substance-dependent people have a tendency to abuse those agents, especially agents with a high abuse potential, such as the benzodiazepines. Pharmacotherapy is of use in the treatment of associated psychiatric disorders, such as major depressive disorders and schizophrenia.

Certain medications may be of use to the sex addict, however, because of their specific effects on reducing the sex drive. Selective serotonin reuptake inhibitors (SSRIs) reduce libido in some persons, a side effect that is used therapeutically. Compulsive masturbation is an example of a behavioral pattern that may benefit from such medication. Medroxyprogesterone acetate diminishes libido in men and thus enables the person better to control sexually addictive behavior.

The use of antiandrogens in women to control hypersexuality has not been sufficiently tested, but since androgenic compounds contribute to the sex drive in women, antiandrogens could be of benefit. Antiandrogenic agents (cyproterone acetate) are not available in the United States but are used in Europe with varying success.

Persistent and Marked Distress about Sexual Orientation

Distress about sexual orientation is characterized by a dissatisfaction with sexual arousal patterns and is usually applied to dissatisfaction with homosexual arousal patterns, a desire to increase heterosexual arousal, and strong negative feelings about being homosexual. A person's occasional statements to the effect that life would be easier if the person were not homosexual do not constitute persistent and marked distress about sexual orientation.

Treatment of sexual orientation distress is controversial. One study reported that with a minimum of 350 hours of psychoanalytic therapy, approximately one-third of 100 bisexual and gay men achieved a heterosexual reorientation at a 5-year follow-up, but this study has been challenged. Behavior therapy and avoidance conditioning techniques have also been used, but with these techniques, behavior may be changed in the laboratory setting but not outside. Prognosis factors weighing in favor of heterosexual reorientation for men include being younger than 35 years, having some experience of heterosexual arousal, and feeling highly motivated to reorient.

Another style of intervention is directed at enabling people with persistent and marked distress about sexual orientation to live comfortably with homosexuality without shame, guilt, anxiety, or depression. Gay counseling centers are engaged with patients in such treatment programs. At present, outcome studies of such centers have not been reported in detail.

As for the treatment of women with persistent and marked distress about sexual orientation, few data are available, and these are primarily single-case studies with variable outcomes.

Gender Identity Disorders

Gender identity is a psychological state that reflects a person's sense of being male or female. It develops in most people by the age of 2 or 3 years and usually corresponds with one's biological sex. Gender identity develops from an innumerable series of cues received from parents and the culture at large that are themselves reactions to the infant's genitalia. Gender role is the external behavioral pattern that reflects a person's inner sense of "I am male" or "I am female." While there is some flexibility regarding what behaviors are considered masculine or feminine, the culture expects men and women (or boys and girls) to have a sense of maleness or femaleness that reflects their anatomical sex. Gender identity disorders involve the persistent desire to be or the insistence that one is of the other sex and extreme discomfort with one's assigned sex and gender role.

EPIDEMIOLOGY

There is little information about the prevalence of gender identity disorders among children, teenagers, and adults. Most estimates of prevalence are based on the number of people seeking sex-reassignment surgery, a number that indicates a male preponderance. The ratios of boys to girls reported in three child-gender-identity clinics were 30 to 1, 17 to 1, and 6 to 1; thus, these clinics had little experience of girls. This disparity may indicate a greater male vulnerability to gender identity disorders or a greater sensitivity to and worry about cross-gender-identified boys than about cross-gender-identified girls in the United States. Studies of boys referred for outpatient psychiatric treatment revealed that up to approximately 50 percent had a significant amount of effeminate behavior. The boys were not referred primarily for problems with gender identity. How many met the criteria for gender identity disorders is unclear.

ETIOLOGY

Biological Factors

Sex steroids influence the expression of sexual behavior in mature men or women; that is, testosterone can increase libido and aggressiveness in women, and estrogen can decrease libido and aggressiveness in men. But masculinity, femininity, and gender identity are more the product of postnatal life events than of prenatal hormonal organization.

The same principle of masculinization or feminization has been applied to the brain. Testosterone affects brain neurons that contribute to the masculinization of the brain in such areas as the hypothalamus. Whether testosterone contributes to so-called masculine or feminine behavioral patterns in gender identity disorders remains a controversial issue. Recent findings point to a difference in the brain of male-to-female transsexuals. In a postmortem sample of six, the red nucleus corresponded in size to that of typical females rather than to typical males; it was not relevant whether the male transsexual was heterosexual or homosexual.

Psychosocial Factors

Children develop a gender identity consonant with their sex of rearing (also known as *assigned sex*). The formation of gender identity is influenced by the interaction of children's temperament and parents' qualities and attitudes. There are culturally acceptable gender roles: boys are not expected to be effeminate, and girls are not expected to be tomboys. There are boys' games (such as cops and robbers) and girls' toys (such as dolls and dollhouses). These roles are learned, although some investigators believe that some boys are temperamentally delicate and sensitive and that some girls are aggressive and energized—traits that are stereotypically known in today's culture as *feminine* and *masculine*, respectively.

The quality of the mother–child relationship in the first years of life is paramount in establishing gender identity. During this period, mothers normally facilitate their children's awareness of and pride in their gender: Children are valued as little boys and girls, but devaluing, hostile mothering can result in gender problems. At the same time, the separation–individuation process is unfolding. When gender problems become associated with separation–individuation problems, the result can be the use of sexuality to remain in relationships characterized by shifts between a desperate infantile closeness and a hostile, devaluing distance.

Some children are given the message that they would be more valued if they adopted the gender identity of the opposite sex. Rejected or abused children may act on such a belief. Gender identity problems can also be triggered by a mother's death, extended absence, or depression, to which a young boy may react by totally identifying with her—that is, by becoming a mother to replace her.

The father's role is also important in the early years, and his presence normally helps the separation–individuation process. Without a father, mother and child may remain overly close. For a girl, the father is normally the prototype of future love objects; for a boy, the father is a model for male identification.

Table 19–1
DSM-IV-TR Diagnostic Criteria for Gender Identity Disorder

A. A strong and persistent cross-gender identification (not merely a desire for any perceived cultural advantages of being the other sex).

In children, the disturbance is manifested by four (or more) of the following:

(1) repeatedly stated desire to be, or insistence that he or she is, the other sex

(2) in boys, preference for cross-dressing or simulating female attire; in girls, insistence on wearing only stereotypical masculine clothing

(3) strong and persistent preferences for cross-sex roles in make-believe play or persistent fantasies of being the other sex

(4) intense desire to participate in the stereotypical games and pastimes of the other sex

(5) strong preference for playmates of the other sex

In adolescents and adults, the disturbance is manifested by symptoms such as a stated desire to be the other sex, frequent passing as the other sex, desire to live or be treated as the other sex, or the conviction that he or she has the typical feelings and reactions of the other sex.

B. Persistent discomfort with his or her sex or sense of inappropriateness in the gender role of that sex.

In children, the disturbance is manifested by any of the following: in boys, assertion that his penis or testes are disgusting or will disappear or assertion that it would be better not to have a penis, or aversion toward rough-and-tumble play and rejection of male stereotypical toys, games, and activities; in girls, rejection of urinating in a sitting position, assertion that she has or will grow a penis, or assertion that she does not want to grow breasts or menstruate, or marked aversion toward normative feminine clothing.

In adolescents and adults, the disturbance is manifested by symptoms such as preoccupation with getting rid of primary and secondary sex characteristics (e.g., request for hormones, surgery, or other procedures to physically alter sexual characteristics to simulate the other sex) or belief that he or she was born the wrong sex.

C. The disturbance is not concurrent with a physical intersex condition.

D. The disturbance causes clinically significant distress or impairment in social, occupational, or other important areas of functioning.

Code based on current age:

Gender identity disorder in children

Gender identity disorder in adolescents or adults

Specify if (for sexually mature individuals):

Sexually attracted to males

Sexually attracted to females

Sexually attracted to both

Sexually attracted to neither

From American Psychiatric Association. *Diagnostic and Statistical Manual of Mental Disorders.* 4th ed. Text rev. Washington, DC: American Psychiatric Association; copyright 2000, with permission.

DIAGNOSIS

According to the fourth revised edition of the *Diagnostic and Statistical Manual of Mental Disorders* (DSM-IV-TR), the essential feature of gender identity disorders is a person's persistent and intense distress about his or her assigned sex and a desire to be, or an insistence that he or she is of, the other sex. As children, both girls and boys show an aversion to normative, stereotypically feminine or masculine clothing and repudiate their respective anatomical characteristics. Table 19–1 lists the DSM-IV-TR criteria for the disorder.

CLINICAL FEATURES

Children

No sharp line can be drawn on the continuum of gender identity disorder between children who should receive a formal diagnosis and those who should not. Girls with the disorder regularly have male companions and an avid interest in sports and rough-and-tumble play; they show no interest in dolls or playing house (unless they play the father or another male role). They may refuse to urinate in a sitting position, claim that they have or will grow a penis, not want to grow breasts or to menstruate, and assert that they will grow up to become a man (not merely to play a man's role).

Boys with the disorder are usually preoccupied with stereotypically female activities. They may have a preference for dressing in girls' or women's clothes or may improvise such items from available material when the genuine articles are not available. (The cross-dressing typically does not cause sexual excitement, as in transvestic fetishism.) They often have a compelling desire to participate in the games and pastimes of girls. Female dolls are often their favorite toys, and girls are regularly their preferred playmates. When playing house, they take a girl's role. Their gestures and actions are often judged to be feminine, and they are usually subjected to male peer group teasing and rejection, a phenomenon that rarely occurs with boyish girls until adolescence. Boys with the disorder may assert that they will grow up to become a woman (not merely in role). They may claim that their penis or testes are disgusting or will disappear or that it would be better not to have a penis or testes. Some children refuse to attend school because of teasing or the pressure to dress in attire stereotypical of their assigned sex. Most children deny being disturbed by the disorder, except that it brings them into conflict with the expectations of their families or peers.

A 5-year-old boy, referred by his general practitioner, was brought for evaluation by both parents. He had been saying either he was a girl or had wanted to be one since age 3. His preferred clothing was that of his sister. He wanted to wear makeup and his mother's jewelry. His favorite toys were dress-up dolls, especially those with long hair. He refused to stand to urinate. In make-believe games he was usually the mommy or a female character. Most of his friends were girls. He showed no interest in sports. All the pictures he drew were of women. The cross-gender behavior was recalled by both parents since the boy was age 2. Neither attempted to interrupt it or redirect his interests until recently, and the boy met their efforts with resistance. They had been advised by a preschool teacher and a regular babysitter to ignore the behavior as it would go away. Neither parent expressed concern that their son would become homosexual, but they are concerned that he may be transsexual.

A 7-year-old girl, referred through her school, had been insisting to other children that she was a boy. Since the age of 2 years she has said that she was a boy and that she did not want to be a girl. Her clothing style preference is that of boys and attempts to make her wear a dress are met with refusal. She watches her father shave and ignores her mother applying makeup. Her friends are boys, and her favorite activities are sports. She has no interest in doll play but loves action and soldier toys and guns. She frequently attempts to urinate while standing.

Adolescents and Adults

There are similar signs and symptoms in adolescents and adults. Adolescents and adults with the disorder manifest a stated desire to be the other sex; they frequently try to pass as a member of the other sex, and they desire to live or to be treated as the other sex. In addition, they desire to acquire the sex characteristics of the opposite sex. They may believe that they were born the wrong sex and may make such characteristic statements as, "I feel that I'm a woman trapped in a male body" or vice versa.

Most retrospective studies of transsexuals report gender identity problems during childhood, but prospective studies of children with gender identity disorders indicate that few become transsexuals and want to change their sex. The disorder is much more common in men (1 per 30,000) than in women (1 per 100,000). Adult transsexuals usually complain that they are uncomfortable wearing the clothes of their assigned sex; therefore, they dress like the other sex dresses and engage in activities associated with the other sex. They find their genitals repugnant, a feeling that may lead to persistent requests for surgery. This desire may override all other wishes.

Men take estrogen to create breasts and other feminine contours, have electrolysis to remove their male hair, and have surgery to remove the testes and the penis and to create an artificial vagina. Women bind their breasts or have a double mastectomy, a hysterectomy, and an oophorectomy; take testosterone to build up muscle mass and deepen the voice; and have surgery in which an artificial phallus is created. These procedures may make a person indistinguishable from members of the other sex. Some investigators describe behavior in sex-reassigned people as almost a caricature of the newly assumed male or female role.

Gender Identity Disorder Not Otherwise Specified

The diagnosis of gender identity disorder not otherwise specified is reserved for people who cannot be classified as having a gender identity disorder with the characteristics just described (Table 19–2). Three examples are listed in DSM-IV-TR: people with intersex conditions and gender dysphoria; adults with transient, stress-related cross-dressing behavior; and people who have a persistent preoccupation with castration or penectomy without a desire to acquire the sex characteristics of the other sex.

Intersex Conditions.   Intersex conditions include a variety of syndromes in which people have gross anatomical or physiological aspects of the opposite sex. They are listed in Table 19–3.

Table 19-2
DSM-IV-TR Diagnostic Criteria for Gender Identity Disorder Not Otherwise Specified

This category is included for coding disorders in gender identity that are not classifiable as a specific gender identity disorder. Examples include

1. Intersex conditions (e.g., partial androgen insensitivity syndrome or congenital adrenal hyperplasia) and accompanying gender dysphoria
2. Transient, stress-related cross-dressing behavior
3. Persistent preoccupation with castration or penectomy without a desire to acquire the sex characteristics of the other sex

From American Psychiatric Association. *Diagnostic and Statistical Manual of Mental Disorders.* 4th ed. Text rev. Washington, DC: American Psychiatric Association; copyright 2000, with permission.

Cross-Dressing.   DSM-IV-TR lists cross-dressing—dressing in clothes of the opposite sex—as a gender identity disorder if it is transient and related to stress. If the disorder is not stress related, people who cross-dress are classified as having transvestic fetishism, which is described as a paraphilia in DSM-IV-TR. An essential feature of transvestic fetishism is that it produces sexual excitement. Stress-related cross-dressing may sometimes produce sexual excitement, but it also reduces a patient's tension and anxiety. Patients may harbor fantasies of cross-dressing but act them out only under stress. Male adult cross-dressers may have the fantasy that they are female, in whole or in part.

Cross-dressing differs from transsexualism in that the patients have no persistent preoccupation with getting rid of their primary and secondary sex characteristics and acquiring the sex characteristics of the other sex. Some people with the disorder once had transvestic fetishism but no longer become sexually aroused by cross-dressing. Other people with the disorder are homosexual men and women who cross-dress. The disorder is most common among female impersonators.

COURSE AND PROGNOSIS

The prognosis for gender identity disorder depends on the age of onset and the intensity of the symptoms. Boys begin to have the disorder before the age of 4 years, and peer conflict develops during the early school years, at about the age of 7 or 8 years. Grossly feminine mannerisms may lessen as boys grow older, especially if attempts are made to discourage such behavior. Cross-dressing may be part of the disorder, and 75 percent of boys who cross-dress begin to do so before age 4. The age of onset is also early for girls, but most give up masculine behavior by adolescence.

In both sexes, homosexuality is likely to develop in one-third to two-thirds of all cases, although, for reasons that are unclear, fewer girls than boys have a homosexual orientation. Steven Levine reported that follow-up studies of gender-disturbed boys consistently indicated that homosexual orientation was the usual adolescent outcome. Transsexualism—that is, the desire for sex-reassignment surgery—occurs in less than 10 percent of cases. Retrospective data on homosexual men indicate a high frequency of cross-gender identifications and feminine gender role behavior during childhood.

Table 19–3
Classification of Intersexual Disorders[a]

Syndrome	Description
Virilizing adrenal hyperplasia (adre-nogenital syndrome)	Results from excess androgens in fetus with XX genotype; most common female intersex disorder; associated with enlarged clitoris, fused labia, hirsutism in adolescence
Turner's syndrome	Results from absence of second female sex chromosome (XO); associated with web neck, dwarfism, cubitus valgus; no sex hormones produced; infertile; usually assigned as females because of female-looking genitals
Klinefelter's syndrome	Genotype is XXY; male habitus present with small penis and rudimentary testes because of low androgen production; weak libido; usually assigned as male
Androgen insensitivity syndrome (testicular-feminizing syndrome)	Congenital X-linked recessive disorder that results in inability of tissues to respond to androgens; external genitals look female and cryptorchid testes present; assigned as females, even though they have XY genotype; in extreme form patient has breasts, normal external genitals, short blind vagina, and absence of pubic and axillary hair
Enzymatic defects in XY genotype (e.g., 5-α-reductase deficiency, 17-hydroxysteroid deficiency)	Congenital interruption in production of testosterone that produces ambiguous genitals and female habitus; usually assigned as female because of female-looking genitalia
Hermaphroditism	True hermaphrodite is rare and characterized by both testes and ovaries in same person (may be 46 XX or 46 XY)
Pseudohermaphroditism	Usually the result of endocrine or enzymatic defect (e.g., adrenal hyperplasia) in persons with normal chromosomes; female pseudohermaphrodites have masculine-looking genitals but are XX; male pseudohermaphrodites have rudimentary testes and external genitals and are XY; assigned as males or females, depending on morphology of genitals

[a]Intersexual disorders include a variety of syndromes that produce persons with gross anatomical or physiological aspects of the opposite sex.

Impaired social and occupational functioning as a result of a person's wanting to participate in the desired (and opposite) gender role is common. Depression is also a common problem, especially if a person feels hopeless about obtaining a sex change with surgery or hormones. Men have been known to castrate themselves, not as a suicide attempt, but as a way of forcing a surgeon to deal with their problem.

TREATMENT

Treatment of gender identity disorders is complex and rarely successful when the goal is to reverse the disorder. Most people with gender identity disorders have fixed ideas and values and are unwilling to change. If and when they enter psychotherapy, it is most often because of depression or anxiety that they

attribute to their condition. Countertransference problems must be addressed assiduously by therapists, many of whom are uncomfortable with patients who have gender identity disorder.

Parents generally bring children with cross-gender behavior patterns to a psychiatrist. Richard Green developed a treatment program designed to inculcate culturally acceptable behavior patterns in boys. Green uses a one-to-one play relationship with children in which adults or peers role-model masculine behavior. Parental counseling in conjunction with group meetings of parents and their children with gender identity disorder is also used. Parents' encouragement of children's atypical behavior (such as dressing a boy in girl's clothing or not cutting his hair) is examined when parents are unaware that they are fostering cross-gender behavior.

Adolescent patients are difficult to treat because of the coexistence of normal identity crises and gender identity confusion. Acting out is common, and adolescents rarely have a strong motivation to alter their stereotypical cross-gender roles. Adult patients generally enter psychotherapy to learn how to deal with their disorder, not to alter it. Therapists usually set a goal of helping patients become comfortable with the gender identity they desire, not of creating a person with a conventional sexual identity. Therapy also explores sex-reassignment surgery and the indications and contraindications for such procedures, which are often impulsively decided on by severely distressed and anxious patients.

Sex-Reassignment Surgery

Surgical treatment is definitive, and because there is no turning back, careful standards preceding the surgery have been developed. Among these standards are the following: Patients must go through a trial of cross-gender living for at least 3 months and sometimes up to 1 year. For some transsexuals, the real-life test may change their minds, because they find it uncomfortable to relate to friends, workers, and lovers in this role. Patients must receive hormone treatments, with estradiol and progesterone in male-to-female changes and testosterone in female-to-male changes. Many transsexuals like the changes that occur in their bodies as a result of this treatment and stop at this point. Approximately 50 percent of transsexuals who meet these criteria go on to sex-reassignment surgery. Outcome studies are highly variable in terms of how success is defined and measured (for example, successful intercourse and body image satisfaction).

Approximately 70 percent of male-to-female and 80 percent of female-to-male sex-reassignment surgery patients report satisfactory results. Unsatisfactory results correlate with a preexisting mental disorder. Suicide in postoperative sex-reassignment surgery patients has been reported in up to 2 percent of all cases. Sex-reassignment surgery is a highly controversial measure that is undergoing much scrutiny.

Hormonal Treatment

Both sexes may be treated with hormones in lieu of surgery. Those who are biologically male take estrogen, and those who are biologically female take testosterone. Patients who take estrogen usually report immediate psychological satisfaction, based on a sense of tranquility, less frequent erections, and fewer sexual drive manifestations than before the hormone treatment. Their new sterility is not of concern to them. After several months, bodily contours become rounded, a limited but pleasing breast enlargement develops, and testicular volume decreases. The quality of the voice does not change. Clinicians must monitor patients for hypertension, hyperglycemia, hepatic dysfunction, and thromboembolic phenomena.

Women who take androgens quickly notice an increased sexual drive, clitoral tingling and enlargement, and, after several months, amenorrhea and hoarseness. If patients undertake weight lifting, a pronounced increase in muscle mass may occur. Depending on the hair distribution already present, patients may have a moderate increase in the amount and coarseness of facial and body hair; some develop frontal balding. Thromboembolic phenomena, hepatic dysfunction, and elevations of cholesterol and triglyceride levels are possible.

Treatment of Intersex Conditions

When intersex conditions are discovered, a panel of pediatric, urological, and psychiatric experts usually determines the sex of rearing on the basis of clinical examination, urological studies, buccal smears, chromosomal analyses, and assessment of the parental wishes.

Education of parents and presentation of the range of options open to them—from in-treatment to surgery—is essential since parents respond to the infant's genitalia in ways that promote the formation of gender identity. Some parents decide

against surgery for ambiguous genitalia but assign the label of boy or girl to the infant on the basis of chromosomal and urological examination. They can then react to the child according to sex role assignment with leeway to adjust the sex assignment should the child act definitively as a member of the sex opposite to the one designated.

If the parents decide on surgery to normalize genital appearance, it is generally undertaken before the age of 3 years. It is easier to assign a child to be female than to assign one to be male because male-to-female genital surgical procedures are far more advanced than are female-to-male procedures. However, that is insufficient reason to assign a chromosomal male to be female.

Treatment of Cross-Dressing

A combined approach, using psychotherapy and pharmacotherapy, is often useful in the treatment of cross-dressing. The stress factors that precipitate the behavior are identified in therapy. The goal is to help patients cope with the stressors appropriately and, if possible, eliminate them. Intrapsychic dynamics about attitudes toward men and women are examined, and unconscious conflicts are identified. Medication, such as antianxiety and antidepressant agents, is used to treat the symptoms. Because cross-dressing may occur impulsively, medications that reinforce impulse control, such as fluoxetine (Prozac), may be helpful. Behavior therapy, aversive conditioning, and hypnosis are alternative methods that may be of use in selected cases.

▲ 20.1 Anorexia Nervosa

In the text revision of the fourth edition of *Diagnostic and Statistical Manual of Mental Disorders* (DSM-IV-TR), anorexia nervosa is characterized as a disorder in which people refuse to maintain a minimally normal weight, intensely fear gaining weight, and significantly misinterpret their body and its shape. DSM-IV-TR also notes that the term anorexia ("lack of appetite") is misleading, because loss of appetite rarely occurs in the early stage of the disorder. Anorexia nervosa is thus characterized by a profound disturbance of body image and the relentless pursuit of thinness, often to the point of starvation. Approximately half of these persons lose weight by drastically reducing their total food intake, and some also develop rigorous exercising programs. The other half of these patients also rigorously diet but lose control and regularly engage in binge eating followed by purging behaviors. Some patients routinely purge after eating small amounts of food.

EPIDEMIOLOGY

Eating disorders of various kinds have been reported in up to 4 percent of adolescent and young adult students. Anorexia nervosa has been reported more frequently over the past several decades than in the past, with increasing reports of the disorder in prepubertal girls and in males. The most common ages of onset of anorexia nervosa are the midteens, but up to 5 percent of anorectic patients have the onset of the disorder in their early 20s. Anorexia nervosa is estimated to occur in approximately 0.5 to 1 percent of adolescent girls. It occurs 10 to 20 times more often in females than in males. The prevalence of young women with some symptoms of anorexia nervosa but who do not meet the diagnostic criteria is estimated to be close to 5 percent.

ETIOLOGY

Biological, social, and psychological factors are implicated in the causes of anorexia nervosa. Some evidence points to higher concordance rates in monozygotic twins than in dizygotic twins. Sisters of patients with anorexia nervosa are likely to be afflicted, but this association may reflect social influences more than genetic factors. Major mood disorders are more common in family members than in the general population. Neurochemically, diminished norepinephrine turnover and activity are suggested by the reduced 3-methoxy-4-hydroxyphenylglycol (MHPG) in the urine and the cerebrospinal fluid (CSF) of some patients with anorexia nervosa. An inverse relation is seen between MHPG and depression in these patients: An increase in MHPG is associated with a decrease in depression.

Biological Factors

Endogenous opioids may contribute to the denial of hunger in patients with anorexia nervosa. Starvation results in many biochemical changes, some of which are also present in depression, such as hypercortisolemia and nonsuppression by dexamethasone. Thyroid function is suppressed as well. These abnormalities are corrected by realimentation. Starvation produces amenorrhea, which reflects lowered hormonal levels (luteinizing, follicle-stimulating, and gonadotropin-releasing hormones). Some anorexia nervosa patients, however, become amenorrheic before significant weight loss. Several computed tomographic (CT) studies reveal enlarged CSF spaces (enlarged sulci and ventricles) in patients with anorexia nervosa during starvation, a finding that is reversed by weight gain. In one positron emission tomographic (PET) scan study, caudate nucleus metabolism was higher in the anorectic state than after realimentation.

Social Factors

Patients with anorexia nervosa find support for their practices in society's emphasis on thinness and exercise. No family constellations are specific to anorexia nervosa, but some evidence indicates that these patients have close but troubled relationships with their parents. In families in which children presented with eating disorders, especially binge eating or purging subtypes, there may be high levels of hostility, chaos, and isolation and low levels of nurturance and empathy. An adolescent with a severe eating disorder may tend to draw attention away from strained marital relationships.

Psychological and Psychodynamic Factors

Anorexia nervosa appears to be a reaction to the demands requiring adolescents to behave more independently and to increase their social and sexual functioning. Patients with the disorder substitute their preoccupations, which are similar to obsessions, with eating and weight gain for other, normal adolescent pursuits. These patients typically lack a sense of autonomy and selfhood. Many experience their bodies as somehow under the control of their parents, so that self-starvation may be an effort to gain validation as a unique and special person. Only through acts of extraordinary self-discipline can an anorectic patient develop a sense of autonomy and selfhood.

Psychoanalytic clinicians who treat patients with anorexia nervosa generally agree that these young patients have been unable to separate psychologically from their mothers. The body may be perceived as though it were inhabited by an introject of an intrusive and unempathic mother. Starvation may unconsciously mean arresting the growth of this intrusive internal object and thereby destroying it. Often, a projective identification process is involved in the interactions between the patient and the patient's family. Many anorectic patients feel that oral desires are greedy and unacceptable; therefore, these desires are projectively disavowed. Other theories have focused on fantasies of oral impregnation. Parents respond to the refusal to eat by becoming frantic about whether the patient is actually eating. The patient can then view the parents as the ones who have unacceptable desires and can projectively disavow them: Others may be voracious and ruled by desire, but not the patient.

DIAGNOSIS AND CLINICAL FEATURES

The onset of anorexia nervosa usually occurs between the ages of 10 and 30 years, although, according to DSM-IV-TR, the most common age of onset is between 14 and 18 years. The DSM-IV-TR diagnostic criteria for anorexia nervosa are given in Table 20.1–1.

The term *anorexia* is a misnomer, because loss of appetite is usually rare until late in the disorder. Evidence that patients are constantly thinking about food is their passions for collecting recipes and for preparing elaborate meals for others. Some patients

Table 20.1–1
DSM-IV-TR Diagnostic Criteria for Anorexia Nervosa

A. Refusal to maintain body weight at or above a minimally normal weight for age and height (e.g., weight loss leading to maintenance of body weight less than 85% of that expected; or failure to make expected weight gain during period of growth, leading to body weight less than 85% of that expected).

B. Intense fear of gaining weight or becoming fat, even though underweight.

C. Disturbance in the way in which one's body weight or shape is experienced, undue influence of body weight or shape on self-evaluation, or denial of the seriousness of the current low body weight.

D. In postmenarcheal females, amenorrhea, i.e., the absence of at least three consecutive menstrual cycles. (A woman is considered to have amenorrhea if her periods occur only following hormone, e.g., estrogen, administration.)

Specify type:

   Restricting type: during the current episode of anorexia nervosa, the person has not regularly engaged in binge-eating or purging behavior (i.e., self-induced vomiting or the misuse of laxatives, diuretics, or enemas)

   Binge-eating/purging type: during the current episode of anorexia nervosa, the person has regularly engaged in binge-eating or purging behavior (i.e., self-induced vomiting or the misuse of laxatives, diuretics, or enemas)

From American Psychiatric Association. *Diagnostic and Statistical Manual of Mental Disorders.* 4th ed. Text rev. Washington, DC: American Psychiatric Association; copyright 2000, with permission.

cannot continuously control their voluntary restriction of food intake and so have eating binges. These binges usually occur secretly and often at night; self-induced vomiting frequently follows an eating binge. Patients abuse laxatives and even diuretics to lose weight, and ritualistic exercising and extensive cycling, walking, jogging, and running are common activities.

Patients with the disorder exhibit peculiar behavior about food. They hide food all over the house and frequently carry large quantities of candies in their pockets and purses. While eating meals, they try to dispose of food in their napkins or hide it in their pockets. They cut their meat into very small pieces and spend a great deal of time rearranging the pieces on their plates. If the patients are confronted with their peculiar behavior, they often deny that their behavior is unusual or flatly refuse to discuss it.

Obsessive-compulsive behavior, depression, and anxiety are other psychiatric symptoms of anorexia nervosa most frequently noted in the literature. Patients tend to be rigid and perfectionist, and somatic complaints, especially epigastric discomfort, are usual. Compulsive stealing, usually of candies and laxatives but occasionally of clothes and other items, is common.

Poor sexual adjustment is frequently described in patients with the disorder. Many adolescent patients with anorexia nervosa have delayed psychosocial sexual development; in adults, a markedly decreased interest in sex often accompanies the onset of the disorder. An unusual minority of anorexia nervosa patients have a premorbid history of promiscuity, substance abuse, or both and during the disorder do not show a decreased interest in sex.

Patients usually come to medical attention when their weight loss becomes apparent. As the weight loss grows profound, physical signs such as hypothermia (as low as 35°C), dependent edema, bradycardia, hypotension, and lanugo (the appearance of neonatal-like hair) appear, and patients show a variety of metabolic changes. Some female patients with anorexia nervosa come to medical attention because of amenorrhea, which often appears before their weight loss is noticeable. Some patients induce vomiting or abuse purgatives and diuretics; such behavior causes concern about hypokalemic alkalosis. Impaired water diuresis may be noted.

Electrocardiographic (ECG) changes, such as flattening or inversion of the T waves, ST segment depression, and lengthening of the QT interval, have been noted in the emaciated stage of anorexia nervosa. ECG changes may also result from potassium loss, which can lead to death. Gastric dilation is a rare complication of anorexia nervosa. In some patients, aortography has shown a superior mesenteric artery syndrome.

Subtypes

DSM-IV-TR identifies two subtypes of anorexia nervosa—the restricting type and the binge-eating/purging type. Binge eating–purging is common among patients with anorexia nervosa and develops in up to 50 percent of them. Each type appears to have distinct historic and clinical features. Those who practice binge eating and purging share many features with people who have bulimia nervosa without anorexia nervosa. Those who binge eat and purge tend to have families in which some members are obese, and they themselves have histories of heavier body weights before the disorder than do people with the restricting type. Binge-eating/purging people are likely to be associated with substance abuse, impulse control disorders, and personality disorders. People with restricting anorexia nervosa limit their food selection, take in as few calories as possible, and often have obsessive-compulsive traits with respect to food and other matters. Both types of people are preoccupied with weight and body image, and both may exercise for hours every day and exhibit bizarre eating behaviors. Both may be socially isolated and have depressive disorder symptoms and diminished sexual interest. Some people with anorexia nervosa may purge but not binge.

DIFFERENTIAL DIAGNOSIS

The differential diagnosis of anorexia nervosa is complicated by patients' denial of the symptoms, the secrecy surrounding their bizarre eating rituals, and their resistance to seeking treatment. Thus, it may be difficult to identify the mechanism of weight loss and the patient's associated ruminative thoughts about distortions of body image.

Clinicians must ascertain that a patient does not have a medical illness that can account for the weight loss (for example, a brain tumor or cancer). Weight loss, peculiar eating behaviors, and vomiting can occur in several mental disorders. Depressive disorders and anorexia nervosa have several features in common, such as depressed feelings, crying spells, sleep disturbance, obsessive ruminations, and occasional suicidal thoughts. The two disorders, however, have several distinguishing features. Generally, a patient with a depressive disorder has a decreased appetite, whereas a patient with anorexia nervosa claims to have a normal appetite and to feel hungry; only in the severe stages of anorexia nervosa do patients actually have a decreased appetite. In contrast to depressive agitation, the hyperactivity seen in anorexia nervosa is planned and ritualistic. The preoccupation with recipes and the caloric content of foods and the preparation of gourmet feasts is typical of patients with anorexia nervosa but is absent in patients with a depressive disorder. And, in depressive disorders, patients have no intense fear of obesity or disturbance of body image.

Weight fluctuations, vomiting, and peculiar food handling may occur in somatization disorder. On rare occasions, a patient fulfills the diagnostic criteria for both somatization disorder and anorexia nervosa; in such a case, both diagnoses should be made. Generally, the weight loss in somatization disorder is not as severe as that in anorexia nervosa, nor does a patient with somatization disorder express a morbid fear of becoming overweight, as is common in the anorexia nervosa patient. Amenorrhea for 3 months or longer is unusual in somatization disorder.

In schizophrenic patients, delusions about food are seldom concerned with caloric content. More likely, they believe the food to be poisoned. Schizophrenic patients are rarely preoccupied with a fear of becoming obese and do not have the hyperactivity that is seen in patients with anorexia nervosa. Schizophrenic patients have bizarre eating habits but not the entire syndrome of anorexia nervosa.

Anorexia nervosa must be differentiated from bulimia nervosa, a disorder in which episodic binge eating, followed by depressive moods, self-deprecating thoughts, and often self-induced vomiting, occurs while patients maintain their weight within a normal range. Patients with bulimia nervosa seldom lose 15 percent of their weight, but the two conditions frequently coexist.

COURSE AND PROGNOSIS

The course of anorexia nervosa varies greatly—spontaneous recovery without treatment, recovery after a variety of treat-

ments, a fluctuating course of weight gains followed by relapses, a gradually deteriorating course resulting in death caused by complications of starvation. A recent study reviewing subtypes of anorexic patients found that restricting-type anorexic patients seemed to be less likely to recover than those who were of the binge-eating/purging type. The short-term response of patients to almost all hospital treatment programs is good. In those who have regained sufficient weight, however, preoccupation with food and body weight often continues, social relationships are often poor, and depression is often present. In general, the prognosis is not good. Studies have shown a range of mortality rates from 5 to 18 percent.

Indicators of a favorable outcome are the admission of hunger, a lessening of denial and immaturity, and improved self-esteem. Such factors as childhood neuroticism, parental conflict, bulimia nervosa, vomiting, laxative abuse, and various behavioral manifestations (such as obsessive-compulsive, hysterical, depressive, psychosomatic, neurotic, and denial symptoms) have been related to poor outcome in some studies but have not been significant in affecting the outcome in other studies.

Ten-year outcome studies in the United States have shown that approximately one-fourth of the patients recover completely and another one-half markedly improve and function fairly well. The other one-fourth includes an overall 7 percent mortality rate and those who are functioning poorly with a chronic underweight condition. Swedish and English studies over a 20- and 30-year period have a mortality rate of 18 percent. Approximately half of anorexia nervosa patients will eventually have the symptoms of bulimia, usually within the first year after the onset of anorexia nervosa.

TREATMENT

In view of the complicated psychological and medical implications of anorexia nervosa, a comprehensive treatment plan, including hospitalization when necessary and both individual and family therapy, is recommended. Behavioral, interpersonal, and cognitive approaches and, in some cases, medication should be considered.

Hospitalization

The first consideration in the treatment of anorexia nervosa is to restore patients' nutritional state; dehydration, starvation, and electrolyte imbalances can lead to serious health compromises and, in some cases, death. The decision to hospitalize a patient is based on the patient's medical condition and the degree of structure needed to ensure patient cooperation. In general, anorexia nervosa patients who are 20 percent below the expected weight for their height are recommended for inpatient programs, and patients who are 30 percent below their expected weight require psychiatric hospitalization that ranges from 2 to 6 months.

Inpatient psychiatric programs for patients with anorexia nervosa generally use a combination of a behavioral management approach, individual psychotherapy, family education and therapy, and, in some cases, psychotropic medications. Successful treatment is promoted by the ability of staff members to maintain a firm yet supportive approach to patients, often through a combination of positive reinforcers (praise) and negative reinforcers (restriction of exercise and purging behavior).

The program must have some flexibility for individualizing treatment to meet patients' needs and cognitive abilities. Patients must become willing participants for treatment to succeed in the long run.

After patients are discharged from the hospital, clinicians usually find it necessary to continue outpatient supervision of the problems identified in the patients and their families.

Psychotherapy

Cognitive-Behavioral Therapy.   Cognitive and behavior therapy principles can be applied in both impatient and outpatient settings. Behavior therapy has been found to be effective for inducing weight gain. Monitoring is an essential component of cognitive-behavioral therapy. Patients are taught to monitor their food intake, their feelings and emotions, their bingeing and purging behaviors, and their problems in interpersonal relationships. Cognitive restructuring is a method that patients are taught to identify autonomic thoughts and to challenge their core beliefs. Problem solving is a specific method whereby patients learn how to think through and devise strategies to cope with their food-related and interpersonal problems. Patients' vulnerability to rely on anorexic behaviors as a means of coping can be reached if they can learn to use these techniques effectively.

Dynamic Psychotherapy.   Dynamic expressive-supportive psychotherapy is sometimes used in the treatment of patients with anorexia nervosa, but patients' resistances may make the process difficult and painstaking. Because patients view their symptoms as constituting the core of their specialness, therapists must avoid excessive investment in trying to change their eating behaviors. The opening phase of the psychotherapy process must be geared to building a therapeutic alliance. Patients may experience early interpretations as though someone else were telling them what they really feel and thereby minimizing and invalidating their own experiences. Therapists who empathize with patients' points of view and take an active interest in what their patients think and feel, however, convey to patients that their autonomy is respected. Above all, psychotherapists must be flexible, persistent, and durable in the face of patients' tendencies to defeat any efforts to help them.

Family Therapy.   A family analysis should be done on all anorexia nervosa patients who are living with their families. On the basis of this analysis, a clinical judgment can be made as to what type of family therapy or counseling is advisable. In some cases, family therapy is not possible, in which case individual therapy is advised to address issues of family relationships. In one controlled family therapy study in London, anorectic patients younger than 18 benefited from family therapy, whereas patients older than 18 did worse in family therapy compared with the control therapy. There are no controlled studies for the combination of individual and family therapy. However, in actual practice, most clinicians provide individual therapy and some form of family counseling in managing anorexia nervosa patients.

Pharmacotherapy

Pharmacological studies have not yet identified any medication resulting in definitive improvement of the core symptoms of anorexia nervosa. Some reports support the use of cyproheptadine (Periactin), a drug with antihistaminic and antiserotonergic properties, for patients with the restricting type of anorexia nervosa. Amitriptyline (Elavil) has also been reported to have some benefit. Other medications that have been tried by patients with anorexia nervosa with variable results include clomipramine (Anafranil), pimozide (Orap), and chlorpromazine (Thorazine). Trials of fluoxetine (Prozac) have resulted in some reports of weight gain, and serotonergic agents may yield positive responses in the future. In anorexia nervosa patients with coexisting depressive disorders, the depressive condition should be treated. Concern exists about the use of tricyclic drugs in low-weight, depressed patients with anorexia nervosa, who may be vulnerable to hypotension, cardiac arrhythmia, and dehydration. Once an adequate nutritional status has been attained, the risks of serious side effects from the tricyclic drugs may decrease; in some cases, the depression improves with weight gain and normalized nutritional status.

▲ 20.2 Bulimia Nervosa and Eating Disorder Not Otherwise Specified

BULIMIA NERVOSA

Bulimia is merely a term that means *binge eating*, which is defined as eating more food than most people in similar circumstances and in a similar period of time, accompanied by a strong sense of losing control. When binge eating occurs in relatively normal-weight or overweight persons who are also excessively concerned with their body shape and weight and who regularly engage in behaviors to counteract the calorie gain in binges, the binge eating is in the context of the disorder known as *bulimia nervosa.*

Epidemiology

Bulimia nervosa is more prevalent than is anorexia nervosa. Estimates of bulimia nervosa range from 1 to 3 percent of young women. Like anorexia nervosa, bulimia nervosa is significantly more common in women than in men, but its onset is often later in adolescence than is the onset of anorexia nervosa. According to the fourth revised edition of the *Diagnostic and Statistical Manual of Mental Disorders* (DSM-IV-TR), the rate of occurrence in males is one-tenth of that in females. The onset may even occur in early adulthood. Occasional symptoms of bulimia nervosa, such as isolated episodes of binge eating and purging, have been reported in up to 40 percent of college women. Bulimia nervosa is often present in normal-weight young women, but sometimes patients have a history of obesity. In industrialized countries, the prevalence is approximately 1 percent of the general population.

Etiology

Biological Factors.   Some investigators have attempted to associate cycles of bingeing and purging with various neurotransmitters. Because antidepressants often benefit patients with bulimia nervosa and because serotonin has been linked to satiety, serotonin and norepinephrine have been implicated. Because plasma endorphin levels are raised in some bulimia nervosa patients who vomit, the feelings of well-being after vomiting that some of these patients experience may be mediated by raised endorphin levels. According to DSM-IV-TR, there is an increased frequency of bulimia nervosa in first-degree relatives of persons with the disorder.

Social Factors.   Patients with bulimia nervosa, like those with anorexia nervosa, tend to be high achievers and to respond to societal pressures to be slender. As with anorexia nervosa patients, many patients with bulimia nervosa are depressed and have increased familial depression, but the families of patients with bulimia nervosa are generally less close and more conflictual than are the families of anorexia nervosa patients. Patients with bulimia nervosa describe their parents as neglectful and rejecting.

Psychological Factors.   Patients with bulimia nervosa, like those with anorexia nervosa, have difficulties with adolescent demands, but bulimia nervosa patients are more outgoing, angry, and impulsive than are anorexia nervosa patients. Alcohol dependence, shoplifting, and emotional lability (including suicide attempts) are associated with bulimia nervosa. These patients generally experience their uncontrolled eating as more ego-dystonic than do anorexia nervosa patients and so more readily seek help.

Patients with bulimia nervosa lack superego control and the ego strength of their counterparts with anorexia nervosa. Their difficulties in controlling their impulses are often manifested by substance dependence and self-destructive sexual relationships, in addition to the binge eating and purging that are the hallmarks of the disorder. Many bulimia nervosa patients have histories of difficulties in separating from caretakers, as manifested by the absence of transitional objects during their early childhood years. Some clinicians have observed that patients with bulimia nervosa use their own bodies as transitional objects. The struggle for separation from a maternal figure is played out in the ambivalence toward food; eating may represent a wish to fuse with the caretaker, and regurgitating may unconsciously express a wish for separation.

Diagnosis and Clinical Features

According to DSM-IV-TR, the essential features of bulimia nervosa are recurrent episodes of binge eating; a sense of lack of control over eating during the eating binges; self-induced vomiting, the misuse of laxatives or diuretics, fasting, or excessive exercise to prevent weight gain; and persistent self-evaluation unduly influenced by body shape and weight (Table 20.2–1). Bingeing usually precedes vomiting by approximately 1 hour.

Vomiting is common and is usually induced by sticking a finger down the throat, although some patients are able to vomit at will. Vomiting decreases the abdominal pain and the feeling of being bloated and allows patients to continue eating without fear of gaining weight. Depression, sometimes called *postbinge anguish*, often follows the episode. During binges, patients eat food that is sweet, high in calories, and generally soft or of

**Table 20.2–1
DSM-IV-TR Diagnostic Criteria for
Bulimia Nervosa**

A. Recurrent episodes of binge eating. An episode of binge eating is characterized by both of the following:
   (1) eating, in a discrete period of time (e.g., within any 2-hour period), an amount of food that is definitely larger than most people would eat during a similar period of time and under similar circumstances
   (2) a sense of lack of control over eating during the episode (e.g., a feeling that one cannot stop eating or control what or how much one is eating)
B. Recurrent inappropriate compensatory behavior in order to prevent weight gain, such as self-induced vomiting; misuse of laxatives, diuretics, enemas, or other medications; fasting; or excessive exercise.
C. The binge eating and inappropriate compensatory behaviors both occur, on average, at least twice a week for 3 months.
D. Self-evaluation is unduly influenced by body shape and weight.
E. The disturbance does not occur exclusively during episodes of anorexia nervosa.
Specify type:
   Purging type: during the current episode of bulimia nervosa, the person has regularly engaged in self-induced vomiting or the misuse of laxatives, diuretics, or enemas
   Nonpurging type: during the current episode of bulimia nervosa, the person has used other inappropriate compensatory behaviors, such as fasting or excessive exercise, but has not regularly engaged in self-induced vomiting or the misuse of laxatives, diuretics, or enemas

From American Psychiatric Association. *Diagnostic and Statistical Manual of Mental Disorders.* 4th ed. Text rev. Washington, DC: American Psychiatric Association; copyright 2000, with permission.

smooth texture, such as cakes and pastry. Some patients prefer bulky foods without regard to taste. The food is eaten secretly and rapidly and is sometimes not even chewed.

Most patients with bulimia nervosa are within their normal weight range, but some may be underweight or overweight. These patients are concerned about their body image and their appearance, worry about how others see them, and are concerned about their sexual attractiveness. Most are sexually active, compared with anorexia nervosa patients, who are not interested in sex. Pica and struggles during meals are sometimes revealed in the histories of patients with bulimia nervosa.

Bulimia nervosa occurs in people with high rates of mood disorders and impulse control disorders. Bulimia nervosa is also reported to occur in those at risk for substance-related disorders and a variety of personality disorders. Patients with bulimia nervosa also have increased rates of anxiety disorders, bipolar I disorder, and dissociative disorders, and histories of sexual abuse.

Subtypes.   There is evidence that bulimia persons who purge differ from binge eaters who do not purge in that the latter tend to have less body-image disturbance and less anxiety concerning eating. Bulimia nervosa patients who do not purge tend to be obese. There are also distinct physiological differences between bulimia patients who purge and those who do not. Because of all these differences, the diagnosis of bulimia nervosa is subtyped into a purging type, for those who regularly engage in self-induced vomiting or the use of laxatives of diuretics, and a nonpurging type, for those who use strict dieting, fasting, or vigorous exercise but do not regularly engage in purging.

Patients with the purging type of bulimia nervosa may be at risk for certain medical complications, such as hypokalemia from vomiting or laxative abuse and hypochloremic alkalosis. Those who vomit repeatedly are at risk for gastric and esophageal tears, although these complications are rare. Patients who purge may have a different course from that of patients who binge and then diet or exercise.

Pathology and Laboratory Examinations

Bulimia nervosa can result in electrolyte abnormalities and various degrees of starvation, although it may not be as obvious as in low-weight patients with anorexia nervosa. Thus, even normal-weight patients with bulimia nervosa should have laboratory studies of electrolytes and metabolism. In general, thyroid function remains intact in bulimia nervosa, but patients may show nonsuppression on the dexamethasone-suppression test (DST). Dehydration and electrolyte disturbances are likely to occur in bulimia nervosa patients who regularly purge. These patients commonly exhibit hypomagnesemia and hyperamylasemia. Although not a core diagnostic feature, many patients with bulimia nervosa have menstrual disturbances. Hypotension and bradycardia occur in some patients.

Differential Diagnosis

The diagnosis of bulimia nervosa cannot be made if the binge eating and purging behaviors occur exclusively during episodes of anorexia nervosa. In such cases, the diagnosis is anorexia nervosa, binge-eating/purging type.

Clinicians must ascertain that patients have no neurological disease, such as epileptic-equivalent seizures, central nervous system (CNS) tumors, Klüver-Bucy syndrome, or Kleine-Levin syndrome.

The pathological features manifested by Klüver-Bucy syndrome are visual agnosia, compulsive licking and biting, examination of objects by the mouth, inability to ignore any stimulus, placidity, altered sexual behavior (hypersexuality), and altered dietary habits, especially hyperphagia. The syndrome is exceedingly rare and is unlikely to cause a problem in differential diagnosis. Kleine-Levin syndrome consists of periodic hypersomnia lasting for 2 to 3 weeks and hyperphagia. As in bulimia nervosa, the onset is usually during adolescence, but the syndrome is more common in men than in women. Patients with borderline personality disorder sometimes binge eat, but the eating is associated with the other signs of the disorder.

Course and Prognosis

In the short run, patients with bulimia nervosa who are able to engage in treatment have reported more than 50 percent improvement in binge eating and purging; among outpatients, improvement seems to last more than 5 years. The patients are not symptom free during periods of improvement, however; bulimia nervosa is a chronic disorder with a waxing and waning course. Some patients with mild courses have long-term remissions. Other patients are disabled by the disorder and have been hospitalized; less than one-third of them are doing well at 3-year follow-up, more than one-third have some improvement in

their symptoms, and approximately one-third have a poor outcome, with chronic symptoms, within 3 years. In a recent study, at 5 to 10 years, approximately half of patients recovered fully from the disorder, whereas 20 percent continued to meet full diagnostic criteria for bulimia nervosa.

The prognosis depends on the severity of the purging sequelae—that is, whether a patient has electrolyte imbalances and to what degree the frequent vomiting results in esophagitis, amylasemia, salivary gland enlargement, and dental caries. In some cases of untreated bulimia nervosa, spontaneous remission occurs in 1 to 2 years.

Treatment

Most patients with uncomplicated bulimia nervosa do not require hospitalization. In general, patients with bulimia nervosa are not as secretive about their symptoms as are patients with anorexia nervosa. Therefore, outpatient treatment is usually not difficult, but psychotherapy is frequently stormy and may be prolonged. Some obese patients with bulimia nervosa who have had prolonged psychotherapy do surprisingly well. In some cases—when eating binges are out of control, outpatient treatment does not work, or a patient exhibits such additional psychiatric symptoms as suicidality and substance abuse—hospitalization may become necessary. In addition, in cases of severe purging, resulting electrolyte and metabolic disturbances may necessitate hospitalization.

Psychotherapy
COGNITIVE-BEHAVIORAL THERAPY.   Cognitive-behavioral therapy should the considered the benchmark, first-line treatment for bulimia nervosa. The data supporting the efficacy of cognitive-behavioral therapy is based on strict adherence to rigorously implemented, highly detailed, manual-guided treatments that include approximately 18 to 20 sessions over 5 to 6 months. Cognitive-behavioral therapy implements a number of cognitive and behavioral procedures to (1) interrupt this self-maintaining behavioral cycle of bingeing and dieting and (2) alter the individual's dysfunctional cognitions and beliefs about food, weight, body image, and overall self-concept.

DYNAMIC PSYCHOTHERAPY.   Psychodynamic treatment of patients with bulimia nervosa has revealed a tendency to concretize introjective and projective defense mechanisms. In a manner analogous to splitting, patients divide food into two categories: items that are nutritious and those that are unhealthy. Food that is designated nutritious may be ingested and retained because it unconsciously symbolizes good introjects, but junk food is unconsciously associated with bad introjects and is therefore expelled by vomiting, with the unconscious fantasy that all destructiveness, hate, and badness are being evacuated. Patients may temporarily feel good after vomiting because of the fantasized evacuation, but the associated feeling of "being all good" is short-lived because it is based on an unstable combination of splitting and projection.

Pharmacotherapy.   Antidepressant medications have been shown to be helpful in bulimia. This includes the serotonin reuptake inhibitors (SSRIs) such as fluoxetine (Prozac). This may be based on elevating central 5-hydroxytryptamine levels. Antide-

**Table 20.2–2
DSM-IV-TR Diagnostic Criteria for Eating Disorder Not Otherwise Specified**

The eating disorder not otherwise specified category is for disorders of eating that do not meet the criteria for any specific eating disorder. Examples include

1. For females, all of the criteria for anorexia nervosa are met except that the individual has regular menses.
2. All of the criteria for anorexia nervosa are met except that, despite significant weight loss, the individual's current weight is in the normal range.
3. All of the criteria for bulimia nervosa are met except that the binge eating and inappropriate compensatory mechanisms occur at a frequency of less than twice a week or for a duration of less than 3 months.
4. The regular use of inappropriate compensatory behavior by an individual of normal body weight after eating small amounts of food (e.g., self-induced vomiting after the consumption of two cookies).
5. Repeatedly chewing and spitting out, but not swallowing, large amounts of food.
6. Binge-eating disorder: recurrent episodes of binge eating in the absence of the regular use of inappropriate compensatory behaviors characteristic of bulimia nervosa.

From American Psychiatric Association. *Diagnostic and Statistical Manual of Mental Disorders.* 4th ed. Text rev. Washington, DC: American Psychiatric Association; copyright 2000, with permission.

**Table 20.2–3
DSM-IV-TR Research Criteria for Binge-Eating Disorder**

A. Recurrent episodes of binge eating. An episode of binge eating is characterized by both of the following:
  (1) eating, in a discrete period of time (e.g., within any 2-hour period), an amount of food that is definitely larger than what most people would eat in a similar period of time under similar circumstances
  (2) a sense of lack of control over eating during the episode (e.g., a feeling that one cannot stop eating or control what or how much one is eating)
B. The binge-eating episodes are associated with three (or more) of the following:
  (1) eating much more rapidly than normal
  (2) eating until feeling uncomfortably full
  (3) eating large amounts of food when not feeling physically hungry
  (4) eating alone because of being embarrassed by how much one is eating
  (5) feeling disgusted with oneself, depressed, or very guilty after overeating
C. Marked distress regarding binge eating is present.
D. The binge eating occurs, on average, at least 2 days a week for 6 months.
  Note: The method of determining frequency differs from that used for bulimia nervosa; future research should address whether the preferred method of setting a frequency threshold is counting the number of days on which binges occur or counting the number of episodes of binge eating.
E. The binge eating is not associated with the regular use of inappropriate compensatory behaviors (e.g., purging, fasting, excessive exercise) and does not occur exclusively during the course of anorexia nervosa or bulimia nervosa.

From American Psychiatric Association. *Diagnostic and Statistical Manual of Mental Disorders.* 4th ed. Text rev. Washington, DC: American Psychiatric Association; copyright 2000, with permission.

pressant medications can reduce binge eating and purging independent of the presence of a mood disorder. Thus, for particularly difficult binge–purge cycles that are not responsive to psychotherapy alone, antidepressants have been successfully used. Imipramine (Tofranil), desipramine (Norpramin), trazodone (Desyrel), and monoamine oxidase inhibitors (MAOIs) have been helpful. In general, most of the antidepressants have been effective at dosages usually given in the treatment of depressive disorders. However, dosages of fluoxetine that are effective in decreasing binge eating may be higher (60 to 80 mg a day) than those used for depressive disorders. In cases of comorbid depressive disorders and bulimia nervosa, medication is helpful. Carbamazepine (Tegretol) and lithium (Eskalith) have not shown impressive results as treatments for binge eating, but they have been used in the treatment of bulimia nervosa patients with comorbid mood disorders, such as bipolar I disorder. There is evidence that the use of antidepressants alone results in a 22 percent rate of abstinence from bingeing and purging. Other studies show that the combination of cognitive-behavioral therapy and medications is the most effective treatment.

EATING DISORDER NOT OTHERWISE SPECIFIED

The DSM-IV-TR diagnostic classification of eating disorder not otherwise specified is a residual category used for eating disorders that do not meet the criteria for a specific eating disorder (Table 20.2–2). Binge-eating disorder—that is, recurrent episodes of binge eating in the absence of the inappropriate compensatory behaviors characteristic of bulimia nervosa (Table 20.2–3)—falls into this category. Such patients are not fixated on body shape and weight.

21 ▲

Normal Sleep and Sleep Disorders

▲ 21.1 Normal Sleep

Sleep is a regular, recurrent, easily reversible state that is characterized by relative quiescence and by a great increase in the threshold of response to external stimuli relative to the waking state. Close monitoring of sleep is an important part of clinical practice; sleep disturbance is often an early symptom of impending mental illness. Some mental disorders are associated with characteristic changes in sleep physiology.

ELECTROPHYSIOLOGY OF SLEEP

Sleep is made up of two physiological states: nonrapid eye movement (NREM) sleep and rapid eye movement (REM) sleep. In NREM sleep, which is composed of stages 1 through 4, most physiological functions are markedly reduced compared with wakefulness. REM sleep is a qualitatively different kind of sleep characterized by a high level of brain activity and physiological activity levels similar to those in wakefulness. Approximately 90 minutes after sleep onset, NREM yields to the first REM episode of the night. This REM latency of 90 minutes is a consistent finding in normal adults: A shortening of REM latency frequently occurs with such disorders as depressive disorders and narcolepsy. The electroencephalogram (EEG) records the rapid conjugate eye movements that are the identifying feature of the sleep state (there are no or few REMs in NREM sleep); the EEG pattern consists of low-voltage, random fast activity with sawtooth waves; the electromyograph (EMG) shows a marked reduction in muscle tone.

In normal people, NREM sleep is a peaceful state relative to waking. The pulse rate is typically slowed five to ten beats a minute below the level of restful waking and is very regular. Respiration is similarly affected, and blood pressure also tends to be low, with few minute-to-minute variations. The resting muscle potential of the body musculature is lower in REM sleep than in a waking state. Episodic, involuntary body movements are present in NREM sleep. There are few REMs, if any, and seldom any penile erections in men. Blood flow through most tissues, including cerebral blood flow, is slightly reduced.

The deepest portions of NREM sleep—stages 3 and 4—are sometimes associated with unusual arousal characteristics. When people are aroused 30 minutes to 1 hour after sleep onset—usually in slow-wave sleep—they are disoriented, and their thinking is disorganized. Brief arousals from slow-wave sleep are also associated with amnesia for events that occur during the arousal. The disorganization during arousal from stage 3 or stage 4 may result in specific problems, including enuresis, somnambulism, and stage 4 nightmares or night terrors.

Polygraphic measures during REM sleep show irregular patterns, sometimes close to aroused waking patterns. Because of this observation, REM sleep has also been termed *paradoxical sleep*. Pulse, respiration, and blood pressure in humans are all high during REM sleep—much higher than during NREM sleep and often higher than during waking. Even more striking than the level or rate is the variability from minute to minute. Brain oxygen use increases during REM sleep. The ventilatory response to increased levels of carbon dioxide (CO_2) is depressed during REM sleep, so that there is no increase in tidal volume as the partial pressure of carbon dioxide (Pco_2) increases. Thermoregulation is altered during REM sleep. In contrast to the homeothermic condition of temperature regulation that is present during wakefulness or NREM sleep, a poikilothermic condition (a state in which animal temperature varies with the changes in the temperature of the surrounding medium) prevails during REM sleep. Poikilothermia, which is characteristic of reptiles, results in a failure to respond to changes in ambient temperature with shivering or sweating, whichever is appropriate to maintaining body temperature. Almost every REM period in men is accompanied by a partial or full penile erection. This finding is of significant clinical value in evaluating the cause of impotence; the nocturnal penile tumescence study is one of the most commonly requested sleep laboratory tests. Another physiological change that occurs during REM sleep is the near-total paralysis of the skeletal (postural) muscles. Because of this motor inhibition, body movement is absent during REM sleep. Probably the most distinctive feature of REM sleep is dreaming. People awakened during REM sleep frequently (60 to 90 percent of the time) report that they had been dreaming. Dreams during REM sleep are typically abstract and surreal. Dreaming does occur during NREM sleep, but it is typically lucid and purposeful.

The cyclical nature of sleep is regular and reliable; a REM period occurs approximately every 90 to 100 minutes during the night (Fig 21.1–1). The first REM period tends to be the shortest, usually lasting less than 10 minutes; the later REM periods may last 15 to 40 minutes each. Most REM periods occur in the last third of the night, whereas most stage 4 sleep occurs in the first third of the night.

These sleep patterns change over a person's life span. In the neonatal period, REM sleep represents more than 50 percent of total sleep time, and the EEG pattern moves from the alert state directly to the REM state without going through stages 1 through 4. Newborns sleep approximately 16 hours a day, with

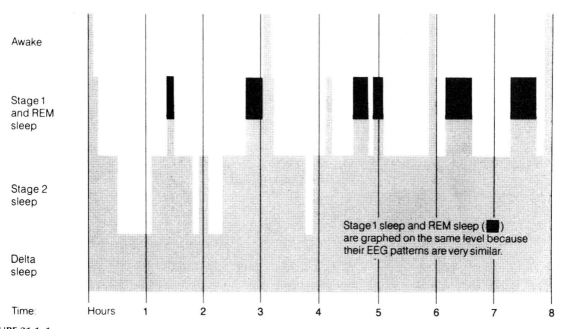

Awake

Stage 1
and REM
sleep

Stage 2
sleep

Stage 1 sleep and REM sleep (■)
are graphed on the same level because
their EEG patterns are very similar.

Delta
sleep

Time: Hours   1   2   3   4   5   6   7   8

FIGURE 21.1–1

Typical sleep pattern of a young human adult. (Reproduced with permission from Hauri P. *The sleep disorders.* Current Concepts, Kalamazoo, MI: Upjohn; 1982:82.)

brief periods of wakefulness. By 4 months of age, the pattern shifts so that the total percentage of REM sleep drops to less than 40 percent, and entry into sleep occurs with an initial period of NREM sleep. By young adulthood, the distribution of sleep stages is as follows:

NREM (75 percent)
Stage 1:   5 percent
Stage 2: 45 percent
Stage 3: 12 percent
Stage 4: 13 percent
REM (25 percent)

This distribution remains relatively constant into old age, although a reduction occurs in both slow-wave sleep and REM sleep in older persons.

SLEEP REGULATION

Most researchers think that there is not one simple sleep control center but a small number of interconnecting systems or centers that are located chiefly in the brainstem and that mutually activate and inhibit one another. Many studies also support the role of serotonin in sleep regulation. Prevention of serotonin synthesis or destruction of the dorsal raphe nucleus of the brainstem, which contains nearly all the brain's serotonergic cell bodies, reduces sleep for a considerable time. Synthesis and release of serotonin by serotonergic neurons are influenced by the availability of amino acid precursors of this neurotransmitter, such as L-tryptophan. Ingestion of large amounts of L-tryptophan (1 to 15 g) reduces sleep latency and nocturnal awakenings. Conversely, L-tryptophan deficiency is associated with less time

spent in REM sleep. Norepinephrine-containing neurons with cell bodies located in the locus ceruleus play an important role in controlling normal sleep patterns. Drugs and manipulations that increase the firing of these noradrenergic neurons produce a marked reduction in REM sleep (REM-off neurons) and an increase in wakefulness. In humans with implanted electrodes (for the control of spasticity), electrical stimulation of the locus ceruleus profoundly disrupts all sleep parameters. Brain acetylcholine is also involved in sleep, particularly in the production of REM sleep.

Disturbances in central cholinergic activity are associated with the sleep changes observed in major depressive disorder. Compared with healthy people and nondepressed psychiatric controls, patients who are depressed have marked disruptions of REM sleep patterns. Administration of a muscarinic agonist, such as arecoline, to depressed patients during the first or second NREM period results in a rapid onset of REM sleep. Depression may be associated with an underlying supersensitivity to acetylcholine. Indeed, approximately half the patients with major depressive disorder experience temporary improvement when they are deprived of sleep or when sleep is restricted. Conversely, reserpine (Serpasil), one of the few drugs that increases REM sleep, also produces depression.

Patients with dementia of the Alzheimer's type have sleep disturbances characterized by reduced REM and slow-wave sleep. The loss of cholinergic neurons in the basal forebrain has been implicated as the cause of these changes. Melatonin secretion from the pineal gland is inhibited by bright light, so the lowest serum melatonin concentrations occur during the day. The suprachiasmatic nucleus of the hypothalamus may act as the anatomical site of a circadian pacemaker that regulates melatonin secretion and the entrainment of the brain to a 24-

hour sleep–wake cycle. Evidence shows that dopamine has an alerting effect. Drugs that increase brain dopamine tend to produce arousal and wakefulness. In contrast, dopamine blockers, such as pimozide (Orap) and the phenothiazines, tend to increase sleep time. A hypothesized homeostatic drive to sleep, perhaps in the form of an endogenous substance—process S—may accumulate during wakefulness and act to induce sleep. Another compound—process C—may act as a regulator of body temperature and sleep duration.

FUNCTIONS OF SLEEP

The functions of sleep have been examined in a variety of ways. Most investigators conclude that sleep serves a restorative, homeostatic function and appears to be crucial for normal thermoregulation and energy conservation. As NREM sleep increases after exercise and starvation, this stage may be associated with satisfying metabolic needs.

Sleep Deprivation

Prolonged periods of sleep deprivation sometimes lead to ego disorganization, hallucinations, and delusions. Depriving people of REM sleep by awakening them at the beginning of REM cycles produces an increase in the number of REM periods and in the amount of REM sleep (rebound increase) when they are allowed to sleep without interruption. REM-deprived patients may exhibit irritability and lethargy. In studies with rats, sleep deprivation produces a syndrome that includes a debilitated appearance, skin lesions, increased food intake, weight loss, increased energy expenditure, decreased body temperature, and death. The neuroendocrine changes include increased plasma norepinephrine and decreased plasma thyroxine levels.

Sleep Requirements

Some people are normally short-sleepers who require fewer than 6 hours of sleep each night to function adequately. Long-sleepers are those who sleep more than 9 hours each night to function adequately. Long-sleepers have more REM periods and more REMs within each period (known as REM density) than do short-sleepers. These movements are sometimes considered a measure of the intensity of REM sleep and are related to the vividness of dreaming. Short-sleepers are generally efficient, ambitious, socially adept, and content. Long-sleepers tend to be mildly depressed, anxious, and socially withdrawn. Increased sleep needs occur with physical work, exercise, illness, pregnancy, general mental stress, and increased mental activity. REM periods increase after strong psychological stimuli, such as difficult learning situations and stress, and after the use of chemicals or drugs that decrease brain catecholamines.

SLEEP–WAKE RHYTHM

Without external clues, the natural body clock follows a 25-hour cycle. The influence of external factors—such as the light–dark cycle, daily routines, meal periods, and other external synchronizers—entrain people to the 24-hour clock. Sleep is also influenced by biological rhythms. Within a 24-hour period, adults sleep once, sometimes twice. This rhythm is not present at birth but develops over the first 2 years of life. In some women, sleep patterns change during the phases of the menstrual cycle. Naps taken at different times of the day differ greatly in their proportions of REM and NREM sleep. In a normal nighttime sleeper, a nap taken in the morning or at noon includes a great deal of REM sleep, whereas a nap taken in the afternoon or the early evening has much less REM sleep. A circadian cycle apparently affects the tendency to have REM sleep. Sleep patterns are not physiologically the same when people sleep in the daytime or during the time when they are accustomed to being awake; the psychological and behavioral effects of sleep differ as well. In a world of industry and communications that often functions on a 24-hour-a-day basis, these interactions are becoming increasingly significant. Even in people who work at night, interference with the various rhythms can produce problems. Conditions in these people's bodies apparently involve long-term cycle disruption and interference.

▲ 21.2 Sleep Disorders

MAJOR SYMPTOMS

Individual sleep requirements vary: Many people are long-sleepers and require 9 to 10 hours of sleep a night, and others are short sleepers, but length of sleep does not always correlate with a sleep disorder. Of interest, however, is a 2002 study of more than 1 million men and women that showed that persons who sleep more than 8.5 hours per night or less than 3.5 hours had a mortality risk 15 percent greater than those who slept an average of 7 hours per night. No reasons were given to explain this statistical finding. It was suggested that short sleepers may have comorbid conditions; but the explanation as yet remains unknown. Four major symptoms characterize most sleep disorders: insomnia, hypersomnia, parasomnia, and sleep–wake schedule disturbance. The symptoms often overlap and are described below.

Insomnia

Insomnia is difficulty in initiating or maintaining sleep. It is the most common sleep complaint and may be transient or persistent.

A brief period of insomnia is most often associated with anxiety, either as a sequela to an anxious experience or in anticipation of an anxiety-provoking experience (e.g., an examination or an impending job interview). In some people, transient insomnia of this kind may be related to grief, loss, or almost any life change or stress. The condition is not likely to be serious, although a psychotic episode or a severe depression sometimes begins with acute insomnia. Specific treatment for the condition is usually not required. When treatment with hypnotic medication is indicated, the physician and the patient should both be clear that the treatment is of short duration and that some symptoms, including a brief recurrence of the insomnia, may be expected when the medication is discontinued.

Persistent insomnia is a fairly common group of conditions in which the problem is most often difficulty in falling asleep rather than in remaining asleep. This insomnia involves two sometimes separable, but often intertwined, problems: somatized tension and anxiety and a conditioned associative response. Patients often have no clear complaint other than insomnia. They may not experience anxiety per se but discharge the anxiety through physiological channels; they may complain chiefly of apprehensive feeling or ruminative thoughts that appear to keep them from falling asleep. Sometimes (but not always), a patient describes the condition's exacerbation at times of stress at work or at home and its remission during vacations.

Hypersomnia

Hypersomnia manifests as excessive amounts of sleep, excessive daytime sleepiness (somnolence), or sometimes both. The term *somnolence* should be reserved for patients who complain of sleepiness and have a clearly demonstrable tendency to fall asleep suddenly in the waking state, who have sleep attacks, and who cannot remain awake; it should not be used for people who are simply physically tired or weary. The distinction, however, is not always clear. Complaints of hypersomnia are much less frequent than are complaints of insomnia, but they are by no means rare if clinicians are alert to them. Narcolepsy is just one well-known condition clearly producing hypersomnia. More than 100,000 narcoleptics are estimated to live in the United States. If substance-related conditions are included, hypersomnia is a common symptom. According to a recent survey, the most common conditions responsible for hypersomnia severe enough to be evaluated by all-night recordings at a sleep disorders center were sleep apnea and narcolepsy.

Transient and situational hypersomnia is a disruption of the normal sleep–wake pattern; it is marked by excessive difficulty in remaining awake and a tendency to remain in bed for unusually long periods or to return to bed to nap frequently during the day. The pattern is experienced suddenly in response to an identifiable recent life change, conflict, or loss. It is seldom marked by definite sleep attacks or unavoidable sleep but, rather, is characterized by tiredness or by falling asleep sooner than usual and by difficulty in arising in the morning.

Parasomnia

Parasomnia is an unusual or undesirable phenomenon that appears suddenly during sleep or that occurs at the threshold between waking and sleeping. Parasomnia usually occurs in stages 3 and 4 and is thus associated with poor recall of the disturbance.

Sleep–Wake Schedule Disturbance.

Sleep–wake schedule disturbance involves the displacement of sleep from its desired circadian period. Patients commonly cannot sleep when they wish to sleep, although they are able to sleep at other times. Correspondingly, they cannot be fully awake when they want to be fully awake, but they are able to be awake at other times. The disturbance does not precisely produce insomnia or somnolence, although the initial complaint is often either insomnia or somnolence; the inabilities to sleep and be awake are elicited only on careful questioning. Sleep–wake schedule disturbance can be considered a misalignment between sleep and wake behaviors. A sleep history questionnaire is helpful in diagnosing a patient's sleep disorder.

CLASSIFICATION

The text revision of the fourth edition of *Diagnostic and Statistical Manual of Mental Disorders* (DSM-IV-TR) classifies sleep disorders on the basis of clinical diagnostic criteria and presumed etiology. The three major categories of sleep disorders in DSM-IV-TR are primary sleep disorders, sleep disorders related to another mental disorder, and other sleep disorders (due to a general medical condition or substance induced). The disorders described in DSM-IV-TR are only a fraction of the known sleep disorders; they provide a framework for a clinical assessment.

PRIMARY SLEEP DISORDERS

Dyssomnias

Primary Insomnia. Primary insomnia is diagnosed when the chief complaint is nonrestorative sleep or a difficulty in initiating or maintaining sleep, and the complaint continues for at least a month (Table 21.2–1). The term *primary* indicates that the insomnia is independent of any known physical or mental condition. Increased nighttime physiological or psychological arousal and negative conditioning for sleep are frequently evident. Patients with primary insomnia are generally preoccupied with getting enough sleep. The more they try to sleep, the greater the sense of frustration and distress and the more elusive sleep becomes.

TREATMENT. Treatment of primary insomnia is among the most difficult problems in sleep disorders. When the conditioned component is prominent, a deconditioning technique may be useful. Patients are asked to use their beds for sleeping and for nothing else; if they are not asleep after 5 minutes in bed, they are instructed to simply get up and do something else. Sometimes, changing to another bed or to another room is useful. When somatized tension or muscle tension is prominent, relaxation tapes, transcendental meditation, and practicing the relaxation response and biofeedback are occasionally helpful. Psychotherapy has not been very useful in the treatment of primary insomnia. Satisfying sexual experiences promote sleep, more so in men than in women.

DRUG THERAPY. Primary insomnia is commonly treated with benzodiazepines, zolpidem (Ambien), zaleplon (Sonata), and other

Table 21.2–1
DSM-IV-TR Diagnostic Criteria for Primary Insomnia

A. The predominant complaint is difficulty initiating or maintaining sleep, or nonrestorative sleep, for at least 1 month.

B. The sleep disturbance (or associated daytime fatigue) causes clinically significant distress or impairment in social, occupational, or other important areas of functioning.

C. The sleep disturbance does not occur exclusively during the course of narcolepsy, breathing-related sleep disorder, circadian rhythm sleep disorder, or a parasomnia.

D. The disturbance does not exclusively occur during the course of another mental disorder (e.g., major depressive disorder, generalized anxiety disorder, a delirium).

E. The disturbance is not due to the direct physiological effects of a substance (e.g., a drug of abuse, a medication) or a general medical condition.

From American Psychiatric Association. *Diagnostic and Statistical Manual of Mental Disorders.* 4th ed. Text rev. Washington, DC: American Psychiatric Association; copyright 2000, with permission.

Table 21.2–2
DSM-IV-TR Diagnostic Criteria for Primary Hypersomnia

A. The predominant complaint is excessive sleepiness for at least 1 month (or less if recurrent) as evidenced by either prolonged sleep episodes or daytime sleep episodes that occur almost daily.

B. The excessive sleepiness causes clinically significant distress or impairment in social, occupational, or other important areas of functioning.

C. The excessive sleepiness is not better accounted for by insomnia and does not occur exclusively during the course of another sleep disorder (e.g., narcolepsy, breathing-related sleep disorder, circadian rhythm sleep disorder, or a parasomnia) and cannot be accounted for by an inadequate amount of sleep.

D. The disturbance does not occur exclusively during the course of another mental disorder.

E. The disturbance is not due to the direct physiological effects of a substance (e.g., a drug of abuse, a medication) or a general medical condition.

Specify if:

Recurrent: if there are periods of excessive sleepiness that last at least 3 days occurring several times a year for at least 2 years

From American Psychiatric Association. *Diagnostic and Statistical Manual of Mental Disorders.* 4th ed. Text rev. Washington, DC: American Psychiatric Association; copyright 2000, with permission.

Table 21.2–3
DSM-IV-TR Diagnostic Criteria for Narcolepsy

A. Irresistible attacks of refreshing sleep that occur daily over at least 3 months.

B. The presence of one or both of the following:

(1) cataplexy (i.e., brief episodes of sudden bilateral loss of muscle tone, most often in association with intense emotion)

(2) recurrent intrusions of elements of rapid eye movement (REM) sleep into the transition between sleep and wakefulness, as manifested by either hypnopompic or hypnagogic hallucinations or sleep paralysis at the beginning or end of sleep episodes

C. The disturbance is not due to the direct physiological effects of a substance (e.g., a drug of abuse, a medication) or another general medical condition.

From American Psychiatric Association. *Diagnostic and Statistical Manual of Mental Disorders.* 4th ed. Text rev. Washington, DC: American Psychiatric Association; copyright 2000, with permission.

hypnotics. Hypnotic drugs should be used with care. Over-the-counter sleep aids have limited effectiveness. Long-acting sleep medications (e.g., flurazepam [Dalmane], quazepam [Doral]) are best for middle-of-the-night insomnia; short-acting drugs (e.g., zolpidem [Ambien], triazolam [Halcion]) are useful for persons who have difficulty falling asleep. In general, sleep medications should not be prescribed for more than 2 weeks because tolerance and withdrawal may result.

Primary Hypersomnia. Primary hypersomnia is diagnosed when no other cause for excessive somnolence occurring for at least 1 month can be found. Some people are long sleepers who, like short sleepers, show a normal variation. Their sleep, although long, is normal in architecture and physiology. Sleep efficiency and the sleep–wake schedule are normal. This patient is without complaints about the quality of sleep, daytime sleepiness, or difficulties with the awake mood, motivation, and performance.

Some people have subjective complaints of feeling sleepy but have no objective findings. They do not have a tendency to fall asleep more often than normal and do not have any objective signs. Clinicians should try to rule out clear-cut causes of excessive somnolence. According to DSM-IV-TR, the disorder should be coded as recurrent if patients have periods of excessive sleepiness lasting at least 3 days and occurring several times a year for at least 2 years (Table 21.2–2).

Treatment. The treatment of primary hypersomnia consists mainly of stimulant drugs, such as amphetamines, given in the morning or evening. Nonsedating antidepressant drugs, such as bupropion (Wellbutrin), and novel stimulants such as modafinil (Provigil) may also be of value in some patients.

Narcolepsy. Narcolepsy consists of excessive daytime sleepiness and abnormal manifestations of rapid eye movement (REM) sleep occurring daily for at least 3 months (Table 21.2–3). These sleep attacks typically occur two to six times a day and last 10 to 20 minutes. They may occur at inappropriate times (e.g., while eating, talking, or driving, and during sex). The REM sleep includes hypnagogic and hypnopompic hallucinations, cataplexy, and sleep paralysis. The appearance of REM sleep within 10 minutes of sleep onset (sleep onset REM periods) is also considered evidence of narcolepsy. The disorder can be dangerous because it can lead to automobile and industrial accidents.

Narcolepsy is not as rare as was once thought. It is estimated to occur in 0.02 to 0.16 percent of adults and shows some familial incidence. Narcolepsy is neither a type of epilepsy nor a psychogenic disturbance. It is an abnormality of the sleep mechanisms—specifically, REM-inhibiting mechanisms—and it has been studied in dogs, sheep, and humans. Narcolepsy can occur at any age, but it most frequently begins in adolescence or young adulthood, generally before the age of 30. The disorder either progresses slowly or reaches a plateau that is maintained throughout life.

Often associated with the problem (close to 50 percent of long-standing cases) is cataplexy, a sudden loss of muscle tone, such as jaw drop, head drop, weakness of the knees, or paralysis of all skeletal muscles with collapse. Patients often remain awake during brief cataplectic episodes; the long episodes usually merge with sleep and show the electroencephalographic (EEG) signs of REM sleep.

Other symptoms include hypnagogic or hypnopompic hallucinations: vivid perceptual experiences, either auditory or visual, occurring at sleep onset or on awakening. Patients are often momentarily frightened, but within a minute or two they return to an entirely normal frame of mind and are aware that nothing was actually there.

Another uncommon symptom is sleep paralysis, most often occurring on awakening in the morning; during the episode, patients are apparently awake and conscious but unable to move a muscle. If the symptom persists for more than a few seconds, as it often does in narcolepsy, it can become extremely uncomfortable. (Isolated brief episodes of sleep paralysis occur in many nonnarcoleptic people.) Patients with narcolepsy report falling asleep quickly at night but often experience broken sleep.

When the diagnosis is not clinically clear, a nighttime polysomnographic recording reveals a characteristic sleep-onset REM period. A test of daytime multipole sleep latency (several recorded naps at 2-hour intervals) shows rapid sleep onset and usually one or more sleep-onset REM periods. A type of human leukocyte antigen called *HLA-DR2* is found in 90 to 100 percent of patients with narcolepsy and only 10 to 35 percent of unaffected persons. One recent study showed that narcolepsy patients are deficient in the neurotransmitter hypocretin, which stimulates appetite and alertness. Another study found that the number of hypocretin neurons (Hrct cells) in narcoleptics is 85 to 95 percent less than in nonnarcoleptic brains.

TREATMENT.   There is no cure for narcolepsy, but symptom management is possible. A regimen of forced naps at a regular time of day occasionally helps patients with narcolepsy, and in some cases, the regimen alone, without medication, can almost cure the patients. When medication is required, stimulants are most commonly used.

Modafinil (Provigil), an α_1-adrenergic receptor agonist, has been approved by the U.S. Food and Drug Administration (FDA) to reduce the number of sleep attacks and to improve psychomotor performance in narcolepsy; this observation suggests the involvement of noradrenergic mechanisms in the disorder. Modafinil lacks some of the adverse side effects of traditional psychostimulants.

Sleep specialists often prescribe tricyclic drugs or selective serotonin reuptake inhibitors (SSRIs) to reduce cataplexy. This approach capitalizes on the REM sleep-suppressant properties of these drugs. Because cataplexy is presumably an intrusion of REM sleep phenomena into the awake state, the rationale is clear. Many reports indicate that imipramine (Tofranil), modafinil, and fluoxetine (Prozac) are quite effective in reducing or eliminating cataplexy. Although drug therapy is the treatment of choice, the overall therapeutic approach should include scheduled naps, lifestyle adjustment, psychological counseling, drug holidays to reduce tolerance, and careful monitoring of drug refills, general health, and cardiac status.

Breathing-Related Sleep Disorder.
Breathing-related sleep disorder is characterized by sleep disruption leading to excessive sleepiness or insomnia that is due to a sleep-related breathing disturbance (Table 21.2–4). Breathing disturbances that may occur during sleep include apneas, hypopneas, and oxygen desaturations. These disturbances invariably cause hypersomnia. Two disorders of the respiratory system that can produce hypersomnia are sleep apnea and central alveolar hypoventilation. Both disorders can also cause insomnia but more commonly produce hypersomnia.

Obstructive Sleep Apnea Syndrome.
Many people—older people and obese people, even those without clinical symptoms—are less likely to have apneic periods in sleep and, in general, more respiratory problems in sleep than when awake. *Sleep apnea* refers to the cessation of airflow at the nose or the mouth. By convention, an apneic period is one that lasts 10 seconds or more. Sleep apnea can be of several distinct types. In pure central sleep apnea, both airflow and respiratory

Table 21.2–4
DSM-IV-TR Diagnostic Criteria for Breathing-Related Sleep Disorder

A. Sleep disruption, leading to excessive sleepiness or insomnia, that is judged to be due to a sleep-related breathing condition (e.g., obstructive or central sleep apnea syndrome or central alveolar hypoventilation syndrome).

B. The disturbance is not better accounted for by another mental disorder and is not due to the direct physiological effects of a substance (e.g., a drug of abuse, a medication) or another general medical condition (other than a breathing-related disorder).

Coding note: Also code sleep-related breathing disorder on Axis III.

From American Psychiatric Association. *Diagnostic and Statistical Manual of Mental Disorders.* 4th ed. Text rev. Washington, DC: American Psychiatric Association; copyright 2000, with permission.

effort (abdomen and chest) cease during the apneic episodes and begin again during arousals. In pure obstructive sleep apnea, airflow ceases but respiratory effort increases during apneic periods; this pattern indicates an obstruction in the airway and increasing efforts by the abdominal and thoracic muscles to force air past the obstruction. Again, the episode ceases with an arousal. The mixed types involve elements of both obstructive and central sleep apnea.

Sleep apnea usually is considered pathological if patients have at least five apneic episodes an hour or 30 apneic episodes during the night. In severe cases of obstructive sleep apnea, patients may have as many as 300 apneic episodes, each followed by an arousal. Thus, almost no normal sleep occurs, even though patients have been in bed and often assume that they have been sleeping for the entire night.

Sleep apnea can be a dangerous condition. It is thought to account for a number of unexplained deaths and crib deaths of infants and children. It is probably also responsible for many pulmonary and cardiovascular deaths in adults and in older people. Episodes of sleep apnea can produce cardiovascular changes, including arrhythmias, and transient alterations in blood pressure for each apneic episode. Long-standing sleep apnea is associated with an increase in pulmonary blood pressure and eventually an increase in systemic blood pressure as well. These cardiovascular changes in sleep apnea may account for a considerable number of cases in which the diagnosis is essential hypertension.

The prevalence of sleep apnea in the population has not been established, but an increasing number of cases are discovered as awareness of its existence grows. In a recent survey of patients with daytime sleepiness whose disorder was serious enough for them to be evaluated polygraphically at a sleep disorders center, 42 percent were found to be suffering from one of the variants of sleep apnea.

A tentative diagnosis of sleep apnea can be made even without polysomnographic recordings. The most characteristic picture is that of middle-aged or older men who report tiredness and inability to stay awake in the daytime, sometimes associated with depression, mood changes, and daytime sleep attacks. They may or may not complain of anything unusual during sleep. When a history is obtained from a spouse or bed partner, it includes reports of loud, intermittent snoring, at times accompanied by gasping. Observers sometimes recall apneic periods when patients appeared to be trying to breathe but were unable to do so. Such patients almost certainly have obstructive sleep apnea. With central or mixed apnea, the complaints are of repeated awakenings during the night, associated with morning headaches and mood changes, but with no difficulty of falling asleep. At onset, the patients may have no complaints at all, although bed partners or roommates report heavy snoring and restless sleep. Obese patients with the disorder are said to have *pickwickian syndrome*.

Patients suspected of having sleep apnea should undergo laboratory recordings. The usual all-night sleep recordings including EEG, electromyogram (EMG), electrocardiogram (ECG), and respiratory tracings of various kinds are useful. Recording airflow and respiratory effort is usually necessary to make a diagnosis. The severity of apneic episodes is determined by using oximetry to measure oxygen saturation during the night. Twenty-four-hour ECG monitoring is sometimes useful to monitor cardiac changes.

Nasal continuous positive airway pressure (nCPAP) is the treatment of choice for obstructive sleep apnea. Other procedures include weight loss, nasal surgery, tracheostomy, and uvulopalatoplasty. Some medications may normalize sleep in patients with apnea. SSRIs and tricyclic antidepressants sometimes help treat sleep apnea by decreasing the amount of time spent in REM sleep, the stage of sleep where apneic episodes most often occur. In addition, theophylline has been shown to decrease the number of episodes of apnea; however, it may interfere with the overall quality of sleep, limiting its general utility. When sleep apnea is established or suspected, patients must avoid the use of sedative medication, including alcohol, because it can considerably exacerbate the condition, which may then become life threatening.

Central Alveolar Hypoventilation.

Central alveolar hypoventilation refers to several conditions marked by impaired ventilation in which the respiratory abnormality appears or greatly worsens only during sleep and in which significant apneic episodes are not present. The ventilatory dysfunction is characterized by inadequate tidal volume or respiratory rate during sleep. Death may occur during sleep (Ondine's curse). Central alveolar hypoventilation is treated with some form of mechanical ventilation (e.g., nasal ventilation).

Circadian Rhythm Sleep Disorder.

Circadian rhythm sleep disorder includes a wide range of conditions involving a misalignment between desired and actual sleep periods. DSM-IV-TR lists four types of circadian rhythm sleep disorder: delayed sleep phase type, jet lag type, shift work type, and unspecified (Table 21.2–5).

DELAYED SLEEP PHASE TYPE.

Delayed sleep phase type of circadian rhythm sleep disorder is marked by sleep and wake times that are intractably later than desired, actual sleep times at virtually the same daily clock hour, no reported difficulty in maintaining sleep once begun, and an inability to advance the sleep phase by enforcing conventional sleep and wake times. The patient's major complaint is often the difficulty of falling asleep at a desired conventional time, and the patient's disorder may appear to be similar to a sleep onset insomnia. Daytime sleepiness often occurs secondary to sleep loss.

Delayed sleep phase type can be treated by gradually delaying the hour of sleep over a period of several days until the desired sleep time is achieved. The strategy works when advancing the sleep time does not

Table 21.2–5
DSM-IV-TR Diagnostic Criteria for Circadian Rhythm Sleep Disorder

A. A persistent or recurrent pattern of sleep disruption leading to excessive sleepiness or insomnia that is due to a mismatch between the sleep–wake schedule required by a person's environment and his or her circadian sleep–wake pattern.

B. The sleep disturbance causes clinically significant distress or impairment in social, occupational, or other important areas of functioning.

C. The disturbance does not occur exclusively during the course of another sleep disorder or other mental disorder.

D. The disturbance is not due to the direct physiological effects of a substance (e.g., a drug of abuse, a medication) or a general medical condition.

Specify type:

Delayed sleep phase type: a persistent pattern of late sleep onset and late awakening times, with an inability to fall asleep and awaken at a desired earlier time

Jet lag type: sleepiness and alertness that occur at an inappropriate time of day relative to local time, occurring after repeated travel across more than one time zone

Shift work type: insomnia during the major sleep period or excessive sleepiness during the major awake period associated with night shift work or frequently changing shift work

Unspecified type

work. The process of sleep phase adjustment can be assisted by the brief use of short-half-life hypnotic agents, such as triazolam, to enforce sleep. Another approach to treating delayed sleep phase type is the use of light therapy. Evening light therapy tends to delay sleep; regular morning light exposure tends to advance sleep.

JET LAG TYPE.

Depending on the length of the east-to-west trip and individual sensitivity, jet lag type usually disappears spontaneously in 2 to 7 days; no specific treatment is required. Some people find that they can prevent the symptoms by altering their mealtimes and sleep times in an appropriate direction before traveling. Others find that what appear to be symptoms of jet lag (fatigue and so on) are actually associated with sleep deprivation and that simply obtaining enough sleep helps. Melatonin taken orally at prescribed times is of use for some persons.

SHIFT WORK TYPE.

Shift work type of circadian rhythm sleep disorder occurs in people who repeatedly and rapidly change their work schedules and occasionally in people with self-imposed chaotic sleep schedules. The most frequent symptom is a period of mixed insomnia and somnolence, but many other symptoms and somatic problems, including peptic ulcer, may be associated with the pattern after some time. Some adolescents and young adults appear to withstand such changes remarkably well and show few symptoms, but older people and those with sensitivity to change are clearly affected.

The symptoms are generally worse the first few days after shifting to a new schedule, but in some people the disrupted sleep–wake patterns persist for a long time. Enforcement of new sleep hours and light therapy may help workers adjust to their new schedules. Many people never adapt completely to unusual shift schedules because they maintain the altered pattern only 5 days a week and return to the prevailing pattern of the rest of the population on days off and on vacations.

Shift work schedules are an important area that has not received sufficient study, especially in view of the unusual shifts and changing

Table 21.2–6
DSM-IV-TR Diagnostic Criteria for Dyssomnia Not Otherwise Specified

The dyssomnia not otherwise specified category is for insomnias, hypersomnias, or circadian rhythm disturbances that do not meet criteria for any specific dyssomnia. Examples include

1. Complaints of clinically significant insomnia or hypersomnia that are attributable to environmental factors (e.g., noise, light, frequent interruptions).

2. Excessive sleepiness that is attributable to ongoing sleep deprivation.

3. "Restless legs syndrome": This syndrome is characterized by a desire to move the legs or arms, associated with uncomfortable sensations typically described as creeping, crawling, tingling, burning, or itching. Frequent movements of the limbs occur in an effort to relieve the uncomfortable sensations. Symptoms are worse when the individual is at rest and in the evening or night, and they are relieved temporarily by movement. The uncomfortable sensations and limb movements can delay sleep onset, awaken the individual from sleep, and lead to daytime sleepiness or fatigue. Sleep studies demonstrate involuntary periodic limb movements during sleep in a majority of individuals with restless legs syndrome. A minority of individuals have evidence of anemia or reduced serum iron stores. Peripheral nerve electrophysiological studies and gross brain morphology are usually normal. Restless legs syndrome can occur in an idiopathic form, or it can be associated with general medical or neurological conditions, including normal pregnancy, renal failure, rheumatoid arthritis, peripheral vascular disease, or peripheral nerve dysfunction. Phenomenologically, the two forms are indistinguishable. The onset of restless legs syndrome is typically in the second or third decade, although up to 20% of individuals with this syndrome may have symptoms before age 10. The prevalence of restless legs syndrome is between 2% and 10% in the general population and as high as 30% in general medical populations. Prevalence increases with age and is equal in males and females. Course is marked by stability or worsening of symptoms with age. There is a positive family history in 50–90% of individuals. The major differential diagnoses include medication-induced akathisia, peripheral neuropathy, and nocturnal leg cramps. Worsening at night and periodic limb movements are more common in restless legs syndrome than in medication-induced akathisia or peripheral neuropathy. Unlike restless legs syndrome, nocturnal leg cramps do not present with the desire to move the limbs nor are there frequent limb movements.

4. Periodic limb movements: Periodic limb movements are repeated low-amplitude brief limb jerks, particularly in the lower extremities. These movements begin near sleep onset and decrease during stage 3 or 4 non–rapid eye movement (NREM) and rapid eye movement (REM) sleep. Movements usually occur rhythmically every 20–60 seconds and are associated with repeated, brief arousals. Individuals are often unaware of the actual movements, but may complain of insomnia, frequent awakenings, or daytime sleepiness if the number of movements is very large. Individuals may have considerable variability in the number of periodic limb movements from night to night. Periodic limb movements occur in the majority of individuals with restless legs syndrome, but they may also occur without the other symptoms of restless legs syndrome. Individuals with normal pregnancy or with conditions such as renal failure, congestive heart failure, and posttraumatic stress disorder may also develop periodic limb movements. Although typical age at onset and prevalence in the general population are unknown, periodic limb movements increase with age and may occur in more than one-third of individuals over age 65. Men are more commonly affected than women.

5. Situations in which the clinician has concluded that a dyssomnia is present but is unable to determine whether it is primary, due to a general medical condition, or substance induced.

From American Psychiatric Association. *Diagnostic and Statistical Manual of Mental Disorders.* 4th ed. Text rev. Washington, DC: American Psychiatric Association; copyright 2000, with permission.

shift schedules that a large proportion of the population now work. People's sensitivities to shifting schedules vary widely, but the bodies of a fair number of people simply do not adapt to shift work; therefore, these people should not be assigned to work in shifts. Temperamentally, some people are "owls," who like to stay up at night and sleep during the day, and others are "larks," who rise early and retire early.

A particular problem occurs in the training of physicians, who are often required to work 36 to 48 hours without sleeping. This condition is dangerous to both doctors and their patients. It behooves medical educators to develop more shifts for doctors in training.

UNSPECIFIED

Advanced Sleep Phase Syndrome. Advanced sleep phase syndrome is characterized by sleep onsets and wake times that are intractably earlier than desired, actual sleep times at virtually the same daily clock hour, no reported difficulty in maintaining sleep once begun, and an inability to delay the sleep phase by enforcing conventional sleep and wake times. Unlike delayed sleep phase type, the condition does not interfere with the work or school day. The major presenting complaint is the inability to stay awake in the evening and to sleep in the morning until desired conventional times.

Disorganized Sleep–Wake Pattern. Disorganized sleep–wake pattern is defined as irregular and variable sleep and waking behavior that

disrupts the regular sleep–wake pattern. The condition is associated with frequent daytime naps at irregular times and excessive bed rest. Sleep at night is not of adequate length, and the condition may seem to be insomnia, although the total amount of sleep in 24 hours is normal for the patient's age.

Dyssomnia Not Otherwise Specified. According to DSM-IV-TR, dyssomnia not otherwise specified includes insomnias, hypersomnias, and circadian rhythm disturbances that do not meet the criteria for any specific dyssomnia (Table 21.2–6).

NOCTURNAL MYOCLONUS. Nocturnal myoclonus consists of highly stereotyped abrupt contractions of certain leg muscles during sleep. Patients lack any subjective awareness of the leg jerks. The condition may be present in approximately 40 percent of people older than 65 years.

The repetitive leg movements occur every 20 to 60 seconds, with extension of the large toe and flexion of the ankle, the knee, and the hips. Frequent awakenings, unrefreshing sleep, and daytime sleepiness are major symptoms. No treatment for nocturnal myoclonus is universally effective. Treatments that may be useful include benzodiazepines, levodopa (Larodopa), quinine, and, in rare cases, opioids.

RESTLESS LEGS SYNDROME. In restless legs syndrome, people feel deep sensations of creeping inside the calves whenever sitting or lying down. The dysesthesias are rarely painful but are agonizingly relentless and cause an almost irresistible urge to move the legs; thus, this syndrome interferes with sleep and with falling asleep. It peaks in middle age and occurs in 5 percent of the population.

The syndrome has no established treatment. Symptoms of restless legs syndrome are relieved by movement and by leg massage. When pharmacotherapy is required, the benzodiazepines, levodopa, quinine, opioids, propranolol (Inderal), valproate (Depakene), and carbamazepine (Tegretol) are of some benefit.

KLEINE-LEVIN SYNDROME. Kleine-Levin syndrome is a relatively rare condition consisting of recurrent periods of prolonged sleep (from which patients may be aroused) with intervening periods of normal sleep and alert waking. During the hypersomniac episodes, wakeful periods are usually marked by withdrawal from social contacts and return to bed at the first opportunity; patients may also display apathy, irritability, confusion, voracious eating, loss of sexual inhibitions, delusions, hallucinations, frank disorientation, memory impairment, incoherent speech, excitation or depression, and truculence. Unexplained fevers have occurred in a few patients.

Kleine-Levin syndrome is uncommon. Approximately 100 cases with features suggesting the diagnosis have been reported. In most cases, several periods of hypersomnia, each lasting for one or several weeks, are experienced by patients over a year. With few exceptions, the first attack occurs between the ages of 10 and 21 years. Rare instances of onset in the fourth and fifth decades of life have been reported. The syndrome appears to be almost invariably self-limited, and enduring remission occurs spontaneously before age 40 in early-onset cases.

MENSTRUAL-ASSOCIATED SYNDROME. Some women experience intermittent marked hypersomnia, altered behavioral patterns, and voracious eating at or shortly before the onset of their menses. Nonspecific EEG abnormalities similar to those associated with Kleine-Levin syndrome have been documented in several instances. Endocrine factors are probably involved, but specific abnormalities in laboratory endocrine measures have not been reported. Increased cerebrospinal fluid (CSF) serotonin levels were identified in one patient.

SLEEP DISTURBANCE IN PREGNANCY. Disturbances in sleep are common in pregnant women. There are several hormonal factors that contribute to this disturbance, including changes in levels of estrogen, progesterone, cortisol, and melatonin from baseline. In addition, changes in maternal respiratory physiology, body habitus, and, in the third trimester, movements of the fetus can all act to diminish the quantity and quality of sleep.

INSUFFICIENT SLEEP. *Insufficient sleep* is defined as an earnest complaint of daytime sleepiness and associated waking symptoms by a person who persistently fails to obtain sufficient daily sleep to support alert wakefulness. The person is voluntarily, but often unwittingly, chronically sleep deprived. The diagnosis can usually be made on the basis of the history, including a sleep log. Some people, especially students and shift workers, who want to maintain an active daytime life and perform their nighttime jobs, may seriously deprive themselves of sleep and thus produce somnolence during waking hours.

SLEEP DRUNKENNESS. Sleep drunkenness is an abnormal form of awakening in which the lack of a clear sensorium in the transition from sleep to full wakefulness is prolonged and exaggerated. A confusion state develops that often leads to individual or social inconvenience and some-

Table 21.2–7
DSM-IV-TR Diagnostic Criteria for Nightmare Disorder

A. Repeated awakenings from the major sleep period or naps with detailed recall of extended and extremely frightening dreams, usually involving threats to survival, security, or self-esteem. The awakenings generally occur during the second half of the sleep period.

B. On awakening from the frightening dreams, the person rapidly becomes oriented and alert (in contrast to the confusion and disorientation seen in sleep terror disorder and some forms of epilepsy).

C. The dream experience, or the sleep disturbance resulting from the awakening, causes clinically significant distress or impairment in social, occupational, or other important areas of functioning.

D. The nightmares do not occur exclusively during the course of another mental disorder (e.g., a delirium, posttraumatic stress disorder) and are not due to the direct physiological effects of a substance (e.g., a drug of abuse, a medication) or a general medical condition.

From American Psychiatric Association. *Diagnostic and Statistical Manual of Mental Disorders.* 4th ed. Text rev. Washington, DC: American Psychiatric Association; copyright 2000, with permission.

times to criminal acts. Essential to the diagnosis is the absence of sleep deprivation. It is a rare condition, and there may be a familial tendency. Before making the diagnosis, clinicians should examine patients' sleep and rule out such conditions as apnea, nocturnal myoclonus, narcolepsy, and an excessive use of alcohol and other substances.

Parasomnias

Nightmare Disorder. Nightmares are long, frightening dreams from which people awaken scared (Table 21.2–7). Like other dreams, nightmares almost always occur during REM sleep and usually after a long REM period late in the night. Some people have frequent nightmares as a lifelong condition; others experience them predominantly at times of stress and illness. Approximately 50 percent of the adult population may report occasional nightmares. No specific treatment is usually required for nightmare disorder. Agents that suppress REM sleep, such as tricyclic drugs, may reduce the frequency of nightmares, and benzodiazepines have also been used. Contrary to popular belief, no harm results from awakening a person who is having a nightmare.

Sleep Terror Disorder. Sleep terror disorder is an arousal in the first third of the night during deep non-REM (NREM) (stages 3 and 4) sleep. It is almost invariably inaugurated by a piercing scream or cry and accompanied by behavioral manifestations of intense anxiety bordering on panic (Table 21.2–8).

Typically, patients sit up in bed with a frightened expression, scream loudly, and sometimes awaken immediately with a sense of intense terror. Patients may remain awake in a disoriented state but more often fall asleep, and, as with sleepwalking, they forget the episodes. A night terror episode after the original scream frequently develops into a sleepwalking episode. Polygraphic recordings of night terrors are somewhat like those of sleepwalking; in fact, the two conditions appear to be

Table 21.2–8
DSM-IV-TR Diagnostic Criteria for Sleep Terror Disorder

A. Recurrent episodes of abrupt awakening from sleep, usually occurring during the first third of the major sleep episode and beginning with a panicky scream.

B. Intense fear and signs of autonomic arousal, such as tachycardia, rapid breathing, and sweating, during each episode.

C. Relative unresponsiveness to efforts of others to comfort the person during the episode.

D. No detailed dream is recalled and there is amnesia for the episode.

E. The episodes cause clinically significant distress or impairment in social, occupational, or other important areas of functioning.

F. The disturbance is not due to the direct physiological effects of a substance (e.g., a drug of abuse, a medication) or a general medical condition.

From American Psychiatric Association. *Diagnostic and Statistical Manual of Mental Disorders.* 4th ed. Text rev. Washington, DC: American Psychiatric Association; copyright 2000, with permission.

Table 21.2–9
DSM-IV-TR Diagnostic Criteria for Sleepwalking Disorder

A. Repeated episodes of rising from bed during sleep and walking about, usually occurring during the first third of the major sleep episode.

B. While sleepwalking, the person has a blank, staring face, is relatively unresponsive to the efforts of others to communicate with him or her, and can be awakened only with great difficulty.

C. On awakening (either from the sleepwalking episode or the next morning), the person has amnesia for the episode.

D. Within several minutes after awakening from the sleepwalking episode, there is no impairment of mental activity or behavior (although there may initially be a short period of confusion or disorientation).

E. The sleepwalking causes clinically significant distress or impairment in social, occupational, or other important areas of functioning.

F. The disturbance is not due to the direct physiological effects of a substance (e.g., a drug of abuse, a medication) or a general medical condition.

From American Psychiatric Association. *Diagnostic and Statistical Manual of Mental Disorders.* 4th ed. Text rev. Washington, DC: American Psychiatric Association; copyright 2000, with permission.

closely related. Night terrors, as isolated episodes, are especially frequent in children. Approximately 1 to 6 percent of children have the disorder, which is more common in boys than in girls and which tends to run in families.

Night terrors may reflect a minor neurological abnormality, perhaps in the temporal lobe or underlying structures, because when night terrors begin in adolescence and young adulthood, they turn out to be the first symptom of temporal lobe epilepsy. In a typical case of night terrors, however, no signs of temporal lobe epilepsy or other seizure disorders are seen either clinically or on EEG recordings.

Although night terrors are closely related to sleepwalking and are occasionally related to enuresis, they are different from nightmares. Night terrors are associated with simply awakening in terror: Patients generally have no dream recall but may occasionally recall a single frightening image.

Specific treatment for night terror disorder is seldom required. Investigation of stressful family situations may be important, and individual or family therapy is sometimes useful. In the rare cases in which medication is required, diazepam (Valium) in small doses at bedtime improves the condition and sometimes completely eliminates the attacks.

Sleepwalking Disorder. Sleepwalking, also known as *somnambulism*, consists of a sequence of complex behaviors that are initiated in the first third of the night during deep NREM (stage 3 and 4) sleep and frequently, although not always, progress—without full consciousness or later memory of the episode—to leaving bed and walking about (Table 21.2–9).

Patients sit up and sometimes perform preservative motor acts, such as walking, dressing, going to the bathroom, talking, screaming, and even driving. The behavior occasionally terminates in an awakening with several minutes of confusion; more frequently, they return to sleep without any recollection of the sleepwalking event. An artificially induced arousal from stage 4 sleep can sometimes produce the condition. For instance, in children, especially those with a history of sleep-walking, an attack can sometimes be provoked by standing them on their feet and thus producing a partial arousal during stage 4 sleep.

Sleepwalking usually begins between ages 4 and 8. Peak prevalence is at approximately 12 years of age. The disorder is more common in boys than in girls, and approximately 15 percent of children have an occasional episode. It tends to run in families. A minor neurological abnormality probably underlies the condition; the episodes should not be considered purely psychogenic, although stressful periods are associated with an increase in sleepwalking in affected people. Extreme tiredness or previous sleep deprivation exacerbates attacks. The disorder is occasionally dangerous because of the possibility of accidental injury. Treatment consists of measures to prevent injury and of drugs that suppress stages 3 and 4 sleep. The sleepwalker may be awakened during the episode without ill effects.

An 11-year-old girl asked her mother to take her to a psychiatrist because she feared she might be "going crazy." Several times during the last 2 months she had awakened confused about where she was until she realized she was on the living room couch or in her little sister's bed, even though she went to bed in her own room. When she recently woke up in her older brother's bedroom, she became very concerned and felt quite guilty about it. Her younger sister said that she had seen the patient walking during the night, looking like a "zombie," that she didn't answer when she called her, and that the patient had done that several times, but usually went back to her bed. The patient feared she might have "amnesia" because she had no memory of anything happening during the night.

There is no history of seizures or of similar episodes during the day. An EEG and physical examination proved normal. The patient's mental status was unremarkable except for some anxiety about her symptoms and the usual early adolescent concerns. School and family functioning were excellent.

DISCUSSION

This girl was not "going crazy" but, rather, was experiencing the characteristic features of sleepwalking disorder: episodes of arising from bed during sleep and walking about, appearing unresponsive during episodes, experiencing amnesia for the episode upon awakening, and exhibiting no evidence of impairment in consciousness several minutes after awakening. Psychomotor epileptic seizures were ruled out by the normal EEG and the absence of any seizure-like behavior during the waking state.

Although the process of dissociation is involved in sleepwalking disorder, because the disturbance begins during sleep, it was classified as a sleep disorder rather than as a dissociative disorder. (From *DSM-IV Casebook*.)

Parasomnia Not Otherwise Specified.   The diagnostic criteria for parasomnia not otherwise specified are given in Table 21.2–10.

SLEEP-RELATED BRUXISM.   Bruxism, or tooth grinding, occurs throughout the night, most prominently in stage 2 sleep. According to dentists, 5 to 10 percent of the population experience bruxism severe enough to produce noticeable damage to teeth. The condition often goes unnoticed by the sleepers, except for an occasional jaw ache in the morning, but bed partners and roommates are consistently awakened by

Table 21.2–10
DSM-IV-TR Diagnostic Criteria for Parasomnia Not Otherwise Specified

The parasomnia not otherwise specified category is for disturbances that are characterized by abnormal behavioral or physiological events during sleep or sleep–wake transitions, but that do not meet criteria for a more specific parasomnia. Examples include

1. REM sleep behavior disorder: motor activity, often of a violent nature, that arises during rapid eye movement (REM) sleep. Unlike sleepwalking, these episodes tend to occur later in the night and are associated with vivid dream recall.
2. Sleep paralysis: an inability to perform voluntary movement during the transition between wakefulness and sleep. The episodes may occur at sleep onset (hypnagogic) or with awakening (hypnopompic). The episodes are usually associated with extreme anxiety and, in some cases, fear of impending death. Sleep paralysis occurs commonly as an ancillary symptom of narcolepsy and, in such cases, should not be coded separately.
3. Situations in which the clinician has concluded that a parasomnia is present but is unable to determine whether it is primary, due to a general medical condition, or substance induced.

From American Psychiatric Association. *Diagnostic and Statistical Manual of Mental Disorders*. 4th ed. Text rev. Washington, DC: American Psychiatric Association; copyright 2000, with permission.

the sound. Treatment consists of a dental bite plate and corrective orthodontic procedures.

RAPID EYE MOVEMENT SLEEP BEHAVIOR DISORDER.   REM sleep behavior disorder is a chronic and progressive condition found mainly in men. It is characterized by the loss of atonia during REM sleep and subsequent emergence of violent and complex behaviors. In essence, patients with the disorder are acting out their dreams. Serious injury to patients or bed partners is a major risk. The development or aggravation of the disorder has been reported in patients with narcolepsy who have been treated with psychostimulants and tricyclic drugs and in patients with depression and obsessive-compulsive disorder (OCD) who have been treated with fluoxetine (Prozac). REM sleep behavior disorder is treated with clonazepam (Klonopin), 0.5 to 2.0 mg a day. Carbamazepine, 100 mg three times a day, is also effective in controlling the disorder.

SLEEPTALKING (SOMNILOQUY).   Sleeptalking is common in children and adults. It has been studied extensively in the sleep laboratory and is found to occur in all stages of sleep. The talking usually involves a few words that are difficult to distinguish. Long episodes of talking involve the sleeper's life and concerns, but sleeptalkers do not relate their dreams during sleep, nor do they often reveal deep secrets. Episodes of sleeptalking sometimes accompany night terrors and sleepwalking. Sleeptalking alone requires no treatment.

SLEEP-RELATED HEAD BANGING (JACTATIO CAPITIS NOCTURNA).   *Sleep-related head banging* is the term for a sleep behavior consisting chiefly of rhythmic to-and-fro head rocking, less commonly of total body rocking, occurring just before or during sleep. Usually, it is observed in the immediate presleep period and is sustained into light sleep. It uncommonly persists into or occurs in deep NREM sleep. Treatment consists of measures to prevent injury.

SLEEP PARALYSIS.   Familial sleep paralysis is characterized by a sudden inability to execute voluntary movements either just at the onset of sleep or on awakening during the night or in the morning.

SLEEP DISORDERS RELATED TO ANOTHER MENTAL DISORDER.   DSM-IV-TR defines a sleep disorder related to another mental disorder as a complaint of sleep disturbance caused by a diagnosable mental disorder but severe enough to merit clinical attention on its own.

Insomnia Related to Another Mental (Axis I or Axis II) Disorder

Insomnia that occurs for at least 1 month and that is clearly related to the psychological and behavioral symptoms of the clinically well-known mental disorders are classified here (Table 21.2–11). The category consists of a heterogeneous group of conditions. The sleep problem is usually, but not always, difficulty in falling asleep and is secondary to anxiety that is part of any of the various mental disorders listed. The insomnia is more common in women than in men. In clear-cut cases in which the anxiety has psychological roots, psychiatric treatment of the anxiety (e.g., individual psychotherapy, group psychotherapy, or family therapy) often relieves the insomnia.

The insomnia associated with major depressive disorder involves relatively normal sleep onset but repeated awakenings during the second half of the night and premature morning

Table 21.2–11
DSM-IV-TR Diagnostic Criteria for Insomnia Related to Another Mental Disorder

A. The predominant complaint is difficulty initiating or maintaining sleep, or nonrestorative sleep, for at least 1 month that is associated with daytime fatigue or impaired daytime functioning.

B. The sleep disturbance (or daytime sequelae) causes clinically significant distress or impairment in social, occupational, or other important areas of functioning.

C. The insomnia is judged to be related to another Axis I or Axis II disorder (e.g., major depressive disorder, generalized anxiety disorder, adjustment disorder with anxiety) but is sufficiently severe to warrant independent clinical attention.

D. The disturbance is not better accounted for by another sleep disorder (e.g., narcolepsy, breathing-related sleep disorder, a parasomnia).

E. The disturbance is not due to the direct physiological effects of a substance (e.g., a drug of abuse, a medication) or a general medical condition.

From American Psychiatric Association. *Diagnostic and Statistical Manual of Mental Disorders.* 4th ed. Text rev. Washington, DC: American Psychiatric Association; copyright 2000, with permission.

awakening, usually with an uncomfortable mood in the morning (morning is the worst time of day for many patients with major depressive disorder). Polysomnography shows reduced stages 3 and 4 sleep, often a short REM latency, and a long first REM period. The use of partial or total sleep deprivation can accelerate the response to antidepressant medication.

Hypersomnia Related to Another Mental (Axis I or Axis II) Disorder

Hypersomnia that occurs for at least 1 month and that is associated with a mental disorder is found in a variety of conditions,

Table 21.2–12
DSM-IV-TR Diagnostic Criteria for Hypersomnia Related to Another Mental Disorder

A. The predominant complaint is excessive sleepiness for at least 1 month as evidenced by either prolonged sleep episodes or daytime sleep episodes that occur almost daily.

B. The excessive sleepiness causes clinically significant distress or impairment in social, occupational, or other important areas of functioning.

C. The hypersomnia is judged to be related to another Axis I or Axis II disorder (e.g., major depressive disorder, dysthymic disorder) but is sufficiently severe to warrant independent clinical attention.

D. The disturbance is not better accounted for by another sleep disorder (e.g., narcolepsy, breathing-related sleep disorder, a parasomnia) or by an inadequate amount of sleep.

E. The disturbance is not due to the direct physiological effects of a substance (e.g., a drug of abuse, a medication) or a general medical condition.

From American Psychiatric Association. *Diagnostic and Statistical Manual of Mental Disorders.* 4th ed. Text rev. Washington, DC: American Psychiatric Association; copyright 2000, with permission.

Table 21.2–13
DSM-IV-TR Diagnostic Criteria for Sleep Disorder Due to a General Medical Condition

A. A prominent disturbance in sleep that is sufficiently severe to warrant independent clinical attention.

B. There is evidence from the history, physical examination, or laboratory findings that the sleep disturbance is the direct physiological consequence of a general medical condition.

C. The disturbance is not better accounted for by another mental disorder (e.g., an adjustment disorder in which the stressor is a serious medical illness).

D. The disturbance does not occur exclusively during the course of a delirium.

E. The disturbance does not meet the criteria for breathing-related sleep disorder or narcolepsy.

F. The sleep disturbance causes clinically significant distress or impairment in social, occupational, or other important areas of functioning.

Specify type:
    Insomnia type: if the predominant sleep disturbance is insomnia
    Hypersomnia type: if the predominant sleep disturbance is hypersomnia
    Parasomnia type: if the predominant sleep disturbance is a parasomnia
    Mixed type: if more than one sleep disturbance is present and none predominates

Coding note: Include the name of the general medical condition on Axis I, e.g., sleep disorder due to chronic obstructive pulmonary disease, insomnia type; also code the general medical condition on Axis III.

From American Psychiatric Association. *Diagnostic and Statistical Manual of Mental Disorders.* 4th ed. Text rev. Washington, DC: American Psychiatric Association; copyright 2000, with permission.

including mood disorders. Excessive daytime sleepiness may be reported in the initial stages of many mild depressive disorders and characteristically in the depressed phase of bipolar I disorder. For a short time, hypersomnia may sometimes be associated with uncomplicated grief. Other mental disorders—such as personality disorders, dissociative disorders, somatoform disorders, dissociative fugue, and amnestic disorders—can produce hypersomnia (Table 21.2–12). Treatment of the primary disorder should result in resolution of the hypersomnia.

OTHER SLEEP DISORDERS

DSM-IV-TR defines a sleep disorder caused by a medical condition as a complaint of sleep disturbance produced by a physiological effect of the medical condition on the sleep–wake system. A substance-induced sleep disorder arises from the use, or the recently discontinued use, of a substance.

Sleep Disorder Due to a General Medical Condition

Any sleep disturbance (e.g., insomnia, hypersomnia, parasomnia, or a combination) can be caused by a general medical condition (Table 21.2–13). Almost any medical condition associated with pain and discomfort (e.g., arthritis or angina) can produce insomnia. Some conditions are associated with insomnia even when pain and discomfort are not specifically present. These conditions include neoplasms, vascular lesions, infections, and degenerative and traumatic conditions. Other conditions, especially endocrine and metabolic diseases, frequently involve some sleep disturbance.

Being aware of the possibility of such conditions and obtaining a good medical history usually lead to a correct diagnosis. The treatment, whenever possible, is treatment of the underlying medical condition.

Sleep-Related Epileptic Seizures. The relation of sleep and epilepsy is complex. Sleep disorders, sleep apnea in particular, can exacerbate seizures. Seizures, in turn, can disrupt sleep structure, particularly REM. When seizures occur almost exclusively during sleep, the condition is called *sleep epilepsy*.

Sleep-Related Cluster Headaches and Chronic Paroxysmal Hemicrania. Sleep-related cluster headaches are agonizingly severe unilateral headaches that often appear during sleep and are marked by an on–off pattern of attacks. Chronic paroxysmal hemicrania is a similar unilateral headache that occurs every day with more frequent but short-lived onsets that are without a preponderant sleep distribution. Both types of vascular headache are examples of sleep-exacerbated conditions and appear in association with REM sleep periods; paroxysmal hemicrania is virtually REM sleep locked.

Sleep-Related Abnormal Swallowing Syndrome. Abnormal swallowing syndrome is a condition during sleep in which inadequate swallowing results in aspiration of saliva, coughing, and choking. It is intermittently associated with brief arousals or awakenings.

Sleep-Related Asthma. Asthma that is exacerbated by sleep in some people may result in significant sleep disturbances.

Sleep-Related Cardiovascular Symptoms. Sleep-related cardiovascular symptoms derive from disorders of cardiac rhythm, myocardial incompetence, coronary artery insufficiency, and blood pressure variability, which may be induced or exacerbated by sleep-altered or sleep-state–modified cardiovascular physiology.

Sleep-Related Gastroesophageal Reflux. Sleep-related gastroesophageal reflux is a disorder in which patients awaken from sleep with burning, substernal pain or a feeling of general pain or tightness in the chest or a sour taste in the mouth. Coughing, choking, and vague respiratory discomfort may also occur repeatedly.

Sleep-Related Hemolysis (Paroxysmal Nocturnal Hemoglobinuria). Paroxysmal nocturnal hemoglobinuria is a rare, acquired, chronic hemolytic anemia in which intravascular hemolysis results in hemoglobinemia and hemoglobinuria. The hemolysis and consequent hemoglobinuria are accelerated during sleep, and the morning urine is colored a brownish red. Hemolysis is linked to the sleep period, even when the period is shifted.

Substance-Induced Sleep Disorder

Any sleep disturbance (e.g., insomnia, hypersomnia, parasomnia, or a combination) can be caused by a substance (Table 21.2–14). According to DSM-IV-TR, clinicians should also specify whether the onset of the disorder occurred during intoxication or withdrawal.

**Table 21.2–14
DSM-IV-TR Diagnostic Criteria for Substance-Induced Sleep Disorder**

A. A prominent disturbance in sleep that is sufficiently severe to warrant independent clinical attention.

B. There is evidence from the history, physical examination, or laboratory findings of either (1) or (2):

(1) the symptoms in Criterion A developed during, or within a month of, substance intoxication or withdrawal

(2) medication use is etiologically related to the sleep disturbance

C. The disturbance is not better accounted for by a sleep disorder that is not substance induced. Evidence that the symptoms are better accounted for by a sleep disorder that is not substance induced might include the following: the symptoms precede the onset of the substance use (or medication use); the symptoms persist for a substantial period of time (e.g., about a month) after the cessation of acute withdrawal or severe intoxication or are substantially in excess of what would be expected given the type or amount of the substance used or the duration of use; or there is other evidence that suggests the existence of an independent non–substance-induced sleep disorder (e.g., a history of recurrent non–substance-related episodes).

D. The disturbance does not occur exclusively during the course of a delirium.

E. The sleep disturbance causes clinically significant distress or impairment in social, occupational, or other important areas of functioning.

Note: This diagnosis should be made instead of a diagnosis of substance intoxication or substance withdrawal only when the sleep symptoms are in excess of those usually associated with the intoxication or withdrawal syndrome and when the symptoms are sufficiently severe to warrant independent clinical attention.

Code [Specific substance]-induced sleep disorder:
Alcohol; amphetamine; caffeine; cocaine; opioid; sedative, hypnotic, or anxiolytic; other [or unknown] substance

Specify type:

Insomnia type: if the predominant sleep disturbance is insomnia

Hypersomnia type: if the predominant sleep disturbance is hypersomnia

Parasomnia type: if the predominant sleep disturbance is a parasomnia

Mixed type: if more than one sleep disturbance is present and none predominates

Specify if:

With onset during intoxication: if the criteria are met for intoxication with the substance and the symptoms develop during the intoxication syndrome

With onset during withdrawal: if criteria are met for withdrawal from the substance and the symptoms develop during, or shortly after, a withdrawal syndrome

From American Psychiatric Association. *Diagnostic and Statistical Manual of Mental Disorders.* 4th ed. Text rev. Washington, DC: American Psychiatric Association; copyright 2000, with permission.

Somnolence related to tolerance or withdrawal from a central nervous system (CNS) stimulant is common in people withdrawing from amphetamines, cocaine, caffeine, and related substances. The somnolence may be associated with severe depression, which occasionally reaches suicidal proportions. The sustained use of CNS depressants, such as alcohol, can cause somnolence. Heavy alcohol use in the evening produces sleepiness and difficulty in arising the next day. This reaction may present a diagnostic problem when patients do not admit to alcohol abuse.

Insomnia is associated with tolerance to or withdrawal from sedative-hypnotic drugs, such as benzodiazepines, barbiturates, and chloral hydrate. With the sustained use of such agents—usually undertaken to treat insomnia arising from a different source—tolerance increases, and the drugs lose their sleep-inducing effects; patients then often increase the dosage. On sudden discontinuation of the drug, severe sleeplessness supervenes, often accompanied by the general features of substance withdrawal. Typically, patients experience a temporary increase in the severity of the insomnia.

Long-term use (more than 30 days) of a hypnotic agent is well tolerated by some patients, but others begin to complain of sleep disturbance, most often multiple brief awakenings during the night. Recordings show a disruption of sleep architecture, reduced stages 3 and 4 sleep, increased stages 1 and 2 sleep, and a fragmentation of sleep throughout the night.

Clinicians should be aware of CNS stimulants as a possible cause of insomnia and should remember that various medications for weight reduction, beverages containing caffeine, and occasionally adrenergic drugs taken by asthmatic patients may all produce this insomnia. Alcohol may help induce sleep but frequently results in nocturnal awakening. Alcohol use during the cocktail hour can produce difficulty in falling asleep later in the evening.

For reasons that are not always clear, a wide variety of drugs occasionally produce sleep problems as a side effect. These drugs include antimetabolites and other cancer chemotherapeutic agents, thyroid preparations, anticonvulsant agents, antidepressant drugs, adrenocorticotropic hormone (ACTH)-like drugs, oral contraceptives, α-methyldopa, and β-adrenergic receptor antagonists.

Other agents do not produce sleep disturbance while being used, but many have this effect after withdrawal. Almost any drug with sedating or tranquilizing agents, including at times the benzodiazepines, the phenothiazines, the sedating tricyclic drugs, and various street drugs, including marijuana and opioids, can have this effect.

Alcohol is a CNS depressant and produces the serious problems of other CNS depressants, both during administration—perhaps related to the development of tolerance—and after withdrawal. The insomnia after long-term alcohol consumption is sometimes severe and lasts for weeks or longer. Clinicians should not give potentially addicting medications to patients who have just recovered from an addiction; if possible, sleeping medications should be avoided.

Among cigarette smokers, the combination of a relaxing ritual and the tendency of low doses of nicotine to cause sedation may actually help sleep, but high doses of nicotine can interfere with sleep, particularly sleep onset. Cigarette smokers typically sleep less than nonsmokers. Nicotine withdrawal may cause drowsiness or arousal.

Impulse-Control Disorders Not Elsewhere Classified

The text revision of the fourth edition of *Diagnostic and Statistical Manual of Mental Disorders* (DSM-IV-TR) lists six categories of impulse-control disorders not classified elsewhere: (1) intermittent explosive disorder, (2) kleptomania, (3) pyromania, (4) pathological gambling, (5) trichotillomania, and (6) impulse-control disorder not otherwise specified (NOS).

Disorders of impulse control have long been recognized. In 1838, Jean Etienne Esquirol proposed the term *monomanic instinctives* to describe behaviors characterized by irresistible urges without apparent motive. Patients with impulse-control disorders do not resist drives or enticements to do something harmful to themselves or to others. They are unable to resist impulses, although they may or may not consciously try to do so, and they may or may not plan their behaviors. Before they act, there is a sense of increasing tension or arousal; afterward there is a sense of pleasure and satisfaction. On occasion, however, there may be feelings of remorse or guilt that disturb the sense of pleasure. Because their behaviors consciously coincide with their desires, their acts are considered ego-syntonic.

ETIOLOGY

Psychodynamic, psychosocial, and biological factors all play an important role in impulse-control disorders; however, the primary causal factor remains unknown. Some impulse-control disorders may have common underlying neurobiological mechanisms. Fatigue, incessant stimulation, and psychic trauma can lower a person's resistance to control impulses.

Psychodynamic Factors

An impulse is a disposition to act to decrease heightened tension caused by the buildup of instinctual drives or by diminished ego defenses against the drives. The impulse disorders have in common an attempt to bypass the experience of disabling symptoms or painful affects by acting on the environment. In his work with adolescents who were delinquent, August Aichhorn described impulsive behavior as related to a weak superego and weak ego structures associated with psychic trauma produced by childhood deprivation.

Otto Fenichel linked impulsive behavior to attempts to master anxiety, guilt, depression, and other painful affects by means of action. He thought that such actions defend against internal danger and they pro-

duce a distorted aggressive or sexual gratification. To observers, impulsive behaviors may appear irrational and motivated by greed, but they may actually be endeavors to find relief from pain.

Heinz Kohut considered many forms of impulse control problems, including gambling, kleptomania, and some paraphiliac behaviors, to be related to an incomplete sense of self. He observed that when patients do not receive the validating and affirming responses that they seek from persons in significant relationships with them, the self might fragment. As a way of dealing with this fragmentation, persons may engage in impulsive behaviors that to others appear self-destructive. Kohut's formulation has some similarities to Donald Winnicott's view that impulsive or deviant behavior in children is a way for them to try to recapture a primitive maternal relationship. Winnicott saw such behavior as hopeful in that the child searches for affirmation and love from the mother rather than abandoning any attempt to win her affection. Several therapists have stressed patients' fixation at the oral stage of development. Patients attempt to master anxiety, guilt, depression, and other painful affects by means of actions, but such actions aimed at obtaining relief seldom succeed even temporarily.

Psychosocial Factors

Psychosocial factors implicated causally in impulse-control disorders are related to early life events. The growing child may have had improper models for identification, such as parents who had difficulty controlling impulses. Other psychosocial factors associated with the disorders include exposure to violence in the home, alcohol abuse, promiscuity, and antisocial behavior.

Biological Factors

Many investigators have focused on possible organic factors in the impulse-control disorders, especially for patients with overtly violent behavior. Experiments have shown that impulsive and violent activity is associated with specific brain regions such as the limbic system. A relation has been found between low cerebrospinal fluid (CSF) levels of 5-hydroxyindoleacetic acid (5-HIAA) and impulsive aggression. Certain hormones, especially testosterone, have also been associated with violent and aggressive behavior. Some reports have described a relation between temporal lobe epilepsy and certain impulsive violent behaviors, as well as an association of aggressive behavior in patients who have histories of head trauma with increased numbers of emergency room visits and other potential organic antecedents. A high incidence of mixed cerebral dominance may be found in some violent populations.

Considerable evidence indicates that the serotonin neurotransmitter system mediates symptoms evident in impulse-control disorders. Brainstem and CSF levels of 5-HIAA are decreased, and serotonin-binding sites are increased in persons who have committed suicide. The dopaminergic and noradrenergic systems have also been implicated in impulsivity.

Impulse-control disorder symptoms may continue into adulthood in persons whose disorder has been diagnosed as childhood attention-deficit/hyperactivity disorder. Lifelong or acquired mental deficiency, epilepsy, and even reversible brain syndromes have long been implicated in lapses in impulse control.

INTERMITTENT EXPLOSIVE DISORDER

Intermittent explosive disorder manifests as discrete episodes of losing control of aggressive impulses; these episodes can result in serious assault or the destruction of property. The aggressiveness expressed is grossly out of proportion to any stressors that may have helped elicit the episodes. The symptoms, which patients may describe as spells or attacks, appear within minutes or hours and, regardless of duration, remit spontaneously and quickly. After each episode, patients usually show genuine regret or self-reproach, and signs of generalized impulsivity or aggressiveness are absent between episodes. The diagnosis of intermittent explosive disorder should not be made if the loss of control can be accounted for by schizophrenia, antisocial or borderline personality disorder, attention-deficit/hyperactivity disorder, conduct disorder, or substance intoxication.

Epidemiology

Intermittent explosive disorder is underreported. The disorder appears to be more common in men than in women. The men are likely to be found in correctional institutions and the women in psychiatric facilities. In one study, approximately 2 percent of all persons admitted to a university hospital psychiatric service had disorders that were diagnosed as intermittent explosive disorder; 80 percent were men.

Evidence indicates that intermittent explosive disorder is more common in first-degree biological relatives of persons with the disorder than in the general population. Many factors other than a simple genetic explanation may be responsible.

Comorbidity

High rates of fire setting in patients with intermittent explosive disorder have been reported. Other disorders of impulse control and substance use, mood, anxiety, and eating disorders have also been associated with intermittent explosive disorder.

Etiology

Psychodynamic Factors. Psychoanalysts have suggested that explosive outbursts occur as a defense against narcissistic injurious events. Rage outbursts serve as interpersonal distance and protect against any further narcissistic injury.

Psychosocial Factors. Typical patients have been described as physically large but dependent men whose sense of masculine identity is poor. A sense of being useless and impotent or of being unable to change the environment often precedes an epi-

sode of physical violence, and a high level of anxiety, guilt, and depression usually follows an episode.

An unfavorable childhood environment often filled with alcohol dependence, beatings, and threats to life is usual in these patients. Predisposing factors in infancy and childhood include perinatal trauma, infantile seizures, head trauma, encephalitis, minimal brain dysfunction, and hyperactivity. Workers who have concentrated on psychogenesis as causing episodic explosiveness have stressed identification with assaultive parental figures as symbols of the target for violence. Early frustration, oppression, and hostility have been noted as predisposing factors. Situations that are directly or symbolically reminiscent of early deprivations (e.g., persons who directly or indirectly evoke the image of the frustrating parent) become targets for destructive hostility.

Biological Factors. Some investigators suggest that disordered brain physiology, particularly in the limbic system, is involved in most cases of episodic violence. Compelling evidence indicates that serotonergic neurons mediate behavioral inhibition. Decreased serotonergic transmission, which can be induced by inhibiting serotonin synthesis or by antagonizing its effects, decreases the effect of punishment as a deterrent to behavior. The restoration of serotonin activity, by administering serotonin precursors such as L-tryptophan or drugs that increase synaptic serotonergic levels, appears to restore control of episodic violent tendencies. Low levels of CSF 5-HIAA have been correlated with impulsive aggression. High CSF testosterone concentrations are correlated with aggressiveness and interpersonal violence in men. Antiandrogenic agents have been shown to decrease aggression.

Familial and Genetic Factors. First-degree relatives of intermittent explosive disorder patients have higher rates of impulse-control disorders, depressive disorders, and substance use disorders. Biological relatives of patients with the disorder were more likely to have histories of temper or explosive outbursts than the general population.

Diagnosis and Clinical Features

The diagnosis of intermittent explosive disorder should be the result of history-taking that reveals several episodes of loss-of-control associated with aggressive outbursts (Table 22–1). One discrete episode does not justify the diagnosis. The histories typically describe a childhood in an atmosphere of alcohol dependence, violence, and emotional instability. Patients' work histories are poor; they report job losses, marital difficulties, and trouble with the law. Most patients have sought psychiatric help in the past, but to no avail. Anxiety, guilt, and depression usually follow an outburst, but this is not a constant finding. Neurological examination sometimes reveals soft neurological signs such as left–right ambivalence and perceptual reversal. Electroencephalographic (EEG) findings are frequently normal or show nonspecific changes.

Physical Findings and Laboratory Examination

Persons with the disorder have a high incidence of soft neurological signs (e.g., reflex asymmetries), nonspecific EEG findings, abnormal neuropsychological testing results (e.g., letter reversal difficulties), and accident proneness. Blood chemistry (liver and thyroid function tests, fasting blood glucose, electrolytes), urinal-

**Table 22–1
DSM-IV-TR Diagnostic Criteria for Intermittent
Explosive Disorder**

A. Several discrete episodes of failure to resist aggressive
impulses that result in serious assaultive acts or destruction
of property.

B. The degree of aggressiveness expressed during the episodes
is grossly out of proportion to any precipitating psychosocial
stressors.

C. The aggressive episodes are not better accounted for by
another mental disorder (e.g., antisocial personality disorder,
borderline personality disorder, a psychotic disorder, a manic
episode, conduct disorder, or attention-deficit/hyperactivity
disorder) and are not due to the direct physiological effects of
a substance (e.g., a drug of abuse, a medication) or a general
medical condition (e.g., head trauma, Alzheimer's disease).

From American Psychiatric Association. *Diagnostic and Statistical Manual of Mental Disorders*. 4th ed. Text rev. Washington, DC: American
Psychiatric Association; copyright 2000, with permission.

ysis (including drug toxicology), and syphilis serology may help
rule out other causes of aggression. Magnetic resonance imagery
(MRI) may reveal changes in the prefrontal cortex, which is associated with loss of impulse control.

Differential Diagnosis

The diagnosis of intermittent explosive disorder can be made
only after disorders associated with the occasional loss of control
of aggressive impulses have been ruled out as the primary cause.
These other disorders include psychotic disorders, personality
change due to a general medical condition, antisocial or borderline personality disorder, and substance intoxication (e.g., alcohol, barbiturates, hallucinogens, and amphetamines), epilepsy,
brain tumors, degenerative diseases, and endocrine disorders.

Conduct disorder is distinguished from intermittent explosive disorder by its repetitive and resistant pattern of behavior,
as opposed to an episodic pattern. Intermittent explosive disorder differs from the antisocial and borderline personality disorders because, in the personality disorders, aggressiveness and
impulsivity are part of patients' characters and thus are present
between outbursts. In paranoid and catatonic schizophrenia,
patients may display violent behavior in response to delusions
and hallucinations, and they show gross impairments in reality
testing. Hostile patients with mania may be impulsively aggressive, but the underlying diagnosis is generally apparent from
their mental status examinations and clinical presentations.

Amok is an episode of acute violent behavior for which the
person claims amnesia. *Amok* is usually seen in southeastern
Asia, but it has been reported in North America. *Amok* is distinguished from intermittent explosive disorder by a single episode and prominent dissociative features.

Course and Prognosis

Intermittent explosive disorder may begin at any stage of life but
usually appears between late adolescence and early adulthood. The
onset may be sudden or insidious, and the course may be episodic
or chronic. In most cases, the disorder decreases in severity with
the onset of middle age, but heightened organic impairment can
lead to frequent and severe episodes.

Treatment

A combined pharmacological and psychotherapeutic approach has
the best chance of success. Psychotherapy with patients who have
intermittent explosive disorder is difficult, however, because of
their angry outbursts. Therapists may have problems with countertransference and limit setting. Group psychotherapy may be helpful, and family therapy is useful, particularly when the explosive
patient is an adolescent or a young adult. A goal of therapy is to
have the patient recognize and verbalize the thoughts or feelings
that precede the explosive outbursts instead of acting them out.

Anticonvulsants have long been used, with mixed results, in
treating explosive patients. Lithium (Eskalith) has been
reported useful in generally lessening aggressive behavior, and
carbamazepine (Tegretol), valproate (Depakene) or divalproex
(Depakote), and phenytoin (Dilantin) have been reported helpful. Some clinicians have also used other anticonvulsants (e.g.,
gabapentin [Neurontin]). Benzodiazepines are sometimes used
but have been reported to produce a paradoxical reaction of
dyscontrol in some cases.

Antipsychotics (e.g., phenothiazines and serotonin-dopamine
antagonists) and tricyclic drugs have been effective in some
cases, but clinicians must then wonder whether schizophrenia or
a mood disorder is the true diagnosis. When there is a likelihood
of subcortical seizure-like activity, medications that lower the
seizure threshold can aggravate the situation. Selective serotonin
reuptake inhibitors (SSRIs), trazodone (Desyrel), and buspirone
(BuSpar) are useful in reducing impulsivity and aggression.

Propranolol (Inderal) and other β-adrenergic receptor antagonists and calcium channel inhibitors have also been effective
in some cases. Some neurosurgeons have performed operative
treatments for intractable violence and aggression. No evidence
indicates that such treatment is effective.

KLEPTOMANIA

The essential feature of kleptomania is a recurrent failure to resist
impulses to steal objects not needed for personal use or for monetary value. The objects taken are often given away, returned surrep-
titiously, or kept and hidden. Persons with kleptomania usually
have the money to pay for the objects they impulsively steal.

Like other impulse-control disorders, kleptomania is characterized by mounting tension before the act, followed by gratification and lessening of tension with or without guilt, remorse,
or depression after the act. The stealing is not planned and does
not involve others. Although the thefts do not occur when
immediate arrest is probable, persons with kleptomania do not
always consider their chances of being apprehended, even
though repeated arrests lead to pain and humiliation.

Epidemiology

The prevalence of kleptomania is not known but is estimated to
be approximately 0.6 percent. The range varies from 3.8 to 24
percent of those arrested for shoplifting. DSM-IV-TR reports
that it occurs in fewer than 5 percent of identified shoplifters.
The male-to-female ratio is 1:3 in clinical samples.

Comorbidity

There is a high comorbidity with other disorders of impulse-control, mood disorders, anxiety disorders, bulimia nervosa, and personality disorders. Many persons with kleptomania have obsessive-compulsive symptoms (e.g., cleaning, hand washing, collecting).

Etiology

Psychosocial Factors. The symptoms of kleptomania tend to appear in times of significant stress (for example, losses, separations, and endings of important relationships). Some psychoanalytic writers have stressed the expression of aggressive impulses in kleptomania; others have discerned a libidinal aspect. Those who focus on symbolism see meaning in the act itself, the object stolen, and the victim of the theft.

Analytic writers have focused on stealing by children and adolescents. Anna Freud pointed out that the first thefts from mother's purse indicate the degree to which all stealing is rooted in the oneness between mother and child. Karl Abraham wrote of the central feeling of being neglected, injured, or unwanted. One theoretician established seven categories of stealing in chronically acting-out children:

1. As a means of restoring the lost mother–child relationship
2. As an aggressive act
3. As a defense against fears of being damaged (perhaps a search by girls for a penis or a protection against castration anxiety in boys)
4. As a means of seeking punishment
5. As a means of restoring or adding to self-esteem
6. In connection with, and as a reaction to, a family secret
7. As excitement (lust angst) and a substitute for a sexual act

One or more of these categories can also apply to adult kleptomania.

Biological Factors. Brain diseases and mental retardation have been associated with kleptomania, as they have with other disorders of impulse control. Focal neurological signs, cortical atrophy, and enlarged lateral ventricles have been found in some patients. Disturbances in monoamine metabolism, particularly of serotonin, have been postulated.

Family and Genetic Factors. In one study, 7 percent of first-degree relatives had obsessive-compulsive disorder. In addition, a higher rate of mood disorders has been reported in family members.

Diagnosis and Clinical Features

The essential feature of kleptomania is recurrent, intrusive, and irresistible urges or impulses to steal unneeded objects (Table 22–2). Patients with kleptomania may also be distressed about the possibility or actuality of being apprehended and may manifest signs of depression and anxiety. Patients feel guilty, ashamed, and embarrassed about their behavior. They often have serious problems with interpersonal relationships and often show signs of personality disturbance. In one study of

Table 22–2
DSM-IV-TR Diagnostic Criteria for Kleptomania

A. Recurrent failure to resist impulses to steal objects that are not needed for personal use or for their monetary value.

B. Increasing sense of tension immediately before committing the theft.

C. Pleasure, gratification, or relief at the time of committing the theft.

D. The stealing is not committed to express anger or vengeance and is not in response to a delusion or a hallucination.

E. The stealing is not better accounted for by conduct disorder, a manic episode, or antisocial personality disorder.

From American Psychiatric Association. *Diagnostic and Statistical Manual of Mental Disorders.* 4th ed. Text rev. Washington, DC: American Psychiatric Association; copyright 2000, with permission.

patients with kleptomania, the frequency of stealing ranged from less than 1 to 120 episodes a month. Most kleptomaniac patients steal from retail stores, but they may also steal from family members in their own households.

Differential Diagnosis

Because most patients with kleptomania are referred for examination in connection with legal proceedings after apprehension, the clinical picture may be clouded by subsequent symptoms of depression and anxiety. Clinicians must differentiate between kleptomania and other forms of stealing. For a diagnosis of kleptomania, stealing must always follow a failure to resist the impulse and the stolen articles must be without immediate usefulness or monetary gain. By contrast, ordinary stealing is usually planned, and the objects are stolen for their use or financial value. Malingerers may try to simulate kleptomania to avoid prosecution. Stealing that occurs in association with conduct disorder, antisocial personality disorder, or a manic episode is clearly related to the pervasive, underlying disorder. Persons with kleptomania do not typically display antisocial behavior other than stealing. Patients with schizophrenia may steal in response to hallucinations and delusions, and patients with cognitive disorders may be accused of stealing when they forget to pay for objects.

Course and Prognosis

Kleptomania may begin in childhood, although most children and adolescents who steal do not become kleptomaniac adults. The onset of the disorder generally is late adolescence. Women are more likely to present for psychiatric evaluation or treatment than are men. Men are more likely to be sent to prison. Men tend to present with the disorder at approximately 50 years of age and women at approximately 35 years of age. In quiescent cases, new bouts of the disorder may be precipitated by loss or disappointment.

The course of the disorder waxes and wanes but tends to be chronic. Persons sometimes have bouts of being unable to resist the impulse to steal, followed by free periods that last for weeks or months. Its spontaneous recovery rate is unknown.

The prognosis with treatment can be good, but few patients come for help of their own accord.

Treatment

Because true kleptomania is rare, reports of treatment tend to be individual case descriptions or a short series of cases. Insight-oriented psychotherapy and psychoanalysis have been successful but depend on patients' motivations. Those who feel guilt and shame may be helped by insight-oriented psychotherapy because of their increased motivation to change their behavior.

Behavior therapy, including systematic desensitization, aversive conditioning, and a combination of aversive conditioning and altered social contingencies, has been reported successful, even when motivation was lacking. The reports cite follow-up studies of up to 2 years. SSRIs, such as fluoxetine (Prozac) and fluvoxamine (Luvox), appear to be effective in some patients with kleptomania. There have also been case reports of successful treatment with tricyclic drugs, trazodone (Desyrel), lithium, valproate (Depakone), naltrexone (ReVia), and electroconvulsive therapy (ECT).

PYROMANIA

Pyromania is the recurrent, deliberate, and purposeful setting of fires. Associated features include tension or affective arousal before setting the fires; fascination with, interest in, curiosity about, or attraction to fire and the activities and equipment associated with fire fighting; and pleasure, gratification, or relief when setting fires or when witnessing or participating in their aftermath. Patients may make considerable advance preparations before starting a fire. Pyromania differs from arson in that the latter is done for financial gain, revenge, or other reasons and is planned beforehand.

Epidemiology

No information is available on the prevalence of pyromania, but only a small percentage of adults who set fires can be classified as having pyromania. The disorder is found far more often in men than in women. Among children who attend outpatient psychiatric clinics, approximately 20 percent have a history of occasional fire setting.

Comorbidity

Persons who set fires are more likely to be mildly retarded than are those in the general population. Some studies have noted an increased incidence of alcohol use disorders in persons who set fires. Fire setters also tend to have a history of antisocial traits, such as truancy, running away from home, and delinquency. Enuresis has been considered a common finding in the history of fire setters, although controlled studies have failed to confirm this. Studies have, however, found an association between cruelty to animals and fire setting. Childhood and adolescent fire setting is often associated with attention-deficit/hyperactivity disorder or adjustment disorders.

Etiology

Psychosocial Factors.   Sigmund Freud saw fire as a symbol of sexuality. He believed the warmth radiated by fire evokes the same sensation that accompanies a state of sexual excitation, and a flame's shape and movements suggest a phallus in activity. Other psychoanalysts have associated pyromania with an abnormal craving for power and social prestige. Some patients with pyromania are volunteer firefighters who set fires to prove themselves brave, to force other firefighters into action, or to demonstrate their power to extinguish a blaze. The incendiary act is a way to vent accumulated rage over frustration caused by a sense of social, physical, or sexual inferiority. Several studies have noted that the fathers of patients with pyromania were absent from the home. Thus, one explanation of fire setting is that it represents a wish for absent father to return home as a rescuer, to put out the fire and to save the child from a difficult existence.

Female fire setters, in addition to being much fewer in number than male fire setters, do not start fires to put firefighters into action as men frequently do. Frequently noted delinquent trends in female fire setters include promiscuity without pleasure and petty stealing, often approaching kleptomania.

Biological Factors.   Significantly low CSF levels of 5-HIAA and 3-methoxy-4-hydroxyphenylglycol (MHPG) have been found in fire setters, which suggests possible serotonergic or adrenergic involvement. The presence of reactive hypoglycemia, based on blood glucose concentrations on glucose tolerance tests, has been put forward as a cause of pyromania. Further studies are needed, however.

Diagnosis and Clinical Features

Persons with pyromania often regularly watch fires in their neighborhoods, frequently set off false alarms, and show interest in firefighting paraphernalia (Table 22–3). Their curiosity is evident, but they show no remorse and may be indifferent to the consequences for life or property. Fire setters may gain satisfaction from the resulting destruction; frequently, they leave obvious clues. Commonly associated features include alcohol intoxication, sexual dysfunctions, below-average intelligence

Table 22–3
DSM-IV-TR Diagnostic Criteria for Pyromania

A. Deliberate and purposeful fire setting on more than one occasion.

B. Tension or affective arousal before the act.

C. Fascination with, interest in, curiosity about, or attraction to fire and its situational contexts (e.g., paraphernalia, uses, consequences).

D. Pleasure, gratification, or relief when setting fires, or when witnessing or participating in their aftermath.

E. The fire setting is not done for monetary gain, as an expression of sociopolitical ideology, to conceal criminal activity, to express anger or vengeance, to improve one's living circumstances, in response to a delusion or hallucination, or as a result of impaired judgment (e.g., in dementia, mental retardation, substance intoxication).

F. The fire setting is not better accounted for by conduct disorder, a manic episode, or antisocial personality disorder.

quotient (IQ), chronic personal frustration, and resentment toward authority figures. Some fire setters become sexually aroused by the fire.

Differential Diagnosis

Clinicians should have little trouble distinguishing between pyromania and the fascination of many young children with matches, lighters, and fire as part of the normal investigation of their environments. Pyromania must also be separated from incendiary acts of sabotage carried out by dissident political extremists or by paid torchers, termed *arsonists* in the legal system.

When fire setting occurs in conduct disorder and antisocial personality disorder, it is a deliberate act, not a failure to resist an impulse. Patients with schizophrenia or mania may set fires in response to delusions or hallucinations. Patients with brain dysfunction (e.g., dementia), mental retardation, or substance intoxication may set fires because of a failure to appreciate the consequences of the act.

Course and Prognosis

While fire setting often begins in childhood, the typical age of onset of pyromania is unknown. When the onset is in adolescence or adulthood, the fire setting tends to be deliberately destructive. Fire setting in pyromania is episodic and may wax and wane in frequency. The prognosis for treated children is good, and complete remission is a realistic goal. The prognosis for adults is guarded, because they frequently deny their actions, refuse to take responsibility, are dependent on alcohol, and lack insight.

Treatment

Little has been written about the treatment of pyromania, and treating fire setters has been difficult because of their lack of motivation. Until research reports the success of any single treatment, an appropriate approach is to use a number of modalities, including behavioral approaches. Because of the recurrent nature of pyromania, any treatment program should include supervision of patients to prevent a repeated episode of fire setting. Incarceration may be the only method of preventing a recurrence. Behavior therapy can then be administered in the institution.

Fire setting by children must be treated with the utmost seriousness. Intensive interventions should be undertaken when possible, but as therapeutic and preventive measures, not as punishment. In the case of children and adolescents, treatment of pyromania or fire setting should include family therapy.

PATHOLOGICAL GAMBLING

Pathological gambling is characterized by persistent and recurrent maladaptive gambling that causes economic problems and significant disturbances in personal, social, or occupational functioning. Aspects of the maladaptive behavior include (1) a preoccupation with gambling; (2) the need to gamble with increasing amounts of money to achieve the desired excitement; (3) repeated unsuccessful efforts to control, cut back or stop gambling; (4) gambling as a way to escape from problems; (5) gambling to recoup losses; (6) lying to conceal the extent of the involvement with gambling; (7) the commission of illegal acts to finance gambling; (8) jeopardizing or losing personal and vocational relationships because of gambling; and (9) a reliance on others for money to pay off debts.

Epidemiology

Up to 3 percent of the general population may be classified as pathological gamblers. In addition, according to DSM-IV-TR, the prevalence of pathological gamblers has been reported to be from 2.8 to 8.0 percent in adolescents and college students. The disorder is more common in men than in women, and the rate is considerably higher in locations where gambling is legal. Approximately one-fourth of pathological gamblers had a parent with a gambling problem; both the fathers of men and the mothers of women with the disorder are more likely to have the disorder than is the population at large. Alcohol dependence is also more common among the parents of pathological gamblers than in the overall population. Women with the disorder are more likely than those not so affected to be married to alcoholic men who are usually absent from the home.

Comorbidity

Rates of other impulse-control disorders, substance-use disorders, mood disorders, attention deficit/hyperactivity disorder, and antisocial, borderline, and narcissistic personality disorders are increased in persons with pathological gambling. Other associated disorders include panic disorder, agoraphobia, obsessive-compulsive disorder, and Tourette's disorder.

Etiology

Psychosocial Factors. Several factors may predispose persons to develop the disorder: loss of a parent by death, separation, divorce, or desertion before a child is 15 years of age; inappropriate parental discipline (absence, inconsistency, or harshness); exposure to, and availability of, gambling activities for adolescents; a family emphasis on material and financial symbols; and a lack of family emphasis on saving, planning, and budgeting.

Psychoanalytic theory has focused on a number of core character difficulties. Freud suggested that compulsive gamblers have an unconscious desire to lose, and they gamble to relieve unconscious feelings of guilt. Another suggestion is that the gamblers are narcissists whose grandiose and omnipotent fantasies lead them to believe they can control events and even predict their outcome. Learning theorists view uncontrolled gambling as resulting from erroneous perceptions regarding control of impulses.

Biological Factors. Several studies have suggested that gamblers' risk-taking behavior may have an underlying neurobiological cause. These theories have centered on both serotonergic and noradrenergic receptor systems. Male pathological gamblers may have subnormal MHPG concentrations in plasma, increased MHPG concentrations in the CSF, and increased urinary output of norepinephrine. Evidence also implicates serotonergic regulatory dysfunction in the pathological gambler. Chronic gamblers

Table 22–4
DSM-IV-TR Diagnostic Criteria for Pathological Gambling

A. Persistent and recurrent maladaptive gambling behavior as indicated by five (or more) of the following:

(1) is preoccupied with gambling (e.g., preoccupied with reliving past gambling experiences, handicapping or planning the next venture, or thinking of ways to get money with which to gamble)

(2) needs to gamble with increasing amounts of money in order to achieve the desired excitement

(3) has repeated unsuccessful efforts to control, cut back, or stop gambling

(4) is restless or irritable when attempting to cut down or stop gambling

(5) gambles as a way of escaping from problems or of relieving a dysphoric mood (e.g., feelings of helplessness, guilt, anxiety, depression)

(6) after losing money gambling, often returns another day to get even ("chasing" one's losses)

(7) lies to family members, therapist, or others to conceal the extent of involvement with gambling

(8) has committed illegal acts such as forgery, fraud, theft, or embezzlement to finance gambling

(9) has jeopardized or lost a significant relationship, job, or educational or career opportunity because of gambling

(10) relies on others to provide money to relieve a desperate financial situation caused by gambling

B. The gambling behavior is not better accounted for by a manic episode.

From American Psychiatric Association. *Diagnostic and Statistical Manual of Mental Disorders.* 4th ed. Text rev. Washington, DC: American Psychiatric Association; copyright 2000, with permission.

have low platelet monoamine oxidase (MAO) activity, a marker of serotonin activity, also linked to difficulties with inhibition. Further studies are needed to confirm these findings.

Diagnosis and Clinical Features

In addition to the features already described, pathological gamblers often appear overconfident, somewhat abrasive, energetic, and free spending. They often show obvious signs of personal stress, anxiety, and depression (Table 22–4). They commonly have the attitude that money is the cause of, and the solution to, all their problems. They make no serious attempt to budget or save money. When their borrowing resources are strained, they are likely to engage in antisocial behavior to obtain money for gambling. Their criminal behavior is typically nonviolent, such as forgery, embezzlement, or fraud, and they consciously intend to return or repay the money. Complications include alienation from family members and acquaintances, the loss of life accomplishments, suicide attempts, and association with fringe and illegal groups. Arrest for nonviolent crimes may lead to imprisonment.

Psychological Testing and Laboratory Examination

Patients with pathological gambling often display high levels of impulsivity on neuropsychological tests. German studies have

demonstrated increased cortisol levels in the saliva of gamblers while they gamble, which can account for the euphoria that occurs during the experience and its addictive potential.

Differential Diagnosis

Social gambling is distinguished from pathological gambling in that the former occurs with friends, on special occasions, and with predetermined acceptable and tolerable losses. Gambling that is symptomatic of a manic episode can usually be distinguished from pathological gambling by the history of a marked mood change and the loss of judgment preceding the gambling.

Manic-like mood changes are common in pathological gambling, but they always follow winning and are usually succeeded by depressive episodes because of subsequent losses. Persons with antisocial personality disorder may have problems with gambling. When both disorders are present, both should be diagnosed.

Course and Prognosis

Pathological gambling usually begins in adolescence for men and late in life for women. The disorder waxes and wanes and tends to be chronic. Four phases are seen in pathological gambling:

1. The winning phase, ending with a big win, equal to approximately a year's salary, which hooks patients. Women usually do not have a big win but use gambling as an escape from problems.

2. The progressive-loss phase, in which patients structure their lives around gambling and then move from being excellent gamblers to being stupid ones who take considerable risks, cash in securities, borrow money, miss work, and lose jobs.

3. The desperate phase, with patients frenziedly gambling with large amounts of money, not paying debts, becoming involved with loan sharks, writing bad checks, and possibly embezzling.

4. The hopeless stage of accepting that losses can never be made up, but the gambling continues because of the associated arousal or excitement. The disorder may take up to 15 years to reach the last phase, but then, within a year or two, patients have deteriorated totally.

Treatment

Gamblers seldom come forward voluntarily to be treated. Legal difficulties, family pressures, or other psychiatric complaints bring gamblers to treatment. Gamblers Anonymous (GA) was founded in Los Angeles in 1957 and modeled on Alcoholics Anonymous (AA); it is accessible, at least in large cities, and is an effective treatment for gambling in some patients. GA is a method of inspirational group therapy that involves public confession, peer pressure, and the presence of reformed gamblers (like sponsors in AA) available to help members resist the impulse to gamble. However, the dropout rate from GA is high. In some cases, hospitalization may help by removing patients from their environments. Insight should not be sought until patients have been away from gambling for

3 months. At this point, patients who are pathological gamblers may become excellent candidates for insight-oriented psychotherapy. Cognitive-behavioral therapy (e.g., relaxation techniques combined with visualization of gambling avoidance) has had some success.

Little is known about the efficacy of pharmacotherapy for treating patients with pathological gambling. One study reported that seven of ten patients remained completely abstinent over 8 weeks after taking fluvoxamine. There have also been case reports of successful treatment with lithium and clomipramine (Anafranil). If gambling is associated with depressive disorders, mania, anxiety, or other mental disorders, pharmacotherapy with antidepressants, lithium, or antianxiety agents is useful.

TRICHOTILLOMANIA

Trichotillomania was first described in 1889 by the French dermatologist Francois Hallopeau. According to DSM-IV-TR, the essential feature of trichotillomania is the recurrent pulling out of hair, which can result in noticeable hair loss. Other clinical symptoms include an increasing sense of tension before pulling the hair and a sense of pleasure, gratification, or relief when pulling out the hair. The diagnosis should not be made if hair pulling is the result of another mental disorder (e.g., disorders manifesting delusions or hallucinations) or a general medical disorder (e.g., a preexisting lesion of the skin).

Epidemiology

Trichotillomania is more common in women than in men but shows no sex difference in children. No information is available on familial patterns, but one study reported that 5 of 19 children had family histories of some form of alopecia. The lifetime prevalence according to DSM-IV-TR is below 1 percent, but this figure may be too low. Trichotillomania may be more common than is now believed, especially if hair pulling without the sense of tension before the pulling and without the sense of relief afterward is considered trichotillomania.

Comorbidity

Persons with trichotillomania have an increased prevalence of mood disorders (e.g., major depressive disorders), anxiety disorders (e.g., obsessive-compulsive disorders, generalized anxiety disorder, social phobia), substance-use disorders, eating disorders, personality disorders (e.g., borderline and obsessive-compulsive disorders), and mental retardation.

Etiology

Although trichotillomania is regarded as multidetermined, its onset has been linked to stressful situations in more than one-fourth of all cases. Disturbances in mother–child relationships, fear of being left alone, and recent object loss are often cited as critical factors contributing to the condition. Substance abuse may encourage development of the disorder. Depressive dynamics are often cited as predisposing factors, but no particular personality trait or disorder characterizes

**Table 22–5
DSM-IV-TR Diagnostic Criteria
for Trichotillomania**

A. Recurrent pulling out of one's hair resulting in noticeable hair loss.

B. An increasing sense of tension immediately before pulling out the hair or when attempting to resist the behavior.

C. Pleasure, gratification, or relief when pulling out the hair.

D. The disturbance is not better accounted for by another mental disorder and is not due to a general medical condition (e.g., a dermatological condition).

E. The disturbance causes clinically significant distress or impairment in social, occupational, or other important areas of functioning.

From American Psychiatric Association. *Diagnostic and Statistical Manual of Mental Disorders.* 4th ed. Text rev. Washington, DC: American Psychiatric Association; copyright 2000, with permission.

patients. Some see self-stimulation as the primary goal of hair pulling.

Trichotillomania is increasingly being viewed as having a biologically determined substrate that may reflect inappropriately released motor activity or excessive grooming behaviors. Biological theories have also pointed to metabolic differences in the serotonin and opioid system. Family members of trichotillomania patients often have a history of tics, impulse-control disorders, and obsessive-compulsive symptoms, further supporting a possible genetic predisposition.

Diagnosis and Clinical Features

Before engaging in the behavior, patients with trichotillomania experience an increasing sense of tension and achieve a sense of release or gratification from pulling out their hair (Table 22–5). All areas of the body may be affected, most commonly the scalp. Other areas involved are eyebrows, eyelashes, and beard; trunk, armpits, and the pubic area are less commonly involved. Hair loss is often characterized by short, broken strands appearing together with long, normal hairs in the affected areas. No abnormalities of the skin or scalp are present.

A 48-year-old woman presented to her internist for a routine physical examination. She became somewhat tearful during the interview, explaining that she was under tremendous pressure at home taking care of her three children and that she recently separated from her husband. During the physical examination, the patient pointed to her head saying that her hair had been falling out during this recent period of stress and that she was somewhat concerned about this. The physician noted that the patient had two distinct areas of hair thinning, one at the vertex of the scalp and one in the frontal region. He also noted that the eyebrow regions were covered with pencil. Otherwise results of the physical examination and routine blood work were normal. He suggested the possibility of a condition other than spontaneous stress-induced hair loss and referred her to a dermatologist. Quite reluctantly, she agreed to the referral.

The patient followed up with the dermatologist, who noted a mixture of long and short hairs in the thinning regions of the scalp. Specimens showed no pathology. When the dermatologist asked the woman whether she might be pulling out her hair, she hesitatingly disclosed that she was. Tearfully, she requested complete confidentiality and asked the physician if he had ever encountered this before. When he reassured her that he had numerous patients with her condition and that treatment was available, she was visibly relieved. (Courtesy of Vivien K. Burt, M.D., and Jeffrey W. Katzman, M.D.)

Pathology and Laboratory Examination

Characteristic histopathological changes in the hair follicle, known as *trichomalacia*, are demonstrated by biopsy and help distinguish trichotillomania from other causes of alopecia.

Differential Diagnosis

Hair pulling may be a wholly benign condition or it may occur in the context of several mental disorders. The phenomenology of trichotillomania and obsessive-compulsive disorder overlap. Like obsessive-compulsive disorder, trichotillomania is often chronic and recognized by patients as undesirable. Unlike those with obsessive-compulsive disorder, patients with trichotillomania do not experience obsessive thoughts, and the compulsive activity is limited to one act, hair pulling. Patients with factitious disorder with predominantly physical signs and symptoms actively seek medical attention and the patient role and deliberately simulate illness toward these ends. Patients who malinger or who have factitious disorder may mutilate themselves to get medical attention, but they do not acknowledge the self-inflicted nature of the lesions. Patients with stereotypical movement disorder have stereotypical and rhythmic movements, and they usually do not seem distressed by their behavior. A biopsy may be necessary to distinguish trichotillomania from alopecia areata and tinea capitis.

Course and Prognosis

The mean age at onset of trichotillomania is in the early teens, most frequently before age 17, but onsets have been reported much later in life. The course of the disorder is not well known; both chronic and remitting forms occur. An early onset (before age 6) tends to remit more readily and responds to suggestion, support, and behavioral strategies. Late onset (after age 13) is associated with an increased likelihood of chronicity and poorer prognosis than the early-onset form. Approximately one-third of persons presenting for treatment report a duration of 1 year or less, whereas in some cases the disorder has persisted for more than two decades.

Treatment

No consensus exists on the best treatment modality for trichotillomania. Treatment usually involves psychiatrists and dermatologists in a joint endeavor. Psychopharmacological methods that have been used to treat psychodermatological disorders include topical steroids and hydroxyzine hydrochloride (Vistaril), an anxiolytic with antihistamine properties; antidepressants; serotonergic agents; and antipsychotics. Whether depression is present or not, antidepressant agents may lead to dermatological improvement. Current evidence strongly points to the efficacy of drugs that alter central serotonin turnover. Patients who respond poorly to SSRIs may improve with augmentation with pimozide (Orap), a dopamine receptor antagonist. A report of successful lithium treatment for trichotillomania cited the possible effect of the drug on aggression, impulsivity, and mood instability as an explanation. Lithium also possesses serotonergic activity. There have been case reports of successful treatment with buspirone, clonazepam (Klonopin), and trazodone. In one placebo-controlled study, patients taking naltrexone had a reduction in symptom severity.

Successful behavioral treatments such as biofeedback, self-monitoring, covert desensitization, and habit reversal have been reported, but most studies have been based on individual cases or small series of cases with relatively short follow-up periods. Further controlled study of the treatments is warranted. Chronic trichotillomania has been treated successfully with insight-oriented psychotherapy. Hypnotherapy and behavior therapy have been mentioned as potentially effective in the treatment of dermatological disorders in which psychological factors may be involved; the skin has been shown to be susceptible to hypnotic suggestion. Most of the work has been research oriented, with little effect on clinical management.

IMPULSE-CONTROL DISORDER NOT OTHERWISE SPECIFIED

The DSM-IV-TR diagnostic category of impulse-control disorder NOS (Table 22–6) is a residual category for disorders of impulse control that do not meet the criteria for a specific impulse-control disorder. Included in this category are such diverse behaviors as compulsive shopping, addiction to video games or the Internet, repetitive self-mutilation, and impulsive sexual behavior.

**Table 22–6
DSM-IV-TR Diagnostic Criteria for Impulse-Control Disorder Not Otherwise Specified**

This category is for disorders of impulse control (e.g., skin picking) that do not meet the criteria for any specific impulse-control disorder or for another mental disorder having features involving impulse control described elsewhere in the manual (e.g., substance dependence, a paraphilia).

From American Psychiatric Association. *Diagnostic and Statistical Manual of Mental Disorders.* 4th ed. Text rev. Washington, DC: American Psychiatric Association; copyright 2000, with permission.

Adjustment Disorders

Adjustment disorders are short-term maladaptive reactions to what a layperson would call a personal calamity but in psychiatric terms would be referred to as a *psychosocial stressor*. An adjustment disorder is expected to remit soon after the stressor ceases or, if it persists, a new level of adaptation is achieved.

According to the text revision of the fourth edition of *Diagnostic and Statistical Manual of Mental Disorders* (DSM-IV-TR), symptoms must appear within 3 months of a stressor's onset. The nature and severity of the stressors are not specified. However, the stressors are more often everyday events that are ubiquitous (e.g., loss of a loved one, change of employment or financial situation) rather than rare, catastrophic events (e.g., natural disasters, violent crimes). The disturbance must not fulfill the criteria for another major psychiatric disorder or bereavement (not considered a mental disorder, although it may be a focus of clinical attention). The symptoms of the disorder usually resolve within 6 months, although they may last longer if produced by a chronic stressor or one with long-lasting consequences.

EPIDEMIOLOGY

According to DSM-IV-TR, the prevalence of the disorder is estimated to be from 2 to 8 percent of the general population. Women are diagnosed twice as often as men, and single women are generally overly represented as most at risk. In children and adolescents, boys and girls are equally diagnosed with adjustment disorders. The disorders may occur at any age but are most frequently diagnosed in adolescents. Among adolescents of either sex, common precipitating stressors are school problems, parental rejection and divorce, and substance abuse. Among adults, common precipitating stressors are marital problems, divorce, moving to a new environment, and financial problems.

Adjustment disorders are one of the most common psychiatric diagnoses for disorders of patients hospitalized for medical and surgical problems. Up to 50 percent of persons with specific medical problems or stressors have been diagnosed with adjustment disorders. Furthermore, 10 to 30 percent of mental health outpatients and up to 12 percent of general hospital inpatients referred for mental health consultations have been diagnosed with adjustment disorders.

ETIOLOGY

By definition, an adjustment disorder is precipitated by one or more stressors. The severity of the stressor or stressors does not always predict the severity of the disorder; the stressor severity is a complex function of degree, quantity, duration, reversibility, environment, and personal context. For example, the loss of a parent is different for a 10-year-old and a 40-year-old. Personality organization and cultural or group norms and values also contribute to the disproportionate responses to stressors.

Stressors may be single, such as a divorce or the loss of a job, or multiple, such as the death of a person important to a patient that coincides with the patient's own physical illness and loss of a job. Stressors may be recurrent, such as seasonal business difficulties, or continuous, such as chronic illness or poverty. A discordant intrafamilial relationship may produce an adjustment disorder that affects the entire family system, or the disorder may be limited to a patient who was perhaps the victim of a crime or who has a physical illness. Sometimes adjustment disorders occur in a group or community setting, and the stressors affect several persons, as in a natural disaster or in racial, social, or religious persecution. Specific developmental stages, such as beginning school, leaving home, getting married, failing to achieve occupational goals, and retiring are often associated with adjustment disorders.

Psychodynamic Factors

Pivotal to understanding adjustment disorder is an understanding of three factors: the nature of the stressor, the conscious and unconscious meanings of the stressor, and the patient's preexisting vulnerability. A concurrent personality disorder or organic impairment may make a person vulnerable to adjustment disorders. Vulnerability is also associated with the loss of a parent during infancy or being reared in a dysfunctional family. Actual or perceived support from key relationships may affect behavioral and emotional responses to stressors.

Psychoanalytic research has emphasized the role of the mother and the rearing environment in a person's later capacity to respond to stress. Particularly important was Donald Winnicott's concept of the *good-enough mother*, a person who adapts to the infant's needs and provides enough support to enable the growing child to tolerate the frustrations in life.

Clinicians must undertake a detailed exploration of a patient's experience of the stressor. Certain patients commonly place all the blame on a particular event when a less obvious event may have had more significant psychological meaning for the patient. Current events may reawaken past traumas or disappointments from childhood, so patients should be encouraged to think about how the current situation relates to similar past events.

Throughout early development, each child develops a unique set of defense mechanisms to deal with stressful events. Because of greater amounts of trauma or greater constitutional vulnerability, some children have less mature defensive constellations than other children. This disadvantage may cause them as adults to react with substantially impaired functioning when they are faced with a loss, a divorce, or a financial setback; those who have developed mature defense mechanisms are less vulnerable and bounce back more quickly from the stressor. Resilience is also crucially determined by the nature of children's early relationships with their parents. Studies of trauma repeatedly indicate that supportive, nurturant relationships prevent traumatic incidents from causing permanent psychological damage.

Psychodynamic clinicians must consider the relation between a stressor and the human developmental life cycle. When adolescents leave home for college, for example, they are at high developmental risk for reacting with a temporary symptomatic picture. Similarly, if the young person who leaves home is the last child in the family, the parents may be particularly vulnerable to a reaction of adjustment disorder. Moreover, middle-aged persons who are confronting their own mortality may be especially sensitive to the effects of loss or death.

Family and Genetic Factors

Some studies suggest that certain persons appear to be at increased risk both for the occurrence of these adverse life events and for the development of pathology once they occur. Findings from a study of more than 2,000 twin pairs indicate that life events and stressors are modestly correlated in twin pairs, with monozygotic twins showing greater concordance than dizygotic twins. Family-environmental and genetic factors each accounted for approximately 20 percent of the variance in that study. Another twin study, which examined genetic contributions to the development of posttraumatic stress disorder symptoms (not necessarily at the level of full disorder, and therefore relevant to adjustment disorders), also concluded that the likelihood of developing symptoms in response to traumatic life events is partially under genetic control.

DIAGNOSIS AND CLINICAL FEATURES

Although, by definition, adjustment disorders follow a stressor, the symptoms do not necessarily begin immediately. Up to 3 months may elapse between a stressor and the development of symptoms. Symptoms do not always subside as soon as the stressor ceases; if the stressor continues, the disorder may be chronic. The disorder may occur at any age, and its symptoms vary considerably, with depressive, anxious, and mixed features most common in adults. Physical symptoms are most common in children and the elderly but may occur in any age group. Manifestations may also include assaultive behavior and reckless driving, excessive drinking, defaulting on legal responsibilities, withdrawal, vegetative signs, insomnia, and suicidal behavior.

Table 23–1
DSM-IV-TR Diagnostic Criteria for Adjustment Disorders

A. The development of emotional or behavioral symptoms in response to an identifiable stressor(s) occurring within 3 months of the onset of the stressor(s).

B. These symptoms or behaviors are clinically significant as evidenced by either of the following:

   (1) marked distress that is in excess of what would be expected from exposure to the stressor

   (2) significant impairment in social or occupational (academic) functioning

C. The stress-related disturbance does not meet the criteria for another specific Axis I disorder and is not merely an exacerbation of a preexisting Axis I or Axis II disorder.

D. The symptoms do not represent bereavement.

E. Once the stressor (or its consequences) has terminated, the symptoms do not persist for more than an additional 6 months.

Specify if:

  Acute: if the disturbance lasts less than 6 months

  Chronic: if the disturbance lasts for 6 months or longer

Adjustment disorders are coded based on the subtype, which is selected according to the predominant symptoms. The specific stressor(s) can be specified on Axis IV.

  With depressed mood

  With anxiety

  With mixed anxiety and depressed mood

  With disturbance of conduct

  With mixed disturbance of emotions and conduct

  Unspecified

From American Psychiatric Association. *Diagnostic and Statistical Manual of Mental Disorders.* 4th ed. Text rev. Washington, DC: American Psychiatric Association; copyright 2000.

The clinical presentations of adjustment disorder can vary widely. DSM-IV-TR lists six adjustment disorders, including an unspecified category (Table 23–1).

Adjustment Disorder with Depressed Mood

In adjustment disorder with depressed mood, the predominant manifestations are depressed mood, tearfulness, and hopelessness. This type must be distinguished from major depressive disorder and uncomplicated bereavement. Adolescents with this type are at increased risk for major depressive disorder in young adulthood.

Adjustment Disorder with Anxiety

Symptoms of anxiety, such as palpitations, jitteriness, and agitation, are present in adjustment disorder with anxiety, which must be differentiated from anxiety disorders.

Adjustment Disorder with Mixed Anxiety and Depressed Mood

In adjustment disorder with mixed anxiety and depressed mood, patients exhibit features of both anxiety and depression that do not meet the criteria for an already established anxiety disorder or depressive disorder.

Adjustment Disorder with Disturbance of Conduct

In adjustment disorder with disturbance of conduct, the predominant manifestation involves conduct in which the rights of others are violated or age-appropriate societal norms and rules are disregarded. Examples of behavior in this category are truancy, vandalism, reckless driving, and fighting. The category must be differentiated from conduct disorder and antisocial personality disorder.

Adjustment Disorder with Mixed Disturbance of Emotions and Conduct

A combination of disturbances of emotions and of conduct sometimes occurs. Clinicians are encouraged to try to make one or the other diagnosis in the interest of clarity.

Adjustment Disorder Unspecified

Adjustment disorder unspecified is a residual category for atypical maladaptive reactions to stress. Examples include inappropriate responses to the diagnosis of physical illness, such as massive denial, severe noncompliance to treatment, and social withdrawal, without significant depressed or anxious mood.

DIFFERENTIAL DIAGNOSIS

Although uncomplicated bereavement can often produce temporarily impaired social and occupational functioning, the person's dysfunction remains within the expectable bounds of a reaction to the loss of a loved one and thus is not considered adjustment disorder. Other disorders from which adjustment disorder must be differentiated include major depressive disorder, brief psychotic disorder, generalized anxiety disorder, somatization disorder, substance-related disorder, conduct disorder, academic problem, occupational problem, identity problem, and posttraumatic stress disorder. These diagnoses should be given precedence in all cases that meet their criteria, even in the presence of a stressor or group of stressors that served as a precipitant. Patients with an adjustment disorder are impaired in social or occupational functioning and show symptoms beyond the normal and expectable reaction to the stressor. Because no absolute criteria help to distinguish an adjustment disorder from another condition, clinical judgment is necessary. Some patients may meet the criteria for both an adjustment disorder and a personality disorder. If the adjustment disorder follows a physical illness, the clinician must make sure that the symptoms are not a continuation or another manifestation of the illness or its treatment.

Acute and Posttraumatic Stress Disorders

In posttraumatic stress disorder or acute stress disorder, the symptoms develop after a traumatic event or events outside the range of normal human experience. The stressors producing this syndrome are expected to cause a psychological reaction in the average person. Persons may experience the stressor alone, as in rape or assault, or in groups, as in military combat or death camps. Mass catastrophes—such as hurricanes, floods, airplane crashes, and bombings—are also iden-

tified as stressors. These stressors contain a psychological component and frequently a concomitant physical component that may directly damage persons' nervous systems. The disorder is more severe and longer lasting when the stressor is of human origin (e.g., rape) than when it is not (e.g., floods). In adjustment disorders, the precipitating stress need not be severe or unusual. Posttraumatic stress disorder is discussed fully in Chapter 13.5.

COURSE AND PROGNOSIS

With appropriate treatment, the overall prognosis of an adjustment disorder is generally favorable. Most patients return to their previous level of functioning within 3 months. Some persons (particularly adolescents) who receive a diagnosis of an adjustment disorder later have mood disorders or substance-related disorders. Adolescents usually require a longer time to recover than adults.

TREATMENT

Psychotherapy

Psychotherapy remains the treatment of choice for adjustment disorders. Group therapy can be particularly useful for patients who have undergone similar stresses—for example, a group of retired persons or patients undergoing renal dialysis. Individual psychotherapy offers the opportunity to explore the meaning of the stressor to the patient so that earlier traumas can be worked through. After successful therapy, patients sometimes emerge from an adjustment disorder stronger than in the premorbid period, although no pathology was evident during that period. Psychotherapy can help persons adapt to stressors that are not reversible or time limited and can serve as a preventive intervention if the stressor does remit. Psychiatrists treating adjustment disorders must be particularly aware of problems of malingering and feigning illness for secondary gain.

Patients with an adjustment disorder that includes a conduct disturbance may have difficulties with the law, authorities, or school. Psychiatrists should not attempt to rescue such patients from the consequences of their actions. Too often, such kindness only reinforces socially unacceptable means of tension reduction and hinders the acquisition of insight and subsequent emotional growth. In these cases, family therapy can help.

Crisis Intervention

Crisis intervention and case management are short-term treatments aimed at helping persons with adjustment disorders resolve their situations quickly by supportive techniques, suggestion, reassurance, environmental modification, and even hospitalization, if necessary. The frequency and length of visits for crisis support vary according to patients' needs; daily sessions may be necessary, sometimes two or three times each day. Flexibility is essential in this approach.

Pharmacotherapy

There are no studies assessing the efficacy of pharmacological interventions in individuals with adjustment disorder, but it may be reasonable to use medication to treat specific symptoms for a brief time. The judicious use of medications can help patients with adjustment disorders, but they should be prescribed for brief periods. Depending on the type of adjustment disorder, a patient may respond to an antianxiety agent or to an antidepressant. Patients with severe anxiety bordering on panic can benefit from anxiolytics such as diazepam (Valium), and those in withdrawn or inhibited states may be helped by a short course of psychostimulant medication. Antipsychotic drugs may be used if there are signs of decompensation or impending psychosis. Selective serotonin reuptake inhibitors (SSRIs) have been found useful in treating symptoms of traumatic grief. Recently, there has been an increase in antidepressant use to augment psychotherapy in patients with adjustment disorders. However, pharmacological intervention in this population is most often used to augment psychosocial strategies rather than serving as the primary modality.

24 ▲

Personality Disorders

Personality has generally been used as a global descriptive label for a person's objectively observable behavior and his or her subjectively reportable inner experience. The wholeness of an individual described in this way represents both the public and the private aspects of his or her life. The word "personality" may have appended to it certain qualifying adjectives with psychiatric significance, such as "passive" or "aggressive," or words without pathological overtones, such as "ambitious" or "religious" or "friendly." A coherent series of such qualifications making up a personality disorder diagnosis implies certain predictions about how a person will behave under given sets of circumstances. It offers the clinician clues about a person's disability and about how he or she may be approached for treatment purposes (i.e., if treatment should be conducted mainly through the use of drugs, surgery, or interviews). Whether used as a psychiatric diagnostic term or as a folk description, the personality label has value for the physician who must deal with the described individual.

CLASSIFICATION

The text revision of the fourth edition of *Diagnostic and Statistical Manual of Mental Disorders* (DSM-IV-TR) defines personality disorders as enduring subjective experiences and behavior that deviate from cultural standards, are rigidly pervasive, have an onset in adolescence or early adulthood, are stable through time, and lead to unhappiness and impairment. When personality traits are rigid, maladaptive, and produce functional impairment of subjective distress, a personality disorder may be diagnosed (Table 24–1).

Personality disorders are grouped into three clusters in DSM-IV-TR. Cluster A covers the paranoid, schizoid, and schizotypal personality disorders; people with these disorders are often perceived as odd and eccentric. Cluster B is made up of the antisocial, borderline, histrionic, and narcissistic personality disorders; people with these disorders often seem dramatic, emotional, and erratic. Cluster C includes the avoidant, dependent, and obsessive-compulsive personality disorders, and a category called personality disorder not otherwise specified (such as passive-aggressive personality disorder and depressive personality disorder); people with those disorders often seem anxious or fearful. Many people exhibit traits that are not limited to a single personality disorder. When a patient meets the criteria for more than one personality disorder, clinicians should diagnose each. Personality disorders are coded on Axis II of DSM-IV-TR.

ETIOLOGY

Genetic Factors

The best evidence that genetic factors contribute to personality disorders comes from investigations of 15,000 pairs of twins in the United States. Among monozygotic twins, the concordance for personality disorders was several times higher than that among dizygotic twins. Moreover, according to one study, monozygotic twins reared apart are about as similar as monozygotic twins reared together. Similarities include multiple measures of personality and temperament, occupational and leisure-time interests, and social attitudes.

Cluster A personality disorders (paranoid, schizoid, and schizotypal) are more common in the biological relatives of patients with schizophrenia than among control groups. More relatives with schizotypal personality disorder occur in the family histories of people with schizophrenia than among control groups. Less correlation exists between paranoid or schizoid personality disorder and schizophrenia.

Cluster B personality disorders (antisocial, borderline, histrionic, and narcissistic) apparently have a genetic base. Antisocial personality disorder is associated with alcohol use disorders. Depression is common in the family backgrounds of patients with borderline personality disorder. These patients have more relatives with mood disorders than do control groups, and people with borderline personality disorder often have mood disorder as well. A strong association is found between histrionic personality disorder and somatization disorder (Briquet's syndrome); patients with each disorder show an overlap of symptoms.

Cluster C personality disorders (avoidant, dependent, obsessive-compulsive, and not otherwise specified) may also have a genetic base. Patients with avoidant personality disorder often have high anxiety levels. Obsessive-compulsive traits are more common in monozygotic twins than in dizygotic twins, and patients with obsessive-compulsive personality disorder show some signs associated with depression—for example, shortened rapid eye movement (REM) latency period and abnormal dexamethasone-suppression test (DST) results.

Biological Factors

Hormones.   People who exhibit impulsive traits also often show increased levels of testosterone, 17-estradiol, and estrone. In nonhuman primates, androgens increase the likelihood of aggression and sexual behavior, but the role of testosterone in

**Table 24–1
DSM-IV-TR General Diagnostic Criteria for a
Personality Disorder**

A. An enduring pattern of inner experience and behavior that deviates markedly from the expectations of the individual's culture. This pattern is manifested in two (or more) of the following areas:
  (1) cognition (i.e., ways of perceiving and interpreting self, other people, and events)
  (2) affectivity (i.e., the range, intensity, lability, and appropriateness of emotional response)
  (3) interpersonal functioning
  (4) impulse control
B. The enduring pattern is inflexible and pervasive across a broad range of personal and social situations.
C. The enduring pattern leads to clinically significant distress or impairment in social, occupational, or other important areas of functioning.
D. The pattern is stable and of long duration, and its onset can be traced back at least to adolescence or early adulthood.
E. The enduring pattern is not better accounted for as a manifestation or consequence of another mental disorder.
F. The enduring pattern is not due to the direct physiological effects of a substance (e.g., a drug of abuse, a medication) or a general medical condition (e.g., head trauma).

From American Psychiatric Association. *Diagnostic and Statistical Manual of Mental Disorders.* 4th ed. Text rev. Washington, DC: American Psychiatric Association; copyright 2000, with permission.

human aggression is unclear. DST results are abnormal in some patients with borderline personality disorder who also have depressive symptoms.

Platelet Monoamine Oxidase.   Low platelet monoamine oxidase (MAO) levels have been associated with activity and sociability in monkeys. College students with low platelet MAO levels report spending more time in social activities than do students with high platelet MAO levels. Low platelet MAO levels have also been noted in some patients with schizotypal disorders.

Smooth Pursuit Eye Movements.   Smooth pursuit eye movements are saccadic (that is, jumpy) in people who are introverted, who have low self-esteem and tend to withdraw, and who have schizotypal personality disorder. These findings have no clinical application, but they do indicate the role of inheritance.

Neurotransmitters.   Endorphins have effects similar to those of exogenous morphine, such as analgesia and the suppression of arousal. High endogenous endorphin levels may be associated with people who are phlegmatic. Studies of personality traits and the dopaminergic and serotonergic systems indicate an arousal-activating function for these neurotransmitters. Levels of 5-hydroxyindoleacetic acid (5-HIAA), a metabolite of serotonin, are low in people who attempt suicide and in patients who are impulsive and aggressive.

Raising serotonin levels with serotonergic agents such as fluoxetine (Prozac) may produce dramatic changes in some

character traits of personality. In many people, serotonin reduces depression, impulsiveness, and rumination and can produce a sense of general well-being. Increased dopamine in the central nervous system, produced by certain psychostimulants (such as amphetamines) can induce euphoria. The effects of neurotransmitters on personality traits have generated much interest and controversy about whether personality traits are inborn or acquired.

Electrophysiology.   Changes in electrical conductance on the electroencephalogram (EEG) occur in some patients with personality disorders, most commonly antisocial and borderline types; these changes appear as slow-wave activity on EEGs.

Psychoanalytic Factors

Sigmund Freud suggested that personality traits are related to a fixation at one psychosexual stage of development. For example, those with an oral character are passive and dependent because they are fixated at the oral stage, when the dependence on others for food is prominent. Those with an anal character are stubborn, parsimonious, and highly conscientious because of struggles over toilet training during the anal period.

Wilhelm Reich subsequently coined the term *character armor* to describe people's characteristic defensive styles for protecting themselves from internal impulses and from interpersonal anxiety in significant relationships. Reich's theory has had a broad influence on contemporary concepts of personality and of personality disorders. For example, each human being's unique stamp of personality is considered largely determined by his or her characteristic defense mechanisms. Each personality disorder in Axis II has a cluster of defenses that help psychodynamic clinicians recognize the type of character pathology present. People with paranoid personality disorder, for instance, use projection, whereas schizoid personality disorder is associated with withdrawal.

When defenses work effectively, people with personality disorders master feelings of anxiety, depression, anger, shame, guilt, and other affects. They often view their behavior as ego-syntonic—that is, it creates no distress for them, even though it may adversely affect others. They may also be reluctant to engage in a treatment process; because their defenses are important in controlling unpleasant affects, they are not interested in surrendering them.

In addition to characteristic defenses in personality disorders, another central feature is internal object relations. During development, particular patterns of self in relation to others are internalized. Through introjection, children internalize a parent or another significant person as an internal presence that continues to feel like an object rather than a self. Through identification, children internalize parents and others in such a way that the traits of the external object are incorporated into the self and the child "owns" the traits. Hence, people with personality disorders are also identified by particular patterns of interpersonal relatedness that stem from these internal object relations patterns.

Defense Mechanisms.   To help those with personality disorders, psychiatrists must appreciate patients' underlying defenses, the unconscious mental processes that the ego uses to resolve conflicts among the four lodestars of the inner life: instinct (wish or need), reality, important people, and conscience. When defenses are most effective, especially in those with personality disorders, they can abolish anxiety and depression. Thus, abandoning a defense increases conscious anxiety and depression—a major reason that those with personality disorders are reluctant to alter their behavior.

Although patients with personality disorders may be characterized by their most dominant or rigid mechanism, each patient uses several defenses. Therefore, the management of defense mechanisms used by patients with personality disorders is discussed here as a general topic and not as an aspect of the specific disorders. Many formulations presented here in the language of psychoanalytic psychiatry can be translated into principles consistent with cognitive and behavioral approaches.

FANTASY. Many people who are often labeled schizoid—those who are eccentric, lonely, or frightened—seek solace and satisfaction within themselves by creating imaginary lives, especially imaginary friends. In their extensive dependence on fantasy, these people often seem to be strikingly aloof. Therapists must understand that the unsociableness of these patients rests on a fear of intimacy. Rather than criticizing them or feeling rebuffed by their rejection, therapists should maintain a quiet, reassuring, and considerate interest without insisting on reciprocal responses. Recognition of patients' fear of closeness and respect for their eccentric ways are both therapeutic and useful.

DISSOCIATION. Dissociation or denial is a Pollyanna-like replacement of unpleasant affects with pleasant ones. People who frequently dissociate are often seen as dramatizing and emotionally shallow; they may be labeled histrionic personalities. They behave like anxious adolescents who, to erase anxiety, carelessly expose themselves to exciting dangers. Accepting such patients as exuberant and seductive is to overlook their anxiety, but confronting them with their vulnerabilities and defects makes them still more defensive. Because they seek appreciation of their courage and attractiveness, therapists should not behave with inordinate reserve. While remaining calm and firm, clinicians should realize that these patients are often inadvertent liars, but they benefit from ventilating their own anxieties and may in the process "remember" what they "forgot." Often therapists deal best with dissociation and denial by using displacement. Thus, clinicians may talk with patients about an issue of denial in an unthreatening circumstance. Empathizing with the denied affect without directly confronting patients with the facts may allow them to raise the original topic themselves.

ISOLATION. Isolation is characteristic of the orderly, controlled people who are often labeled obsessive-compulsive personalities. Unlike those with histrionic personality, people with obsessive-compulsive personality remember the truth in fine detail but without affect. In a crisis, patients may show an intensification of self-restraint, overly formal social behavior, and obstinacy. Patients' quests for control may annoy clinicians or make them anxious. Often, such patients respond well to precise, systematic, and rational explanations and value efficiency, cleanliness, and punctuality as much as they do clinicians' effective responsiveness. Whenever possible, therapists should allow such patients to control their own care and should not engage in a battle of wills.

PROJECTION. In projection, patients attribute their own unacknowledged feelings to others. Patients' excessive fault-finding and sensitivity to criticism may appear to therapists as prejudiced, hypervigilant injustice collecting, but should not be met by defensiveness and argument.

Instead, clinicians should frankly acknowledge even minor mistakes on their part and should discuss the possibility of future difficulties. Strict honesty, concern for patients' rights, and maintaining the same formal, concerned distance as with patients who use fantasy defenses are all helpful. Confrontation guarantees a lasting enemy and an early termination of the interview. Therapists need not agree with patients' injustice collecting but should ask whether both can agree to disagree.

The technique of counterprojection is especially helpful. Clinicians acknowledge and give paranoid patients full credit for their feelings and perceptions; they neither dispute patients' complaints nor reinforce them but agree that the world described by patients is conceivable. Interviewers can then talk about real motives and feelings, misattributed to someone else, and begin to cement an alliance with patients.

SPLITTING. In splitting, people toward whom patients' feelings are or have been ambivalent are divided into good and bad. For example, in an inpatient setting, a patient may idealize some staff members and uniformly disparage others. This defense behavior can be highly disruptive on a hospital ward and can ultimately provoke the staff to turn against the patient. When staff members anticipate the process, discuss it at staff meetings, and gently confront the patient with the fact that no one is all good or all bad, the phenomenon of splitting can be dealt with effectively.

PASSIVE AGGRESSION. People with passive-aggressive defense turn their anger against themselves. In psychoanalytic terms this phenomenon is called *masochism* and includes failure, procrastination, silly or provocative behavior, self-demeaning clowning, and frankly self-destructive acts. The hostility in such behavior is never entirely concealed. Indeed, in a mechanism such as wrist cutting, others feel as much anger as if they themselves had been assaulted and view the patient as a sadist, not a masochist. Therapists can best deal with passive aggression by helping patients to ventilate their anger.

ACTING OUT. In acting out, patients directly express unconscious wishes or conflicts through action to avoid being conscious of either the accompanying idea or the affect. Tantrums, apparently motiveless assaults, child abuse, and pleasureless promiscuity are common examples. Because the behavior occurs outside reflective awareness, acting out often appears to observers to be unaccompanied by guilt, but when acting out is impossible, the conflict behind the defense may be accessible. Faced with acting out, either aggressive or sexual, in an interview situation, a clinician must recognize that the patient has lost control, that anything the interviewer says will probably be misheard, and that getting the patient's attention is of paramount importance. Depending on the circumstances, a clinician's response may be, "How can I help you if you keep screaming?" or, if the patient's loss of control seems to be escalating, "If you continue screaming, I'll leave." An interviewer who feels genuinely frightened of the patient can simply leave and, if necessary, ask for help from ward attendants or the police.

PROJECTIVE IDENTIFICATION. The defense mechanism of projective identification appears mainly in borderline personality disorder and consists of three steps: An aspect of the self is projected onto someone else; the projector tries to coerce the other person to identify with what has been projected; and the recipient of the projection and the projector feel a sense of oneness or union.

PARANOID PERSONALITY DISORDER

People with paranoid personality disorder are characterized by long-standing suspiciousness and mistrust of people in general.

They refuse responsibility for their own feelings and assign responsibility to others. They are often hostile, irritable, and angry. Bigots, injustice collectors, pathologically jealous spouses, and litigious cranks often have paranoid personality disorder.

Epidemiology

The prevalence of paranoid personality disorder is 0.5 to 2.5 percent of the general population. Those with the disorder rarely seek treatment themselves; when referred to treatment by a spouse or an employer, they can often pull themselves together and appear undistressed. Relatives of patients with schizophrenia show a higher incidence of paranoid personality disorder than do controls. The disorder is more common in men than in women and does not appear to have a familial pattern. The prevalence among people who are homosexual is no higher than usual, as was once thought, but is believed to be higher among minority groups, immigrants, and people who are deaf than it is in the general population.

Diagnosis

On psychiatric examination, patients with paranoid personality disorder may be formal in manner and act baffled about having to seek psychiatric help. Muscular tension, an inability to relax, and a need to scan the environment for clues may be evident, and patients' manner is often humorless and serious. Although some premises of their arguments may be false, their speech is goal directed and logical. Their thought content shows evidence of projection, prejudice, and occasional ideas of reference. The DSM-IV-TR diagnostic criteria are listed in Table 24–2.

Clinical Features

The essential feature of people with paranoid personality disorder is a pervasive and unwarranted tendency, which begins by early adulthood and appears in a variety of contexts, to interpret other people's actions as deliberately demeaning or threatening. Almost invariably, those with the disorder expect to be exploited or harmed by others in some way. They frequently dispute, without any justification, friends' or associates' loyalty or trustworthiness. Such people are often pathologically jealous and for no reason question the fidelity of their spouses or sexual partners. People with this disorder externalize their own emotions and use the defense of projection: They attribute to others the impulses and thoughts that they are unable to accept in themselves. Ideas of reference and logically defended illusions are common.

Persons with paranoid personality disorder are affectively restricted and appear to be unemotional. They pride themselves on being rational and objective, but such is not the case. They lack warmth and are impressed with, and pay close attention to, power and rank; they express disdain for those who are seen as weak, sickly, impaired, or in some way defective. In social situations, people with paranoid personality disorder may appear business-like and efficient, but they often generate fear or conflict in others.

Differential Diagnosis

Paranoid personality disorder can usually be differentiated from delusional disorder by the absence of fixed delusions. Unlike

Table 24–2
DSM-IV-TR Diagnostic Criteria for Paranoid Personality Disorder

A. A pervasive distrust and suspiciousness of others such that their motives are interpreted as malevolent, beginning by early adulthood and present in a variety of contexts, as indicated by four (or more) of the following:

   (1) suspects, without sufficient basis, that others are exploiting, harming, or deceiving him or her

   (2) is preoccupied with unjustified doubts about the loyalty or trustworthiness of friends or associates

   (3) is reluctant to confide in others because of unwarranted fear that the information will be used maliciously against him or her

   (4) reads hidden demeaning or threatening meanings into benign remarks or events

   (5) persistently bears grudges, i.e., is unforgiving of insults, injuries, or slights

   (6) perceives attacks on his or her character or reputation that are not apparent to others and is quick to react angrily or to counterattack

   (7) has recurrent suspicions, without justification, regarding fidelity of spouse or sexual partner

B. Does not occur exclusively during the course of schizophrenia, a mood disorder with psychotic features, or another psychotic disorder and is not due to the direct physiological effects of a general medical condition.

Note: If criteria are met prior to the onset of schizophrenia, add "premorbid," e.g., "paranoid personality disorder (premorbid)."

From American Psychiatric Association. *Diagnostic and Statistical Manual of Mental Disorders.* 4th ed. Text rev. Washington, DC: American Psychiatric Association; copyright 2000, with permission.

people with paranoid schizophrenia, those with personality disorders have no hallucinations or formal thought disorder. Paranoid personality disorder can be distinguished from borderline personality disorder because paranoid patients are rarely capable of overly involved, tumultuous relationships with others. Paranoid patients lack the long history of antisocial behavior of people with antisocial character. People with schizoid personality disorder are withdrawn and aloof and do not have paranoid ideation.

Course and Prognosis

Adequate and systematic long-term studies of paranoid personality disorder have not been conducted. In some, paranoid personality disorder is lifelong; in others it is a harbinger of schizophrenia. In still others, paranoid traits give way to reaction formation, appropriate concern with morality, and altruistic concerns as they mature or as stress diminishes. In general, however, those with paranoid personality disorder have lifelong problems working and living with others. Occupational and marital problems are common.

Treatment

Psychotherapy.   Psychotherapy is the treatment of choice. Therapists should be straightforward in all their dealings with these patients. If a therapist is accused of an inconsistency or fault, such as lateness for an appointment, honesty and an apology are preferable to a defensive explanation. Therapists must remember that trust and toleration of intimacy are troubled areas for patients with the disorder. Individual psychotherapy thus requires a professional and not overly warm style from therapists. Clinicians' overzealous use of interpretation—especially interpretation about deep feelings of dependence, sexual concerns, and wishes for intimacy—significantly increase patients' mistrust. Paranoid patients usually do not do well in group psychotherapy, although it can be useful for improving social skills and diminishing suspiciousness through role playing. Many cannot tolerate the intrusiveness of behavior therapy, also used for social skills training.

Pharmacotherapy.   Pharmacotherapy is useful in dealing with agitation and anxiety. In most cases, an antianxiety agent such as diazepam (Valium) is sufficient, but it may be necessary to use an antipsychotic, such as thioridazine (Mellaril) or haloperidol (Haldol), in small dosages and for brief periods to manage severe agitation or quasi-delusional thinking. The antipsychotic drug pimozide (Orap) has been successfully used to reduce paranoid ideation in some patients.

SCHIZOID PERSONALITY DISORDER

Schizoid personality disorder is diagnosed in patients who display a lifelong pattern of social withdrawal. Their discomfort with human interaction, their introversion, and their bland, constricted affect are noteworthy. People with schizoid personality disorder are often seen by others as eccentric, isolated, or lonely.

Epidemiology

The prevalence of schizoid personality disorder is not clearly established, but the disorder may affect 7.5 percent of the general population. The sex ratio of the disorder is unknown; some studies report a 2:1 male-to-female ratio. People with the disorder tend to gravitate toward solitary jobs that involve little or no contact with others. Many prefer night work to day work, so that they need not deal with many people.

Diagnosis

On an initial psychiatric examination, patients with schizoid personality disorder may appear ill at ease. They rarely tolerate eye contact, and interviewers may surmise that such patients are eager for the interview to end. Their affect may be constricted, aloof, or inappropriately serious, but underneath the aloofness, sensitive clinicians can recognize fear. These patients find it difficult to be lighthearted: Their efforts at humor may seem adolescent and off the mark. Their speech is goal directed, but they are likely to give short answers to questions and to avoid spontaneous conversation. They may occasionally use unusual figures of speech, such as an odd metaphor, and may be fascinated with inanimate objects or metaphysical constructs. Their mental content may reveal an unwarranted sense of intimacy with people they do not know well or whom they have not seen for a long time. Their sensorium is intact, their memory functions well, and their proverb interpretations are abstract. The DSM-IV-TR diagnostic criteria are listed in Table 24–3.

Table 24–3
DSM-IV-TR Diagnostic Criteria for Schizoid Personality Disorder

A. A pervasive pattern of detachment from social relationships and a restricted range of expression of emotions in interpersonal settings, beginning by early adulthood and present in a variety of contexts, as indicated by four (or more) of the following:

(1) neither desires nor enjoys close relationships, including being part of a family

(2) almost always chooses solitary activities

(3) has little, if any, interest in having sexual experiences with another person

(4) takes pleasure in few, if any, activities

(5) lacks close friends or confidants other than first-degree relatives

(6) appears indifferent to the praise or criticism of others

(7) shows emotional coldness, detachment, or flattened affectivity

B. Does not occur exclusively during the course of schizophrenia, a mood disorder with psychotic features, another psychotic disorder, or a pervasive developmental disorder and is not due to the direct physiological effects of a general medical condition.

Note: If criteria are met prior to the onset of schizophrenia, add "premorbid," e.g., "schizoid personality disorder (premorbid)."

From American Psychiatric Association. *Diagnostic and Statistical Manual of Mental Disorders.* 4th ed. Text rev. Washington, DC: American Psychiatric Association; copyright 2000, with permission.

Clinical Features

Persons with schizoid personality disorder seem to be cold and aloof; they display a remote reserve and show no involvement with everyday events and the concerns of others. Patients appear quiet, distant, seclusive, and unsociable. They may pursue their own lives with remarkably little need or longing for emotional ties and are the last to be aware of changes in popular fashion.

The life histories of such people reflect solitary interests and success at noncompetitive, lonely jobs that others find difficult to tolerate. Their sexual lives may exist exclusively in fantasy, and he or she may postpone mature sexuality indefinitely. Men may not marry because they are unable to achieve intimacy; women may passively agree to marry an aggressive man who wants the marriage. People with schizoid personality disorder usually reveal a lifelong inability to express anger directly. They are able to invest enormous affective energy in nonhuman interests such as mathematics and astronomy, and they may be very attached to animals. Dietary and health fads, philosophical movements, and social improvement schemes, especially those that require no personal involvement, often engross them.

Although people with schizoid personality disorder appear self-absorbed and lost in daydreams, they have a normal capacity to recognize reality. Because aggressive acts are rarely included in their repertoire of usual responses, most threats, real or imagined, are dealt with by fantasied omnipotence or resignation. They are often seen as aloof, yet such people can sometimes conceive, develop, and give to the world genuinely original, creative ideas.

Differential Diagnosis

In contrast to patients with schizophrenia and schizotypal personality disorder, patients with schizoid personality disorder do not have schizophrenic relatives, and they may have successful, if isolated, work histories. They also differ from patients with schizophrenia by exhibiting no thought disorder or delusional thinking. Although patients with paranoid personality disorder share many traits with those with schizoid personality disorder, the former exhibit more social engagement, a history of aggressive verbal behavior, and a greater tendency to project their feelings onto others. If just as emotionally constricted, patients with obsessive-compulsive and avoidant personality disorders experience loneliness as dysphoric, possess a richer history of past object relations, and do not engage as much in autistic reverie. Theoretically, the chief distinction between a patient with schizotypal personality disorder and one with schizoid personality disorder is that a schizotypal patient is more similar to a patient with schizophrenia in oddities of perception, thought, behavior, and communication. Patients with avoidant personality disorder are isolated but strongly wish to participate in activities, a characteristic absent in those with schizoid personality disorder.

Course and Prognosis

The onset of schizoid personality disorder usually occurs in early childhood. Like all personality disorders, schizoid personality disorder is long lasting, but not necessarily lifelong. The proportion of patients who incur schizophrenia is unknown.

Treatment

Psychotherapy. The treatment of patients with schizoid personality disorder is similar to that of those with paranoid personality disorder. Schizoid patients' tendencies toward introspection, however, are consistent with psychotherapists' expectations, and schizoid patients may become devoted, if distant, patients. As trust develops, schizoid patients may, with great trepidation, reveal a plethora of fantasies, imaginary friends, and fears of unbearable dependence—even of merging with the therapist.

In group therapy settings, patients with schizoid personality disorder may be silent for long periods; nonetheless, they do become involved. The patients should be protected against aggressive attack by group members for their proclivity to be silent. With time the group members become important to schizoid patients and may provide the only social contact in their otherwise isolated existence.

Pharmacotherapy. Pharmacotherapy with small dosages of antipsychotics, antidepressants, and psychostimulants has been effective in some patients. Serotonergic agents may make patients less sensitive to rejection. Benzodiazepines may be of use to diminish interpersonal anxiety.

SCHIZOTYPAL PERSONALITY DISORDER

Persons with schizotypal personality disorder are strikingly odd or strange, even to laypersons. Magical thinking, peculiar notions, ideas of reference, illusions, and derealization are part of a schizotypal person's everyday world.

Table 24–4
DSM-IV-TR Diagnostic Criteria for Schizotypal Personality Disorder

A. A pervasive pattern of social and interpersonal deficits marked by acute discomfort with, and reduced capacity for, close relationships as well as by cognitive or perceptual distortions and eccentricities of behavior, beginning by early adulthood and present in a variety of contexts, as indicated by five (or more) of the following:

(1) ideas of reference (excluding delusions of reference)

(2) odd beliefs or magical thinking that influences behavior and is inconsistent with subcultural norms (e.g., superstitiousness, belief in clairvoyance, telepathy, or "sixth sense"; in children and adolescents, bizarre fantasies or preoccupations)

(3) unusual perceptual experiences, including bodily illusions

(4) odd thinking and speech (e.g., vague, circumstantial, metaphorical, overelaborate, or stereotyped)

(5) suspiciousness or paranoid ideation

(6) inappropriate or constricted affect

(7) behavior or appearance that is odd, eccentric, or peculiar

(8) lack of close friends or confidants other than first-degree relatives

(9) excessive social anxiety that does not diminish with familiarity and tends to be associated with paranoid fears rather than negative judgments about self

B. Does not occur exclusively during the course of schizophrenia, a mood disorder with psychotic features, another psychotic disorder, or a pervasive developmental disorder.

Note: If criteria are met prior to the onset of schizophrenia, add "premorbid," e.g., "schizotypal personality disorder (premorbid)."

From American Psychiatric Association. *Diagnostic and Statistical Manual of Mental Disorders.* 4th ed. Text rev. Washington, DC: American Psychiatric Association; copyright 2000, with permission.

Epidemiology

This disorder occurs in approximately 3 percent of the population. The sex ratio is unknown. There is a greater association of cases among the biological relatives of patients with schizophrenia than among controls, and a higher incidence among monozygotic twins than among dizygotic twins (33 percent versus 4 percent in one study).

Diagnosis

Schizotypal personality disorder is diagnosed on the basis of the patients' peculiarities of thinking, behavior, and appearance. Taking a history may be difficult because of the patient's unusual way of communicating. The DSM-IV-TR diagnostic criteria for schizotypal personality disorder are given in Table 24–4.

Clinical Features

In patients with schizotypal personality disorder, thinking and communicating are disturbed. Although frank thought disorder is absent, their speech may be distinctive or peculiar, may have meaning only to them, and may often need interpretation. Like patients with schizophrenia, those with schizotypal personality disorder may not know their own feelings and yet are exquisitely sensitive to, and aware of, the feelings of others, especially negative affects like anger. These patients may be superstitious or claim powers of clairvoyance and may believe that they have other special powers of thought and insight. Their inner world may be filled with vivid imaginary relationships and child-like fears and fantasies. They may admit to perceptual illusions or macropsia and confess that other people seem to be wooden and all the same.

Because people with schizotypal personality disorder have poor interpersonal relationships and may act inappropriately, they are isolated and have few, if any, friends. Patients may show features of borderline personality disorder, and indeed, both diagnoses can be made. Under stress, patients with schizotypal personality disorder may decompensate and have psychotic symptoms, but these are usually of brief duration. In patients with severe cases of the disorder, anhedonia and severe depression may be present.

Differential Diagnosis

Theoretically, people with schizotypal personality disorder can be distinguished from those with schizoid and avoidant personality disorders by the presence of oddities in their behavior, thinking, perception, and communication, and perhaps by a clear family history of schizophrenia. Patients with schizotypal personality disorder can be distinguished from those with schizophrenia by their absence of psychosis. If psychotic symptoms do appear, they are brief and fragmentary. Some patients meet the criteria for both schizotypal personality disorder and borderline personality disorder. Patients with paranoid personality disorder are characterized by suspiciousness but lack the odd behavior of patients with schizotypal personality disorder.

Course and Prognosis

A long-term study by Thomas McGlashan reported that 10 percent of those with schizotypal personality disorder eventually committed suicide. Retrospective studies have shown that many patients thought to have had schizophrenia actually had schizotypal personality disorder, and according to current clinical thinking, the schizotype is the premorbid personality of the patient with schizophrenia. Some, however, maintain a stable schizotypal personality throughout their lives and marry and work in spite of their oddities.

Treatment

Psychotherapy. The principles of treatment of schizotypal personality disorder are no different from those of schizoid personality disorder, but clinicians must deal sensitively with the former. These patients have peculiar patterns of thinking, and some are involved in cults, strange religious practices, and the occult. Therapists must not ridicule such activities or be judgmental about these beliefs or activities.

Pharmacotherapy. Antipsychotic medication may be useful in dealing with ideas of reference, illusions, and other symptoms of the disorder and can be used in conjunction with psychotherapy. Antidepressants are of use when a depressive component of the personality is present.

ANTISOCIAL PERSONALITY DISORDER

Antisocial personality disorder is an inability to conform to the social norms that ordinarily govern many aspects of people's adolescent and adult behavior. Although characterized by continual antisocial or criminal acts, the disorder is not synonymous with criminality.

Epidemiology

The prevalence of antisocial personality disorder is 3 percent in men and 1 percent in women. It is most common in poor urban areas and among mobile residents of these areas. Boys with the disorder come from larger families than do girls with the disorder. The onset of the disorder is before the age of 15. Girls usually have symptoms before puberty, and boys even earlier. In prison populations, the prevalence of antisocial personality disorder may be as high as 75 percent. A familial pattern is present in that the disorder is five times more common among first-degree relatives of men with the disorder than among controls.

Diagnosis

Patients with antisocial personality disorder can fool even the most experienced clinicians. In an interview, patients can appear composed and credible, but beneath the veneer (or, to use Hervey Cleckley's term, *the mask of sanity*), there is tension, hostility, irritability, and rage. A stress interview, in which patients are vigorously confronted with inconsistencies in their histories, may be necessary to reveal the pathology.

A diagnostic workup should include a thorough neurological examination. Because patients often show abnormal EEG results and soft neurological signs suggestive of minimal brain damage in childhood, these findings can be used to confirm the clinical impression. The DSM-IV-TR diagnostic criteria are listed in Table 24–5.

Clinical Features

Patients with antisocial personality disorder can often seem to be normal and even charming and ingratiating. Their histories, however, reveal many areas of disordered life functioning. Lying, truancy, running away from home, thefts, fights, substance abuse, and illegal activities are typical experiences that patients report as beginning in childhood. These patients often impress opposite-sex clinicians with the colorful, seductive aspects of their personalities, but same-sex clinicians may regard them as manipulative and demanding. Patients with antisocial personality disorder exhibit no anxiety or depression, a lack that may seem grossly incongruous with their situations, although suicide threats and somatic preoccupations may be common. Their own explanations of their antisocial behavior make it seem mindless, but their mental content reveals the complete absence of delusions and other signs of irrational thinking. In fact, they frequently have a heightened sense of reality testing and often impress observers as having good verbal intelligence.

Table 24–5
DSM-IV-TR Diagnostic Criteria for Antisocial Personality Disorder

A. There is a pervasive pattern of disregard for and violation of the rights of others occurring since age 15 years, as indicated by three (or more) of the following:
 (1) failure to conform to social norms with respect to lawful behaviors as indicated by repeatedly performing acts that are grounds for arrest
 (2) deceitfulness, as indicated by repeated lying, use of aliases, or conning others for personal profit or pleasure
 (3) impulsivity or failure to plan ahead
 (4) irritability and aggressiveness, as indicated by repeated physical fights or assaults
 (5) reckless disregard for safety of self or others
 (6) consistent irresponsibility, as indicated by repeated failure to sustain consistent work behavior or honor financial obligations
 (7) lack of remorse, as indicated by being indifferent to or rationalizing having hurt, mistreated, or stolen from another
B. The individual is at least age 18 years.
C. There is evidence of conduct disorder with onset before age 15 years.
D. The occurrence of antisocial behavior is not exclusively during the course of schizophrenia or a manic episode.

From American Psychiatric Association. *Diagnostic and Statistical Manual of Mental Disorders.* 4th ed. Text rev. Washington, DC: American Psychiatric Association; copyright 2000, with permission.

Those with this disorder do not tell the truth and cannot be trusted to carry out any task or adhere to any conventional standard of morality. Promiscuity, spouse abuse, child abuse, and drunk driving are common events in their lives. A notable finding is a lack of remorse for these actions; that is, they appear to lack a conscience.

Mr. Y is a 26-year-old man who is transferred from a prison to a psychiatric unit as a result of a suicide attempt. Mr. Y has a history of three previous suicide attempts and multiple problems with the law. From information contained in the patient's social services, medical, and legal records, the clinician is able to piece together Mr. Y's history.

Mr. Y's mother was a prostitute and drug addict, and he never knew his father. He had a history of very serious conduct problems from a young age. He began getting into fights with other children almost from the day he began school and was caught torturing animals on a number of occasions when he was in elementary school. When he was 9 years old, Mr. Y threw his baby brother out of the window of their first floor apartment, causing multiple fractures. During his childhood, Mr. Y spent several years in a group home and stayed in many foster homes, but these placements were never successful. He would occasionally stay with his maternal grandmother, who was taking care of up to eight other grandchildren at the same time. Mr. Y began using drugs at age 10.

In early adolescence, Mr. Y joined a gang where he became involved in selling drugs and running numbers. He fathered his first child at the age of 13. Before he was 17, he was arrested on a variety of charges that included theft, possession of illegal drugs, and assault, but, because of his age, he received a series of suspended sentences. He was constantly truant from school and finally dropped out permanently at age 15. At that time, he began living on the street with other friends from his gang who were also engaged in using and selling drugs. At age 17, he was sentenced to 2 years in prison for stabbing someone in a fight in a bar. During this imprisonment, he attempted suicide by hanging himself with an article of clothing. As a result of this, he was transferred to the infirmary for several weeks and did not have to participate in his work detail.

By the time Mr. Y was 23, he had fathered five children, none of whom he sees or supports. When he is not crossed, Mr. Y is a manipulative person who can be charming, funny, and gregarious. When he is on drugs or when he does not get his way, however, he can become coldly furious and ruthlessly destructive.

Mr. Y has been treated for a series of drug overdoses, several of which were intentional. He has been hospitalized in psychiatric facilities on three occasions because of depression and suicide attempts. This is the fourth such hospitalization. Mr. Y's behavior follows a characteristic pattern during these hospitalizations. Initially, he seems to blossom and get better right away and is helpful with staff and patients. Soon, however, Mr. Y begins stirring up trouble on the ward and leading the other patients in revolt concerning smoking privileges, passes, and the need for medication. On one occasion during his most recent hospitalization, he was caught having intercourse with a 60-year-old female patient. (From DSM-IV Case Studies.)

Differential Diagnosis

Antisocial personality disorder can be distinguished from illegal behavior in that antisocial personality disorder involves many areas of a person's life. When antisocial behavior is the only manifestation, patients are classified in the DSM-IV-TR category of additional conditions that may be a focus of clinical attention—specifically, adult antisocial behavior. Dorothy Lewis found that many of these people have a neurological or mental disorder that has been either overlooked or undiagnosed. More difficult is the differentiation of antisocial personality disorder from substance abuse. When both substance abuse and antisocial behavior begin in childhood and continue into adult life, both disorders should be diagnosed. When, however, the antisocial behavior is clearly secondary to premorbid alcohol abuse or other substance abuse, the diagnosis of antisocial personality disorder is not warranted.

In diagnosing antisocial personality disorder, clinicians must adjust for the distorting effects of socioeconomic status, cultural background, and sex. Furthermore, the diagnosis of antisocial personality disorder is not warranted when mental retardation, schizophrenia, or mania can explain the symptoms.

Course and Prognosis

Once an antisocial personality disorder develops, it runs an unremitting course, with the height of antisocial behavior usually occurring in late adolescence. The prognosis is variable. Some reports indicate that symptoms decrease as people grow older. Many patients have somatization disorder and multiple physical complaints. Depressive disorders, alcohol use disorders, and other substance abuse are common.

Treatment

Psychotherapy.   If patients with antisocial personality disorder are immobilized (for example, placed in hospitals), they often become amenable to psychotherapy. When patients feel that they are among peers, their lack of motivation for change disappears. Perhaps for this reason self-help groups have been more useful than have jails in alleviating the disorder.

Before treatment can begin, firm limits are essential. Therapists must find ways of dealing with patients' self-destructive behavior. And to overcome patients' fear of intimacy, therapists must frustrate patients' desire to run from honest human encounters. In doing so, a therapist faces the challenge of separating control from punishment and of separating help and confrontation from social isolation and retribution.

Pharmacotherapy.   Pharmacotherapy is used to deal with incapacitating symptoms such as anxiety, rage, and depression, but because patients are often substance abusers, drugs must be used judiciously. If a patient shows evidence of attention-deficit/hyperactivity disorder, psychostimulants such as methylphenidate (Ritalin) may be of use. Attempts have been made to alter catecholamine metabolism with drugs and to control impulsive behavior with antiepileptic drugs, for example, carbamazepine (Tegretol), valproate (Depakote), especially if abnormal wave forms are noted on an EEG. β-Adrenergics have been used to reduce aggression.

BORDERLINE PERSONALITY DISORDER

Patients with borderline personality disorder stand on the border between neurosis and psychosis and are characterized by extraordinarily unstable affect, mood, behavior, object relations, and self-image. The disorder has also been called *ambulatory schizophrenia*, as-if personality (a term coined by Helene Deutsch), pseudoneurotic schizophrenia (described by Paul Hoch and Phillip Politan), and psychotic character disorder (described by John Frosch).

Epidemiology

No definitive prevalence studies are available, but borderline personality disorder is thought to be present in approximately 1 to 2 percent of the population and is twice as common in women as in men. An increased prevalence of major depressive disorder, alcohol use disorders, and substance abuse is found in first-degree relatives of people with borderline personality disorder.

Table 24–6
DSM-IV-TR Diagnostic Criteria for Borderline Personality Disorder

A pervasive pattern of instability of interpersonal relationships, self-image, and affects, and marked impulsivity beginning by early adulthood and present in a variety of contexts, as indicated by five (or more) of the following:

(1) frantic efforts to avoid real or imagined abandonment. **Note:** Do not include suicidal or self-mutilating behavior covered in Criterion 5.

(2) a pattern of unstable and intense interpersonal relationships characterized by alternating between extremes of idealization and devaluation

(3) identity disturbance: markedly and persistently unstable self-image or sense of self

(4) impulsivity in at least two areas that are potentially self-damaging (e.g., spending, sex, substance abuse, reckless driving, binge eating). **Note:** Do not include suicidal or self-mutilating behavior covered in Criterion 5.

(5) recurrent suicidal behavior, gestures, or threats, or self-mutilating behavior

(6) affective instability due to a marked reactivity of mood (e.g., intense episodic dysphoria, irritability, or anxiety usually lasting a few hours and only hours and only rarely more than a few days)

(7) chronic feelings of emptiness

(8) inappropriate, intense anger or difficulty controlling anger (e.g., frequent displays of temper, constant anger, recurrent physical fights)

(9) transient, stress-related paranoid ideation or severe dissociative symptoms

From American Psychiatric Association. *Diagnostic and Statistical Manual of Mental Disorders.* 4th ed. Text rev. Washington, DC: American Psychiatric Association; copyright 2000, with permission.

Diagnosis

According to DSM-IV-TR, the diagnosis of borderline personality disorder can made by early adulthood when patients show at least five of the criteria listed in Table 24–6.

Biological studies may aid in the diagnosis; some patients with borderline personality disorder show shortened REM latency and sleep continuity disturbances, abnormal DST results, and abnormal thyrotropin-releasing hormone (TRH) test results. Those changes, however, are also seen in some cases of depressive disorders.

Clinical Features

Persons with borderline personality disorder almost always appear to be in a state of crisis. Mood swings are common: Patients can be argumentative at one moment, depressed at the next, and later complain of having no feelings.

Patients may have short-lived psychotic episodes (so-called micropsychotic episodes) rather than full-blown psychotic breaks, and the psychotic symptoms of these patients are almost always circumscribed, fleeting, or doubtful. The behavior of patients with borderline personality disorder is highly unpredictable, and their achievements are rarely at the level of their abilities. The painful nature of their lives is reflected in repetitive self-destructive acts. Such patients may slash their wrists and perform other self-mutilations to elicit help from others, to express anger, or to numb themselves to overwhelming affect.

Because they feel both dependent and hostile, people with this disorder have tumultuous interpersonal relationships. They can be dependent on those to whom they are close and when frustrated can express enormous anger toward their intimate friends. Patients with borderline personality disorder cannot tolerate being alone, and they prefer a frantic search for companionship, no matter how unsatisfactory, to their own company. To assuage loneliness, if only for brief periods, they accept a stranger as a friend or behave promiscuously. They often complain about chronic feelings of emptiness and boredom and the lack of a consistent sense of identity (identity diffusion); when pressed, they often complain about how depressed they usually feel despite the flurry of other affects.

Most therapists agree that these patients show ordinary reasoning abilities on structured tests, such as the Wechsler Adult Intelligence Scale, and show deviant processes only on unstructured projective tests, such as the Rorschach test.

Functionally, patients with borderline personality disorder distort their relationships by considering each person to be either all good or all bad. The patient sees people as either nurturing attachment figures or as hateful and sadistic figures who deprive him or her of security needs and threaten him or her with abandonment whenever they feel dependent. As a result of this splitting, the good person is idealized, and the bad person devalued. Shifts of allegiance from one person or group to another are frequent. Otto Kernberg found that the defense mechanism of projective identification occurs in patients with borderline personality disorder. Therapists must be aware of this process so that they can act neutrally toward such patients.

Some clinicians use the concepts of panphobia, pananxiety, panambivalence, and chaotic sexuality to delineate these patients' characteristics.

Differential Diagnosis

The disorder is differentiated from schizophrenia on the basis of the borderline patient's lack of prolonged psychotic episodes, thought disorder, and other classic schizophrenic signs. Patients with schizotypal personality disorder show marked peculiarities of thinking, strange ideation, and recurrent ideas of reference. Those with paranoid personality disorder are marked by extreme suspiciousness. Patients with borderline personality disorder generally have chronic feelings of emptiness and short-lived psychotic episodes; they act impulsively and demand extraordinary relationships; they may mutilate themselves and make manipulative suicide attempts.

Course and Prognosis

This disorder is fairly stable; patients change little over time. Longitudinal studies show no progression toward schizophrenia, but patients have a high incidence of major depressive disorder episodes. The diagnosis is usually made before the age of 40, when patients are attempting to make occupational, marital, and other choices and are unable to deal with the normal stages of the life cycle.

Treatment

Psychotherapy.   Psychotherapy for patients with borderline personality disorder is an area of intensive investigation and has been the treatment of choice. For best results, pharmacotherapy has been added to the treatment regimen.

Psychotherapy is difficult for patients and therapists alike. Patients regress easily, act out their impulses, and show labile or fixed negative or positive transferences, which are difficult to analyze. Projective identification may also cause countertransference problems when a therapist is unaware that patients are unconsciously trying to coerce him or her to act out a particular behavior. Splitting as a defense mechanism causes patients to alternately love and hate therapists and others in the environment. A reality-oriented approach is more effective than in-depth interpretations of the unconscious.

Therapists have used behavior therapy to control patients' impulses and angry outbursts and to reduce their sensitivity to criticism and rejection. Social skills training, especially with videotape playback, is helpful to enable patients to see how their actions affect others and thereby to improve their interpersonal behavior.

Patients with borderline personality disorder often do well in a hospital setting in which they receive intensive psychotherapy on both an individual basis and a group basis. In a hospital they can also interact with trained staff members from a variety of disciplines and can be provided with occupational, recreational, and vocational therapy. Such programs are especially helpful when the home environment is detrimental to a patient's rehabilitation because of intrafamilial conflicts or other stresses such as parental abuse. Within the protected environment of the hospital, patients who are excessively impulsive, self-destructive, or self-mutilating can be given limits, and their actions can be observed. Under ideal circumstances, patients remain in the hospital until they show marked improvement, up to 1 year in some cases. Patients can then be discharged to special support systems such as day hospitals, night hospitals, and halfway houses.

A particular form of psychotherapy called dialectical behavior therapy (DBT) has been used for borderline patients, especially those with parasuicidal behavior such as frequent cutting. For a further discussion of DBT, see Section 31.6.

Pharmacotherapy.   Pharmacotherapy is useful to deal with specific personality features that interfere with patients' overall functioning. Antipsychotics have been used to control anger, hostility, and brief psychotic episodes. Antidepressants improve the depressed mood common in patients with borderline personality disorder. The MAO inhibitors (MAOIs) have been effective in modulating impulsive behavior in some patients. Benzodiazepines, particularly alprazolam (Xanax), help anxiety and depression, but other patients show a disinhibition with this class of drugs. Anticonvulsants such as carbamazepine (Tegretol) may improve global functioning for some patients. Serotonergic agents such as fluoxetine (Prozac) have been helpful in some cases.

HISTRIONIC PERSONALITY DISORDER

Persons with histrionic personality disorder are excitable and emotional and behave in a colorful, dramatic, extroverted fashion. Accompanying their flamboyant aspects, however, is often an inability to maintain deep, long-lasting attachments.

Epidemiology

According to DSM-IV-TR, limited data from general population studies suggest a prevalence of histrionic personality disorder of approximately 2 to 3 percent. Rates of approximately 10 to 15 percent have been reported in inpatient and outpatient mental health settings when structured assessment is used. The disorder is diagnosed more frequently in women than in men. Some studies have found an association with somatization disorder and alcohol-use disorders.

Diagnosis

In interviews, patients with histrionic personality disorder are generally cooperative and eager to give a detailed history. Gestures and dramatic punctuation in their conversations are common; they may make frequent slips of the tongue, and their language is colorful. Affective display is common, but, when pressed to acknowledge certain feelings (such as anger, sadness, and sexual wishes), they may respond with surprise, indignation, or denial. The results of the cognitive examination are usually normal, although a lack of perseverance may be shown on arithmetic or concentration tasks, and the patient's forgetfulness of affect-laden material may be astonishing. The DSM-IV-TR diagnostic criteria are listed in Table 24–7.

Clinical Features

People with histrionic personality disorder show a high degree of attention-seeking behavior. They tend to exaggerate their thoughts and feelings and make everything sound more important than it really is. They display temper tantrums, tears, and

Table 24–7
DSM-IV-TR Diagnostic Criteria for Histrionic Personality Disorder

A pervasive pattern of excessive emotionality and attention seeking, beginning by early adulthood and present in a variety of contexts, as indicated by five (or more) of the following:

(1) is uncomfortable in situations in which he or she is not the center of attention

(2) interaction with others is often characterized by inappropriate sexually seductive or provocative behavior

(3) displays rapidly shifting and shallow expression of emotions

(4) consistently uses physical appearance to draw attention to self

(5) has a style of speech that is excessively impressionistic and lacking in detail

(6) shows self-dramatization, theatricality, and exaggerated expression of emotion

(7) is suggestible, i.e., easily influenced by others or circumstances

(8) considers relationships to be more intimate than they actually are

From American Psychiatric Association. *Diagnostic and Statistical Manual of Mental Disorders.* 4th ed. Text rev. Washington, DC: American Psychiatric Association; copyright 2000, with permission.

accusations when they are not the center of attention or are not receiving praise or approval.

Seductive behavior is common in both sexes. Sexual fantasies about people with whom patients are involved are common, but patients are inconsistent about verbalizing these fantasies and may be coy or flirtatious rather than sexually aggressive. In fact, histrionic patients may have a psychosexual dysfunction: Women may be anorgasmic, and men may be impotent. Their need for reassurance is endless: They may act on their sexual impulses to reassure themselves that they are attractive to the other sex. Their relationships tend to be superficial, however, and they can be vain, self-absorbed, and fickle. Their strong dependence needs make them overly trusting and gullible.

The major defenses of patients with histrionic personality disorder are repression and dissociation. Accordingly, such patients are unaware of their true feelings and are unable to explain their motivations. Under stress, reality testing easily becomes impaired.

Differential Diagnosis

Distinguishing between histrionic personality disorder and borderline personality disorder is difficult, but in borderline personality disorder, suicide attempts, identity diffusion, and brief psychotic episodes are more likely. Although both conditions may be diagnosed in the same patient, clinicians should separate the two. Somatization disorder (Briquet's syndrome) may occur in conjunction with histrionic personality disorder. Patients with brief psychotic disorder and dissociative disorders may warrant a coexisting diagnosis of histrionic personality disorder.

Course and Prognosis

With age, people with histrionic personality disorder show fewer symptoms, but because they lack the energy of earlier years, the difference in number of symptoms may be more apparent than real. People with this disorder are sensation seekers and may get into trouble with the law, abuse substances, and act promiscuously.

Treatment

Psychotherapy.   Patients with histrionic personality disorder are often unaware of their own real feelings; clarification of their inner feelings is an important therapeutic process. Psychoanalytically oriented psychotherapy, whether group or individual, is probably the treatment of choice for histrionic personality disorder.

Pharmacotherapy.   Pharmacotherapy can be adjunctive when symptoms are targeted (such as the use of antidepressants for depression and somatic complaints, antianxiety agents for anxiety, and antipsychotics for derealization and illusions).

NARCISSISTIC PERSONALITY DISORDER

Persons with narcissistic personality disorder are characterized by a heightened sense of self-importance and grandiose feelings of uniqueness.

**Table 24–8
DSM-IV-TR Diagnostic Criteria for Narcissistic
Personality Disorder**

A pervasive pattern of grandiosity (in fantasy or behavior), need for admiration, and lack of empathy, beginning by early adulthood and present in a variety of contexts, as indicated by five (or more) of the following:

(1) has a grandiose sense of self-importance (e.g., exaggerates achievements and talents, expects to be recognized as superior without commensurate achievements)

(2) is preoccupied with fantasies of unlimited success, power, brilliance, beauty, or ideal love

(3) believes that he or she is "special" and unique and can only be understood by, or should associate with, other special or high-status people (or institutions)

(4) requires excessive admiration

(5) has a sense of entitlement, i.e., unreasonable expectations of especially favorable treatment or automatic compliance with his or her expectations

(6) is interpersonally exploitative, i.e., takes advantage of others to achieve his or her own ends

(7) lacks empathy: is unwilling to recognize or identify with the feelings and needs of others

(8) is often envious of others or believes that others are envious of him or her

(9) shows arrogant, haughty behaviors or attitudes

From American Psychiatric Association. *Diagnostic and Statistical Manual of Mental Disorders.* 4th ed. Text rev. Washington, DC: American Psychiatric Association; copyright 2000, with permission.

Epidemiology

According to DSM-IV-TR, estimates of the prevalence of narcissistic personality disorder range from 2 to 16 percent in the clinical population and less than 1 percent in the general population. People with the disorder may impart to their children an unrealistic sense of omnipotence, grandiosity, beauty, and talent; thus, offspring of such parents may have a higher-than-usual risk for developing the disorder themselves. The number of cases of narcissistic personality disorder reported is increasing steadily.

Diagnosis

Table 24–8 gives the DSM-IV-TR diagnostic criteria for narcissistic personality disorder.

Clinical Features

Persons with narcissistic personality disorder have a grandiose sense of self-importance; they consider themselves special and expect special treatment. Their sense of entitlement is striking. They handle criticism poorly and may become enraged when someone dares to criticize them, or they may appear completely indifferent to criticism. People with this disorder want their own way and are frequently ambitious to achieve fame and fortune. Their relationships are fragile, and they can make others furious by their refusal to obey conventional rules of behavior. Interpersonal exploitiveness is commonplace. They are unable to show empathy and feign sympathy only to achieve their selfish ends. Because of their fragile self-esteem, they are prone to depression.

Interpersonal difficulties, occupational problems, rejection, and loss are among the stresses that narcissists commonly produce by their behavior—stresses they are least able to handle.

Differential Diagnosis

Borderline, histrionic, and antisocial personality disorders often accompany narcissistic personality disorder so that a differential diagnosis is difficult. Patients with narcissistic personality disorder have less anxiety than do those with borderline personality disorder; their lives tend to be less chaotic, and they are less likely to attempt suicide. Patients with antisocial personality disorder have a history of impulsive behavior, often associated with alcohol or other substance abuse, that frequently gets them into trouble with the law. Patients with histrionic personality disorder show features of exhibitionism and interpersonal manipulativeness that are similar to those of patients with narcissistic personality disorder.

Course and Prognosis

Narcissistic personality disorder is chronic and difficult to treat. Patients with the disorder must constantly deal with blows to their narcissism resulting from their own behavior or from life experience. Aging is handled poorly; patients value beauty, strength, and youthful attributes, to which they cling inappropriately. They may be more vulnerable, therefore, to midlife crises than are other groups.

Treatment

Psychotherapy.   Because patients must renounce their narcissism to make progress, the treatment of narcissistic personality disorder is difficult. Psychiatrists such as Otto Kernberg and Heinz Kohut have advocated using psychoanalytic approaches to effect change, but much research is required to validate the diagnosis and to determine the best treatment.

Some clinicians advocate group therapy for their patients who learn how to share with others and under ideal circumstances can develop an empathic response to others.

Pharmacotherapy.   Lithium (Eskalith) has been used with patients whose clinical picture includes mood swings. Because patients with narcissistic personality disorder tolerate rejection poorly and are prone to depression, antidepressants, especially serotonergic drugs, may also be of use.

AVOIDANT PERSONALITY DISORDER

Persons with avoidant personality disorder show an extreme sensitivity to rejection and may lead a socially withdrawn life. Although shy, they are not asocial and show a great desire for companionship, but they need unusually strong guarantees of uncritical acceptance. Such people are commonly described as having an inferiority complex.

Epidemiology

Avoidant personality disorder is common: The prevalence of the disorder is 1 to 10 percent of the general population. No

**Table 24–9
DSM-IV-TR Diagnostic Criteria for Avoidant
Personality Disorder**

A pervasive pattern of social inhibition, feelings of inadequacy, and hypersensitivity to negative evaluation, beginning by early adulthood and present in a variety of contexts, as indicated by four (or more) of the following:

(1) avoids occupational activities that involve significant inter-personal contact, because of fears of criticism, disapproval, or rejection

(2) is unwilling to get involved with people unless certain of being liked

(3) shows restraint within intimate relationships because of the fear of being shamed or ridiculed

(4) is preoccupied with being criticized or rejected in social situations

(5) is inhibited in new interpersonal situations because of feel-ings of inadequacy

(6) views self as socially inept, personally unappealing, or infe-rior to others

(7) is unusually reluctant to take personal risks or to engage in any new activities because they may prove embarrassing

From American Psychiatric Association. *Diagnostic and Statistical Man-ual of Mental Disorders.* 4th ed. Text rev. Washington, DC: American Psychiatric Association; copyright 2000, with permission.

information is available on sex ratio or familial pattern. Infants classified as having a timid temperament may be more prone to the disorder than are those high on activity–approach scales.

Diagnosis

In clinical interviews, patients' most striking aspect is anxiety about talking with an interviewer. Their nervous and tense man-ner appears to wax and wane with their perception of whether an interviewer likes them. Patients seem vulnerable to the inter-viewer's comments and suggestions and may regard a clarifica-tion or an interpretation as a criticism. The DSM-IV-TR diagnostic criteria for avoidant personality disorder are listed in Table 24–9.

Clinical Features

Hypersensitivity to rejection by others is the central clinical feature of avoidant personality disorder, and their main person-ality trait is timidity. People with the disorder desire the warmth and security of human companionship but justify their avoid-ance of relationships by their alleged fear of rejection. When talking with someone, they express uncertainty, show a lack of self-confidence, and may speak in a self-effacing manner. Because they are hypervigilant about rejection, they are afraid to speak up in public or to make requests of others. They are apt to misinterpret other people's comments as derogatory or ridi-culing. The refusal of any request leads them to withdraw from others and to feel hurt.

In the vocational sphere, patients with avoidant personality disorder often take jobs on the sidelines. They rarely attain much personal advancement or exercise much authority but seem shy and eager to please. These people are generally

unwilling to enter relationships unless they are given an unusu-ally strong guarantee of uncritical acceptance. Consequently, they often have no close friends or confidants.

Differential Diagnosis

Patients with avoidant personality disorder desire social interac-tion, unlike patients with schizoid personality disorder, who want to be alone. Patients with avoidant personality disorder are not as demanding, irritable, or unpredictable as are those with borderline and histrionic personality disorders. Avoidant personality disorder and dependent personality disorder are similar. Patients with dependent personality disorder are presumed to have a greater fear of being abandoned or unloved than do those with avoidant per-sonality disorder, but the clinical picture may be indistinguishable.

Course and Prognosis

Many people with avoidant personality disorder are able to function in a protected environment. Some marry, have chil-dren, and live their lives surrounded only by family members. Should their support system fail, however, they are subject to depression, anxiety, and anger. Phobic avoidance is common, and patients with the disorder may give histories of social pho-bia or incur social phobia in the course of their illness.

Treatment

Psychotherapy.   Psychotherapeutic treatment depends on solidifying an alliance with patients. As trust develops, a thera-pist must convey an accepting attitude toward the patient's fears, especially the fear of rejection. The therapist eventually encourages a patient to move out into the world to take what are perceived as great risks of humiliation, rejection, and failure. But therapists should be cautious when giving assignments to exercise new social skills outside therapy; failure may reinforce a patient's already poor self-esteem. Group therapy may help patients understand the effects of their sensitivity to rejection on themselves and others. Assertiveness training is a form of behavior therapy that may teach patients to express their needs openly and to enlarge their self-esteem.

Pharmacotherapy.   Pharmacotherapy has been used to manage anxiety and depression when they are associated with the disorder. Some patients are helped by β-adrenergic receptor antagonists, such as atenolol (Tenormin), to manage autonomic nervous system hyperactivity, which tends to be high in patients with avoidant personality disorder, especially when they approach feared situations. Serotonergic agents may help rejec-tion sensitivity.

Theoretically, dopaminergic drugs might cause more nov-elty-seeking behavior in these patients; however, it is important that the patient be psychologically prepared for any new experi-ence that might occur as a result.

DEPENDENT PERSONALITY DISORDER

Persons with dependent personality disorder subordinate their own needs to those of others, get others to assume responsibil-ity for major areas of their lives, lack self-confidence, and may

Table 24–10
DSM-IV-TR Diagnostic Criteria for Dependent Personality Disorder

A pervasive and excessive need to be taken care of that leads to submissive and clinging behavior and fears of separation, beginning by early adulthood and present in a variety of contexts, as indicated by five (or more) of the following:

(1) has difficulty making everyday decisions without an excessive amount of advice and reassurance from others

(2) needs others to assume responsibility for most major areas of his or her life

(3) has difficulty expressing disagreement with others because of fear of loss of support or approval. **Note:** Do not include realistic fears of retribution

(4) has difficulty initiating projects or doing things on his or her own (because of a lack of self-confidence in judgment or abilities rather than a lack of motivation or energy)

(5) goes to excessive lengths to obtain nurturance and support from others, to the point of volunteering to do things that are unpleasant

(6) feels uncomfortable or helpless when alone because of exaggerated fears of being unable to care for himself or herself

(7) urgently seeks another relationship as a source of care and support when a close relationship ends

(8) is unrealistically preoccupied with fears of being left to take care of himself or herself

From American Psychiatric Association. *Diagnostic and Statistical Manual of Mental Disorders.* 4th ed. Text rev. Washington, DC: American Psychiatric Association; copyright 2000, with permission.

experience intense discomfort when alone for more than a brief period. The disorder has been called *passive-dependent personality*. Freud described an oral-dependent personality dimension characterized by dependence, pessimism, fear of sexuality, self-doubt, passivity, suggestibility, and lack of perseverance; his description is similar to the DSM-IV-TR categorization of dependent personality disorder.

Epidemiology

Dependent personality disorder is more common in women than in men. One study diagnosed 2.5 percent of all personality disorders as falling into this category. It is more common in young children than in older ones. People with chronic physical illness in childhood may be most prone to the disorder.

Diagnosis

In interviews, patients appear to be compliant. They try to cooperate, welcome specific questions, and look for guidance. The DSM-IV-TR diagnostic criteria for dependent personality disorder are listed in Table 24–10.

Clinical Features

Dependent personality disorder is characterized by a pervasive pattern of dependent and submissive behavior. People with the disorder cannot make decisions without an excessive amount of advice and reassurance from others. They avoid positions of responsibility and become anxious if asked to assume a leader-

ship role. They prefer to be submissive. When on their own, they find it difficult to persevere at tasks but may find it easy to perform these tasks for someone else.

Because people with the disorder do not like to be alone, they seek out others on whom they can depend; their relationships are thus distorted by their need to be attached to another person. In *folie à deux* (shared psychotic disorder), one member of the pair usually suffers from dependent personality disorder; the submissive partner takes on the delusional system of the more aggressive, assertive partner on whom he or she is dependent.

Pessimism, self-doubt, passivity, and fears of expressing sexual and aggressive feelings all typify the behavior of people with dependent personality disorder. An abusive, unfaithful, or alcoholic spouse may be tolerated for long periods in order not to disturb the sense of attachment.

Differential Diagnosis

The traits of dependence are found in many psychiatric disorders so that differential diagnosis is difficult. Dependence is a prominent factor in patients with histrionic and borderline personality disorders, but those with dependent personality disorder usually have a long-term relationship with one person, rather than a series on whom they are dependent, and they do not tend to be overtly manipulative. Patients with schizoid and schizotypal personality disorders may be indistinguishable from those with avoidant personality disorder. Dependent behavior may occur in patients with agoraphobia, but these patients tend to have a high level of overt anxiety or even panic.

Course and Prognosis

Little is known about the course of dependent personality disorder. There tends to be impaired occupational functioning, as people with the disorder lack the ability to act independently and without close supervision. Social relationships are limited to those on whom they can depend, and many suffer physical or mental abuse because they cannot assert themselves. They risk major depressive disorder if they sustain the loss of the person on whom they are dependent, but with treatment the prognosis is favorable.

Treatment

Psychotherapy. The treatment of dependent personality disorder can often be successful. Insight-oriented therapies enable patients to understand the antecedents of their behavior, and, with the support of a therapist, patients can become more independent, assertive, and self-reliant. Behavioral therapy, assertiveness training, family therapy, and group therapy have all been used, with successful outcomes in many cases.

A pitfall in treatment may arise when a therapist encourages a patient to change the dynamics of a pathological relationship (for example, supports a physically abused wife in seeking help from the police). At this point, patients may become anxious and unable to cooperate in therapy; they may feel torn between complying with the therapist and losing a pathological external relationship. Therapists must show great respect for these patients' feelings of attachment, no matter how pathological these feelings may seem.

Pharmacotherapy.   Pharmacotherapy has been used to deal with specific symptoms such as anxiety and depression, which are common associated features of dependent personality disorder. Patients who experience panic attacks or who have high levels of separation anxiety may be helped by imipramine (Tofranil). Benzodiazepines and serotonergic agents have also been useful. If a patient's depression or withdrawal symptoms respond to psychostimulants, they may be used.

OBSESSIVE-COMPULSIVE PERSONALITY DISORDER

Obsessive-compulsive personality disorder is characterized by emotional constriction, orderliness, perseverance, stubbornness, and indecisiveness. The essential feature of the disorder is a pervasive pattern of perfectionism and inflexibility. This disorder is also know as *anancastic personality disorder*.

Epidemiology

The prevalence of obsessive-compulsive personality disorder is unknown. It is more common in men than in women and is diagnosed most often in oldest children. The disorder also occurs more frequently in first-degree biological relatives of people with the disorder than in the general population. Patients often have backgrounds characterized by harsh discipline. Freud hypothesized that the disorder is associated with difficulties in the anal stage of psychosexual development, generally around the age of 2, but in various studies this theory has not been validated.

Diagnosis

In interviews, patients with obsessive-compulsive personality disorder may have a stiff, formal, and rigid demeanor. Their affect is not blunted or flat but can be described as constricted. They lack spontaneity, and their mood is usually serious. Such patients may be anxious about not being in control of the interview. Their answers to questions are unusually detailed. The defense mechanisms they use are rationalization, isolation, intellectualization, reaction formation, and undoing. The DSM-IV-TR diagnostic criteria for obsessive-compulsive personality disorder are listed in Table 24–11.

Clinical Features

Persons with obsessive-compulsive personality disorder are preoccupied with rules, regulations, orderliness, neatness, details, and the achievement of perfection. These traits account for the general constriction of the entire personality. They insist that rules be followed rigidly and are unable to tolerate what they perceive to be infractions. Accordingly, they lack flexibility and are intolerant. They are capable of prolonged work, provided it is routinized and does not require changes to which they cannot adapt.

People with obsessive-compulsive personality disorder have limited interpersonal skills. They are formal and serious and often lack a sense of humor. They alienate people, are unable to compromise, and insist that others submit to their needs. They are, however, eager to please those whom they see as more

Table 24–11
DSM-IV-TR Diagnostic Criteria for Obsessive-Compulsive Personality Disorder

A pervasive pattern of preoccupation with orderliness, perfectionism, and mental and interpersonal control, at the expense of flexibility, openness, and efficiency, beginning by early adulthood and present in a variety of contexts, as indicated by four (or more) of the following:

(1) is preoccupied with details, rules, lists, order, organization, or schedules to the extent that the major point of the activity is lost

(2) shows perfectionism that interferes with task completion (e.g., is unable to complete a project because his or her own overly strict standards are not met)

(3) is excessively devoted to work and productivity to the exclusion of leisure activities and friendships (not accounted for by obvious economic necessity)

(4) is overconscientious, scrupulous, and inflexible about matters of morality, ethics, or values (not accounted for by cultural or religious identification)

(5) is unable to discard worn-out or worthless objects even when they have no sentimental value

(6) is reluctant to delegate tasks or to work with others unless they submit to exactly his or her way of doing things

(7) adopts a miserly spending style toward both self and others; money is viewed as something to be hoarded for future catastrophes

(8) shows rigidity and stubbornness

From American Psychiatric Association. *Diagnostic and Statistical Manual of Mental Disorders.* 4th ed. Text rev. Washington, DC: American Psychiatric Association; copyright 2000, with permission.

powerful than themselves, and they carry out these people's wishes in an authoritarian manner. Because they fear making mistakes, they are indecisive and ruminate about making decisions. Although a stable marriage and occupational adequacy are common, people with obsessive-compulsive personality disorder have few friends. Anything that threatens to upset their perceived stability or the routine of their lives can precipitate a great deal of anxiety otherwise bound up in the rituals that they impose on their lives and try to impose on others.

Differential Diagnosis

When recurrent obsessions or compulsions are present, obsessive-compulsive disorder should be noted on Axis I. Perhaps the most difficult distinction is between outpatients with some obsessive-compulsive traits and those with obsessive-compulsive personality disorder. The diagnosis of personality disorder is reserved for those patients with significant impairments in their occupational or social effectiveness. In some cases, delusional disorder coexists with personality disorders and should be noted.

Course and Prognosis

The course of obsessive-compulsive personality disorder is variable and unpredictable. From time to time, people may develop obsessions or compulsions in the course of their disorder. Some adolescents with obsessive-compulsive personality disorder evolve into warm, open, and loving adults; in others, the disorder can be either the harbinger of schizophrenia or—decades later and exacerbated by the aging process—major depressive disorder.

Persons with obsessive-compulsive personality disorder may flourish in positions demanding methodical, deductive, or detailed work, but they are vulnerable to unexpected changes, and their personal lives may remain barren. Depressive disorders, especially those of late onset, are common.

Treatment

Psychotherapy. Unlike patients with the other personality disorders, those with obsessive-compulsive personality disorder are often aware of their suffering, and they seek treatment on their own. Overtrained and oversocialized, these patients highly value free association and nondirective therapy. Treatment, however, is often long and complex, and countertransference problems are common.

Group therapy and behavior therapy occasionally offer certain advantages. In both contexts it is easy to interrupt the patients in the midst of their maladaptive interactions or explanations. Preventing the completion of their habitual behavior raises patients' anxiety and leaves them susceptible to learning new coping strategies. Patients can also receive direct rewards for change in group therapy, something less often possible in individual psychotherapies.

Pharmacotherapy. Clonazepam (Klonopin), a benzodiazepine with anticonvulsant use, has reduced symptoms in patients with severe obsessive-compulsive disorder. Whether it is of use in the personality disorder is unknown. Clomipramine (Anafranil) and such serotonergic agents as fluoxetine, usually at dosages of 60 to 80 mg a day, may be of use if obsessive-compulsive signs and symptoms break through. Mixed selective serotonin reuptake inhibitors (SSRIs) and serotonin agonists such as nefazodone (Serzone) may be useful.

PERSONALITY DISORDER NOT OTHERWISE SPECIFIED

In DSM-IV-TR, this category of personality disorder not otherwise specified is reserved for disorders that do not fit into any of the previously described personality disorder categories. Passive-aggressive personality disorder and depressive personality disorder (described below) are now listed as examples of personality disorder not otherwise specified. A narrow spectrum of behavior or a particular trait—such as oppositionalism, sadism, or masochism—can also be classified in this category. A patient with features of more than one personality disorder but without the complete criteria of any one disorder can be assigned this classification. The DSM-IV-TR criteria for personality disorder not otherwise specified are presented in Table 24–12.

Passive-Aggressive Personality Disorder

Persons with passive-aggressive personality disorder are characterized by covert obstructionism, procrastination, stubbornness, and inefficiency. Such behavior is a manifestation of passively expressed underlying aggression. In DSM-IV-TR, the disorder is also called *negativistic personality disorder*.

Table 24–12
DSM-IV-TR Diagnostic Criteria for Personality Disorder Not Otherwise Specified

This category is for disorders of personality functioning that do not meet criteria for any specific personality disorder. An example is the presence of features of more than one specific personality disorder that do not meet the full criteria for any one personality disorder ("mixed personality"), but that together cause clinically significant distress or impairment in one or more important areas of functioning (e.g., social or occupational). This category can also be used when the clinician judges that a specific personality disorder that is not included in the classification is appropriate. Examples include depressive personality disorder and passive-aggressive personality disorder.

From American Psychiatric Association. *Diagnostic and Statistical Manual of Mental Disorders.* 4th ed. Text rev. Washington, DC: American Psychiatric Association; copyright 2000, with permission.

Epidemiology. No data are available about the epidemiology of the disorder. Sex ratio, familial patterns, and prevalence have not been adequately studied.

Diagnosis. The criteria for passive-aggressive disorder are presented in Table 24–13.

Clinical Features. Passive-aggressive personality disorder patients characteristically procrastinate, resist demands for adequate performance, find excuses for delays, and find fault with those on whom they depend; yet they refuse to extricate themselves from the dependent relationships. They usually lack assertiveness and are not direct about their own needs and wishes. They fail to ask needed questions about what is expected of them and may become anxious when forced to succeed or when their usual defense of turning anger against themselves is removed.

Table 24–13
DSM-IV-TR Research Criteria for Passive-Aggressive Personality Disorder

A. A pervasive pattern of negativistic attitudes and passive resistance to demands for adequate performance, beginning by early adulthood and present in a variety of contexts, as indicated by four (or more) of the following:

   (1) passively resists fulfilling routine social and occupational tasks

   (2) complains of being misunderstood and unappreciated by others

   (3) is sullen and argumentative

   (4) unreasonably criticizes and scorns authority

   (5) expresses envy and resentment toward those apparently more fortunate

   (6) voices exaggerated and persistent complaints of personal misfortune

   (7) alternates between hostile defiance and contrition

B. Does not occur exclusively during major depressive episodes and is not better accounted for by dysthymic disorder.

From American Psychiatric Association. *Diagnostic and Statistical Manual of Mental Disorders.* 4th ed. Text rev. Washington, DC: American Psychiatric Association; copyright 2000, with permission.

In interpersonal relationships, these people attempt to manipulate themselves into a position of dependence, but others often experience this passive, self-detrimental behavior as punitive and manipulative. People with this disorder expect others to do their errands and to carry out their routine responsibilities. Friends and clinicians may become enmeshed in trying to assuage the patient's many claims of unjust treatment. The close relationships of people with passive-aggressive personality disorder, however, are rarely tranquil or happy. Because they are bound to their resentment more closely than to their satisfaction, they may never even formulate goals for finding enjoyment in life. People with the disorder lack self-confidence and are typically pessimistic about the future.

Differential Diagnosis. Passive-aggressive personality disorders must be differentiated from histrionic and borderline personality disorders. Patients with passive-aggressive personality disorder, however, are less flamboyant, dramatic, affective, and openly aggressive than are those with histrionic and borderline personality disorders.

Course and Prognosis. In a follow-up study averaging 11 years of 100 passive-aggressive inpatients, Ivor Small found that the disorder was associated with alcohol abuse and depression in approximately 50 percent of patients. Others were irritable, anxious, and had somatic complaints. Without treatment, the prognosis is guarded.

Treatment. Patients with passive-aggressive personality disorder who receive supportive psychotherapy have good outcomes, but psychotherapy for these patients has many pitfalls. To fulfill their demands is often to support their pathology, but to refuse their demands is to reject them. Therapy sessions can thus become a battleground on which a patient expresses feelings of resentment against a therapist on whom the patient wishes to become dependent. With these patients, clinicians must treat suicide gestures as any covert expression of anger and not as object loss in major depressive disorder. Therapists must point out the probable consequences of passive-aggressive behaviors as they occur. Such confrontations may be more helpful than a correct interpretation in changing patients' behavior.

Antidepressants should be prescribed only when clinical indications of depression and the possibility of suicide exist. Depending on the clinical features, some patients have responded to benzodiazepines and psychostimulants.

Depressive Personality Disorder

Persons with depressive personality disorder are characterized by lifelong traits that fall along the depressive spectrum. They are pessimistic, anhedonic, duty bound, self-doubting, and chronically unhappy. The disorder is newly classified in DSM-IV-TR, but melancholic personality was described by early 20th century European psychiatrists such as Ernst Kretschmer.

Epidemiology. Because depressive personality disorder is a new category, no epidemiological data are available. On the basis of the prevalence of depressive disorders in the overall population, however, depressive personality disorder seems to be common, to occur equally in men and women, and to occur in families in which depressive disorders are found.

Etiology. The cause of depressive personality disorder is unknown, but the same factors involved in dysthymic disorder and major depressive disorder may be at work. Psychological theories involve early loss, poor parenting, punitive superegos, and extreme feelings of guilt. Biological theories involve the hypothalamic-pituitary-adrenal-thyroid axis, including the noradrenergic and serotonergic amine systems. Genetic predisposition, as indicated by Stella Chess's studies of temperament, may also play a role.

Diagnosis and Clinical Features. A classic description of depressive personality was provided in 1963 by Arthur Noyes and Laurence Kolb:

> They feel but little of the normal joy of living and are inclined to be lonely and solemn, to be gloomy, submissive, pessimistic, and self-deprecatory. They are prone to express regrets and feelings of inadequacy and hopelessness. They are often meticulous, perfectionistic, overconscientious, preoccupied with work, feel responsibility keenly, and are easily discouraged under new conditions. They are fearful of disapproval, tend to suffer in silence and perhaps to cry easily, although usually not in the presence of others. A tendency to hesitation, indecision, and caution betrays an inherent feeling of insecurity.

More recently, Hagop Akiskal described seven groups of depressive traits: quiet, introverted, passive, and nonassertive; gloomy, pessimistic, serious, and incapable of fun; self-critical, self-reproachful, and self-derogatory; skeptical, critical of others, and hard to please; conscientious, responsible, and self-disciplined; brooding and given to worry; preoccupied with negative events, feelings of inadequacy, and personal shortcomings.

Patients with depressive personality disorder complain of chronic feelings of unhappiness. They admit to low self-esteem and find it difficult to find anything in their lives about which they are joyful, hopeful, or optimistic. They are self-critical and derogatory and are likely to denigrate their work, themselves, and their relationships with others. Their physiognomy often reflects their mood—poor posture, depressed facies, hoarse voice, and psychomotor retardation. The DSM-IV-TR criteria are listed in Table 24–14.

Differential Diagnosis. Dysthymic disorder is a mood disorder characterized by greater fluctuation in mood than occurs in depressive personality disorder. The personality disorder is chronic and lifelong, whereas dysthymic disorder is episodic, can occur at any time, and usually has a precipitating stressor. The depressive personality can be conceptualized as part of a spectrum of affective conditions in which dysthymic disorder and major depressive disorder are more severe variants. Patients with avoidant personality disorder are introverted and dependent but tend to be more anxious than depressed, compared with people with depressive personality disorder.

Course and Prognosis. People with depressive personality disorder may be at great risk for dysthymic disorder and major depressive disorder. In a recent study by Donald Klein and Gregory Mills, subjects with depressive personality exhibited significantly higher rates of current mood disorder, lifetime mood disorder, major depression, and dysthymia than did subjects without depressive personality.

Table 24–14
DSM-IV-TR Research Criteria for Depressive Personality Disorder

A. A pervasive pattern of depressive cognitions and behaviors beginning by early adulthood and present in a variety of contexts, as indicated by five (or more) of the following:
  (1) usual mood is dominated by dejection, gloominess, cheerlessness, joylessness, unhappiness
  (2) self-concept centers around beliefs of inadequacy, worth-lessness, and low self-esteem
  (3) is critical, blaming, and derogatory toward self
  (4) is brooding and given to worry
  (5) is negativistic, critical, and judgmental toward others
  (6) is pessimistic
  (7) is prone to feeling guilty or remorseful
B. Does not occur exclusively during major depressive episodes and is not better accounted for by dysthymic disorder.

From American Psychiatric Association. *Diagnostic and Statistical Manual of Mental Disorders.* 4th ed. Text rev. Washington, DC: American Psychiatric Association; copyright 2000, with permission.

Treatment. Psychotherapy is the treatment of choice for depressive personality disorder. Patients respond to insight-oriented psychotherapy, and because their reality testing is good, they are able to gain insight into the psychodynamics of their illness and to appreciate its effects on their interpersonal relationships. Treatment is likely to be long term. Cognitive therapy helps patients understand the cognitive manifestations of their low self-esteem and pessimism. Group psychotherapy and interpersonal therapy are also useful. Some people respond to self-help measures.

Psychopharmacological approaches include the use of antidepressant medications, especially such serotonergic agents as sertraline (Zoloft), 50 mg a day. Some patients respond to small dosages of psychostimulants, such as amphetamine, 5 to 15 mg a day. In all cases, psychopharmacological agents should be combined with psychotherapy to achieve maximum effects.

Sadomasochistic Personality Disorder

Some personality types are characterized by elements of sadism or masochism or a combination of both. Sadomasochistic personality disorder is listed here because it is of major clinical and historical interest in psychiatry. It is not an official diagnostic category in DSM-IV-TR or its appendix, but it can be diagnosed as personality disorder not otherwise classified.

Sadism is the desire to cause others pain by being either sexually abusive or generally physically or psychologically abusive. It is named after the Marquis de Sade, a late 18th century writer of erotica describing people who experienced sexual pleasure while inflicting pain on others. Freud believed that sadists ward off castration anxiety and are able to achieve sexual pleasure only when they can do to others what they fear will be done to them.

Masochism, named after Leopold von Sacher-Masoch, a 19th century German novelist, is the achievement of sexual gratification by inflicting pain on the self. So-called moral masochists generally seek humiliation and failure rather than physical pain. Freud believed that masochists' ability to achieve orgasm is disturbed by anxiety and guilt feelings about sex, which are alleviated by suffering and punishment.

Clinical observations indicate that elements of both sadistic and masochistic behavior are usually present in the same person. Treatment with insight-oriented psychotherapy, including psychoanalysis, has been effective in some cases. As a result of therapy, patients become aware of the need for self-punishment secondary to excessive unconscious guilt and also come to recognize their repressed aggressive impulses, which originate in early childhood.

Sadistic Personality Disorder

Sadistic personality disorder is not included in DSM-IV-TR, but it still appears in the literature and may be of descriptive use. Beginning in early adulthood, people with sadistic personality disorder show a pervasive pattern of cruel, demeaning, and aggressive behavior that is directed toward others. Physical cruelty or violence is used to inflict pain on others and not to achieve another goal, such as mugging a person in order to steal. People with the disorder like to humiliate or demean people in front of others and have usually treated or disciplined people uncommonly harshly, especially children. In general, people with sadistic personality disorder are fascinated by violence, weapons, injury, or torture. To be included in this category, such people cannot be motivated solely by the desire to derive sexual arousal from their behavior; if they are so motivated, the paraphilia of sexual sadism should be diagnosed.

PERSONALITY CHANGE DUE TO A GENERAL MEDICAL CONDITION

Personality change due to a general medical condition is characterized by a marked change in personality style and traits from a previous level of functioning. Patients must show evidence of a causative organic factor antedating the onset of the personality change.

Etiology

Structural damage to the brain is usually the cause of the personality change, and head trauma is probably the most common cause. Cerebral neoplasms and vascular accidents, particularly of the temporal and frontal lobes, are also common causes.

Diagnosis and Clinical Features

A change in personality from previous patterns of behavior or an exacerbation of previous personality characteristics is notable. Impaired control of the expression of emotions and impulses is a cardinal feature. Emotions are characteristically labile and shallow, although euphoria or apathy may be prominent. The euphoria may mimic hypomania, but true elation is absent, and patients may admit to not really feeling happy. There is a hollow and silly ring to their excitement and facile jocularity, particularly when the frontal lobes are involved (called *witzelsucht* in German). Also associated with damage to the frontal lobes, the so-called frontal lobe syndrome, is prominent indifference and apathy, characterized by a lack of concern for events in the immediate environment. Temper outbursts with little or no provocation may occur, especially after alcohol ingestion, and may result in violent behavior. The expression of impulses may be manifested by inappropriate jokes, a coarse manner, improper sexual advances, and antisocial conduct resulting in conflicts with the law, such as assaults on others, sexual misdemeanors, and shoplifting. Foresight and the ability to anticipate the social or legal consequences of actions are typically diminished.

Persons with personality change due to a general medical condition have a clear sensorium. Mild disorders of cognitive function often coexist but do not amount to intellectual deterioration. Patients may be inattentive, which may account for disorders of recent memory. With some prodding, however, patients are likely to recall what they claim to have forgotten. The diagnosis should be suspected in patients who show marked changes in behavior or personality involving emotional lability and impaired impulse control, who have no history of mental disorder, and whose personality changes occur abruptly or over a relatively brief time.

Differential Diagnosis

A personality change may herald a cognitive disorder that will eventually evolve into dementia. In these cases, as deterioration begins to encompass significant memory and cognitive deficits, the diagnosis of the disorder changes from personality change caused by a general medical condition to dementia. In differentiating the specific syndrome from other disorders in which personality change may occur—such as schizophrenia, delusional disorder, mood disorders, and impulse control disorders—physicians must consider the most important factor, the presence in the personality change disorder of a specific organic causative factor.

Course and Prognosis

Both the course and the prognosis of personality change due to a general medical condition depend on its cause. If the disorder is the result of structural damage to the brain, the disorder tends to persist. The disorder may follow a period of coma and delirium in cases of head trauma or vascular accident and may be permanent. The personality change may evolve into dementia in cases of brain tumor, multiple sclerosis (MS), and Huntington's disease. Personality changes produced by chronic intoxication, medical illness, or drug therapy (such as levodopa [Larodopa] for parkinsonism) may be reversed if the underlying cause is treated. Some patients require custodial care, or at least close supervision, to meet their basic needs, avoid repeated conflicts with the law, and protect themselves and their families from the hostility of others and from destitution resulting from impulsive and ill-considered actions.

Treatment

Management of personality change disorder involves treatment of the underlying organic condition when possible. Psychopharmacological treatment of specific symptoms may be indicated in some cases, such as imipramine or fluoxetine for depression.

Patients with severe cognitive impairment or weakened behavioral controls may need counseling to help avoid difficulties at work or to prevent social embarrassment. As a rule, patients' families need emotional support and concrete advice on how to help minimize patients' undesirable conduct. Alcohol should be avoided, and social engagements should be curtailed when patients have tendencies to act in a grossly offensive manner.

25 ◭

Psychological Factors Affecting Medical Condition and Psychosomatic Medicine

Psychosomatic medicine emphasizes the unity of mind and body and the interaction between them. It assumes that psychological factors are important in the development of all diseases; however, its role in the predisposition, initiation, progression, or exacerbation of a disease or reaction to a disease is open to debate and varies from disorder to disorder.

The text revision of the fourth edition of *Diagnostic and Statistical Manual of Mental Disorders* (DSM-IV-TR) does not use the term *psychosomatic*. Instead, it describes psychological factors affecting medical conditions as "one or more psychological or behavioral problems that adversely and significantly affect the course or outcome of a general medical condition, or that significantly increase a person's risk of an adverse outcome." Nevertheless, few would disagree that psychological or behavioral factors play a role in almost every medical condition.

CLASSIFICATION

The DSM-IV-TR diagnostic criteria for psychological factors affecting medical condition are presented in Table 25–1. Excluded are (1) classic mental disorders that have physical symptoms as part of the disorder (e.g., conversion disorder, in which a physical symptom is produced by psychological conflict); (2) somatization disorder, in which the physical symptoms are not based on organic pathology; (3) hypochondriasis, in which patients have an exaggerated concern with their health; (4) physical complaints that are frequently associated with mental disorders (e.g., dysthymic disorder, which usually has such somatic accompaniments as muscle weakness, asthenia, fatigue, and exhaustion); and (5) physical complaints associated with substance-related disorders (e.g., coughing associated with nicotine dependence).

STRESS THEORY

In the 1920s, Walter Cannon (1875–1945) conducted the first systematic study of the relation of stress to disease. He demonstrated that stimulation of the autonomic nervous system readied the organism for the "fight or flight" response characterized by hypertension, tachycardia, and increased cardiac output. This was useful in the animal who could fight or flee, but in the

person who could do neither by virtue of being civilized, the ensuing stress resulted in disease (e.g., produced hypertension).

In the 1950s, Harold Wolff (1898–1962) observed that the physiology of the gastrointestinal tract appeared to correlate with specific emotional states. Hyperfunction was associated with hostility, and hypofunction with sadness. Wolff regarded such reactions as nonspecific, believing that the patient's reaction is determined by the general life situation and perceptual appraisal of the stressful event. Earlier, William Beaumont (1785–1853), an American military surgeon, had a patient named Alexis St. Martin, who became famous because of a gunshot wound that resulted in a permanent gastric fistula. Beaumont noted that during highly charged emotional states, the mucosa could become either hyperemic or blanch, indicating that blood flow to the stomach was influenced by emotions.

Hans Selye (1907–1982) developed a model of stress that he called the *general adaptation syndrome*. It consisted of three phases: (1) the alarm reaction; (2) the stage of resistance, in which adaptation is ideally achieved; and (3) the stage of exhaustion, in which acquired adaptation or resistance may be lost. He considered stress a nonspecific bodily response to any demand caused by either pleasant or unpleasant conditions. Selye believed that stress, by definition, need not always be unpleasant. He called unpleasant stress "distress." Accepting both types of stress—pleasant or unpleasant—requires adaptation.

Neurotransmitter Responses to Stress

Stressors activate noradrenergic systems in the brain (most notably in the locus ceruleus) and cause release of catecholamines from the autonomic nervous system. Stressors also activate serotonergic systems in the brain, as evidenced by increased serotonin turnover. Recent evidence suggests that although glucocorticoids tend to enhance overall serotonin functioning, there may be differences in glucocorticoid regulation of serotonin-receptor subtypes, which may have implications for serotonergic functioning in depression and related illnesses. For example, glucocorticoids may increase serotonin 5-HT_2-mediated actions, thus contributing to the intensification of actions of these receptor types, which have been implicated in the pathophysiology of major depressive disorder. Stress also

Table 25–1
DSM-IV-TR Diagnostic Criteria for Psychological Factors Affecting General Medical Condition

A. A general medical condition (coded on Axis III) is present.
B. Psychological factors adversely affect the general medical condition in one of the following ways:
   (1) the factors have influenced the course of the general medical condition as shown by a close temporal association between the psychological factors and the development or exacerbation of, or delayed recovery from, the general medical condition
   (2) the factors interfere with the treatment of the general medical condition
   (3) the factors constitute additional health risks for the individual
   (4) stress-related physiological responses precipitate or exacerbate symptoms of the general medical condition
Choose name based on the nature of the psychological factors (if more than one factor is present, indicate the most prominent):

   Mental disorder affecting . . . [indicate the general medical condition] (e.g., an Axis I disorder such as major depressive disorder delaying recovery from a myocardial infarction)

   Psychological symptoms affecting . . . [indicate the general medical condition] (e.g., depressive symptoms delaying recovery from surgery; anxiety exacerbating asthma)

   Personality traits or coping style affecting . . . [indicate the general medical condition] (e.g., pathological denial of the need for surgery in a patient with cancer; hostile, pressured behavior contributing to cardiovascular disease)

   Maladaptive health behaviors affecting . . . [indicate the general medical condition] (e.g., overeating; lack of exercise; unsafe sex)

   Stress-related physiological response affecting . . . [indicate the general medical condition] (e.g., stress-related exacerbations of ulcer, hypertension, arrhythmia, or tension headache)

   Other or unspecified psychological factors affecting . . . [indicate the general medical condition] (e.g., interpersonal, cultural, or religious factors)

From American Psychiatric Association. *Diagnostic and Statistical Manual of Mental Disorders.* 4th ed. Text rev. Washington, DC: American Psychiatric Association; copyright 2000, with permission.

increases dopaminergic neurotransmission in mesoprefrontal pathways.

Amino acid and peptidergic neurotransmitters are also intricately involved in the stress response. Studies have shown that corticotropin-releasing factor (CRF) (as a neurotransmitter, not just as a hormonal regulator of hypothalamic-pituitary-adrenal axis functioning), glutamate (through N-methyl-D-aspartate [NMDA] receptors), and γ-aminobutyric acid (GABA) all play important roles in generating the stress response or in modulating other stress-responsive systems such as dopaminergic and noradrenergic brain circuitry.

Endocrine Responses to Stress

In response to stress, CRF is secreted from the hypothalamus into the hypophysial-pituitary-portal system. CRF acts at the anterior pituitary to trigger release of adrenocorticotropic hormone (ACTH). Once ACTH is released, it acts at the adrenal cortex to stimulate the synthesis and release of glucocorticoids. Glucocorticoids themselves have myriad effects within the body, but their actions can be summarized in the short term as

promoting energy use, increasing cardiovascular activity (in the service of the "flight-or-fight" response), and inhibiting functions such as growth, reproduction, and immunity.

This hypothalamic-pituitary-adrenal axis is subject to tight negative feedback control by its own end products (i.e., ACTH and cortisol) at multiple levels, including the anterior pituitary, the hypothalamus, and such suprahypothalamic brain regions as the hippocampus. In addition to CRF, numerous secretagogues (i.e., substances that elicit ACTH release) exist that can bypass CRF release and act directly to initiate the glucocorticoid cascade. Examples of such secretagogues include catecholamines, vasopressin, and oxytocin. Interestingly, different stressors (e.g., cold stress versus hypotension) trigger different patterns of secretagogue release, again demonstrating that the notion of a uniform stress response to a generic stressor is an oversimplification.

Immune Response to Stress

Part of the stress response consists of the inhibition of immune functioning by glucocorticoids. This inhibition may reflect a compensatory action of the hypothalamic-pituitary-adrenal axis to mitigate other physiological effects of stress. Conversely, stress can also cause immune activation through a variety of pathways. CRF itself can stimulate norepinephrine release via CRF receptors located on the locus ceruleus, which activates the sympathetic nervous system, both centrally and peripherally, and increases epinephrine release from the adrenal medulla. In addition, there are direct links of norepinephrine neurons that synapse upon immune target cells. Thus, in the face of stressors there is also profound immune activation, including the release of humoral immune factors (cytokines) such as interleukin-1 (IL-1) and IL-6. These cytokines can themselves cause further release of CRF, which in theory serves to increase glucocorticoid effects and thereby self-limits the immune activation.

Vicissitudes of Life

A life event or situation, pleasant or unpleasant (Selye's distress), often occurring by chance, generates challenges to which the person must adequately respond. Thomas Holmes and Richard Rahe constructed a social readjustment rating scale after asking hundreds of persons from varying backgrounds to rank the relative degree of adjustment required by changing life events. Holmes and Rahe listed 43 life events associated with varying amounts of disruption and stress in average persons' lives; for example, the death of a spouse, 100 life-change units; divorce, 73 units; marital separations, 65 units; and the death of a close family member, 63 units (Table 25–2). Accumulation of 200 or more life-change units in a single year increases the risk of developing a psychosomatic disorder in that year. Of interest, persons who face general stresses optimistically, rather than pessimistically, are less apt to experience psychosomatic disorders; if they do, they are more apt to recover easily.

SPECIFIC DISORDERS

Below are listed some specific disorders associated with the cardiovascular, gastrointestinal, and other bodily systems that are associated with psychological sequela. In some cases, stress may precipitate or exacerbate the disorder. Almost any organ

Table 25–2
Social Readjustment Rating Scale

Life Event	Mean Value
1. Death of spouse	100
2. Divorce	73
3. Marital separation from mate	65
4. Detention in jail or other institution	63
5. Death of a close family member	63
6. Major personal injury or illness	53
7. Marriage	50
8. Being fired at work	47
9. Marital reconciliation with mate	45
10. Retirement from work	45
11. Major change in the health or behavior of a family member	44
12. Pregnancy	40
13. Sexual difficulties	39
14. Gaining a new family member (through birth, adoption, oldster moving in, etc.)	39
15. Major business readjustment (merger, reorganization, bankruptcy, etc.)	39
16. Major change in financial state (a lot worse off or a lot better off than usual)	38
17. Death of a close friend	37
18. Changing to a different line of work	36
19. Major change in the number of arguments with spouse (either a lot more or a lot less than usual regarding child rearing, personal habits, etc.)	35
20. Taking on a mortgage greater than $10,000 (purchasing a home, business, etc.)[a]	31
21. Foreclosure on a mortgage or loan	30
22. Major change in responsibilities at work (promotion, demotion, lateral transfer)	29
23. Son or daughter leaving home (marriage, attending college, etc.)	29
24. In-law troubles	29
25. Outstanding personal achievement	28
26. Wife beginning or ceasing work outside the home	26
27. Beginning or ceasing formal schooling	26
28. Major change in living conditions (building a new home, remodeling, deterioration of home or neighborhood)	25
29. Revision of personal habits (dress, manners, associations, etc.)	24
30. Troubles with the boss	23
31. Major change in working hours or conditions	20
32. Change in residence	20
33. Changing to a new school	20
34. Major change in usual type or amount of recreation	19
35. Major change in church activities (a lot more or a lot less than usual)	19
36. Major change in social activities (clubs, dancing, movies, visiting, etc.)	18
37. Taking on a mortgage or loan less than $10,000 (purchasing a car, TV, freezer, etc.)	17
38. Major change in sleeping habits (a lot more or a lot less sleep or change in part of day when asleep)	16
39. Major change in number of family get-togethers (a lot more or a lot less than usual)	15
40. Major change in eating habits (a lot more or a lot less food intake or very different meal hours or surroundings)	15
41. Vacation	15
42. Christmas	12
43. Minor violations of the law (traffic tickets, jaywalking, disturbing the peace, etc.)	11

[a]This figure no longer has any relevance in the light of inflation; what is significant is the total amount of debt from all sources.

Reprinted with permission from Holmes T. Life situations, emotions, and disease. *Psychosom Med.* 1978;9:747.

system in the body can be affected, and the disorders mentioned are representative and by no means definitive.

Gastroesophageal Reflux Disease (GERD)

GERD is the most common disorder of the esophagus and accounts for most over-the-counter antacid consumption. The predominant symptom is heartburn, which may be accompanied by regurgitation and pain. Multiple factors in addition to stress appear to be important in the generation of reflux: (1) presence of a hiatal hernia, (2) effectiveness of the lower esophageal sphincter in blocking the reflux of stomach acid, (3) effectiveness of the esophagus in clearing and neutralizing reflux, (4) ability of the esophagus to protect itself against acid and pepsin, and (5) delayed gastric emptying and acid hypersecretion. Up to 80 percent of patients with GERD have a hiatal hernia. However, 50 percent of patients with a hiatal hernia do not have GERD. Psychological distress increases symptom severity in patients prone to this disease. In a survey of GERD sufferers, excessive stress, too much excitement, family arguments, and temporary depression were felt to trigger symptoms.

Peptic Ulcer Disease

Peptic ulcer refers to mucosal ulceration involving the distal stomach or proximal duodenum. Symptoms of peptic ulcer disease include a gnawing or burning epigastric pain that occurs 1 to 3 hours after meals and is relieved by food or antacids. Accompanying symptoms can include nausea, vomiting, dyspepsia, or signs of gastrointestinal bleeding such as hematemesis or melena.

Early theories identified excess gastric acid secretion as the most important etiological factor, but the importance of infection with *Helicobacter pylori* is now acknowledged. *H. pylori* is associated with 95 to 99 percent of duodenal ulcers and 70 to 90 percent of gastric ulcers. Antibiotic therapy that targets *H. pylori* results in much higher healing and cure rates than antacid and histamine inhibitor therapy used alone.

Early studies of peptic ulcer disease suggested that psychological factors had a role in the production of ulcer vulnerability, mediated through the increased gastric acid excretion associated with psychological stress. Studies of prisoners of war during World War II documented rates of peptic ulcer formation twice as high as in controls. Psychosocial factors may be involved in the clinical expression of symptoms, possibly by reducing immune responses, resulting in vulnerability to *H. pylori* infection.

Ulcerative Colitis

Ulcerative colitis is an inflammatory bowel disease of unknown cause affecting primarily the large intestine. The predominant symptom is bloody diarrhea. Extracolonic manifestations can include uveitis, iritis, skin diseases, and primary sclerosing cholangitis. Diagnosis is made mainly by colonoscopy or proctoscopy. Surgical resection of portions of the large bowel or entire bowel can result in cure for some patients. Studies of patients with ulcerative colitis have shown a predominance of obsessive-compulsive traits. They are neat, orderly, punctual, and have difficulty expressing anger. There is wide variation, however, in the psychiatric picture of patients with this disorder.

Crohn's Disease

Crohn's disease is an inflammatory bowel disease affecting primarily the small intestine and colon. Common symptoms include diarrhea, abdominal pain, and weight loss. It is less prevalent than ulcerative colitis. The course is chronic, often with periods of remission followed by periods of acute symptoms. Treatment consists of the use of antibiotic agents, immunosuppressive drugs, and corticosteroids. A study of psychiatric symptoms in Crohn's disease before the onset of physical symptoms found higher rates (23 percent) of preexisting panic disorder than in control subjects and subjects with ulcerative colitis.

Coronary Heart Disease

Psychiatric disorders frequently occur as complications or comorbid conditions in persons with cardiovascular disease. Depression, anxiety, delirium, and cognitive disorders are especially prevalent. Surveys of ambulatory cardiology patients with documented heart disease indicate that 5 to 10 percent have anxiety disorders (predominantly panic attacks and phobias) and 10 to 15 percent have mood disorders (predominantly depressive episodes, minor depression, or dysthymia). Major depressive disorder occurs in 15 to 20 percent of patients after myocardial infarction.

Because autonomic cardiac modulation is profoundly sensitive to acute emotional stress such as intense anger, fear, or sadness, it is not surprising that acute emotions, especially anxiety, affect the heart. Instances of sudden cardiac death related to sudden emotional distress have been noted throughout history in all cultures. High levels of anxiety symptoms are associated with a tripling of risk of sudden cardiac death and also raise the risk of future coronary events in patients with myocardial infarction by two to five times that for nonanxious patients who have had heart attacks. Risk is increased in both the immediate postinfarction period and over 18-month follow-up.

Hostility and Type A Behavior Pattern.
The relation between a behavior pattern characterized by easily aroused anger, impatience, hostility, competitive striving, and time urgency (type A) and coronary heart disease dominated studies in psychosomatic cardiology in the 1970s and 1980s. Several large prospective epidemiological studies found the type A pattern to be associated with a nearly twofold increased risk of incident myocardial infarction and coronary disease–related mortality. Hostility as the core component of the type A concept has received considerable empirical support as the most important predictor of coronary heart disease; low hostility is associated with low coronary disease risk. Hostility is associated with increased levels of circulating catecholamines and increased lipid concentrations—risk factors for disease. Adrenergic receptor function is down-regulated in hostile men, presumably an adaptive response to heightened sympathetic-adrenergic drive and chronic overproduction of catecholamines resulting from chronic and frequent anger. Conversely, submissiveness has been found to protect against coronary disease risk in women.

Acute Mental Stress.
States of fear, excitement, and acute anger reduce blood flow through atherosclerotic coronary segments and provoke coronary spasm, thus causing abnormal left ventricular wall motion and electrocardiographic (ECG) evidence of myocardial ischemia. Acute mental stress may cause angina in the presence of normal coronary arteries, as a result of coronary artery spasm. Studies indicate that relaxation training can alter autonomic activation during mental stress, implying a potential therapeutic role for such training in stress-induced ischemia.

Valvular Heart Disease and Anxiety Disorders

The relation between valvular heart disease and psychiatric disorder has been of considerable interest over the past several decades. In panic disorder, mitral valve prolapse is detected in 10 to 25 percent of patients

studied with echocardiography. However, prolapse also occurs in a substantial portion of the population without panic disorder, and the nature of the relation remains uncertain. The subjective experience of valve prolapse (palpitations, fluttering, and chest pressure) may trigger panic sensations; alternatively, the association may be purely coincidental.

Coronary Artery Bypass Graft Surgery

Coronary artery bypass graft surgery is one of the most frequently performed surgeries in the United States. Psychiatric complications after this surgery have been noted since its inception and persist despite improvements in cardiopulmonary bypass anesthetic and surgical technique. Persistent, subtle, memory and cognitive impairment may occur after this surgery. In a recent study of more than 2,100 elective coronary artery bypass graft surgical patients at 24 centers, clinical observation yielded an adverse neurological event rate of 6.1 percent. Death, focal neurological impairment (stroke), or stupor occurred in 3.1 percent; these events were predicted by older age, proximal aortic atherosclerosis, and prior history of neurological disease. Nonspecific impairment in intellectual function occurred in 2.6 percent, and seizures in 0.4 percent. Risk factors of these events were older age, systolic hypertension at admission, pulmonary disease, and excessive alcohol use.

Mild-to-moderate depression occurs in approximately one-third of patients after coronary bypass surgery but may remit within weeks to months. Depressive symptoms are present in almost 40 percent of coronary artery bypass graft patients 6 months after surgery. Patients who remain depressed exhibited increased mortality at 3-year follow-up.

Hypertension

Hypertension is a disease characterized by an elevated blood pressure of 160/95 mm Hg or above. It is primary (essential hypertension of unknown etiology) or secondary to a known medical illness. Some patients have labile blood pressure (e.g., "white coat" hypertension, in which elevations occur only in a physician's office and are related to anxiety). Personality profiles associated with essential hypertension include persons who have a general readiness to be aggressive that they try to control, albeit unsuccessfully.

Asthma

Asthma is a chronic, episodic illness characterized by extensive narrowing of the tracheobronchial tree. Symptoms include coughing, wheezing, chest tightness, and dyspnea. Nocturnal symptoms and exacerbations are common. Although patients with asthma are characterized as having excessive dependency needs, no specific personality type has been identified; however, up to 30 percent of persons with asthma meet the criteria for panic disorder or agoraphobia. The fear of dyspnea may directly trigger asthma attacks, and high levels of anxiety are associated with increased rates of hospitalization and asthma-associated mortality. Certain personality traits in asthma patients are associated with greater use of corticosteroids and bronchodilators and longer hospitalizations than would be predicted from pulmonary function alone. These traits include intense fear, emotional lability, sensitivity to rejection, and lack of persistence in difficult situations.

Family members of patients with severe asthma tend to have higher-than-predicted prevalence rates of mood disorders, posttraumatic stress disorder, substance use, and antisocial personality disorder. How these conditions contribute to the genesis or maintenance of asthma in an individual patient is unknown. The familial and current social environment may interact with a genetic predisposition for asthma to influence the timing and severity of the clinical picture. This interaction may be especially insidious in adolescents whose need for, and fear of, emotional separation from the family often become entangled in battles over medication adherence as well as other modes of diligent self-care.

Hyperventilation Syndrome

Patients with hyperventilation syndrome breathe rapidly and deeply for several minutes, often unaware that they are doing so. They soon complain of feelings of suffocation, anxiety, giddiness, and lightheadedness. Tetany, palpitations, chronic pain, and paresthesias about the mouth and in the fingers and toes are associate symptoms. Finally, syncope may occur. The symptoms are caused by an excessive loss of CO_2 resulting in respiratory alkalosis. Cerebral vasoconstriction results from low cerebral tissue P_{CO_2}.

The attack can be aborted by having patients breathe into a paper (not plastic) bag or hold their breath for as long as possible, which raises the plasma P_{CO_2}. Another useful treatment technique is to have patients deliberately hyperventilate for 1 or 2 minutes and then describe the syndrome to them. This can also be reassuring to patients who fear they have a progressive, if not fatal, disease.

Hyperthyroidism

Hyperthyroidism, or thyrotoxicosis, results from overproduction of thyroid hormone by the thyroid gland. The most common cause is exophthalmic goiter, also called *Graves' disease*. Toxic nodular goiter causes another 10 percent of cases among middle-aged and elderly patients. Physical signs of hyperthyroidism include increased pulse, arrhythmias, elevated blood pressure, fine tremor, heat intolerance, excessive sweating, weight loss, tachycardia, menstrual irregularities, muscle weakness, and exophthalmos. Psychiatric features include nervousness, fatigue, insomnia, mood lability, and dysphoria. Speech may be pressured, and patients may exhibit a heightened activity level. Cognitive symptoms include a short attention span, impaired recent memory, and an exaggerated startle response. Patients with severe cases may exhibit visual hallucinations, paranoid ideation, and delirium. While some symptoms of hyperthyroidism resemble those of a manic episode, an association between hyperthyroidism and mania has rarely been observed; however, both disorders may exist in the same patient.

Hypothyroidism

Hypothyroidism results from inadequate synthesis of thyroid hormone and is categorized as either overt or subclinical. In overt hypothyroidism, thyroid hormone concentrations are abnormally low, thyroid-stimulating hormone (TSH) levels are elevated, and patients are symptomatic; in subclinical hypothyroidism, patients have normal thyroid hormone concentrations but elevated TSH levels.

Psychiatric symptoms of hypothyroidism include depressed mood, apathy, impaired memory, and other cognitive defects. Also, hypothyroidism may contribute to treatment-refractory depression. A psychotic syndrome of auditory hallucinations and paranoia, named "myxedema madness," has been described in some patients. Urgent psychiatric treatment is necessary for patients presenting with severe psychiatric symptoms (e.g., psychosis or suicidal depression). Psychotropic agents should be given at low doses initially, as the reduced metabolic rate of hypothyroid patients may reduce breakdown and result in higher concentrations of medications in blood, as in the following case.

A 45-year-old male with bipolar I disorder had been well on lithium monotherapy for 5 years, but over the course of several months he became increasingly withdrawn and reported fatigue and poor concentration. The patient's family noted that he was forgetful and uncharacteristically listless and apathetic. No stressors were identified, and the patient's lithium concentration was therapeutic. His TSH concentration was elevated, at 14 mEq/L. The patient was treated with levothyroxine 0.05 mg and within 6 weeks experienced improved energy and a subjective return to baseline cognitive functioning. His TSH 8 weeks after initiation of thyroid replacement therapy was normal. (Courtesy of Victoria C. Hendrick, M.D., and Thomas R. Garrick, M.D.)

Subclinical Hypothyroidism

Subclinical hypothyroidism may produce depressive symptoms and cognitive deficits, although they are less severe than those produced by overt hypothyroidism. The lifetime prevalence of depression in patients with subclinical hypothyroidism is approximately double that in the general population. These patients display a lower response rate to antidepressants and a greater likelihood of responding to liothyronine (Cytomel) augmentation than euthyroid patients with depression.

Diabetes Mellitus

Diabetes mellitus is a disorder of metabolism and the vascular system, manifested by disturbances in the body's handling of glucose, lipid, and protein. It results from impaired insulin secretion or action. Heredity and family history are important in the onset of diabetes; however, sudden onset is often associated with emotional stress, which disturbs the homeostatic balance in persons who are predisposed to the disorder. Psychological factors that seem significant are those provoking feelings of frustration, loneliness, and dejection. Patients with diabetes must usually maintain some dietary control over their diabetes. When they are depressed and dejected, they often overeat or overdrink self-destructively and cause their diabetes to get out of control. This reaction is especially common in patients with juvenile, or type I, diabetes. Terms such as *oral, dependent, seeking maternal attention*, and *excessively passive* have been applied to persons with this condition.

Supportive psychotherapy helps achieve cooperation in the medical management of this complex disease. Therapists should encourage patients to lead as normal a life as possible, recognizing that they have a chronic but manageable disease. In known diabetes patients, ketoacidosis can produce some violence and confusion. More commonly, hypoglycemia (often occurring when a diabetic patient drinks alcohol) can produce severe anxiety states, confusion, and disturbed behavior. Inappropriate behavior due to hypoglycemia must be distinguished from that due to simple drunkenness.

Adrenal Disorders

Cushing's syndrome results from adrenocortical hyperfunction and can develop from either excessive secretion of ACTH (which stimulates the adrenal gland to produce cortisol) or from adrenal pathology (e.g., a cortisol-producing adrenal tumor). *Addison's disease* results from decreased pituitary secretion of ACTH, with a drop in cortisol production. Psychiatric symptoms are common in both conditions and vary from severe depression to elation with or without evidence of psychotic features.

Atopic Dermatitis

Atopic dermatitis (also called *atopic eczema* or *neurodermatitis*) is a chronic skin disorder characterized by pruritus and inflammation (eczema), which often begins as an erythematous, pruritic, maculopapular eruption. Atopic dermatitis patients tend to be more anxious and depressed than clinical and disease-free control groups. Anxiety or depression exacerbates atopic dermatitis by eliciting scratching behavior, and depressive symptoms appear to amplify the itch perception. Studies of children with atopic dermatitis found that those with behavior problems had more severe illness. In families that encouraged independence, children had less severe symptoms, whereas parental overprotectiveness reinforced scratching.

Psoriasis

Psoriasis is a chronic, relapsing disease of the skin, with lesions characterized by silvery scales with a glossy, homogeneous erythema under the scales. It is difficult to control the adverse effect of psoriasis on quality of life. It can lead to stress that can in turn trigger more psoriasis. Patients often describe disease-related stress resulting from the cosmetic disfigurement and social stigma of psoriasis, rather than stressful major life events. Psoriasis-related stress may have more to do with psychosocial difficulty inherent in the interpersonal relationships of patients with psoriasis than with the severity or chronicity of psoriasis activity.

Controlled studies have found that psoriatic patients have high levels of anxiety and depression and significant comorbidity with a wide array of personality disorders, including schizoid, avoidant, passive-aggressive, and obsessive-compulsive personality disorders. Patients' self-report of psoriasis severity correlated directly with depression and suicidal ideation, and comorbid depression reduced the threshold for pruritus in psoriasis patients. Heavy alcohol consumption (more than 80 grams of ethanol daily) by male psoriasis patients may predict a poor treatment outcome.

Psychogenic Excoriation

Psychogenic excoriations (also called *psychogenic pruritus*) are lesions caused by scratching or picking in response to an itch or other skin sensation or because of an urge to remove an irregularity on the skin from preexisting dermatoses such as acne. Lesions are typically found in areas that the patient can easily reach (e.g., the face, upper back, and the upper and lower extremities) and are a few millimeters in diameter and weeping, crusted, or scarred, with occasional postinflammatory hypopigmentation or hyperpigmentation. The behavior in psychogenic excoriation sometimes resembles obsessive-compulsive disorder in that it is repetitive, ritualistic, and tension reducing, and patients attempt (often unsuccessfully) to resist excoriating. The skin is an important erogenous zone, and Freud believed it susceptible to unconscious sexual impulses.

Pruritus Vulvae

Specific physical causes, either localized or generalized, may be demonstrable in pruritus vulvae, and the presence of glaring psychopathology in no way lessens the need for adequate medical investigation. In some patients, pleasure derived from rubbing and scratching is conscious—they realize it is a symbolic form of masturbation—but more often than not the pleasure element is repressed. Some patients may give a long history of sexual frustration, which was frequently intensified at the time of the onset of the pruritus.

Hyperhidrosis

States of fear, rage, and tension can induce increased sweat secretion that appears primarily on the palms, the soles, and the axillae. The sensitivity of sweating in response to emotion serves as the basis for measurement of sweat by the galvanic skin response (an important tool of psychosomatic research), biofeedback, and the polygraph (lie detector test). Under conditions of prolonged emotional stress, excessive sweating (hyperhidrosis) may lead to secondary skin changes, rashes, blisters, and infections; therefore, hyperhidrosis may underlie several other dermatological conditions that are not primarily related to emotions. Basically, hyperhidrosis may be viewed as an anxiety phenomenon mediated by the autonomic nervous system, and it must be differentiated from drug-induced states of hyperhidrosis.

Rheumatoid Arthritis

Rheumatoid arthritis is a disease characterized by chronic musculoskeletal pain arising from inflammation of the joints. The disorder's significant causative factors are hereditary, allergic, immunological, and psychological.

Stress may predispose patients to rheumatoid arthritis and other autoimmune diseases by immune suppression. Depression is comorbid with rheumatoid arthritis in approximately 20 percent of individuals. Those who get depressed are more likely to be unmarried, have a longer duration of illness, and have a higher occurrence of medical comorbidities. Individuals with rheumatoid arthritis and depression commonly demonstrate poorer functional status, more reported painful joints, more pronounced experience of pain, more health care use, more bed days, and more inability to work than patients with similar objective measures of arthritic activity without depression.

Psychotropic agents may be of use in some patients. Sleep, which is often disrupted by pain, can be assisted by the combination of a nonsteroidal antiinflammatory drug (NSAID) and trazodone (Desyrel) or mirtazapine (Remeron), with appropriate cautionary advice regarding orthostatic hypotension. Tricyclic drugs exert mild antiinflammatory effects independent of their mood-altering benefit; however, anticholinergic effects (prominent among the tricyclic drugs and also present with some serotonergic agents) can aggravate dry oral and ocular membranes in some patients with the disorder.

Systemic Lupus Erythematosus

Systemic lupus erythematosus is a connective tissue disease of unclear etiology, characterized by recurrent episodes of destructive inflammation of several organs including the skin, joints, kidneys, blood vessels, and central nervous system (CNS). This disorder is highly unpredictable, often incapacitating, and potentially disfiguring, and its treatment requires administration of potentially toxic drugs. The psychiatrist can assist in promoting positive interactions between patients and the program staff and ensuring a tolerant attitude on the part of these staff members. Supportive psychotherapy can help patients acquire the knowledge and maturity necessary to deal with the disorder as effectively as possible.

Low Back Pain

Low back pain affects almost 15 million Americans and is one of the major reasons for days lost from work and for disability claims paid to workers by insurance companies. Signs and symptoms vary from patient to patient, most often consisting of excruciating pain, restricted movement, paraesthesias, and weakness or numbness, all of which may be accompanied by anxiety, fear, or even panic. The areas most affected are the lower lumbar, lumbosacral, and sacroiliac regions. It is often accompanied by sciatica, with pain radiating down one or both buttocks or following the distribution of the sciatic nerve. Although low back pain may be caused by a ruptured intervertebral disk, a fracture of the back, congenital defects of the lower spine, or a ligamentous muscle strain, many instances are psychosomatic. Examining physicians should be particularly alert to patients who give a history of minor back trauma followed by severe disabling pain. Patients with low back pain often report that the pain began at a time of psychological trauma or stress, but others (perhaps 50 percent) develop pain gradually over a period of months. Patients' reactions to the pain are disproportionately emotional, with excessive anxiety and depression. Furthermore, the distribution of the pain rarely follows a normal neuroanatomical distribution and may vary in location and intensity.

There are two approaches to treatment. In the first or conventional method, treatment is symptomatic. Analgesics such as aspirin (up to 4 g a day) can be used for pain. Muscle relaxants such as diazepam (Valium; 2.5 to 5 mg every 4 to 6 hours for 2 or 3 days) are used to reduce muscle spasms and anxiety. Physical therapy is prescribed for the person in severe pain with restricted movement. Some patients respond to relaxation therapy and biofeedback. Many techniques have been proposed to treat low back pain, most of which are untested and unproved in overall effectiveness. These include various forms of massage, acupressure, acupuncture, injections of anesthetics or steroids, traction, bed rest, electrical stimulation, ultrasound, and hot packs and cold packs.

The second approach, developed by John Sarno, is psycho-educational. This treatment is based on the premise that the back is structurally sound without any abnormality to account for symptoms. To assure both patient and doctor, a careful physical examination is recommended, including a neurological examination and magnetic resonance imaging (MRI) if necessary. An MRI study that shows some abnormality does not automatically implicate it as the cause of the pain. To the contrary, normal changes in spinal morphology occur with age, and most such patients are asymptomatic. Additionally, many patients who have MRI studies show spinal abnormalities as an incidental finding and have never complained of back pain. These include bulging or herniated intravertebral disks, osteophytes, spinal stenosis, and other osteoarthritic changes, but they are not responsible for pain or any neurological symptom.

According to Sarno, the pathophysiology involved is vasospasm of blood vessels that supply the involved muscle, nerve, or tendon. Vasospasm is mediated by the autonomic nervous system, which is extraordinarily sensitive to changes in emotional tone, chronic emotional stress, and unconscious affects. The ischemia and oxygen deprivation cause pain in the areas involved. An analogy can be drawn to the vasospasm of coronary arteries that cause angina.

Treatment includes educating patients about the physiological component (vasospasm) and helping them understand the working of the mind and conflicts that arise from unconscious affects, especially that of rage. The patient understands that the mind is substituting physical pain for emotional pain so that the conscious mind does not have to deal with conflict. Physical activity should be resumed as quickly as possible, and treatments such as spinal manipulation and mandatory physical therapy sessions used minimally, if at all.

HEADACHES

Headaches are the most common neurological symptom and one of the most common medical complaints. Every year, approximately 80 percent of the population suffers from at least one headache and 10 to 20

percent go to physicians with headache as their primary complaint. Headaches are also a major cause of absenteeism from work and avoidance of social and personal activities.

Most headaches are not associated with significant organic disease; many persons are susceptible to headaches at times of emotional stress. Moreover, in many psychiatric disorders, including anxiety and depressive disorders, headache is frequently a prominent symptom. Patients with headaches are often referred to psychiatrists by primary care physicians and neurologists after extensive biomedical workups that often include MRI of the head. Most workups for common headache complaints have negative findings, and such results may be frustrating for both patient and physician. Physicians not well versed in psychological medicine may attempt to reassure such patients by telling them that there is no disease. But their reassurance may have the opposite effect—it may increase patients' anxiety and even escalate into a disagreement about whether the pain is real or imagined. Psychological stress usually exacerbates headaches, whether their primary underlying cause is physical or psychological.

Migraine (Vascular) and Cluster Headaches

Migraine (vascular) headache is a paroxysmal disorder characterized by recurrent unilateral headaches, with or without related visual and gastrointestinal disturbances (e.g., nausea, vomiting, and photophobia). They are probably caused by a functional disturbance in the cranial circulation. Migraines can be precipitated by cycling estrogen, which may account for their higher prevalence in women. Stress is also a precipitant, and many persons with migraine are overly controlled, perfectionists, and unable to suppress anger. Cluster headaches are related to migraines, they are unilateral, occur up to eight times a day, and are associated with miosis, ptosis, and diaphoresis.

Migraines and cluster headaches are best treated during the prodromal period with ergotamine tartrate (Cafergot) and analgesics. Prophylactic administration of propranolol or verapamil (Isoptin) is useful when the headaches are frequent. Sumatriptan (Imitrex) is indicated for the short-term treatment of migraine and can abort attacks. Selective serotonin reuptake inhibitors (SSRIs) are also useful for prophylaxis. Psychotherapy to diminish the effects of conflict and stress and certain behavioral techniques (e.g., biofeedback) have been reported to be useful.

Tension (Muscle Contraction) Headaches

Emotional stress is often associated with prolonged contraction of head and neck muscles, which over several hours may constrict the blood vessels and result in ischemia. A dull, aching pain, sometimes feeling like a tightening band, often begins suboccipitally and may spread over the head. The scalp may be tender to the touch, and in contrast to a migraine, the headache is usually bilateral and not associated with prodromata, nausea, or vomiting. Tension headaches may be episodic or chronic and need to be differentiated from migraine headaches, especially with and without aura.

Tension headaches are frequently associated with anxiety and depression and occur to some degree in approximately 80 percent of persons during periods of emotional stress. Tense, high-strung, competitive personalities are especially prone to the disorder. In the initial state, persons may be treated with antianxiety agents, muscle relaxants, and massage or heat application to the head and the neck; antidepressants may be prescribed when an underlying depression is present. Psychotherapy is an effective treatment for persons chronically afflicted by tension headaches. Learning to avoid or cope better with tension is the most effective long-term management approach. Biofeedback using electromyogram

(EMG) feedback from the frontal or temporal muscles may help some patients. Relaxation exercises and meditation also benefit some patients.

Psycho-Oncology

Psycho-oncology seeks to study both the impact of cancer on psychological functioning and the role that psychological and behavioral variables may play in cancer risk and survival. A hallmark of psycho-oncology research has been intervention studies that attempt to influence the course of illness in patients with cancer. A landmark study by David Spiegel found that women with metastatic breast cancer who received weekly group psychotherapy survived an average of 18 months longer than control patients randomly assigned to routine care. While this study requires replication, there was no doubt that even if longevity was not extended, the quality of life was improved. In another study, patients with malignant melanoma who received structured group intervention exhibited a statistically significant lower recurrence of cancer and a lower mortality rate than patients who did not receive such therapy. The malignant melanoma patients who received the group intervention also exhibited significantly more large granular lymphocytes and natural killer (NK) cells as well as indications of increased NK cell activity, suggesting an increased immune response. Another study used a group behavioral intervention (relaxation, guided imagery, and biofeedback training) for patients with breast cancer, who demonstrated higher NK cell activity and lymphocyte mitogen responses than the controls.

Because new treatment protocols have in many cases transformed cancer from an incurable to frequently chronic and often curable disease, the psychiatric aspects of cancer—the reactions to both the diagnosis and the treatment—are increasingly important. At least half of the 1 million persons who contracted cancer in the United States in 1987 were alive 5 years later. Currently, an estimated 3 million cancer survivors have no evidence of the disease.

Approximately half of all cancer patients have mental disorders. The largest group are those with adjustment disorder (68 percent), and major depressive disorder (13 percent) and delirium (8 percent) are the next most common diagnoses.

When persons learn that they have cancer, their psychological reactions include fear of death, disfigurement, and disability; fear of abandonment and loss of independence; fear of disruption in relationships, role functioning, and financial standings; and denial, anxiety, anger, and guilt. Although suicidal thoughts and wishes are frequent in persons with cancer, the actual incidence of suicide is only slightly higher than that in the general population. Psychiatrists should make a careful assessment of psychiatric and medical issues in every patient. Special attention should be given to family factors, in particular, preexisting intrafamily conflicts, family abandonment, and family exhaustion.

TREATMENT

Psychiatric Aspects

Treatment of psychosomatic disorders from a psychiatric viewpoint is a difficult task. Psychiatrists must focus therapy on understanding the motivations and mechanisms of disturbed functioning and helping patients realize the nature of their illness and the implications of its costly adaptive patterns. These insights should produce changed and healthier patterns of behavior.

Patients with psychosomatic disorders are usually more reluctant to deal with their emotional problems than patients with other psychiatric problems. Psychosomatic patients try to avoid responsibility for their illness by isolating the diseased organ and presenting it to the doctor for diagnosis and cure. They may be satisfying an infantile need to be cared for passively, while denying that they are adults, with all the attendant stresses and conflicts.

Medical Aspects

Internists' treatment of psychosomatic disorders should follow the established rules for medical management. Generally, internists should spend as much time as possible with a patient and listen sympathetically to the many complaints; they must be reassuring and supportive. Before performing a physically manipulative procedure—particularly if it is painful, such as a colonoscopy—the internist should explain to a patient just what to expect. The explanation allays the patient's anxiety, makes the patient more cooperative, and actually facilitates the examination.

Patients' attitudes toward taking drugs may also affect the outcome of the psychosomatic treatment. For example, patients with diabetes who do not accept their illness and who have self-destructive impulses of which they are unaware may purposely not control their diet and, as a result, end up in a hyperglycemic coma. Others use their illness as a welcome punishment for guilt or as a way to avoid responsibility. Therapy in such cases must strive to help patients minimize their fears and focus on self-care and reestablishment of a healthy body image.

Behavioral Change

A major role of psychiatrists and other physicians working with psychosomatic patients is mobilizing the patient to change behavior in ways that optimize the process of healing. This may require a general change in lifestyle (e.g., taking vacations) or a more specific behavioral change (e.g., giving up smoking). Whether or not this occurs depends in large measure on the quality of the relationship between doctor and patient. Failure of the physician to establish good rapport accounts for much of the ineffectiveness in getting patients to change.

Rapport is the spontaneous, conscious feeling of harmonious responsiveness between patient and doctor. It implies understanding and trust between the two. With rapport, patients feel accepted, even though they may think their assets outnumber their liabilities. Frequently, the physician is the person to whom the patient can talk about things he or she cannot talk about with anyone else. Most patients feel that they can trust physicians, especially psychiatrists, to keep secrets. This confidence must not be betrayed. Feeling that someone knows, understands, and accepts them is a source of strength that may enable patients to embark on a healthy course of action such as enrolling in Alcoholics Anonymous (AA) or changing eating habits.

OTHER TYPES OF THERAPY FOR PSYCHOSOMATIC DISORDERS

Group Psychotherapy and Family Therapy

The group approach offers interpersonal contact with others suffering from the same illness and provides support for patients who fear the threat of isolation and abandonment. Family therapy offers hope of a change in the relationship between family members who are often stressed and reactively hostile to the sick member.

Relaxation Techniques

Edmund Jacobson in 1938 developed a method called *progressive muscle relaxation* to teach relaxation without using instrumentation as is used in biofeedback. Patients were taught to relax muscle groups such as those involved in "tension headaches." When they encountered, and were aware of, situations that caused tension in their muscles, the patients were trained to relax. This method is a type of systematic desensitization—a type of behavior therapy.

Herbert Benson in 1975 used concepts developed from transcendental meditation in which a patient maintained a more passive attitude, allowing relaxation to occur on its own. Benson derived his techniques from various Eastern religions and practices, such as yoga. All of these techniques have in common a position of comfort, a peaceful environment, a passive approach, and a pleasant mental image on which one can concentrate.

Hypnosis

Hypnosis is effective in smoking cessation and dietary change augmentation. It is used in combination with aversive imagery (e.g., cigarettes taste obnoxious). Some patients exhibit a moderately high relapse rate and may require repeated programs of hypnotic therapy (usually three to four sessions).

Biofeedback

Neal Miller in 1969 published his pioneering paper "Learning of Visceral and Glandular Responses," in which he reported that in animals, various visceral responses regulated by the involuntary autonomic nervous system could be modified by learning accomplished through operant conditioning carried out in the laboratory. This led to humans being able to learn to control certain involuntary physiological responses (called *biofeedback*), such as blood vessel vasoconstriction, cardiac rhythm, and heart rate. These physiological changes seem to play a significant role in the development and treatment or cure of certain psychosomatic disorders. Such studies did, in fact, confirm that conscious learning could control heart rate and systolic pressure in humans.

Biofeedback and related techniques have been useful in tension headaches, migraine headaches, and Raynaud's disease. Although biofeedback techniques initially produced encouraging results in treating essential hypertension, relaxation therapy has produced more significant long-term effects than biofeedback.

Acupressure and Acupuncture

Acupressure and acupuncture are Chinese healing techniques that are mentioned in ancient medical texts dating back to 3000 BC. A basic tenet of Chinese medicine is the belief that vital energy (qi or chi) flows along specific pathways (meridians), which have approximately 350 points (acupoints), whose manipulation corrects imbalances by stimulating or removing blockages to energy flow. Another fundamental concept is the idea of two opposing energy fields (yin and yang), which must be in balance for health to be sustained. In acupressure, the acupoints are manipulated by the fingers; in acupuncture, sterilized silver or gold needles (some the diameter of a human hair) are inserted into the skin to varying depths (0.5 mm to 1.5 cm) and are rotated or left in place for varying periods to correct any imbalance of qi.

Acupuncture techniques have been used in almost all of the disorders mentioned in this section with variable results.

26

Psychiatry and Reproductive Medicine

Pregnant women undergo marked psychological changes. Their attitudes toward pregnancy reflect deeply felt beliefs about all aspects of reproduction, including whether the pregnancy was planned and whether the baby is wanted. The relationship with the infant's father, the age of the mother, and her sense of identity also affect the woman's reaction to prospective motherhood. Prospective fathers also face psychological challenges.

Psychologically healthy women often find pregnancy a means of self-realization. Many women report that being pregnant is a creative act gratifying a fundamental need. Other women use pregnancy to diminish self-doubts about femininity or to reassure themselves that they can function as women in the most basic sense. Still others view pregnancy negatively; they may fear childbirth or feel inadequate about mothering.

During early stages of their own development, women must undergo the experience of separating from their mothers and of establishing an independent identity; this experience later affects their own success at mothering. If a woman's mother was a poor role model, a woman's sense of maternal competence may be impaired, and she may lack confidence before and after her baby's birth. Women's unconscious fears and fantasies during early pregnancy often center on the idea of fusion with their own mothers.

MATERNAL–FETAL ATTACHMENT

Psychological attachment to the fetus begins in utero, and by the beginning of the second trimester, most women have a mental picture of the infant. Even before being born, the fetus is viewed as a separate being, endowed with a prenatal personality. Many mothers talk to their unborn children. Recent evidence suggests that emotional talk with the fetus is related not only to early mother–infant bonding but also to the mother's efforts to have a healthy pregnancy—for example, by giving up cigarettes and caffeine. According to psychoanalytic theorists, the child-to-be is a blank screen on which a mother projects her hopes and fears. In rare instances, these projections account for postpartum pathological states, such as a mother's wanting to harm her infant, whom she views as a hated part of herself. Normally, however, giving birth to a child fulfills a woman's need to create and nurture life.

Fathers are also profoundly affected by pregnancy. Impending parenthood demands a synthesis of such developmental issues as gender role and identity, separation-individuation from a man's own father, sexuality, and, as Erik Erikson proposed, generativity. Pregnancy fantasies in men and wishes to give birth in boys reflect early identifications with their mothers as well as the wish to be as powerful and creative as they perceive mothers to be. For some men, getting a woman pregnant is proof of their potency, a dynamic that plays a large part in adolescent fatherhood.

PARTURITION

Fears regarding pain and bodily harm during delivery are universal and, to some extent, warranted. Preparation for childbirth affords a sense of familiarity and can ease anxieties, which facilitates delivery. Continuous emotional support during labor reduces the rate of cesarean section and forcep deliveries, the need for anesthesia, the use of oxytocin, and the duration of labor. A technically difficult or even painful delivery, however, does not appear to influence the decision to bear additional children.

Men's responses to pregnancy and labor have not been well studied, but the recent trend toward inclusion of fathers in the birth process eases their anxieties and elicits a fuller sense of participation. Fathers do not parent the same way as mothers, and new mothers often need to be encouraged to respect these differences and view them positively.

DEPRESSION AND PSYCHOSIS IN THE POSTPARTUM PERIOD

Approximately 20 to 40 percent of women report some emotional disturbance or cognitive dysfunction in the postpartum period. Many experience so-called "baby blues," a normal state of sadness, dysphoria, frequent tearfulness, and clinging dependence. These feelings, which may last several days, have been ascribed to rapid changes in women's hormonal levels, the stress of childbirth, and the awareness of the increased responsibility that motherhood brings.

Postpartum depression is characterized by a depressed mood, excessive anxiety, and insomnia. The onset is within 3 to 6 months after delivery. Table 26–1 differentiates postpartum "baby blues" from postpartum depression.

In rare cases (1 to 2 in 1,000 deliveries), a woman's postpartum depression is characterized by depressed feelings and suicidal ideation. In severe cases, the depression may reach psychotic proportions, with hallucinations, delusions, and thoughts of infanticide. Although previous psychiatric prob-

Table 26–1
Comparison of "Baby Blues" and Postpartum Depression

Characteristic	"Baby Blues"	Postpartum Depression
Incidence	50% of women who give birth	10% of women who give birth
Time of onset	3–5 days after delivery	Within 3–6 mo after delivery
Duration	Days to weeks	Months to years, if untreated
Associated stressors	No	Yes, especially lack of support
Sociocultural influence	No; present in all cultures and socio-economic classes	Strong association
History of mood disorder	No association	Strong association
Family history of mood disorder	No association	Some association
Tearfulness	Yes	Yes
Mood lability	Yes	Often present, but sometimes mood is uniformly depressed
Anhedonia	No	Often
Sleep disturbance	Sometimes	Nearly always
Suicidal thoughts	No	Sometimes
Thoughts of harming the baby	Rarely	Often
Feelings of guilt, inadequacy	Absent or mild	Often present and excessive

Reproduced with permission from Miller LJ. How "baby blues" and postpartum depression differ. *Women's Psychiatric Health.* 1995:13. © 1995, The KSF Group.

lems put women at risk for postpartum disturbances, there is evidence to suggest that postpartum mood disorder is a specific concept, distinct from other psychiatric diagnoses. Others argue that these mood disorders are not a distinct entity but are part of a bipolar spectrum as reflected in the classification in the text revision of the fourth edition of *Diagnostic and Statistical Manual of Mental Disorders* (DSM-IV-TR). Women with severe postpartum depressions are at high risk for future episodes, and failure to treat may contribute to long-term treatment refractory mood disorders. See Section 11.4 for a further discussion of this disorder.

A syndrome has been described in fathers characterized by mood changes during their wives' pregnancies or after the babies are born. Such a father is affected by several factors: added responsibility, diminished sexual outlet, decreased attention from his wife, and the belief that the child is a binding force in an unsatisfactory marriage.

Miss S, aged 16, thought she had become pregnant after her first coital experience, which occurred without contraception. Shortly after she read about the signs and symptoms of pregnancy, her menses stopped. She related that she felt tingling in her breasts, which she believed were enlarged. She also reported nausea and vomiting in the morning, which was observed by her mother. On examination, the uterus was enlarged, breasts were developed with dark areola and contained milk, and a pigmented line was observed from the umbilicus to the pubis. The abdomen was not enlarged, but she believed she felt fetal movement. A pregnancy test had negative results and the patient was so informed; however, she could not be dissuaded of her belief that she was pregnant. She entered psychotherapy, and within 2 months her menses returned and she accepted the fact that she was not pregnant.

PSEUDOCYESIS

Pseudocyesis (false pregnancy) is the development of the classic symptoms of pregnancy—amenorrhea, nausea, breast enlargement and pigmentation, abdominal distention, and labor pains—in a nonpregnant woman. Pseudocyesis demonstrates the ability of the psyche to dominate the soma, probably via central input at the level of the hypothalamus. Predisposing psychological processes are thought to include a pathological wish for and fear of pregnancy; ambivalence or conflict regarding gender, sexuality, or childbearing; and a grief reaction to loss following a miscarriage, tubal ligation, or hysterectomy. The patient may have a true somatic delusion that is not subject to reality testing, but often a negative pregnancy test result or pelvic ultrasound scan leads to resolution. Psychotherapy is recommended during or after a presentation of pseudocyesis to evaluate and treat the underlying psychological dysfunction. A related event, *couvade*, occurs in some cultures in which the father of the child undergoes a simulated labor, as though he were giving birth. In those societies, *couvade* is a normal phenomenon.

HYPEREMESIS GRAVIDARUM

Hyperemesis gravidarum is differentiated from morning sickness in that vomiting is chronic, persistent, and frequent, leading to ketosis, acidosis, weight loss, and dehydration. The prognosis is excellent for both mother and fetus with prompt treatment. Most women can be treated as outpatients with change to smaller meals, discontinuation of iron supplements, and avoiding certain foods. In severe cases, hospitalization may be necessary. Although the cause is unknown, there may be a psychological component. Women with histories of anorexia nervosa or bulimia nervosa may be at risk.

PICA

Pica is the repeated ingestion of nonnutritive substances, such as dirt, clay, starch, sand, and feces. This eating disorder is most often seen in young children but is common in pregnant women in some subcultures, most notably among African-American women in the rural South, where the eating of clay or starch (for example, Argo) may occur. The cause of pica is unknown.

GRIEF REACTIONS AND PERINATAL DEATH

Perinatal death is defined as death sometime between the 20th week of gestation and the first month of life and includes spontaneous abortion (miscarriage), fetal demise, stillbirth, and neonatal death. In previous years, the intense bond between the expectant or new parent and the fetus or neonate was underestimated, but perinatal loss is now recognized as a significant trauma for both parents. Parents who experience such a loss go through a period of mourning much like that experienced when any loved one is lost.

Intrauterine fetal death, which can occur at any time during the pregnancy, is an emotionally traumatic experience. In the early months of pregnancy, a woman is usually unaware of fetal death and learns of it only from her doctor. Later in pregnancy, after fetal movements and heart tones have been experienced, a woman may be able to detect fetal demise. When given the diagnosis of fetal death, most women want the dead fetus removed; depending on the trimester, labor may be induced, or the woman may have to wait for the spontaneous expulsion of the uterine contents. Many couples view sexual relations during the period of waiting not only as undesirable but as psychologically unacceptable as well.

A sense of loss also accompanies the birth of a stillborn child as well as an induced abortion of an abnormal fetus detected by antenatal diagnosis. Psychological attachment to a child begins before birth, and grief and mourning occur after a loss at any time. The grief experienced after a third-trimester loss, however, is generally greater than that experienced after a first-trimester loss. Some parents do not wish to view a stillborn child, and their wishes should be respected. Others wish to hold the stillborn, and this act can assist the mourning process. A subsequent pregnancy may diminish overt feelings of grief but does not eliminate the need to mourn. So-called replacement children are at risk for overprotection and future emotional problems.

27

Relational Problems

DEFINITION

According to the text revision of the fourth edition of *Diagnostic and Statistical Manual of Mental Disorders* (DSM-IV-TR), relational problems are patterns of interaction between members of a relational unit that are associated with symptoms or significant impairment in functioning in one or more individual members or with significant impairment in the functioning of the relational unit itself. DSM-IV-TR distinguishes five categories of relational problems. The first category, relational problem related to a mental or general medical condition, deals with the association between relationships and health. The other categories focus on problems in specific relational units: parent–child relational problem, partner relational problem, sibling relational problem, and relational problem not otherwise specified.

EPIDEMIOLOGY

No reliable figures are available on the prevalence of relational problems. One can assume they are ubiquitous; however, most relational problems resolve without professional intervention. The nature, frequency, and effects of the problem on those involved are elements that need to be taken into account before a diagnosis of relational problem is made. For example, divorce, which occurs in just under 50 percent of marriages, is a problem between partners that is resolved through the legal remedy of divorce and need not be diagnosed as a relational problem. However, if the persons are unable to resolve the disputation between them and continue to live together in a sadomasochistic or pathologically depressed relationship with unhappiness and abuse, then they should be so labeled. Relationship problems that cannot be resolved by friends, family, or clergy of the persons involved will need professional intervention by psychiatrists, clinical psychologists, social workers, and other mental health professionals.

RELATIONAL PROBLEM RELATED TO A MENTAL DISORDER OR GENERAL MEDICAL CONDITION

According to DSM-IV-TR, clinicians should use the category of relational problems related to a mental disorder or general medical condition when the focus of clinical attention is a pattern of impaired interaction associated with a mental disorder or a general medical condition in a family member.

Adults must often assume the responsibility of caring for aging parents while they are still caring for their own children, and this dual obligation can create stress. When adults take care of their parents, both parties must adapt to a reversal of their former roles, and the caretakers not only face the potential loss of their parents, but also must cope with evidence of their own mortality.

Some caretakers abuse their aging parents—a problem that is now receiving attention. Abuse is most likely to occur when the caretaking offspring have substance abuse problems, are under economic stress, and have no relief from their caretaking duties, or when the parent is bedridden or has a chronic illness requiring constant nursing attention. More women are abused than are men, and most abuse occurs in people over age 75.

The development of a chronic illness in a family member stresses the family system and requires adaptation on the part of the sick person and the other family members. The person who has become sick must frequently face a loss of autonomy, an increased sense of vulnerability, and sometimes a taxing medical regimen. The other family members must experience the loss of the person as he or she was before the illness, and they usually have substantial caretaking responsibility—for example, in debilitating neurological diseases, including dementia of the Alzheimer's type, and in diseases such as acquired immune deficiency syndrome (AIDS) and cancer. In these cases, the whole family must deal with the stress of prospective death as well as the current illness. Some families use the anger engendered by such situations to create support organizations, increase public awareness of the disease, and rally around the sick member. But chronic illness frequently produces depression in family members and may cause them to withdraw from or to attack one another. The burden of caring for ill family members falls disproportionately on the women in a family—mothers, daughters, and daughters-in-law.

Chronic emotional illness also requires major adaptations by families. For instance, family members may react with chaos or fear to the psychotic productions of a family member with schizophrenia. The schizophrenic person's regression, exaggerated emotions, frequent hospitalizations, and economic and social dependence can stress the family system. Family members may react with hostile feelings (referred to as *expressed emotion*) that are associated with a poor prognosis for the person who is sick. Similarly, a family member with bipolar I disorder can disrupt a family, particularly during manic episodes.

Family devastation can occur when illness suddenly strikes a previously healthy person, when illness occurs earlier than expected in the life cycle (some impairment of physical capacities is expected in old age, although many older people are healthy), when illness affects the economic stability of the family, and when little can be done to improve or ease the condition of the sick family member.

PARENT–CHILD RELATIONAL PROBLEM

According to DSM-IV-TR, this diagnosis applies to cases in which the focus of clinical attention is a pattern of interaction between parent and child associated with clinically significant impairment in individual or family functioning or with clinically significant symptoms. Examples include impaired communication, overprotection, and inadequate discipline.

Difficulties in many situations stress the usual parent–child interaction. In a family in which the parents are divorced, parent–child problems may arise in the relationship with either the custodial or the noncustodial parent. The remarriage of a divorced or widowed parent can also lead to a parent–child problem. The resentment of a stepparent by a stepchild and the favoring of a natural child are usual reactions in a new family's initial phases of adjustment. When a second child is born, both familial stress and happiness may result, although happiness is the dominant emotion in most families. The birth of a child can also be troublesome when parents had adopted a child in the belief that they were infertile.

Other situations that may produce a parent–child problem are the development of fatal, crippling, or chronic illness, such as leukemia, epilepsy, sickle-cell anemia, or spinal cord injury, in either parent or child. The birth of a child with congenital defects, such as cerebral palsy, blindness, and deafness, may also produce parent–child problems. These situations, which are not rare, challenge the emotional resources of those involved. Parents and child must face present and potential loss and must adjust their day-to-day lives physically, economically, and emotionally. These situations can strain the healthiest families and produce parent–child problems not just with the sick person but also with the unaffected family members. In a family with a severely sick child, parents may resent, prefer, or neglect the other children because the ill child requires so much time and attention.

Parents with children who have emotional disorders face particular problems, depending on the child's illness. In families with a schizophrenic child, family treatment is beneficial and improves the social adjustment of the patient. Similarly, family therapy is of use if there is a child with a mood disorder. In families with a substance-abusing child or adolescent, involvement of the family is crucial to help provide control of the drug-seeking behavior and to allow family members to verbalize feelings of frustration and anger that are invariably present.

Normal developmental crises can also be related to parent–child problems. For instance, adolescence is a time of frequent conflict, as the adolescent resists rules and demands increasing autonomy, while at the same time eliciting protective control by displaying immature and dangerous behavior.

The parents of sons aged 18, 15, and 11 years presented with distress about the behavior of their middle child. The family had been cohesive with satisfactory relationships among all members until 6 months prior to this consultation.

At that time the 15-year-old began seeing a girl from a comparatively unsupervised household. Frequent arguments had developed between parents and son regarding going out on school nights, curfews, and neglect of schoolwork. The son's combativeness and lowered academic achievement upset his parents a great deal. They had not experienced similar conflicts with their oldest child. However, the adolescent maintained a good relationship with his siblings and friends, was not a behavior problem at school, continued to participate on the school basketball team, and was not a substance user.

Day Care Centers

Quality of care during the first 3 years of life is crucial to neuropsychological development. A 1997 study from the National Institute of Child Health and Human Development indicated that day care was not harmful to children, provided that the caregivers and day care teachers provided consistent, empathetic, nurturing care. Unfortunately, not all day care centers can meet that level of care, especially those located in poor urban areas. Children receiving less-than-optimal care show decreased intellectual and verbal skills that indicate delayed neurocognitive development. They may also become irritable, anxious, or depressed, which interferes with the parent–child bonding experience, and they are less assertive and less effectively toilet trained by the age of 5.

Currently, more than 55 percent of women are in the work force, many of whom have no choice but to place their children in day care centers. Approximately 40 percent of entering medical students are women; unfortunately, very few medical centers make adequate provisions for on-site day care centers for their students or staff. Similarly, corporations need to provide on-site, high-quality care for the children of their employees. Not only will that approach benefit the children, but corporate economic benefits will accrue as a result of reduced absenteeism, increased productivity, and happier working mothers. Such programs have the added benefit of decreasing stresses on marriages.

PARTNER RELATIONAL PROBLEM

According to DSM-IV-TR, clinicians should use this category when the focus of clinical attention is a pattern of interaction between the spouses or partners. These patterns are characterized by negative communication (such as criticisms), distorted communication (such as unrealistic expectations), or noncommunication (such as withdrawal), associated with clinically significant impairment in individual or family functioning or symptoms in one or both partners.

When people have partner relational problems, psychiatrists must assess whether a patient's distress arises from the relationship or from a mental disorder. Mental disorders are more common in single people—those who never married or who are widowed, separated, or divorced—than among married people. Clinicians should evaluate developmental, sexual, and occupational and relationship histories, for purposes of diagnosis.

Marriage demands a sustained level of adaptation from both partners. In a troubled marriage, a therapist can encourage the partners to explore areas such as the extent of communication between the partners, their handling of finances, and the couple's sexual interaction. The birth of a child, an abortion or miscarriage, economic stresses, episodes of illness, major career changes, and any situations that involve a significant change in marital roles can precipitate stressful periods in a relationship. Illness in a child exerts the greatest strain on a marriage, and marriages in which a child has died through illness or accident more often than not end in divorce. Complaints of life-long anorgasmia or impotence by marital partners are usually indicative of intrapsychic problems, although sexual dissatisfaction is involved in many cases of marital maladjustment.

Adjustment to marital roles can be a problem when partners are of different backgrounds and have grown up with different value systems. Problems involving conflicts in values, adjustment to new roles, and poor communication are most effectively handled when therapist and partners examine the couple's relationship, as in marital therapy.

SIBLING RELATIONAL PROBLEM

According to DSM-IV-TR, clinicians should use this category when the focus of clinical attention is a pattern of sibling interaction associated with clinically significant impairment in individual or family functioning or symptoms in one or more siblings. Problems arising from sibling rivalry can occur with the birth of a child and can recur as the children grow up. Competition among children for the attention, affection, and esteem of their parents is a fact of family life. This rivalry can extend to others who are not siblings and can remain a factor in normal and abnormal compet-

itiveness throughout life. In some families, children receive labels early in life, such as "the good child" or "the black sheep," and they may turn these labels into self-fulfilling prophesies. In good sibling relationships, the pleasures of companionship and the bonds created by kinship and shared experiences outweigh feelings of rivalry.

RELATIONAL PROBLEM NOT OTHERWISE SPECIFIED

Racial and religious prejudices can cause problems in interpersonal relationships. Some social scientists believe that racism and religious bigotry have only a weak psychological base, and they emphasize social and class factors as causative. Other investigators view prejudice as a learned attitude and consider it a cultural variant. Several psychiatrists think that people are motivated to change their prejudices only if they see them as part of a mental disorder. When prejudice is a maladaptive defense built to protect the prejudiced person from profound feelings of inadequacy, it involves the projection of unwanted and devalued attributes onto the blamed group.

In the workplace, sexual harassment is often a combination of inappropriate sexual interactions, displays of power and dominance, and expressions of negative gender stereotypes. Relational difficulties resulting from sexual harassment can be classified under this diagnosis.

Problems Related to Abuse or Neglect

The text revision of the fourth edition of *Diagnostic and Statistical Manual of Mental Disorders* (DMS-IV-TR) specifies five problems related to abuse or neglect, which are listed in Table 28–1. Physical abuse of adult includes spouse or partner abuse and abuse of elderly person. Sexual abuse of adult includes rape, sexual coercion, and sexual harassment.

CHILD ABUSE AND NEGLECT

Children who have been physically or sexually abused exhibit many psychiatric disturbances, including anxiety, aggressive behavior, paranoid ideation, posttraumatic stress disorder, depressive disorders, and an increased risk of suicidal behavior. Abuse seems to increase the risk of psychiatric disturbances in already vulnerable children, and abused children of parents with psychopathology are more likely to experience a mental disorder than are children of psychiatrically disturbed parents who are not abused. Children who have been sexually abused reportedly have an increased frequency of poor self-esteem, depression, dissociative disorders, and substance abuse. Chronic maltreatment appears to promote aggressive and violent behavior in vulnerable children. The child who is the object of physical abuse is also known as *the battered child*.

Epidemiology

According to the National Committee for the Prevention of Child Abuse, approximately 3 million cases of child abuse and neglect were reported to public social service agencies in 1994; of this number, approximately 1 million cases were substantiated. Each year in the United States, child abuse and neglect cause 2,000 to 4,000 deaths, and each year 150,000 to 200,000 new cases of sexual abuse are reported. An estimated one of every three to four girls and an estimated one of every seven to eight boys will be sexually assaulted by the age of 18 years. The actual occurrence rates are likely to be higher than these estimates because many maltreated children go unrecognized and many are reluctant to report the abuse. Of these children who are physically abused, 32 percent are younger than 5 years of age; 27 percent are between 5 and 9 years of age; 27 percent are between 10 and 14 years of age; and 14 percent are between 15 and 18 years of age. More than 50 percent of all abused and neglected children were born prematurely or had low birth weights. Most child maltreatment is at the hands of parents (75

percent), other relatives (15 percent), or an unrelated caretaker (10 percent).

Sexual attacks on children by groups of other children have recently increased. Of 1,600 young offenders whose cases of sexual abuse of other children were analyzed by a university abuse-prevention center, more than 25 percent had started before the age of 12 years. Group leaders had often been abused themselves. However, followers seemed to succumb to peer pressure and to a society that glamorizes violence and links violence with sex.

Etiology

Many factors contribute to child abuse and neglect. Abusive parents have themselves often been victims of physical and sexual abuse and of long-term exposure to violent home lives of pain and physical torment, which are powerful promoters of aggression. Thus, parents brought up in abusive families may continue the abuse tradition with their children. In some cases, adults believe that their methods are acceptable ways of teaching discipline. In other cases, parents are ambivalent about their methods of abusive parenting but find themselves without coping mechanisms and so fall into behaviors similar to those of their own parents.

Stressful living conditions, such as overcrowding and poverty, can contribute to aggressive behavior and may contribute to physical abuse toward children. Social isolation, the lack of a support system, and parental substance abuse increase the potential for abusive and neglectful treatment of children. When such environmental crises as unemployment, housing problems, and lack of finances heighten stress levels in vulnerable families, neglect or abuse may ensue. Mental disorders can play a role in child abuse and neglect insofar as a parent's judgment and thought processes may be impaired. Parents who are depressed, psychotic, or who have severe personality disorders may view their children as bad or as trying to drive them crazy.

Certain characteristics may increase a child's vulnerability to neglect and physical and sexual abuse. Children who are premature, mentally retarded, or physically disabled and those who cry excessively or are unusually demanding—the so-called difficult child—may be at high risk for abuse or neglect. Many abused children are perceived by their parents as being different, slow in development, bad, selfish, or hard to discipline. Children who are hyperactive are particularly vulnerable to abuse, especially when they are born to parents with limited capacities for nurturant behavior.

Table 28–1
DSM-IV-TR Problems Related to Abuse or Neglect

Physical abuse of child
This category should be used when the focus of clinical attention is physical abuse of a child.

Sexual abuse of child
This category should be used when the focus of clinical attention is sexual abuse of a child.

Neglect of child
This category should be used when the focus of clinical attention is child neglect.

Physical abuse of adult
This category should be used when the focus of clinical attention is physical abuse of an adult (e.g., spouse beating, abuse of elderly parent).

Sexual abuse of adult
This category should be used when the focus of clinical attention is sexual abuse of an adult (e.g., sexual coercion, rape).

Reprinted with permission from American Psychiatric Association. *Diagnostic and Statistical Manual of Mental Disorders.* 4th ed. Copyright, Washington, DC: American Psychiatric Association; 1994.

The perpetrator of physical abuse is more often the mother than the father. One parent is usually the active batterer, and the other passively accepts the battering. Of a group of perpetrators studied, 80 percent were regularly living in the homes of the children they abused. More than 80 percent of the children studied were living with married parents, and approximately 20 percent were living with a single parent. The average age of a mother who abuses her children is reported to be around 26 years; the father's average age is 30 years. Many abused children come from poor homes, and the families tend to be socially isolated.

Abusive parents have inappropriate expectations of their children, with a reversal of dependence needs. Parents treat an abused child as if the child were older than the parents. A parent often turns to the child for reassurance, nurturing, comfort, and protection and expects a loving response. Ninety percent of such parents were severely physically abused by their own mothers or fathers.

Men usually perpetrate sexual abuse, although women acting in concert with men or alone are also involved, especially in child pornography. Men are the perpetrators in approximately 95 percent of cases of sexual abuse of girls and approximately 80 percent of cases of sexual abuse of boys. Perpetrators of sexual abuse are usually known to the child and in many cases have been victims of physical or sexual abuse. In some circumstances, pedophilia is a factor: The adult perpetrator is more aroused by children than by adult partners. Many times, however, the perpetrator has no preference for child sexual partners. In some cases, sexual abuse is mixed with physical abuse.

Diagnosis and Clinical Features

Physical Abuse of Child. Clinicians must always consider physical abuse when a child shows bruises or injuries that cannot be adequately explained or that are incompatible with the history that the parent gives. Suspicious physical indicators are bruises and marks that form symmetrical patterns, such as injuries to both sides of the face and regular patterns on the back, buttocks, and thighs; accidental injuries are unlikely to result in symmetrical patterns. Bruises may have the shape of the instrument used to make them, such as a belt buckle or a cord. Burns by cigarettes result in symmetrical, round scars, and immersions in boiling water produce burns that look like socks or gloves or that are doughnut-shaped. Physical aggression can cause multiple and spiral fractures, especially in a young baby; retinal hemorrhages in an infant may be due to shaking.

Children repeatedly brought to hospitals for treatment of peculiar or puzzling problems by overly cooperative parents may be victims of Munchausen syndrome by proxy, that is, factitious disorder: In this abuse scenario, a parent repeatedly inflicts illness on or causes injury to a child—by injecting toxins or by inducing the child to ingest drugs or toxins so as to cause diarrhea, dehydration, or other symptoms—and then eagerly seeks medical attention. Because the pathological parents are stealthy and superficially compliant, this diagnosis is difficult to make.

Behaviorally, abused children may appear withdrawn and frightened or may show aggressive behavior and labile mood. They often exhibit depression, poor self-esteem, and anxiety. They may try to physically cover up injuries and are usually reticent to disclose the abuse for fear of retaliation. Abused children often show some delay in developmental milestones, may have difficulties with peer relationships, and may engage in self-destructive or suicidal behaviors.

A 16-month-old boy was brought to the hospital emergency room because of burns from scalding water. The child had patches of erythema on his abdomen, down the sides of his legs, and on the medial aspect of his upper arms. The diapered area had been protected from the heat. While the emergency room staff proceeded with their assessment and treatment, the child abuse consultant interviewed the parents separately. The father reported that he had been trying to heat a baby bottle by placing it in the bathtub and running hot water on it. The father returned in a few minutes and found the toddler, who apparently had climbed into the tub, in about 2 inches of hot water. The mother confirmed that she had been busy and had asked the father to heat the bottle in the bathtub. The consultant thought that the pattern of the burns was consistent with the story; the pattern did not look like that seen in forcible submersion. Although the parents' accounts were unusual, they corroborated each other and were consistent with the injuries. The consultant concluded that this was not likely to be child abuse but might constitute negligence. The consultant notified child protective services. (Courtesy of Bessel A. van der Kolk, M.D.)

Sexual Abuse of Child. Most cases of sexual abuse involving children are never revealed because of the victim's feelings of guilt, shame, ignorance, and tolerance, compounded by some physicians' reluctance to recognize and report sexual abuse, the court's insistence on strict rules of evidence, and families' fears of dissolution if the sexual abuse is discovered.

Despite their familial roles, sexual abusers often threaten to hurt, kill, or abandon the children if the events are disclosed.

No specific behavioral manifestations prove that sexual abuse has taken place, but children may exhibit many possible significant behaviors. Young children who have a detailed knowledge of sexual acts have usually witnessed or participated in sexual behavior. Young sexually abused children often exhibit their sexual knowledge through play and may initiate sexual behaviors with their peers. Aggressive behavior is common among abused children. Children who are extremely fearful of adults, particularly men, may have been subjected to sexual abuse. Clinicians should listen carefully to children who report sexual assaults even when parts of their stories are not consistent. When a child begins to disclose information about sexual assaults, retractions and contradictions are typical, and anxiety may prevent full disclosure.

The diagnosis of sexual abuse in children is full of pitfalls. An estimated 2 to 8 percent of allegations of sexual abuse are false. A much higher percentage of reports cannot be substantiated. Many investigations are hastily done or carried out by inexperienced evaluators. In custody cases, an allegation of sexual abuse can be a maneuver to limit a parent's visitation rights. Alleged sexual abuse of a preschool-age child is particularly difficult to evaluate because of the child's immature cognitive and language development. The use of anatomically correct dolls has grown in popularity, but the use of such dolls is controversial. Patient and careful evaluations by experienced, objective professionals are necessary, and leading questions must be avoided. Children under the age of 3 years are unlikely to produce a verbal memory of past trauma or abuses, but their experience may be reflected in play or fantasies. Some abused children meet the DSM-IV-TR diagnostic criteria for posttraumatic stress disorder.

Depressive feelings, usually combined with shame, guilt, and a sense of permanent damage, are commonly reported among children who have been sexually abused. Adolescents who have undergone sexual abuse are said to show high rates of poor impulse control and self-destructive and suicidal behaviors. Posttraumatic stress disorder and dissociative disorders are common in adults who have been sexually abused as children. Sexual abuse is a common preexisting factor in the development of dissociative identity disorder (also known as *multiple personality disorder*). Signs of dissociation are described as periods in which the children are amnestic, do not feel the pain, or feel that they are somewhere else. Borderline personality disorder has been reported in some patients with histories of sexual abuse. Substance abuse has also been reported with high frequency among adolescents and adults who were sexually abused as children.

INCEST. Incest is defined as the occurrence of sexual relations between close blood relatives. A broader definition describes incest as sexual intercourse between participants who are related to each other by a formal or informal kinship bond that is culturally regarded as a bar to sexual relations. For example, sexual relations between stepparents and stepchildren or among stepsiblings are usually considered incestuous, even though no blood relationships exist.

Sociologists have underlined the role of incest prohibitions as socialization factors, and biological factors also support the taboo. Inbreeding groups risk unmasking lethal or detrimental recessive genes and the progeny of inbred groups are generally less fit than are less closely related offspring. Anthropologists have observed that different cultures have different types of incest taboos.

Fathers, stepfathers, uncles, and older siblings most commonly abuse children. A passive, sick or absent, or somehow incapacitated mother, a daughter who takes on a maternal role in the family, a father who abuses alcohol, and overcrowding are common features of father–daughter incest in many homes. Mother–son incest is the strongest and most nearly universal taboo, and this form of incest is rarer than any other. Such behavior usually indicates a more severe psychopathology in the participants than is the case in father–daughter and sibling incest.

Accurate figures on the incidence of incest are difficult to obtain because of families' shame and embarrassment. Girls are victims more often than are boys; in the United States, approximately 15 million women have been the objects of incestuous attention, and one-third of all sexually abused people have been molested before the age of 9.

Incestuous behavior is reported much more frequently among families of low socioeconomic status than among other families. This difference may be caused by greater contact with reporting officials such as welfare workers, public health personnel, and law enforcement agents and does not truly reflect a higher incidence in these families. Incest is more easily hidden by economically stable families than by those of low socioeconomic status.

Social, cultural, physiological, and psychological factors all contribute to the breakdown of the incest taboo. Incestuous behavior has been associated with alcohol abuse, overcrowding, increased physical proximity, and rural isolation that prevents adequate extrafamilial contacts. Some communities tolerate incestuous behavior more than does the whole of society. Major mental disorders and intellectual deficiencies can contribute to clinical incest. Some family therapists view incest as a defense designed to maintain a dysfunctional family unit. The older and stronger participant in incestuous behavior is usually male.

Homosexual Incest. Father–son and mother–daughter incest are rarely reported, but a family in which same-sex incest occurs is usually highly disturbed, with a violent, alcohol-dependent, or antisocial father; a dependent or disabled mother who is unable to protect her children; and an absence of the usual family roles and individual identities. A son involved in father–son incest is frequently the eldest child, and, if there is a daughter, the father often sexually abuses her as well. Fathers in this situation do not necessarily have any other history of homosexual behavior. Sons may experience homicidal or suicidal ideation and may first consult or be sent to a psychiatrist because of self-destructive behavior.

STATUTORY RAPE. Intercourse is unlawful between a man older than 16 years of age and a woman under the age of consent, which varies from 14 to 21 years, depending on the jurisdiction. Thus, a man of 18 and a girl of 15 may have consensual intercourse, yet the man may be held for statutory rape. Statutory rape may vary dramatically from other types of rape in being nonassaultive and nonviolent, and it is not a deviant act unless the age discrepancy is sufficient for the man to be defined as a pedophile, which is usually when the girl is less than 13 years old. Parents of the consenting girl, rather than the girl herself, usually press charges of statutory rape.

Neglect of Child.

A maltreated child often shows no obvious signs of being battered but has multiple minor physical evidences of emotional and, at times, nutritional deprivation, neglect, and abuse. A maltreated child, often brought to a hospital or to a private physician, has a history of failure to thrive, malnutrition, poor skin hygiene, irritability, withdrawal, and other signs of psychological and physical neglect.

Children who have been neglected may show overt failure to thrive at less than 1 year of age. Their physical and emotional development is drastically impaired; they may be physically small and unable to display appropriate social interaction. Hunger, chronic infections, poor hygiene, inappropriate dress, and eventual malnutrition may all be evident. Behaviorally, children who are chronically neglected can be indiscriminately affectionate, even with strangers, or socially unresponsive, even in familiar situations. Neglected children may be runaways or exhibit conduct disorder.

An extreme form of failure to thrive in children of 5 years or older is psychosocial dwarfism, in which a chronically deprived child does not grow and develop, even when offered adequate amounts of food. Such children have normal proportions but are exceedingly small for their age. They often have reversible endocrinological changes resulting in decreased growth hormone, and they cease to grow for a time. Behaviorally, children with this disorder exhibit bizarre eating behaviors and disturbed social relationships. Binge eating, the ingestion of garbage or inedible substances, the drinking of toilet water, and induced vomiting have been reported.

Parents who neglect their children are often overwhelmed, depressed, isolated, and impoverished. Unemployment, the absence of a two-parent family, and substance abuse may exacerbate the situation. There are several possible prototypes of neglectful mothers. Some young, inexperienced, socially isolated, and ignorant mothers may temporarily be unable to care for their children. Other neglectful mothers are chronically passive and withdrawn women who may have been raised in chaotic, abusive, and neglectful homes. In these cases, once the situation comes to the attention of a child protective agency, the mother often accepts help. Mothers with major mental disorders who view their children as evil or as purposely driving them crazy are difficult to help.

Pathology and Laboratory Examination.   Although no definitive laboratory tests are available to help clinicians diagnose child physical or sexual abuse or neglect, a physical examination to identify physical stigma is indicated when abuse is suspected. In cases of failure to thrive, endocrinological screening is indicated. An external genital examination is indicated in cases of suspected child sexual abuse to identify scars, tears, and genital infections. X-ray evidence of fractures may be present in various stages of reparative changes, but when no fractures or dislocations are apparent on examination, bone repair may become evident within weeks after the specific bone trauma.

Differential Diagnosis

Parental feuding and custody disputes are among the factors that complicate identifying and substantiating of abuse and neglect situations. When marital discord is severe, children are often caught in the line of fire. A mother who is overwhelmingly hostile toward a separated father may be convinced and may convince a child that the father is abusive. In some cases, parents have gone so far as to fabricate entire abuse scenarios and to coach children to repeat them. In other instances, parents may refuse to accept the possibility that a spouse or close rela-

tive is the perpetrator of abuse, may repeatedly insist that a child stop telling lies, and may coerce a child into retracting the disclosures. In either scenario, the child suffers profoundly, and the alleged abuse situation is never disentangled.

When a child speaks in a manner consistent with his or her language development stage and does not use rehearsed-sounding, adultlike phrasing, the abuse allegations may be true. Distress, the display of precocious sexual behavior, and a knowledge of or preoccupation with sexual material also support the possibility of sexual abuse. A child who has not been abused but who is coached to report sexual or physical abuse is also placed under unbearable duress. Therefore, clinicians must recognize that severe chronic parental conflict discord in which a child is caught can be as destructive as physical and sexual abuse.

Course and Prognosis

The outcome of cases of child physical and sexual abuse and neglect is multifactorial, depending on the severity, duration, and nature of the abuse, and on the child's vulnerabilities. Children who already suffer from mental retardation, pervasive developmental disorders, physical disabilities, disruptive behavior, and attention-deficit disorders are likely to have a poorer outcome than are children unhampered by mental or physical disorders. Children who are abused for long periods, from the time they are babies or toddlers into adolescence, are likely to be more profoundly damaged than are those who have experienced only brief episodes of abuse. The development of mental disorders—such as major depressive disorder, suicidal behavior, posttraumatic stress disorder, dissociative identity disorder, and substance abuse—further complicates the long-term prognosis, as does the nature of the relationship between victim and abuser and the adult support figures available to children after disclosure. The best outcomes occur when children are cognitively intact, the abuse is recognized and interrupted in an early phase, and the entire family is capable of participating in treatment.

Treatment

Child.   The first part of treating child abuse and neglect is to ensure the child's safety and well-being. Children may need to be removed from abusive or neglectful families to ensure their protection; yet, on an emotional level, a child may feel additionally vulnerable in an unfamiliar setting. Because of the high risk for psychiatric symptoms in abused and neglected children, a comprehensive psychiatric evaluation is in order. Next, along with providing specific treatments for any mental disorders present, a therapist may have to deal with the immediate situation and the long-term implications of the abuse or neglect. Therapists must address several psychotherapeutic issues: dealing with the child's fears, anxieties, and self-esteem; building a trusting adult relationship in which the child is not exploited or betrayed; and ultimately gaining a helpful perspective of the factors contributing to the child's victimization at home.

Ideally, each abused and neglected child should receive an intervention plan based on the assessment of the factors responsible for parents' psychopathology. The plan should include an overall prognosis for parents' achieving adequate parenting skills; the time estimated to achieve meaningful change in parents' ability to parent; an estimate of whether the parent's dysfunction is confined to this child or involves other children, whether the parents' overall malfunctioning, if that is the case, is short-term or long-term, and whether a mother's malfunctioning is confined to infants as opposed to older children (that is, when the incidence of abuse is inversely related to a child's age); willingness of those involved to participate in the intervention plan; the availability of personnel and physical resources to implement the various intervention strategies; and the risk of the child sustaining additional physical or sexual abuse by remaining in the home.

Parents.   On the basis of the information obtained, several options can be selected to improve parents' functioning: eliminate or diminish the social or environmental stresses; lessen the adverse psychological effects of social factors on the parents; reduce the demands on the mother to a level within her capacity through day care placement of the child or the provision of a housekeeper or baby-sitter; provide emotional support, encouragement, sympathy, stimulation, instruction in maternal care, and aid in learning to plan for, assess, and meet the needs of the infant (supportive casework); and resolve or diminish the parents' inner psychic conflicts (psychotherapy).

Incestuous Behavior.   The first step in the treatment of incestuous behavior is its disclosure. Once a breakthrough of family members' denial, collusion, and fear has been achieved, incest is unlikely to recur. When the participants suffer from severe psychopathology, treatment must be directed toward the underlying illness. Family therapy is useful to reestablish the group as a functioning unit and to develop healthier role definitions for each member. While the participants are learning to develop internal restraints and appropriate ways to gratify their needs, the external control provided by therapy helps prevent further incestuous behavior. At times, legal agencies must help enforce external controls.

Reporting.   In cases of suspected child abuse and neglect, physicians should diagnose the suspected maltreatment; secure the child's safety by admitting the child to a hospital or by arranging out-of-home placement; report the case to the appropriate social service department, child protection unit, or central registry; make an assessment with the help of a history, a physical examination, a skeletal survey, and photographs; request a social worker's report and appropriate surgical and medical consultations; confer with members of a child abuse committee within 72 hours; arrange a program of care for the child and the parents; and arrange for social service follow-up. Among those generally included as mandated child-abuse reporters are physicians, psychologists, school officials, police officers, hospital personnel engaged in the treatment of patients, district attorneys, and providers of child day care and foster care.

Prevention.   To prevent child abuse and neglect, clinicians must identify those families at high risk and intervene before a child becomes a victim. Once high-risk families have been identified, a comprehensive program should include psychiatric monitoring of the families, including the identified high-risk child. Families can be educated to recognize when they are being neglectful or abusive, and alternative coping strategies can be suggested.

In general, child abuse and neglect prevention and treatment programs should try to prevent the separation of parents and children if possible, prevent the placement of children in institutions, encourage the parents' attainment of self-care status, and encourage the family's attainment of self-sufficiency. As a last resort and to prevent further abuse and neglect, children may have to be removed from families who are unwilling or unable to profit from the treatment program. In cases of sexual abuse, the licensing of day care centers and the psychological screening of people who work in them should be mandatory to prevent further abuses. Education of the medical profession, members of allied health fields, and all who come in contact with children aid in early detection. And providing support services to stressed families aids in preventing the problem in the first place.

PHYSICAL ABUSE OF ADULT

Spouse Abuse

Spouse abuse is estimated to occur in 2 to 12 million families in the United States. This aspect of domestic violence has been recognized as a severe problem, largely because of recent cultural emphasis on civil rights and the work of feminist groups, but the problem itself is long standing.

The major problem in spouse abuse is wife abuse. One study estimated that there are 1.8 million battered wives in the United States, excluding divorced women and women battered on dates. Wife beating occurs in families of every racial and religious background and in all socioeconomic strata. It is most frequent in families with problems of substance abuse, particularly alcohol and crack abuse. Behavioral, cultural, intrapsychic, and interpersonal factors all contribute to the problem. Abusive men are likely to have come from violent homes where they witnessed wife beating or were abused themselves as children. The act itself is reinforcing; once a man has beaten his wife, he is likely to do so again. Abusive husbands tend to be immature, dependent, nonassertive, and to suffer from strong feelings of inadequacy.

The husband's aggression is bullying behavior designed to humiliate their wives and to build up their own low self-esteem. Impatient, impulsive, abusive husbands physically displace aggression provoked by others onto their wives. The abuse is most likely to occur when a man feels threatened or frustrated at home, at work, or with his peers. The dynamics include identification with an aggressor (father, boss), testing behavior (Will she stay with me, no matter how I treat her?), distorted desires to express manhood, and dehumanization of women. As in rape, aggression is deemed permissible when a woman is perceived as property. Approximately 50 percent of battered wives grew up in violent homes, and their most common trait is dependence.

The Surgeon General's office has identified pregnancy as a high-risk period for battering; 15 to 25 percent of pregnant women are physically abused while pregnant, and the abuse often results in birth defects. Hot lines, emergency shelters for women, and other organizations (such as the National Coalition Against Domestic Violence) have been established to aid battered wives and to educate the public. One major problem of abused women has been finding a place to go when they leave home, frequently in fear of their lives.

Battering is often severe, involving broken limbs, broken ribs, internal bleeding, and brain damage. When an abused wife tries to leave her husband, he often becomes doubly intimidating and threatens to "get" her. If the woman has small children to care for, her problem is compounded. The abusive husband wages a conscious campaign to isolate his wife and make her feel worthless. Women face risks when they leave an abusive husband; they have a 75 percent greater chance of being killed by their batterers than do women who stay.

Some men feel remorse and guilt after an episode of violent behavior and so become particularly loving. If this behavior gives the wife hope, she remains until the next, inevitable occurring cycle of violence.

When a man is convinced that a woman will no longer tolerate the situation and when she begins to exert control over his behavior, change is initiated. By leaving for a prolonged period, if she is physically and economically able to do so, and by making therapy for the man a condition of return, a woman can begin a cycle of improvement. Family therapy is effective in treating the problem, usually in conjunction with social and legal agencies. With men who are relatively less impulsive, external controls, such as calling the neighbors or the police, may be sufficient to stop the behavior.

Some husband-beating wives have also been reported. Husbands complain of fear of ridicule if they expose the problem; they fear charges of counterassault and often feel unable to leave the situation because of financial difficulties. Husband abuse has also been reported when a frail, elderly man is married to a much younger woman.

Elder Abuse

An estimated 10 percent of persons above 64 years of age are abused. *Elder abuse* is defined by the American Medical Association (AMA) as "an act or omission which results in harm or threatened harm to the health or welfare of an elderly person." Mistreatment includes abuse and neglect—physically, psychologically, financially, and materially. Sexual abuse does occur. Acts of omission include withholding food, medicine, clothing, and other necessities.

Family conflicts and other problems often underlie elder abuse. The victims tend to be very old and frail. They often live with their assailants, who may be financially dependent on the victims. Both the victim and the perpetrator tend to deny or minimize the presence of abuse. Interventions include providing legal services, housing, and medical, psychiatric, and social services.

SEXUAL ABUSE OF ADULT

Rape

The conventional definition of rape is the perpetration of an act of sexual intercourse with a woman against her will and consent, whether her will is overcome by force or fear resulting from the threat of force or by drugs or intoxicants; or when, because of mental deficiency, she is incapable of exercising rational judgment, or when she is below an arbitrary age of consent. Rape, however, can occur between married partners and between people of the same sex. The crime of rape requires only slight penile penetration of the victim's outer vulva; full erection and ejaculation are unnecessary for defining the crime.

Forced acts of fellatio and anal penetration, although they frequently accompany rape, are legally considered sodomy.

The problem of rape is most appropriately discussed under the heading of aggression. Rape is an act of violence and humiliation that happens to be expressed through sexual means. Rape expresses power or anger; sex is rarely the dominant issue because sexuality is used in the service of nonsexual needs.

Rape of Women.   In recent research, male rapists are categorized into separate groups: sexual sadists, who are aroused by the pain of their victims; exploitive predators, who use their victims as objects for their gratification in an impulsive way; inadequate men, who believe that no woman would voluntarily sleep with them and who are obsessed with fantasies about sex; and men for whom rape is a displaced expression of anger and rage. Some believe that the anger was originally directed toward a wife or mother, but feminist theory proposes that a woman serves as an object for the displacement of aggression that a rapist cannot express directly toward other men. Women are considered men's property or vulnerable possessions, a rapist's instrument for revenge against other men.

Rape often occurs as an accompaniment to another crime. Rapists always threaten their victims with fists, a knife, or a gun, and frequently harm them in nonsexual ways as well. Victims may be beaten, wounded, and killed.

Statistics show that most men who commit rapes are between 25 and 44 years of age; 51 percent are white and tend to rape white victims, 47 percent are black and tend to rape black victims, and the remaining 2 percent come from all other races. Alcohol is involved in 34 percent of all forcible rapes.

According to the Federal Bureau of Investigation (FBI), there are between 95,000 and 100,000 forcible rapes reported to law enforcement in the United States each year. Rape, however, is a highly underreported crime: An estimated four to five out of ten rapes are reported. The underreporting is attributed to victims' feelings of shame and to the belief that there is no recourse through the legal system.

People who are raped can be of any age. Cases have been reported in which the victims were as young as 15 months and as old as 82 years, but women age 16 to 24 are at highest risk. Rape most commonly occurs in a woman's own neighborhood, frequently inside or near her own home. Most rapes are premeditated; approximately half are committed by strangers and half by men known, to varying degrees, by the victims. Seven percent of all rapes are perpetrated by close relatives of the victim; 10 percent of rapes involve more than one attacker.

A woman being raped is frequently in a life-threatening situation. During the rape, she experiences shock and fright approaching panic; her prime motivation is to stay alive. In most cases, rapists choose victims slightly smaller than themselves. Rapists may urinate or defecate on their victims, ejaculate into their faces and hair, force anal intercourse, and insert foreign objects into their vaginas and rectums.

After a rape, a woman often experiences shame, humiliation, confusion, fear, and rage. The type and duration of the reaction are variable, but women report that the effects last for a year or longer. Many women experience the symptoms of posttraumatic stress disorder. Some women, particularly those who have always felt sexually adequate, are able to resume sexual relations with men; but others become phobic about sexual interaction or have such symptoms as vaginismus. Few women emerge from the assault completely unscathed. The manifestations and the degree of damage depend on the violence of the attack itself, the vulnerability of the woman, and the support system available to her immediately after the attack.

A rape victim fares best when she receives immediate support and is able to ventilate her fear and rage to loving family members, sympathetic physicians, and law enforcement officials. Knowing that she has socially acceptable means of recourse, such as the arrest and conviction of the rapist, can help a rape victim.

Unless a woman has a severe underlying disorder, therapy is usually supportive in approach and focuses on restoring a victim's sense of adequacy and control over her life; it also aims to relieve the feelings of helplessness, dependence, and obsession with the assault that frequently follow rape. Group therapy with homogeneous groups of people who have been raped is a particularly effective form of treatment.

In addition to the physical and psychological trauma experienced when they are assaulted, rape victims until recently also faced skepticism from those to whom they reported the crime (if they had sufficient strength to do so) or accusations of having provoked or desired the assault. In reality, the National Commission on the Causes and Prevention of Violence found discernible victim participation in rape in only 4.4 percent of all cases. This statistic is lower than that of any other crime of violence. The education of police officers and the assignment of policewomen to deal with rape victims have helped increase reporting the crime. Rape crisis centers and telephone hot lines are available for immediate aid and information for victims. Volunteer groups work in emergency rooms in hospitals and with physician education programs to assist in the treatment of victims.

Legally, women no longer must prove in court that they actively struggled against a rapist, and testimony about a victim's previous sexual history has been declared inadmissible as evidence in several states. Because penalties for first-time rapists have been reduced, juries are likely to consider a conviction. In some states, wives can now prosecute husbands for rape.

Date Rape.   *Date* or *acquaintance rape* is a term applied to rapes in which the rapist is known to the victim. The assault can occur on a first date or after the man and woman have known each other for many months. Considerable data on date rape have been gathered from college populations. In one study, 38 percent of male students said that they would commit rape if they thought they could get away with it, and 11 percent stated that they had committed rape; 16 percent of female students said that they had

been raped by men they knew or were dating. In addition to suffering the symptoms of all rape survivors, victims of date rape berate themselves for exercising poor judgment in their choice of male friends and are more likely to blame themselves for provoking the rapist than are other victims. Many colleges and universities have set up programs for rape prevention and for counseling those who have been assaulted.

Rape of Men.   In some states the definition of rape is being changed to substitute the word *person* for *female.* In most states, male rape is legally defined as sodomy. Homosexual rape is much more frequent among men than among women and occurs frequently in closed institutions such as prisons and maximum-security hospitals.

The dynamics are identical to those of heterosexual rape. The crime enables the rapist to discharge aggression and to aggrandize himself. The victim is usually smaller than the rapist, is always perceived as passive and unmanly (weaker), and is used as an object. A rapist selecting a male victim may be heterosexual, bisexual, or homosexual. The most common act is anal penetration of the victim; the second most common is fellatio.

Homosexual-rape victims often feel, as do raped women, that they have been irreparably damaged. Some also fear that they will become homosexual because of the attack.

Sexual Coercion

Sexual coercion is a term used to describe incidents in which one person dominates another by force or compels the other person to perform a sexual act.

Stalking.   *Stalking* is defined as a pattern of harassing or menacing behavior coupled with a threat to do harm. Some stalkers continue that activity for years; others for only a few months. In all instances stalkers should be reported to law enforcement agencies as the best means of deterrent. Most stalkers are men, but women who stalk are just as likely to violently attack their victims as are men.

Sexual Harassment.   *Sexual harassment* refers to sexual advances, request for sexual favors, verbal or physical conduct of a sexual nature—all of which are unwelcomed by the victim. In more than 95 percent of cases the perpetrator is a man; the victim, a woman. In the case of a man being harassed, it is usually by another man. A woman sexually harassing a man is a rare event.

Additional Conditions That May Be a Focus of Clinical Attention

The conditions discussed in this section are not considered true mental disorders, but are problems that have led people to come into contact with the mental health care system. Once in the system, people with a condition that may be a focus of clinical attention should have a thorough neuropsychiatric evaluation, which may or may not uncover a mental disorder. These categories are of clinical interest to psychiatrists because they may accompany mental illness or may be early harbingers of underlying mental disorders.

There are 13 conditions that make up the diagnostic category of additional disorders that may be a focus of clinical attention. Nine of these conditions are discussed in this chapter: bereavement, occupational problems, adult antisocial behavior, malingering, phase of life problem, noncompliance with treatment for a mental disorder, religious or spiritual problem, acculturation problem, and age-associated memory decline (four other conditions included in the text revision of the fourth edition of *Diagnostic and Statistical Manual of Mental Disorders* [DSM-IV-TR] are discussed in Chapter 48: borderline intellectual functioning, academic problem, childhood or adolescent antisocial behavior, and identity problem).

BEREAVEMENT

Normal bereavement begins immediately after or within a few months of the loss of a loved one. Feelings of sadness, preoccupation with thoughts about the deceased, tearfulness, irritability, insomnia, and difficulties in concentrating and carrying out daily activities are some typical signs and symptoms. On the basis of cultural group, bereavement is limited to a varying time, usually 6 months; but it may be longer. Normal bereavement, however, can lead to a full depressive disorder that requires treatment.

DSM-IV-TR includes the following description of bereavement:

This category can be used when the focus of clinical attention is a reaction to the death of a loved one. As part of their reaction to the loss, some grieving individuals present with symptoms characteristic of a Major Depressive Episode (e.g., feelings of sadness and associated symptoms such as insomnia, poor appetite, and weight loss). The diagnosis of Major Depressive Disorder is generally not given unless the symptoms are still present 2 months after the loss. However, the presence of certain symptoms that are not characteristic of a "normal" grief reaction may

be helpful in differentiating bereavement from a Major Depressive Episode. These include (1) guilt about things other than actions taken or not taken by the survivor at the time of the death; (2) thoughts of death other than the survivor feeling that he or she would be better off dead or should have died with the deceased person; (3) morbid preoccupation with worthlessness; (4) marked psychomotor retardation; (5) prolonged and marked functional impairment; and (6) hallucinatory experiences other than thinking that he or she hears the voice of, or transiently sees the image of, the deceased person.

OCCUPATIONAL PROBLEM

Occupational or industrial psychiatry is that area of psychiatry specifically concerned with vocational maladjustment and the psychiatric aspects of problems at work. The practical symptoms of job dissatisfaction are mistakes at work, accident-proneness, absenteeism, and sabotage. The psychiatric symptoms include insecurity, reduced self-esteem, anger, and resentment at having to work.

DSM-IV-TR includes the following statement about occupational problem:

This category can be used when the focus of clinical attention is an occupational problem that is not due to a mental disorder or, if it is due to a mental disorder, is sufficiently severe to warrant independent clinical attention. Examples include job dissatisfaction and uncertainty about career choices.

People are particularly vulnerable to occupational problems at several points in their working lives—on entry into the working world, at times of promotion or transfer, during periods of unemployment, and at retirement. Specific situations—such as having too much or too little to do, being subjected to conflicting demands, feeling distracted by family problems, having responsibility without authority, and working for demanding and unhelpful managers—also create occupational distress.

Career Choices and Changes

The choice of a career is a major life decision. A significant number of young people follow in their parents' footsteps, but many others are unsure of what to do and try several jobs before settling on an occupation. Disadvantaged youngsters frequently have little choice about a career. When young adults have a poor education and lack training and skills, even overwhelming ambition rarely leads them out of poverty or into occupational satisfaction. In discussing career choices with a patient, a psychiatrist should explore special talents and interests, childhood goals, the patient's models, family influences, future expectations, work and academic histories, and motivation to work.

Distress about work is readily understood when an employee has been fired, demoted, or passed over for promotion. Some people experience problems after they win professional advancement. Anxiety about assuming new responsibilities and the fact that people may be promoted to jobs that are beyond their capacities are among the reasons for this reaction.

Adjusting to retirement is most difficult for those unprepared for it. Adverse reactions occur when a person is forced to retire prematurely or because of illness. Retirement is also a problem for people whose identity is based primarily on occupational status and income. Retirement may pose a greater hardship for women than for men in some cases. Women face a longer retirement period owing to their greater life expectancy, are more likely to be alone (widowed) during their retirement years, and are usually poorer and have lower retirement incomes than do men.

Vocational Rehabilitation

Rehabilitation is often necessary for those traumatized by stresses in the workplace, or who have had to take a leave of absence because of medical or psychiatric reasons, or who have been fired. Individual or group counseling enables people to improve personal relationships, raise self-esteem, or learn new work skills. Patients with schizophrenia may benefit from sheltered workshops in which they perform work that is geared to their level of function. Some patients with schizophrenia or autism do well in tasks that are repetitive or require obsessive concern with details.

ADULT ANTISOCIAL BEHAVIOR

Characterized by activities that are illegal or immoral or both, antisocial behavior usually begins in childhood and often persists throughout life.

DSM-IV-TR includes the following statements about adult antisocial behavior:

> This category can be used when the focus of clinical attention is adult antisocial behavior that is not due to a mental disorder (e.g., Conduct Disorder, Antisocial Personality Disorder, or an Impulse-Control Disorder). Examples include the behavior of some professional thieves, racketeers, or dealers in illegal substances.

Major symptoms of the disorder are a history of arrests, impulsiveness, pathological lying, alcohol abuse, and difficulties in work and relationships. The term *antisocial behavior* somewhat confusingly applies both to people's actions that are not due to a mental disorder and to actions by those who never received a neuropsychiatric workup to determine the presence or absence of a mental disorder.

Epidemiology

Depending on the criteria and the sampling, estimates of the prevalence of adult antisocial behavior range from 5 to 15 percent of the population. Within prison populations, investigators report prevalence figures of between 20 and 80 percent. Men account for more adult antisocial behavior than do women.

Etiology

Antisocial behaviors in adulthood are characteristic of a variety of people, ranging from those with no demonstrable psychopathology to those who are severely impaired and suffer from psychotic disorders, cognitive disorders, and retardation, among other conditions. A comprehensive neuropsychiatric assessment of antisocial adults is indicated and may reveal potentially treatable psychiatric and neurological impairments that can easily be overlooked. Only in the absence of mental disorders can patients be categorized as displaying adult antisocial behavior. Adult antisocial behavior may be influenced by genetic and social factors.

Genetic Factors.   Data supporting the genetic transmission of antisocial behavior are based on studies that find a 60 percent concordance rate in monozygotic twins and approximately a 30 percent concordance rate in dizygotic twins. Adoption studies show a high rate of antisocial behavior in the biological relatives of adoptees identified with antisocial behavior and a high incidence of antisocial behavior in the adopted-away offspring of those with antisocial behavior. The prenatal and perinatal periods of those who subsequently display antisocial behavior often are associated with low birth weight, mental retardation, and prenatal exposure to alcohol and other drugs of abuse.

Social Factors.   Studies showed that in neighborhoods in which families with low socioeconomic status (SES) predominate, the sons of unskilled workers are more likely to commit more offenses, and more serious criminal offenses, than are the sons of middle-class and skilled workers, at least during adolescence and early adulthood. These data are not as clear for women, but the findings are generally similar in studies from many countries. Areas of family training differ by SES group. Middle-SES parents tend to use love-oriented techniques in discipline. They withdraw affection rather than impose physical punishment, which is commonly associated with low SES groups. Negative parental attitudes toward aggressive behavior, attempts to curb aggressive behavior, and the ability to communicate the parents' values are more characteristic of middle and high SES groups. Adult antisocial behavior is associated with the use and abuse of alcohol and other substances and also with the easy availability of handguns.

Diagnosis and Clinical Features

The diagnosis of adult antisocial behavior is one of exclusion. Substance dependence in such behavior often makes it difficult to separate the antisocial behavior related primarily to substance dependence from disordered behaviors that occurred either before substance use or during episodes unrelated to substance dependence.

During the manic phases of bipolar I disorder, certain aspects of behavior, such as wanderlust, sexual promiscuity, and financial difficulties, can be similar to adult antisocial behavior. Patients with schizophrenia may have episodes of adult antisocial behavior, but the symptom picture is usually clear, especially regarding thought disorder, delusions, and hallucinations on the mental status examination.

Neurological conditions may be associated with adult antisocial behavior, and electroencephalograms (EEGs), computed tomography (CT) scans, magnetic resonance imaging (MRI), and complete neurological examinations are indicated. Temporal lobe epilepsy should be considered in the differential diagnosis. When a clear-cut diagnosis of temporal lobe epilepsy or encephalitis can be made, the disorder may be considered to contribute to the adult antisocial behavior. Abnormal EEG findings are prevalent among violent offenders: An estimated 50 percent of aggressive criminals have abnormal EEG findings.

Adult antisocial behavior must be distinguished from antisocial personality disorder, which is discussed in Chapter 24.

Treatment

In general, therapists are pessimistic about treating adult antisocial behavior. They have little hope of changing a pattern that has been present almost continuously throughout a person's life. Psychotherapy has not been effective, and no major breakthroughs with biological treatments, including medications, have occurred.

Therapists show more enthusiasm for the use of therapeutic communities and other forms of group treatment, even though the data provide little basis for optimism. Many adult criminals who are incarcerated and in institutional settings have shown some response to group therapy approaches. The history of violence, criminality, and antisocial behavior has shown that such behaviors seem to decrease after age 40. Recidivism in criminals, which can reach 90 percent in some studies, also decreases in middle age.

MALINGERING

Malingering is characterized by the voluntary production and presentation of false or grossly exaggerated physical or psychological symptoms. Patients always have an external motivation that falls into one of three categories: to avoid difficult or dangerous situations, responsibilities, or punishment; to receive compensation, free hospital room and board, a source of drugs, or haven from the police; and to retaliate when the patient feels guilt or suffers a financial loss, legal penalty, or job loss. The presence of a clearly definable goal is the main factor that differentiates malingering from factitious disorders.

Epidemiology

The incidence of malingering is unknown, but it is common and occurs most frequently in settings with a preponderance of men—the military, prisons, factories, and other industrial settings—although the condition also occurs in women.

Diagnosis and Clinical Features

DSM-IV-TR includes the following remarks about malingering:

> The essential feature of Malingering is the intentional production of false or grossly exaggerated physical or psychological symptoms, motivated by external incentives such as avoiding military duty, avoiding work, obtaining financial compensation, evading criminal prosecution, or obtaining drugs. Under some circumstances, malingering may represent adaptive behavior—for example, feigning illness while a captive of the enemy during wartime.

Malingering should be strongly suspected if any combination of the following is noted:

1. Medicolegal context of presentation (e.g., the person is referred by an attorney to the clinician for examination)
2. Marked discrepancy between the person's claimed stress or disability and the objective findings
3. Lack of cooperation during the diagnostic evaluation and in complying with the prescribed treatment regimen
4. The presence of antisocial personality disorder

Many malingerers express mostly subjective, vague, ill-defined symptoms—for example, headache; pains in the neck, lower back, chest, or abdomen; dizziness; vertigo; amnesia; anxiety; and depression—and the symptoms often have a family history, in all likelihood not medically caused but incredibly difficult to refute. Malingerers may complain bitterly and describe how much the symptoms impair their normal function and how much they dislike the symptoms. The patients may use the best doctors who are the most trusted (and perhaps most gullible) and promptly and willingly pay all their bills, even if excessive, to impress the doctors with their integrity. To seem credible, malingerers must report the symptoms but tell their physicians as little as possible. If they do describe all the symptoms of a disease, the symptoms are said to come and go. Malingerers are often preoccupied with compensation rather than cure and have a knowledge of the law and precedents relative to their claims.

Objective tests—such as audiometry, brainstem audiometry, auditory and visually evoked potentials, galvanic skin response, electromyography (EMG), and nerve conduction studies—may be helpful in sorting out auditory, labyrinthine, ophthalmological, neurological, and other problems.

Differential Diagnosis

Malingering differs from factitious disorder in that the motivation for the symptom production in malingering is an external incentive (e.g., insurance payments), whereas in factitious disorder, external incentives are absent. Evidence of an intrapsychic need to maintain the sick role (e.g., to satisfy dependency needs) suggests factitious disorder. Malingering is differentiated from somatoform disorders by the intentional production of symptoms and by the obvious, external incentives associated with it. In malingering, in contrast to some somatoform disorders such as conversion disorder, symptom relief is not often obtained by suggestion or hypnosis.

Treatment

A patient suspected of malingering should be thoroughly and objectively evaluated, and the physician should refrain from showing any suspicion. If a clinician becomes angry (a common response to malingerers), a confrontation may occur with two consequences: The doctor–patient relationship is disrupted and no further positive intervention is possible; the patient will be even more guarded, and proof of deception may become virtually impossible. If the patient is accepted and not discredited, subsequent patient hospital or outpatient observation may reveal the versatility of the symptoms, which are consistently present only when patients know that they are being observed. Preserving the doctor–patient relationship is often essential to diagnosis and long-term treatment. Careful evaluation usually reveals the relevant issue without the need for a confrontation. It is usually best to use an intensive treatment approach as though the symptoms were real. The symptoms can then be given up in response to treatment, without the patient's losing face.

PHASE OF LIFE PROBLEM

DSM-IV-TR includes the following description of phase of life problem:

> This category can be used when the focus of clinical attention is a problem associated with a particular developmental phase or some other life circumstance that is not due to a mental disorder or, if it is due to a mental disorder, is sufficiently severe to warrant independent clinical attention. Examples include problems associated with entering school, leaving parental control, starting a new career, and changes involved in marriage, divorce, and retirement.

External events are most likely to overwhelm people's adaptive capacities when they are unexpected or numerous—that is, a number of stresses occurring within a short time—when the strain is chronic and unremitting, or when one loss heralds a myriad of concomitant adjustments that strain people's recuperative powers.

The strains most likely to produce anxiety and depression relate to major life-cycle changes: marriage, occupation, and parenthood. These events affect both men and women, but women, those in low SES groups, and minorities seem particularly vulnerable to adverse reactions. Again, the change creates significant strain when it is unexpected and when it involves not only adjustment to a loss (a spouse or a job) but also the need to adjust to a new status that entails further hardships and problems.

In general, people are able to adjust to life changes if they have mature defense mechanisms such as altruism, humor, and capacity for sublimation. Flexibility, reliability, strong family ties, regular employment, adequate income, job satisfaction, a pattern of regular recreation and social participation, realistic goals, and a history of adequate performance—in short, a full and satisfying life—create resilience to deal with life changes.

NONCOMPLIANCE WITH TREATMENT

In DSM-IV-TR, the following statement appears:

> This category can be used when the focus of clinical attention is noncompliance with an important aspect of the treatment for a mental disorder or a general medical condition. The reasons for noncompliance may include discomfort resulting from treatment (e.g., medication side effects), expense of treatment, decisions based on personal value judgments of religious or cultural beliefs about the advantages and disadvantages of the proposed treatment, maladaptive personality traits or coping styles (e.g., denial of illness), or the presence of a mental disorder (e.g., Schizophrenia, Avoidant Personality Disorder). This category should be used only when the problem is sufficiently severe to warrant independent clinical attention.

RELIGIOUS AND SPIRITUAL PROBLEM

In DSM-IV-TR, the following statement appears:

> This category can be used when the focus of clinical attention is a religious or spiritual problem. Examples include distressing experiences that involve loss or questioning of faith, problems associated with conversion to a new faith, or questioning other spiritual values which may not necessarily be related to an organized church or religious institution.

From the psychological point of view, perhaps the most striking feature of religion is its universality. There are few societies in which religion plays no significant role, and there are relatively few people who, at one time or another, have not experienced some religious stirring. From this universality, one must infer that religion performs an adaptive function that is invoked to satisfy one or more universal human needs.

Pastoral Counseling

The pastoral function of the clergy in the United States extends to assisting the individual members of the religious congregation to deal with serious problems that they cannot resolve alone and that may cause anguish and damage. The pastoral function includes visiting the ill, comforting the mourner, encouraging the widow, and helping the orphan. The term *counseling* involves consultation for the purpose of helping the troubled person solve a specific presenting problem. It may be a marital problem, a parent–child problem, a problem of conflict among siblings, or a complaint of feeling guilt or anxiety.

Cults

Cults are charismatic groups that can affect participants in adverse ways, which may eventually bring them into contact with the mental health care system. Cults are characterized by an intensely held belief system and ideology imposed on members, by a high level of group cohesion serving to prevent members' freedom of choice to leave the group, and by a profound influence on the members' behavior, possibly inducing psychiatric symptoms, producing overt psychotic disorders.

Most potential cult members are in their adolescence or otherwise struggling with establishing their own identities. They are drawn to a cult, which holds out the false promise of emotional well-being and purports to offer the sense of direction for which the people are searching. Cult members are encouraged to proselytize and to draw new members into the group. They are often encouraged to break with family members and friends and to socialize only with other group members. Cults are invariably led by charismatic personalities, who are often ruthless in their quest for financial, sexual, and power gains. Cult leaders usually demand conformity to the cult's ideological belief system, which may have strong religious or quasi-religious overtones. Exit therapy has been developed to guide cult members out of the group in cases where lingering emotional ties to people outside the cult can be mobilized.

ACCULTURATION PROBLEM

In DSM-IV-TR, the following statement about the acculturation problem appears:

> This category can be used when the focus of clinical attention is a problem involving adjustment to a different culture (e.g., following migration).

Periods of cultural transition, with changing mores and fluidity of role definition, may increase people's vulnerability to life strain. Extreme cultural transition can create a condition of severe distress, also called *culture shock*, which occurs when a person is suddenly thrust into an alien culture or has divided loyalties to two different cultures. In a less extreme form, culture shock occurs when young men and women enter the army, when people change jobs, when families move or undergo a significant change in income, when children first go to school, and when inner-city children are bused to middle-class schools.

AGE-RELATED COGNITIVE DECLINE

DSM-IV-TR includes the following comment:

> This category can be used when the focus of clinical attention is an objectively identified decline in cognitive functioning consequent to the aging process that is within normal limits given the

person's age. Individuals with this condition may report problems remembering names or appointments or may experience difficulty in solving complex problems. This category should be considered only after it has been determined that the cognitive impairment is not attributable to a specific mental disorder or neurological condition.

Cognitive decline is lower in persons who exercise, do not smoke, drink little or no alcohol, and who challenge their intellect at work or play (e.g., crossword puzzles). The ability to learn new material is maintained through old age; the major change, however, is that it takes longer and requires more practice than in young persons.

30

Emergency Psychiatric Medicine

▲ 30.1 Psychiatric Emergencies

Emergency psychiatry has become a subspecialty of general psychiatry requiring specific skills to deal with situations for which immediate therapeutic intervention frequently is necessary. The widening scope of emergency psychiatry goes beyond general psychiatric practice to include such specialized problems as the abuse of substances, children, and spouses; the violence of suicide, homicide, and rape; and such social issues as homelessness, aging, competence, and acquired immune deficiency syndrome (AIDS). Emergency psychiatrists must be up-to-date on medicolegal issues and managed care.

EPIDEMIOLOGY

Psychiatric emergency rooms are used equally by men and women and more by single than married people. Approximately 20 percent of these patients are suicidal and approximately 10 percent are violent. The most common diagnoses are mood disorders (including depressive disorders and manic episodes), schizophrenia, and alcohol dependence. Approximately 40 percent of all patients seen in psychiatric emergency rooms require hospitalization. Most visits occur during the night hours, but there is no usage difference based on the day of the week or the month of the year. Contrary to popular belief, studies have not found a higher-than-usual use of psychiatric emergency rooms during a full moon or during the Christmas season.

EMERGENCY PSYCHIATRIC INTERVIEW

An emergency interview is similar to a standard psychiatric interview except for the time limitation imposed by the other patients waiting to be seen and by the potential sense of urgency in assessing the risk to the patient or others. Usually, a physician focuses on the presenting complaint and the reasons that the patient has come to the emergency room. The time constraint requires that a clinician structure the interview, particularly with patients who may respond with long, rambling accounts of their illnesses. If friends, relatives, or the police accompany the patient, a supplemental history

should be obtained from them, especially if the patient is mute, negativistic, uncooperative, or otherwise unable to give a coherent history.

Patients may be highly motivated to reveal themselves to gain relief from suffering, but they may also be both consciously and unconsciously motivated to conceal innermost feelings that they perceive to be shameful or threatening. If a patient has been brought to the hospital involuntarily, willingness or ability to cooperate may be impaired. A psychiatrist's relationship with a patient strongly influences what the patient does and does not say, even within the context of a first interview in an emergency room; therefore, a large portion of the psychiatric emergency interview involves the specific and sophisticated techniques of listening, observation, and interpretation that provide the foundation of psychiatric training overall. Being straightforward, honest, calm, and nonthreatening is very important, as is the ability to convey to patients the idea that the clinician is in control and will act decisively to protect them from hurting themselves or others.

Sometimes people contact the emergency room by telephone. In such cases, a psychiatrist should obtain the number from which the call is made and the exact address. If the call is interrupted, the psychiatrist will be able to direct help to the patient. If the patient is alone and the psychiatrist ascertains that the patient is in danger, the police should be alerted. If possible, an assistant should call the police on another line while the psychiatrist keeps the patient engaged until help arrives. The patient should not be told to drive alone to the hospital, but an emergency medical team or mobile crisis unit should be dispatched to bring the patient to the hospital.

The greatest potential error in emergency room psychiatry is overlooking a physical illness as the cause of an emotional illness. Head traumas, medical illnesses, substance abuse (including alcohol), cerebrovascular diseases, metabolic abnormalities, and medications may all cause abnormal behavior, and psychiatrists should take concise medical histories that concentrate on these areas.

Range of Problems

A wide range of conditions may account for the emergency room visit. The most common complaints are depression (especially with suicidal ideation) and anxiety. The most common behavioral patterns are violent or assaultive acts, suicidal attempts, and disorganized behavior—the last usually associated with schizophrenia, bipolar disorder, or substance abuse.

Violence

Violence is physical aggression inflicted by one person on another. When it is directed toward oneself, it is referred to as *self-mutilation* or *suicidal behavior*. Violence can be due to a wide range of psychiatric disorders, but it may also occur in normal people who cannot cope with life stresses in less severe ways. As mentioned above, violence and threats of violence are frequently encountered in psychiatric emergency settings. The physician and the staff members must know how to rapidly initiate a procedure for the prevention of escalating violence. The procedure may involve behavioral, pharmacological, and psychosocial interventions.

CLINICAL FEATURES AND DIAGNOSIS

The psychiatric conditions most commonly associated with violence include such psychotic disorders as schizophrenia and mania (particularly if the patient is paranoid or is experiencing command hallucinations), intoxication with alcohol and drugs, withdrawal from alcohol and sedative-hypnotics, catatonic excitement, agitated depression, personality disorders that are characterized by rage and poor impulse control (for example, borderline and antisocial personality disorders), and organic disorders (especially those with frontal and temporal lobe involvement).

Other risk factors for violence include a statement of intent, a specific plan, the availability of the means of violence, male sex, young age (15 to 24 years), low socioeconomic status (SES), poor social support system, history of violence, other antisocial acts, poor impulse control, history of suicide attempts, and recent stressors. A history of violence is the best predictor of violence. Additional important factors include a history of childhood victimization; childhood history of the triad of bed-wetting, fire-setting, and cruelty to animals; criminal records; military or police service; reckless driving; and family history of violence.

The first goal with the potentially violent patient is the prevention of immediate violence. The next objective is to make a diagnosis that will lead to a treatment plan, including measures to minimize the likelihood of subsequent violence.

EVALUATION AND TREATMENT

The clinician should assume that violence is always a possibility and never be surprised by sudden violent acts. If a weapon is found, it should always be surrendered to a security guard. Potentially violent patients should not be interviewed alone or in an office with the door closed. The clinician should be alert for signs of impending violence, such as the clenching of teeth and fists, verbal threats (menacing), the availability of weapons or objects potentially usable as weapons (for example, a fork, an ice pick, an ashtray), psychomotor agitation (considered by many to be an important indicator), alcohol or drug intoxication, paranoid delusions, and command hallucinations.

Sufficient staff members should be on hand to safely restrain the patient if needed. Constant observation may be necessary to detain the violent patient, and involuntary hospitalization to stabilize the patient is a common outcome.

Drug Treatment

Drug treatment depends on the specific diagnosis. Benzodiazepines and antipsychotics are used most often for tranquilization. Haloperidol (Haldol) given at 5 mg by mouth or intramuscularly (IM) or lorazepam (Ativan) 2 mg by mouth or IM may be tried initially. If the patient is already taking an antipsychotic, more of the same drug may be given. If the patient's agitation has not decreased in 20 to 30 minutes, the dose may be repeated. Benzodiazepines may be ineffective in patients who are tolerant and may cause disinhibition, which can potentially worsen the violence. Avoid antipsychotics in patients at risk for seizures. For patients with epilepsy, an anticonvulsant—for example, carbamazepine (Tegretol)—may be effective.

Rapid Tranquilization.   Antipsychotic medication can be given rapidly at 30- to 60-minute intervals to achieve the quickest therapeutic result possible. The procedure is useful for agitated patients and for those in excited states. The drugs of choice for rapid tranquilization are haloperidol and other high-potency antipsychotics. In adults, 5 to 10 mg of haloperidol can be given orally or IM and repeated in 20- to 30-minute intervals until a patient becomes calm. Some patients may experience mild extrapyramidal symptoms within the first 24 hours after rapid tranquilization; although the side effects are rare, psychiatrists should not overlook them. In general, most patients respond before a total dose of 50 mg is given. The goal is not to produce sedation or somnolence; rather, a patient should be able to cooperate in the assessment process and, ideally, be able to provide some explanation of the agitated behavior. Agitated or panic-stricken patients can be treated with small doses of lorazepam, 2 to 4 mg intravenously (IV) or IM, which can be repeated if necessary in 20 to 30 minutes until quieted down. Extrapyramidal emergencies respond to benztropine (Cogentin), 2 mg orally or IM, or diphenhydramine (Benadryl), 50 mg IM or IV. Some patients respond to diazepam (Valium), 5 to 10 mg orally or IV.

Restraints

Restraints are used when patients are so dangerous to themselves or others that they pose a severe threat that cannot be controlled in any other way. Patients may be restrained temporarily to receive medication or for long periods if medication cannot be used. Most often, patients in restraints quiet down after a time. On a psychodynamic level, such patients may even welcome the control of their impulses provided by restraints.

Disposition

In some cases, the usual option to admit or to discharge the patient is not felt to be optimal. Suspected toxic psychoses, brief decompensations in a patient with a personality disorder, and adjustment reactions to traumatic events, for example, may be best managed in an extended-observation setting. Allowing the patient additional time in a secure environment can result in sufficient improvement or clarification of the issues to make traditional inpatient treatment unnecessary. Also, doing so can spare the patient the trauma and the stigma of a psychiatric admission and can free up bed space for more needy patients. Crisis intervention for victims of rape and other traumas can also be done in an extended-observation setting.

When the decision is to admit the patient to the hospital, it is preferable to do so on a voluntary status. Allowing patients that option gives them a sense of control over their lives and of participation in the treatment decisions. Patients who clearly meet involuntary admission criteria on the basis of dangerousness to themselves or to others cannot leave the hospital without further review and can always be converted to involuntary status if warranted.

Other Disorders

Table 30.1–1 lists (in alphabetic order) a broad range of problems that are seen in the emergency room. Some are induced by underlying medical disease or substance abuse. Others are the direct result of a major mental disorder or similar stressful situation that causes personality disorganization and aberrant behavior. Suicide is covered comprehensively in the next section (30.2).

Table 30.1–1
Common Psychiatric Emergencies

Syndrome	Emergency Manifestations	Treatment Issues
Abuse of child or adult	Signs of physical trauma	Management of medical problems; psychiatric evaluation; report to authorities
Acquired immune deficiency syndrome (AIDS)	Changes in behavior secondary to organic causes; changes in behavior secondary to fear and anxiety; suicidal behavior	Management of neurological illness; management of psychological concomitants; reinforcement of social support
Adolescent crises	Suicidal attempts and ideation; substance abuse, truancy, trouble with law, pregnancy, running away; eating disorders; psychosis	Evaluation of suicidal potential, extent of substance abuse, family dynamics; crisis-oriented family and individual therapy; hospitalization if necessary; consultation with appropriate extrafamilial authorities
Agoraphobia	Panic; depression	Alprazolam (Xanax), 0.25 mg to 2 mg; propranolol (Inderal); antidepressant medication
Agranulocytosis (clozapine [Clozaril]-induced)	High fever, pharyngitis, oral and perianal ulcerations	Discontinue medication immediately; administer granulocyte colony-stimulating factor
Akathisia	Agitation, restlessness, muscle discomfort; dysphoria	Reduce antipsychotic dosage; propranolol (30 to 120 mg a day); benzodiazepines; diphenhydramine (Benadryl) orally or IV; benztropine (Cogentin) IM
Alcohol-related emergencies		
Alcohol delirium	Confusion, disorientation, fluctuating consciousness and perception, autonomic hyperactivity; may be fatal	Chlordiazepoxide (Librium); haloperidol (Haldol) for psychotic symptoms may be added if necessary
Alcohol intoxication	Disinhibited behavior, sedation at high doses	With time and protective environment, symptoms abate
Alcohol persisting amnestic disorder	Confusion, loss of memory even for all personal identification data	Hospitalization; hypnosis; amobarbital (Amytal) interview; rule out organic cause
Alcohol persisting dementia	Confusion, agitation, impulsivity	Rule out other causes for dementia; no effective treatment; hospitalization if necessary
Alcohol psychotic disorder with hallucinations	Vivid auditory (at times visual) hallucinations with affect appropriate to content (often fearful); clear sensorium	Haloperidol for psychotic symptoms
Alcohol seizures	Grand mal seizures; rarely status epilepticus	Diazepam (Valium), phenytoin (Dilantin); prevent by using chlordiazepoxide (Librium) during detoxification
Alcohol withdrawal	Irritability, nausea, vomiting, insomnia, malaise, autonomic hyperactivity, shakiness	Fluid and electrolytes maintained; sedation with benzodiazepines; restraints; monitoring of vital signs; 100 mg thiamine IM
Idiosyncratic alcohol intoxication	Marked aggressive or assaultive behavior	Generally no treatment required other than protective environment
Korsakoff's syndrome	Alcohol stigmata, amnesia, confabulation	No effective treatment; institutionalization often needed
Wernicke's encephalopathy	Oculomotor disturbances, cerebellar ataxia; mental confusion	Thiamine, 100 mg IV or IM, with $MgSO_4$ given before glucose loading
Amphetamine (or related substance) intoxication	Delusions, paranoia; violence; depression (from withdrawal); anxiety, delirium	Antipsychotics; restraints; hospitalization if necessary; no need for gradual withdrawal; antidepressants may be necessary
Anorexia nervosa	Loss of 25% of body weight of the norm for age and sex	Hospitalization; electrocardiogram (ECG), fluid and electrolytes; neuroendocrine evaluation
Anticholinergic intoxication	Psychotic symptoms, dry skin and mouth, hyperpyrexia, mydriasis, tachycardia, restlessness, visual hallucinations	Discontinue drug, IV physostigmine (Antilirium), 0.5 to 2 mg, for severe agitation or fever, benzodiazepines; antipsychotics contraindicated

(continued)

Table 30.1–1 (continued)

Syndrome	Emergency Manifestations	Treatment Issues
Anticonvulsant intoxication	Psychosis; delirium	Dosage of anticonvulsant is reduced
Benzodiazepine intoxication	Sedation, somnolence, and ataxia	Supportive measures; flumazenil (Romazicon), 7.5 to 45 mg a day, titrated as needed, should be used only by skilled personnel with resuscitative equipment available
Bereavement	Guilt feelings, irritability; insomnia; somatic complaints	Must be differentiated from major depressive disorder; antidepressants not indicated; benzodiazepines for sleep; encouragement of ventilation
Borderline personality disorder	Suicidal ideation and gestures; homicidal ideations and gestures; substance abuse; micropsychotic episodes; burns, cut marks on body	Suicidal and homicidal evaluation (if great, hospitalization); small dosages of antipsychotics; clear follow-up plan
Brief psychotic disorder	Emotional turmoil, extreme lability; acutely impaired reality testing after obvious psychosocial stress	Hospitalization often necessary; low dosage of antipsychotics may be necessary but often resolves spontaneously
Bromide intoxication	Delirium; mania; depression; psychosis	Serum levels obtained (>50 mg a day); bromide intake discontinued; large quantities of sodium chloride IV or orally; if agitation, paraldehyde or antipsychotic is used
Caffeine intoxication	Severe anxiety, resembling panic disorder; mania; delirium; agitated depression; sleep disturbance	Cessation of caffeine-containing substances; benzodiazepines
Cannabis intoxication	Delusions; panic; dysphoria; cognitive impairment	Benzodiazepines and antipsychotics as needed; evaluation of suicidal or homicidal risk; symptoms usually abate with time and reassurance
Catatonic schizophrenia	Marked psychomotor disturbance (either excitement or stupor); exhaustion; can be fatal	Rapid tranquilization with antipsychotics; monitor vital signs; amobarbital may release patient from catatonic mutism or stupor but can precipitate violent behavior
Cimetidine psychotic disorder	Delirium; delusions	Reduce dosage or discontinue drug
Clonidine withdrawal	Irritability; psychosis; violence; seizures	Symptoms abate with time, but antipsychotics may be necessary; gradual lowering of dosage
Cocaine intoxication and withdrawal	Paranoia and violence; severe anxiety; manic state; delirium; schizophreniform psychosis; tachycardia, hypertension, myocardial infarction, cerebrovascular disease; depression and suicidal ideation	Antipsychotics and benzodiazepines; antidepressants or ECT for withdrawal depression if persistent; hospitalization
Delirium	Fluctuating sensorium; suicidal and homicidal risk; cognitive clouding; visual, tactile, and auditory hallucinations; paranoia	Evaluate all potential contributing factors and treat each accordingly; reassurance, structure, clues to orientation; benzodiazepines and low-dosage, high-potency antipsychotics must be used with extreme care because of their potential to act paradoxically and increase agitation
Delusional disorder	Most often brought in to emergency room involuntarily; threats directed toward others	Antipsychotics if patient will comply (IM if necessary); intensive family intervention; hospitalization if necessary
Dementia	Unable to care for self; violent outbursts; psychosis; depression and suicidal ideation; confusion	Small dosages of high-potency antipsychotics; clues to orientation; organic evaluation, including medication use; family intervention
Depressive disorders	Suicidal ideation and attempts; self-neglect; substance abuse	Assessment of danger to self; hospitalization if necessary; nonpsychiatric causes of depression must be evaluated
L-Dopa intoxication	Mania; depression; schizophreniform disorder; may induce rapid cycling in patients with bipolar I disorder	Lower dosage or discontinue drug
Dystonia, acute	Intense involuntary spasm of muscles of neck, tongue, face, jaw, eyes, or trunk	Decrease dosage of antipsychotic; benztropine or diphenhydramine IM
Group hysteria	Groups of people exhibit extremes of grief or other disruptive behavior	Group is dispersed with help of other health care workers; ventilation, crisis-oriented therapy; if necessary, small dosages of benzodiazepines
Hallucinogen-induced psychotic disorder with hallucinations	Symptom picture is result of interaction of type of substance, dose taken, duration of action, user's premorbid personality, setting; panic; agitation; atropine psychosis	Serum and urine screens; rule out underlying medical or mental disorder; benzodiazepines (2 to 20 mg) orally; reassurance and orientation; rapid tranquilization; often responds spontaneously

(continued)

Table 30.1–1 (*continued*)

Syndrome	Emergency Manifestations	Treatment Issues
Homicidal and assaultive behavior	Marked agitation with verbal threats	Seclusion, restraints, medication
Homosexual panic	Not seen with men or women who are comfortable with their sexual orientation; occurs in those who adamantly deny having any homoerotic impulses; impulses are aroused by talk, a physical overture, or play among same-sex friends, such as wrestling, sleeping together, or touching each other in a shower or hot tub; panicked person sees others as sexually interested in him or her and defends against them	Ventilation, environmental structuring, and, in some instances, medication for acute panic (e.g., alprazolam, 0.25 to 2 mg) or antipsychotics may be required; opposite-sex clinician should evaluate the patient whenever possible, and the patient should not be touched save for the routine examination; patients have attacked physicians who were examining an abdomen or performing a rectal examination (e.g., on a man who harbors thinly veiled unintegrated homosexual impulses)
Hypertensive crisis	Life-threatening hypertensive reaction secondary to ingestion of tyramine-containing foods in combination with MAOIs; headache, stiff neck, sweating, nausea, vomiting	α-Adrenergic blockers (e.g., phentolamine [Regitine]); nifedipine (Procardia) 10 mg orally; chlorpromazine (Thorazine); make sure symptoms are not secondary to hypotension (side effect of monoamine oxidase inhibitors [MAOIs] alone)
Hyperthermia	Extreme excitement or catatonic stupor or both; extremely elevated temperature; violent hyperagitation	Hydrate and cool; may be drug reaction, so discontinue any drug; rule out infection
Hyperventilation	Anxiety, terror, clouded consciousness; giddiness, faintness; blurring vision	Shift alkalosis by having patient breathe into paper bag; patient education; antianxiety agents
Hypothermia	Confusion; lethargy; combativeness; low body temperature and shivering; paradoxical feeling of warmth	IV fluids and rewarming; cardiac status must be carefully monitored; avoidance of alcohol
Incest and sexual abuse of child	Suicidal behavior; adolescent crises; substance abuse	Corroboration of charge; protection of victim; contact social services; medical and psychiatric evaluation; crisis intervention
Insomnia	Depression and irritability; early morning agitation; frightening dreams; fatigue	Hypnotics only in short term; e.g., triazolam (Halcion), 0.25 to 0.5 mg, at bedtime; treat any underlying mental disorder; rules of sleep hygiene
Intermittent explosive disorder	Brief outbursts of violence; periodic episodes of suicide attempts	Benzodiazepines or antipsychotics for short term; long-term evaluation with computed tomography (CT) scan, sleep-deprived electroencephalogram (EEG), glucose tolerance curve
Jaundice	Uncommon complication of low-potency phenothiazine use (e.g., chlorpromazine)	Change drug to low dosage of a low-potency agent in a different class
Leukopenia and agranulocytosis	Side effects within the first 2 months of treatment with antipsychotics	Patient should call immediately for sore throat, fever, etc., and obtain immediate blood count; discontinue drug; hospitalize if necessary
Lithium toxicity	Vomiting; abdominal pain; profuse diarrhea; severe tremor, ataxia; coma; seizures; confusion; dysarthria; focal neurological signs	Lavage with wide-bore tube; osmotic diuresis; medical consultation; may require ICU treatment
Major depressive episode with psychotic features	Major depressive episode symptoms with delusions; agitation, severe guilt; ideas of reference; suicide and homicide risk	Antipsychotics plus antidepressants; evaluation of suicide and homicide risk; hospitalization and ECT if necessary
Manic episode	Violent, impulsive behavior; indiscriminate sexual or spending behavior; psychosis; substance abuse	Hospitalization; restraints if necessary; rapid tranquilization with antipsychotics; restoration of lithium levels
Marital crises	Precipitant may be discovery of an extramarital affair, onset of serious illness, announcement of intent to divorce, or problems with children or work; one or both members of the couple may be in therapy or may be psychiatrically ill; one spouse may be seeking hospitalization for the other	Each should be questioned alone regarding extramarital affairs, consultations with lawyers regarding divorce, and willingness to work in crisis-oriented or long-term therapy to resolve the problem; sexual, financial, and psychiatric treatment histories from both, psychiatric evaluation at the time of presentation; may be precipitated by onset of untreated mood disorder or affective symptoms caused by medical illness or insidious-onset dementia; referral for management of the illness reduces immediate stress and enhances the healthier spouse's coping capacity; children may give insights available only to someone intimately involved in the social system

(continued)

Table 30.1–1 (*continued*)

Syndrome	Emergency Manifestations	Treatment Issues
Migraine	Throbbing, unilateral headache	Sumatriptan (Imitrex), 6 mg IM
Mitral valve prolapse	Associated with panic disorder; dyspnea and palpitations; fear and anxiety	Echocardiogram; alprazolam or propranolol
Neuroleptic malignant syndrome	Hyperthermia; muscle rigidity; autonomic instability; parkinsonian symptoms; catatonic stupor; neurological signs; 10% to 30% fatality; elevated creatine phosphokinase	Discontinue antipsychotic; IV dantrolene (Dantrium); bromocriptine (Parlodel) orally; hydration and cooling; monitor CPK levels
Nitrous oxide toxicity	Euphoria and light-headedness	Symptoms abate without treatment within hours of use
Nutmeg intoxication	Agitation; hallucinations; severe headaches; numbness in extremities	Symptoms abate within hours of use without treatment
Opioid intoxication and withdrawal	Intoxication can lead to coma and death; withdrawal is not life-threatening	IV naloxone, narcotic antagonist; urine and serum screens; psychiatric and medical illnesses (e.g., AIDS) may complicate picture
Panic disorder	Panic, terror; acute onset	Must differentiate from other anxiety-producing disorders, both medical and psychiatric; ECG to rule out mitral valve prolapse; propranolol (10 to 30 mg); alprazolam (0.25 to 2.0 mg); long-term management may include an antidepressant
Paranoid schizophrenia	Command hallucinations; threat to others or themselves	Rapid tranquilization; hospitalization; long-acting depot medication; threatened persons must be notified and protected
Parkinsonism	Stiffness, tremor, bradykinesia, flattened affect, shuffling gait, salivation, secondary to antipsychotic medication	Oral antiparkinsonian drug for 4 weeks to 3 months; decrease dosage of the antipsychotic
Perioral (rabbit) tremor	Perioral tumor (rabbit-like facial grimacing) usually appearing after long-term therapy with antipsychotics	Decrease dosage or change to a medication in another class
Phencyclidine (or phencyclidine-like intoxication)	Paranoid psychosis; can lead to death; acute danger to self and others	Serum and urine assay; benzodiazepines may interfere with excretion; antipsychotics may worsen symptoms because of anticholinergic side effects; medical monitoring and hospitalization for severe intoxication
Phenelzine-induced psychotic disorder	Psychosis and mania in predisposed people	Reduce dosage or discontinue drug
Phenylpropanolamine toxicity	Psychosis; paranoia; insomnia; restlessness; nervousness; headache	Symptoms abate with dosage reduction or discontinuation (found in over-the-counter diet aids and oral and nasal decongestants)
Phobias	Panic, anxiety; fear	Treatment same as for panic disorder
Photosensitivity	Easy sunburning secondary to use of antipsychotic medication	Patient should avoid strong sunlight and use high-level sunscreens
Pigmentary retinopathy	Reported with dosages of thioridazine (Mellaril) of 800 mg a day or above	Remain below 800 mg a day of thioridazine
Postpartum psychosis	Childbirth can precipitate schizophrenia, depression, reactive psychoses, mania, and depression; affective symptoms are most common; suicide risk is reduced during pregnancy but increased in the postpartum period	Danger to self and others (including infant) must be evaluated and proper precautions taken; medical illness presenting with behavioral aberrations is included in the differential diagnosis and must be sought and treated; care must be paid to the effects on father, infant, grandparents, and other children
Posttraumatic stress disorder	Panic, terror; suicidal ideation; flashbacks	Reassurance; encouragement of return to responsibilities; avoid hospitalization if possible to prevent chronic invalidism; monitor suicidal ideation
Priapism (trazodone [Desyrel]-induced)	Persistent penile erection accompanied by severe pain	Intracorporeal epinephrine; mechanical or surgical drainage
Propranolol toxicity	Profound depression; confusional states	Reduce dosage or discontinue drug; monitor suicidality

(*continued*)

Table 30.1–1 (*continued*)

Syndrome	Emergency Manifestations	Treatment Issues
Rape	Not all sexual violations are reported; silent rape reaction is characterized by loss of appetite, sleep disturbance, anxiety, and, sometimes, agoraphobia; long periods of silence, mounting anxiety, stuttering, blocking, and physical symptoms during the interview when the sexual history is taken; fear of violence and death and of contracting a sexually transmitted disease or being pregnant	Rape is a major psychiatric emergency; victim may have enduring patterns of sexual dysfunction; crisis-oriented therapy, social support, ventilation, reinforcement of healthy traits, and encouragement to return to the previous level of functioning as rapidly as possible; legal counsel; thorough medical examination and tests to identify the assailant (e.g., obtaining samples of pubic hairs with a pubic hair comb, vaginal smear to identify blood antigens in semen); if a woman, methoxy-progesterone or diethylstilbestrol orally for 5 days to prevent pregnancy; if menstruation does not commence within one week of cessation of the estrogen, all alternatives to pregnancy, including abortion, should be offered; if the victim has contracted a venereal disease, appropriate antibiotics; witnessed written permission is required for the physician to examine, photograph, collect specimens, and release information to the authorities; obtain consent, record the history in the patient's own words, obtain required tests, record the results of the examination, save all clothing, defer diagnosis, and provide protection against disease, psychic trauma, and pregnancy; men's and women's responses to rape affectively are reported similarly, although men are more hesitant to talk about homosexual assault for fear they will be assumed to have consented
Reserpine intoxication	Major depressive episodes; suicidal ideation; nightmares	Evaluation of suicidal ideation; lower dosage or change drug; antidepressants or ECT may be indicated
Schizoaffective disorder	Severe depression; manic symptoms; paranoia	Evaluation of dangerousness to self or others; rapid tranquilization if necessary; treatment of depression (antidepressants alone can enhance schizophrenic symptoms); use of antimanic agents
Schizophrenia	Extreme self-neglect; severe paranoia; suicidal ideation or assaultiveness; extreme psychotic symptoms	Evaluation of suicidal and homicidal potential; identification of any illness other than schizophrenia; rapid tranquilization
Schizophrenia in exacerbation	Withdrawn; agitation; suicidal and homicidal risk	Suicide and homicide evaluation; screen for medical illness; restraints and rapid tranquilization if necessary; hospitalization if necessary; reevaluation of medication regimen
Sedative, hypnotic, or anxiolytic intoxication and withdrawal	Alterations in mood, behavior, thought—delirium; derealization and depersonalization; untreated, can be fatal; seizures	Naloxone (Narcan) to differentiate from opioid intoxication; slow withdrawal with phenobarbital (Luminal) or sodium thiopental or benzodiazepine; hospitalization
Seizure disorder	Confusion; anxiety; derealization and depersonalization; feelings of impending doom; gustatory or olfactory hallucinations; fugue-like state	Immediate EEG; admission and sleep-deprived and 24-hour EEG; rule out pseudoseizures; anticonvulsants
Substance withdrawal	Abdominal pain; insomnia, drowsiness; delirium; seizures; symptoms of tardive dyskinesia may emerge; eruption of manic or schizophrenic symptoms	Symptoms of psychotropic drug withdrawal disappear with time or disappear with reinstitution of the substance; symptoms of antidepressant withdrawal can be successfully treated with anticholinergic agents, such as atropine; gradual withdrawal of psychotropic substances over two to four weeks generally obviates development of symptoms
Sudden death associated with antipsychotic medication	Seizures; asphyxiation; cardiovascular causes; postural hypotension; laryngeal-pharyngeal dystonia; suppression of gag reflex	Specific medical treatments
Sudden death of psychogenic origin	Myocardial infarction after sudden psychic stress; voodoo and hexes; hopelessness, especially associated with serious physical illness	Specific medical treatments; folk healers
Suicide	Suicidal ideation; hopelessness	Hospitalization, antidepressants
Sympathomimetic withdrawal	Paranoia; confusional states; depression	Most symptoms abate without treatment; antipsychotics; antidepressants if necessary

(*continued*)

Table 30.1–1 (*continued*)

Syndrome	Emergency Manifestations	Treatment Issues
Tardive dyskinesia	Dyskinesia of mouth, tongue, face, neck, and trunk; choreoathetoid movements of extremities; usually but not always appearing after long-term treatment with antipsychotics, especially after a reduction in dosage; incidence highest in the elderly and brain-damaged; symptoms are intensified by antiparkinsonian drugs and masked but not cured by increased dosages of antipsychotic	No effective treatment reported; may be prevented by prescribing the least amount of drug possible for as little time as is clinically feasible and using drug-free holidays for patients who need to continue taking the drug; decrease or discontinue drug at first sign of dyskinetic movements
Thyrotoxicosis	Tachycardia; gastrointestinal dysfunction; hyperthermia; panic, anxiety, agitation; mania; dementia; psychosis	Thyroid function test (T_3, T_4, thyroid-stimulating hormone [TSH]); medical consultation
Toluene abuse	Anxiety; confusion; cognitive impairment	Neurological damage is nonprogressive and reversible if toluene use is discontinued early
Vitamin B_{12} deficiency	Confusion; mood and behavior changes; ataxia	Treatment with vitamin B_{12}
Volatile nitrates	Alternations of mood and behavior; light-headedness; pulsating headache	Symptoms abate with cessation of use; combined with sildenafil (Viagra) can be fatal and must be avoided.

▲ 30.2 Suicide

The word *suicide* is derived from Latin for "self-murder." If successful, it is a fatal act that represents the person's wish to die. There is a range, however, between thinking about suicide and acting it out. Some persons have ideas of suicide that they will never act upon; some plan for days, weeks, or even years before acting; and others take their lives seemingly on impulse, without premeditation.

EPIDEMIOLOGY

Each year more than 30,000 persons die by suicide in the United States. The number of attempted suicides is approximately 650,000. There are approximately 85 suicides a day in this country—about 1 every 20 minutes. The suicide rate in the United States has averaged 12.5 per 100,000 in the 20th century, with a high of 17.4 per 100,000 during the Great Depression of the 1930s. From 1983 to 1998, the overall suicide rate remained relatively stable, whereas the rate for 15- to 24-year-olds has increased two- to threefold. Suicide is currently ranked the ninth overall cause of death in this country, after heart disease, cancer, cerebrovascular disease, chronic obstructive pulmonary disease, accidents, pneumonia, influenza, and diabetes mellitus.

U.S. suicide rates are at the midpoint of the rates for industrialized countries as reported to the United Nations. Internationally, suicide rates range from highs of more than 25 per 100,000 persons in Scandinavia, Switzerland, Germany, Austria, the Eastern European countries (the so-called suicide belt), and Japan, to fewer than 10 per 100,000 in Spain, Italy, Ireland, Egypt, and the Netherlands. The prime suicide site of the world is the Golden Gate Bridge in San Francisco, with more than 800 suicides since the bridge opened in 1937.

Risk Factors

Sex.   Men commit suicide more than four times as often as women, a rate that is stable over all ages. Women, however, are four times more likely to attempt suicide than men.

Age.   Suicide rates increase with age and underscore the significance of the midlife crisis. Among men, suicides peak after age 45; among women, the greatest number of completed suicides occurs after age 55. Rates of 40 per 100,000 population occur in men age 65 and older. Older persons attempt suicide less often than younger persons but are more often successful. Although they are only 10 percent of the total population, older persons account for 25 percent of suicides. The rate for those 75 years or older is more than three times the rate among young persons.

The suicide rate, however, is rising most rapidly among young persons, particularly in men 15 to 24 years old, and the rate is still rising. The suicide rate for females in the same age group is increasing more slowly than that for males. Among men 25 to 34 years old, the suicide rate increased almost 30 percent over the past decade. Suicide is the third leading cause of death in the 15- to 24-year-old age group, after accidents and homicides, and attempted suicides in this age group number between 1 million and 2 million annually. Most suicides now occur among those aged 15 to 44.

Race.   Two of every three suicides are white males. The rate of suicide among whites has been nearly twice that among all other groups; these figures, however, are now questionable, as the suicide rate among blacks is rising. The suicide rate for white males (19.6 per 100,000 persons) is 1.6 times that for black males (12.5), 4 times that for white women (4.8), and 8.2 times that for black women (2.4). Among young persons who live in inner cities and certain Native American and Inuit groups, suicide rates have greatly exceeded the national rate.

Suicide rates among immigrants are higher than those in the native-born population.

Religion.   Historically, suicide rates among Roman Catholic populations have been lower than rates among Protestants and Jews. The degree of orthodoxy and integration may be a more accurate measure of risk in this category than simple institutional religious affiliation.

Marital Status.   Marriage reinforced by children seems to lessen the risk of suicide significantly. The suicide rate is 11 per 100,000 for married persons; single, never-married persons register an overall rate nearly double that. Previously married persons, however, show sharply higher rates than those who never married: 24 per 100,000 among persons who are widowed, and 40 per 100,000 among those who are divorced, with divorced men registering 69 suicides per 100,000, compared with 18 per 100,000 for divorced women. Suicide occurs more frequently than usual in persons who are socially isolated and have a family history of suicide (attempted or real). Persons who commit so-called anniversary suicides take their lives on the day a member of their family did.

Occupation.   The higher a person's social status, the greater the risk of suicide, but a fall in social status also increases the risk. Work, in general, protects against suicide. Among occupational rankings, professionals, particularly physicians, have traditionally been considered to be at the greatest risk of suicide, but the best recent studies have found no increased suicide risk for male physicians in the United States. Their annual suicide rate is approximately 36 per 100,000, which is the same as that for white men over 25 years of age. Recent U.K. and Scandinavian data, by contrast, show that the suicide rate for male physicians is two to three times that found in the general male population of the same age. Special at-risk populations are musicians, dentists, law enforcement officers, lawyers, and insurance agents. Suicide is higher among the unemployed than among employed persons. The suicide rate increases during economic recessions and depressions and times of high unemployment and decreases during times of high employment and during wars.

Physician Suicides.   Female physicians have a higher risk of suicide than other women. In the United States, the annual suicide rate for female physicians is approximately 41 per 100,000, compared with 12 per 100,000 among all white women over 25 years of age. Similarly, in England and Wales, the suicide rate for unmarried female physicians is 2.5 times that among unmarried women in the general population, although it is comparable to that of other groups of professional women.

Studies show that physicians who commit suicide have a mental disorder. The most common mental disorders among physicians and among physician suicide victims are depressive disorders and substance dependence. Some evidence indicates that female physicians have an unusually high lifetime risk for mood disorders, which may be the major determinant of the elevated suicide risk. Often, a physician who commits suicide has experienced recent professional, personal, or family difficulties. Both male and female physicians commit suicide significantly more often by substance overdoses and less often by firearms than persons in the general population; drug availability and knowledge about toxicity are important factors in physician suicides.

Among physicians, psychiatrists are considered to be at greatest risk, followed by ophthalmologists and anesthesiologists, but the trend is toward an equalization among all specialties.

Methods.   Men's higher rate of successful suicide is related to the methods they use: firearms, hanging, or jumping from high places. Women more commonly take an overdose of psychoactive substances or a poison, but their use of firearms is increasing. In states with gun control laws, the use of firearms has decreased as a method of suicide. Globally, the most common method of suicide is hanging.

Physical Health.   The relation of physical health and illness to suicide is significant. Previous medical care appears to be a positively correlated risk indicator of suicide: 32 percent of all persons who commit suicide have had medical attention within 6 months of death. Postmortem studies show that a physical illness is present in some 25 to 75 percent of all suicide victims, and a physical illness is estimated to be an important contributing factor in up to 50 percent of suicides.

Factors associated with illness and contributing to both suicides and suicide attempts are loss of mobility, especially when physical activity is important to occupation or recreation; disfigurement, particularly among women; and chronic, intractable pain. In addition to the direct effects of illness, the secondary effects—for example, disruption of relationships and loss of occupational status—are poor prognostic factors.

Certain drugs can produce depression, which may lead to suicide in some cases. Among these drugs are reserpine (Serpasil), corticosteroids, antihypertensives, and some anticancer agents.

Mental Health.   Highly significant psychiatric factors in suicide include substance abuse, depressive disorders, schizophrenia, and other mental disorders. Almost 95 percent of all persons who commit or attempt suicide have a diagnosed mental disorder. Depressive disorders account for 80 percent of this figure, schizophrenia accounts for 10 percent, and dementia or delirium for 5 percent. Among all persons with mental disorders, 25 percent are also alcohol dependent and have dual diagnoses. Persons with delusional depression are at highest risk of suicide. The suicide risk in persons with depressive disorders is approximately 15 percent, and 25 percent of all those with a history of impulsive behavior or violent acts are also at high risk of suicide. Previous psychiatric hospitalization for any reason increases the risk of suicide.

Among adults who commit suicide, significant differences between young and old exist for both psychiatric diagnoses and antecedent stressors. A study in San Diego, California, showed that diagnoses of substance abuse and antisocial personality disorder occurred most often among suicides under 30 years of age, and diagnoses of mood disorders and cognitive disorders most often among suicides ages 30 and over. Stressors associated with suicide in those under age 30 were separation, rejection, unemployment, and legal troubles; illness stressors most often occurred among suicide victims who were older than 30.

Psychiatric Patients.   Psychiatric patients' risk for suicide is 3 to 12 times that of nonpatients. The degree of risk varies, depending on age, sex, diagnosis, and inpatient or outpatient status. After adjustment for age, male and female psychiatric patients who have at some time been inpatients have five and ten times higher suicide risks, respectively, than their counterparts in the general population. For male and female outpatients who have never been admitted to a hospital for psychiatric treatment, the suicide risks are three and four times greater, respectively, than those of their counterparts in the general population. The higher suicide risk for psychiatric patients who have been inpatients reflects the fact that patients with severe mental disorders tend to be hospitalized—for example, patients with depressive disorder who require electroconvulsive therapy (ECT). The psychiatric diagnosis with greatest risk of suicide in both sexes is a mood disorder.

In one study, the mean age of male suicides was 29.5 years and that of women 38.4 years. The relative youthfulness of these suicide cases was due partly to the fact that two early-onset, chronic mental disorders—schizophrenia and recurrent major depressive disorder—accounted for just over half of these suicides.

A small, but significant, percentage of psychiatric patients who commit suicide do so while they are inpatients. Most of these do not kill themselves in the psychiatric ward itself but on the hospital grounds, while on a pass or weekend leave, or when absent without leave.

For both sexes, the suicide risk is highest in the first week of the psychiatric admission; after 3 to 5 weeks, inpatients have the same risk as the general population. The inpatient rates of suicide do not rise uniformly with age, as in the general population; in fact, the rates for female psychiatric patients fall with advancing age, mainly because older persons who are suicidal do not seek medical aid. Times of staff rotation, particularly of the psychiatric residents, are periods associated with inpatient suicides. Epidemics of inpatient suicides tend to be associated with periods of ideological change on the ward, staff disorganization, and staff demoralization.

Among psychiatric outpatients, the period after discharge is a time of increased suicide risk. A follow-up study of 5,000 patients discharged from an Iowa psychiatric hospital showed that in the first 3 months after discharge, the rate of suicide for female patients was 275 times that of all Iowa women; the rate of suicide for male patients was 70 times that of all Iowa men.

Patients, especially those with panic disorder, who frequent emergency services, also have an increased suicide risk. One study reported that such patients have a suicide rate more than seven times the age-adjusted and sex-adjusted rate for the general population (but the rate is similar to that of other clinical psychiatric populations). The two main risk groups are patients with depressive disorders, schizophrenia, and substance abuse, and patients who make repeated visits to the emergency room. Thus, mental health professionals working in emergency services must be well trained in taking patients' psychiatric histories, examining their mental states, assessing suicidal risk, and making appropriate dispositions. They must also be aware of the need to contact patients at risk who fail to keep follow-up appointments.

DEPRESSIVE DISORDERS.   Mood disorders are the diagnoses most commonly associated with suicide. As the suicide risk in depressive disorders rises mainly when patients are depressed, the psychopharmacological advances of the past 25 years may have reduced the suicide risk among patients with depressive disorder. Nevertheless, the age-

adjusted suicide rates for patients with mood disorders have been estimated to be 400 per 100,000 for male patients and 180 per 100,000 for female patients.

More patients with depressive disorders commit suicide early in the illness rather than later; more men than women commit suicide; and the chance of depressed persons killing themselves increases if they are single, separated, divorced, widowed, or recently bereaved. Depressive disorder patients in the community who commit suicide tend to be middle aged or older.

A few studies have investigated which patients with mood disorders have an increased suicide risk. These studies indicate that social isolation enhances suicidal tendencies among depressed patients. This finding is in accord with the data from epidemiological studies showing that persons who commit suicide may be poorly integrated into society. Suicide among depressed patients is likely at the onset or the end of a depressive episode. As with other psychiatric patients, the months after discharge from a hospital are a time of high risk. Studies show that one-third or more of depressed patients who commit suicide do so within 6 months of leaving a hospital; presumably they have relapsed.

Regarding outpatient treatment, most depressed suicidal patients had a history of therapy; however, less than half were receiving psychiatric treatment at the time of suicide. Of those who were in treatment, studies have shown that it was less than adequate. For example, most patients who received antidepressants were prescribed subtherapeutic doses of the medication.

SCHIZOPHRENIA.   The suicide risk is high among patients with schizophrenia: Up to 10 percent die by committing suicide. In the United States, an estimated 4,000 schizophrenic patients commit suicide each year. The onset of schizophrenia is typically in adolescence or early adulthood, and most of these patients who commit suicide do so during the first few years of their illness; therefore, schizophrenic patients who commit suicide are young.

Approximately 75 percent of all schizophrenic suicides are committed by unmarried men, and approximately 50 percent have made a previous suicide attempt. Depressive symptoms are closely associated with their suicides. Hospital-based studies have reported that depressive symptoms were present during the last period of contact in at least two-thirds of patients with schizophrenia who committed suicide; only a small percentage committed suicide because of hallucinated instructions or a need to escape persecutory delusions. Up to 50 percent of suicides among patients with schizophrenia occur during the first few weeks and months after discharge from a hospital; only a minority commit suicide while inpatients.

ALCOHOL DEPENDENCE.   Up to 15 percent of all alcohol-dependent persons commit suicide. The suicide rate for those who are alcoholic is estimated to be approximately 270 per 100,000 annually; in the United States, between 7,000 and 13,000 alcohol-dependent persons commit suicide each year.

Approximately 80 percent of all alcohol-dependent suicide victims are male, a percentage that largely reflects the sex ratio for alcohol dependence. Alcohol-dependent suicide victims tend to be white, middle aged, unmarried, friendless, socially isolated, and currently drinking. Up to 40 percent have made a previous suicide attempt. Up to 40 percent of all suicides by persons who are alcohol dependent occur within a year of the patient's last hospitalization; older alcohol-dependent patients are at particular risk during the postdischarge period.

Studies show that many alcohol-dependent patients who eventually commit suicide are rated depressed during hospitalization and that up to two-thirds are assessed as having mood disorder symptoms during the period in which they commit suicide. As many as 50 percent of all alcohol-dependent suicide victims have experienced the loss of a close, affectionate relationship during the previous year. Such interpersonal losses and other types of undesirable life events are probably brought about by the alcohol dependence and contribute to the development of the mood disorder symptoms, which are often present in the weeks and months before the suicide.

The largest group of male alcohol-dependent patients are those with an associated antisocial personality disorder. Studies show that such patients are particularly likely to attempt suicide; to abuse other substances; to exhibit impulsive, aggressive, and criminal behaviors; and to be found among alcohol-dependent suicide victims.

OTHER SUBSTANCE DEPENDENCE. Studies in various countries have found an increased suicide risk among those who abuse substances. The suicide rate for persons who are heroin dependent is approximately 20 times the rate for the general population. Adolescent girls who use intravenous (IV) substances also have a high suicide rate. The availability of a lethal amount of substances, IV use, associated antisocial personality disorder, a chaotic lifestyle, and impulsivity are some of the factors that predispose substance-dependent persons to suicidal behavior, particularly when they are dysphoric, depressed, or intoxicated.

PERSONALITY DISORDERS. A high proportion of those who commit suicide have various associated personality difficulties or disorders. Having a personality disorder may be a determinant of suicidal behavior in several ways: by predisposing to major mental disorders like depressive disorders or alcohol dependence; by leading to difficulties in relationships and social adjustment; by precipitating undesirable life events; by impairing the ability to cope with a mental or physical disorder; and by drawing persons into conflicts with those around them, including family members, physicians, and hospital staff members.

An estimated 5 percent of patients with antisocial personality disorder commit suicide. Suicide is three times more common among prisoners than among the general population. More than one-third of prisoner suicides have had past psychiatric treatment, and half have made a previous suicide threat or attempt, often in the previous 6 months.

ANXIETY DISORDER. Unsuccessful suicide attempts are made by almost 20 percent of patients with a panic disorder and social phobia. If depression is an associated feature, however, the risk of success rises.

Previous Suicidal Behavior.
A past suicide attempt is perhaps the best indicator that a patient is at increased risk of suicide. Studies show that approximately 40 percent of depressed patients who commit suicide have made a previous attempt. The risk of a second suicide attempt is highest within 3 months of the first attempt.

Depression is associated not only with completed suicide, but also with serious attempts at suicide. The clinical feature most often associated with the seriousness of the intent to die is a diagnosis of a depressive disorder. This is shown by studies that relate the clinical characteristics of suicidal patients with various measures of the medical seriousness of the attempt or of the intent to die. Also, intent-to-die scores correlate significantly with both suicide risk scores and the number and severity of depressive symptoms. The attempters rated as having high suicide intent are more often male, older, single or separated, and living alone than those with low intent. In other words, depressed patients who seriously attempt suicide more closely resemble suicide victims than they do suicide attempters.

ETIOLOGY

Sociological Factors

Durkheim's Theory. The first major contribution to the study of the social and cultural influences on suicide was made at the end of the 19th century by the French sociologist Émile Durkheim. In an attempt to explain statistical patterns, Durkheim divided suicides into three social categories: egoistic, altruistic, and anomic. Egoistic suicide applies to those who are not strongly integrated into any social group. The lack of family integration explains why unmarried persons are more vulnerable to suicide than married ones and why couples with children are the best-protected group. Rural communities have more social integration than urban areas and thus less suicide. Protestantism is a less cohesive religion than Roman Catholicism, and so Protestants have a higher suicide rate than Catholics.

Altruistic suicide applies to those prone to suicide stemming from their excessive integration into a group, with suicide being the outgrowth of the integration—for example, a Japanese soldier who sacrifices his life in battle. Anomic suicide applies to persons whose integration into society is disturbed so that they cannot follow customary norms of behavior. Anomie explains why a drastic change in economic situation makes persons more vulnerable than they were before their change in fortune. In Durkheim's theory, anomie also refers to social instability and a general breakdown of society's standards and values.

Psychological Factors

Freud's Theory. Sigmund Freud offered the first important psychological insight into suicide. He described only one patient who made a suicide attempt, but he saw many depressed patients. In his paper "Mourning and Melancholia," Freud stated his belief that suicide represents aggression turned inward against an introjected, ambivalently cathected love object. Freud doubted that there would be a suicide without an earlier repressed desire to kill someone else.

Menninger's Theory. Building on Freud's ideas, Karl Menninger, in *Man Against Himself*, conceived of suicide as inverted homicide because of a patient's anger toward another person. This retroflexed murder is either turned inward or used as an excuse for punishment. He also described a self-directed death instinct (Freud's concept of Thanatos) plus three components of hostility in suicide: the wish to kill, the wish to be killed, and the wish to die.

Recent Theories. Contemporary suicidologists are not persuaded that a specific psychodynamic or personality structure is associated with suicide. They believe that much can be learned about the psychodynamics of suicidal patients from their fantasies about what would happen and what the consequences would be if they commit suicide. Such fantasies often include wishes for revenge, power, control, or punishment; atonement, sacrifice, or restitution; escape or sleep; rescue, rebirth, reunion with the dead; or a new life. The suicidal patients most likely to act out suicidal fantasies may have lost a love object or received a narcissistic injury, may experience overwhelming affects like rage and guilt, or may identify with a suicide victim. Group dynamics underlie mass suicides like those at Masada, at Jonestown, and by the Heaven's Gate cult.

Depressed persons may attempt suicide just as they appear to be recovering from their depression. A suicide attempt can cause a long-standing depression to disappear, especially if it fulfills a patient's need for punishment. Of equal relevance, many suicide patients use a preoccupation with suicide as a way of fighting off intolerable depression and a sense of hopelessness. In fact, a study by Aaron Beck showed that hopelessness was one of the most accurate indicators of long-term suicidal risk.

Biological Factors.
Diminished central serotonin plays a role in suicidal behavior. A group at the Karolinska Institute in Sweden were the first to note that low concentrations of the serotonin metabolite 5-hydroxyindoleacetic acid (5-HIAA) in the lumbar cerebrospinal fluid (CSF) were associated with suicidal behavior. This finding has been replicated many times and in different diagnostic groups. Postmortem neurochemical studies have reported modest decreases in serotonin itself or 5-HIAA in either the brainstem or the frontal cortex of suicide victims. Postmortem receptor studies have reported significant changes in presynaptic and postsynaptic serotonin binding sites in suicide victims. Taken together, these CSF, neurochemical, and receptor studies support the hypothesis that reduced central serotonin is associated with suicide. Recent studies also report some changes in the noradrenergic system of suicide victims.

Low concentrations of 5-HIAA in CSF also predict future suicidal behavior. For example, the Karolinska group examined completed suicide in a sample of 92 depressed patients who had attempted suicide. They found that 8 of the 11 patients who committed suicide within 1 year belonged to the subgroup with below-median concentrations of 5-HIAA in CSF. The suicide risk in that subgroup was 17 percent, compared with 7 percent among those with above-median concentrations of 5-HIAA in CSF. Also, the cumulative number of patient-months survived during the first year after attempted suicide was significantly lower in the subgroup with low 5-HIAA concentrations. The Karolinska group concluded that low 5-HIAA concentrations in CSF predict short-range suicide risk in the high-risk group of depressed patients who have attempted suicide. Low 5-HIAA concentrations in CSF have also been demonstrated in adolescents who kill themselves.

Genetic Factors.
Suicidal behavior, like other psychiatric disorders, tends to run in families. In psychiatric patients, a family history of suicide increases the risk of attempted suicide and that of completed suicide in most diagnostic groups.

TWIN STUDIES. A landmark study in 1991 investigated 176 twin pairs in which one twin had committed suicide. In nine of these twin pairs, both twins had committed suicide. Seven of these nine pairs concordant for suicide were found among the 62 monozygotic pairs, while two pairs concordant for suicide were found among the 114 dizygotic twin pairs. This twin group difference for concordance for suicide (11.3 versus 1.8 percent) is statistically significant ($P < .01$).

Another study collected a group of 35 twin pairs in which one twin had committed suicide, and the living co-twin was interviewed. Ten of the 26 living monozygotic co-twins had themselves attempted suicide, compared with zero of the nine living dizygotic co-twins ($P < .04$). Although monozygotic and dizygotic twins may have some differing developmental experiences, these results show that monozygotic twin pairs have significantly higher concordance for both suicide and attempted suicide, which suggests that genetic factors may play a role in suicidal behavior.

MOLECULAR GENETIC STUDIES. Tryptophan hydroxylase (TPH) is an enzyme involved in the biosynthesis of serotonin. A polymorphism in the human TPH gene has been identified, with two alleles—*U* and *L*. Because low concentrations of 5-HIAA in CSF are associated with suicidal behavior, it was hypothesized that such individuals may have alterations in genes controlling serotonin synthesis and metabolism. It was found that impulsive alcoholics, who had low CSF 5-HIAA concentrations, had more *LL* and *UL* genotypes. Furthermore, a history of suicide attempts was significantly associated with TPH genotype in all the violent alcoholics; 34 of the 36 violent subjects who attempted suicide had either the *UL* or *LL* genotype. Thus, it was concluded that the presence of the *L* allele was associated with an increased risk of suicide attempts.

Also, a history of multiple suicide attempts was found most often in subjects with the *LL* genotype and, to a lesser extent, among those with the *UL* genotype. This led to the suggestion that the *L* allele was associated with repetitive suicidal behavior. The presence of one *TPH*L* allele may indicate a reduced capacity to hydroxylate tryptophan to 5-hydroxytryptophan in the synthesis of serotonin, producing low central serotonin turnover and thus a low concentration of 5-HIAA in CSF.

Parasuicidal Behavior.
Parasuicide is a term introduced to describe patients who injure themselves by self-mutilation (e.g., cutting the skin) but who usually do not wish to die. Studies show that approximately 4 percent of all patients in psychiatric hospitals have cut themselves; the female-to-male ratio is almost 3 to 1. The incidence of self-injury in psychiatric patients is estimated to be more than 50 times that in the general population. Psychiatrists note that so-called cutters have cut themselves over several years. Self-injury is found in approximately 30 percent of all abusers of oral substances and 10 percent of all IV users admitted to substance-treatment units.

These patients are usually in their 20s and may be single or married. Most cut delicately, not coarsely, usually in private with a razor blade, knife, broken glass, or mirror. The wrists, arms, thighs, and legs are most commonly cut; the face, breasts, and abdomen are cut infrequently. Most persons who cut themselves claim to experience no pain and give reasons such as anger at themselves or others, relief of tension, and the wish to die. The great majority are classified as having personality disorders and are significantly more introverted, neurotic, and hostile than controls. Alcohol abuse and other substance abuse are common, and most cutters have attempted suicide. Self-mutilation has been viewed as localized self-destruction, with mishandling of aggressive impulses caused by a person's unconscious wish to punish himself or herself or an introjected object.

PREDICTION

Clinicians must assess an individual patient's risk for suicide on the basis of a clinical examination. Suicide is grouped into high-risk–related and low-risk–related factors (Table 30.2–1).

Table 30.2–1
Evaluation of Suicide Risk

Variable	High Risk	Low Risk
Demographic and social profile		
Age	Over 45 years	Below 45 years
Sex	Male	Female
Marital status	Divorced or widowed	Married
Employment	Unemployed	Employed
Interpersonal relationship	Conflictual	Stable
Family background	Chaotic or conflictual	Stable
Health		
Physical	Chronic illness	Good health
	Hypochondriac	Feels healthy
	Excessive substance intake	Low substance use
Mental	Severe depression	Mild depression
	Psychosis	Neurosis
	Severe personality disorder	Normal personality
	Substance abuse	Social drinker
	Hopelessness	Optimism
Suicidal activity		
Suicidal ideation	Frequent, intense, prolonged	Infrequent, low intensity, transient
Suicide attempt	Multiple attempts	First attempt
	Planned	Impulsive
	Rescue unlikely	Rescue inevitable
	Unambiguous wish to die	Primary wish for change
	Communication internalized (self-blame)	Communication externalized (anger)
	Method lethal and available	Method of low lethality or not readily available
Resources		
Personal	Poor achievement	Good achievement
	Poor insight	Insightful
	Affect unavailable or poorly controlled	Affect available and appropriately controlled
Social	Poor rapport	Good rapport
	Socially isolated	Socially integrated
	Unresponsive family	Concerned family

Reprinted with permission from Adam K. Attempted suicide. *Psychiatr Clin North Am.* 1985;8:183.

High-risk characteristics include more than 45 years of age, male gender, alcohol dependence (the suicide rate is 50 times higher in alcohol-dependent persons than in those who are not alcohol dependent), violent behavior, previous suicidal behavior, and previous psychiatric hospitalization.

TREATMENT

Most suicides among psychiatric patients are preventable, as indicated by the evidence that inadequate assessment or treatment is often associated with suicide. Some patients experience suffering so great and intense, or so chronic and unresponsive to treatment, that their eventual suicides may be perceived as inevitable. Fortunately, such patients are relatively uncommon. Other patients have severe personality disorders, are highly impulsive, and commit suicide spontaneously, often when dysphoric or intoxicated or both.

The evaluation for suicide potential involves a complete psychiatric history; a thorough examination of the patient's mental state; and an inquiry about depressive symptoms, suicidal thoughts, intents, plans, and attempts. Taken together, a

lack of future plans, giving away personal property, making a will, and having recently experienced a loss imply increased risk of suicide. The decision to hospitalize a patient depends on diagnosis, severity of the depression and suicidal ideation, the patient's and the family's coping abilities, the patient's living situation, availability of social support, and the absence or presence of risk factors for suicide.

Inpatient versus Outpatient Treatment

Whether to hospitalize patients with suicidal ideation is the most important clinical decision to be made. Not all such patients require hospitalization; some may be treated on an outpatient basis. But the absence of a strong social support system, a history of impulsive behavior, and a suicidal plan of action are indications for hospitalization. To decide whether outpatient treatment is feasible, clinicians should use a straightforward clinical approach: They should ask patients considered suicidal to agree to call when they become uncertain about their ability to control their suicidal impulses. Patients who can make such an agreement with a doctor with whom they have a relationship reaffirm the belief that they have sufficient strength to control such impulses and to seek help.

In return for a patient's commitment, clinicians should be available to the patient 24 hours a day. If a patient who is considered seriously suicidal cannot make the commitment, immediate emergency hospitalization is indicated; both the patient and the patient's family should be so advised. If, however, the patient is to be treated on an outpatient basis, the therapist should note the patient's home and work telephone numbers for emergency reference; occasionally, a patient hangs up unexpectedly during a late-night call or gives only a name to the answering service. If the patient refuses hospitalization, the family must take the responsibility to be with the patient 24 hours a day.

Many psychiatrists believe that any patient who has attempted suicide, despite its lethality, should be hospitalized. Although most of these patients voluntarily enter a hospital, the danger to self is one of the few clear-cut indications currently acceptable in all states for involuntary hospitalization. In a hospital, patients can receive antidepressant or antipsychotic medications as indicated; individual therapy, group therapy, and family therapy are available; and patients receive the hospital's social support and sense of security. Other therapeutic measures depend on patients' underlying diagnoses. For example, if alcohol dependence is an associated problem, treatment must be directed toward alleviating that condition.

Although patients classified as acutely suicidal may have favorable prognoses, chronically suicidal patients are difficult to treat, and they exhaust the caretakers. Constant observation by special nurses, seclusion, and restraints cannot prevent suicide when a patient is resolute. ECT may be necessary for some severely depressed patients, who may require several treatment courses.

Useful measures for the treatment of depressed suicidal inpatients include searching patients and their belongings on arrival in the ward for objects that may be used for suicide and repeating the search at times of exacerbation of the suicidal ideation. Ideally, suicidal depressed inpatients should be treated on a locked ward where the windows are shatterproof, and the patient's room should be located near the nursing station to maximize observation by the nursing staff. The treatment team must assess how much to restrict the patient and whether to make regular checks or use continuous direct observation. Vigorous treatment with antidepressant or antipsychotic medication should be initiated.

Supportive psychotherapy by a psychiatrist shows concern and may alleviate some of a patient's intense suffering. Some patients may be able to accept the idea that they are suffering from a recognized illness and that they will probably make a complete recovery. Patients should be dissuaded from making major life decisions while they are suicidally depressed, because such decisions are often morbidly determined and may be irrevocable. The consequences of such bad decisions can cause further anguish and misery when the patient has recovered.

Patients recovering from a suicidal depression are at particular risk. As the depression lifts, patients become energized and are thus able to put their suicidal plans into action (paradoxical suicide). Sometimes, depressed patients, with or without treatment, suddenly appear to be at peace with themselves because they have reached a secret decision to commit suicide. Clinicians should be especially suspicious of such a dramatic clinical change, which may portend a suicide attempt. Although rare, some patients lie to the psychiatrist about their suicidal intent, thus subverting the most careful clinical assessment.

A patient may commit suicide even when in the hospital. According to one survey, approximately 1 percent of all suicides were committed by patients who were being treated in general medical-surgical or psychiatric hospitals, but the annual suicide rate in psychiatric hospitals is only 0.003 percent.

Legal and Ethical Factors. Liability issues stemming from suicides in psychiatric hospitals frequently involve questions about a patient's rate of deterioration, the presence during hospitalization of clinical signs indicating risk, and psychiatrists' and staff members' awareness of, and response to, these clinical signs.

In approximately half of cases in which suicides occur while patients are on a psychiatric unit, a lawsuit results. Courts do not require zero suicide rates, but do require periodic patient evaluation for suicidal risk, formulation of a treatment plan with a high level of security, and having staff members follow the treatment plan.

Aiding and abetting a suicide adds another dimension to the legal and ethical issues; some court decisions have held that although neither suicide nor attempted suicide is punishable, anyone who assists in the act may be punished. (Physician-assisted suicide is discussed in Chapter 51.)

31 ▲

Psychotherapies

▲ 31.1 Psychoanalysis and Psychoanalytic Psychotherapy

PSYCHOANALYSIS

Psychoanalysis emphasizes the conflict between unconscious drives and moral judgments that patients may make about their impulses. That conflict accounts for the phenomenon of repression, which is regarded as pathological. Free association—in which patients say whatever comes into their minds—allows repressed memories to be recovered and thereby contributes to cure. In *The Interpretation of Dreams*, Sigmund Freud (1856–1939) described the *topographical model* of the mind as consisting of conscious, preconscious, and unconscious. The conscious mind was conceptualized as awareness; the preconscious, as thoughts and feelings that are easily available to consciousness; and the unconscious, as thoughts and feelings that cannot be made conscious without overcoming strong resistances. The unconscious contains nonverbal forms of thought function and gives rise to dreams, parapaxes (slips of the tongue), and psychological symptoms.

Goal

The chief requirement of psychoanalysis is the gradual integration of the previously repressed material into the total structure of the personality. It is a slow process, requiring the analyst to maintain a balance between the interpretation of unconscious material and the patient's ability to deal with increased awareness. If the work proceeds too rapidly, the patient may experience the analysis as a new trauma. The work of analysis initially is preparing the patient to deal with the anxiety-producing material that has been uncovered. The patient is taught to be aware of innermost thoughts and feelings and to recognize the natural resistances to the mind's willingness or ability to deal directly with noxious psychic material. The patient and the analyst seldom follow a straight path to insight. Instead, the process of analysis is more like putting together pieces of an immense and complicated jigsaw puzzle.

Analytic Setting

The usual analytic setting is for the patient to lie on a couch or sofa, behind which the analyst sits, partially or totally outside the patient's field of vision. The couch helps the analyst pro-duce the controlled regression that favors the emergence of repressed material. The patient's reclining position in the presence of an attentive analyst almost re-creates symbolically the early parent–child situation, which varies from patient to patient. The position also helps the patient focus on inner thoughts, feelings, and fantasies, which can then become the focus of free associations. Moreover, the use of the couch introduces an element of sensory deprivation because the patient's visual stimuli are limited and analysts' verbalizations are relatively few. That state promotes regression. There has been some disagreement, however, about the use of the couch as always characteristic of psychoanalysis. Otto Fenichel stated that whether the patient lies down or sits and whether certain rituals of procedure are used do not matter. The best condition is the one most appropriate to the analytic task.

Role of the Analyst

For the most part, the analyst's activity is limited to timely interpretation of the patient's associations. Ideally, analysts—who have undergone a personal psychoanalysis as part of their training—are able to maintain an attitude of benevolent objectivity or neutrality toward the patient, trying not to impose their own personalities or systems of values. Nevertheless, it is not possible or desirable for the analyst to be a so-called blank screen, *tabula rasa*, or analyst incognito. A real relationship underlies the analytic setting, and the handling of the real relationship may make the difference between success and failure in treatment.

Treatment Methods

Fundamental Rule of Psychoanalysis. The fundamental or basic rule is that the patient agrees to be completely honest with the analyst and tell everything without selection. Freud referred to the technique that allowed for such honesty as a *free association*.

Free Association. In free association, patients say everything that comes to mind without any censoring, regardless of whether they believe the thought to be unacceptable, unimportant, or embarrassing. Associations are directed by three kinds of unconscious forces: The pathogenic conflicts of the neurosis, the wish to get well, and the wish to please the analyst. The interplay among those factors becomes complex. For example, a thought or an impulse that is unacceptable to patients and that is a part of their neuroses may conflict with their wishes to please the analyst, who, they assume, also finds the impulse unacceptable. But if patients follow the fundamental rule, they overcome the resistance.

Free-Floating Attention.
The analysts' counterpart to the patients' free association is a special way of listening called *free-floating attention*. Analysts allow the patients' associations to stimulate their own associations and are thereby able to discern a theme in the patients' free associations that may be reflected back to the patients then or at some later time. Analysts' careful attention to their own subjective experiences is an indispensable part of analysis.

Rule of Abstinence.
By following the rule of abstinence, the patient is able to delay gratifying any instinctual wishes so as to talk about them in treatment. The tension thus engendered produces relevant associations that the analyst uses to increase the patient's awareness. The rule does not refer to sexual abstinence but, rather, to not allowing the treatment setting to gratify the patient's infantile longing for love and affection.

Analytic Process

Transference.
A major criterion by which psychoanalysis can be differentiated in principle from other forms of psychotherapy is the management of the transference. Indeed, as mentioned above, psychoanalysis has been defined as the analysis of transference.

Transference concerns the patient's feelings and behaviors toward the analyst that are based on infantile wishes the patient has toward parents or parental figures. Those feelings are unconscious but are revealed in the so-called *transference neurosis*, in which patients struggle to gratify their unconscious infantile wishes through the analyst. The transference may be positive, in which the analyst needs to be seen as a person of exceptional worth, ability, and character; or it may be negative, in which the analyst becomes the embodiment of what the patient experienced or feared from parental figures in the past. Negative transferences can be expressed and experienced in highly labile and volatile ways, especially in patients whose personalities are described as borderline or narcissistic. Both situations reflect the patient's need to repeat unresolved childhood conflicts.

The analyst's role is to help the patient gain true insight into the distortions of transference and, through insight, to increase the patient's capacity for gratifying relationships based on mature and realistic expectations, rather than on irrational, childhood-derived fantasies.

Countertransference.
Just as the term "transference" is used to encompass the patient's total range of feelings for and against the analyst, "countertransference" encompasses a broad spectrum of the analyst's reactions to the patient. Countertransference has unconscious components based on conflicts of which the analyst is not aware. Ideally, the analyst ought to be aware of countertransference issues, which may interfere with the analyst's ability to remain detached and objective. The analyst should remove such impediments by either further analysis or self-analysis. However, with some patients or groups of patients, a particular analyst does not work well, and the experienced clinician, recognizing that fact, refers such patients to a colleague.

Therapeutic Alliance.
In addition to transferential and countertransferential issues, a real relationship between the analyst and the patient involves two adults entering into a joint venture, referred to as the *therapeutic* or *working alliance*. Both commit themselves to exploring the patient's problems, to establishing mutual trust, and to cooperating with each other to achieve a realistic goal of cure or the amelioration of symptoms. Studies have shown that a strong therapeutic alliance is associated with best treatment outcomes.

Interpretation.
In psychoanalysis, the analyst provides the patient with interpretations about psychological events that were neither previously understood by nor meaningful to the patient. The transference constitutes a major frame of reference for interpretation. A complete psychoanalytic interpretation includes meaningful statements of current conflicts and the historical factors that influenced them. However, such complete interpretations constitute a relatively small part of the analysis. Most interpretations are limited in scope and deal with matters of immediate concern.

Interpretations must be well-timed. The analyst may have a formulation in mind, but the patient may not be prepared to deal with it directly because of a variety of factors, such as anxiety level, negative transference, and external life stress. The analyst may decide to wait until the patient can fully understand the interpretation. The proper timing of the interpretation requires great clinical skill.

DREAM INTERPRETATION.
In his classic work *The Interpretation of Dreams*, Freud referred to the dream as the "royal road to the unconscious." The *manifest content* of a dream is what the dreamer reports. The *latent content* is the unconscious meaning of the dream after the condensations, substitutions, and symbols are analyzed. The dream arises from what Freud referred to as the *day's residue* (that is, the events of the preceding day that stimulated the patient's unconscious mind). Dreams may serve as a wish-fulfillment mechanism and as a way of mastering anxiety about a life event.

Freud outlined several technical procedures to use in dream interpretations: (1) have the patient associate to elements of the dream in the order in which they occurred, (2) have the patient associate to a particular dream element that the patient or the therapist chooses, (3) disregard the content of the dream, and ask the patient what events of the previous day could be associated with the dream (the day's residue), and (4) avoid giving any instructions, and leave it to the dreamer to begin. The analyst uses the patient's associations to find a clue to the workings of the unconscious mind.

Resistance.
Freud believed that unconscious ideas or impulses are repressed and prevented from reaching awareness because they are unacceptable to consciousness for some reason. He referred to that phenomenon as *resistance*, which has to be overcome if the analysis is to proceed. Resistance may sometimes be a conscious process manifested by withholding relevant information. Other examples of resistance are remaining silent for a long time, being late or missing appointments, and paying bills late or not at all. The signs of resistance are legion, and almost any feature of the analytic situation can be used in resistance. Freud once said that any treatment can be considered psychoanalysis that works by undoing resistance and interpreting transferences.

INDICATIONS FOR TREATMENT

The primary indications for psychoanalysis are long-standing psychological conflicts that have produced a symptom or disorder. The connection between the conflict and the symptom may be direct or indirect. Psychoanalysis is considered effective in treating certain anxiety disorders, such as phobias and obsessive-compulsive disorder, mild depressive disorders (dysthymic disorder), some personality disorders, and some impulse-control and sexual disorders. More important than diagnosis, however, is the patient's ability to form an analytic pact and to maintain a commitment to a progressively deepening analytic process that brings about internal change through increasing self-awareness. Freud believed that the patient also has to be able to form a strong transference attachment to the analyst (i.e., *transference neurosis*), without which analysis is not possible. That excluded most psychotic patients because of the difficulty they have in forming the affective and realistic bonds that are essential to the development and the resolution of the transference neurosis. The ego of the patient in analysis must be able to tolerate frustration without responding with some serious form of acting out or shifting from one pathological pattern to another. That excludes most substance-dependent patients, who are regarded as unsuitable because their egos are unable to tolerate the frustration and the emotional demands of psychoanalysis.

CONTRAINDICATIONS FOR TREATMENT

The various contraindications to psychoanalysis are relative, but each must be considered before embarking on a course of treatment.

Age

Traditionally, many analysts believed that most adults over 40 lack sufficient flexibility for major personality changes. However, analysts now believe that more important than age is the patient's individual capacity for thoughtful introspection and desire for change. The ideal candidates are generally young adults. Children are unable to follow the rule of free association, but, with modification of technique (for example, play therapy), they have been successfully analyzed.

Intelligence

Patients must be intelligent enough to be able to understand the procedure and to cooperate in the process.

Life Circumstances

If the patient's life situation cannot be modified, analysis may only make it worse. For example, it can be hazardous to create goals for patients who are unable to fulfill them because of external limitations.

Antisocial Personality Disorder

Clinicians and researchers seem to agree that the absence of relatedness to others is the single most negative predictor of psychotherapy response. The true antisocial personality is a person who may benefit from certain types of therapy, such as group therapy with other antisocial personalities, but who is not suited for analytically oriented psychotherapy. Personality traits such as sadistic cruelty to others, total absence of remorse, and lack of emotional attachment are the key distinguishing features that lead to an inability to engage in therapy. An extremely intelligent person with antisocial personality disorder can be expert at sabotaging therapy; and a mildly retarded antisocial personality may not have the cognitive ability to engage in the psychoanalysis.

Time Constraints

Unless the patient has time to participate and to wait for change, another type of therapy should be considered. The constraint applies especially to emergency symptoms and to those that the patient can no longer tolerate, including those that are dangerous (for example, strong suicide impulses).

Nature of the Relationship

The analysis of friends, relatives, and acquaintances is contraindicated because it distorts the transference and the analyst's objectivity.

Other Contraindications

Some patients work better with some analysts than with others. Sometimes that determination can be made after a single consultation, but often a trial analysis of several sessions is necessary. That time also allows patients to see whether they wish to continue. Experience has shown that it does not matter whether the analyst is a man or a woman, although some patients may initially prefer to see one or the other, a preference that is eventually understood as the analysis proceeds.

DYNAMICS OF THERAPEUTIC RESULTS

The process of improvement and cure involves the release of repression safely and effectively. The structural apparatus of the mind—id, ego, and superego—are modified. The ego is able to deal with repression impulses and is finally in a position to accept or renounce them.

Analysis helps reduce the intensity of the conflicts and helps find acceptable ways of handling impulses that cannot be reduced. Instead of an acceptable method of channeling unmodified infantile strivings, the drives' primary-process quality itself is lessened, and they become adapted to reality. The ultimate goal is the elimination of symptoms, thereby increasing the patient's capacity for work, enjoyment, and self-understanding.

Few long-term outcome studies of psychoanalysis have been conducted because of the complex patient–therapist variables. Nevertheless, psychoanalysis is effective under the proper circumstances for many disorders.

PSYCHOANALYTIC PSYCHOTHERAPY

Psychoanalytic psychotherapy is therapy based on psychoanalytic formulations that have been modified conceptually and technically. Unlike psychoanalysis, which has as its ultimate concern the uncovering and the subsequent working through of infantile conflicts as they arise in the transference neurosis, psychoanalytic psychotherapy takes as its focus the patient's current conflicts and current dynamic patterns—that is, the analysis of the patient's problems with other persons and with themselves. Also unlike psychoanalysis, which has as its technique the use of free association and the analysis of the transference neurosis, psychoanalytic psychotherapy is characterized by interviewing and discussion techniques that infrequently use free association. And again unlike psychoanalysis, psychoanalytic psychotherapy usually limits its work on transference to a discussion of the patient's reactions to the psychiatrist and others. The reaction to the psychiatrist is not interpreted as much as it is in psychoanalysis. Nevertheless, transference attitude and responses to the therapist may arise from time to time and can be used productively. For example, spontaneous transference in the therapeutic situation may give valuable clues to patients' behavior in extratherapeutic situations and, at times, to their childhood. Those transferences may tell the therapist the probable focus for the patient at any given time, inside or outside the treatment relationship.

TREATMENT TECHNIQUES

One way in which psychoanalytic psychotherapy differs from classic psychoanalysis is that the former does not usually use a couch. The stimulation of temporary regressive patterns of feelings and thinking, which is valuable to psychoanalysis, is much less necessary in psychoanalytic psychotherapy, with its focus on current dynamic patterns. In psychoanalytic psychotherapy, the patient and the therapist are usually in full view of each other, which may make the therapist seem real and not a composite of projected fantasies. That type of therapy is much more flexible than psychoanalysis, and it may be used in conjunction with psychotropic medication more often than is psychoanalysis.

Psychoanalytic psychotherapy can range from a single supportive interview, centering on a current but pressing problem, to many years of treatment, with one to three interviews a week of varying length. In contrast to psychoanalysis, psychoanalytic psychotherapy treats most of the disorders in the field of psychopathology.

Role of Insight

Insight is patients' understanding of their psychological functioning and personalities. The clinician should specify the area or the level of understanding or experience into which the patient is to achieve insight. In insight-oriented therapy (such as psychoanalytic or psychodynamic psychotherapy), the psychiatrist emphasizes the value of new insights into the current dynamics of patients' feelings, responses, behavior, and, especially, current relationships with other persons. To a smaller extent, the emphasis is on the value of developing some insight into patients' responses to the therapist and responses in childhood.

Insight-oriented therapy is the treatment of choice for a patient who has adequate ego strength but who, for one reason or another, should not or cannot undergo psychoanalysis.

The therapy's effectiveness does not depend solely on the insights developed or used. The patient's therapeutic response is also based on such factors as the ventilation of feelings in a nonjudgmental but limit-setting atmosphere, identification with the therapist, and other relationship factors. A therapeutic relationship does not require an indiscriminate acceptance of all that a patient says and does. At times, the therapist must intervene on the side of a relatively weak ego by giving unmistakable evidence that the patient could try to achieve a better adjustment or by setting realistic limits to the patient's maladaptive behavior. In so doing, therapists try to be guided by their dynamic assessments of the situation and not by their countertransference responses.

Inevitably, the therapist's attitudes and responses to the patient are different from those of important figures in the patient's childhood. At times, the therapist discusses those differences. Patients may come to see that they have generalized their parents' attitudes as being universal and have generalized their own responses; thus, their responses to all parental or significant figures have become automatic.

Insight-oriented psychotherapy is frequently complicated by spontaneous strong transferences to the therapist that at times threaten to disrupt the treatment. The insight-oriented therapist must decide, on the basis of an understanding of each individual patient, how to respond to those transference reactions. If the patient is highly introspective and psychologically minded, the therapist may choose to make relatively deep transference interpretations (for example, relating the reactions to significant childhood fantasies). If the patient is fragile and not capable of tolerating an interpretation that is perceived as emotionally threatening, the therapist may choose to remain relatively superficial in approach (for example, relating the reactions to current, reality-based feelings).

Supportive Psychotherapy

Supportive psychotherapy (also called *relationship-oriented psychotherapy*) offers the patient support by an authority figure during a period of illness, turmoil, or temporary decompensation. It also has the goal of restoring and strengthening the patient's defenses and integrating capacities that have been impaired. It provides a period of acceptance and dependence for a patient who needs help in dealing with guilt, shame, and anxiety and in meeting the frustration or the external pressures that may be too great to handle.

Supportive therapy uses a number of methods, either singly or in combination, including (1) warm, friendly, strong leadership, (2) gratification of dependence needs, (3) support in the ultimate development of legitimate independence, (4) help in the development of pleasurable sublimations (for example, hobbies), (5) adequate rest and diversion, (6) removal of excessive external strain if possible, (7) hospitalization when indicated, (8) medication to alleviate symptoms, and (9) guidance and advice in dealing with current issues.

One of the greatest dangers lies in the possibility of fostering too great a regression and too strong a dependence. From the beginning, the psychiatrist must plan to work persistently to enable the patient to assume independence. But some patients require supportive therapy indefinitely, often with just the goal of maintaining a marginal adjustment that enables them to function in society.

The expression of emotion is an important part of supportive psychotherapy. The verbalization of unexpressed strong emotions may bring considerable relief. The goal of such talking out is not primarily to gain insight into the unconscious

Table 31.1–1
Scope of Psychoanalytic Practice: A Clinical Continuum[a]

Feature	Psychoanalysis	Psychoanalytic Psychotherapy	
		Expressive Mode	Supportive Mode
Frequency	Regular four to five times a week: 50-minute hour	Regular one to three times a week: half to full hour	Flexible one time a week or less; or as needed, half to full hour
Duration	Long-term: usually 3 to 5+ years	Short-term or long-term: several sessions to months or years	Short-term or intermittent long-term; single session to lifetime
Setting	Patient primarily on couch with analyst out of view	Patient and therapist face-to-face; occasional use of couch	Patient and therapist face-to-face; couch contraindicated
Modus operandi	Systematic analysis of all (positive and negative) transference and resistance; primary focus on analyst and intrasession events; transference neurosis facilitated; regression encouraged	Partial analysis of dynamics and defenses; focus on current interpersonal events and transference to others outside sessions; analysis of negative transference; positive transference left unexplored unless it impedes progress; limited regression encouraged	Formation of therapeutic alliance and real object relationship; analysis of transference contraindicated with rare exceptions; focus on conscious external events; regression discouraged
Analyst–therapist role	Absolute neutrality; frustration of patient; reflector–mirror role	Modified neutrality; implicit gratification of patient and great activity	Neutrality suspended; limited explicit gratification, direction, and disclosure
Mutative change agents	Insight predominates within relatively deprived environment	Insight within empathic environment; identification with benevolent object	Auxiliary or surrogate ego as temporary substitute; holding environment; insight to degree possible
Patient population	Neuroses; mild character psychopathology	Neuroses; mild to moderate character psychopathology, especially narcissistic and borderline personality disorders	Severe character disorders; latent or manifest psychoses; acute crises; physical illness
Patient requisites	High motivation; psychological-mindedness; good previous object relationships; ability to maintain transference neurosis; good frustration tolerance	High to moderate motivation and psychological-mindedness; ability to form therapeutic alliance; some frustration tolerance	Some degree of motivation and ability to form therapeutic alliance
Basic goals	Structural reorganization of personality; resolution of unconscious conflicts; insight into intrapsychic events; symptom relief an indirect result	Partial reorganization of personality and defenses; resolution of preconscious and conscious derivatives of conflicts; insight into current interpersonal events; improved object relations; symptom relief a goal or prelude to further exploration	Reintegration of self and ability to cope; stabilization or restoration of preexisting equilibrium; strengthening defenses; better adjustment or acceptance of pathological symptom relief and environmental restructuring as primary goals
Major techniques	Free association method predominates; fully dynamic interpretation (including confrontation, clarification, and working through), with emphasis on genetic reconstruction	Limited free association; confrontation, clarification, and partial interpretation predominate, with emphasis on here-and-now interpretation and limited genetic interpretation	Free association method contraindicated; suggestions (advice) predominates; abreaction useful; confrontation, clarification, and interpretation in the here and now secondary; genetic interpretation contraindicated
Adjunct treatment	Primarily avoided; if applied, all negative and positive meanings and implications thoroughly analyzed	May be necessary (e.g., psychotropic drugs as temporary measure); if applied, negative implications explored and diffused	Often necessary (e.g., psychotropic drugs, family therapy, rehabilitative therapy, or hospitalization) if applied, positive implications are emphasized

[a]This division is not categorical; all practice resides on a clinical continuum.
Table by Toksoz Byram Karasu, M.D.

dynamic patterns than may be intensifying current responses. Rather, the reduction of inner tension and anxiety may result from the expression of emotion, and its subsequent discussion may lead to insight into a current problem and objectivity in evaluating it.

Corrective Emotional Experience.   The relationship between the therapist and the patient gives the therapist an opportunity to display behavior different from the destructive or unproductive behavior of the patient's parents. At times, such experiences seem to neutralize or reverse some of the effects of the parents' mistakes. If the patient had overly authoritarian parents, the therapist's friendly, flexible, nonjudgmental, nonauthoritarian—but at times firm and limit-setting—attitude means that the patient has an opportunity to adjust to, be led by, and identify with a new type of parent figure. Franz Alexander called that process a *corrective emotional experience.*

Providing a corrective emotional experience in psychotherapy is suitable for a variety of psychogenic illnesses. For example, it may be useful when a patient resists an insight-oriented psychotherapy or is considered too emotionally disturbed for such a procedure. Supportive therapy may be chosen when the diagnostic assessment indicates that a gradual maturing process, based on the elaboration of new foci for identification, is the most promising path toward improvement. Table 31.1–1 outlines a comparison and description of the types of therapies discussed in this section.

▲ 31.2 Brief Psychotherapy

The brief psychotherapies are an important component of current methods to treat a variety of mental disorders. Short-term treatment methods (also called *time-limited psychotherapy*) not only help people deal with current problems and crises. They are also useful for major mental disorders such as depression, anxiety, and posttraumatic stress disorder, among others. Derived from psychoanalytic and learning theories, these therapies have their own treatment techniques and specific criteria for selecting patients. Short-term therapies have gained widespread popularity, partly because of the great pressure on health care professionals to contain treatment costs. It is also easier to evaluate treatment efficacy by comparing groups of people who have undergone short-term therapy for mental illness with control groups than it is to measure the results of long-term psychotherapy. Thus, short-term therapies have been the subject of much research, especially on outcome, and have been found to be effective.

BRIEF PSYCHOTHERAPY

History

In 1946, Franz Alexander and Thomas French identified most of the basic characteristics of brief psychotherapy. They described a therapeutic experience designed to put patients at ease, to manipulate the transference, and to flexibly use trial interpretations. Alexander and French emphasized developing a corrective emotional experience capable of repairing traumatic events of the past and convincing patients that new ways of thinking, feeling, and behaving are possible. At about the same time, Eric Lindemann established a consultation service at the Massachusetts General Hospital in Boston for people experiencing a crisis. He developed new treatment methods to deal with these situations and eventually applied these techniques to people who were not in crisis but who were experiencing various kinds of emotional distress. Since then, the field has been influenced by many workers such as David Malan and Michael Balint in England, Peter Sifneos and Myrna Weissman in

America, and Habib Davanloo in Canada. Their work is discussed below.

Types

Brief Focal Psychotherapy (Tavistock-Malan). Brief focal psychotherapy was originally developed in the 1950s by the Michael Balint team at the Tavistock Clinic in London. Malan, a member of the team, reported the results of the therapy. Malan's selection criteria for treatment included eliminating absolute contraindications, rejecting patients for whom certain dangers seemed inevitable, clearly assessing patients' psychopathology, and determining patients' capacities to consider problems in emotional terms, face disturbing material, respond to interpretations, and endure the stress of the treatment. Malan found that high motivation invariably correlated with successful outcome. Contraindications to treatment were serious suicidal attempts, substance dependence, chronic alcohol abuse, incapacitating chronic obsessional symptoms, incapacitating chronic phobic symptoms, and gross destructive or self-destructive acting out.

REQUIREMENTS AND TECHNIQUES. In Malan's routine, therapists should identify the transference early and interpret it and the negative transference. They should then link the transferences to patients' relationships to their parents. Both patients and therapists should be willing to become deeply involved and to bear the ensuing tension. Therapists should formulate circumscribed focus and set a termination date in advance, and patients should work through grief and anger about termination. An experienced therapist should allow approximately 20 sessions as an average length for the therapy; a trainee should allow about 30 sessions. Malan himself did not exceed 40 interviews with his patients.

Time-Limited Psychotherapy (Boston University–Mann). A psychotherapeutic model of exactly 12 interviews focusing on a specified central issue was developed at Boston University by James Mann and his colleagues in the early 1970s. In contrast with Malan's emphasis on clear-cut selection and rejection criteria, Mann has not been as explicit about the appropriate candidates for time-limited psychotherapy. Mann considered determining a patient's central conflict reasonably correctly and exploring young people's maturational crises with many psychological and somatic complaints to be the major emphases of his theory. Mann's exceptions, similar to his rejection criteria, include people with major depressive disorder that interferes with the treatment agreement, those with acute psychotic states, and desperate patients who need, but cannot tolerate, object relations.

REQUIREMENTS AND TECHNIQUES. Mann's technical requirements included strict limitation to 12 sessions, positive transference predominating early, specification and strict adherence to a central issue involving transference, positive identification, making separation a maturational event for patients, and the absolute prospect of termination to avoid development of dependence. The role of the therapist is active; he or she clarifies present and past experiences and resistances and educates patients through direct information, reeducation, and manipulation. The conflicts likely to be encountered included independence versus dependence, activity versus passivity, unresolved or delayed grief, and adequate verses inadequate self-esteem.

Short-Term Dynamic Psychotherapy (McGill University–Davanloo).

As conducted by Habib Davanloo at McGill University, short-term dynamic psychotherapy encompasses nearly all varieties of brief psychotherapy and crisis intervention. Patients treated in Davanloo's series are classified as those whose psychological conflicts are predominantly oedipal, those whose conflicts are not oedipal, and those whose conflicts have more than one focus. Davanloo also devised a specific psychotherapeutic technique for patients with severe, long-standing neurotic problems, specifically those with incapacitating obsessive-compulsive disorders and phobias.

Davanloo's selection criteria emphasize the evaluation of those ego functions of primary importance to psychotherapeutic work: the establishment of a psychotherapeutic focus, the psychodynamic formulation of patients' psychological problems, the ability to have emotional interaction with evaluators, the history of give-and-take relationships with a significant person in patients' life, patients' ability to experience and tolerate anxiety, guilt, and depression; patients' motivations for change, patients' psychological-mindedness, and patients' ability to respond to interpretation and to link evaluators with people in the present and past. Both Malan and Davanloo emphasized patients' responses to interpretation as an important selection and prognostic criterion.

REQUIREMENTS AND TECHNIQUES. The highlights of Davanloo's psychotherapeutic approach are flexibility (therapists should adapt the technique to patients' needs), control of patients' regressive tendencies, active intervention so as not to allow patients to develop overdependence on a therapist, and patients' intellectual insight and emotional experiences in the transference. These emotional experiences become corrective as a result of the interpretation.

Short-Term Anxiety-Provoking Psychotherapy (Harvard University–Sifneos).

Sifneos developed short-term anxiety-provoking psychotherapy at the Massachusetts General Hospital in Boston during the 1950s. He used the following criteria for selection: a circumscribed chief complaint (implying a patient's ability to select one of a variety of problems to be given top priority and the patient's desire to resolve the problem in treatment), one meaningful or give-and-take relationship during early childhood, the ability to interact flexibly with an evaluator and to express feelings appropriately, above-average psychological sophistication (implying not only above-average intelligence but also an ability to respond to interpretations), a specific psychodynamic formulation (usually a set of psychological conflicts underlying a patient's difficulties and centering on an oedipal focus), a contract between therapist and patient to work on the specified focus and the formulation of minimal expectations of outcome, and good-to-excellent motivation for change and not just for symptom relief.

REQUIREMENTS AND TECHNIQUES. Treatment can be divided into four major phases: patient-therapist encounter, early therapy, height of treatment, and evidence of change and termination. Therapists use the following techniques during the four phases.

Patient–Therapist Encounter. A therapist establishes a working alliance by using the patient's quick rapport with and positive feelings for the therapist that appear in this phase. Judicious use of open-ended and forced-choice questions enables the therapist to outline and concentrate on a therapeutic focus. The therapist specifies the minimum expectations of outcome to be achieved by the therapy.

Early Therapy. In transference, feelings for the therapist are clarified as soon as they appear, a technique that leads to the establishment of a true therapeutic alliance.

Height of the Treatment. This phase emphasizes active concentration on the oedipal conflicts that have been chosen as the therapeutic focus for the therapy; repeated use of anxiety-provoking questions and confrontations; avoidance of pregenital characterological issues, which the patient uses defensively to avoid dealing with the therapist's anxiety-provoking techniques; avoidance at all costs of a transference neurosis; repetitive demonstration of the patient's neurotic ways or maladaptive patterns of behavior; concentration on the anxiety-laden material, even before the defense mechanisms have been clarified; repeated demonstrations of parent-transference links by the use of properly timed interpretations based on material given by the patient; establishment of a corrective emotional experience; encouragement and support of the patient, who becomes anxious while struggling to understand the conflicts; new learning and problem-solving patterns; and repeated presentations and recapitulations of the patient's psychodynamics until the defense mechanisms used in dealing with oedipal conflicts are understood.

Evidence of Change and Termination of Psychotherapy. This phase emphasizes the tangible demonstration of change in the patient's behavior outside therapy, evidence that adaptive patterns of behavior are being used, and initiation of talk about terminating the treatment.

Outcome

The outcomes of these brief treatments have been investigated more extensively than has any other form of psychotherapy. Contrary to prevailing ideas that the therapeutic factors in psychotherapy are nonspecific, controlled studies and other assessment methods (for example, interviews with unbiased evaluators, patients' self-evaluations) point to the importance of the specific techniques used. The capacity for genuine recovery in certain patients is far greater than was thought. A certain type of patient receiving brief psychotherapy can benefit greatly from a practical working through of his or her nuclear conflict in the transference. Such patients can be recognized in advance through a process of dynamic interaction, because they are responsive and motivated and able to face disturbing feelings and because a circumscribed focus can be formulated for them. The more radical the technique in terms of transference, depth of interpretation, and the link to childhood, the more radical the therapeutic effects will be. For some disturbed patients, a carefully chosen partial focus can be therapeutically effective.

INTERPERSONAL PSYCHOTHERAPY

Interpersonal psychotherapy (ITP), a time-limited treatment for major depressive disorder, was developed in the 1970s, defined in a manual, and tested in randomized clinical trials by the late Gerald L. Klerman and Myrna Weissman. Based on the ideas of Harry Stack Sullivan and the interpersonal school, ITP generally deals with current rather than past interpersonal relationships, focusing on the patient's immediate social context. It attempts to intervene in symptom formation and social dysfunction associated with depression. It assumes a connection between the onset of mood disorders (and perhaps other psychiatric disorders) and the interpersonal context in which they occur.

Requirements and Techniques

As short-term treatment for depression, ITP consists of three phases. The first phase generally consists of the first one to three sessions. Its goals are to gather psychiatric history, establish a diagnosis, and introduce the framework for treatment. The psychiatric history explores current social functioning. Particular attention is paid to gathering extensive information about interpersonal events that may have precipitated the depressive episode. The patient's current and past significant interpersonal relationships, including the family of origin, friendships, and community relations, are also reviewed during this first phase. The data gleaned from this review are used to identify one of four problem areas that will guide the therapy: unresolved grief, social role disputes, social role transitions, and interpersonal deficits. Psychiatric diagnosis is informed by standard criteria. Decisions about the concomitant use of medication are based on the severity of the symptoms, past response to interventions, and patient preference. The patient is placed in the sick role; the therapist explicitly discusses the diagnosis of depression and its attendant symptoms as well as explains what the patient can expect from treatment. The depressive syndrome is then related to the patient's main interpersonal theme, which is related to the syndrome's onset.

The middle phase of treatment is directed toward resolving the problem area. Specific goals and strategies are used for each of the four areas. For a patient whose main problem area is unresolved grief, the goals of treatment are to facilitate the mourning process and assist the patient in finding new activities and relationships to offset the loss. In the treatment of interpersonal role disputes, the dispute is identified, a plan of action is chosen, and a satisfactory resolution is sought through the modification of expectations or improved communication. If resolution proves impossible, clients are encouraged to consider terminating that plan of action in favor of finding better ones. For depression associated with role transitions, the patient is helped to mourn and accept the loss of the old role. Efforts are directed to helping the patient regard the new role as more positive than the old one. Self-esteem is enhanced by focusing on the new skills that are mastered in learning the new role. Finally, when interpersonal deficits are the core theme, the therapist encourages the patient to establish relationships and diminish social isolation.

Each session begins with the question "How have things been since we last met?" to focus on current mood states and their association with recent interactions. The basic techniques for handling each problem area are clarifying positive and negative feeling states, identifying past models for relationships, and guiding and encouraging the patient in examining and choosing alternative courses of action.

Interpersonal psychotherapy has been used across a variety of depressed populations: geriatric, adolescent, HIV-infected, dysthymic disorder, bipolar disorder, and depressed patients with marital problems. It has also been used for non-mood psychiatric conditions such as substance abuse and bulimia nervosa.

Ms. A, a 29-year-old never-married vice president in a successful business, presented with a 9-month history of depression complicated by panic attacks. She described her involvement in a relationship with her superior at work, which they both desired but which work policy forbade. Her symptoms emerged under the pressure she felt to resolve this situation, from which she saw no way out. Neither she nor her boyfriend, Bob, wanted to leave their jobs, and neither wanted to end the relationship. Yet exposure of their secret threatened both their jobs.

In this context Ms. A developed the full spectrum of symptoms of major depressive disorder, with a Hamilton Rating Scale for Depression score of 28 on presentation, including intermittent panic attacks and suicidal ideation without attempts. Her work and mood suffered. She had a family history of depression and alcoholism but had no prior symptoms, and she did not drink. She had been in twice-weekly psychodynamic psychotherapy for 2 years, starting after the breakup of a previous relationship. She felt that this therapy had increased her self-understanding but had not helped her symptoms. She had considered but declined to take antidepressant medication, feeling it would not resolve her dilemma.

Although quite depressed, Ms. A quickly agreed that she was in a depressive episode and was able to relate it to her interpersonal situation. This had some aspects of a role transition—a change in her personal and work roles—but was best characterized as a role dispute with Bob: What did she want to happen, and what options did she have to negotiate its happening? A 12-week time limit was set for treatment. Her interpersonal therapist focused on helping her explore various options. She developed a resume and went to a headhunter to seek new job possibilities, although she was ambivalent at leaving her hard-earned and promising post. Role-playing helped her discuss the situation and its possibilities with her lover. Subsequent encounters with Bob better defined the nature of their agreements and differences.

Simply defining the problem and mobilizing Ms. A to constructive action improved her mood and yielded a greater sense of mastery of her situation. ITP also helped her develop interpersonal skills; although Ms. A was appropriately assertive in her work role, she was far more pliant and submissive in her personal relationships, a problem that emerged in reviewing her interpersonal inventory of past romances. Depressive symptoms steadily subsided, but the turning point came in the sixth week of ITP when, after considerable exploration and role-playing in therapy, Ms. A told her boyfriend that she had decided she could not give up her job; either they would have to end the relationship, or he would have to move. He initially said that his own job came first. But several days later he recanted, saying how much he loved her and that he would try to find a new job himself. Her symptoms resolved. Shortly thereafter, a wonderful prospect appeared for Ms. A, in effect giving her a promotion at a different, related company and allowing the relationship to continue overtly. She attributed her symptomatic improvement to her newly firm stand, not to the job change. On 6-month follow-up, she remained euthymic without panic attacks and felt she was holding her own in a relationship that was going more smoothly than previous relationships ever had. (Courtesy of Myrna M. Weissman, M.D., and John C. Markowitz, Ph.D.)

Results

The efficacy of IPT or a treatment for acute depression has been demonstrated in several randomized trials. In one study, ITP was comparable to imipramine (Tofranil) in depressed patients and combined drug-ITP treatment was better than either alone. ITP also improves interpersonal relationships and social functioning, which are not addressed in psychopharmacologic treatment. Trials are under way in other depressive disorders such as dysthymia, postpartum depression, eating disorders, and borderline personally disorders. ITP has not been of use when compared with standard treatment for opioid- and cocaine-dependent patients. Monthly maintenance ITP has been used successfully in patient recurrences of depressive episodes in some patients.

▲ 31.3 Group Psychotherapy, Combined Individual and Group Psychotherapy, and Psychodrama

GROUP PSYCHOTHERAPY

Group psychotherapy is a treatment in which carefully selected people who are emotionally ill meet in a group guided by a trained therapist and help one another effect personality change. By using a variety of technical maneuvers and theoretical constructs, the leader directs group members' interactions to bring about changes.

Group psychotherapy encompasses the theoretical spectrum of therapies in psychiatry: supportive, structured, limit-setting (for example, groups with chronically psychotic people), cognitive-behavioral, interpersonal, family, and analytically oriented groups. Compared with individual therapies, two of the main strengths of group therapy are the opportunity for immediate feedback from a patient's peers and the chance for both patient and therapist to observe a patient's psychological, emotional, and behavioral responses to a variety of people, who elicit a variety of transferences.

Patient Selection

To determine a patient's suitability for group psychotherapy, a therapist needs a great deal of information, which is gathered in a screening interview. The psychiatrist should take a psychiatric history and perform a mental status examination to obtain certain dynamic, behavioral, and diagnostic information.

Authority Anxiety.   Those patients whose primary problem is their relationship to authority and who are extremely anxious in the presence of authority figures may or may not do well in group therapy because they are more comfortable in a group than in a dyadic (one-to-one) setting. Patients with a great deal of authority anxiety may be blocked, anxious, resistant, and unwilling to verbalize thoughts and feelings in an individual setting, generally for fear of the therapist's censure or disapproval. Thus, they may welcome the suggestion of

group psychotherapy to avoid the scrutiny of the dyadic situation. Conversely, if a patient reacts negatively to the suggestion of group psychotherapy or openly resists the idea, the therapist should consider the possibility that the patient has a high degree of peer anxiety.

> Ms. B was referred to group treatment after her fifth serious suicide attempt; each of which had occurred during the absence of her individual therapist. She came to the group most reluctantly, fearful that she was going to be dropped off in the group and abandoned. She viewed the group leader with much distrust but found three members of the group who could empathize with her plight and who had also suffered similar self-destructive incidents and could help her move away from taking action. Her presence in the group was stormy and embattled for years, but eventually she became a strong proponent of group treatment. Notably, she was never hospitalized after joining the group. Finally, she concluded her individual work and remained in the group with the full agreement of both therapists. (Courtesy of Anne Alonso, Ph.D.)

Peer Anxiety.   Patients with conditions such as borderline and schizoid personality disorders who have destructive relationships with their peer groups or who have been extremely isolated from peer group contact generally react negatively or anxiously when placed in a group setting. When such patients can work through their anxiety, however, group therapy can be beneficial.

Diagnosis.   The diagnosis of patients' disorders is important in determining the best therapeutic approach and in evaluating patients' motivations for treatment, capacities for change, and personality structure strengths and weaknesses. There are few contraindications to group therapy. Antisocial patients generally do poorly in a heterogeneous group setting because they cannot adhere to group standards; but if the group is composed of other antisocial patients, they may respond better to peers than to perceived authority figures. Depressed patients profit from group therapy after they have established a trusting relationship with the therapist. Patients who are actively suicidal or severely depressed should not be treated solely in a group setting. Manic patients are disruptive but, once under pharmacological control, do well in the group setting. Patients who are delusional and who may incorporate the group into their delusional system should be excluded, as should patients who pose a physical threat to other members because of uncontrollable aggressive outbursts.

Preparation

Patients prepared by a therapist for a group experience tend to continue in treatment longer and report less initial anxiety than do those who are not so prepared. The preparation consists of a therapist's explaining, before the first session, the procedure in as much detail as possible and answering the patient's questions.

Size.   Group therapy has been successful with as few as three members and as many as 15, but most therapists consider eight to ten members the optimal size. There may be insufficient interaction with fewer members unless they are especially verbal, and with more than ten members the interaction may be too great for the members or the therapist to follow.

Frequency and Length of Sessions.

Most group psychotherapists conduct group sessions once a week. Maintaining continuity in sessions is important. When there are alternate sessions, the group meets twice a week, once with and once without the therapist. Group sessions generally last anywhere from one to two hours, but the time limit set should be constant.

Homogeneous versus Heterogeneous Groups.

Most therapists believe that groups should be as heterogeneous as possible to ensure maximum interaction. Members with different diagnostic categories and varied behavioral patterns, from all races, social levels, and educational backgrounds, and of varying ages and both sexes should be brought together. Patients between ages 20 and 65 can be effectively included in the same group. Age differences aid in developing of parent–child and brother–sister models, and patients have the opportunity to relive and rectify interpersonal difficulties that may have appeared insurmountable.

Both children and adolescents are best treated in groups composed mostly of people in their own age groups. Some adolescent patients are capable of assimilating the material of an adult group, regardless of content, but they should not be deprived of a constructive peer experience that they may otherwise not have.

Open versus Closed Groups.

Closed groups have a set number and composition of patients. If members leave, no new members are accepted. In open groups, membership is more fluid, and new members are taken on whenever old members leave.

Mechanisms

Group Formation.

Each patient approaches group therapy differently, and in this sense groups are microcosms. Patients use typical adaptive abilities, defense mechanisms, and ways of relating, and when these tactics are ultimately reflected back to them by the group, patients learn to be introspective about their personality functioning. A process inherent in group formation requires that patients suspend their previous ways of coping. In entering the group, they allow their executive ego functions—reality testing, adaptation to and mastery of the environment, and perception—to be assumed to some degree by the collective assessment provided by the total membership, including the leader.

Therapeutic Factors.

Table 31.3–1 outlines 20 significant therapeutic factors that account for change in group psychotherapy.

Role of the Therapist

Although opinions differ about how active or passive a group therapist should be, the consensus is that the therapist's role is primarily facilitative. Ideally, the group members themselves are the primary source of cure and change. The climate produced by the therapist's personality is a potent agent of change. The therapist is more than an expert applying techniques; he or she exerts a personal influence that taps such variables as empathy, warmth, and respect.

Inpatient Group Psychotherapy

Group therapy is an important part of hospitalized patients' therapeutic experiences. Groups may be organized in many ways on a ward. In a community meeting, an entire inpatient unit meets with all the staff members (for example, psychiatrists, psychologists, and nurses). In team meetings, 15 to 20 patients and staff members meet; a regular or small group composed of eight to ten patients may meet with one or two therapists, as in traditional group therapy. Although the goals of each group vary, they all have common purposes: to increase patients' awareness of themselves through their interactions with the other group members, who provide feedback about their behavior; to provide patients with improved interpersonal and social skills; to help the members adapt to an inpatient setting; and to improve communication between patients and staff. In addition, one type of group meeting is attended only by inpatient hospital staff and is meant to improve communication among the staff members and to provide mutual support and encouragement in their day-to-day work with patients. Community meetings and team meetings are more helpful for dealing with patient treatment problems than they are for providing insight-oriented therapy, which is the province of the small-group therapy meeting.

Self-Help Groups

Self-help groups are composed of people who are trying to cope with a specific problem or life crisis. Usually organized with a particular task in mind, such groups do not attempt to explore individual psychodynamics in great depth or to change personality functioning significantly. But self-help groups have improved the emotional health and well-being of many persons.

A distinguishing characteristic of the self-help groups is their homogeneity. The members have the same disorders and share their experiences—good and bad, successful and unsuccessful—with one another. By so doing, they educate each other, provide mutual support, and alleviate the sense of alienation usually felt by people drawn to this kind of group.

Self-help groups emphasize cohesion, which is exceptionally strong in these groups. Because of the group members' similar problems and symptoms, they develop a strong emotional bond. Each group may have its unique characteristics, to which the members can attribute magical qualities of healing. Examples of self-help groups are Alcoholics Anonymous (AA), Gamblers Anonymous (GA), and Overeaters Anonymous (OA).

Self-help groups and therapy groups have begun to converge: Self-help groups have enabled their members to give up patterns of unwanted behavior; therapy groups have helped their members understand why and how they got to be the way they were or are.

COMBINED INDIVIDUAL AND GROUP PSYCHOTHERAPY

In combined individual and group psychotherapy, patients individually see a therapist and also take part in group sessions. The therapist for the group and individual sessions is usually the same person. Groups can vary in size from 3 to 15 members, but the most helpful size is eight to ten. Patients must attend all group sessions. Attendance at individual sessions is also important, and the failure to attend either group or individual sessions should be examined as part of the therapeutic process.

Table 31.3–1
Twenty Therapeutic Factors in Group Psychotherapy

Factor	Definition
Abreaction	A process by which repressed material, particularly a painful experience or conflict, is brought back to consciousness. In the process, the person not only recalls but relives the material, which is accompanied by the appropriate emotional response; insight usually results from the experience.
Acceptance	The feeling of being accepted by other members of the group; differences of opinion are tolerated, and there is an absence of censure.
Altruism	The act of one member helping another; putting another person's need before one's own and learning that there is value in giving to others. The term was originated by Auguste Comte (1798–1857), and Sigmund Freud believed it was a major factor in establishing group cohesion and community feeling.
Catharsis	The expression of ideas, thoughts, and suppressed material that is accompanied by an emotional response that produces a state of relief in the patient.
Cohesion	The sense that the group is working together toward a common goal; also referred to as a sense of "we-ness"; believed to be the most important factor related to positive therapeutic effects.
Consensual validation	Confirmation of reality by comparing one's own conceptualizations with those of other group members; interpersonal distortions are thereby corrected. The term was introduced by Harry Stack Sullivan; Trigant Burrow had used the phrase "consensual observation" to refer to the same phenomenon.
Contagion	The process in which the expression of emotion by one member stimulates the awareness of a similar emotion in another member.
Corrective familial experience	The group re-creates the family of origin for some members who can work through original conflicts psychologically through group interaction (e.g., sibling rivalry, anger toward parents).
Empathy	The capacity of a group member to put himself or herself into the psychological frame of reference of another group member and thereby understand his or her thinking, feeling, or behavior.
Identification	An unconscious defense mechanism in which the person incorporates the characteristics and the qualities of another person or object into his or her ego system.
Imitation	The conscious emulation or modeling of one's behavior after that of another (also called *role modeling*); also known as spectator therapy, as one patient learns from another.
Insight	Conscious awareness and understanding of one's own psychodynamics and symptoms of maladaptive behavior. Most therapists distinguish two types: (1) intellectual insight—knowledge and awareness without any changes in maladaptive behavior; (2) emotional insight—awareness and understanding leading to positive changes in personality and behavior.
Inspiration	The process of imparting a sense of optimism to group members; the ability to recognize that one has the capacity to overcome problems; also known as instillation of hope.
Interaction	The free and open exchange of ideas and feelings among group members; effective interaction is emotionally charged.
Interpretation	The process during which the group leader formulates the meaning or significance of a patient's resistance, defenses, and symbols; the result is that the patient has a cognitive framework within which to understand his or her behavior.
Learning	Patients acquire knowledge about new areas, such as social skills and sexual behavior; they receive advice, obtain guidance, and attempt to influence and are influenced by other group members.
Reality testing	Ability of the person to evaluate objectively the world outside the self; includes the capacity to perceive oneself and other group members accurately. *See also* Consensual validation.
Transference	Projection of feelings, thoughts, and wishes onto the therapist, who has come to represent an object from the patient's past. Such reactions, while perhaps appropriate for the condition prevailing in the patient's earlier life, are inappropriate and anachronistic when applied to the therapist in the present. Patients in the group may also direct such feelings toward one another, a process called *multiple transferences*.
Universalization	The awareness of the patient that he or she is not alone in having problems; others share similar complaints or difficulties in learning; the patient is not unique.
Ventilation	The expression of suppressed feelings, ideas, or events to other group members; the sharing of personal secrets that ameliorate a sense of sin or guilt (also referred to as *self-disclosure*).

Combined therapy is a particular treatment modality, not a system by which individual therapy is augmented by an occasional group session or a group therapy in which a participant meets alone with a therapist from time to time. Rather, it is an ongoing plan in which the group experience interacts meaningfully with the individual sessions and in which reciprocal feedback helps form an integrated therapeutic experience. Although the one-to-one doctor–patient relationship makes possible a deep examination of the transference reaction for some patients, it may not provide the corrective emotional experi-

ences necessary for therapeutic change for other patients. The group gives patients a variety of people with whom they can have transferential reactions. In the microcosm of the group, patients can relive and work through familial and other important influences.

Most workers in the field believe that combined therapy has the advantages of both dyadic and group settings, without sacrificing the qualities of either. Generally, the dropout rate in combined therapy is lower than that in group therapy alone. In many cases, combined therapy appears to bring problems to the surface and to resolve them more quickly than may be possible with either method alone.

PSYCHODRAMA

Psychodrama is a method of group psychotherapy originated by the Viennese-born psychiatrist Jacob Moreno in which personality makeup, interpersonal relationships, conflicts, and emotional problems are explored by means of special dramatic methods. Therapeutic dramatization of emotional problems includes the protagonist or patient, the person who acts out problems with the help of auxiliary egos, people who enact varying aspects of the patient, and the director, psychodramatist, or therapist, the person who guides those in the drama toward the acquisition of insight.

Techniques

The psychodrama may focus on any special area of functioning (a dream, a family, or a community situation), a symbolic role, an unconscious attitude, or an imagined future situation. Such symptoms as delusions and hallucinations can also be acted out in the group. Techniques to advance the therapeutic process and to increase productivity and creativity include the soliloquy (a recital of overt and hidden thoughts and feelings), role reversal (the exchange of the patient's role for the role of a significant person), the double (an auxiliary ego acting as the patient), the multiple double (several egos acting as the patient did on varying occasions), and the mirror technique (an ego imitating the patient and speaking for him or her). Other techniques include the use of hypnosis and psychoactive drugs to modify the acting behavior in various ways.

▲ 31.4 Family Therapy and Couples Therapy

FAMILY THERAPY

Family therapy is any intervention that focuses on altering the interactions among family members and attempts to improve the functioning of the family as a unit of individual members of the family. The clinician conducting family therapy attempts to interrupt rigid intergenerational patterns that cause distress within or between individuals. Family therapy can address the concerns of any family member, yet it is most likely to influence children, whose daily reality is directly affected by family context.

Theoretical Issues

According to family systems theory, family units act as though each has its own homeostasis of interacting that must be maintained at any cost. Family therapy aims to bring to light the often hidden patterns that maintain the group's balance and to help the group understand the purposes of the pattern. Family therapists generally think that one family member has been labeled as the patient whom the family identifies as "the one who is the problem, is to blame, and needs help." A family therapist's goal is to help a family understand that the identified patient's symptoms in fact serve the crucial function of maintaining the family's homeostasis. The process of family therapy helps reveal a family's repetitious and ultimately predictable communication patterns that sustain and reflect the identified patient's behavior.

Inherent in family systems theory is the belief, to one degree or another, that a marital relationship strongly influences the nature of a family's system of homeostasis. One influential family therapist has expressed this concept by describing the marital dyad as the "architects of the family."

Techniques

Initial Consultation. Family therapy is familiar enough to the general public for families with a high level of conflict to request it specifically. When the initial complaint is about an individual family member, however, pretreatment work may be needed. Underlying resistance to a family approach typically includes fears by parents that they will be blamed for their child's difficulties, that the entire family will be pronounced sick, that a spouse will object, and that open discussion of one child's misbehavior will have a negative influence on siblings. Refusal by an adolescent or young adult patient to participate in family therapy is frequently a disguised collusion with the fears of one or both parents.

Interview Technique. The special quality of a family interview springs from two important facts: A family comes to treatment with its history and dynamics firmly in place. To a family therapist, the established nature of the group, more than the symptoms, constitutes the clinical problem. Family members usually live together and, at some level, depend on one another for their physical and emotional well-being. Whatever transpires in the therapy session is known to all. Central principles of technique also derive from these facts. For example, the therapist must carefully channel the catharsis of anger by one family member toward another. The person who is the object of the anger will react to the attack, and the anger may escalate into violence and fracture relationships, with one or more member withdrawing from therapy. For another example, free association is inappropriate in family therapy because it can encourage one person to dominate a session. Thus, therapists must always control and direct the family interview.

Virginia Satir recommended initiating at least the first two sessions of family therapy with a family-life chronology. The technique reflects many family therapy paradigms.

Frequency and Length of Treatment. Unless an emergency arises, sessions are usually held no more than once a week. Each session, however, may require as much as 2 hours. Long sessions can include an intermission to give the therapist time to organize the material and plan a response. A flexible schedule is necessary when geography or personal circumstances make it physically difficult for the family to get together. The length of treatment depends not only on the nature of the problem but also on the therapeutic model. Therapists who exclusively use problem-solving models may accomplish their goals in a few sessions while therapists using growth-oriented models may work with a family for years and may schedule sessions at long intervals.

Modifications of Techniques

Family Group Therapy.   Family group therapy combines several families into a single group. Families share mutual problems and compare their interactions with those of the other families in the group. Treatment of schizophrenia has been effective in multiple family groups. Parents of disturbed children may also meet together to share their situations.

Social Network Therapy.   In social network therapy, the social community or network of a disturbed patient meets in group sessions with the patient. The network includes those with whom the patient comes into contact in daily life, not only the immediate family but also relatives, friends, tradespersons, teachers, and co-workers.

Paradoxical Therapy.   In this approach, which evolved from the work of Gregory Bateson, a therapist suggests that the patient intentionally engage in the unwanted behavior (called the *paradoxical injunction*), and, for example, avoid a phobic object or perform a compulsive ritual. Although paradoxical therapy and the use of paradoxical injunctions are relatively new, the therapy can create new insights for some patients. It is used in individual therapy as well as in family therapy.

Reframing.   Reframing, also known as *positive connotation*, is a relabeling of all negatively expressed feelings or behavior as positive. When the therapist attempts to get family members to view behavior from a new frame of reference, "This child is impossible" becomes "This child is desperately trying to distract and protect you from what he or she perceives as an unhappy marriage." Reframing is an important process that allows family members to view themselves in new ways that can produce change.

Goals

Family therapy has several goals: to resolve or reduce pathogenic conflict and anxiety within the matrix of interpersonal relationships; to enhance the perception and fulfillment by family members of one another's emotional needs; to promote appropriate role relationships between the sexes and generations; to strengthen the capacity of individual members and the family as a whole to cope with destructive forces inside and outside the surrounding environment; and to influence family identity and values so that members are oriented toward health and growth. The therapy ultimately aims to integrate families into the large systems of society, extended family, community groups, and social systems such as schools, medical facilities, and social, recreational, and welfare agencies.

COUPLES (MARITAL) THERAPY

Couples or marital therapy is a form of psychotherapy designed to psychologically modify the interaction of two people who are in conflict with each other over one parameter or a variety of parameters—social, emotional, sexual, or economic. In couples therapy, a trained person establishes a therapeutic contract with a patient-couple and, through definite types of communication, attempts to alleviate the disturbance, to reverse or change maladaptive patterns of behavior, and to encourage personality growth and development.

Marriage counseling may be considered more limited in scope than marriage therapy: Only a particular familial conflict is discussed, and the counseling is primarily task oriented, geared to solving a specific problem such as child rearing. Marriage therapy, by contrast, emphasizes restructuring a couple's interaction and sometimes explores the psychodynamics of each partner. Both therapy and counseling stress helping marital partners to cope effectively with their problems. Most important is the definition of appropriate and realistic goals, which may involve extensive reconstruction of the union or problem-solving approaches or a combination of both.

Types of Therapy

Individual Therapy.   In individual therapy, the partners may consult different therapists, who do not necessarily communicate with each other and indeed may not even know each other. The goal of treatment is to strengthen each partner's adaptive capacities. At times, only one of the partners is in treatment; and in such cases, it is often helpful for the person who is not in treatment to visit the therapist. The visiting partner may give the therapist data about the patient that may otherwise be overlooked, overt or covert anxiety in the visiting partner as a result of change in the patient can be identified and dealt with, irrational beliefs about treatment events can be corrected, and conscious or unconscious attempts by the partner to sabotage the patient's treatment can be examined.

Individual Couples Therapy.   In individual couples therapy, each partner is in therapy, which is either concurrent, with the same therapist, or collaborative, with each partner seeing a different therapist.

Conjoint Therapy.   Conjoint therapy is the most common treatment method in couples therapy, in which either one or two therapists treat the partners in joint sessions. Cotherapy with therapists of both sexes prevents a particular patient from feeling ganged up on when confronted by two members of the opposite sex.

Four-Way Session.   In a four-way session, each partner is seen by a different therapist, with regular joint sessions in which all four people participate. A variation of the four-way session is the roundtable interview, developed by William Masters and Virginia Johnson for the rapid treatment of sexually dysfunctional couples. Two patients and two opposite-sex therapists meet regularly.

Group Psychotherapy.   Group therapy for couples allows a variety of group dynamics to affect the participants. Groups usually consist of three to four couples and one or two therapists. The couples identify with one another and recognize that others have similar problems, each gains support and empathy from fellow group members of the same or opposite sex, they explore sexual attitudes and have an opportunity to gain new information from their peer groups, and each receives specific feedback about his or her behavior, either negative or positive, that may have more meaning and be better assimilated coming from a neutral nonspouse member, for example, than from the spouse or the therapist.

Combined Therapy. *Combined therapy* refers to all or any of the preceding techniques used concurrently or in combination. Thus, a particular patient-couple may begin treatment with one or both partners in individual psychotherapy, continue in conjoint therapy with the partner, and terminate therapy after a course of treatment in a married couples group. The rationale for combined therapy is that no single approach to marital problems has been shown to be superior to another. A familiarity with a variety of approaches thus allows therapists a degree of flexibility that provides maximum benefit for couples in distress.

Indications

Whatever the specific therapeutic technique, initiation of couples therapy is indicated when individual therapy has failed to resolve the relationship difficulties, when the onset of distress in one or both partners is clearly a relational problem, and when couples therapy is requested by a couple in conflict. Problems in communication between partners are a prime indication for couples therapy. In such instances, one spouse may be intimidated by the other, may become anxious when attempting to tell the other about thoughts or feelings, or may project unconscious expectations onto the other. The therapy is geared toward enabling each partner to see the other realistically.

Conflicts in one or several areas, such as the partners' sexual life, are also indications for treatment. Similarly, difficulty in establishing satisfactory social, economic, parental, or emotional roles implies that a couple needs help. Clinicians should evaluate all aspects of the marital relationship before attempting to treat only one problem, which could be a symptom of a pervasive marital disorder.

Contraindications

Contraindications for couples therapy include patients with severe forms of psychosis, particularly patients with paranoid elements and those in whom the marriage's homeostatic mechanism is a protection against psychosis, marriages in which one or both partners really want to divorce, and marriages in which one spouse refuses to participate because of anxiety or fear.

Goals

Nathan Ackerman defined the aims of couples therapy as follows: The goals of therapy for partner relational problems are to alleviate emotional distress and disability and to promote the levels of well-being of both partners together and of each as an individual. Ideally, therapists move toward these goals by strengthening the shared resources for problem solving, by encouraging the substitution of adequate controls and defenses for pathogenic ones, by enhancing both the immunity against the disintegrative effects of emotional upset and the complementarity of the relationship, and by promoting the growth of the relationship and of each partner.

Couples therapy does not ensure the maintenance of any marriage or relationship. Indeed, in certain instances it may show the partners that they are in a nonviable union that should be dissolved. In these cases, couples may continue to meet with therapists to work through the difficulties of separating and obtaining a divorce, a process that has been called *divorce therapy*.

▲ 31.5 Biofeedback

Biofeedback relies on instrumentation to measure moment-to-moment physiological processes. It provides patients with information about their performance in various situations. Using this "feedback," it is possible to control physiological functions so as to change them. Biofeedback is based on the idea that the autonomic nervous system can come under voluntary control through operant conditioning. The benefits of biofeedback may be augmented by the relaxation that patients are trained to facilitate.

THEORY

Neal Miller demonstrated the medical potential of biofeedback by showing that the normally involuntary autonomic nervous system can be operantly conditioned, by using appropriate feedback. By means of instruments, patients acquire information about the status of involuntary biological functions, such as skin temperature and electrical conductivity, muscle tension, blood pressure, heart rate, and brain wave activity. Patients then learn to regulate one or more of these biological states that affect symptoms. For example, a person can learn to raise the temperature of his or her hands to reduce the frequency of migraines, palpitations, or angina pectoris. Presumably, patients lower the sympathetic activation and voluntarily self-regulate arterial smooth muscle vasoconstrictive tendencies.

METHODS
Instrumentation

The feedback instrument used depends on the patient and the specific problem. The most effective instruments are the electromyogram (EMG), which measures the electrical potentials of muscle fibers; the electroencephalogram (EEG), which measures alpha waves that occur in relaxed states; the galvanic skin response gauge (GSR), which shows decreased skin conductivity during a relaxed state; and the thermistor, which measures skin temperature (which drops during tension because of peripheral vasoconstriction). Patients are attached to one of the measuring instruments to measure a physiological function and translate the measurement into an audible or visual signal that patients use to gauge their responses. For example, in the treatment of bruxism, an EMG is attached to the masseter muscle. The EMG emits a high tone when the muscle is contracted and a low tone when at rest. Patients can learn to alter the tone to indicate relaxation. Patients receive feedback about the masseter muscle, the tone reinforces the learning, and the condition ameliorates—all these events interacting synergistically.

Many less specific clinical applications—such as treating insomnia, improving athletic performance, achieving altered states of consciousness, and supplementing psychotherapy for anxiety associated with somatoform disorders—use a model in which frontalis muscle EMG biofeedback is combined with thermal biofeedback and verbal instructions in progressive relaxation.

Relaxation Therapy

Progressive relaxation was developed by Edmund Jacobson, M.D., in 1929. Learning relaxation involves cultivating a muscle sense. To develop the muscle sense, patients are taught to isolate and contract specific muscles or muscle groups, one at a time.

Joseph Wolpe.   Joseph Wolpe chose progressive relaxation as a response incompatible with anxiety when designing his systematic desensitization treatment (discussed below). Instructions to relax and tense specific muscle groups are given. Once the patients have mastered this procedure (typically after three sessions), they practice relaxation by recall (i.e., without tensing the muscles).

Autogenic Training

Autogenic training is a method of self-suggestion that originated in Germany. It involves the patients directing their attention to specific bodily areas and hearing themselves think certain phrases reflecting a relaxed state. In the original German version, patients progressed through six themes over many sessions. Autogenic relaxation is an American modification of autogenic training, in which all six areas are covered in one session.

RESULTS

Biofeedback and progressive relaxation have been shown to be effective treatment methods for a broad range of disorders. They form one basis of behavioral medicine in which the patient changes (or learns how to change) behavior that contributes to illness. They form a basis upon which many complementary and alternative medical procedures are effective (e.g., yoga) in which relaxation is an important component. Relaxation also informs more mainstream treatments such as hypnosis.

▲ 31.6 Behavior Therapy

Behavior therapy represents clinical applications of the principles developed in learning theory. Behavioral psychology, or behaviorism, arose in the early 20th century in reaction to the method of introspection that dominated psychology at the time. John B. Watson, the father of behaviorism, had initially studied animal psychology. This background made it a small conceptual leap to argue that psychology should concern itself only with publicly observable phenomena (i.e., overt behavior). According to behavioristic thinking, since mental content is not publicly observable, it cannot be subjected to rigorous scientific inquiry. Consequently, behaviorists developed a focus on overt behaviors and their environmental influences.

Today, different behavioral schools continue to share a focus on verifiable behavior. Behavioral views differ from cognitive views in holding that physical rather than mental events control behavior. According to behaviorism, mental phenomena or speculations about them have little or no scientific interest.

SYSTEMATIC DESENSITIZATION

Developed by Joseph Wolpe, systematic desensitization is based on the behavioral principle of counterconditioning, whereby a person overcomes maladaptive anxiety elicited by a situation or an object by approaching the feared situation gradually and in a psy-

chophysiological state that inhibits anxiety. In systematic desensitization, patients attain a state of complete relaxation and are then exposed to the stimulus that elicits the anxiety response. The negative reaction of anxiety is inhibited by the relaxed state, a process called *reciprocal inhibition*. Rather than use actual situations or objects that elicit fear, patients and therapists prepare a graded list or hierarchy of anxiety-provoking scenes associated with a patient's fears. The learned relaxation state and the anxiety-provoking scenes are systematically paired in treatment. Thus, systematic desensitization consists of three steps: relaxation training, hierarchy construction, and desensitization of the stimulus.

Relaxation Training

Relaxation produces physiological effects opposite those of anxiety: slow heart rate, increased peripheral blood flow, and neuromuscular stability. A variety of relaxation methods have been developed. Some, such as yoga and Zen, have been known for centuries. Most methods use so-called progressive relaxation developed by the psychiatrist Edmund Jacobson. Patients relax major muscle groups in a fixed order, beginning with the small muscle groups of the feet and working cephalad or vice versa. Some clinicians employ hypnosis to facilitate relaxation or use tape-recorded exercise to allow patients to practice relaxation on their own. Mental imagery is a relaxation method in which patients are instructed to imagine themselves in a place associated with pleasant, relaxed memories. Such images allow patients to enter a relaxed state or experience, as Herbert Benson termed it, the *relaxation response*.

The physiological changes that take place during relaxation are the opposite of those induced by the adrenergic stress responses that are part of many emotions. Muscle tension, respiration rate, heart rate, blood pressure, and skin conductance decrease. Finger temperature and blood flow to the finger usually increase. Relaxation increases respiratory heart rate variability, an index of parasympathetic tone.

Hierarchy Construction

When constructing a hierarchy, clinicians determine all the conditions that elicit anxiety, and then patients create a hierarchy list of 10 to 12 scenes in order of increasing anxiety. For example, an acrophobic hierarchy may begin with a patient's imagining standing near a window on the second floor and end with being on the roof of a 20-story building, leaning on a guard rail and looking straight down.

Desensitization of the Stimulus

In the final step, called *desensitization*, patients proceed systematically through the list from the least to the most anxiety-provoking scene while in a deeply relaxed state. The rate at which patients progress through the list is determined by their responses to the stimuli. When patients can vividly imagine the most anxiety-provoking scene of the hierarchy with equanimity, they experience little anxiety in the corresponding real-life situation.

Adjunctive Use of Drugs

Clinicians have used various drugs to hasten relaxation, but drugs should be used cautiously and only by clinicians trained and experienced in potential adverse effects. Either the ultrarapidly acting barbiturate sodium methohexital (Brevital) or diazepam (Valium) is given intravenously in subanesthetic doses. If the procedural details are carefully followed, almost all patients find the procedure pleasant, with few unpleasant side effects. The advantages of pharmacological desensitization are that preliminary training in relaxation can be shortened, almost all patients are able to become adequately relaxed, and the treatment itself seems to proceed more rapidly than without the drugs.

Indications

Systematic desensitization works best when there is a clearly identifiable anxiety-provoking stimulus. Phobias, obsessions, compulsions, and certain sexual disorders have been successfully treated with the technique.

THERAPEUTIC GRADED EXPOSURE

Therapeutic graded exposure is similar to systematic desensitization except that relaxation training is not involved and treatment is usually carried out in a real-life context. This means that the individual must be brought in contact with (i.e., be exposed to) the warning stimulus to learn firsthand that no dangerous consequences will ensue. Exposure is graded according to a hierarchy. Patients afraid of cats, for example, might progress from looking at a picture of a cat to holding one.

FLOODING

Flooding (sometimes called *implosion*) is similar to graded exposure in that it involves exposing the patient to the feared object in vivo; however, there is no hierarchy. Flooding is based on the premise that escaping from an anxiety-provoking experience reinforces the anxiety through conditioning. Thus, clinicians can extinguish the anxiety and prevent the conditioned avoidance behavior by not allowing patients to escape the situation. Clinicians encourage patients to confront feared situations directly, without a gradual buildup as in systematic desensitization or graded exposure. No relaxation exercises are used, as in systematic desensitization. Patients experience fear, which gradually subsides after a time. The success of the procedure depends on patients' remaining in the fear-generating situation until they are calm and feeling a sense of mastery. Prematurely withdrawing from the situation or prematurely terminating the fantasized scene is equivalent to an escape, which then reinforces both the conditioned anxiety and the avoidance behavior and produces the opposite of the desired effect. In a variant, called *imaginal flooding*, the feared object or situation is confronted only in the imagination rather than in real life. Many patients refuse flooding because of the psychological discomfort involved. It is also contraindicated in patients for whom intense anxiety would be hazardous (for example, patients with heart disease or fragile psychological adaptation). The technique works best with specific phobias.

The patient was a 33-year-old female with social fears of eating in public. In particular, she was afraid of being observed by others when chewing and swallowing, particularly at dinner parties. A contrived situation was arranged in which the patient came to the session with a prepared meal and drink. She entered a conference room in which five persons in professional attire were already seated along a table.

The patient was instructed to eat her meal in front of these individuals. Between bites, she was instructed to look at them often, and they had been instructed to avoid staring contests. She was not to distract herself from her anxiety symptoms. She was to eat her meal slowly, paying attention to the behavior of the observers and to her anxiety symptoms (e.g., dry mouth or difficulty swallowing). No conversation between the patient and observers was permitted. The observers would look at her and observe her chewing and swallowing behaviors, at times writing comments in a notebook. Occasionally observers would communicate by whispering to each other, exchanging written notes, or giving knowing glances and smiles.

The only other communication occurred between the patient and therapist, and this was limited to the patient providing her subjective units of distress rating. The session lasted 90 minutes. Note that this situation may seem quite traumatizing. However, because the exposure session is long and continues until ratings decline, the patient becomes desensitized. (Courtesy of Rolf G. Jacob, M.D., and William H. Pelham, M.D.)

EXPOSURE TO STIMULI PRESENTED IN VIRTUAL REALITY

Advances in computer technology have made it possible to present environmental cues in virtual reality for exposure treatment. Beneficial effects have been reported with virtual reality exposure of patients with height phobia, fear of flying, spider phobia, and claustrophobia. A great deal of experimental work is being done in the field. One model uses an avatar of the patient walking through a crowded supermarket filled with other avatars as a way of conquering agoraphobia.

ASSERTIVENESS TRAINING

To be assertive requires that people have confidence in their judgment and sufficient self-esteem to express their opinions. Assertiveness and social skills training teach people how to respond appropriately in social situations, to express their opinions in acceptable ways, and to achieve their goals. A variety of techniques, including role modeling, desensitization, and positive reinforcement (reward of desired behavior), are used to increase assertiveness. Social skills training deals with assertiveness but also attends to a variety of real-life tasks, such as food shopping, looking for work, interacting with other people, and overcoming shyness.

AVERSION THERAPY

When a noxious stimulus (punishment) is presented immediately after a specific behavioral response, theoretically the response is eventually inhibited and extinguished. Many types of noxious stimuli are used: electric shocks, substances that induce vomiting, corporal punishment, and social disapproval. The negative stimulus is paired with the behavior, which is thereby suppressed. The unwanted behavior may disappear after a series of such sequences. Aversion therapy has been used for alcohol abuse, paraphilias, and other behaviors with impulsive or compulsive qualities, but this therapy is controversial for many reasons. For example, punishment does not always lead to the expected decrease in response and can sometimes be positively reinforcing. Aversion therapy has been used with good effect in some cultures in the treatment of opioid addicts.

EYE MOVEMENT DESENSITIZATION AND REPROCESSING (EMDR)

Saccadic eye movements are rapid oscillations of the eyes that occur when a person tracks an object that is moved back and forth across the line of vision. If saccades are induced while the person is imagining or thinking about an anxiety-producing event, a few studies have demonstrated that a positive thought or image can be induced that results in decreased anxiety. EMDR has been used in posttraumatic stress disorders and phobias.

POSITIVE REINFORCEMENT

When a behavioral response is followed by a generally rewarding event such as food, avoidance of pain, or praise, it tends to be strengthened and to occur more frequently than before the reward. This principle has been applied in a variety of situations. On inpatient hospital wards, patients with mental disorders receive a reward for performing a desired behavior, such as tokens that they may use to purchase luxury items or certain privileges. The process, known as *token economy*, has been successful in altering behavior. Table 31.6–1 gives a summary of some clinical applications of behavior therapy.

DIALECTICAL BEHAVIOR THERAPY (DBT)

DBT has been used successfully in patients with borderline personality disorder and parasuicidal behavior. It is eclectic, drawing on methods from supportive, cognitive, and behavioral therapies. Some elements are derived from Franz Alexander's view of therapy as a corrective emotional experience, and also from certain Eastern philosophical schools (e.g., Zen). Patients are seen weekly, with the goal of improving interpersonal skills and decreasing self-destructive behavior by means of techniques involving advice, use of metaphor, storytelling, and confrontation, among others. Borderline patients especially are helped to deal with the ambivalent feelings that are characteristic of the disorder. Marsha Linehan, Ph.D., developed the treatment method, based on her theory that borderline patients are unable to identify emotional experiences and cannot tolerate frustration or rejection. As with other behavioral approaches, DBT assumes all behavior (including thoughts and feelings) are learned and the borderline patient behaves in ways that reinforce or even reward his or her behavior, regardless of how maladaptive it is.

Functions of DBT

As described by its originator, there are five essential "functions" in treatment: (1) to enhance and expand the patient's repertoire of skillful behavioral patterns, (2) to improve patient motivation to change by reducing reinforcement of maladaptive behavior, including dysfunctions (cognitions and emotions), (3) to ensure that new behavioral patterns generalize from the therapeutic to the natural environment, (4) to structure the environment so that

Table 31.6–1
Some Common Clinical Applications of Behavior Therapy

Disorder	Comments
Agoraphobia	Graded exposure and flooding can reduce the fear of being in crowded places. About 60% of patients so treated improve. In some cases the spouse can serve as the model while accompanying the patient into the fear situation; however, the patient cannot get a secondary gain by keeping the spouse nearby and displaying symptoms.
Alcohol dependence	Aversion therapy in which the alcohol-dependent patient is made to vomit (by adding an emetic to the alcohol) every time a drink is ingested is effective in treating alcohol dependence.
Anorexia nervosa	Observe eating behavior; contingency management; record weight.
Bulimia nervosa	Record bulimic episodes; log moods.
Hyperventilation	Hyperventilation test; controlled breathing; direct observation.
Other phobias	Systematic desensitization has been effective in treating phobias, such as fears of heights, animals, and flying.
Paraphilias	Electric shocks or other noxious stimuli can be applied at the time of a paraphilic impulse, and eventually the impulse subsides.
Schizophrenia	The token economy procedure, in which tokens are awarded for desirable behavior and can be used to buy ward privileges, has been useful in treating inpatient schizophrenia patients.
Sexual dysfunctions	Sex therapy, developed by William Masters and Virginia Johnson, is a behavior therapy technique used for various sexual dysfunctions, especially male erectile disorder, orgasm disorders, and premature ejaculation.
Shy bladder	Inability to void in a public bathroom; relaxation exercises.
Type A behavior	Physiological assessment; muscle relaxation, biofeedback (on EMG)

effective behaviors, rather than dysfunctional behaviors, are reinforced, and (5) to enhance the motivation and capabilities of the therapist so that effective treatment is rendered. Therapy is conducted in both individual or group behavioral skills training sessions. Homework assignments and coaching in person and by telephone are part of the treatment. Environmental structuring may occur by having family members come to treatment with the patient, by changing the environment so it supports and reinforces therapeutic improvements, or by training the patient in how to intervene in his or her own environment. Finally, therapist capabilities and motivations are addressed through weekly team meetings aimed at improving therapists' skills and motivation and reducing burn-out.

In studies evaluating the effect of DBT for patients with borderline personality disorder, there were positive findings: Patients had a low dropout rate from treatment; there was a lower incidence of parasuicidal behaviors; there was a reduction in self-report of angry affect and improved social adjustment and work performance. The method is now being applied to other disorders, including substance abuse, eating disorder, and posttraumatic stress disorder.

▲ 31.7 Cognitive Therapy

Cognitive therapy—according to its originator, Aaron Beck—is "based on an underlying theoretical rationale that an individual's affect and behavior are largely determined by the way in which he structures the world." A person's structuring of the world is based on cognitions (verbal or pictorial ideas available to consciousness), which are based on assumptions (schemas developed from previous experiences). According to Beck,

> If a person interprets all his experiences in terms of whether he is competent and adequate, his thinking may be dominated by the schema, "Unless I do everything perfectly, I'm a failure." Consequently, he reacts to situations in terms of adequacy even when they are unrelated to whether or not he is personally competent.

GENERAL CONSIDERATIONS

Cognitive therapy is a short-term structure therapy that uses active collaboration between patient and therapist to achieve its therapeutic goals, which are oriented toward current problems and their resolution. Therapy is usually conducted on an individual basis, although group methods are sometimes helpful. A therapist may also prescribe drugs in conjunction with therapy.

Depressive disorders (with or without suicidal ideation) have been the main focus of cognitive therapy; however, cognitive therapy is also used with other conditions, such as panic disorder, obsessive-compulsive disorder, paranoid personality disorder, and somatoform disorders. The treatment of depression can serve as a paradigm of the cognitive approach.

COGNITIVE THEORY OF DEPRESSION

According to the cognitive theory of depression, cognitive dysfunctions are the core of depression, and affective and physical changes and other associated features of depression are consequences of cognitive dysfunctions. For example, apathy and low energy are results of a person's expectation of failure in all areas. Similarly, paralysis of will stems from a person's pessimism and feelings of hopelessness. The cognitive triad of depression is a negative self-perception whereby people see themselves as defective, inadequate, deprived, worthless, and undesirable; they have a tendency to experience the world as negative, demanding, and self-defeating and to expect failure and punishment; and they have an expectation of continued hardship, suffering, deprivation, and failure.

The goal of therapy is to alleviate depression and to prevent its recurrence by helping patients to identify and test negative cognitions, to develop alternative and more flexible schemas, and to rehearse both new cognitive and behavioral responses. Changing the way persons think can alleviate the depressive disorder.

STRATEGIES AND TECHNIQUES

Therapy is relatively short and lasts up to approximately 25 weeks. If a patient does not improve in this time, the diagnosis should be reevaluated. Maintenance therapy can be carried out over years. As with other psychotherapies, therapists' attributes are important to successful therapy. They must exude warmth, understand the life experience of each patient, and be truly genuine and honest with themselves and with their patients. Therapists must be able to relate skillfully and interactively with their patients. Cognitive therapists set the agenda at the beginning of each session, assign homework to be performed between sessions, and teach new skills. Therapist and patient actively collaborate. The three components of cognitive therapy are didactic aspects, cognitive techniques, and behavioral techniques.

Didactic Aspects

The therapy's didactic aspects include explaining to patients the cognitive triad, schemas, and faulty logic. Therapists must tell patients that they will formulate hypotheses together and test them over the course of the treatment. Cognitive therapy requires a full explanation of the relationship between depression and thinking, affect, and behavior, as well as the rationale for all aspects of treatment. This explanation contrasts with psychoanalytically oriented therapies, which require little explanation.

Cognitive Techniques

The therapy's cognitive approach includes four processes: eliciting automatic thoughts, testing automatic thoughts, identifying maladaptive underlying assumptions, and testing the validity of maladaptive assumptions.

Eliciting Automatic Thoughts.
Automatic thoughts, also called *cognitive distortions*, are cognitions that intervene between external events and a person's emotional reaction to the event. As an example, the belief that "people will laugh at me when they see how badly I bowl" is an automatic thought that occurs to someone who has been asked to go bowling and responds negatively. Another example is a person's thinking that "she doesn't like me" when someone passes the person in the hall without saying hello. Every psychopathological disorder has its own specific cognitive profile of distorted thought, which, if known, provides a framework for specific cognitive interventions.

Testing Automatic Thoughts.
Acting as a teacher, a therapist helps a patient test the validity of automatic thoughts. The goal is to encourage the patient to reject inaccurate or exaggerated automatic thoughts after careful examination. Patients often blame themselves when things that may well have been outside their control go awry. The therapist reviews the entire situation with the patient and helps reattribute the blame or cause of the unpleasant events. Generating alternative explanations for events is another way of undermining inaccurate and distorted automatic thoughts.

Identifying Maladaptive Assumptions.
As patient and therapist continue to identify automatic thoughts, patterns usually become apparent. The patterns represent rules or maladaptive general assumptions that guide a patient's life. Samples of such rules are "In order to be happy, I must be perfect" and "If anyone doesn't like me, I'm not lovable." Such rules inevitably lead to disappointments and failure and ultimately to depression.

Testing the Validity of Maladaptive Assumptions.
Testing the accuracy of maladaptive assumptions is similar to testing the validity of automatic thoughts. In a particularly effective test, therapists ask patients to defend the validity of their assumptions. For example, patients may state that they should always work up to their potential, and a therapist may ask, "Why is that so important to you?"

Behavioral Techniques

Behavioral and cognitive techniques go hand in hand: Behavioral techniques test and change maladaptive and inaccurate cognitions. The overall purposes of such techniques are to help patients understand the inaccuracy of their cognitive assumptions and learn new strategies and ways of dealing with issues.

Among the behavioral techniques in cognitive therapy are scheduling activities, mastery and pleasure, graded task assignments, cognitive rehearsal, self-reliance training, role playing, and diversion techniques. Scheduling activities on an hourly basis is one of the first things done in therapy. Patients keep records of the activities and review them with the therapist. In addition to scheduling activities, patients are asked to rate the amount of mastery and pleasure their activities bring them. Patients are often surprised to learn that they have much more mastery of activities and enjoy them more than they had thought.

To simplify the situation and to allow for mini-accomplishments, therapists often break tasks into subtasks, as in graded task assignments, so as to demonstrate to patients that they can succeed. In cognitive rehearsal, patients imagine and rehearse the various steps in meeting and mastering a challenge.

Patients, especially inpatients, are encouraged to become self-reliant by doing such simple things as making their own beds, doing their own shopping, and preparing their own meals. This process is called *self-reliance training*. Role-playing is a particularly powerful and useful technique to elicit automatic thoughts and to learn new behaviors. Diversion techniques are useful in helping patients get through difficult times and include physical activity, social contact, work, play, and visual imagery.

Imagery

The effect of imagery on behavior was first discussed by Paul Schilder in his book, *The Image and Appearance of the Human Body*. Schilder described images as having physiological components: When people visualize themselves running, they subliminally activate the same muscles used in running and this reaction can be measured with electromyography (EMG). This phenomenon is used in sports training, in which athletes visualize every conceivable event in a performance and develop a muscle memory for each activity. A combination of behavioral and cognitive theories can help to master anxiety or to deal with feared situations.

Thought stoppage can treat impulsive or obsessive behavior. For instance, patients imagine a stop sign with a police officer nearby or another image that evokes inhibition at the same time that they recognize an impulse or obsession that is alien to the ego. Similarly, obesity can be treated by having patients visualize themselves as thin, athletic, trim, and well muscled and then training them to evoke this image whenever they have an urge to eat. Hypnosis or autogenic training can enhance such imagery. In a technique called *guided imagery*, therapists encourage patients to have fantasies that can be interpreted as wish fulfillments or attempts to master disturbing affects or impulses.

EFFICACY

Cognitive therapy can be used alone in the treatment of mild to moderate depressive disorders or in conjunction with antidepressant medication for major depressive disorder. Studies have clearly shown that cognitive therapy is effective and in some cases is superior or equal to medication alone. It is one of the most useful psychotherapeutic interventions currently available for depressive disorders and shows promise in the treatment of other disorders.

Cognitive therapy has also been studied as a way of increasing compliance with lithium (Eskalith) in patients with bipolar I disorder and as an adjunct in treating withdrawal from heroin.

▲ 31.8 Hypnosis

Herbert Spiegel defines *hypnosis* as a state of heightened focal concentration and receptivity. It is typified by a feeling of involuntariness; movements seem automatic, and suggested perceptions can alter or replace ordinary ones. Hypnosis has also been described as an altered state of consciousness, a dissociated state, and a state of regression.

Martin Orne defined *hypnosis* as a state or condition in which a person can respond to appropriate suggestions by experiencing alterations of perceptions, memory, or mood. The essential feature of hypnosis is the subjective experimental change. A pioneer in clinical hypnotic induction, Milton Erickson, described the process of a clinical trance as "a free period in which individuality can flourish."

Hypnotherapists perceive clinical hypnosis and therapeutic trance as extensions of common processes in everyday life. Daydreaming and inner preoccupation, during which people seemingly automatically go through the motions of a daily routine, are typical examples. During such periods, people spontaneously focus attention inward, just as in a trance state a patient is induced to be receptive to inner experiences. The primary view shared by hypnotherapists and other psychotherapists is an appreciation and understanding of the dynamics of unconscious processes in behavior.

HISTORY

The Austrian physician Friedrich Anton Mesmer (1734–1815) originated the phenomenon of hypnosis, which he called *mesmerism* and believed to be the result of "animal magnetism" or an invisible fluid passing between subject and mesmerizer. A Scottish physician, James Braid (1795–1860), first used the term *hypnosis* (from *hypnos*, the Greek word for "sleep") in the 1840s, to refer to what he thought was a specific state of sleep. In the late 19th century, the French neurologist Jean-Martin Charcot (1825–1893) considered hypnotism a special physiological state. His contemporary Hippolyte-Marie Bernheim (1840–1919) believed it to be a psychological state of heightened suggestibility.

Sigmund Freud, who had studied with Charcot, used hypnosis early in his career to help patients recover repressed memories. Freud noted that patients relived traumatic events while under hypnosis, a process known as *abreaction*. Freud later replaced hypnosis with the technique of free association.

Today, hypnosis is used as a form of therapy (hypnotherapy), a method of investigation to recover lost memories, and a research tool.

NEUROPHYSIOLOGIC CORRELATES OF HYPNOSIS

There are no specific neurophysiological findings in a person who is in a hypnotized state. Unlike sleep, in which there are typical encephalographic (EEG) changes, the EEG of a hypnotized person is more similar to that of a fully awake and attentive individual. Some researchers have found increased alpha activity, but this is not a consistent finding. Positron emission tomography (PET) studies have shown some changes in the frontal cortex of hypnotized subjects.

HYPNOTIC CAPACITY AND INDUCTION

Therapists can use several specific procedures to help patients be hypnotized and respond to suggestion. These procedures capitalize on naturally occurring hypnosis-like phenomena that most people have probably experienced. But because these experiences are rarely talked about, patients find them fascinating. For example, when discussing hypnosis with a patient, a therapist may ask: "Have you ever had the experience of driving home while thinking about an issue that preoccupies you and suddenly realize that, although you have arrived safe and sound, you can't recall having driven past familiar landmarks? It's as if you had been asleep, and yet you stopped at all the red lights, and you avoided collisions. You were somehow traveling on automatic pilot." Most people resonate to this experience and are usually happy to describe similar personal experiences.

When patients realize that they have probably undergone hypnosis-like episodes, they can understand that they have the capacity to use the hypnotic mode, which is merely an extension of such states. Although the episodes were not necessarily hypnotic states, the extent to which a person experiences them is correlated with hypnotizability.

TRANCE STATE

People under hypnosis are said to be in a trance state, which may be light, medium, or heavy (deep). In a light trance, there are changes in motor activity: People's muscles can feel relaxed, the hands can levitate, and paresthesia can be induced. A medium trance is characterized by diminished pain sensation and partial or complete amnesia. A deep trance is associated with induced visual or auditory experiences and deep anesthesia. Time distortion occurs at all trance levels but is most profound in the deep trance.

In posthypnotic suggestion, a person is instructed to perform a simple act or to experience a particular sensation after awakening from the trance state. The suggestion may cause a person to perceive a bad taste to cigarettes or to a particular food and thus can aid in treating nicotine dependence or obesity. Posthypnotic suggestions are associated with deep trance states.

HYPNOTHERAPY

Patients in hypnotic trances can recall memories that are unavailable to consciousness in the nonhypnotic state. In therapy, such memories can corroborate psychoanalytic hypotheses about a patient's dynamics or can enable a patient to use such memories as a catalyst for new associations. Some patients can induce age regression, during which they reexperience events that occurred earlier in life. Whether the patient experiences the events as they actually occurred is controversial, but the material elicited can be used to further the therapy. Patients in a trance state may describe an event with an intensity similar to its original occurrence (abreaction) and can feel a sense of relief as a result. Trance states play a role in treating of amnestic disorders and dissociative fugue, although clinicians should be aware that quickly bringing repressed memory into consciousness may be hazardous and may overwhelm the patient with anxiety.

Indications and Uses

Hypnosis has been used, with varying degrees of success, to control obesity and substance-related disorders such as alcohol abuse and nicotine dependence. Major surgery has been performed with no anesthetic except hypnosis. Hypnosis has also been applied to managing chronic pain disorder, asthma, warts, pruritus, aphonia, and conversion disorder. Patients can easily achieve relaxation with hypnosis, so that they can deal with phobias by controlling their anxiety. Hypnosis can also induce relaxation in systematic desensitization.

Contraindication

Hypnotized patients are in a state of atypical dependence on a therapist; they may develop a strong transference, characterized by a positive attachment that must be respected and interpreted. In other instances, a negative transference may erupt in patients who are fragile or who have difficulty in testing reality. Patients who have problems with basic trust, such as those with paranoia or patients who dislike giving up control, such as those who are obsessive-compulsive, are not good candidates for hypnosis. A secure ethical value system is important to all therapy and particularly to hypnotherapy, in which patients (especially those in a deep trance) are extremely suggestible and malleable. There is controversy about whether patients can perform acts during a trance state that they otherwise find repugnant or that run contrary to their moral code. Fears about hypnosis still exist, generally due to misinformation.

▲ 31.9 Psychosocial Treatment and Rehabilitation

Psychosocial treatment and rehabilitation refer to the use of various methods to enable people who are severely mentally ill to develop social and vocational skills for independent living. Such treatment is carried out at many sites: hospitals, outpatient clinics, mental health centers, day hospitals, and home or social clubs.

SOCIAL SKILLS TRAINING

Social skills are interpersonal behaviors required for community survival, for independence, and for establishing, maintaining, and deepening supportive, socially rewarding relationships. Severe mental disorders such as schizophrenia disrupt one or more affective, cognitive, verbal, and behavioral domains of functioning and impair people's potential for enjoying and sustaining interpersonal relationships, which are the essence of social life. Clinicians have developed treatment packages termed *social skills training*, which have proved effective for patients with schizophrenia to remediate deficits in social behaviors.

Methods

Role-playing is the vehicle used to assess a patient's pretreatment social competence and to train targeted behavioral excesses or deficits during treatment. Training scenes are selected either on the basis of an individual's past difficulties or of problems that apply to most of the psychiatric population to which the patient belongs. Training sessions vary in length from 45 to 90 minutes, depending on the number of patients participating and on their levels of functioning. Although the group format provides vicarious learning opportunities through observation of other patients' behavior as well as through reinforcement by peers, the group experience is sometimes supplemented by individual training; such training allows more intensive focus on a single patient's behavior and provides an opportunity for more practice in sessions.

Social skills training programs for schizophrenics cover conversation skills, conflict management skills, assertiveness skills, community living skills, friendship and dating skills, work and vocational skills, and medication management skills. Each of these skills has several components. For example, assertiveness skills include making requests,

refusing requests, making complaints, responding to complaints, expressing unpleasant feelings, asking for information, making apologies, letting someone know you are afraid, and refusing alcohol and street drugs. Each component involves specific steps. Conflict management includes skills in negotiating, compromising, tactful disagreeing, responding to untrue accusations, and leaving overly stressful situations. Table 31.9–1 outlines social skills training for schizophrenia patients.

Goals

In a treatment setting, there are four major goals of social skills training: (1) improve social skills in specific situations, (2) moderate generalization of acquired skills to similar situations, (3) acquisition or relearning of social and conversational skills, and (4) decrease social anxiety. Learning, however, is tedious or almost nonexistent when patients are floridly ill with positive symptoms and high levels of distractibility.

Some findings limit the applicability of social skills training. It is more difficult to teach complex conversational skills than to teach briefer, more discrete verbal and nonverbal responses in social situations. Because complex behaviors are more critical for generating social support in the community, methods have been developed to improve the learning and durability of conversational skills. These training methods, focusing on training in social skills and information-processing skills, are discussed below.

Training in Social Perception Skills.   Recently, efforts have been made to develop strategies for training patients in affect and social cue recognition. Patients with chronic psychotic disorders such as schizophrenia often have difficulty perceiving and interpreting the subtle affective and cognitive cues that are critical elements of communication. Social perception abilities are considered the first step in effective interpersonal problem solving; difficulties in this area are likely to lead to a cascade of deficits in social behavior. Training skills in social perception address these deficits and help provide a foundation for developing more specific social and coping skills.

Table 31.9–1
Social Skills Training in Schizophrenia Patients

Skills	Component Behaviors
Initiating positive comments	
Listening empathically	
Making positive requests for action	
Expressing negative feelings directly	
Coping with unexpected hostility and withdrawal	
Acknowledging pleasing events	Look at the other person
	Pleasant facial expression
	Warm tone of voice
	Say what the other person did or said and how that pleased you
Problem solving	Pinpoint the problem
	Share ownership of the problem
	Generate alternatives
	Weigh pros and cons of each alternative
	Choose a reasonable alternative
	Plan how to implement
	Review and reward progress and efforts

Courtesy of Robert Paul Liberman, M.D.

Despite attending several social gatherings, Matt felt apart from the rest of the group. He reported that these events seemed like "a jumble of sights and sounds." His therapist, recognizing Matt's difficulty with social perception, gave him a series of questions designed to help him organize and give meaning to the social stimuli he encountered. For example, when Matt was confused about a conversation someone was having with him, he would ask himself, "What is this person's short-term goal? At what level of disclosure should I be? Should I be talking now or listening?" Identifying the rules and goals of a particular social interaction provided a template for Matt to recognize and react to a greater variety of social cues, thus enhancing his behavioral repertoire. (Courtesy of Robert Paul Liberman, M.D., Alex Kopelowicz, M.D., and Thomas E. Smith, M.D.)

Information-Processing Model of Training.   Methods of training that follow a cognitive perspective teach patients to use a set of generative rules that can be adapted for use in various situations. For example, a six-step problem-solving strategy has developed as an outline for helping patients overcome interpersonal dilemmas: (1) adopt a problem-solving attitude, (2) identify the problem, (3) brainstorm alternative solutions, (4) evaluate solutions and pick one to implement, (5) plan the implementation and carry it out, and (6) evaluate the efficacy of the effort and, if ineffective, choose another alternative. While the stepwise, structured, linear process of problem solving occurs intuitively, without conscious awareness in normal persons, it can be a useful interpersonal crutch to help cognitively impaired mental patients cope with the information needed to fill their social and personal needs.

MILIEU THERAPY

The locus of milieu is a living, learning, or working environment. The defining characteristics of treatment are the use of a team to provide treatment and the time the patient spends in the environment. Recent adaptations of milieu therapy have included 24-hour-a-day programs that are situated in community locales frequented by patients and that provide in vivo support, case management, and training in living skills.

Most milieu therapy programs emphasize group and social interaction; rules and expectations are mediated by peer pressure for normalization of adaptation. When patients are viewed as responsible human beings, the patient role becomes blurred. Milieu therapy stresses a patient's rights to goals and to have freedom of movement and informal relationship with staff; it also emphasizes interdisciplinary participation and goal-oriented, clear communication.

Token Economy

The use of tokens, points, or credits as secondary or generalized reinforcers can be seen as normalizing a mental hospital or day hospital environment with a program mimicking society's use of money to meet instrumental needs. Token economies establish the rules and culture of a hospital inpatient unit or partial hospitalization program, offering coherence and consistency to the interdisciplinary team as it struggles to promote therapeutic progress in difficult patients. These programs are challenging to establish, however, and their widespread dissemination has suffered because of the organizational prerequisites and the additional resources and rewards needed to create a truly positively reinforcing environment.

PSYCHOSOCIAL CLUBHOUSES AND SELF-HELP PROGRAMS

Psychosocial self-help emerged during the late 1940s when ex-patients began to meet together in so-called social clubs to satisfy their needs for acceptance and emotional support. Emphasizing self-help, mutual interdependence, and reliance on assets, the movement led to the establishment of Fountain House and hundreds of cloned offspring throughout the United States. Instead of thinking of themselves as patients, they became members and formed groups and teams to accomplish tasks, plan activities, and solve problems; and in so doing, the quality of their lives improved. Creating their own social support network, members of psychosocial clubs design activities that build experiences of mutual ownership and needs. Staff members, primarily nonprofessionals or those trained in vocational rehabilitation, provide positive, accepting reactions and require members to obtain psychiatric treatment, such as medication, elsewhere. Thus, the club has rehabilitation goals, not clinical goals. During the day, members of the club spend time engaging in activities such as chores, operating a snack bar, assisting each other in banking and budgeting, visiting friends who are hospitalized, printing a newspaper, helping each other with entitlements from social agencies, manning a thrift shop, working the switchboard, or refurbishing cooperative apartments.

VOCATIONAL TRAINING

An important part of psychosocial rehabilitation is enabling people to work. Job placements are located in normal places of business, from large corporations to small businesses; they are at the entry level and require minimal training or skills. These transitional jobs are opportunities to work temporarily en route to full-time employment elsewhere or to longer-term employment in the entry-level position. The number of transitional employment programs in the United States has grown to over 100, with over 500 employers involved in providing wages in excess of $4 million. An 18-month follow-up evaluation of people working in transitional jobs revealed that 16 percent were employed independently on a full-time basis, and an additional 45 percent continued part-time work in the transitional program or were attending school or other training programs. Only 2 percent were in psychiatric hospitals at the time of the 18-month follow-up.

32

Biological Therapies

▲ 32.1 General Principles of Psychopharmacology

The numerous pharmacological agents used to treat psychiatric disorders are referred to by three general terms that are used interchangeably: *psychotropic drugs*, *psychoactive drugs*, and *psychotherapeutic drugs*. Traditionally, those agents were divided into four categories: (1) antipsychotic drugs or neuroleptics, used to treat psychosis; (2) antidepressant drugs, used to treat depression; (3) antimanic drugs, or mood stabilizers, used to treat bipolar disorder; and (4) antianxiety drugs, or anxiolytics, used to treat anxious states. That division, however, is less valid now than it was in the past for the following reasons:

1. Many drugs of one class are used to treat disorders previously assigned to another class. For example, many antidepressant drugs are used to treat anxiety disorders, and some antianxiety drugs are used to treat psychoses, depressive disorders, and bipolar disorders.
2. Drugs from all four categories are used to treat disorders not previously treatable by drugs—for example, eating disorders, panic disorder, and impulse-control disorders.
3. Drugs such as clonidine (Catapres), propranolol (Inderal), verapamil (Isoptin, Calan), and gabapentin (Neurontin) can treat a variety of psychiatric disorders effectively and do not fit easily into the traditional classification of drugs.
4. Some descriptive psychopharmacological terms overlap in meaning. For example, anxiolytics decrease anxiety, sedatives produce a calming or relaxing effect, and hypnotics produce sleep. However, most anxiolytics function as sedatives and at high doses can be used as hypnotics, and all hypnotics can be used for daytime sedation at low doses.

For these reasons, in the sections that follow, each drug is discussed according to its pharmacological category. Each drug is described in terms of its pharmacological actions, including pharmacodynamics and pharmacokinetics. Indications, contraindications, drug–drug interactions, and adverse effects are also discussed.

PHARMACOLOGICAL ACTIONS

Pharmacokinetic interactions concern how the body handles a drug. Pharmacodynamic interactions concern the effects of drugs on the biological activities of the body.

Pharmacodynamics

The major pharmacodynamic considerations include receptor mechanisms, the dose-response curve, the therapeutic index, and the development of tolerance, dependence, and withdrawal phenomena. The *receptor* for a drug can be defined generally as the cellular component to which the drug binds and through which the drug initiates its pharmacodynamic effects on the body. A drug can be an agonist for a receptor and stimulate the specific biological activity of the receptor or an antagonist that inhibits the biological activity. Some drugs are classified as partial agonists because they cannot fully activate a specific receptor. The receptor site for a psychopharmacological drug is often the receptor for an endogenous neurotransmitter. For example, most antipsychotic medications are receptor antagonists at the dopamine type 2 (D_2) receptor. However, this may not be true for other psychotherapeutic drugs (e.g., lithium [Eskalith], which may act by inhibiting the enzyme inositol 1-phosphatase).

The dose-response curve plots the drug concentration against the effects of the drug. The *potency* of a drug refers to the relative dose required to achieve certain effects. Haloperidol (Haldol), for example, is more potent than chlorpromazine (Thorazine) because approximately 5 mg of haloperidol is required to achieve the same therapeutic effect as 100 mg of chlorpromazine. However, both these drugs are equal in their *clinical efficacy*—that is, the maximum clinical response achievable by administration of a drug.

The adverse effects of most drugs are often a direct result of their primary pharmacodynamic effects. *Therapeutic index* is a relative measure of the toxicity or safety of a drug and is defined as the ratio of the median toxic dose to the median effective dose. The *median toxic dose* is the dose at which 50 percent of patients experience a specific toxic effect, and the *median effective dose* is the dose at which 50 percent of patients have a specified therapeutic effect. The therapeutic index for haloperidol and cardiovascular effects is quite high, as evidenced by the wide range of dosages in which haloperidol is prescribed. Conversely, the therapeutic index for lithium is quite low, thus requiring careful monitoring of serum lithium levels in patients given the drug. Both interindividual and intraindividual variations can affect the response to a specific drug. An individual patient may be hyporeactive, normally reactive, or hyperreactive to a drug. For example, some patients require 150 mg a day of imipramine (Tofranil), whereas others may require 300 mg a day. Idiosyncratic drug responses occur when a patient experiences a particularly unusual or rare effect from a drug. For example, some patients become quite agitated when given a benzodiazepine, such as diazepam (Valium).

A person may become less responsive to a particular drug as it is administered over time, a process that is referred to as the development of *tolerance*. The development of tolerance may sometimes be associated with the appearance of physical dependence on the drug. In a parallel fashion, pharmacokinetic drug interactions concern the effects of drugs on the plasma concentrations of one another, and pharmacodynamic drug interactions concern the effects of drugs on the receptor activities of one another.

Pharmacokinetics

Absorption. Psychotherapeutic drugs reach the brain through the bloodstream. Orally administered drugs dissolve in the fluid of the gastrointestinal (GI) tract, depending on their lipid solubility and the GI tract's local pH, motility, and surface area, and are then absorbed into the blood.

Stomach acidity may be reduced by gastric ion pump inhibitors, such as omeprazole (Prilosec) and lansoprazole (Prevacid); by histamine H_2 receptor blockers, such as cimetidine (Tagamet), famotidine (Pepcid), nizatidine (Axid), and ranitidine (Zantac); or by antacids. Gastric and intestinal motility may be slowed by anticholinergic drugs or increased by dopamine receptor antagonists, such as metoclopramide (Reglan).

Under favorable conditions, parenteral administration can achieve therapeutic plasma concentrations more rapidly than oral administration. However, if a drug is emulsified in an insoluble carrier matrix, intramuscular (IM) administration can sustain the drug's gradual release for several weeks. Such formulations are called *depot* preparations. Intravenous (IV) administration is the quickest route for achieving therapeutic blood concentrations, but it also carries the highest risk of sudden and life-threatening adverse effects.

Distribution and Bioavailability. Drugs that circulate bound to plasma proteins are called *protein bound*, and those that circulate unbound are called *free*. Only the free fraction can pass through the blood–brain barrier. The *distribution* of a drug to the brain is governed by the brain's regional blood flow, the blood–brain barrier, and the drug's affinity for its receptors in the brain. High cerebral blood flow, high lipid solubility, and high receptor affinity promote the therapeutic actions of the drug. A drug's *volume of distribution* is a measure of the apparent space in the body available to contain the drug, which can vary with age, sex, adipose tissue content, and disease state.

Bioavailability refers to the fraction of the total amount of administered drug that can subsequently be recovered from the bloodstream. Bioavailability is an important variable, because Food and Drug Administration (FDA) regulations specify that the bioavailability of a generic formulation can differ from that of the brand-name formulation by no more than a specific amount.

Metabolism and Excretion

Metabolic Routes. The four major metabolic routes for drugs are *oxidation*, *reduction*, *hydrolysis*, and *conjugation*. Metabolism usually yields inactive metabolites that are more polar and therefore more readily excreted. However, metabolism also transforms many inactive prodrugs into therapeutically active metabolites. The liver is the principal site of *metabolism*, and bile, feces, and urine are the major routes of *excretion*. Psychotherapeutic drugs are also excreted in sweat, saliva, tears, and breast milk.

Quantitation of Metabolism and Excretion. Four important quantities regarding metabolism and excretion are time of peak plasma concentration, half-life, first-pass effect, and clearance. The time between the administration of a drug and the appearance of *peak plasma concentrations* varies depending on the route of administration and rate of absorption. A drug's *half-life* is the amount of time it takes for metabolism and excretion to reduce a particular plasma concentration by half. A drug administered steadily at time intervals shorter than its half-life will reach 97 percent of its steady-state plasma concentration after five half-lives. The *first-pass effect* refers to the initial metabolism of orally administered drugs within the portal circulation of the liver and is quantitated as the fraction of absorbed drug reaching the systemic circulation unmetabolized. *Clearance* is a measure of the amount of the drug excreted from the body in a specific period of time.

Cytochrome P450 Enzymes. Most psychotherapeutic drugs are oxidized by the hepatic cytochrome P450 (CYP) enzyme system, which is so named because it absorbs light strongly at a wavelength of 450 nm. The human CYP enzymes comprise several distinct families and subfamilies. In the CYP nomenclature, the family is denoted by a numeral, the subfamily by a capital letter, and the individual member of the subfamily by a second numeral (e.g., 2D6). Persons with genetic polymorphisms in the CYP genes that encode inefficient versions of CYP enzymes are considered "poor metabolizers."

The CYP enzymes are responsible for the inactivation of most psychotherapeutic drugs. These enzymes act primarily in the endoplasmic reticulum of the hepatocytes and the cells of the intestine. Thus, cellular pathophysiology, such as that caused by viral hepatitis or cirrhosis, may affect the efficiency of drug metabolism by the CYP enzymes.

There are three ways in which drug interactions influence the CYP system:

1. Induction. Expression of the CYP genes may be induced by alcohol, by certain drugs (barbiturates, anticonvulsants), or by smoking. For example, an inducer of CYP 3A4, such as cimetidine, may increase the metabolism and decrease the plasma concentrations of a substrate of 3A4, such as alprazolam (Xanax).
2. Noncompetitive inhibition. Certain drugs that are not substrates for a particular enzyme may nonetheless indirectly inhibit the enzyme and slow its metabolism of other drug substrates. For example, concurrent administration of a CYP 2D6 inhibitor, such as fluoxetine (Prozac), may inhibit the metabolism and thus raise the plasma concentrations of CYP 2D6 substrates, including amitriptyline (Elavil). If one CYP enzyme is inhibited, then its substrate accumulates until it is metabolized by an alternate CYP enzyme.
3. Competitive inhibition. Concurrent administration of two or more substrates for a particular enzyme may produce competitive inhibition of the enzyme, but such interactions are not usually clinically relevant. For example, clomipramine (Anafranil) and theophylline (Theo-Dur, Slo-bid) are both substrates of CYP 1A2, but their concurrent administration has little effect on their respective plasma concentrations.

CLINICAL GUIDELINES

Physicians who practice clinical psychopharmacology require skill as both diagnosticians and psychotherapists, knowledge of

Patients generally have less trouble with adverse effects if they have been told to expect them. Psychiatrists can explain the appearance of adverse effects as evidence that the drug is working. But clinicians should distinguish between probable or expected adverse effects and rare or unexpected ones.

DISCONTINUATION (WITHDRAWAL) SYNDROMES

The transient emergence of mild symptoms upon discontinuation or reduction of dosage is associated with a number of drugs, including paroxetine (Paxil), venlafaxine (Effexor), sertraline (Zoloft), fluvoxamine (Luvox), and the tricyclic and tetracyclic drugs. More severe discontinuation symptoms are associated with lithium (rebound mania), dopamine-receptor antagonists (tardive dyskinesias), and benzodiazepines (anxiety and insomnia). One such syndrome occurs with the withdrawal of selective serotonin reuptake inhibitors (SSRIs)—the serotonin discontinuation syndrome. It consists of agitation, nausea, dysequilibrium, and dysphoria. The syndrome is more likely to occur if the plasma half-life of the agent is brief, if the drug is taken for at least 2 months, or if higher dosages are used. The symptoms are time limited and can be minimized by gradually reducing the dosage.

DRUG INTERACTIONS

In addition to the CYP-induced drug interactions mentioned above, drug interactions with other causes may increase or decrease the activity of both the psychiatric drug and any other medications the patient is taking. In some cases, this may increase the risk of adverse reactions, and clinicians should be fully aware of all of the possible interactions before exposing patients to more than one drug at a time. Drug interactions are frequently used to augment the desired therapeutic benefit by influencing distinct pharmacodynamic sites of action. For example, in the treatment of depression, SSRIs, which raise synaptic serotonin levels, may be mixed with bupropion (Wellbutrin), which has little serotonergic activity but is highly active on the norepinephrine and dopamine systems. The resulting mixture of activities may be a more powerful antidepressant than either drug alone. Augmentation strategies should avoid duplication of pharmacodynamic activity, should not pair an agonist with an antagonist of the same receptor, and should be approached with caution to avoid potentially dangerous adverse effects. For example, mixing a tricyclic drug and a monoamine oxidase inhibitor (MAOI) is reasonable, since each drug affects distinct cellular sites, but it is also perilous because it may cause a hypertensive crisis. In general, drugs with few adverse effects make the best candidates for augmentation strategies.

Drug interactions may be either pharmacokinetic or pharmacodynamic, and they vary greatly in their potential to cause serious problems. An additional consideration is phantom drug interactions. A patient who was taking only drug A may later receive both drug A and drug B. The clinician may notice some effect and attribute it to the induction of metabolism. What may have happened is that the patient was more compliant at one point in the observation period than in another, or there may have been some other effect of which the clinician was unaware. The clinical literature can contain reports of phantom drug interactions that are rare or nonexistent.

Other interactions are true but unproved, although reasonably plausible. Still other interactions have some modest effects and are well documented, and some clinically important drug interactions are well studied and well proved. But clinicians must remember that animal pharmacokinetic data cannot always be generalized readily to humans; in vitro data do not necessarily replicate the results obtained under in vivo conditions; single-case reports can contain misleading information; and studies of acute conditions should not be regarded uncritically as relevant to chronic, steady-state conditions.

Informed clinicians need to keep these considerations in mind and focus on clinically important interactions, not on those that may be mild, unproved, or entirely phantom. At the same time, clinicians should maintain an open and receptive attitude toward the possibility of pharmacokinetic and pharmacodynamic drug interactions.

INTOXICATION AND OVERDOSE

Adverse effects may occur with any drug. Although most are mild and transitory, some are severe and lethal. The prescribing psychiatrist or physician must be vigilant in determining the emergence of toxicity or signs of overdose. The toxic dose for one person may be lethal in another person, depending on such factors as route of administration, rate of absorption, interaction with other drugs, and age and general health of the patient. One must also remember that a patient may have ingested more than one substance, so the clinical picture may represent polysubstance abuse. Treatment must be adjusted accordingly, and a history (from other persons) should be obtained and all drugs should be inspected. The beginning of this book contains illustrations of the various drugs used in psychiatry, which can be useful.

An attempt by a patient to commit suicide by taking an overdose of a prescribed medication is an extreme event. Some are more lethal than others in overdose. Barbiturates, for example, have a higher potential for lethality than SSRIs, and the doctor must be aware of which drugs are more potentially lethal. It is good clinical practice to write nonrefillable prescriptions for small quantities of drugs when suicide is a consideration. In extreme cases, the doctor should verify that patients are taking the medication and not hoarding the pills for a later overdose attempt. Patients may attempt suicide just as they appear to be getting better. Clinicians, therefore, should continue to be careful about prescribing large quantities of medication until the patient has almost completely recovered.

Another consideration is the possibility of an accidental overdose, particularly by children in the household. Patients should be advised to keep psychotherapeutic medications clearly labeled and in a safe place.

▲ 32.2 Medication-Induced Movement Disorders

The text revision of the fourth edition of *Diagnostic and Statistical Manual of Mental Disorders* (DSM-IV-TR) includes in the category of "medication-induced movement disorders" not only such disorders but also any medication-induced adverse effect that becomes a focus of clinical attention. The most common neuroleptic-related movement disorders are parkinsonism, acute dystonia, and acute akathisia. Neuroleptic malignant syndrome is a life-threatening and often misdiagnosed condition. Neuroleptic-induced tardive dyskinesia is a late-appearing adverse effect of neuroleptic drugs and can be irreversible; but recent data indicate that the syndrome, although still serious and potentially disabling, is less pernicious than was previously thought in patients taking dopamine receptor antagonists and occurs only rarely in patients taking serotonin-dopamine antagonists (SDAs).

NEUROLEPTIC-INDUCED PARKINSONISM

Neuroleptic-induced parkinsonism is characterized principally by the triad of resting tremor, rigidity, and bradykinesia (referred to in DSM-IV-TR as *akinesia*). The typical parkinsonian tremor oscillates at a steady rate of 3 to 6 cycles per second, and it may be suppressed by intended movement. Rigidity is a disorder of muscle tone—that is, the underlying tension involuntarily present in the muscles. Disorders of tone can result in either hypertonia (rigidity) or hypotonia. The hypertonia associated with neuroleptic-induced parkinsonism is of either the lead-pipe type, in which tone is continuously elevated, or the cogwheel type, in which a tremor is superimposed on rigidity. Cogwheel rigidity is revealed when an examiner rotates the hand around the axis of the wrist and encounters a regular rhythmical, ratchet-like resistance. The syndrome of bradykinesia can include a patient's mask-like facial appearance, decreased accessory arm movements when the patient walks, and a characteristic difficulty in initiating movement. The so-called *rabbit syndrome* is a tremor affecting the lips and perioral muscles; it is most commonly considered part of the syndrome of neuroleptic-induced parkinsonism, although it often appears later in treatment than other symptoms. Other parkinsonian features include slowed thinking, worsening of negative symptoms, excessive salivation, drooling, shuffling gait, micrographia, seborrhea, and dysphoria.

The pathophysiology of neuroleptic-induced parkinsonism involves the blockade of dopamine type 2 (D_2) receptors in the caudate at the termination of the nigrostriatal dopamine neurons, the same neurons that degenerate in idiopathic Parkinson's disease. Patients who are elderly and female are at the highest risk for neuroleptic-induced parkinsonism. More than 50 percent of patients treated with long-term, high-potency dopamine receptor antagonists may develop neuroleptic-induced parkinsonism at some point in their course of medication. Functional neuroimaging studies have shown that parkinsonism is seen with 80 percent or higher occupancy of D_2 receptors in the caudate. By the same method, antipsychotic efficacy was seen with only 50 to 75 percent D_2 receptor occupancy.

Treatment

Once parkinsonian symptoms appear, the three steps in treatment are reducing the dosage of the neuroleptic, instituting antiextrapyramidal system medications, and (possibly) changing the neuroleptic. The SDAs are a recommended alternative to the dopamine receptor antagonists for patients with neuroleptic-induced movement disorders. Studies show that the inci-

dence of drug-induced parkinsonism is low for the SDAs and for low-potency dopamine receptor antagonists, such as thioridazine (Mellaril). Extrapyramidal symptoms are associated with dosages of risperidone (Risperdal) in excess of the recommended maximum dose of 4 to 6 mg a day. The common development of tolerance to the parkinsonian adverse effects of these drugs is poorly understood. Once treatment is initiated, therefore, clinicians should attempt to reduce or stop the antiextrapyramidal system medications after 14 to 21 days of treatment to assess whether the medications are still necessary.

NEUROLEPTIC MALIGNANT SYNDROME

Neuroleptic malignant syndrome is a life-threatening complication of antipsychotic treatment and can occur anytime during the course of treatment. The symptoms include muscular rigidity and dystonia (hence the classification of the disorder as a movement disorder), akinesia, mutism, obtundation, and agitation. The autonomic symptoms include high fever, sweating, and increased blood pressure and heart rate. The neuroleptic malignant syndrome may also be precipitated in patients with Parkinson's disease by abrupt withdrawal of the dopamine precursor levodopa, which suggests that the syndrome may be one possible result of a precipitous reduction in dopamine receptor activation. The prevalence of neuroleptic malignant syndrome is estimated to be 0.02 to 2.4 percent of patients exposed to dopamine receptor antagonists.

Treatment

In addition to supportive medical treatment, the most commonly used medications for the condition are dantrolene (Dantrium) and bromocriptine (Parlodel), although amantadine (Symmetrel) is sometimes used. Bromocriptine and amantadine possess direct dopamine receptor agonist effects and may serve to overcome the antipsychotic-induced dopamine receptor blockade. Mortality rates are reported to be 10 to 20 percent. The lowest effective dosage of antipsychotic drug should be used to reduce the chance of neuroleptic malignant syndrome. Antipsychotic drugs with anticholinergic effects seem less likely to cause neuroleptic malignant syndrome.

NEUROLEPTIC-INDUCED ACUTE DYSTONIA

Dystonias are brief or prolonged contractions of muscles that result in obviously abnormal movements or postures, including oculogyric crises, tongue protrusion, trismus, torticollis, laryngeal-pharyngeal dystonias, and dystonic postures of the limbs and trunk. The development of dystonic symptoms is characterized by their early onset during the course of treatment with neuroleptics and their high incidence in men, in patients younger than age 30, and in patients given high dosages of high-potency medications. The pathophysiological mechanism for dystonias is not clearly understood, although changes in neuroleptic concentrations and the resulting changes in homeostatic mechanisms within the basal ganglia may be the major causes of dystonias.

Treatment

Treatment of dystonias should be immediate; the most common agents are anticholinergic or antihistaminergic drugs. If a patient fails to respond to three doses of these drugs within 2 hours, the clinician should consider other causes for the dystonic movements. After resolution of the acute episode, oral anticholinergic agents should be given, and their effects reassessed every 2 weeks.

NEUROLEPTIC-INDUCED ACUTE AKATHISIA

Akathisia is characterized by subjective feelings of restlessness, objective signs of restlessness, or both. Examples include a sense of anxiety, inability to relax, jitteriness, pacing, rocking motions while sitting, and rapid alternation of sitting and standing. Akathisia can often be misdiagnosed as anxiety or as increased psychotic agitation, and it may result in an increase in the dosage of antipsychotic medication, which actually exacerbates the condition. Middle-aged women are at increased risk of akathisia, and the time course is similar to that for neuroleptic-induced parkinsonism. Akathisia has been associated with the use of a wide range of psychiatric drugs, including antipsychotics, antidepressants, and sympathomimetics. A recent report associates akathisia with a poor treatment outcome.

Treatment

The three basic steps in the treatment of akathisia are reducing neuroleptic medication dosage, attempting treatment with appropriate drugs, and considering changing the neuroleptic. The most efficacious drugs in the treatment of akathisia are the β-adrenergic receptor antagonists, although anticholinergic drugs, benzodiazepines, and cyproheptadine (Periactin) may benefit some patients. Patients may be less likely to experience akathisia while receiving low-potency neuroleptics—for example, thioridazine—than while receiving high-potency neuroleptics—for example, haloperidol (Haldol); the SDAs are associated with a low incidence of akathisia.

NEUROLEPTIC-INDUCED TARDIVE DYSKINESIA

Neuroleptic-induced tardive dyskinesia is a late-appearing disorder of involuntary, choreoathetoid movements. The most common movements involve the orofacial region along with choreoathetoid movements of the fingers and toes. Athetoid movements of the head, neck, and hips also occur in seriously affected patients. In the most serious cases, patients may have breathing and swallowing irregularities that result in aerophagia, belching, and grunting. The Abnormal Involuntary Movement Scale (AIMS), administered every 3 to 6 months to patients who are taking antipsychotic drugs, is an effective diagnostic tool for tardive dyskinesia (Table 32.2–1).

The risk factors for tardive dyskinesia, which occurs in up to 25 percent of patients treated with dopamine receptor antagonists for over 4 years, include long-term treatment with neuroleptics, increasing age, female sex, the presence of a mood disorder, and the presence of a cognitive disorder. Tardive dystonia may appear after several years of exposure to neuroleptics, is more common in younger patients, and may coexist with tardive dyskinesia. It is characterized by sustained or slow involuntary movements of the neck, trunk, face, or limbs.

Table 32.2–1
Abnormal Involuntary Movement Scale (AIMS) Examination Procedure

Patient identification:_____ Date:_____
Rated by:

Either before or after completing the examination procedure, observe the patient unobtrusively at rest (e.g., in waiting room).

The chair to be used in this examination should be a hard, firm one without arms.

After observing the patient, he or she may be rated on a scale of 0 (none), 1 (minimal), 2 (mild), 3 (moderate), and 4 (severe) according to the severity of symptoms.

Ask the patient whether there is anything in his/her mouth (i.e., gum, candy, etc.) and if there is to remove it.

Ask the patient about the current condition of his/her teeth. Ask the patient if he/she wears dentures. Do teeth or dentures bother the patient now?

Ask the patient whether he/she notices any movement in mouth, face, hands, or feet. If yes, ask to describe and to what extent they currently bother the patient or interfere with his/her activities.

0 1 2 3 4	Have the patient sit in chair with hands on knees, legs slightly apart, and feet flat on floor. (Look at entire body for movements while in this position.)
0 1 2 3 4	Ask the patient to sit with hands hanging unsupported. If male, between legs; if female and wearing a dress, hanging over knees. (Observe hands and other body areas.)
0 1 2 3 4	Ask the patient to open mouth. (Observe tongue at rest within mouth.) Do this twice.
0 1 2 3 4	Ask the patient to protrude tongue. (Observe abnormalities of tongue movement.) Do this twice.
0 1 2 3 4	Ask the patient to tap thumb, with each finger, as rapidly as possible for 10–15 seconds; separately with right hand, then with left hand. (Observe facial and leg movements.)
0 1 2 3 4	Flex and extend patient's left and right arms. (One at a time.)
0 1 2 3 4	Ask the patient to stand up. (Observe in profile. Observe all body areas again, hips included.)
0 1 2 3 4	Ask the patient to extend both arms outstretched in front with palms down. (Observe trunk, legs, and mouth.)[a]
0 1 2 3 4	Have the patient walk a few paces, turn and walk back to chair. (Observe hands and gait.) Do this twice.[a]

[a]Activated movements.

Treatment

Although various treatments for tardive dyskinesia have been unsuccessful, the course of tardive dyskinesia is considered less relentless than was previously thought. The SDAs are associated with an extremely low risk of developing tardive dyskinesia and therefore present an effective treatment approach. Patients with tardive dyskinesia frequently experience an exacerbation of their symptoms when the dopamine receptor antagonist is withheld, whereas substitution of an SDA may limit the abnormal movements without worsening the progression of the dyskinesia. Before the appearance of the antipsychotics in the 1950s, clinicians noted that 1 to 5 percent of psychiatric inpatients with schizophrenia developed movements resembling tardive dyskinesia. This observation suggests that not all cases of tardive dyskinesia should necessarily be attributed to antipsychotics. Nevertheless, the treatment is the same whatever the cause.

MEDICATION-INDUCED POSTURAL TREMOR

Tremor is defined as a rhythmical alteration in movement that usually exceeds 1 beat per second. Typically, tremors decrease during periods of relaxation and sleep and increase during periods of anger and increased tension. These characteristics sometimes mistakenly lead inexperienced clinicians to assume that a patient is faking the tremor. Whereas all the DSM-IV-TR diagnoses previously discussed specifically include an association with neuroleptics, DSM-IV-TR acknowledges that a range of psychiatric medications can produce tremor—most notably lithium (Eskalith), antidepressants, and valproate (Depakene)—and still other psychiatric medications are associated with the induction of tremor.

The treatment of tremor involves four general steps. First, the lowest possible dosage of the psychiatric drug should be used. Second, patients should minimize their caffeine and alcohol consumption. Third, the psychiatric drug should be taken at bedtime to minimize the amount of daytime tremor. Fourth, β-adrenergic receptor antagonists can be given to treat drug-induced tremors. Carbamazepine (Tegretol) has also been found to be of use in some cases.

MEDICATION-INDUCED MOVEMENT DISORDER NOT OTHERWISE SPECIFIED

Although neuroleptics are the psychiatric drugs most commonly associated with movement disorders, almost all the most commonly used psychiatric drugs can produce movement disorders in some patients. Furthermore, many nonpsychiatric drugs can produce movement disorders, and patients who are treated with both psychiatric and nonpsychiatric drugs may experience additive effects of these medications on their movement disorders. DSM-IV-TR also defines the diagnostic category as including movement disorders other than those already specified. Such movement disorders include tardive dystonia, tardive Tourette's syndrome, tardive myoclonus, tardive akathisia, and tardive parkinsonism.

ADVERSE EFFECTS OF MEDICATION NOT OTHERWISE SPECIFIED

This category allows clinicians to record the adverse effects of medications, other than movement symptoms, which become a focus of treatment. Examples of such adverse effects include priapism, severe hypotension, and cardiac abnormalities.

▲ 32.3.1 α₂-Adrenergic Receptor Agonists: Clonidine and Guanfacine

Clonidine (Catapres) and guanfacine (Tenex) are presynaptic α₂-adrenergic receptor agonists approved for use as antihypertensive agents. Stimulation of α₂-adrenergic receptors reduces the firing rate of noradrenergic neurons and reduces plasma concentrations of norepinephrine. Because of the widespread actions of the noradrenergic system, clonidine has also been adopted for use as a psychopharmacological agent. The most important clinical applications in psychiatry are as therapy for attention-deficit/hyperactivity disorder, opioid withdrawal, Tourette's disorder, and suppression of agitation in posttraumatic stress disorder. Their role as a treatment for selected mental disorders is generally limited to instances in which other interventions have failed to ameliorate symptoms adequately.

PHARMACOLOGICAL ACTIONS

Clonidine and guanfacine are well absorbed from the gastrointestinal (GI) tract and reach peak plasma levels 1 to 3 hours after oral administration. The half-life of clonidine is 6 to 20 hours and that of guanfacine is 10 to 30 hours.

The agonist effects of clonidine and guanfacine on presynaptic α₂-adrenergic receptors in the sympathetic nuclei of the brain result in a decrease in the amount of norepinephrine released from the presynaptic nerve terminals. This generally resets the body's sympathetic tone to a lower level and decreases arousal.

EFFECTS ON SPECIFIC ORGANS AND SYSTEMS

Both clonidine and guanfacine reduce peripheral sympathetic tone, lower diastolic and systolic blood pressure, and cause bradycardia. Activation of central α₂-receptors results in a sleep-like state in animal studies. Both cause sedation and sleep in humans. Both increase slow-wave sleep, reduce rapid eye movement (REM) sleep time and percentage, and increase REM latency. The effects on the GI tract are minimal, with some reduction in basal gastric acid secretion. There is little effect on renal function.

THERAPEUTIC INDICATIONS

Withdrawal from Opioids, Alcohol, Benzodiazepines, or Nicotine

Clonidine and guanfacine are effective in reducing the autonomic symptoms of rapid opioid withdrawal (e.g., hypertension, tachycardia, dilated pupils, sweating, lacrimation, and rhinorrhea) but not the associated subjective sensations. Clonidine administration (0.1 to 0.2 mg two to four times a day) is initiated prior to detoxification and is then tapered off over 1 to 2 weeks.

Clonidine and guanfacine can reduce symptoms of alcohol and benzodiazepine withdrawal, including anxiety, diarrhea, and tachycardia. Clonidine and guanfacine can reduce craving, anxiety, and irritability symptoms of nicotine withdrawal. The transdermal patch formulation of clonidine is associated with better long-term compliance for purposes of detoxification than the tablet formulation is.

Tourette's Disorder

Clonidine and guanfacine are effective drugs for the treatment of Tourette's disorder. Most clinicians begin treatment for Tourette's disorder with the standard dopamine receptor antagonists, haloperidol (Haldol) and pimozide (Orap), and the serotonin-dopamine antagonists (SDAs), risperidone (Risperdal) and olanzapine (Zyprexa). However, if concerned about the adverse effects of these drugs, the clinician may begin treatment with clonidine or guanfacine. The starting dosage of clonidine for a child is 0.05 mg a day; it can be raised to 0.3 mg a day in divided doses. Three months are needed before the beneficial effects of clonidine can be seen in Tourette's disorder. Response rates of 0 to 70 percent have been reported.

Other Tic Disorders

Clonidine and guanfacine reduce the frequency and severity of tics in persons with tic disorder, with or without comorbid attention-deficit/hyperactivity symptoms.

Hyperactivity and Aggression in Children

Clonidine and guanfacine can be useful alternatives for the treatment of attention-deficit/hyperactivity disorder. They are used in place of sympathomimetics and antidepressants, which may produce paradoxical worsening of hyperactivity in some children with mental retardation, aggression, or features on the spectrum of autism. Clonidine and guanfacine can improve mood, reduce activity level, and improve social adaptation. Some multiply impaired children may respond favorably to clonidine, while others may simply become sedated. The starting dosage is 0.05 mg a day; it can be raised to 0.3 mg a day in divided doses. The efficacy of clonidine and guanfacine for control of hyperactivity and aggression often diminishes over several months of use.

Clonidine or guanfacine can be combined with methylphenidate (Ritalin) or dextroamphetamine (Dexedrine, Dextrostat) to treat hyperactivity and inattentiveness, respectively. A small number of cases have been reported of sudden death of children taking clonidine together with methylphenidate; however, it has not been conclusively demonstrated that these medications contributed to those deaths. Clinicians should explain to the family that the efficacy and safety of this combination have not been investigated in controlled trials. Periodic cardiovascular assessments, including vital signs and electrocardiograms (ECGs), are warranted if this combination is used.

Posttraumatic Stress Disorder

Acute exacerbations of posttraumatic stress disorder may be associated with hyperadrenergic symptoms, such as hyperarousal, exaggerated startle response, insomnia, vivid nightmares, tachycardia, agitation, hypertension, and perspiration. These symptoms may respond to the use of clonidine or (especially for overnight benefit) guanfacine.

Other Disorders

Other potential indications for clonidine include other anxiety disorders (panic disorder, phobias, obsessive-compulsive disorder, and generalized anxiety disorder) and mania, in which it may be synergistic with lithium (Eskalith) or carbamazepine (Tegretol). Anecdotal reports have noted the efficacy of clonidine in schizophrenia and tardive dyskinesia. A clonidine patch can reduce the hypersalivation and dysphagia caused by clozapine (Clozaril). Isolated reports describe successful use of clonidine in premenstrual syndrome and restless legs syndrome.

PRECAUTIONS AND ADVERSE REACTIONS

The most common adverse effects associated with clonidine are dry mouth and eyes, fatigue, sedation, dizziness, nausea, hypotension, and constipation, which result in discontinuation of therapy by approximately 10 percent of all persons taking the drug. Some persons also experience sexual dysfunction. Tolerance may develop to these adverse effects. A similar but milder adverse effect profile is seen with guanfacine, especially at doses of 3 mg or more per day. Clonidine and guanfacine should not be taken by adults with a blood pressure below 90/60 or with cardiac arrhythmias, especially bradycardia. Development of bradycardia warrants gradual, tapered discontinuation of the drug. Clonidine in particular is associated with sedation, and tolerance does not usually develop to this adverse effect. Uncommon central nervous system (CNS) adverse effects of clonidine include insomnia, anxiety, and depression; rare CNS adverse effects include vivid dreams, nightmares, and hallucinations. Fluid retention associated with clonidine treatment can be treated with diuretics. The transdermal patch formulation of clonidine can cause local skin irritation, which can be minimized by rotating the sites of application.

Overdose

Persons who take an overdose of clonidine can present with coma and constricted pupils, symptoms similar to those of an opioid overdose. Other symptoms of overdose are decreased blood pressure, pulse, and respiratory rates. Guanfacine overdose produces a milder version of these symptoms. Clonidine and guanfacine should be used with caution in persons with heart disease, any type of vascular disease, renal disease, Raynaud's syndrome, or a history of depression. Clonidine and guanfacine should be avoided during pregnancy and by nursing mothers. Elderly persons are more sensitive to the drug than younger adults. Children are susceptible to the same adverse effects as adults.

Withdrawal

Abrupt discontinuation of clonidine use can cause anxiety, restlessness, perspiration, tremor, abdominal pain, palpitations, headache, and a dramatic rise in blood pressure. These symptoms may appear approximately 20 hours after the last dose of clonidine and thus may be seen if one or two doses are skipped. A similar set of symptoms occasionally occurs 2 to 4 days after discontinuation of guanfacine, but the usual course is a gradual return to baseline blood pressure over 2 to 4 days. Because of the possibility of discontinuation symptoms, dosages of clonidine and guanfacine should be tapered down slowly.

DRUG–DRUG INTERACTIONS

Coadministration of clonidine or guanfacine and tricyclic drugs can inhibit the hypotensive effects of both. Trazodone (Desyrel) can potentially produce hypotension and sedation when combined with clonidine. Any antihypertensive agent or drug that causes hypotension as a side effect may amplify blood pressure drops if coadministered with these drugs. They may also enhance the CNS depressive effects of barbiturates, alcohol, and other sedative-hypnotic agents. Concomitant use of β-adrenergic receptor antagonists can increase the severity of rebound phenomena, including hypertension, when clonidine use is discontinued. Yohimbine (Yocon), an α_2-adrenergic receptor antagonist, blocks the pharmacological effects of clonidine. The reported sudden deaths of children taking concurrent methylphenidate and clonidine remain unexplained. They may represent isolated instances of children with preexisting cardiovascular abnormalities who either experienced adverse events unrelated to medication or had reactions to the clonidine alone.

LABORATORY INTERFERENCES

No known laboratory interferences are associated with the use of clonidine or guanfacine.

Dosage and Clinical Guidelines

Clonidine is available in 0.1-, 0.2-, and 0.3-mg tablets. The usual starting dosage is 0.1 mg orally twice a day; the dosage can be raised by 0.1 mg a day to an appropriate level (up to 1.2 mg per day). Clonidine must always be tapered when it is discontinued, to avoid rebound hypertension, which may occur approximately 20 hours after the last clonidine dose. A weekly transdermal formulation of clonidine is available at doses of 0.1, 0.2, and 0.3 mg per day. The usual starting dosage is a 0.1-mg-per-day patch, which is changed each week for adults and every 5 days for children; the dosage can be increased every 1 to 2 weeks. Transition from the oral to the transdermal formulations should be accomplished gradually, by overlapping them for 3 to 4 days.

Guanfacine is available in 1- and 2-mg tablets. The usual starting dose is 1 mg before sleep, and this may be increased to 2 mg before sleep after 3 to 4 weeks, if necessary. Regardless of the indication for which clonidine or guanfacine is being used, the drug should be withheld if a person becomes hypotensive (blood pressure below 90/60).

▲ 32.3.2 β-Adrenergic Receptor Antagonists

The β-adrenergic receptor antagonists, which are variously referred to as β-*blockers* and β-*antagonists,* represent an important psychopharmacological intervention—the reduction of adrenergic receptor activation. β-Adrenergic receptor antagonists are commonly used in medical practice for their peripheral effects in the treatment of hypertension, angina, certain cardiac arrhythmias, and the symptoms of hyperthyroidism, but the drugs are also used for their central actions in the treatment of migraine. Their effectiveness as peripherally and centrally acting agents has been well demonstrated for social phobia (e.g., performance anxiety), lithium-induced postural tremor, control of aggressive behavior, and neuroleptic-induced acute akathisia.

PHARMACOLOGICAL ACTIONS

The β-adrenergic receptor antagonists differ with regard to lipophilicities, metabolic routes, β-receptor selectivity, and half-lives (Table 32.3.2–1). The absorption of β-receptor antagonists from the gastrointestinal (GI) tract is variable. The agents that are most soluble in lipids (i.e., are lipophilic) are likely to cross the blood–brain barrier and enter the brain; agents that are least lipophilic are less likely to enter the brain. When central nervous system (CNS) effects are desired, a lipophilic drug may be preferred; when only peripheral effects are desired, a less lipophilic drug may be indicated.

EFFECTS ON SPECIFIC ORGANS AND SYSTEMS

β_1-Receptors modulate chronotropic and inotropic cardiac functions. They have a marked blood-pressure-lowering effect in patients with hypertension and produce bradycardia. β_2-Receptors modulate bronchodilatation and vasodilation. For this reason, β_1-selective drugs are preferable in the treatment of patients with asthma and other obstructive pulmonary diseases; the blockade of the pulmonary β_2-receptors blocks the bronchodilating effects of epinephrine. Some experts, however, would never use β-adrenergic receptor antagonists in patients with asthma but might substitute a benzodiazepine for the same indication.

THERAPEUTIC INDICATIONS
Anxiety Disorders

Propranolol (Inderal) is useful for the treatment of social phobia, primarily of the performance type (e.g., disabling anxiety before a musical performance). Data are also available for its use in treatment of panic disorder, posttraumatic stress disorder, and generalized anxiety disorder. In social phobia, the common treatment approach is to take 10 to 40 mg of propranolol 20 to 30 minutes before the anxiety-provoking situation. Persons may try a test run of one of the β-adrenergic receptor antagonists before using it to prepare for an anxiety-provoking situation to ensure that they do not experience any adverse effects from the drug or the dose. β-Adrenergic receptor antagonists may blunt cognition in some persons. They are less effective for the treatment of panic disorder than benzodiazepines or selective serotonin reuptake inhibitors (SSRIs).

Lithium-Induced Postural Tremor

β-Adrenergic receptor antagonists are beneficial for lithium-induced postural tremor and other medication-induced postural tremors—for example, those induced by the tricyclic drugs and valproate (Depakene). The initial approach to this movement disorder includes lowering the dose of lithium (Eskalith), eliminating aggravating factors such as caffeine, and administering lithium at bedtime. However, if these interventions are inadequate, propranolol in the range of 20 to 160 mg a day, given two or three times daily, is generally effective for the treatment of lithium-induced postural tremor.

Neuroleptic-Induced Acute Akathisia

Many studies have shown that β-adrenergic receptor antagonists can be effective in the treatment of neuroleptic-induced acute

Table 32.3.2–1
β-Adrenergic Drugs Used in Psychiatry

Generic Name	Trade Name	Lipophilic	Metabolism	Receptor Selectivity	Half-Life (h)	Usual Starting Dosage (mg)	Usual Maximum Dosage (mg)
Propranolol	Inderal	Yes	Hepatic	$\beta_1 = \beta_2$	3–6	10–20 bid or tid	30–140 bid
Nadolol	Corgard	No	Renal	$\beta_1 = \beta_2$	14–24	40 od	30–240 od
Pindolol	Visken	Intermediate	Hepatic	$\beta_1 = \beta_2$	3–4	5 bid	30 bid
Labetalol	Normodyne, Trandate	Intermediate	Hepatic	$\beta_1 = \beta_2$	4–6	100 bid	400–800 tid
Metoprolol	Lopressor	Yes	Hepatic	$\beta_1 > \beta_2$	3–4	50 bid	75–150 bid
Atenolol	Tenormin	No	Renal	$\beta_1 > \beta_2$	5–8	50 od	50–100 od
Acebutolol	Sectral	No	Hepatic	$\beta_1 > \beta_2$	3–4	400 od	600 bid

akathisia. Most clinicians believe that β-adrenergic receptor antagonists are more effective for this indication than anticholinergics and benzodiazepines. β-Adrenergic receptor antagonists are not effective in the treatment of such neuroleptic-induced movement disorders as acute dystonia and parkinsonism.

Aggression and Violent Behavior

β-Adrenergic receptor antagonists may be effective in reducing the number of aggressive and violent outbursts in persons with impulse disorders, schizophrenia, and aggression associated with brain injuries such as trauma, tumors, anoxic injury, encephalitis, alcohol dependence, and degenerative disorders (e.g., Huntington's disease). Many studies have added a β-adrenergic receptor antagonist to the ongoing therapy (e.g., antipsychotics, anticonvulsants, lithium), making it difficult to distinguish additive effects from independent effects. Propranolol dosages for this indication range from 50 to 800 mg a day.

Alcohol Withdrawal

Propranolol has been reported to be useful as an adjuvant to benzodiazepines but not as a sole agent in the treatment of alcohol withdrawal. The following dose schedule is suggested: no propranolol for a pulse rate below 50; 50 mg of propranolol for a pulse rate between 50 and 80; and 100 mg of propranolol for a pulse rate of 80 or above.

Antidepressant Augmentation

Pindolol (Visken) has been used to augment and hasten the antidepressant effects of SSRIs, tricyclic drugs, and electroconvulsive therapy (ECT). Small studies have shown that pindolol administered at the onset of antidepressant therapy may shorten the usual 2- to 4-week latency of antidepressant response by several days. Because the β-adrenergic receptor antagonists may induce depression in some persons, augmentation strategies with these drugs must be further clarified in controlled trials.

Other Disorders

A number of case reports and controlled studies have reported data indicating that β-adrenergic receptor antagonists may be of modest benefit to persons with schizophrenia and with manic symptoms. It has also been used in some patients with stuttering.

PRECAUTIONS AND ADVERSE REACTIONS

The β-adrenergic receptor antagonists are contraindicated for use in persons with asthma, insulin-dependent diabetes, congestive heart failure, significant vascular disease, persistent angina, and hyperthyroidism. They are contraindicated in diabetic persons because the drugs antagonize the normal physiological response to hypoglycemia. The β-adrenergic receptor antagonists can worsen atrioventricular (A-V) conduction defects and lead to complete A-V heart block and death. If the clinician decides that the risk-benefit ratio warrants a trial of a β-adrenergic receptor antagonist in a person with one of these coexisting medical conditions, a β_1-selective agent should be the first choice. All currently available β-adrenergic receptor antagonists are excreted in breast milk and should be administered with caution to nursing women.

The most common adverse effects of β-adrenergic receptor antagonists are hypotension and bradycardia. In persons at risk for these adverse effects, a test dosage of 20 mg a day of propranolol can be given to assess their reaction to the drug. Depression has been associated with lipophilic β-receptor antagonists such as propranolol, but it is probably rare. Nausea, vomiting, diarrhea, and constipation may also be caused by treatment with these agents. Serious CNS adverse effects (e.g., agitation, confusion, and hallucinations) are rare.

DRUG–DRUG INTERACTIONS

Concomitant administration of propranolol results in increased plasma concentrations of antipsychotics, anticonvulsants, theophylline (Theo-Dur, Slo-Bid), and levothyroxine (Synthroid). Other β-adrenergic receptor antagonists possibly have similar effects. The β-adrenergic receptor antagonists that are eliminated by the kidneys may have similar effects on drugs that are also eliminated by the renal route. Barbiturates, phenytoin (Dilantin), and cigarette smoking increase the elimination of β-adrenergic receptor antagonists that are metabolized by the liver. Several reports have associated hypertensive crises and bradycardia with the coadministration of β-adrenergic receptor antagonists and monoamine oxidase inhibitors (MAOIs). Depressed myocardial contractility and A-V nodal conduction may occur from concomitant administration of a β-adrenergic receptor antagonist and calcium channel inhibitors.

LABORATORY INTERFERENCES

The β-adrenergic receptor antagonists do not interfere with standard laboratory tests.

Dosage and Clinical Guidelines

Propranolol is available in 10-, 20-, 40-, 60-, 80-, and 90-mg tablets; 4-, 8-, and 80-mg/mL solutions; and 60-, 80-, 120-, and 160-mg sustained-release capsules. Nadolol (Corgard) is available in 20-, 40-, 80-, 120-, and 160-mg tablets. Pindolol is available in 5- and 10-mg tablets. Labetalol (Normodyne, Trandate) is available in 100-, 200-, and 300-mg tablets. Metoprolol (Lopressor, Toprol) is available in 50- and 100-mg tablets; and in 50-, 100-, and 200-mg sustained-release tablets. Atenolol (Tenormin) is available in 25-, 50-, and 100-mg tablets. Acebutolol (Sectral) is available in 200- and 400-mg capsules.

For the treatment of chronic disorders, propranolol administration is usually initiated at 10 mg by mouth three times a day or 20 mg by mouth twice daily. The dosage can be raised by 20 to 30 mg a day until a therapeutic effect begins to emerge. The dosage should be leveled off at the appropriate range for the disorder under treatment. The treatment of aggressive behavior sometimes requires dosages up to 800 mg a day, and therapeutic effects may not be seen until the person has been receiving the maximal dosage for 4 to 8 weeks. As mentioned, for treatment of social phobia, primarily the performance type, the patient should take 10 to 40 mg of propranolol 20 to 30 minutes before the performance.

Pulse and blood pressure should be taken regularly, and the drug should be withheld if the pulse rate is below 50 or the systolic blood pressure is below 90. Drug use should be temporarily discontinued if it produces severe dizziness, ataxia, or wheezing. Treatment with β-adrenergic receptor antagonists should never be discontinued abruptly. Propranolol use should be tapered by 60 mg a day until a dosage of 60 mg a day is reached, after which the dosage should be tapered by 10 to 20 mg a day every 3 or 4 days.

▲ 32.3.3 Amantadine

Amantadine (Symmetrel) is used primarily for the treatment of medication-induced movement disorders, such as neuroleptic-induced parkinsonism. It is also used as an antiviral agent for the prophylaxis and treatment of influenza A infection.

PHARMACOLOGICAL ACTIONS

Amantadine is well absorbed from the gastrointestinal (GI) tract after oral administration, reaches peak plasma concentrations in approximately 2 to 3 hours, has a half-life of approximately 12 to 18 hours, and attains steady-state concentrations after approximately 4 to 5 days of therapy. Amantadine is excreted unmetabolized in the urine. Plasma concentrations of amantadine can be as much as twice as high in elderly persons as in younger adults. Patients with renal failure accumulate amantadine in their bodies.

Amantadine augments dopaminergic neurotransmission in the central nervous system (CNS). The precise mechanism for this effect is unknown, but it may involve dopamine release from presynaptic vesicles, blocking reuptake of dopamine into presynaptic nerve terminals, or an agonist effect on postsynaptic dopamine receptors.

EFFECTS ON SPECIFIC ORGANS AND SYSTEMS

Amantadine is associated with CNS and GI adverse effects at high doses.

THERAPEUTIC INDICATIONS

The primary indication for amantadine in psychiatry is for the treatment of extrapyramidal signs and symptoms, such as parkinsonism, akinesia, and so-called rabbit syndrome (focal perioral tremor of the choreoathetoid type) caused by the administration of dopamine receptor antagonist drugs (e.g., haloperidol [Haldol]). Amantadine is as effective as the anticholinergics (e.g., benztropine [Cogentin]) for these indications and results in improvement in approximately one-half of all persons who take it. However, amantadine is not generally considered as effective as the anticholinergics for the treatment of acute dystonic reactions and is not effective in treating tardive dyskinesia and akathisia.

Amantadine is a reasonable compromise for persons with extrapyramidal symptoms who would be sensitive to additional anticholinergic effects, particularly those taking a low-potency dopamine receptor antagonist or the elderly. Elderly persons are prone to anticholinergic adverse effects in both the CNS, such as anticholinergic delirium, and in the peripheral nervous system, such as urinary retention. Amantadine is associated with less memory impairment than the anticholinergics are. Amantadine is reportedly of benefit in treating some selective serotonin reuptake inhibitor (SSRI)–associated side effects, such as lethargy, fatigue, anorgasmia, and ejaculatory inhibition. It is used in general medical practice for the treatment of parkinsonism of all causes, including idiopathic parkinsonism.

PRECAUTIONS AND ADVERSE EFFECTS

The most common CNS effects are mild dizziness, insomnia, and impaired concentration (dosage related), which occur in 5 to 10 percent of persons. Irritability, depression, anxiety, dysarthria, and ataxia occur in 1 to 5 percent of persons. More severe CNS adverse effects, including seizures and psychotic symptoms, have been reported. Nausea is the most common peripheral adverse effect of amantadine. Headache, loss of appetite, and blotchy spots on the skin have also been reported.

Livedo reticularis of the legs (a purple discoloration of the skin, caused by dilation of blood vessels) has been reported in up to 5 percent of persons who take the drug for over a month. It usually diminishes with elevation of the legs and resolves in almost all cases when drug use is terminated.

Amantadine is relatively contraindicated in persons with renal disease or a seizure disorder. It should be used with caution in persons with edema or cardiovascular disease. Some evidence indicates that amantadine is teratogenic, and thus it should not be taken by pregnant women. Because amantadine is excreted in milk, women who are breast-feeding should not take the drug.

Suicide attempts with amantadine overdosages are life-threatening. Symptoms can include toxic psychoses (confusion, hallucinations, aggressiveness) and cardiopulmonary arrest. Emergency treatment beginning with gastric lavage is indicated.

DRUG INTERACTIONS

Coadministration of amantadine with phenelzine (Nardil) or other monoamine oxidase inhibitors (MAOIs) may significantly increase resting blood pressure. The coadministration of amantadine with CNS stimulants can result in insomnia, irritability, nervousness, and possibly seizures or irregular heartbeat. Amantadine should not be coadministered with anticholinergics because adverse effects such as confusion, hallucinations, nightmares, dryness of mouth, and blurred vision may be exacerbated.

DOSAGE AND CLINICAL GUIDELINES

Amantadine is available in 100-mg capsules and as a 50 mg/5 mL syrup. The usual starting dosage of amantadine is 100 mg given orally twice a day, although the dosage can be cautiously increased up to 200 mg given orally twice a day if indicated. Amantadine should be used in persons with renal impairment only in consultation with the physician treating the renal condition. If amantadine is successful in the treatment of the drug-induced extrapyramidal symptoms, it should be continued for 4 to 6 weeks and then discontinued to see whether the person has become tolerant to the neurological adverse effects of the antipsychotic medication. Amantadine use should be tapered over 1 to 2 weeks once a decision has been made to discontinue use of the drug. Persons taking amantadine should not drink alcoholic beverages.

▲ 32.3.4 Anticholinergics

In the clinical practice of psychiatry, the anticholinergic drugs have their primary use as treatments for medication-induced movement disorders, particularly neuroleptic-induced parkinsonism, neuroleptic-induced acute dystonia, and medication-induced postural tremor. The anticholinergic drugs may also be of limited use in the treatment of neuroleptic-induced acute akathisia. Before the introduction of levodopa (Larodopa), the anticholinergic drugs were commonly used in the treatment of idiopathic Parkinson's disease.

The common use of the term *anticholinergic drugs* is misleading. There are two general types of acetylcholine receptors: the muscarinic receptors and the nicotinic receptors. The muscarinic receptors are G protein–linked receptors, and the nicotinic receptors are ligand-gated ion channels. The anticholinergic drugs discussed in this section are specific for the muscarinic receptors and, thus, are also referred to as *antimuscarinic drugs*.

PHARMACOLOGICAL ACTIONS

All anticholinergic drugs are well absorbed from the gastrointestinal (GI) tract after oral administration, and all are lipophilic enough to enter the central nervous system (CNS). Trihexyphenidyl (Artane) and benztropine (Cogentin) reach peak plasma concentrations in 2 to 3 hours after oral administration and have a duration of action of 1 to 12 hours. Benztropine is absorbed equally rapidly by intramuscular (IM) and intravenous (IV) administration; IM administration is preferred because of its low risk for adverse effects.

All six anticholinergic drugs listed in this chapter block muscarinic acetylcholine receptors, and benztropine and ethopropazine (Parsidol) also have some antihistaminergic effects. None of the available anticholinergic drugs has any effects on the nicotinic acetylcholine receptors. Of the six drugs, trihexyphenidyl is the most stimulating, perhaps acting through dopaminergic neurons, and benztropine is the least stimulating and, thus, carries the least abuse potential.

EFFECTS ON SPECIFIC ORGANS AND SYSTEMS

The antimuscarinic activity of the anticholinergic drugs discussed here affects the functioning of the autonomic ganglia and most commonly affects the GI tract, the heart, the bladder, and other parasympathetic functions.

THERAPEUTIC INDICATIONS

The primary indication for the use of anticholinergics in psychiatric practice is for the treatment of *neuroleptic-induced parkinsonism*, characterized by tremor, rigidity, cogwheeling, bradykinesia, sialorrhea, stooped posture, and festination. All the available anticholinergics are equally effective in the treatment of parkinsonian symptoms. Neuroleptic-induced parkinsonism is most common in the elderly and is most frequently seen with high-potency dopamine receptor antagonists, for example, haloperidol (Haldol). The onset of symptoms usually occurs after 2 or 3 weeks of treatment. The incidence of neuroleptic-induced parkinsonism is significantly lower with the newer antipsychotic drugs of the serotonin-dopamine antagonist (SDA) class.

Another indication is for the treatment of *neuroleptic-induced acute dystonia*, which is most common in young men. The syndrome often occurs early in the course of treatment, is commonly associated with high-potency dopamine receptor antagonists (e.g., haloperidol), and most commonly affects the muscles of the neck, tongue, face, and back. Anticholinergic drugs are effective in both short-term treatment of dystonias and prophylaxis against neuroleptic-induced acute dystonias.

Akathisia is characterized by a subjective and objective sense of restlessness, anxiety, and agitation. Although a trial of anticholinergics for the treatment of neuroleptic-induced acute akathisia is reasonable, these drugs are not generally considered as effective as the β-adrenergic receptor antagonists, the benzodiazepines, and clonidine (Catapres).

PRECAUTIONS AND ADVERSE REACTIONS

The adverse effects of the anticholinergic drugs result from blockade of muscarinic acetylcholine receptors. Anticholinergic drugs should be used cautiously, if at all, by persons with prostatic hypertrophy, urinary retention, and narrow-angle glaucoma. The anticholinergics are occasionally used as drugs of abuse because of their mild mood-elevating properties.

The most serious adverse effect associated with anticholinergic toxicity is anticholinergic intoxication, which can be characterized by delirium, coma, seizures, agitation, hallucinations,

Table 32.3.4–1
Anticholinergic Drugs

Generic Name	Brand Name	Tablet Size	Injectable	Usual Daily Oral Dose	Short-Term IM or IV Dose
Benztropine	Cogentin	0.5, 1, 2 mg	1 mg/mL	1–4 mg one to three times	1–2 mg
Biperiden	Akineton	2 mg	5 mg/mL	2 mg one to three times	2 mg
Ethopropazine	Parsidol	10, 50 mg	—	50–100 mg one to three times	—
Orphenadrine	Norflex, Dispal	100 mg	30 mg/mL	50–100 mg three times	60 mg IV given over 5 min
Procyclidine	Kemadrin	5 mg	—	2.5–5 mg three times	—
Trihexy-phenidyl	Artane, Trihex-ane, Trihexy-5	2.5 mg elixir 2 mg per 5 mL	—	2–5 mg two to four times	—

severe hypotension, supraventricular tachycardia, and peripheral manifestations—flushing, mydriasis, dry skin, hyperthermia, and decreased bowel sounds. Treatment should begin by immediate discontinuation of all anticholinergic drugs. The syndrome of anticholinergic intoxication can be diagnosed and treated with physostigmine (Antilirium, Eserine), an inhibitor of anticholinesterase, 1 to 2 mg IV (1 mg every 2 minutes) or IM every 30 or 60 minutes. Treatment with physostigmine should be used only in severe cases and only when emergency cardiac monitoring and life-support services are available, because physostigmine can lead to severe hypotension and bronchial constriction.

DRUG–DRUG INTERACTIONS

The most common drug–drug interactions with the anticholinergics occur when they are coadministered with psychotropics that also have high anticholinergic activity, such as dopamine receptor antagonists, tricyclic and tetracyclic drugs, and monoamine oxidase inhibitors (MAOIs). Many other prescription drugs and over-the-counter cold preparations also induce significant anticholinergic activity. The coadministration of those drugs can result in a life-threatening anticholinergic intoxication syndrome. Anticholinergic drugs can also delay gastric emptying, thereby decreasing the absorption of drugs that are broken down in the stomach and usually absorbed in the duodenum (e.g., levodopa and dopamine receptor antagonists).

LABORATORY INTERFERENCES

No laboratory interferences have been associated with anticholinergics.

DOSAGE AND CLINICAL GUIDELINES

The six anticholinergic drugs discussed in this chapter are available in a range of preparations (Table 32.3.4–1).

▲ 32.3.5 Antihistamines

Certain antihistamines (antagonists of histamine H_1 receptors) are used in clinical psychiatry to treat neuroleptic-induced parkinsonism and neuroleptic-induced acute dystonia and also as hypnotics and anxiolytics. Diphenhydramine (Benadryl) is used to treat neuroleptic-induced parkinsonism and neuroleptic-induced acute dystonia and sometimes as a hypnotic. Hydroxyzine hydrochloride (Atarax) and hydroxyzine pamoate (Vistaril) are used as anxiolytics. Promethazine (Phenergan) is used for its sedative and anxiolytic effects. Cyproheptadine (Periactin) has been used for the treatment of anorexia nervosa and inhibited male and female orgasm caused by serotonergic agents. So-called second-generation H_1 receptor antagonists—fexofenadine (Allegra), loratadine (Claritin), and cetirizine (Zyrtec)—are not used in psychiatry.

PHARMACOLOGICAL ACTIONS

The H_1 antagonists used in psychiatry are well absorbed from the gastrointestinal (GI) tract. The antiparkinsonian effects of intramuscular (IM) diphenhydramine have their onset in 15 to 30 minutes, and the sedative effects of diphenhydramine peak in 1 to 3 hours. The sedative effects of hydroxyzine and promethazine begin after 20 to 60 minutes and last for 4 to 6 hours. Because all three drugs are metabolized in the liver, persons with hepatic disease, such as cirrhosis, may attain high plasma concentrations with long-term administration. Cyproheptadine is well absorbed after oral administration, and its metabolites are excreted in the urine.

Activation of H_1 receptors stimulates wakefulness; therefore, receptor antagonism causes sedation. All four agents also possess some antimuscarinic cholinergic activity. Cyproheptadine is unique among the drugs, since it has both potent antihistamine and serotonin 5-HT_2 receptor antagonist properties.

EFFECTS ON SPECIFIC ORGANS AND SYSTEMS

The effects of the antihistamines on the central nervous system (CNS) include sedation and antagonism of dopamine type 2 (D_2) receptor blockade–induced movement disorders. The antihistamines may also reduce the symptoms of motion sickness in some patients. Peripherally, histamine triggers capillary permeability and stimulates the release of mediators of inflammation.

THERAPEUTIC INDICATIONS

Antihistamines are useful as a treatment for neuroleptic-induced parkinsonism, neuroleptic-induced acute dystonia, and neuroleptic-induced akathisia. They are an alternative to anticholinergics and amantadine for these purposes. The antihistamines are rela-

Table 32.3.5–1
Dosage and Administration of Traditional Antihistamines Used in Psychiatry

Drugs	Route	Preparation	Dosage
Diphenhy-dramine (Benadryl)	po	Capsules and tablets: 25 mg, 50 mg elixir and syrup: 12.5 mg/5 mL	Adults: 25–50 mg 3–4 times daily Usual sleep-aid dose: 50 mg hs Children: 5 mg/kg/24 h in 4 divided doses, not to exceed 300 mg/day
	IM (deep)	Solution: 10 mg/mL, 50 mg/mL	Adults: 10–50 mg IV or deep IM may use 100 mg if required, maximum daily dose 400 mg: for dystonic reactions, 50 mg IV over 2–3 min Children: 5 mg/kg/24 h (maximum 300 mg/day)
Hydroxyzine (Atarax, Vistaril)	po	Hydrochloride syrup: 10 mg/5 mL Tablets: 10 mg, 25 mg, 50 mg, 100 mg Pamoate suspension: 25 mg/5 mL Capsules: 25 mg, 50 mg, 100 mg	Adults: 25–100 mg qid Children: under 6: 50 mg/24 h in 3–4 divided doses over 6: 50–100 mg/day in 3–4 divided doses
	IM	Hydrochloride solution: 25 mg/mL, 50 mg/mL	Adults: 50–100 mg q4–6h prn for sedation Children: 0.5 mg/lb of body weight
Promethazine (Phenergan)	po	Syrup: 6.25 mg/5 mL, 25 mg/5 mL Tablets: 12.5 mg, 25 mg, 50 mg	Adults: 25–50 mg for sedation Children: 12.5–25 mg hs for nighttime and preoperative sedation
	pr	Suppositories: 50 mg, 25 mg, 12.5 mg	
	IM	Solution: 25 mg/mL and 50 mg/mL	
Cyrohepta-dine (Peri-actin)	po	Tablets: 4 mg Syrup: 2 mg/5 mL	Adult: usually 4–20 mg/day (may require up to 32 mg/day) for allergies, not to exceed 0.5 mg/kg/day: for antidepressant-induced anorgasmia: 4–16 mg, either in divided daily doses or approximately 1–2 h prior to coitus Children: for allergies, approximately 0.25 mg/kg/day 2–6 yr old: 2 mg po 2–3 times daily; maximum 12 mg/day 7–14 yr old: 4 mg po 2–3 times daily; maximum 16 mg/day

tively safe hypnotics, but they are not superior to the benzodiazepines, which have been much better studied in terms of efficacy and safety. The antihistamines have not been proved effective for long-term anxiolytic therapy; therefore, either the benzodiazepines, buspirone (BuSpar), or selective serotonin reuptake inhibitors (SSRIs) are preferable for such treatment. Cyroheptadine is sometimes used to treat impaired orgasms, especially delayed orgasm resulting from treatment with serotonergic drugs.

Because it promotes weight gain, cyroheptadine may be of some use in the treatment of eating disorders, such as anorexia nervosa. Cyroheptadine can reduce recurrent nightmares with posttraumatic themes. The antiserotonergic activity of cyroheptadine may counteract the serotonin syndrome caused by concomitant use of multiple serotonin-activating drugs, such as SSRIs and monoamine oxidase inhibitors (MAOIs).

PRECAUTIONS AND ADVERSE REACTIONS

Antihistamines are commonly associated with sedation, dizziness, and hypotension, all of which can be severe in elderly persons, who are also likely to suffer from the anticholinergic effects of those drugs. Paradoxical excitement and agitation are adverse effects seen in a small number of persons. Poor motor coordination can result in accidents; therefore, persons should be warned about driving and operating machinery. Other common adverse effects include epigastric distress, nausea, vomiting, diarrhea, and constipation. Because of mild anticholinergic activity, some persons experience dry mouth, urinary retention, blurred vision, and constipation. For this reason also, antihistamines should be used only at very low doses, if at all, by per-

sons with narrow-angle glaucoma or obstructive GI, prostate, or bladder conditions. A central anticholinergic syndrome with psychosis may be induced by either cyroheptadine or diphenhydramine. The use of cyroheptadine in some persons has been associated with weight gain, which may contribute to its reported efficacy in some persons with anorexia nervosa.

In addition to the above adverse effects, antihistamines have some potential for abuse. The coadministration of antihistamines and opioids can increase the euphoria experienced by persons with substance dependence. Overdoses of antihistamines can be fatal. Antihistamines are excreted in breast milk, so their use should be avoided by nursing mothers. Because of some potential for teratogenicity, pregnant women should also avoid use of antihistamines.

DRUG–DRUG INTERACTIONS

The sedative property of antihistamines can be additive with that of other CNS depressants, such as alcohol, other sedative-hypnotic drugs, and many psychotropic drugs, including tricyclic drugs and dopamine receptor antagonists. The anticholinergic activity can also be additive with that of other anticholinergic drugs and can sometimes result in severe anticholinergic symptoms or intoxication. The beneficial effects of SSRIs can be antagonized by cyroheptadine.

LABORATORY INTERFERENCES

H_1 antagonists may eliminate the wheal and induration that form the basis of allergy skin tests. Promethazine may interfere with pregnancy tests and may increase blood glucose concentrations. Diphenhydramine may yield a false-positive urine test result for phencyclidine (PCP). Hydroxyzine use can falsely elevate the results of certain tests for urinary 17-hydroxycorticosteroids.

DOSAGE AND CLINICAL GUIDELINES

The antihistamines are available in a variety of preparations (Table 32.3.5–1). IM injections should be deep, since superficial administration can cause local irritation.

Intravenous (IV) administration of 25 to 50 mg of diphenhydramine is an effective treatment for neuroleptic-induced acute dystonia, which may immediately disappear. Treatment with 25 mg three times a day—up to 50 mg four times a day if necessary—can be used for neuroleptic-induced parkinsonism, akinesia, and buccal movements. Diphenhydramine can be used as a hypnotic at a 50-mg dose for mild transient insomnia. Doses of 100 mg have not been shown to be superior to doses of 50 mg, but they produce more anticholinergic effects than doses of 50 mg.

Hydroxyzine is most commonly used as a short-term anxiolytic. Hydroxyzine should not be given IV, since it is irritating to the blood vessels. Dosages of 50 to 100 mg given orally four times a day for long-term treatment or 50 to 100 mg IM every 4 to 6 hours for short-term treatment are usually effective.

SSRI-induced anorgasmia may sometimes be reversed with 4 to 16 mg a day of cyproheptadine taken by mouth 1 or 2 hours before anticipated sexual activity. A number of case reports have reported that cyproheptadine may be of some use in the treatment of eating disorders, such as anorexia nervosa. Cyproheptadine is available in 4-mg tablets and a 2 mg/5 mL solution. Children and elderly patients are more sensitive to the effects of antihistamines than are young adults.

▲ 32.3.6 Barbiturates and Similarly Acting Drugs

The use of barbiturates and similar compounds such as meprobamate (Miltown) has been practically eliminated by the benzodiazepines, other anxiolytics such as buspirone (BuSpar), and the hypnotics zolpidem (Ambien) and zaleplon (Sonata). The newer agents have a lower abuse potential and a higher therapeutic index than the barbiturates; nevertheless, the barbiturates and similarly acting drugs still have a role in the treatment of certain mental disorders.

PHARMACOLOGICAL ACTIONS

The barbiturates are well absorbed after oral administration. The binding of barbiturates to plasma proteins is high, but lipid solubility varies. The individual barbiturates are metabolized by the liver and excreted by the kidneys. The half-lives of specific barbiturates range from 1 to 120 hours. The mechanism of action of barbiturates involves the γ-aminobutyric acid (GABA) receptor–benzodiazepine receptor–chloride ion channel complex.

EFFECTS ON SPECIFIC ORGANS AND SYSTEMS

The barbiturates have their major effects on the central nervous system (CNS), although significant effects also occur in the liver and can occur in the cardiovascular system. In the CNS, barbiturates are associated with the inhibition of the reticular activating system. Respiratory depression can arise, which can be additive to that of other respiratory depressants (e.g., alcohol). In the liver, barbiturate use can double the induction of metabolic liver enzymes and thus lower the plasma levels of both the barbiturates and other drugs metabolized in the liver. Although at low dosages barbiturates have a relatively safe cardiovascular profile, at high dosages they may impair cardiac contractility or evoke cardiac arrhythmias. Barbiturate administration rarely causes potentially fatal laryngospasm, a potential adverse event that may guide clinicians to use benzodiazepines, rather than barbiturates, in most situations (e.g., drug-assisted interviewing).

THERAPEUTIC INDICATIONS

Electroconvulsive Therapy

Methohexital (Brevital) is commonly used as an anesthetic agent for electroconvulsive therapy (ECT). It carries lower cardiac risks than other barbiturate anesthetics. Used intravenously (IV), methohexital produces rapid unconsciousness and because of rapid redistribution has a brief duration of action (5 to 7 minutes). Typical dosing for ECT is 0.7 to 1.2 mg/kg. Methohexital may also be used to abort prolonged seizures in ECT or to limit postictal agitation.

Seizures

Phenobarbital (Solfoton, Luminal), the most commonly used barbiturate for treatment of seizures, has indications for the treatment of generalized tonic-clonic and simple partial seizures. Parenteral barbiturates are used in the emergency management of seizures independent of cause. Intravenous phenobarbital should be administered slowly, 10 to 20 mg/kg, for status epilepticus.

Narcoanalysis

Amobarbital (Amytal) has been used historically as a diagnostic aid in a number of clinical conditions, including conversion reactions, catatonia, hysterical stupor, and unexplained muteness, and to differentiate stupor of depression, schizophrenia, and structural brain lesions.

The "Amytal interview" is performed by placing the patient in a reclining position and administering amobarbital IV, 50 mg a minute. Infusion is continued until lateral nystagmus is sustained or drowsiness is noted, usually at 75 to 150 mg. Following this, 25 to 50 mg may be administered every 5 minutes to maintain narcosis. The patient should rest for 15 to 30 minutes after the interview before attempting to walk.

Sleep

The barbiturates reduce sleep latency and the number of awakenings during sleep, though tolerance to these effects generally develops within 2 weeks. Discontinuation of barbiturates often leads to rebound increases on electroencephalogram (EEG) measures of sleep and worsening of the insomnia.

Withdrawal from Sedative Hypnotics

Barbiturates are sometimes used to determine the extent of tolerance to barbiturates or other hypnotics to guide detoxification. Once intoxication has resolved, a test dose of pentobarbital (200 mg) is given orally. An hour later the patient is examined. Tolerance and dose requirements are determined by the extent to which the patient is affected. If the patient is not sedated, another 100 mg of pentobarbital may be administered every 2 hours, up to three times (maximum, 500 mg over 6 hours). The amount needed for mild intoxication corresponds to the approximate daily dose of barbiturate used. Phenobarbital (30 mg) may then be substituted for each 100 mg of pentobarbital. This daily dose requirement may be administered in divided doses and gradually tapered by 10 percent a day, with adjustments made according to withdrawal signs.

PRECAUTIONS AND ADVERSE REACTIONS

Some adverse effects of barbiturates are similar to those of benzodiazepines, including paradoxical dysphoria, hyperactivity, and cognitive disorganization. Rare adverse effects associated with barbiturate use include the development of Stevens-Johnson syndrome, megaloblastic anemia, and neutropenia.

A major difference between the barbiturates and the benzodiazepines is the low therapeutic index of the barbiturates. An overdose of barbiturates can easily prove fatal. In addition to narrow therapeutic indexes, the barbiturates are associated with a signifi-

cant risk of abuse potential and the development of tolerance and dependence. Barbiturate intoxication is manifested by confusion, drowsiness, irritability, hyporeflexia or areflexia, ataxia, and nystagmus. The symptoms of barbiturate withdrawal are similar to, but more marked than, those of benzodiazepine withdrawal.

Because of some evidence of teratogenicity, barbiturates should not be used by pregnant women or women who are breast-feeding. Barbiturates should be used with caution by patients with a history of substance abuse, depression, diabetes, hepatic impairment, renal disease, severe anemia, pain, hyperthyroidism, or hypoadrenalism. Barbiturates are also contraindicated in patients with acute intermittent porphyria, impaired respiratory drive, or limited respiratory reserve.

DRUG–DRUG INTERACTIONS

The primary area for concern about drug interactions is the potentially additive effects of respiratory depression. Barbiturates should be used with great caution with other prescribed CNS drugs (including antipsychotic and antidepressant drugs) and nonprescribed CNS agents (e.g., alcohol). Caution must also be exercised when prescribing barbiturates to patients who are taking other drugs that are metabolized in the liver, especially cardiac drugs and anticonvulsants. Because individual patients have a wide range of sensitivities to barbiturate-induced enzyme induction, one cannot predict how much the metabolism of concurrently administered medications will be affected. Drugs that may have their metabolism enhanced by barbiturate administration include opioids, antiarrhythmic agents, antibiotics, anticoagulants, anticonvulsants, antidepressants, β-adrenergic receptor antagonists, dopamine receptor antagonists, contraceptives, and immunosuppressants.

Table 32.3.6–1
Barbiturate Dosages

Drug	Selected Preparations[a,b]	Daily Dosage Range (Sedative[c]/Hypnotic)	Anticonvulsant	Pediatric
Amobarbital	30, 200 mg	100–200 mg[c]/50–300 mg	65–500 mg (IV)	2–6 mg/kg up to 100 mg
Aprobarbital	40 mg/5 mL	40–160 mg[c]/40–120 mg	Not established	Not established
Butabarbital	30 mg/5 mL 15, 30, 50, 100 mg	45–120 mg[c]/50–100 mg	Not established	2–6 mg/kg (max 100 mg)
Mephobarbital	32, 50, 100 mg	66–300 mg[c]/100 mg	200–600 mg	16–32 mg three to four times daily (≤ age 5) 32–64 mg three to four times daily (> age 5)
Methohexital	500 mg/50 mL (I)	0.7–1.2 mg/kg for ECT	Not established	Not established
Pentobarbital	50, 100 mg 50 mg/mL (I) 20 mg/mL 30, 60, 120, 200 mg (r)	60–100 mg[c]/100–150 mg	100 mg IV at 1-min intervals up to 500 mg	2–6 mg/kg up to 100 mg
Phenobarbital	8, 15, 30, 60, 100 mg 30, 60, 65, 130 mg/mL (I) 20 mg/5 mL	30–120 mg[c]/100–300 mg	100–300 mg IV up to 600 mg/day 60–250 mg/day oral	1–3 mg/kg
Secobarbital	100 mg 50 mg/mL (I)	100–300 mg[c]/100 mg	5.5 mg/kg intravenous, may repeat every 3–4 hours	3–5 mg/kg

[a]Other preparations are available.
[b]Dosages are oral form (tablets or capsules) unless specified: I, injection; r, rectal suppository.
[c]Sedative dosage is equal to the hypnotic dosage, but should be split 3 to 4 times daily.

LABORATORY INTERFERENCES

No known laboratory interferences are associated with the administration of barbiturates.

DOSAGE AND CLINICAL GUIDELINES

Barbiturates and other drugs described below begin to act within 1 to 2 hours of administration. The dosages of barbiturates vary (Table 32.3.6–1), and treatment should begin with low dosages that are increased to achieve a clinical effect. Children and older persons are more sensitive to the effects of barbiturates than young adults. The most commonly used barbiturates are available in a variety of dose forms. Barbiturates with half-lives in the 15- to 40-hour range are preferable, because long-acting drugs tend to accumulate in the body. Clinicians should instruct patients clearly about the adverse effects and the potential for dependence associated with barbiturates.

Although determining plasma concentrations of barbiturates is rarely necessary in psychiatry, monitoring phenobarbital concentrations is standard practice when the drug is used as an anticonvulsant. The therapeutic blood concentrations for phenobarbital in this indication range from 15 to 40 mg/L, although some patients may experience significant adverse effects in that range.

Barbiturates are contained in combination products with which the clinician should be familiar.

OTHER SIMILARLY ACTING DRUGS

A number of agents that act similarly to the barbiturates are used in the treatment of anxiety and insomnia. Four such available drugs are paraldehyde (Paral), ethchlorvynol (Placidyl), meprobamate, and glutethimide (Doriden). These drugs are rarely used because of their abuse potential and potentially toxic effects. The reader is referred to a standard textbook of pharmacology for information about these medications.

▲ 32.3.7 Benzodiazepines

This section covers three areas: (1) the benzodiazepines, a group of compounds that enhance the activity of the $GABA_A$ receptor by binding to the benzodiazepine receptor site; (2) zolpidem (Ambien) and zaleplon (Sonata), benzodiazepine agonists at the type 2 benzodiazepine receptor (BZ_2) site; and (3) flumazenil (Romazicon), a benzodiazepine receptor antagonist. The benzodiazepine receptor agonists are primarily indicated for treating anxiety and insomnia; flumazenil is primarily indicated for treating benzodiazepine overdose.

Benzodiazepines are the drugs of choice for management of acute anxiety and agitation. Because of the risk of psychological dependence, long-term use of benzodiazepines should be carefully monitored.

PHARMACOLOGICAL ACTIONS

With the exception of clorazepate (Tranxene), all the benzodiazepines are completely absorbed unchanged from the gastrointestinal (GI) tract. The absorption, the attainment of peak concentrations, and the onset of action are quickest for diazepam (Valium), lorazepam (Ativan), alprazolam (Xanax), triazolam (Halcion), and estazolam (ProSom). The rapid onset of effects is important to persons who take a single dose of a benzodiazepine to calm an episodic burst of anxiety or to fall asleep rapidly. Several benzodiazepines are effective following intravenous (IV) injection, whereas only lorazepam and midazolam (Versed) have rapid and reliable absorption following intramuscular (IM) administration.

Diazepam, chlordiazepoxide (Librium), clonazepam (Klonopin), clorazepate, flurazepam (Dalmane), prazepam (Centrax), quazepam (Doral), and halazepam (Paxipam) have plasma half-lives of 30 to more than 100 hours and are, therefore, the longest-acting benzodiazepines. The plasma half-life of these compounds can be as high as 200 hours in persons whose metabolism is genetically slow. Because attainment of steady-state plasma concentrations of the drugs can take up to 2 weeks, persons may experience symptoms and signs of toxicity after only 7 to 10 days of treatment with a dosage that seemed initially to be in the therapeutic range.

The half-lives of lorazepam, oxazepam (Serax), temazepam (Restoril), and estazolam are between 8 and 30 hours. Alprazolam has a half-life of 10 to 15 hours, and triazolam has the shortest half-life (2 to 3 hours) of all the orally administered benzodiazepines.

The advantages of long–half-life drugs over short–half-life drugs include less frequent dosing, less variation in plasma concentration, and less severe withdrawal phenomena. The disadvantages include drug accumulation, increased risk of daytime psychomotor impairment, and increased daytime sedation. The advantages of the short–half-life drugs over the long–half-life drugs include no drug accumulation and less daytime sedation. The disadvantages include more frequent dosing and earlier and more severe withdrawal syndromes. Rebound insomnia and anterograde amnesia are considered more of a problem with the short–half-life drugs than with the long–half-life drugs. (Table 32.3.7–1 lists the half-lives of the drugs.)

Zolpidem and zaleplon are rapidly and well absorbed after oral administration, though absorption can be delayed by as much as 1 hour if they are taken with food. Zolpidem reaches peak plasma concentrations in 1.6 hours and has a half-life of 2.6 hours. Zaleplon reaches peak plasma concentrations in 1 hour and has a half-life of 1 hour. The rapid metabolism and lack of active metabolites of zolpidem and zaleplon avoid the accumulation of potentially toxic compounds often seen with long-term use of benzodiazepines.

Benzodiazepines activate all three specific γ-aminobutyric acid–benzodiazepine (GABA-BZ) binding sites of the $GABA_A$ receptor, which opens chloride channels and reduces the rate of neuronal and muscle firing. Because of the wide tissue distribution of $GABA_A$ receptors, benzodiazepines have sedative, muscle relaxant, and anticonvulsant effects. Zolpidem and zaleplon selectively activate only one of the benzodiazepine binding sites, which may account for their selective sedative effects and relative lack of muscle relaxant and anticonvulsant effects.

EFFECTS ON SPECIFIC ORGANS AND SYSTEMS

In addition to the central nervous system (CNS) effects on anxiety and sleep, benzodiazepines are effective anticonvulsants. They are

Table 32.3.7–1
Half-Lives, Doses, and Preparations of Benzodiazepine Receptor Agonists and Antagonists

Drug	Dose Equivalents	Half-Life (h)	Rate of Absorption	Usual Adult Dosage	Dose Preparations
Agonists					
Clonazepam	0.5	Long (metabolite, >20)	Rapid	1–6 mg/d bid	0.5-, 1.0-, and 2.0-mg tablets
Diazepam	5	Long (>20) (Nordazepam—long, >20)	Rapid	4–40 mg/d bid to qid	2-, 5-, and 10-mg tablets (slow-release 15-mg capsules)
Alprazolam	0.25	Intermediate (6–20)	Medium	0.5–10 mg/d bid to qid	0.25-, 0.5-, 1.0-, and 2.0-mg tablets
Lorazepam	1	Intermediate (6–20)	Medium	1–6 mg/d tid	0.5-, 1.0-, and 2.0-mg tablets; 2, 4 mg/mL parenteral
Oxazepam	15	Intermediate (6–20)	Slow	30–120 mg/d tid or qid	10-, 15-, and 30-mg capsules (15-mg tablets)
Temazepam	5	Intermediate (6–20)	Medium	7.5–30 mg/d hs	7.5-, 15-, and 30-mg capsules
Chlordiaze-poxide	10	Intermediate (6–20) (Demethylchlordiazepoxide—intermediate, 6–20) (Demoxepam—long, >20) (Nordazepam—long, >20)	Medium	10–150 mg tid or qid	5-, 10-, and 25-mg tablets or capsules
Flurazepam	5	Short (<6) (N-hydroxyethylflurazepam—short, <6) (N-desalkylflurazepam—long, >20)	Rapid	15–30 mg hs	15- and 30-mg capsules
Triazolam	0.1–0.03	Short (<6)	Rapid	0.125 mg or 0.250 mg hs	0.125- or 0.250-mg tablets
Clorazepate	7.5	Short (<6) Nordazepam—long, >20)	Rapid	15–60 mg bid or qid	3.75-, 7.5-, and 15-mg tablets (slow-release 11.25- and 22.5-mg tablets)
Halazepam	20	Short (<6) (Nordazepam—long, >20)	Medium	60–160 mg/d tid or qid	20- and 40-mg tablets
Prazepam	10	Short (<6) (Nordazepam—long, >20)	Slow	30 mg/d (20–60 mg/d) qid or tid	5-, 10-, or 20-mg capsules
Estazolam	0.33	Intermediate (6–20) (4-hydroxyestazolam—intermediate 6–20)	Rapid	1.0 or 2.0 hs	1- and 2-mg tablets
Quazepam	5	Long (>20) (2-oxoquazepam-N-desalkylflurazepam—long, >20)	Rapid	7.5 or 15 mg hs	7.5- and 15-mg tablets
Midazolam	1.25–1.7	Short (<6)	Rapid	5 to 50 mg parenteral	5 mg/mL parenteral, 1-, 2-, 5-, and 10-mL vials
Zolpidem	2.5	Short (<6)	Rapid	5 mg or 10 mg hs	5- and 10-mg tablets
Zaleplon	2.5	Short (1)	Rapid	10 mg hs	5- and 10-mg capsules
Antagonist					
Flumazenil	0.05	Short (<6)	Rapid	0.2 to 0.5 mg/min injection over 3–10 min (total, 1–5 mg)	0.1 mg/mL (5- and 10-mL vials)

also effective skeletal muscle relaxants, primarily through their ability to inhibit spinal polysynaptic afferent pathways, although monosynaptic afferent pathways may also be affected.

THERAPEUTIC INDICATIONS

Anxiety

Generalized anxiety disorder, adjustment disorder with anxiety, and other anxiety states are the major clinical applications for benzodiazepines in psychiatry and general medical practice.

Most patients should be treated for a predetermined, specific, and relatively brief period. Some patients with generalized anxiety disorder may warrant maintenance treatment with benzodiazepines. The selective serotonin reuptake inhibitors (SSRIs) are effective antianxiety agents that lack abuse potential, although their antianxiety effects require 2 to 4 weeks to develop.

Mixed Anxiety-Depressive Disorder

Alprazolam is indicated for the treatment of anxiety associated with depression. The availability of several antidepressant drugs with more favorable safety profiles makes alprazolam a second-line drug for this indication; however, some patients respond to this medication when other drugs have had minimal effects.

Panic Disorder and Social Phobia

The two high-potency benzodiazepines, alprazolam and clonazepam, are effective for two anxiety disorders, panic disorder with or without agoraphobia and social phobia. The Food and Drug Administration (FDA) has approved the use of alprazolam for the treatment of panic disorder. The dosage guidelines for the use of alprazolam in panic disorder are similar to those for depression, discussed below. Paroxetine (Paxil) and sertraline (Zoloft) have also been approved by the FDA for treatment of panic disorder. Because SSRIs may not be fully effective for 2 to 4 weeks after initiation of treatment, coadministration of a high-potency benzodiazepine for the first 2 to 4 weeks of use of the SSRI can provide rapid control of anxiety.

Obsessive-Compulsive Disorder and Posttraumatic Stress Disorder

Benzodiazepines, especially clonazepam, which has serotonergic properties, may treat the anxiety component of obsessive-compulsive disorder. Clonazepam may be effective for certain patients who do not respond to clomipramine (Anafranil). Benzodiazepines may also be used to augment clomipramine or the SSRIs, and they may help reduce hyperarousal in posttraumatic stress disorder.

Insomnia. Flurazepam, temazepam, quazepam, estazolam, and triazolam are the benzodiazepines approved for use as hypnotics. The benzodiazepine hypnotics differ principally in their half-lives; flurazepam has the longest half-life, and triazolam has the shortest. Flurazepam may be associated with minor cognitive impairment on the day after its administration, and triazolam may be associated with mild rebound anxiety. Temazepam or estazolam may be a reasonable compromise for the average adult patient. Because of its high specificity for the BZ_1 receptor, quazepam may be associated with few adverse cognitive effects, but quazepam shares the final metabolite with flurazepam—desalkylflurazepam (half-life of approximately 100 hours)—and, therefore, may be associated with daytime impairment when used for a long time. Estazolam produces rapid onset of sleep and a hypnotic effect for 6 to 8 hours. All the benzodiazepines produce a moderate decrease in rapid eye movement (REM) sleep, although their use is not associated with REM rebound. Generally, the benzodiazepines are associated with a decrease in stage 3 and stage 4 sleep, although the significance of this is not known. Benzodiazepines alone generally should not be taken for long periods of time, to limit the risk of development of dependence. Longer-term treatment of insomnia should include behavioral modification, relaxation techniques, and exploration of the underlying causes of insomnia, such as anxiety or depression.

The sole indication for zolpidem and zaleplon is insomnia, but the spectrum of their psychological effects closely resembles that of benzodiazepines. Zolpidem, and particularly zaleplon, are usually not associated with rebound insomnia after the discontinuation of their use for short periods. Use of zolpidem and zaleplon for periods longer than 1 month is not associated with delayed emergence of adverse effects.

Depression

Unique among the benzodiazepines, alprazolam has antidepressant effects equal to those of the tricyclic drugs, but alprazolam is not effective with seriously depressed inpatients. The efficacy of alprazolam in depressive disorders may reflect its potency; the antidepressant effects of other benzodiazepines may be evident only at doses that also induce sedation or sleep. The starting dosage of alprazolam for the treatment of depression should be 1 to 1.5 mg a day and should be raised by 0.5 mg a day every 3 or 4 days. The maximal dosage is usually 4 mg a day, although some investigators and clinicians have used dosages as high as 10 mg a day. The use of high dosages is controversial because of the possibility of withdrawal symptoms. Clinicians must taper, rather than abruptly stop, alprazolam use, usually at the rate of 0.5 mg a day every 3 to 4 days.

Bipolar I Disorder

Clonazepam is effective in the management of manic episodes and as an adjuvant to lithium (Eskalith) therapy in lieu of antipsychotics. As an adjuvant to lithium, clonazepam may result in increased time between cycles and fewer-than-usual depressive episodes. The other high-potency benzodiazepine, alprazolam, may be as effective as clonazepam for this indication, which is not recognized by the FDA, and alprazolam should be considered a second-line treatment.

Akathisia

Standard anticholinergic drugs—for example, benztropine (Cogentin)—are often ineffective in treating neuroleptic-induced acute akathisia. The first-line drug for akathisia is most commonly a β-adrenergic receptor antagonist—for example, propranolol (Inderal). Several studies have found, however, that benzodiazepines are also effective in treating some patients with akathisia.

Parkinson's Disease

A small number of persons with idiopathic Parkinson's disease will respond to long-term use of zolpidem with reduced bradykinesia and rigidity. Zolpidem dosages of 10 mg four times daily may be tolerated without sedation for several years.

Other Psychiatric Indications

Clonazepam augmentation may accelerate, but not potentiate, the antidepressant effects of fluoxetine (Prozac). Chlordiazepoxide is used to manage the symptoms of alcohol withdrawal. The benzodiazepines (especially IM lorazepam) are used to manage both substance-induced (except amphetamine) and psychotic agitation in the emergency room. A few studies report the use of high dosages of benzodiazepines in schizophrenia patients who had not responded to antipsychotics or who were unable to take the traditional drugs because of adverse effects. The successful use of IM lorazepam for the treatment of catatonia has been reported. Benzodiazepines have also been used instead of amobarbital (Amytal) for drug-assisted interviewing.

Flumazenil for Benzodiazepine Overdose

Flumazenil is used to reverse the adverse psychomotor, amnestic, and sedative effects of benzodiazepine receptor agonists, including benzodiazepines, zolpidem, and zaleplon. Flumazenil is administered IV and has a half-life of 7 to 15 minutes. The most common adverse effects of flumazenil are nausea, vomiting, dizziness, agitation, emotional lability, cutaneous vasodilation, injection-site pain, fatigue, impaired vision, and headache. The most common serious adverse effect associated with use of flumazenil is the precipitation of seizures, which is especially likely to occur in persons with seizure disorders, those who are physically dependent on benzodiazepines, or those who have ingested large quantities of benzodiazepines. Flumazenil alone may impair memory retrieval.

In mixed-drug overdosage, the toxic effects (e.g., seizures and cardiac arrhythmias) of other drugs (e.g., tricyclic drugs) may emerge with the reversal of the benzodiazepine effects of flumazenil. For example, seizures caused by an overdosage of tricyclic drugs may have been partially treated in a person who had also taken an overdosage of benzodiazepines. With flumazenil treatment, the tricyclic-induced seizures or cardiac arrhythmias may appear and result in a fatal outcome. Flumazenil does not reverse the effects of ethanol, barbiturates, or opioids.

PRECAUTIONS AND ADVERSE REACTIONS

The most common adverse effect of benzodiazepines is drowsiness, which occurs in approximately 10 percent of all patients. Because of this adverse effect, patients should be advised to be careful while driving or using machinery when taking the drugs. Drowsiness can occur the day after the use of a benzodiazepine for insomnia the previous night, so-called residual daytime sedation. Some patients also experience dizziness (less than 1 percent) and ataxia (less than 2 percent). These symptoms can result in falls and hip fractures, especially in elderly patients. The most serious adverse effects of benzodiazepines occur when other sedative substances, such as alcohol, are taken concurrently. The combinations can result in marked drowsiness, disinhibition, or even respiratory depression. Other relatively rare adverse effects have been mild cognitive deficits that may impair job performance in patients who are taking benzodiazepines. Anterograde amnesia has also been associated with benzodiazepines, particularly high-potency benzodiazepines. A rare, paradoxical increase in aggression has been reported in patients given benzodiazepines, although this effect may be most common in patients with brain damage. Allergic reactions to the drugs are also rare, but a few studies report maculopapular rashes and generalized itching. The symptoms of benzodiazepine intoxication include confusion, slurred speech, ataxia, drowsiness, dyspnea, and hyporeflexia.

Triazolam has received significant attention in the media because of an alleged association with serious aggressive behavioral manifestations, which were associated with doses greater than 1 mg, which is twice the recommended maximum dose. Although little evidence supports the association, the Upjohn Company, which manufactures triazolam, has issued a statement emphasizing that the drug is best used as a short-term (fewer than 10 days) treatment of insomnia, that physicians should carefully evaluate the emergence of any abnormal thinking or behavioral changes in patients treated with triazolam, and that they should consider all appropriate potential causes.

Patients with hepatic disease and elderly patients are particularly likely to have adverse effects and toxicity from the benzodiazepines, especially when the drugs are administered in repeated or high doses, because of these patients' impaired metabolism of the compounds. Benzodiazepines can significantly impair respiration in patients with chronic obstructive pulmonary disease and sleep apnea. Benzodiazepines should be used with caution in patients with a history of substance abuse, cognitive disorders, renal disease, hepatic disease, porphyria, CNS depression, and myasthenia gravis.

Some data indicate that benzodiazepines are teratogenic; therefore, their use during pregnancy is not advised. Moreover, the use of benzodiazepines in the third trimester can precipitate a withdrawal syndrome in newborns. The drugs are secreted in the breast milk in sufficient concentrations to affect neonates. Benzodiazepines may cause dyspnea, bradycardia, and drowsiness in nursing babies.

Zolpidem and zaleplon are generally well tolerated. At zolpidem dosages of 10 mg per day and zaleplon dosages above 10 mg per day, a small number of persons experience dizziness, drowsiness, dyspepsia, or diarrhea. Zolpidem and zaleplon are secreted in breast milk and are, therefore, contraindicated for use by nursing mothers. The dosage of zolpidem and zaleplon should be reduced in the elderly and in persons with hepatic impairment. In rare cases, zolpidem may cause hallucinations, which can last up to 1 hour in some persons. Coadministration of zolpidem and SSRIs may extend the duration of hallucinations in susceptible patients to 1 to 7 hours.

Tolerance, Dependence, and Withdrawal

When benzodiazepines are used for short periods (1 to 2 weeks) in moderate dosages, they usually cause no significant tolerance, dependence, or withdrawal effects. The short-acting benzodiazepines (e.g., triazolam) may be an exception, as some patients have reported increased anxiety the day after taking a single dose of the drug. Some patients also report a tolerance for the anxiolytic effects of benzodiazepines and require increased dosages to maintain the clinical remission of symptoms. There is also a cross-tolerance among most of the classes of antianxiety drugs, with the notable exception of buspirone (BuSpar) and the SSRIs.

The appearance of a withdrawal syndrome, also called a *discontinuation syndrome*, depends on the length of time a patient has taken a benzodiazepine, the dosage the patient has been taking, the rate at which drug use is tapered, and the half-life of the compound. Abrupt discontinuation of benzodiazepine use, particularly those with short half-lives, is associated with severe withdrawal symptoms. Serious symptoms may include depression, paranoia, delirium, and seizures. The incidence of the syndrome is controversial, but some features of the syndrome may occur in as many as 50 percent of patients treated with the drugs. A severe withdrawal syndrome develops only in patients who have taken high dosages for long periods. The appearance of the syndrome may be delayed for 1 or 2 weeks in patients who had been taking 2-keto benzodiazepines with long half-lives.

Alprazolam use seems to be particularly associated with an immediate, severe withdrawal syndrome, and it should be tapered gradually. A recent study comparing simple tapering of alprazolam use with tapering plus cognitive, anticipatory guidance regarding the alprazolam discontinuation effects found that patients were much more likely to remain off alprazolam indefinitely if they have been fully warned to expect the signs and symptoms of discontinuation. This is important because a significant percentage of patients who use alprazolam for long periods cannot successfully discontinue taking it.

Zolpidem and zaleplon can produce a mild withdrawal syndrome lasting 1 day after prolonged use at higher therapeutic dosages. Rarely, a person taking zolpidem has self-titrated the daily dosage up to 300 to 400 mg a day. Abrupt discontinuation of such a high dosage of zolpidem may cause withdrawal symptoms for 4 or more days. Tolerance does not develop to the sedative effects of zolpidem and zaleplon.

DRUG–DRUG INTERACTIONS

The most common and potentially serious benzodiazepine receptor agonist interaction is excessive sedation and respiratory depression occurring when benzodiazepines, zolpidem, or zaleplon are administered concomitantly with other CNS depressants, such as alcohol, barbiturates, tricyclic and tetracyclic drugs, dopamine receptor antagonists, opioids, and antihistamines. Ataxia and dysarthria may be likely to occur when lithium, antipsychotics, and clonazepam are combined. The combination of benzodiazepines and clozapine (Clozaril) has been reported to cause delirium and should be avoided. Cimetidine (Tagamet), disulfiram (Antabuse), isoniazid (Nydrazid), estrogen, and oral contraceptives increase the plasma concentrations of diazepam, chlordiazepoxide, clorazepate, flurazepam, prazepam, and halazepam. Cimetidine increases the plasma concentrations of zaleplon. The plasma concentrations of triazolam and alprazolam are increased to potentially toxic concentrations by nefazodone (Serzone) and fluvoxamine (Luvox). The manufacturer of nefazodone recommends that the dosage of triazolam be lowered by 75 percent and the dosage of alprazolam lowered by 50 percent, when given concomitantly with nefazodone. Over-the-counter preparations of kava plant, advertised as a "natural tranquilizer," can potentiate the action of benzodiazepine receptor agonists through synergistic overactivation of GABA receptors. Carbamazepine (Tegretol) can lower the plasma concentration of alprazolam. Antacids and food may decrease the plasma concentrations of benzodiazepines, and smoking may increase the metabolism of benzodiazepines. Rifampin (Rifadin), phenytoin (Dilantin), carbamazepine, and phenobarbital (Solfoton, Luminal) significantly increase the metabolism of zaleplon. The benzodiazepines may increase the plasma concentrations of phenytoin and digoxin (Lanoxin). SSRIs may prolong and exacerbate the severity of zolpidem-induced hallucinations.

Laboratory Interferences

No known laboratory interferences are associated with the use of benzodiazepine receptor agonists or antagonists.

DOSAGE AND ADMINISTRATION

Benzodiazepines

Benzodiazepines are categorized as short-, intermediate-, or long-acting drugs. Their sedative and anxiolytic effects appear within 30 to 60 minutes of administration and terminate as soon as the drugs are excreted. This is in contrast to the antianxiety effects of the serotonergic drugs, which may take 2 to 4 weeks to develop.

The clinical decision to treat an anxious patient with a benzodiazepine should be carefully considered. Medical causes of anxiety (e.g., thyroid dysfunction, caffeinism, and medications) should be ruled out. Benzodiazepine use should be started at a low dosage, and the patient should be instructed about the drug's sedative properties and abuse potential. An estimated length of therapy should be decided at the beginning of therapy, and the need for continued therapy should be reevaluated at least monthly because of the problems associated with long-term use.

Duration of Treatment. Benzodiazepines can be used to treat illnesses other than anxiety disorders. In such cases, the duration of treatment should generally be similar to that for the standard drugs used to treat these disorders. The use of benzodiazepines over a long period for chronically anxious patients is often valuable, although controversial. In his 1980 textbook on drug treatment in psychiatry, Donald Klein stated, "There are many reports of patients maintained on benzodiazepines for years with apparent benefit and without the development of tolerance. Nonetheless, it is dubious practice to prescribe such medications indefinitely without accompanying psychotherapy."

Discontinuation of Therapy. Benzodiazepine withdrawal syndrome occurs when patients discontinue benzodiazepines abruptly; 90 percent of patients after long-term use experience some symptoms of withdrawal on discontinuation if the drug is tapered slowly. Benzodiazepine withdrawal syndrome consists of anxiety, nervousness, diaphoresis, restlessness, irritability, fatigue, light-headedness, tremor, insomnia, and weakness. The higher the dose and the shorter the half-life, the more severe the withdrawal symptoms can be.

When the medication is to be discontinued, drug use must be tapered slowly (25 percent a week); otherwise, symptoms are likely to recur or rebound. Monitoring of any withdrawal symptoms (possibly with a standardized rating scale) and psychological support for the patient aid successful discontinuation of benzodiazepine use. Concurrent use of carbamazepine during discontinuation of benzodiazepine use reportedly permits more rapid and better tolerated withdrawal than a gradual taper alone. The dosage range of carbamazepine used to facilitate withdrawal is 400 to 500 mg a day. Some clinicians report particular difficulty in tapering and discontinuing alprazolam use, particularly with patients who have been receiving high dosages for long periods. There have been reports of successful discontinuation of alprazolam use by switching to clonazepam, which is then gradually withdrawn.

Choice of Drug and Potency. The wide range of benzodiazepines is available in an equally wide range of formulations (see Table 32.3.7–1). The drugs differ primarily in their half-lives. Another difference is in the rate of onset of their potency and anxiolytic effects. *Potency* is a general term used to express the pharmacological activity of a drug. Some benzodiazepines are more potent than others, in that a relatively smaller dose of one compound will achieve the same effect as a larger dose of another. For example, 0.25 mg of clonazepam achieves the same effect as 5 mg of diazepam; thus, clonazepam is considered a high-potency benzodiazepine. Conversely, oxazepam has an approximate dose equivalence of 15 mg and is a low-potency drug. The four high-potency benzodiazepines—alprazolam, triazolam, estazolam, and clonazepam—are the drugs most likely to be effective for new applications such as depression, bipolar I disorder, panic disorder, and the phobias.

Drug Combinations.   The most common drug combinations with benzodiazepines involve antipsychotics and antidepressants, in addition to the benzodiazepine's obvious use as adjuvant hypnotics. The combination of a benzodiazepine and an antidepressant may be indicated in the treatment of markedly anxious depressed patients and patients with panic disorder. Several reports indicate that the combined use of alprazolam and an antipsychotic may further reduce psychotic symptoms in patients who did not respond adequately to the antipsychotic alone. The combined use of benzodiazepines and tricyclic drugs may improve compliance by reducing the subjective side effects and immediately reducing anxiety and insomnia. The combination, however, may also cause excessive sedation and cognitive impairment and may even exacerbate the depression, and it adds significantly to the lethality of an overdose.

Zolpidem and Zaleplon

Zolpidem is available in 5- and 10-mg tablets. A single 10-mg dose is the usual dose for the treatment of insomnia and is also the maximum daily dose. A single dose of zolpidem can be expected to provide 5 hours of sleep with minimal residual impairment. For persons over age 65 or persons with hepatic impairment, an initial dose of 5 mg is advised.

Zaleplon is available in 5- and 10-mg capsules. A single 10-mg dose is the usual adult dose. The dose can be increased to a maximum of 20 mg as tolerated. A single dose of zaleplon can be expected to provide 4 hours of sleep with minimal residual impairment. For persons over age 65 or persons with a hepatic impairment, an initial dose of 5 mg is advised.

▲ 32.3.8 Bupropion

Bupropion (Wellbutrin, Zyban) is a first-line agent for treatment of depression and smoking cessation. It generally is more effective against symptoms of depression than those of anxiety, and it is quite effective in combination with selective serotonin reuptake inhibitors (SSRIs). Smoking cessation is most successful when bupropion (called Zyban for this indication) is used in combination with behavioral modification techniques.

Bupropion is a unique antidepressant with a highly favorable profile of adverse effects. Of particular note among antidepressants, it is associated with little inhibition of sexual function. It also carries a higher likelihood of weight loss than weight gain. It possesses some dopaminergic effects and may serve as a mild psychostimulant as well as an antidepressant.

PHARMACOLOGICAL ACTIONS

Bupropion is well absorbed from the gastrointestinal (GI) tract. Peak plasma concentrations of bupropion are usually reached within 2 hours

of oral administration, and peak levels of the sustained-release version are seen after 3 hours. The mean half-life of the compound is 12 hours, ranging from 8 to 40 hours.

The mechanism of action for the antidepressant effects of bupropion is poorly understood. It was initially thought that bupropion acts through the blockade of dopamine reuptake. However, central nervous system (CNS) concentrations of bupropion are probably not sufficient to result in significant dopamine reuptake inhibition. Nonetheless, some data indicate that bupropion exerts its antidepressant effects by increasing the functional efficiency of noradrenergic systems. Regarding the effects of bupropion on smoking cessation, it is a noncompetitive inhibitor of nicotinic acetylcholine receptors and thus may interfere with the addictive actions of nicotine.

EFFECTS ON SPECIFIC ORGANS AND SYSTEMS

Except for its CNS effects, bupropion is nearly devoid of activity in human organs. No evidence has been found for significant effects of bupropion on liver, cardiac, or renal function, although the dosage of bupropion should be adjusted downward in patients with liver and renal impairment. It may increase blood pressure in previously hypertensive patients. Rare cases of lymphadenopathy, anemia, and pancytopenia have been reported, although their association with bupropion use is uncertain and routine monitoring of blood is not indicated. Bupropion does not affect sexual functioning. It has been associated with weight changes, more often with weight loss than with weight gain. There have been reports of rashes and pruritus in a few patients.

THERAPEUTIC INDICATIONS

Depression

The therapeutic efficacy of bupropion in depression is well established in both outpatient and inpatient settings. Improved sleep early in the course of treatment is seen less often with bupropion than with some other antidepressants, because of its lack of sedation; however, it does not disrupt sleep architecture as much as the SSRIs. It is also of use in hypoactive sexual desire that may accompany depression.

Bupropion in combination with lithium (Eskalith) is effective and well tolerated in some persons with refractory depression, but this combination may rarely cause CNS toxicity, including seizures.

Bipolar Disorders

Bupropion may be less likely than tricyclics to precipitate mania in persons with bipolar I disorder, although it is not free of this risk. It may be less likely than other antidepressants to exacerbate or induce rapid-cycling bipolar II disorder.

Attention-Deficit/Hyperactivity Disorder

Bupropion is a major second-line agent, after the sympathomimetics, for treatment of attention-deficit/hyperactivity disorder (ADHD). It can be nearly as efficacious as methylphenidate (Ritalin) for childhood and adult ADHD. Bupropion is an appropriate choice for persons with comorbid ADHD and depression or persons with comorbid ADHD, conduct disorder, or substance abuse.

Cocaine Detoxification

Some clinicians have reported that bupropion can be used to reduce the cravings for cocaine in persons who have withdrawn from the substance.

Smoking Cessation

Bupropion is indicated for use in combination with behavioral modification programs for smoking cessation. Success of smoking cessation efforts is best associated with a high degree of motivation and structured behavioral support. Bupropion and nicotine substitutes (Nicoderm, Nicotrol) individually increase the success rate, and they act synergistically in combination.

PRECAUTIONS AND ADVERSE REACTIONS

The most common adverse effects associated with use of bupropion are headache, insomnia, upper respiratory complaints, and nausea. Restlessness, agitation, and irritability may also occur. Most likely because of its potentiating effects on dopaminergic neurotransmission, bupropion has rarely been associated with psychotic symptoms, including hallucinations, delusions, and catatonia, as well as delirium. Most notable about bupropion is the absence of significant drug-induced orthostatic hypotension, weight gain, daytime drowsiness, and anticholinergic effects. Some persons, however, may experience dry mouth or constipation, and weight loss may occur in approximately 25 percent of persons. Bupropion causes no significant cardiovascular or clinical laboratory changes.

A major advantage of bupropion over SSRIs is that bupropion is virtually devoid of any adverse effects on sexual functioning, whereas the SSRIs are associated with such effects in up to 80 percent of persons. Some persons taking bupropion experience increased sexual responsiveness and even spontaneous orgasm.

At dosages of 300 mg a day or less of the sustained-release preparation, the incidence of seizures is 0.05 percent, which is no worse than the incidence of seizures with other antidepressants. The risk of seizures increases to approximately 0.1 percent with doses above 400 mg a day. Risk factors for seizures, such as past history of seizures, use of alcohol, recent benzodiazepine withdrawal, organic brain disease, head trauma, or epileptiform discharges on electroencephalography (EEG), warrant critical examination of the decision to use bupropion.

Because high dosages (more than 400 mg a day) of bupropion may be associated with a euphoric feeling, bupropion may be relatively contraindicated in persons with histories of substance abuse. The use of bupropion by pregnant women has not been studied and is not recommended. Because bupropion is secreted in breast milk, the use of bupropion by nursing women is not recommended.

Overdoses with bupropion are associated with a generally favorable outcome, except in the cases of huge doses and mixed-drug overdoses. Seizures occur in approximately one-third of all overdoses, and fatalities can involve uncontrollable seizures, bradycardia, and cardiac arrest. In general, however, bupropion is safer in overdose cases than other antidepressants are, with the possible exception of the SSRIs.

Drug–Drug Interactions

Bupropion should not be used concurrently with monoamine oxidase inhibitors (MAOIs) because of the possibility of inducing a hypertensive crisis, and at least 14 days should pass after discontinuation of MAOI use before treatment with bupropion is initiated. Addition of bupropion may permit persons taking antiparkinsonian medications to lower the doses of their dopaminergic drugs. However, delirium, psychotic symptoms, and dyskinetic movements may be associated with coadministration of bupropion and dopaminergic agents such as levodopa (Larodopa), pergolide (Permax), ropinirole (Requip), pramipexole (Mirapex), amantadine (Symmetrel), and bromocriptine (Parlodel).

The combination of bupropion and fluoxetine (Prozac) is one of the most effective and well-tolerated treatments for all types of depression, but a few case reports indicate that panic, delirium, or seizures may be associated with this combination. Patients with panic disorder are sensitive to the activating effects of bupropion and may have their anxiety exacerbated.

Carbamazepine (Tegretol) may decrease plasma concentrations of bupropion, and bupropion may increase plasma concentrations of valproic acid (Depakene).

LABORATORY INTERFERENCES

Bupropion may give a false-positive result on urinary amphetamine screens. No other reports have appeared of laboratory interferences clearly associated with bupropion treatment. Clinically nonsignificant changes in the electrocardiogram (ECG) (premature beats and nonspecific ST-T changes) and decreases in the white blood cell count (by approximately 10 percent) have been reported in a small number of persons.

DOSAGE AND CLINICAL GUIDELINES

Bupropion is available in 75- and 100-mg tablets, and sustained-release bupropion is available in 100-, 150-, and 200-mg tablets. Treatment should be initiated in the average adult with 100 mg orally twice a day or 150 mg of the sustained-release version once a day. On the fourth day of treatment, the dosage can be raised to 100 mg three times a day or 300 mg a day of the sustained-release formulation taken in the morning or in two divided doses. Since 300 mg is the recommended dosage, the person should be maintained on this dosage for several weeks before increasing the dosage further. Because of the risk of seizures, dosage increases should never exceed 100 mg in a 3-day period; a single dose of bupropion should never exceed 150 mg, and a single dose of sustained-release bupropion should never exceed 300 mg. The total daily dosage should not exceed 450 mg of the immediate-release formulation or 400 mg of the sustained-release version.

For smoking cessation, the patient should start taking 150 mg a day of sustained-release bupropion 10 to 14 days before quitting smoking. On the fourth day, the dosage should be increased to 150 mg twice daily. Treatment generally lasts 7 to 12 weeks.

▲ 32.3.9 Buspirone and Gepirone

BUSPIRONE

Buspirone (BuSpar) is indicated for the treatment of anxiety disorders. Unlike the benzodiazepines and the barbiturates, buspirone does not have sedative, hypnotic, muscle-relaxant, or anticonvulsant effects; carries a low potential for abuse; and is not associated with withdrawal phenomena or cognitive impairment.

PHARMACOLOGICAL ACTIONS

Buspirone is well absorbed from the gastrointestinal (GI) tract and is unaffected by food intake. The drug reaches peak plasma levels in 60 to 90 minutes after oral administration. The short half-life (2 to 11 hours) necessitates dosing three times daily. In contrast to benzodiazepines and barbiturates, which act on the γ-aminobutyric acid (GABA)-associated chloride ion channel, buspirone has no effect on that receptor mechanism. Rather, buspirone acts as an agonist or partial agonist on serotonin 5-HT$_{1A}$-receptors. Buspirone also has activity at 5-HT$_2$ and dopamine type 2 (D$_2$) receptors, although the significance of the effects at these receptors is unknown. At D$_2$ receptors, it has properties of both an agonist and an antagonist. The fact that buspirone takes 2 to 3 weeks to exert its therapeutic effects implies that whatever its initial effects, the therapeutic effects may involve the modulation of several neurotransmitters and intraneuronal mechanisms.

EFFECTS ON SPECIFIC ORGANS AND SYSTEMS

The effects of buspirone on organs other than the brain are minimal. The drug has no significant effects on the respiratory system, heart, vascular system, blood, smooth muscles, or autonomic nervous system.

THERAPEUTIC INDICATIONS

Generalized Anxiety Disorder

Buspirone is safe and effective for treatment of generalized anxiety disorder. Compared with benzodiazepines, buspirone is generally more effective for symptoms of anger and hostility, equally effective for psychic symptoms of anxiety, and less effective for somatic symptoms of anxiety. The full benefit of buspirone is evident usually at dosages above 30 mg a day. Buspirone offers several advantages over the benzodiazepines in long-term use, including lack of development of withdrawal symptoms upon discontinuation and less need to return to benzodiazepines once the initial course of drug treatment is terminated. Buspirone is not associated with any abuse potential, even in groups at high risk for addictive behavior.

Compared with the benzodiazepines, buspirone has a delayed onset of action and lacks any euphoric effect. Unlike benzodiazepines, buspirone has no immediate effects, and the patient should be told that a full clinical response may take 2 to 4 weeks. If an immediate response is needed, the patient can start treatment with a benzodiazepine and then be withdrawn from the drug after buspirone's effects begin. Sometimes the sedative effects of benzodiazepines, which are not found with buspirone, are desirable; however, these sedative effects may impair motor performance and cause cognitive deficits.

Other Disorders

Buspirone is not effective in the treatment of panic disorder or social phobia; however, it may reduce the increased arousal and flashbacks associated with posttraumatic stress disorder. Evidence of the efficacy of high-dosage buspirone (30 to 90 mg a day) for depressive disorders is mixed. Buspirone is sometimes used to augment serotonergic antidepressant drugs for major depressive and obsessive-compulsive disorders.

Because buspirone does not act on the GABA-chloride ion channel complex, the drug is not recommended for the treatment of withdrawal from benzodiazepines, alcohol, or sedative-hypnotic drugs, except as treatment of comorbid anxiety symptoms.

Buspirone can effectively reduce aggression and anxiety in persons with organic brain disease or traumatic brain injury. It may also reduce comorbid oppositional-defiant symptoms, aggressive behavior, hyperactivity, impulsivity, inattention, and mood in children with attention-deficit/hyperactivity disorder (ADHD). Buspirone may also reduce hyperactivity associated with autistic spectrum disorders.

Buspirone may be beneficial for treatment of the physical and psychic symptoms of premenstrual dysphoric disorder. At higher dosages, buspirone may ameliorate the sexual inhibition of the selective serotonin reuptake inhibitors (SSRIs). It is also used to treat SSRI-induced bruxism.

PRECAUTIONS AND ADVERSE REACTIONS

The most common adverse effects of buspirone are headache, nausea, dizziness, and (rarely) insomnia. No sedation is associated with buspirone. Some persons may report a minor feeling of restlessness, although that symptom may reflect an incompletely treated anxiety disorder. No deaths have been reported from overdoses of buspirone, and the median lethal dose (LD$_{50}$) is estimated to be 160 to 550 times the recommended daily dose. Buspirone should be used with caution by persons with hepatic and renal impairment, pregnant women, and nursing mothers. It can be used safely by the elderly.

DRUG–DRUG INTERACTIONS

Coadministration of buspirone and haloperidol (Haldol) results in increased blood concentrations of haloperidol. Buspirone should not be used with monoamine oxidase inhibitors (MAOIs) to avoid hypertensive episodes, and a 2-week washout period should pass between the discontinuation of MAOI use and the initiation of treatment with buspirone. Erythromycin (E-mycin), itraconazole (Sporanox), nefazodone (Serzone), and grapefruit juice may raise plasma concentrations of buspirone.

LABORATORY INTERFERENCES

Single doses of buspirone can cause transient elevations in growth hormone, prolactin, and cortisol concentrations, although the effects are not clinically significant.

DOSAGE AND CLINICAL GUIDELINES

Buspirone is available in single-scored 5- and 10-mg tablets and triple-scored 15- and 30-mg tablets; treatment is usually initiated with either 5 mg orally three times daily or 7.5 mg orally twice daily. The dosage can be raised 5 mg every 2 to 4 days to the usual dosage range of 15 to 60 mg a day.

Switching from a Benzodiazepine to Buspirone

Buspirone is as effective as the benzodiazepines in the treatment of anxiety in persons who have never received benzodiazepines; however, buspirone does not achieve the same response in patients who have received benzodiazepines in the past. This is probably due to the absence of the immediate mildly euphoric and sedative effects of the benzodiazepines. The most common clinical problem, therefore, is how to initiate buspirone therapy in a person who is currently taking benzodiazepines. There are two alternatives. First, the clinician can start buspirone treatment gradually while the benzodiazepine is being withdrawn. Second, the clinician can start buspirone treatment and bring the person up to a therapeutic dosage for 2 to 3 weeks while that person is still receiving the regular dosage of the benzodiazepine, and then slowly taper the benzodiazepine dosage. Coadministration of buspirone and benzodiazepines may be effective in the treatment of anxiety disorders that have not responded to treatment with either drug alone.

GEPIRONE

Gepirone (Ariza) is a pyridinyl piperazine partial 5-HT_{1A} receptor agonist related to buspirone that is used as an antidepressant and anxiolytic. Generalized anxiety disorder patients show a delayed anxiolytic response similar to that seen with buspirone. Mechanism-of-action studies have demonstrated that gepirone, compared to buspirone, possesses a much greater selectivity for 5-HT_{1A} receptors over D_2 receptors. Long-term studies have shown that gepirone has a differential action at presynaptic (agonist) and postsynaptic (partial agonist) 5-HT_{1A} receptors. It has minimal receptor affinity for histamine and other receptor types.

Common adverse events include dizziness, paresthesias, palpitations, headache, nausea, nervousness, and insomnia. There are no clinically relevant changes in blood pressure, heart rate, cardiac conduction, or laboratory parameters. Gepirone has no detectable inhibition of CYP 450 enzymes.

Gepirone is used once daily in the form of extended-release tablets. Dose titration is necessary, with a starting dosage of 20 mg a day, increased over several weeks up to 80 mg a day if necessary.

▲ 32.3.10 Calcium Channel Inhibitors

The calcium channel inhibitors are variously referred to as *calcium channel antagonists*, *calcium channel blockers*, and *organic calcium channel inhibitors*. The calcium channel inhibitors were first developed as cardiac drugs to treat hypertension, angina, and specific types of cardiac arrhythmias.

Calcium channel inhibitors are used in psychiatry as antimanic agents for persons who do not respond well to first-line agents such as lithium (Eskalith), valproic acid (Depakene), carbamazepine (Tegretol), or other anticonvulsants. Calcium channel inhibitors include nifedipine (Procardia, Adalat), nimodipine (Nimotop), isradipine (DynaCirc), amlodipine (Norvasc, Lotrel), nicardipine (Cardene), nisoldipine (Sular), nitrendipine, and verapamil (Calan). They are used for control of mania and ultradian bipolar disorder (mood cycling in less than 24 hours).

PHARMACOLOGICAL ACTIONS

The calcium channel inhibitors are well absorbed from the gastrointestinal (GI) tract, with significant first-pass hepatic metabolism. Considerable intraindividual and interindividual variations are seen in the plasma concentrations of the drugs after a single dose. The half-life of verapamil after the first dose is 2 to 8 hours; the half-life increases to 5 to 12 hours after the first few days of therapy. The half-lives of the other calcium channel blockers range from 1 to 2 hours for nimodipine and isradipine, to 30 to 50 hours for amlodipine. The calcium channel inhibitors inhibit the influx of calcium into neurons through L-type (long-acting) voltage-dependent calcium channels.

EFFECTS ON SPECIFIC ORGANS AND SYSTEMS

The major effects of calcium channel inhibitors are on the vasculature, which responds with vasodilation to the calcium channel inhibitors. Diuresis also occurs. The calcium channel inhibitors interfere with atrioventricular (AV) conduction and can lead to AV heart block, especially in elderly patients.

THERAPEUTIC INDICATIONS

Bipolar Disorder

There are mixed reports about the efficacy of verapamil for both short-term and maintenance treatment of bipolar disorders, to be used after trials of lithium, carbamazepine, and valproate. The other drugs, such as nimodipine, isradipine, and amlodipine, may be particularly effective in the treatment of manic episodes and of rapid-cycling or ultrarapid-cycling bipolar disorders. The clinician should begin treatment with a short-acting drug such as nimodipine or isradipine, beginning with a low dosage and increasing the dosage every 4 to 5 days until a clinical response is seen or adverse effects appear. Once symptoms are controlled, a longer-acting drug, such as amlodipine, can be substituted as maintenance therapy. Failure to respond to verapamil does not exclude a favorable response to one of the other drugs.

Recurrent Brief Depressive Disorder

Calcium channel inhibitors may be effective for persons with recurrent brief depressive disorder; however, more trials are needed.

Other Psychiatric Indications

Calcium channel inhibitors may be beneficial in Tourette's disorder, Huntington's disease, Alzheimer's disease, panic disorder, premenstrual dysphoric disorder, and intermittent explosive disorder. Well-controlled studies have found a lack of efficacy for calcium channel inhibitors in schizophrenia, tardive dyskinesia, and major depression.

PRECAUTIONS AND ADVERSE REACTIONS

The most common adverse effects associated with calcium channel inhibitors are those due to vasodilation: dizziness, headache, tachycardia, nausea, dysesthesias, and peripheral edema. Verapamil and diltiazem (Cardizem) in particular can cause hypotension, bradycardia, and AV heart block, which necessitates close monitoring and sometimes discontinuation of the drugs. In all patients with cardiovascular disease, the drugs should be used with caution. Other common adverse effects include constipation, fatigue, rash, coughing, and wheezing. Adverse effects noted with diltiazem include hyperactivity, akathisia, and parkinsonism; with verapamil, delirium, hyperprolactinemia, and galactorrhea; with nimodipine, a subjective sense of chest tightness and skin flushing; and with nifedipine, depression. The drugs have not been evaluated for safety in pregnant women and are best avoided. Because the drugs are secreted in breast milk, nursing mothers should also avoid the drugs.

DRUG–DRUG INTERACTIONS

Calcium channel inhibitors should not be used by persons taking β-adrenergic receptor antagonists, hypotensives (e.g., diuretics, vasodilators, and angiotensin-converting enzyme inhibitors), or antiarrhythmic drugs (e.g., quinidine [Cardioquin] and digoxin [Lanoxin]). Verapamil and diltiazem but not nifedipine have been reported to precipitate carbamazepine-induced neurotoxicity. Cimetidine (Tagamet) has been reported to increase plasma concentrations of nifedipine and diltiazem. Some patients who are treated with lithium and calcium channel inhibitors concurrently may be at increased risk for the signs and symptoms of neurotoxicity, and deaths have occurred.

LABORATORY INTERFERENCES

No known laboratory interferences are associated with the use of calcium channel inhibitors.

DOSAGE AND CLINICAL GUIDELINES

Verapamil is available in 40-, 80-, and 120-mg tablets; 120-, 180-, and 240-mg sustained-release tablets; and 100-, 120-, 180-, 200-, 240-, 300-, and 360-mg sustained-release capsules. The starting dosage is 40 mg orally three times a day and can be raised in increments every 4 to 5 days up to 80 to 120 mg three times a day. The patient's blood pressure, pulse, and electrocardiogram (ECG) (in patients older than 40 years or with a history of cardiac illness) should be routinely monitored.

Nifedipine is available in 10- and 20-mg capsules and 30-, 60-, and 90-mg extended-release tablets. Administration should be started at 10 mg orally three or four times a day and can be increased up to a maximum dosage of 120 mg a day.

Nimodipine is available in 30-mg capsules. It has been used at 60 mg every 4 hours for ultrarapid-cycling bipolar disorder, and sometimes briefly at up to 630 mg per day.

Isradipine is available in 2.5- and 5-mg capsules and 5- or 10-mg controlled-release tablets. Administration should be started at 2.5 mg a day and can be increased up to a maximum of 15 mg a day in divided doses.

Amlodipine is available in 2.5-, 5-, and 10-mg tablets. Administration should start at 5 mg once at night and can be increased to a maximum dosage of 10 to 15 mg a day.

Diltiazem is available in 30-, 60-, 90-, and 120-mg tablets; 60-, 90-, 120-, 180-, 240-, 300-, and 360-mg extended-release capsules; and 60-, 90-, 120-, 180-, 240-, 300-, and 360-mg extended-release tablets. Administration should start with 30 mg orally four times a day and can be increased up to a maximum of 360 mg a day.

Elderly persons are more sensitive to the calcium channel inhibitors than younger adults. No specific information is available regarding the use of the agents for children.

▲ 32.3.11 Carbamazepine

Carbamazepine (Tegretol) is effective for the treatment of acute mania and for the prophylactic treatment of bipolar I disorder. It is a first-line agent for these disorders along with lithium (Eskalith) and valproic acid (Depakene). Carbamazepine is also used to treat partial and generalized-onset epilepsy and trigeminal neuralgia. A congener, oxcarbazepine (Trileptal), is also available for use in bipolar disorder.

PHARMACOLOGICAL ACTIONS

Carbamazepine is absorbed slowly and erratically from the gastrointestinal (GI) tract, and absorption is enhanced when the drug is taken with meals. Peak plasma concentrations are reached 2 to 8 hours after a single dose, and steady-state levels are reached after 2 to 4 days on a steady dosage. The suspension formulation is absorbed somewhat faster, and the extended-release formulation somewhat slower, than the standard formulation. The half-life of carbamazepine at the initiation of treatment has a wide range; after 1 month of administration the half-life decreases to a range of 12 to 17 hours because of the induction of hepatic enzymes, which reach their maximum level after approximately 1 month of therapy. The extended-release formulation permits achievement of smooth steady-state concentrations with twice-daily dosing. Carbamazepine is metabolized in the liver, and the 10,11-epoxide metabolite is active as an anticonvulsant; its activity in the treatment of bipolar disorders is unknown.

The anticonvulsant effects of carbamazepine are attributed mainly to binding to voltage-dependent sodium channels in the inactive state and prolonging their inactivation. This secondarily reduces voltage-dependent calcium channel activation and, therefore, synaptic transmission. Additional effects include reduction of currents through N-methyl-D-aspartate (NMDA) glutamate-receptor channels, competitive antagonism of adenosine A_1 receptors, and potentiation of central nervous system (CNS) catecholamine neurotransmission. Whether any or all of these mechanisms also result in mood stabilization is not known.

EFFECTS ON SPECIFIC ORGANS AND SYSTEMS

Besides the effects on the CNS, carbamazepine has its most significant effects on the hematopoietic system. Carbamazepine is associated with a benign and often transient decrease in the white blood cell count, with values usually remaining above 3,000. The decrease is thought to be due to the inhibition of colony-stimulating factor in bone marrow, an effect that can be reversed by the coadministration of lithium, which stimulates the colony-stimulating factor. The benign suppression of white blood cell production must be differentiated from the potentially fatal adverse effects of agranulocytosis, pancytopenia, and aplastic anemia.

As reflected by its use in treating diabetes insipidus, carbamazepine apparently has a vasopressin-like effect on the vasopressin receptor and sometimes causes the development of water intoxication or hyponatremia, particularly in elderly patients. This adverse effect can be treated with demeclocycline (Declomycin) or lithium. Another endocrine effect associated with carbamazepine is an increase in urinary free cortisol.

Carbamazepine induces several hepatic enzymes and may thus interfere with the metabolism of various other drugs. The effects of carbamazepine on the cardiovascular system are minimal. It does decrease atrioventricular (A-V) conduction, and thus the use of carbamazepine is contraindicated in patients with A-V heart blocks.

Carbamazepine may cause a rash, which may be transient even if the drug is continued, but may lead to serious and potentially life-threatening dermatological conditions on rare occasions. Other system-specific allergic reactions have been reported, and rarely, a lupus-like disorder has been associated with use of carbamazepine.

THERAPEUTIC INDICATIONS

Bipolar Disorder

Manic Episodes. Carbamazepine is effective in the treatment of acute mania, with efficacy comparable to that of lithium and antipsychotics. Carbamazepine is also effective in the prophylaxis of both manic and depressive episodes in bipolar disorders, after lithium and valproic acid. Carbamazepine is an effective antimanic agent in 50 to 70 percent of persons within 2 to 3 weeks of initiation, and it may be effective in some persons who are not responsive to lithium, such as those with dysphoric mania, rapid cycling, or a negative family history of mood disorders. The antimanic effects of carbamazepine can be augmented by concomitant administration of lithium, valproic acid, thyroid hormones, dopamine receptor antagonists, or serotonin-dopamine antagonists. Some persons may respond to carbamazepine but not lithium or valproic acid, and vice versa. Tolerance for the antimanic effects of carbamazepine can develop in some persons.

Depressive Episodes. The available data indicate that carbamazepine is an effective treatment for depression in some persons. Approximately 25 to 30 percent of depressed persons respond to carbamazepine. That percentage is significantly smaller than the 60 to 70 percent response rate for standard antidepressants. Nevertheless, carbamazepine is an alternative drug for depressed persons who have not responded to conventional treatments, including electroconvulsive therapy (ECT) or who have marked or rapid periodicity in their depressive episodes.

Schizophrenia and Schizoaffective Disorder

Carbamazepine is effective in the treatment of schizophrenia and schizoaffective disorder. Persons with prominent positive symptoms (e.g., hallucinations) may be likely to respond, as are persons who display impulsive aggressive outbursts.

Impulse-Control Disorders

Carbamazepine is effective in controlling impulsive, aggressive behavior in nonpsychotic persons of all ages, including children and the elderly. Other drugs for impulse-control disorders, particularly intermittent explosive disorder, include lithium, propranolol (Inderal), and antipsychotics. Because of the risk of serious adverse effects with carbamazepine, treatment with other agents is warranted before initiating a trial with carbamazepine.

Carbamazepine is also effective in controlling nonacute agitation and aggressive behavior in schizophrenic persons. Diagnoses to be ruled out before initiating treatment with carbamazepine include akathisia and neuroleptic malignant syndrome. Clinically, lorazepam (Ativan) is more effective than carbamazepine for the control of acute agitation.

Posttraumatic Stress Disorder

Carbamazepine has been suggested, along with antidepressants, benzodiazepines, lithium, β-adrenergic receptor antagonists, and α_2-adrenergic receptor agonists, as a treatment for posttraumatic stress disorder (PTSD). Carbamazepine is particularly useful for management of agitation and aggression in PTSD.

Alcohol and Benzodiazepine Withdrawal

Carbamazepine is as effective as the benzodiazepines in the control of symptoms associated with alcohol withdrawal. It may also assist in withdrawal from chronic alcohol or benzodiazepine use, especially in seizure-prone persons. However, the lack of any advantage of carbamazepine over the benzodiazepines for alcohol withdrawal and the potential risk of adverse effects with carbamazepine limit the clinical usefulness of this application.

PRECAUTIONS AND ADVERSE REACTIONS

Although the drug's hematological effects are not dose related, most of the adverse effects of carbamazepine are correlated with plasma concentrations above 9 mg/mL. The rarest but most serious adverse effects of carbamazepine are blood dyscrasias, hepatitis, and exfoliative dermatitis. Otherwise, carbamazepine is relatively well tolerated by persons except for mild GI and CNS effects that can be significantly reduced if the dosage is increased slowly and minimal effective plasma concentrations are maintained.

Blood Dyscrasias

Severe blood dyscrasias (aplastic anemia, agranulocytosis) occur in approximately 1 in 125,000 persons treated with carbamazepine. There does not appear to be a correlation between the degree of benign white blood cell suppression (leukopenia), which is seen in 1 to 2 percent of persons, and the emergence of life-threatening blood dyscrasias. Persons should be warned that the emergence of such symptoms as fever, sore throat, rash, petechiae, bruising, and easy bleeding can potentially herald a serious dyscrasia and should cause them to seek medical evaluation immediately. Routine hematological monitoring in carbamazepine-treated persons is recommended at 3, 6, 9, and 12 months. If there is no significant evidence of bone marrow suppression by that time, many experts would reduce the monitoring interval. However, even assiduous monitoring may fail to detect severe blood dyscrasias before they cause symptoms.

Hepatitis

Within the first few weeks of therapy, carbamazepine can cause both a hepatitis associated with increases in liver enzymes, particularly transaminases, and a cholestasis associated with elevated bilirubin and alkaline phosphatase. Mild transaminase elevations warrant observation only, but persistent elevations that exceed three times the upper limit of normal indicate discontinuation of carbamazepine. Hepatitis can recur if the drug is reintroduced to the person and can result in death.

Exfoliative Dermatitis

A benign pruritic rash occurs in 10 to 15 percent of persons treated with carbamazepine, usually within the first few weeks of treatment. Approximately three persons per million per week may experience life-threatening dermatological syndromes, including exfoliative dermatitis, erythema multiforme, Stevens-Johnson syndrome, and toxic epidermal necrolysis. The possible emergence of these serious dermatological problems causes most clinicians to discontinue carbamazepine use in a person who develops any type of rash. If carbamazepine seems to be the only effective drug for a person who has a benign rash with carbamazepine treatment, a retrial of the drug can be undertaken with pretreatment of the person with prednisone (40 mg a day) in an attempt to treat the rash, although other symptoms of an allergic reaction (e.g., fever and pneumonitis) may develop, even with steroid pretreatment. The risk of drug rash is approximately equal between valproic acid and carbamazepine in the first 2 months of use but is subsequently much higher for carbamazepine.

Gastrointestinal Effects

The most common adverse effects of carbamazepine are nausea, vomiting, gastric distress, constipation, diarrhea, and anorexia. The severity of the adverse effects is reduced if the dosage of carbamazepine is increased slowly and kept at the minimal effective plasma concentration. Unlike lithium and valproate, carbamazepine does not appear to cause weight gain.

Central Nervous System Effects

Acute confusional states can occur with carbamazepine alone but occur most often in combination with lithium or antipsychotic drugs. Elderly persons and persons with cognitive disorders are at increased risk for CNS toxicity from carbamazepine. The symptoms of CNS toxicity include dizziness, ataxia, clumsiness, sedation, diplopia, hyperreflexia, clonus, and tremor. These symptoms can be reduced by slow upward titration of the dosage. The incidence of cognitive disturbances about equals that with carbamazepine, lithium, and valproic acid.

Other Adverse Effects

Carbamazepine decreases cardiac conduction (although less than the tricyclic drugs do) and thus can exacerbate preexisting cardiac disease. Carbamazepine should be used with caution in persons with glaucoma, prostatic hypertrophy, diabetes, or a history of alcohol abuse. Carbamazepine occasionally activates vasopressin-receptor function, which results in a condition resembling the syndrome of secretion of inappropriate antidiuretic hormone (SIADH), characterized by hyponatremia and, rarely, water intoxication. This is the opposite of the renal effects of lithium (i.e., nephrogenic diabetes insipidus). Augmentation of lithium with carbamazepine does not reverse the lithium effect, however. Emergence of confusion, severe weakness, or headache in a person taking carbamazepine should prompt measurement of serum electrolytes. Carbamazepine use rarely elicits an immune hypersensitivity response consisting of fever, rash, eosinophilia, and possibly fatal myocarditis.

Some evidence indicates that minor cranial facial abnormalities, fingernail hypoplasia, and spina bifida in infants may be associated with maternal use of carbamazepine during pregnancy. Therefore, pregnant women should not use carbamazepine unless absolutely necessary. The risk of neural tube defects can be reduced by maternal intake of folic acid 1 to 4 mg daily for at least 3 months prior to conception. Carbamazepine is secreted in breast milk, but its use during breast-feeding is considered safe by the American Academy of Pediatrics.

DRUG–DRUG INTERACTIONS

Principally because it induces several hepatic enzymes, carbamazepine may interact with many drugs. For the most part, addition of carbamazepine lowers the plasma concentrations of affected drugs, and monitoring for decreased clinical effects is frequently indicated. Coadministration with lithium, antipsychotic drugs, verapamil (Calan), or nifedipine (Procardia) can precipitate carbamazepine-induced CNS adverse effects. Carbamazepine can decrease the concentrations of oral contraceptives in blood, resulting in breakthrough bleeding and uncertain prophylaxis against pregnancy. Carbamazepine should not be administered with monoamine oxidase inhibitors (MAOIs), which should be discontinued at least 2 weeks before initiating treatment with carbamazepine. Carbamazepine may significantly induce the metabolism of bupropion (Wellbutrin).

LABORATORY INTERFERENCES

Carbamazepine treatment is associated with a transient decrease in thyroid hormones (thyroxine [T_4] and triiodothyronine [T_3]) without an associated increase in thyroid-stimulating hormone (TSH). Carbamazepine is also associated with an increase in total serum cholesterol, primarily by increasing high-density lipoproteins. The thyroid and cholesterol effects are not clinically significant. Carbamazepine may interfere with the dexamethasone-suppression test and may also cause false-positive pregnancy test results.

DOSAGE AND CLINICAL GUIDELINES

Carbamazepine can be used alone or with an antipsychotic drug for the treatment of manic episodes, although carbamazepine-induced CNS adverse effects (drowsiness, dizziness, ataxia) are likely to occur with this combination of drugs. Persons who do not respond to lithium alone may respond when carbamazepine is added to the lithium treatment. If a person then responds, an attempt should be made to withdraw the lithium to assess whether the person can be treated successfully with carbamazepine alone. When lithium and carbamazepine are used together, the clinician should minimize or discontinue any antipsychotics, sedatives, or anticholinergic drugs the person may be taking to reduce the risks for adverse effects associated with taking multiple drugs. The combination of lithium and carbamazepine must be monitored closely for CNS toxicity, which may be fatal if not properly treated. Lithium and the carbamazepine should both be used at standard therapeutic plasma concentrations before a trial of combined therapy is considered to have been a therapeutic failure. A 3-week trial of carbamazepine at therapeutic plasma concentrations usually suffices to determine whether the drug will be effective in the treatment of acute mania; a longer trial is necessary to assess efficacy in the treatment of depression. Carbamazepine is also used in combination with valproic acid, another anticonvulsant that is effective in bipolar disorders. When carbamazepine and valproate are used in combination, the dosage of carbamazepine should be decreased, because valproate displaces carbamazepine binding on proteins, and the dosage of valproate may need to be increased.

Pretreatment Medical Evaluation

The person's medical history should include information about preexisting hematological, hepatic, and cardiac diseases, because all three can be relative contraindications for carbamazepine treatment. Persons with hepatic disease require only one-third to one-half the usual dosage; the clinician should be cautious about raising the dosage in such persons and should do so only slowly and gradually. The laboratory examination should include a complete blood count with platelet count, liver function tests, serum electrolytes, and an electrocardiogram (ECG) in persons older than 40 years or with a preexisting cardiac disease. An electroencephalogram (EEG) is not necessary before the initiation of treatment, but it may be helpful in some cases for the documentation of objective changes correlated with clinical improvement.

Initiation of Treatment

Carbamazepine is available in 100- and 200-mg tablets and as a 100 mg/5 mL suspension. The usual starting dosage is 200 mg orally two times a day; however, with titration, three-times-a-day

dosing is optimal. An extended-release version suitable for twice-a-day maintenance dosing is available in 100-, 200-, and 400-mg tablets. Carbamazepine should be taken with meals, and the drug should be stored in a cool, dry place. Carbamazepine can lose one-third of its potency when stored in a humid environment, such as a bathroom. In a hospital setting with seriously ill persons, the dosage can be raised by not more than 200 mg a day until a dosage of 600 to 1,200 mg a day is reached. This relatively rapid titration, however, is often associated with adverse effects and may adversely affect compliance with the drug. In less ill persons and in outpatients, the dosage should be raised no more quickly than 200 mg every 2 to 7 days to minimize the occurrence of minor adverse effects such as nausea, vomiting, drowsiness, and dizziness. When discontinuing treatment with carbamazepine, the clinician generally should taper the dosage, although the drug can safely be stopped abruptly in most persons.

Blood Concentrations

The anticonvulsant blood concentration range for carbamazepine is 4 to 12 µg/mL, and this range should be reached before determining that carbamazepine is not effective in the treatment of a mood disorder. It is clinically prudent to come up to that range gradually, since the person is likely to tolerate a gradual increase of carbamazepine better than a rapid increase. The clinician should titrate carbamazepine up to the highest well-tolerated dosage before deciding that the drug is ineffective. Plasma concentrations should be determined when a person has been receiving a steady dosage for at least 5 days. Blood for the determination of plasma levels is drawn in the morning, before the first daily dose of carbamazepine is taken. The total daily dosage necessary to achieve plasma concentrations in the usual therapeutic range varies from 400 to 1,600 mg a day, with a mean around 1,000 mg a day.

Routine Laboratory Monitoring

The most serious potential effects of carbamazepine are agranulocytosis and aplastic anemia. Although it has been suggested that complete laboratory blood assessments be performed every 2 weeks for the first 2 months of treatment and quarterly thereafter, this conservative approach may not be justified by a cost-benefit analysis and may not detect a serious blood dyscrasia before it occurs. The Food and Drug Administration (FDA) has revised the package insert for carbamazepine to suggest that blood monitoring be performed at the discretion of the physician. Education about the signs and the symptoms of a developing hematological problem is probably more effective than frequent blood monitoring in protecting against blood dyscrasias. It has also been suggested that liver and renal function tests be conducted quarterly, although the benefit of conducting tests this frequently has been questioned. It seems reasonable, however, to assess hematological status, along with liver and renal functions, whenever a routine examination of the person is being conducted.

The following laboratory values should prompt the physician to discontinue carbamazepine treatment and to consult a hematologist: total white blood cell count below 3,000/mm^3, erythrocyte count below 4.0×10^6 per mm^3, neutrophil count below 1,500/mm^3, hematocrit less than 32 percent, hemoglobin less than 11 g per 100 mL, platelet count below 100,000/mm^3, reticulocyte count below 0.3 percent, and a serum iron concentration below 150 mg per 100 mL.

▲ 32.3.12 Chloral Hydrate

Chloral hydrate, in use since 1869, is one of the oldest sedative-hypnotic drugs. It is rarely used because there are safer options, such as the benzodiazepines.

PHARMACOLOGICAL ACTIONS

Chloral hydrate is well absorbed from the gastrointestinal (GI) tract. The parent compound is metabolized within minutes by the liver to the active metabolite trichloroethanol, which has a half-life of 8 to 11 hours. A dose of chloral hydrate induces sleep in approximately 30 to 60 minutes and maintains sleep for 4 to 8 hours. It probably potentiates γ-aminobutyric acid (GABA)-ergic neurotransmission, which suppresses neuronal excitability.

EFFECTS ON SPECIFIC ORGANS AND SYSTEMS

In addition to its central nervous system (CNS) effects, chloral hydrate has effects on the GI system and the skin. The GI effects include nonspecific irritation, nausea, vomiting, flatulence, and an unpleasant taste. The dermatological effects, although uncommon, include rashes, urticaria, purpura, eczema, and erythema multiforme. The dermatological lesions are sometimes accompanied by fever.

THERAPEUTIC INDICATIONS

The major indication for chloral hydrate is insomnia. Whether chloral hydrate affects rapid eye movement (REM) sleep is controversial, but patients experience no REM rebound after discontinuation of chloral hydrate therapy.

PRECAUTIONS AND ADVERSE REACTIONS

The most common GI adverse effects are nausea, vomiting, and diarrhea. Patients should be warned that they may experience residual daytime sedation and impaired motor coordination. Chloral hydrate should be avoided in patients with severe renal, cardiac, or hepatic disease or with porphyria. The drug may aggravate GI inflammatory conditions. Chloral hydrate should not be used during pregnancy or by nursing women.

In addition to the development of tolerance, chloral hydrate dependence can occur, with symptoms similar to those of alcohol dependence. The symptoms of intoxication include confusion, ataxia, dysarthria, bradycardia, arrhythmia, and severe drowsiness. The lethal adult dose of chloral hydrate has ranged between 5 and 40 g; thus the drug is a particularly poor choice for potentially suicidal patients. The lethality of the drug is potentiated by other CNS depressants, including alcohol. With long-term use and overdose, gastritis and gastric ulceration can develop. Hepatic and renal damage can follow overdose attempts, which may result in jaundice and albuminuria.

DRUG–DRUG INTERACTIONS

Because of metabolic interference, chloral hydrate should be strictly avoided with alcohol, a notorious concoction known as a "Mickey Finn." Use of chloral hydrate less than 24 hours before receiving intravenous furosemide (Lasix) can cause diaphoresis, flushes, and unsteady blood pressure. Chloral hydrate may displace warfarin (Coumadin) from plasma proteins and enhance anticoagulant activity; this combination should be avoided.

LABORATORY INTERFERENCES

Chloral hydrate administration can lead to false-positive results for urine glucose determinations that use cupric sulfate (e.g., Clinitest) but not in tests that use glucose oxidase (e.g., Clinistix and Tes-Tape). Chloral hydrate may also interfere with the determination of urinary catecholamines and 17-hydroxycorticosteroids.

DOSAGE AND CLINICAL GUIDELINES

Chloral hydrate is available in 500-mg capsules, 500 mg per 5 mL solution, and 324-, 500-, and 648-mg rectal suppositories. The standard dose of chloral hydrate is 500 to 2,000 mg at bedtime. Because the drug is a GI irritant, it should be administered with water, milk, other liquids, or antacids to decrease gastric irritation.

▲ 32.3.13 Cholinesterase Inhibitors

Four drugs have been approved by the Food and Drug Administration (FDA) for treatment of Alzheimer's disease and similar disorders with cognitive deficits: tacrine (Cognex), rivastigmine (Exelon), galantamine (Reminyl), and donepezil (Aricept). These drugs are cholinesterase inhibitors, which reduce intrasynaptic cleavage and inactivation of acetylcholine and thus potentiate cholinergic neurotransmission, which in turn tends to produce modest improvement in memory and goal-directed thought.

At one time tacrine was the only drug available, but several untoward effects, especially hepatic toxicity that required weekly blood tests, rendered it useful to only a minority of patients with Alzheimer's disease. Later, donepezil was approved, which has a simpler dosage regimen, has fewer adverse effects, and does not require weekly blood tests. Rivastigmine and galantamine followed, also with a safer profile. Other similar agents are in the investigational stages of development but are not yet available for use in the United States, including sustained-release physostigmine salicylate (Synapton), suronacrine, eptastigmine, and metrifonate. These drugs are considered most useful for patients who have mild to moderate memory loss but nevertheless have enough of their basal forebrain cholinergic neurons to benefit from augmentation of cholinergic neurotransmission.

Memantine, an N-methyl-D-aspartate (NMDA) receptor antagonist, is under investigation. It is not a cholinesterase inhibitor and works by protecting neurons from excessive stimulation by glutamate, a possible factor in the cause of Alzheimer's disease.

Memantine is discussed separately below. It is used in Alzheimer's disease and has a different mechanism of action.

PHARMACOLOGICAL ACTIONS

All of the cholinesterase inhibitors are readily absorbed from the gastrointestinal (GI) tract. Peak plasma concentrations differ slightly but are reached approximately 3 to 4 hours after oral dosing. The half-life of donepezil is 70 hours in the elderly, and it is taken only once daily. Steady-state levels are achieved within approximately 2 weeks. Presence of stable alcoholic cirrhosis reduces clearance of donepezil by 20 percent. Rivastigmine and galantamine reach peak plasma concentrations in 1 hour. The actions of both drugs may be delayed by up to 90 minutes if taken with food. The half-life of rivastigmine is 1 hour, but because it remains bound to cholinesterases, a single dose is therapeutically active for 10 hours, and it is taken twice daily.

Peak plasma concentrations of tacrine are reached approximately 90 minutes after oral dosing. The half-life of tacrine is approximately 2 to 4 hours, thereby necessitating four-times-daily dosing; galantamine has a half-life of approximately 7 hours and is given twice daily.

Galantamine is an agonist at nicotinic sites without producing desensitization, as well as a cholinesterase inhibitor. This ability to enhance the sensitivity of the acetylcholine receptor is possessed only by galantamine and physostigmine. The mechanism of action is analogous to that of benzodiazepines at the γ-aminobutyric acid (GABA) A site. Consequently, the drug has an in vivo cholinomimetic activity that is even stronger than its acetylcholinesterase inhibitory properties alone would predict.

The primary mechanism of action of cholinesterase inhibitors is reversible, nonacylating inhibition of acetylcholinesterase and butyrylcholinesterase, the enzymes that catabolize acetylcholine in the central nervous system (CNS). The enzyme inhibition increases synaptic concentrations of acetylcholine, especially in the hippocampus and cerebral cortex. Unlike tacrine, which is nonselective for all forms of acetylcholinesterase, donepezil appears to be selectively active within the CNS and to have little activity in the periphery. Donepezil's favorable adverse effect profile appears to correlate with its lack of inhibition of cholinesterases in the GI tract. Rivastigmine and galantamine appear to have somewhat more peripheral activity than donepezil and are thus more likely to cause GI adverse effects than donepezil is.

EFFECTS ON SPECIFIC ORGANS AND SYSTEMS

In addition to its effects on cognitive performance, tacrine affects the liver and the parasympathetic nervous system. Tacrine is associated with an increase in hepatic enzymes—serum glutamic-oxaloacetic transaminase (SGOT) and serum glutamic-pyruvic transaminase (SGPT)—in 25 to 30 percent of patients. Because of its cholinomimetic properties, tacrine causes activation of the parasympathetic nervous system, which results in all the usual signs and symptoms of muscarinic activity: nausea, vomiting, diarrhea, and other autonomic symptoms. The other drugs in this class have little or no hepatotoxic effect, although they may produce GI activation with nausea, vomiting, and anorexia.

THERAPEUTIC INDICATIONS

Donepezil, rivastigmine, galantamine, and tacrine are effective for the treatment of cognitive impairment in dementia of the Alzheimer's type. Based on numerous well-controlled studies, the cholinesterase inhibitors in long-term use slow the progression of memory loss and diminish apathy, depression, hallucinations, anxiety, euphoria, and purposeless motor behaviors. Functional autonomy (i.e., the ability to carry out the activities of daily living) is less well preserved. Some persons note immediate improvement in memory, mood, psychotic symptoms, and interpersonal skills. Others note little initial benefit but are able to retain their cognitive and adaptive faculties at a relatively stable level for many months. Use of cholinesterase inhibitors may delay or reduce the need for nursing home placement.

Donepezil may be beneficial for the treatment of dementia due to diffuse Lewy body disease and for treatment of cognitive deficits due to traumatic brain injury. Donepezil is under study for treatment of cognitive impairment less severe than that due to Alzheimer's disease. People with multiinfarction and other types of dementias may not respond to acetylcholinesterase inhibitors. Occasionally, cholinesterase inhibitors elicit an idiosyncratic catastrophic reaction, with signs of grief and agitation, which is self-limited once the drug is discontinued. Use of cholinesterase inhibitors to improve cognition by nondemented individuals should be discouraged.

PRECAUTIONS AND ADVERSE REACTIONS

Donepezil

Donepezil is generally well tolerated at recommended dosages. Less than 3 percent of persons taking donepezil experience nausea, diarrhea, and vomiting. These mild symptoms are more common with a 10-mg dose than with a 5-mg dose, and they tend to resolve after 3 weeks of continued use. Donepezil may cause weight loss. Donepezil treatment has been infrequently associated with bradyarrhythmias, especially in persons with underlying cardiac disease. A small number of persons experience syncope.

Rivastigmine

Rivastigmine is generally well tolerated, but recommended dosages may need to be scaled back in the initial period of treatment to limit GI and CNS adverse effects. These mild symptoms are more common at dosages above 6 mg a day, and they tend to resolve once the dosage is lowered. The most common adverse effects associated with rivastigmine are nausea, vomiting, dizziness, headache, diarrhea, abdominal pain, anorexia, fatigue, and somnolence. Rivastigmine may cause weight loss, but it does not appear to cause hepatic, renal, hematological, or electrolyte abnormalities.

Galantamine

Galantamine is well tolerated and at 8 mg a day produced improved cognition in patients with mild or moderate impairment. With higher doses (24 mg a day) the risk of adverse effects, including syncope, increases. Adverse effects are primarily GI, are dose related, and in approximately 5 percent of patients lead to discontinuation of use of the drug.

Tacrine

Tacrine is cumbersome to titrate and use, and it poses the risk of potentially significant elevations in hepatic transaminase levels in

25 to 30 percent of persons, nausea and vomiting in approximately 20 percent of persons, and diarrhea and other cholinergic symptoms in approximately 11 percent of persons. Aside from elevated transaminase levels, the most common specific adverse effects associated with tacrine treatment are nausea, vomiting, myalgia, anorexia, and rash, but only nausea, vomiting, and anorexia are clearly related to the dosage. Transaminase elevations characteristically develop during the first 6 to 12 weeks of treatment, and cholinergically mediated events are dosage related. Because of the high risk of hepatotoxicity and the availability of newer and safer drugs in this class, tacrine is rarely, if ever, used.

DRUG–DRUG INTERACTIONS

The metabolism of donepezil may be increased by phenytoin (Dilantin), carbamazepine (Tegretol), dexamethasone (Decadron), rifampin (Rifadin), or phenobarbital (Solfoton). All cholinesterase inhibitors should be used cautiously with drugs that also possess cholinomimetic activity, such as succinylcholine (Anectine) or bethanechol (Urecholine). Coadministration of cholinesterase inhibitors and drugs that have cholinergic antagonist activity (e.g., tricyclic drugs) is probably counterproductive. Donepezil is highly protein bound, but it does not displace other protein-bound drugs, such as furosemide (Lasix), digoxin (Lanoxin), or warfarin (Coumadin). Rivastigmine circulates mostly unbound to serum proteins and has no significant known drug interactions. Coadministration of paroxetine (Paxil) and erythromycin increases the blood level of galantamine. Except for tacrine, some of these drugs inhibit the metabolic pathways of the cytochrome P450 isoenzymes, but this has no clinical significance.

LABORATORY INTERFERENCES

No laboratory interferences have been associated with any of the cholinesterase inhibitors.

DOSAGE AND CLINICAL GUIDELINES

Before the initiation of treatment with cholinesterase inhibitors, potentially treatable causes of dementia should be ruled out and the diagnosis of dementia of the Alzheimer's type should be established with a thorough neurological evaluation. Detailed neuropsychological testing can detect early signs of Alzheimer's disease. Psychiatric evaluation also should focus on depression, anxiety, and psychosis.

Donepezil is available in 5- and 10-mg tablets. Treatment should be initiated at 5 mg each night. If well tolerated and of some discernible benefit after 4 weeks, the dosage should be increased to a maintenance dosage of 10 mg each night. Donepezil absorption is unaffected by meals.

Rivastigmine is available in 1.5-, 3-, 4.5-, and 6-mg capsules. The recommended initial dosage is 1.5 mg twice daily for a minimum of 2 weeks, after which increases of 1.5 mg a day can be made at intervals of at least 2 weeks to a target dosage of 6 mg a day, taken in two equal doses. If tolerated, the dosage may be further titrated upward to a maximum of 6 mg twice daily. The risk of adverse GI events can be reduced by administration of rivastigmine with food.

Galantamine is available in 4-, 8-, and 12-mg tablets and a 4-mg/mL oral solution. The recommended starting dose is 4 mg twice a day. After 4 weeks, the dose should be increased to 8 mg twice a day (16 mg per day). If tolerated, a further increase to 12 mg twice a day may be attempted after a minimum of 4 weeks of the previous dose. Administration with meals may limit adverse GI complaints. For patients with renal impairment a dose greater than 16 mg a day should be avoided.

Tacrine is available in 10-, 20-, 30-, and 40-mg capsules. Before the initiation of tacrine treatment, a complete physical and laboratory examination should be conducted, with special attention to liver function tests and baseline hematological indexes. Treatment should be initiated at 10 mg four times a day and then raised by increments of 10 mg a dose every 6 weeks up to 160 mg a day; the person's tolerance of each dosage is indicated by the absence of unacceptable adverse effects and lack of elevation of alanine aminotransferase (ALT) activity. Tacrine should be given four times daily—ideally 1 hour before meals, since the absorption of tacrine is reduced by approximately 25 percent when it is taken during the first 2 hours after meals. As mentioned above, because of the high risk of hepatotoxicity, tacrine is no longer recommended, especially since the newer compounds are equally effective and without risk.

MEMANTINE

Memantine is an N-methyl-D-aspartate (NMDA) receptor antagonist. The mechanism of action by which memantine is thought to produce clinical effects is distinctly different from the agents currently available to treat Alzheimer's disease, all of which modulate concentrations of the neurotransmitter acetylcholine.

By blocking the NMDA receptor, memantine is able to protect neurons from excessive stimulation by the excitatory neurotransmitter glutamate, without interfering with the role of glutamate, in normal neuronal functioning. Glutamate plays an integral role in neural pathways associated with learning and memory, perhaps affecting the movement of electrical signals across nearly 70 percent of the CNS's excitatory synapses. Excessive amounts of glutamate can, however, damage cells by causing too much excitation. The excitotoxicity produced by glutamate is hypothesized to be responsible for the neuronal cell death observed in Alzheimer's as well as other neurodegenerative disorders. Memantine, known as Akatinol, is currently used in Europe.

▲ 32.3.14 Dantrolene

Dantrolene (Dantrium) is a direct-acting skeletal muscle relaxant. In contemporary clinical psychiatry, dantrolene is one of the potentially effective treatments for neuroleptic malignant syndrome, catatonia, and serotonin syndrome.

PHARMACOLOGICAL ACTIONS

Approximately one-third of orally administered dantrolene is slowly absorbed from the gastrointestinal (GI) tract. At sufficient dosages, consistent plasma concentrations can be maintained. Peak blood concentrations are seen approximately 5 hours after oral administration. The elimination half-life of dantrolene is approximately 9 hours. Dantrolene is largely protein bound, metabolized by the liver, and excreted in the urine. Dantrolene produces skeletal muscle relaxation by directly affecting the contractile response of the muscles at the site beyond the myoneural junction. The skeletal muscle relaxant effect is the basis of its efficacy in reducing the muscle destruction and hyperthermia associated with neuroleptic malignant syndrome.

EFFECTS ON SPECIFIC ORGANS AND SYSTEMS

The skeletal muscle relaxant effect of dantrolene can cause muscle weakness and such symptoms as slurring of speech and drooling. Dantrolene also has effects on the GI system (e.g., diarrhea) and the nervous system (e.g., headache and depression) and possibly toxic effects on hepatocytes, as indicated by an association with elevated liver function test results.

THERAPEUTIC INDICATIONS

The primary psychiatric indication for intravenous (IV) dantrolene is muscle rigidity in neuroleptic malignant syndrome. Dantrolene is almost always used in conjunction with appropriate supportive measures and a dopamine receptor agonist—for example, bromocriptine (Parlodel). Approximately 80 percent of all patients with neuroleptic malignant syndrome who received dantrolene apparently benefited clinically from the drug. Muscle relaxation and general and dramatic improvement in symptoms can appear within minutes of IV administration, although in most cases the beneficial effects can take several hours to appear. Dantrolene has been used in efforts to treat other psychiatric conditions characterized by life-threatening muscle rigidity, such as catatonia and serotonin syndrome.

PRECAUTIONS AND ADVERSE REACTIONS

Muscle weakness, drowsiness, dizziness, light-headedness, nausea, diarrhea, malaise, and fatigue are the most common adverse effects of dantrolene. These effects are generally transient. The central nervous system (CNS) effects of dantrolene can include speech disturbances (which may also reflect its effects on the muscles of speech), headaches, visual disturbances, altered taste, depression, confusion, hallucinations, nervousness, and insomnia. Many serious adverse effects of dantrolene are associated with long-term treatment, rather than with its short-term use in treating neuroleptic malignant syndrome. Dantrolene should be used with caution by patients with hepatic, renal, and chronic lung diseases. Dantrolene can cross the placenta and is thus contraindicated for pregnant women and should not be used by nursing mothers except in emergency situations, such as neuroleptic malignant syndrome. Data are not available about the use of dantrolene by older patients, and no unique problems have been associated with its use by children.

DRUG–DRUG INTERACTIONS

The risk of liver toxicity may be increased for patients also taking estrogens. Dantrolene should be used with caution by patients who are using other drugs that produce drowsiness, most notably the benzodiazepines. In the case of neuroleptic malignant syndrome, however, the general guidelines for dantrolene must be weighed against the severity of the syndrome. Dantrolene should not be

given intravenously in combination with calcium channel inhibitors. Concomitant administration of dantrolene and theophylline (Theo-Dur, Slo-Bid) in animals has caused seizures and death.

LABORATORY INTERFERENCES

No known laboratory interferences are associated with dantrolene, although experience with its use in patients with neuroleptic malignant syndrome is still limited.

DOSAGE AND ADMINISTRATION

In addition to the immediate discontinuation of antipsychotic drugs, medical support to cool the patient, and monitoring of vital signs and renal output, dantrolene can be given in dosages of 1 mg/kg orally 4 times daily or 1 to 5 mg/kg IV to reduce muscle spasms in patients with neuroleptic malignant syndrome. Although some clinicians have recommended low dosages because of the adverse effects, other clinicians indicate that dosages of 10 mg/kg a day are most likely to be effective. Intravenous administration of dantrolene relaxes muscle tension within several minutes. Dantrolene is supplied as 25-, 50-, and 100-mg capsules and in a 20-mg parenteral preparation for reconstitution with 60 mL of sterile water.

▲ 32.3.15 Disulfiram

Disulfiram (Antabuse) is used to ensure abstinence in the treatment of alcohol dependence. Its main effect is to produce a rapid and violently unpleasant reaction in a person who ingests even a small amount of alcohol while taking disulfiram. Because of the risk of severe and even fatal disulfiram–alcohol reactions, disulfiram therapy is used less often today than previously.

PHARMACOLOGICAL ACTIONS

Disulfiram is almost completely absorbed from the gastrointestinal (GI) tract after oral administration. It is metabolized in the liver and excreted in the urine. It is lipid soluble and has an estimated half-life of 60 to 120 hours. One or 2 weeks may be needed before disulfiram is totally eliminated from the body after the last dose has been taken.

Disulfiram is an aldehyde dehydrogenase inhibitor that interferes with the metabolism of alcohol and produces thereby a marked increase in blood acetaldehyde levels. The accumulation of acetaldehyde (to a level up to 10 times higher than occurs in the normal metabolism of alcohol) produces a wide array of unpleasant reactions called the *disulfiram–alcohol reaction*, characterized by nausea, throbbing headache, vomiting, hypotension, flushing, sweating, thirst, dyspnea, tachycardia, chest pain, vertigo, and blurred vision. The reaction occurs almost immediately after the ingestion of one alcoholic drink and may last up to 30 minutes.

THERAPEUTIC INDICATIONS

The primary indication for disulfiram use is as an aversive conditioning treatment for alcohol dependence. Either the fear of having a disulfiram–alcohol reaction or the memory of having had one is meant to condition the patient not to use alcohol. Some clinicians induce a disulfiram–alcohol reaction in patients at the beginning of therapy to convince the patients of the severe unpleasantness of the symptoms. This practice is not recommended, however, as a disulfiram–alcohol reaction can lead to cardiovascular collapse. A graphic description of the severity and unpleasantness of the disulfiram–alcohol reaction usually suffices to discourage patients from imbibing alcohol. Disulfiram treatment should be combined with such treatments as psychotherapy, group therapy, and support groups like Alcoholics Anonymous (AA). The treatment of alcohol dependence requires careful monitoring, since a patient can simply decide not to take the disulfiram; compliance with the medication should be checked if possible.

PRECAUTIONS AND ADVERSE REACTIONS

With Alcohol Consumption

The intensity of the disulfiram–alcohol reaction varies with each patient. In extreme cases, it is marked by respiratory depression, cardiovascular collapse, myocardial infarction, convulsions, and death. Therefore, disulfiram is contraindicated for patients with a significant pulmonary or cardiovascular disease. In addition, disulfiram should be used with caution, if at all, by patients with nephritis, brain damage, hypothyroidism, diabetes, hepatic disease, seizures, polydrug dependence, or an abnormal electroencephalogram (ECG). Most fatal reactions occur in patients who are taking more than 500 mg a day of disulfiram and who consume more than 3 ounces of alcohol. The treatment of a severe disulfiram–alcohol reaction is primarily supportive to prevent shock.

Without Alcohol Consumption

The adverse effects of disulfiram in the absence of alcohol consumption include fatigue, dermatitis, impotence, optic neuritis, a variety of mental changes, acute polyneuropathy, and hepatic damage. A metabolite of disulfiram inhibits dopamine hydroxylase and thus potentially exacerbates psychosis in patients with psychotic disorders.

DRUG–DRUG INTERACTIONS

Disulfiram increases the blood concentration of diazepam (Valium), chlordiazepoxide (Librium), paraldehyde (Paral), phenytoin (Dilantin), caffeine, theophylline (Theo-Dur, Slo-Bid), tetrahydrocannabinol (the active ingredient in marijuana), barbiturates, anticoagulants, isoniazid (Nydrazid, Rifamate), and tricyclic drugs. Concomitant administration of disulfiram and tranylcypromine (Parnate) causes seizures and death in animals.

LABORATORY INTERFERENCES

In rare instances, disulfiram has been reported to decrease the uptake of iodine-131 and protein-bound iodine test results. In research settings, disulfiram may reduce urinary concentrations of homovanillic acid, the major metabolite of dopamine, because of its inhibition of dopamine hydroxylase.

DOSAGE AND ADMINISTRATION

Disulfiram is supplied in tablets of 250 and 500 mg. The usual initial dosage is 500 mg a day taken by mouth for the first 1 or 2 weeks, followed by a maintenance dosage of 250 mg a day. The dosage should not exceed 500 mg a day. The maintenance dosage range is 125 to 500 mg a day.

Patients must be instructed that the ingestion of even the smallest amount of alcohol brings on a disulfiram–alcohol reaction, with all its unpleasant effects. Patients should also be warned against ingesting any alcohol-containing preparations, such as cough drops, tonics of any kind, and alcohol-containing foods and sauces. Some reactions have occurred in men who used alcohol-based aftershave lotions and inhaled the fumes; therefore, precautions must be explicit and should include any topically applied preparations containing alcohol, such as perfume.

Disulfiram should not be administered until patients have abstained from alcohol for at least 12 hours. Disulfiram can cause an unpleasant reaction within 15 minutes after the first dose in a person who has even tiny serum concentrations of unmetabolized alcohol. Patients should be warned that the disulfiram–alcohol reaction may occur as long as 1 or 2 weeks after the last dose of disulfiram. Patients should carry identification cards describing the disulfiram–alcohol reaction and listing the name and the telephone number of the physician to be called.

▲ 32.3.16 Dopamine Receptor Agonists and Precursors: Bromocriptine, Levodopa, Pergolide, Pramipexole, and Ropinirole

Dopamine receptor agonists and precursors increase the amount of dopamine in the brain. They are used to treat various adverse effects of antipsychotic drugs, including (1) parkinsonism, (2) extrapyramidal symptoms, (3) akinesia, (4) focal perioral tremors, (5) hyperprolactinemia, (6) galactorrhea, and (7) neuroleptic malignant syndrome. The drugs in this class most commonly prescribed are bromocriptine (Parlodel), levodopa (Larodopa), and carbidopa-levodopa (Sinemet). New dopamine receptor agonists include ropinirole (Requip), pramipexole (Mirapex), and pergolide (Permax), which are better tolerated than bromocriptine.

PHARMACOLOGICAL ACTIONS

Levodopa, or L-dopa, is rapidly absorbed after oral administration, and peak plasma levels are reached after 30 to 120 minutes. The half-life of levodopa is 90 minutes. Absorption of levodopa can be significantly reduced by changes in gastric pH and by ingestion with meals. Bromocriptine, pergolide, and ropinirole are rapidly absorbed but undergo first-pass metabolism such that only approximately 30 to 55 percent of the dosage is bioavailable. Peak concentrations are achieved 1½ to 3 hours after oral administration. Pergolide has a half-life of about 27 hours, and a single dose has 5 to 6 hours of clinical activity. The half-life of ropinirole is 6 hours. Pramipexole is rapidly absorbed with little first-pass metabolism and reaches peak concentrations in 2 hours. Its half-life is 8 hours.

Once levodopa enters the dopaminergic neurons of the CNS, it is converted by dopa decarboxylase into the neurotransmitter dopamine. Bromocriptine, pergolide, ropinirole, and pramipexole act directly on dopamine receptors. Dopamine, pramipexole, and ropinirole bind approximately 20 times more selectively to dopamine D_3 than D_2 receptors; the corresponding ratio for pergolide is 5, and for bromocriptine is less than 2. Levodopa, pramipexole, and ropinirole have no significant activity at nondopaminergic receptors, but pergolide and bromocriptine bind to serotonin 5-HT$_1$ and 5-HT$_2$, and α_1-, α_2-, and β-adrenergic receptors.

EFFECTS ON SPECIFIC ORGANS AND SYSTEMS

Dopamine activity affects many organ systems in addition to the CNS. Because of the role of dopamine in the maintenance of blood pressure, these drugs are commonly associated with hypertension, although hypotension has been reported in some patients. Dopaminergic activity can also affect heart rate and rhythm. The gastrointestinal (GI) system is also sensitive to dopaminergic drugs and frequently causes symptoms of GI distress, especially nausea.

THERAPEUTIC INDICATIONS
Medication-Induced Movement Disorders

Dopamine receptor agonists are used for the treatment of medication-induced parkinsonism, extrapyramidal symptoms, akinesia, and focal perioral tremors. Their use has diminished sharply, however, because the incidence of medication-induced movement disorders is much lower with the use of the newer, atypical antipsychotics (serotonin-dopamine antagonists [SDAs]).

For the treatment of medication-induced movement disorders, most clinicians rely on anticholinergics, amantadine (Symmetrel), and antihistamines because they are equally effective and have few adverse effects. Bromocriptine remains in use in the treatment of neuroleptic malignant syndrome; however, the incidence of this disorder is diminishing with the decreasing use of dopamine receptor antagonists.

Dopamine receptor agonists are also used to counteract the hyperprolactinemic effects of dopamine receptor antagonists, which result in the side effects of amenorrhea and galactorrhea. Dopamine receptor agonists may reduce the pharmacological effects of cocaine but are not effective in reducing the craving for cocaine associated with withdrawal.

Sexual Dysfunction

All dopamine receptor agonists can improve erectile dysfunction. However, they are rarely used because therapeutic dosages frequently cause intolerable adverse effects, and sildenafil (Viagra) is better tolerated and more effective. Sublingual apomorphine (Uprima) may find a therapeutic niche in treatment of erectile dysfunction in men in whom sildenafil is contraindicated due to use of nitrate-containing medications. However, the safety of

coadministration of apomorphine and nitrates has not yet been determined.

PRECAUTIONS AND ADVERSE REACTIONS

Adverse effects are common with dopamine receptor agonists, thus limiting the usefulness of these drugs. Adverse effects are dosage dependent and include nausea, vomiting, orthostatic hypotension, headache, dizziness, and cardiac arrhythmias. To reduce the risk of orthostatic hypotension, the initial dosage of all dopamine receptor agonists should be quite low, with incremental increases in dosage at intervals of at least 1 week. These drugs should be used with caution in persons with hypertension, cardiovascular disease, and hepatic disease. After long-term use, persons, and particularly elderly persons, may experience choreiform and dystonic movements and psychiatric disturbances, including hallucinations, delusions, confusion, depression, and mania and other behavioral changes.

Long-term use of bromocriptine and pergolide can produce retroperitoneal and pulmonary fibrosis, pleural effusions, and pleural thickening. In general, ropinirole and pramipexole have a similar but much milder adverse effect profile than levodopa, bromocriptine, and pergolide. Pramipexole and ropinirole may cause irresistible sleep attacks that occur suddenly, without warning, and have caused motor vehicle accidents. The most common adverse effects of apomorphine are nausea, orthostatic hypotension, sedation, bradycardia, syncope, perspiration, and vomiting. Apomorphine's sedative effects are exacerbated by concurrent use of alcohol or other CNS depressants. Dopamine receptor agonists are contraindicated during pregnancy and for nursing mothers especially, because they inhibit lactation.

DRUG–DRUG INTERACTIONS

Dopamine receptor antagonists are capable of reversing the effects of dopamine receptor agonists, but this is not usually clinically significant. The concurrent use of tricyclic drugs and dopamine receptor agonists has been reported to cause symptoms of neurotoxicity, such as rigidity, agitation, and tremor. They may also potentiate the hypotensive effects of diuretics and other antihypertensive medications. Dopamine receptor agonists should not be used in conjunction with monoamine oxidase inhibitors (MAOIs), including selegiline (Eldepryl), and MAOI use should be discontinued at least 2 weeks before the initiation of dopamine receptor agonist therapy.

Benzodiazepines, phenytoin (Dilantin), and pyridoxine may interfere with the therapeutic effects of dopamine receptor agonists. Ergot alkaloids and bromocriptine should not be used concurrently, as they may cause hypertension and myocardial infarction. Progestins, estrogens, and oral contraceptives may interfere with the effects of bromocriptine and may raise plasma concentrations of ropinirole. Ciprofloxacin (Cipro) can raise plasma concentrations of ropinirole, and cimetidine (Tagamet) can raise plasma concentrations of pramipexole.

LABORATORY INTERFERENCES

Levodopa administration has been associated with false reports of elevated serum and urinary uric acid concentrations, urinary glucose test results, urinary ketone test results, and urinary cat-

Table 32.3.16–1
Available Preparations of Dopamine Receptor Agonists and Carbidopa

Generic Name	Trade Name	Preparations
Bromocriptine	Parlodel	2.5-, 5-mg tablets
Carbidopa	Lodosyn	25 mg[a]
Levodopa	Larodopa	100-, 250-, 500-mg tablets
Levodopa-carbidopa (cocareldopa)	Sinemet, Atamet	100/10-, 100/25-, 250/25-mg tablets; 100/25-, 200/50-mg extended-release tablets
Pergolide	Permax	0.05-, 0.25-, and 1-mg tablets
Pramipexole	Mirapex	0.125-, 0.25-, 0.5-, 1-, 1.5-mg tablets
Ropinirole	Requip	0.25-, 0.5-, 1-, 2-, 5-mg tablets

[a]Drug only available directly through the manufacturer.

echolamine concentrations. No laboratory interferences have been associated with the administration of the other dopamine receptor agonists.

DOSAGE AND CLINICAL GUIDELINES

Table 32.3.16–1 lists the various dopamine receptor agonists and their formulations. For the treatment of antipsychotic-induced parkinsonism, the clinician should start with a 100-mg dose of levodopa three times a day, which may be increased until the person has functionally improved. The maximum dosage of levodopa is 2,000 mg a day, but most persons respond to dosages below 1,000 mg per day. The dosage of the carbidopa component of the levodopa-carbidopa formulation should total at least 75 mg a day.

The dosage of bromocriptine for mental disorders is uncertain, although it seems prudent to begin with low dosages (1.25 mg twice daily) and to increase the dosage gradually. Bromocriptine is usually taken with meals to help reduce the likelihood of nausea.

The starting dosage of pergolide is 0.05 mg daily, which can be increased by 0.1 to 0.15 mg a day every 3 days for four increments, then by 0.25 mg per day every 3 days divided into three equal daily dosages, until therapeutic benefit or adverse effects emerge. The average dosage for treatment of idiopathic Parkinson's disease is 3 mg per day, and the maximum dosage is 5 mg per day.

The starting dosage of pramipexole is 0.125 mg three times daily, which is increased to 0.25 mg three times daily in the second week and is increased by 0.25 mg per dose each week until therapeutic benefit or adverse effects emerge. Persons with idiopathic Parkinson's disease usually experience benefit at a total daily dose of 1.5 mg, and the maximum daily dose is 4.5 mg.

For ropinirole, the starting dosage is 0.25 mg three times daily and is increased by 0.25 mg per dose each week to a total daily dose of 3 mg, then by 0.5 mg per dose each week to a total daily dose of 9 mg, then by 1 mg per dose each week to a maximum dosage of 24 mg a day, until therapeutic benefit or adverse effects emerge. The average daily dose for persons with idiopathic Parkinson's disease is approximately 16 mg.

Sublingual apomorphine for treatment of erectile dysfunction has been tested in 2- and 4-mg formulations. It is taken at least 15 minutes before initiation of sexual intercourse. Clinical guidelines regarding the minimum time interval between doses are not yet available.

▲ 32.3.17 Dopamine Receptor Antagonists: Typical Antipsychotics

The dopamine receptor antagonists discussed in this section are so named because they are high-affinity antagonists of dopamine receptors. Other terms used to refer to these drugs are *typical*, *traditional*, or *conventional antipsychotics*. They are used in the treatment of schizophrenia and other psychotic disorders. The dopamine receptor antagonists include chlorpromazine (Thorazine), thioridazine (Mellaril), fluphenazine (Prolixin), and haloperidol (Haldol), among many others (Table 32.3.17–1).

A new class of antipsychotic agents, the serotonin-dopamine antagonists (SDAs), also called *newer*, *novel*, *emerging*, or *atypical antipsychotics*, has appeared, which has fewer neurological adverse effects than the dopamine receptor antagonists and is effective against a broader range of psychotic symptoms. Differentiating the two classes of antipsychotics—dopamine receptor antagonists and SDAs—is increasingly important, since they have different mechanisms of action and different clinical effects. The SDAs are covered in Section 32.3.27.

PHARMACOLOGICAL ACTIONS

Most dopamine receptor antagonists are incompletely absorbed after oral administration, although liquid preparations are absorbed more efficiently than other formulations. The half-lives of these drugs range from 10 to 20 hours, and all can be given in one daily oral dose once the person is in a stable condition and has adjusted to any adverse effects. Many drugs are also available in parenteral forms that can be given intramuscularly in emergency situations, resulting in more rapid and more reliable attainment of therapeutic plasma concentrations than is possible with oral administration. Peak plasma concentrations are usually reached 1 to 4 hours after oral administration and 30 to 60 minutes after parenteral administration.

The typical antipsychotic drugs appear to reduce psychotic symptoms by inhibiting dopamine binding to dopamine D_2 receptors. The antipsychotic effects appear to derive from inhibition of dopaminergic neurotransmission in the mesocortical dopamine projection, while the parkinsonian adverse effects result from blockade of the nigrostriatal pathway. Inhibition of the tuberoinfundibular tract is responsible for the endocrine effects of the drugs. The drugs reduce psychotic symptoms due to either a primary psychiatric disorder, such as schizophrenia, or another medical condition.

EFFECTS ON SPECIFIC ORGANS AND SYSTEMS

Most dopamine receptor antagonists have significant effects on other receptors, including adrenergic, cholinergic, and histaminergic receptors. The other receptor effects affect organs and systems

Table 32.3.17–1
Dopamine Receptor Antagonist Drugs, Trade Names, Potencies, and Dosages

Generic Name	Trade Name	Potency[a] (mg of Drug Equivalent to 100 mg Chlorpromazine)	Usual Adult Dosage Range (mg/day)	Usual Single IM Dosage (mg)
Phenothiazines				
Aliphatic				
Chlorpromazine	Thorazine	100—low	300–800	25–50
Triflupromazine	Vesprin	25–50—low	100–150	20–60
Promazine	Sparine	40—low	40–800	50–150
Piperazine				
Prochlorperazine	Compazine	15—medium	40–150	10–20
Perphenazine	Trilafon	10—medium	8–40	5–10
Trifluoperazine	Stelazine	3–5—high	6–20	1–2
Fluphenazine	Prolixin, Permitil	1.5–3—high	1–20	2–5
Acetophenazine	Tindal (no longer manufactured)	25—medium	60–120	—
Butaperazine	Repoise (not sold in U.S.)	10—medium	—	—
Carphenazine	Proketazine (not sold in U.S.)	25—medium	—	—
Piperidine				
Thioridazine[c]	Mellaril	100—low	200–700[b]	—
Mesoridazine	Serentil	50—low	75–300	25
Piperacetazine	Quide (not sold in U.S.)	10—medium	—	—
Thioxanthenes				
Chlorprothixene	Taractan (no longer manufactured)	50—low	50–400	25–50
Thiothixene	Navane	2–5—high	6–30	2–4
Dibenzoxazepine				
Loxapine	Loxitane	10–15—medium	60–100	12.5–50
Dihydroindole				
Molindone	Moban	6–10—medium	50–100	—
Butyrophenones				
Haloperidol	Haldol	2–5—high	6–20	2–6
Droperidol	Inapsine	10—medium	—	—
Diphenylbutylpiperidine				
Pimozide[c]	Orap	1—high	1–10	—

[a]Recommended adult dosages are 200 to 400 mg per day of chlorpromazine or an equivalent amount of another drug.
[b]Maximum 800 mg.
[c]Second-line drug because of cardiotoxicity.

in various ways in addition to the brain. Perhaps the most significant effects involve the heart and the vascular system. Many dopamine receptor antagonist drugs, particularly the low-potency drugs, decrease cardiac contractility, increase atrial and ventricular conduction times, and increase the length of refractory periods. The α_1-adrenergic antagonist activity can result in vasodilation and orthostatic (postural) hypotension. The major effect on the gastrointestinal system is mediated by the drug's blockade of muscarinic cholinergic receptors, which results in dry mouth and constipation, especially with clozapine (Clozaril) and the low-potency drugs. The dopamine receptor antagonist drugs as a class can have various effects on the skin (e.g., rashes, photosensitivities, and discoloring), although these effects are uncommon. A transient decrease in leukopoiesis commonly results from dopamine receptor antagonist treatment.

THERAPEUTIC INDICATIONS

Primary Psychotic Disorders

Dopamine receptor antagonists are effective in both short-term and long-term management of schizophrenia, schizophreniform

disorder, schizoaffective disorder, delusional disorder, brief psychotic disorder, manic episodes, and major depressive disorder with psychotic features. They both reduce acute symptoms and prevent future exacerbations.

Schizophrenia.   In general, the dopamine receptor antagonists are thought to be more effective in the treatment of the positive symptoms of schizophrenia (e.g., hallucinations, delusions, and agitation) than in the treatment of the negative symptoms (e.g., emotional withdrawal and ambivalence) or the cognitive dissociations. The dopamine receptor antagonists themselves may also contribute to the negative symptoms. It is also generally believed that paranoid symptoms are treated more effectively than nonparanoid symptoms and that women are more responsive than men. Some persons do not respond to any of the dopamine receptor antagonists but may show improvement with the SDAs, which also have been demonstrated to improve negative and cognitive as well as positive symptoms.

Bipolar Disorders.   Antipsychotics are often used in combination with antimanic drugs to treat psychosis or manic excitement in bipolar I disorder. The standard drugs for treatment of bipolar disorder, lithium (Eskalith), carbamazepine (Tegretol), and valproate (Depakene), generally have a slower onset of action than do antipsychotics in the treatment of the acute symptoms. The general practice is to use combination therapy at the initiation of treatment and then gradually withdraw the antipsychotics.

Persons with schizoaffective disorder and delusional disorder often respond favorably to treatment with dopamine receptor antagonists. Some persons with borderline personality disorder who have marked psychotic symptoms as part of their disorder respond at least partially to antipsychotic drugs, although these persons in particular also require psychotherapeutic treatment.

Secondary Psychoses

The dopamine receptor antagonists are generally effective in the treatment of psychotic symptoms associated with an organic cause (i.e., tumors). Agitation and psychosis associated with such neurological conditions as dementia of the Alzheimer's type also respond to antipsychotic treatment.

Severe Agitation and Violent Behavior

Dopamine receptor antagonists are used to treat persons who are severely agitated and violent, although other drugs such as benzodiazepines are also effective for the immediate control of such behavior. Symptoms such as extreme irritability, lack of impulse control, severe hostility, gross hyperactivity, and agitation respond to short-term treatment with dopamine receptor antagonists.

PRECAUTIONS AND ADVERSE REACTIONS
Nonneurological Adverse Effects

Cardiac Effects. Low-potency dopamine receptor antagonists are more cardiotoxic than high-potency dopamine receptor antagonists are. Chlorpromazine use prolongs the QT and PR intervals, blunts the T waves, and depresses the ST segment. Thioridazine use, in particular, markedly affects the T wave and is associated with malignant arrhythmias, such as torsades de pointes, perhaps explaining why overdoses of piperidine phenothiazines may be the most lethal of this group of drugs. When QT intervals exceed 0.44 ms, there is some correlation with an increased risk for sudden death, possibly secondary to ventricular tachycardia or ventricular fibrillation.

Sudden Death. The cardiac effects of dopamine receptor antagonists have been hypothesized to be related to sudden death in patients treated with the drugs. But careful evaluation of the literature indicates that it is premature to attribute the sudden deaths to dopamine receptor antagonist drugs used alone. Supporting this view is the observation that the introduction of dopamine receptor antagonists had no effect on the incidence of sudden death in patients with schizophrenia. In addition, both low-potency and high-potency drugs were involved in the reported cases. Furthermore, many reports concerned patients with other medical problems who were also treated with several other drugs. Pimozide use prolongs the QT

interval, an effect that is potentiated during concomitant administration of macrolide antibiotics, which inhibit the metabolism of pimozide by the hepatic enzyme cytochrome P450 isoenzyme 3A3/4 (CYP 3A3/4). At least two deaths have been attributed to cardiotoxicity as a result of simultaneous administration of pimozide and clarithromycin (Biaxin). The Food and Drug Administration (FDA) has therefore recently contraindicated the use of pimozide with clarithromycin, erythromycin, azithromycin (Zithromax), and dirithromycin (Dynabac).

Orthostatic (Postural) Hypotension. Orthostatic (postural) hypotension is mediated by adrenergic blockade and is most common with low-potency dopamine receptor antagonists, particularly chlorpromazine, thioridazine, chlorprothixene (Taractan), and clozapine. It occurs most frequently during the first few days of treatment, and tolerance is rapidly developed for the adverse effects. The chief dangers of orthostatic hypotension are that the patients may faint, fall, and injure themselves, although such occurrences are uncommon.

Hematological Effects. An often transient leukopenia with a white blood cell (WBC) count of approximately 3,500 is a common but not serious problem. Agranulocytosis is a life-threatening hematological problem that occurs most often with chlorpromazine use but is seen with almost all dopamine receptor antagonists. Agranulocytosis occurs most frequently during the first 3 months of treatment and with an incidence of approximately 1 in 10,000 patients treated with dopamine receptor antagonists.

Peripheral Anticholinergic Effects. Peripheral anticholinergic effects are common and consist of dry mouth and nose, blurred vision, constipation, urinary retention, and mydriasis. Some patients also have nausea and vomiting.

Endocrine Effects. Blockade of the dopamine receptors in the tuberoinfundibular tract results in the increased secretion of prolactin, which can result in breast enlargement, galactorrhea, and impotence in men and amenorrhea and inhibited orgasm in women. The SDAs, in contrast, are not particularly associated with increased prolactin levels and may be the drug of choice for patients in whom increased prolactin release results in disturbing effects. Type II diabetes has reportedly been associated with the long-term use of both typical and atypical antipsychotics.

Weight Gain. A common adverse effect of treatment with dopamine receptor antagonists is weight gain, which can be significant in some cases. Molindone (Moban) and, perhaps, loxapine (Loxitane) are not associated with the symptom and may be indicated when weight gain is a serious health hazard or a reason for noncompliance. Type II diabetes may be a product of weight gain in some patients.

Dermatological Effects. Allergic dermatitis and photosensitivity occur in a small percentage of patients, most commonly in those taking low-potency drugs, particularly chlorpromazine. A variety of skin eruptions—urticarial, maculopapular, petechial, and edematous—have also been reported. The eruptions occur early in treatment, generally in the first few weeks, and remit spontaneously.

Ophthalmological Effects. Thioridazine is associated with irreversible pigmentation of the retina when given in dosages of more than 800 mg a day. An early symptom of this effect can sometimes be nocturnal confusion related to difficulty with night vision. The pigmentation is similar to that seen in retinitis pigmentosa; it can progress even after the thioridazine is stopped and can finally result in blindness. The pigmentation is not reversible.

Jaundice. Obstructive or cholestatic jaundice is a rare adverse effect of dopamine receptor antagonist treatment. The adverse effect usually occurs in the first month of treatment and is heralded by symptoms of upper abdominal pain, nausea and vomiting, a flu-like syndrome, fever, rash, eosinophilia, bilirubin in the urine, and increased serum bilirubin, alkaline phosphatase, and hepatic transaminases. If jaundice occurs, clinicians generally discontinue the medication.

Neurological Adverse Effects

The dopamine receptor antagonist drugs, especially the typical or old ones, are associated with a number of uncomfortable extrapyramidal neurological adverse effects and several potentially serious ones. Many of the neurological adverse effects are severe enough to warrant attention as separate problems that require their own treatment plans. The recognition that the treatment-emergent adverse effects are of significant clinical importance is reflected in the text revision of the fourth edition of *Diagnostic and Statistical Manual of Mental Disorders* (DSM-IV-TR) by the inclusion of a separate group of medication-induced movement disorders (see Section 32.2). The common occurrence of uncomfortable neurological adverse effects—particularly parkinsonism, tremor, akathisia, and dystonia—prompted the search for new antipsychotic drugs that are not likely to cause medication-induced movement disorders. The SDAs are less likely than the dopamine receptor antagonist drugs to cause these movement disorders. Of the adverse effects next described, for example, only akathisia is significantly more common in patients treated with SDAs than in patients treated with placebo.

Pregnancy and Lactation

If possible, dopamine receptor antagonists should be avoided during pregnancy, particularly in the first trimester, unless the benefit outweighs the risk. In fact, however, very few data indicate a correlation between the presence of congenital malformations in infants and the use of dopamine receptor antagonists during pregnancy, except perhaps for chlorpromazine. Some data do indicate that the use of dopamine receptor antagonists during pregnancy may result in decreased dopamine receptors in the neonate, increased cholesterol, and perhaps behavioral disturbances. Nevertheless, dopamine receptor antagonist use in the second and third trimesters is probably relatively safe. High-potency dopamine receptor antagonists are preferable to low-potency drugs, as the low-potency drugs are associated with hypotension.

Haloperidol and phenothiazines pass into breast milk. Whether loxapine, molindone, and pimozide pass into breast milk is not known, although they probably do. Women who are taking dopamine receptor antagonists should not breast-feed their infants, as the available data do not prove the practice safe.

LABORATORY INTERFERENCES

Dopamine receptor antagonist drugs have been reported to interfere with some laboratory tests. Chlorpromazine and perphenazine have been reported to cause both false-positive and false-negative results in immunological pregnancy tests and falsely elevated bilirubin (with reagent test strips) and urobilinogen (with Ehrlich's reagent test) values. Dopamine receptor antagonist drugs have also been associated with an abnormal shift in results of the glucose tolerance test, although this shift may reflect the effects of the drugs on the glucose-regulating system. Phenothiazines have also been reported to interfere with the measurement of steroid metabolism.

DOSAGE AND ADMINISTRATION

Dopamine receptor antagonists may have a calming and sedating effect within 1 hour of administration, but improvement in the full range of positive psychotic symptoms usually appears within 1 to 2 weeks of onset of treatment, and a therapeutic trial in severely or chronically ill patients requires 6 weeks. Continuing improvement in symptoms is seen over the first 3 to 12 months of use. These drugs are remarkably safe in short-term use, and, if necessary, clinicians can administer the drugs without conducting a physical or laboratory examination of the patient.

Choice of Drug

Although the potencies of the dopamine receptor antagonists vary widely, all available typical dopamine receptor antagonists are equally efficacious in the treatment of schizophrenia. Data support the conclusion that SDAs may be more effective than other antipsychotic drugs for the treatment of the negative symptoms of schizophrenia. With the dopamine receptor antagonist drugs, no type of schizophrenia and no particular symptoms are most effectively treated by any single class of dopamine receptor antagonists. The SDAs have become the drugs of first choice in the treatment of schizophrenia if their possibly superior efficacies with negative symptoms and their superior safety profiles continue to be confirmed in wide clinical testing.

SDAs such as clozapine, olanzapine (Zyprexa), sertindole (Serlect), and others are less likely to raise prolactin levels than are dopamine receptor antagonists. Clozapine and olanzapine have significant anticholinergic effects, however, and may cause sedation. In the future, the dopamine receptor antagonists may be reserved for those patients who tolerate them with minimal adverse effects, for economic reasons, or for the fact that they are available in depot forms.

Short-Term Treatment. The equivalent of 5 to 10 mg of haloperidol is a reasonable dose for an adult patient in an acute state. A geriatric patient may benefit from as little as 1 mg of haloperidol. The administration of more than 50 mg of chlorpromazine in one injection may result in serious hypotension. Intramuscular (IM) administration of the dopamine receptor antagonists results in peak plasma levels in approximately 30 minutes, versus 90 minutes by the oral route. Doses of dopamine receptor antagonists for IM administration are approximately half the doses given by the oral route. In a short-term treatment setting, patients should be observed for 1 hour after the first dose of dopamine receptor antagonist medication. After that time, most clinicians administer a second dose of a dopamine receptor antagonist or a sedative agent (e.g., a benzodiazepine) to achieve effective behavioral control. Possible sedatives include lorazepam (Ativan, 2 mg IM) and amobarbital (Amytal, 50 to 250 mg IM).

Treatment Effects.   Agitation and excitement are usually the first symptoms to improve with dopamine receptor antagonist treatment. Approximately 75 percent of patients with a short history of illness have significant improvement in their psychosis. Patients with a long history of illness may need a full 6 weeks of treatment to evaluate the extent of the improvement in psychotic symptoms. Data indicate that psychotic symptoms, both positive and negative, continue to improve 3 to 12 months after the initiation of treatment.

The equivalent of 10 to 20 mg of haloperidol or 400 mg of chlorpromazine a day is adequate treatment for most patients with schizophrenia. Some research studies indicate that in a significant proportion of patients, 5 mg of haloperidol or 200 mg of chlorpromazine may, in fact, be just as effective as higher doses. It is reasonable to give dopamine receptor antagonist drugs in divided doses when initiating treatment, to minimize the peak plasma levels and to reduce the incidence of adverse effects. The total daily dose can subsequently be consolidated into a single daily dose after the first or second week of treatment. The single daily dose is usually given at bedtime to help induce sleep and to reduce the incidence of adverse effects. This practice may increase the risk of elderly patients falling if they get out of bed during the night. The sedative effects of dopamine receptor antagonists last only a few hours, in contrast to the antipsychotic effects, which last for 1 to 3 days.

Maintenance Treatment.   The first 3 to 6 months after a psychotic episode are usually considered a period of stabilization for the patient. After that time, the dosage of the dopamine receptor antagonist can be decreased approximately 20 percent every 6 months until the minimum effective dosage is found. A patient is usually maintained on antipsychotic medications for 1 to 2 years after the first psychotic episode. Antipsychotic treatment is often continued for 5 years after a second psychotic episode, and lifetime maintenance is considered after the third psychotic episode, although attempts to reduce the daily dosage can be made every 6 to 12 months.

Dopamine receptor antagonist drugs are effective in controlling psychotic symptoms, but patients may report that they prefer being off the drugs, because they feel better without them. This problem may be less common with the new antipsychotic drugs, such as clozapine, risperidone (Risperdal), and olanzapine (Zyprexa). Normal persons who have taken dopamine receptor antagonist drugs report a sense of dysphoria. Clinicians must discuss maintenance medication with the patient and take into account the patient's wishes, the severity of their illnesses, and the quality of their support systems.

Long-Acting Depot Medications.   Because some patients with schizophrenia do not comply with oral dopamine receptor antagonist regimens, long-acting depot preparations may be needed. A clinician usually administers the IM preparations once

every 1 to 4 weeks, and thus knows immediately when a patient has missed a dose of medication. Two depot preparations (a decanoate and an enanthate) of fluphenazine (Prolixin, Permitil) and a decanoate preparation of haloperidol are available in the United States. The preparations are injected IM into an area of large muscle tissue, from which they are absorbed slowly into the blood.

Treatment-Resistant Persons.   Various studies indicate that 10 to 35 percent of persons with schizophrenia fail to obtain significant benefit from the antipsychotic drugs. Persons are often defined as treatment-resistant if they have failed at least two adequate trials of antipsychotics from two pharmacological classes. Adequate trials are usually defined as at least 6 weeks of daily doses equivalent to 20 mg of haloperidol or 1,000 mg of chlorpromazine. It is useful to determine plasma concentrations for such persons, since one possibility is that they are slow metabolizers who are grossly overmedicated with a particular drug. More likely, however, they simply do not respond to the typical antipsychotic drugs. Studies have shown that up to two-thirds of nonresponders to typical antipsychotic drugs may respond to SDAs.

▲ 32.3.18 Lithium

Lithium (Eskalith, Lithobid, Lithonate) is the most commonly used short-term, long-term, and prophylactic treatment for bipolar I disorder. It is also used as an adjunctive medication in the treatment of major depressive disorder, schizoaffective disorder, therapy-resistant schizophrenia, anorexia nervosa, and bulimia nervosa and for control of chronic aggression in both children and adults.

PHARMACOLOGICAL ACTIONS

After ingestion, lithium is completely absorbed by the gastrointestinal (GI) tract. Serum levels peak in 1 to 1 1/2 hours for standard preparations and in 4 to 4 1/2 hours for controlled-release preparations. Lithium does not bind to plasma proteins, is not metabolized, and is distributed nonuniformly throughout body water. Lithium does not cross the blood–brain barrier rapidly, a fact that perhaps explains why an overdose is not usually a problem and why long-term lithium intoxication takes time to resolve completely. The half-life of lithium is approximately 20 hours, and equilibrium is reached after 5 to 7 hours of regular intake. Lithium is almost entirely eliminated by the kidneys. Because lithium is absorbed by the proximal tubules, lithium clearance is approximately one-fifth of creatinine clearance. Renal clearance of lithium decreases with renal insufficiency (common in older persons) and in the puerperium and increases during pregnancy. Lithium is excreted in breast milk and in insignificant amounts in the feces and perspiration.

The therapeutic mechanism of action for lithium remains uncertain. The similarity of the lithium ion to the sodium, potassium, calcium, and magnesium ions may be related to its therapeutic effects.

EFFECTS ON SPECIFIC ORGANS AND SYSTEMS

Lithium most commonly affects the thyroid, heart, kidneys, and hematopoietic system. Lithium impedes the release of thyroid hormones from the thyroid and can result in hypothyroidism or goiter; the disorder affects women more than men. Lithium also impairs sinus node function, which can result in heart block in susceptible persons. Lithium reduces the ability of the kidneys to concentrate urine. Although this effect is usually not clinically significant, it is not always reversible after discontinuing lithium use. Pathological nonspecific interstitial fibrosis has been reported as a postmortem finding in some persons who were treated with lithium for a long time, but this is an unusual outcome. The major effect of lithium on the hematopoietic system is a clinically nonsignificant increase in leukocyte production.

THERAPEUTIC INDICATIONS

Bipolar I Disorder

Lithium has proved effective in both the short-term treatment and the prophylaxis of bipolar I disorder in approximately 70 to 80 percent of patients. Both manic and depressive episodes respond to lithium treatment alone. Lithium should also be considered as a potential treatment for patients with severe cyclothymic disorder.

Manic Episodes. Approximately 80 percent of manic patients respond to lithium treatment, although the response to lithium alone can take 1 to 3 weeks of treatment at therapeutic concentrations. Because of the delay in response to lithium alone, benzodiazepines—for example, clonazepam (Klonopin) and lorazepam (Ativan)—or antipsychotics are used for the first 1 to 3 weeks to obtain immediate relief from the mania. Predictors of a poor response to lithium in the treatment of manic episodes include mixed and dysphoric manic episodes (which may occur in up to 40 percent of patients), rapid cycling, and coexisting substance-related disorders. Lithium is effective as long-term prophylaxis of both manic and depressive episodes in approximately 70 to 80 percent of persons with bipolar I disorder.

Depressive Episodes. Lithium is effective in the treatment of major depressive disorder and depression associated with bipolar I disorder. Because antidepressants can trigger mania in persons with bipolar disorders, lithium monotherapy is an ideal treatment for both mania and depression in persons with bipolar disorder. Lithium may also be prescribed with an antidepressant for long-term maintenance of persons with bipolar disorder. Tricyclic and tetracyclic drugs are considered more likely to trigger severe mania than are bupropion (Wellbutrin) or selective serotonin reuptake inhibitors (SSRIs). Augmentation of lithium therapy with valproate (Depakene) or carbamazepine (Tegretol) is usually well tolerated, with little risk of precipitation of mania.

Schizophrenia. The symptoms of one-fifth to one-half of all patients with schizophrenia are further reduced when lithium is coadministered with their antipsychotic drug. The therapeutic benefit of lithium does not seem to be correlated with the absence or presence of affective symptoms in these patients. Some schizophrenia patients who cannot take antipsychotic drugs may benefit from lithium treatment alone. The intermittent aggressive outbursts of some patients with schizophrenia may also be reduced by lithium treatment.

Schizoaffective Disorder and Schizophrenia

Among persons with schizoaffective disorder, those with predominant mood symptoms—either bipolar type or depressive type—are more likely to respond to lithium than those with predominant psychotic symptoms. Serotonin-dopamine antagonists (SDAs) and dopamine receptor antagonists are the treatments of choice for persons with schizoaffective disorder, whereas lithium is a useful augmentation agent, particularly for persons whose symptoms are resistant to treatment with SDAs and dopamine receptor antagonists. Lithium augmentation of SDA or dopamine receptor antagonist treatment, however, may be effective for persons with schizoaffective disorder, even in the absence of a prominent mood disorder component.

Aggression

Lithium has been used to treat aggressive outbursts in patients with schizophrenia, prison inmates, children with conduct disorder, and mentally retarded patients. Less success has been reported in the treatment of aggressiveness associated with head trauma and epilepsy. Other drugs for the treatment of aggression include anticonvulsants, β-adrenergic receptor antagonists, and antipsychotics. The treatment of aggressive patients requires a flexible approach in the use of these drugs along with psychosocial and behavioral treatment strategies.

Maintenance

Maintenance treatment with lithium markedly decreases the frequency, the severity, and the duration of manic and depressive episodes in persons with bipolar I disorder. Lithium provides relatively more effective prophylaxis for mania than for depression, and supplemental antidepressant strategies may be necessary either intermittently or continuously. Lithium maintenance is almost always indicated after the second episode of bipolar I disorder depression or mania and should be considered after the first episode for adolescents or for persons who have a family history of bipolar I disorder. Others who benefit from lithium maintenance are those who have poor support systems, had no precipitating factors for the first episode, have a high suicide risk, had a sudden onset of the first episode, or had a first episode of mania. Clinical studies have shown that lithium reduces the incidence of suicide in bipolar I disorder patients sixfold or sevenfold. Lithium is also effective treatment for persons with severe cyclothymic disorder.

Initiating maintenance therapy after the first manic episode is considered wise on the basis of several observations. First, each episode of mania increases the risk of subsequent episodes. Second, among persons responsive to lithium, relapses are 30 times more likely after lithium use is discontinued. Third, case reports describe persons who initially responded to lithium, discontinued taking it, and then had a relapse but no longer responded to lithium in subsequent episodes. Continued maintenance treatment with lithium is often associated with increasing efficacy and reduced mortality. Therefore, an episode of depression or mania that occurs after a relatively short time of lithium maintenance does not necessarily represent treatment failure. However, lithium treatment alone may begin to lose its effectiveness after several years of successful use. If this occurs, then supplemental treatment with an anticonvulsant may be useful.

Maintenance lithium dosages often can be adjusted to achieve a plasma concentration somewhat lower than that needed for treatment of acute mania. If lithium use is to be discontinued, then the dosage should be slowly tapered. Abrupt discontinuation of lithium therapy is associated with increased risk of recurrence of manic and depressive episodes.

PRECAUTIONS AND ADVERSE EFFECTS

The most common adverse effects from lithium treatment are increased thirst, polyuria, gastric distress, weight gain, tremor, fatigue, and mild cognitive impairment. Gastric distress may include nausea, vomiting, and diarrhea and can often be reduced by further dividing the dosage, administering the lithium with food, or switching among the various lithium preparations. Weight gain and edema can be impossible to treat except by encouraging the patient to eat less and to exercise moderately. The tremor affects mostly the fingers and sometimes can be worse at peak levels of the drug. It can be reduced by further dividing the dosage. Propranolol (Inderal) (30 to 120 mg a day in divided doses) reduces the tremor significantly in most patients. The fatigue and mild cognitive impairment may decrease with time. Rare neurological adverse effects include symptoms of mild parkinsonism, ataxia, and dysarthria. Patients with brain impairment are at risk of neurotoxicity. Lithium may exacerbate Parkinson's disease. Lithium should be used with caution in diabetic patients, as it may induce seizures or exacerbate a seizure disorder. Dehydrated, debilitated, and medically ill patients are susceptible to adverse effects and toxicity. Leukocytosis is a common benign effect of lithium treatment.

Gastrointestinal Effects

GI symptoms can include nausea, decreased appetite, vomiting, and diarrhea and can be diminished by dividing the dosage, administering the lithium with food, or switching to another lithium preparation. The lithium preparation least likely to cause diarrhea is lithium citrate. Some lithium preparations contain lactose, which can cause diarrhea in lactose-intolerant persons. Persons taking slow-release formulations of lithium who experience diarrhea due to unabsorbed medication in the lower part of the GI tract may experience less diarrhea with standard-release preparations. Diarrhea may also respond to antidiarrheal preparations such as loperamide (Imodium, Kaopectate), bismuth subsalicylate (Pepto-Bismol), or diphenoxylate with atropine (Lomotil). Weight gain results from a poorly understood effect of lithium on carbohydrate metabolism and can also result from lithium-induced edema.

Neurological Effects

Tremor. A lithium-induced postural tremor may occur that is usually 8 to 12 Hz and is most notable in outstretched hands, especially in the fingers, and during tasks involving fine manipulations. The tremor can be reduced by dividing the daily dosage, using a sustained-release formulation, reducing caffeine intake, reassessing the concomitant use of other medicines, and treating comorbid anxiety. β-Adrenergic receptor antagonists, such as propranolol, 30 to 120 mg a day in divided doses, and primidone (Mysoline), 50 to 250 mg a day, are usually effective in reducing the tremor. In persons with hypokalemia, potassium supplemen-

tation may improve the tremor. When a person taking lithium has a severe tremor, the possibility of lithium toxicity should be suspected and evaluated.

> After 19 years of successful lithium maintenance, a 37-year-old woman was switched to carbamazepine because of polyuria and proteinuria. Only in retrospect did she and her physicians become aware of the cognitive dulling and impaired concentration that had been present during her many years of lithium use.

Cognitive Effects. Lithium use has been associated with dysphoria, lack of spontaneity, slowed reaction times, and impaired memory. The presence of these symptoms should be noted carefully, because they are a frequent cause of noncompliance. The differential diagnosis for such symptoms should include depressive disorders, hypothyroidism, hypercalcemia, other illnesses, and other drugs. Some, but not all, persons have reported that fatigue and mild cognitive impairment decrease with time.

Other Neurological Effects. Uncommon neurological adverse effects include symptoms of mild parkinsonism, ataxia, and dysarthria, although the last two symptoms may also be due to lithium intoxication. Lithium is (rarely) associated with development of peripheral neuropathy, benign intracranial hypertension (pseudotumor cerebri), findings resembling myasthenia gravis, and increased risk of seizures.

Renal Effects

The most common adverse renal effect of lithium is polyuria with secondary polydipsia. The symptom is a particular problem in 25 to 35 percent of persons taking lithium, who may have a urine output of more than 3 L a day (normal, 1 to 2 L a day). The polyuria primarily results from lithium antagonism to the effects of antidiuretic hormone, which thus causes diuresis. When polyuria is a significant problem, the person's renal function should be evaluated and followed up with 24-hour urine collections for creatinine clearance determinations. Treatment consists of fluid replacement, the use of the lowest effective dosage of lithium, and single daily dosing of lithium.

The most serious renal adverse effects, which are rare and associated with continuous lithium administration for 10 years or more, involve appearance of nonspecific interstitial fibrosis, associated with a gradual decrease in glomerular filtration rate, increased serum creatinine concentrations, and (rarely) renal failure. Lithium occasionally is associated with nephrotic syndrome and features of distal renal tubular acidosis. It is prudent to check the serum creatinine concentration, urine chemistries, and 24-hour urine volume of persons taking lithium annually.

> A 55-year-old man, successfully stabilized on lithium for 22 years, experienced a gradual increase in serum creatinine to 2.4 mg/dL (normal range, 0.6 to 1.3 mg/dL). A thorough evaluation by a nephrologist produced no another explanation, and lithium was felt to be the most likely cause.

Thyroid Effects

Lithium affects thyroid function, causing a generally benign and often transient diminution in the concentrations of circulating thyroid hormones. Reports have attributed goiter (5 percent of persons), benign reversible exophthalmos, hyperthyroidism, and hypothyroidism (7 to 10 percent of persons) to lithium treatment. Lithium-induced hypothyroidism is more common in women (14 percent) than in men (4.5 percent). Women are at highest risk during the first 2 years of treatment. Persons taking lithium to treat bipolar disorder are twice as likely to develop hypothyroidism if they develop rapid cycling. Approximately 50 percent of persons receiving long-term lithium treatment have laboratory abnormalities, such as an abnormal thyrotropin-releasing hormone (TRH) response, and approximately 30 percent have elevated concentrations of thyroid-stimulating hormone (TSH). If symptoms of hypothyroidism are present, replacement with levothyroxine (Synthroid) is indicated. Even in the absence of hypothyroid symptoms, some clinicians treat persons with significantly elevated TSH concentrations with levothyroxine. In lithium-treated persons, TSH concentrations should be measured every 6 to 12 months. Lithium-induced hypothyroidism should be considered when evaluating depressive episodes that emerge during lithium therapy.

Cardiac Effects

The cardiac effects of lithium, which resemble those of hypokalemia on the electrocardiogram (ECG), are caused by the displacement of intracellular potassium by the lithium ion. The most common changes on the ECG are T wave flattening or inversion. The changes are benign and disappear after the lithium is excreted from the body. Nevertheless, baseline ECGs are essential and should be repeated annually.

Because lithium also depresses the pacemaking activity of the sinus node, lithium treatment can result in sinus dysrhythmias, heart block, and episodes of syncope. Lithium treatment, therefore, is contraindicated in persons with sick sinus syndrome. In rare cases, ventricular arrhythmias and congestive heart failure have been associated with lithium therapy. Lithium cardiotoxicity is more prevalent in persons on a low-salt diet, those taking certain diuretics or angiotensin-converting enzyme inhibitors, and those with fluid-electrolyte imbalances or any renal insufficiency.

Dermatological Effects

Several cutaneous adverse effects, which may be dose dependent, have been associated with lithium treatment. The most prevalent effects include acneiform, follicular, and maculopapular eruptions; pretibial ulcerations; and worsening of psoriasis. Alopecia has also been reported. Many of those conditions respond favorably to changing to another lithium preparation and taking the usual dermatological measures. Lithium concentrations should be monitored if tetracycline is used for the treatment of acne, because it can increase the retention of lithium. Occasionally, aggravated psoriasis or acneiform eruptions may force the discontinuation of lithium treatment.

Lithium Toxicity and Overdoses

The early signs and symptoms of lithium toxicity include neurological symptoms, such as coarse tremor, dysarthria, and ataxia; GI symptoms; cardiovascular changes; and renal dysfunction.

The later signs and symptoms include impaired consciousness, muscular fasciculations, myoclonus, seizures, and coma. Risk factors include exceeding the recommended dosage; reduced excretion due to renal impairment, a low-sodium diet, or drug interaction; and dehydration. Elderly persons are more vulnerable to the effects of increased serum lithium concentrations. The higher the lithium concentration and the longer the lithium concentration has been high, the worse are the symptoms of lithium toxicity. Lithium toxicity is a medical emergency, since it can result in permanent neuronal damage and death.

The treatment of lithium toxicity involves discontinuing the lithium and treating the dehydration. Unabsorbed lithium can be removed from the GI tract by ingestion of polystyrene sulfonate (Kayexalate) or polyethylene glycol solution (GoLYTELY) but not activated charcoal. Ingestion of a single large dose may create clumps of medication in the stomach, which can be removed by gastric lavage with a wide-bore tube. The value of forced diuresis is still debated. In the most serious cases, hemodialysis is the most effective means of rapid removal of excessive amounts of serum lithium. Postdialysis serum lithium concentrations may rise as lithium is redistributed from tissues to blood, and repeat dialysis may be needed. Neurological improvement may lag behind clearance of serum lithium by several days, because lithium crosses the blood–brain barrier slowly.

Adolescents

The serum lithium concentration for adolescents is similar to that for adults. Although the adverse-effect profile is similar in adolescents and adults, weight gain and acne associated with lithium use can be particularly troublesome to an adolescent.

Elderly Persons

Lithium is a safe and effective drug for the elderly. However, the treatment of elderly persons taking lithium may be complicated by the presence of other medical illnesses, decreased renal function, special diets that affect lithium clearance, and generally increased sensitivity to lithium. Elderly persons should initially be given low dosages, their dosages should be switched less frequently than those of younger persons, and a longer time must be allowed for renal excretion to equilibrate with absorption before lithium can be assumed to have reached its steady-state concentrations.

In general, the elderly should be started on lower-than-usual dosages, with dosage changes occurring less frequently than in younger patients. The elimination half-life of lithium increases with age, and the time required to reach steady state is much longer in the elderly. If lithium use is stopped, levels fall more slowly and the resolution of adverse effects and toxicity may be prolonged.

A 60-year-old man was treated with 900 mg a day of lithium carbonate. The dosage was continued unchanged for 10 years, despite laboratory evidence of gradually increasing serum lithium and creatinine concentrations. Even as the clinical symptoms of toxicity were being reported, a thiazide diuretic was added to treat hypertension. Three weeks later, the patient was hospitalized with a serum lithium concentration of 4.2 mEq/L and marked neurological impairment that never fully resolved.

Pregnant Women

Lithium should not be administered to pregnant women in the first trimester because of the risk of birth defects. The most common malformations involve the cardiovascular system, most commonly Ebstein's anomaly of the tricuspid valves. The risk of Ebstein's malformation in lithium-exposed fetuses is 1 in 1,000, which is 20 times the risk in the general population. The possibility of fetal cardiac anomalies can be evaluated with fetal echocardiography. The teratogenic risk of lithium (4 to 12 percent) is higher than that for the general population (2 to 3 percent) but appears to be lower than that associated with use of valproate or carbamazepine. A woman who continues to take lithium during pregnancy should use the lowest effective dosage. The maternal lithium concentration must be monitored closely during pregnancy and especially after pregnancy, because of the significant decrease in renal lithium excretion in the first few days after delivery. Adequate hydration can reduce the risk of lithium toxicity during labor. Lithium prophylaxis is recommended for all women with bipolar disorder as they enter the postpartum period. Lithium is excreted into breast milk and should be taken by a nursing mother only after careful evaluation of potential risks and benefits. Signs of lithium toxicity in infants include lethargy, cyanosis, abnormal reflexes, and sometimes hepatomegaly.

Miscellaneous Effects

Lithium should be used with caution in diabetic persons, who should monitor their blood glucose concentrations carefully to avoid diabetic ketoacidosis. Benign, reversible leukocytosis is commonly associated with lithium treatment. Dehydrated, debilitated, and medically ill persons are most susceptible to adverse effects and toxicity.

DRUG–DRUG INTERACTIONS

Lithium has been used successfully with dopamine receptor antagonists for many years. However, coadministration of higher dosages of dopamine receptor antagonists and lithium may result in a synergistic increase in the symptoms of lithium-induced neurological adverse effects. This interaction may occur with use of any dopamine receptor antagonist.

Coadministration of lithium and anticonvulsants—including carbamazepine, valproate, and clonazepam—may increase lithium concentrations and aggravate lithium-induced neurological adverse effects. Used wisely, however, the coadministration of lithium and anticonvulsants can benefit some persons therapeutically. Treatment with the combination should be initiated at slightly lower dosages than usual, and dosages should be increased gradually. Changes from one treatment for mania to another should be made carefully, with as little temporal overlap between the drugs as possible.

Most diuretics (e.g., thiazide and potassium sparing) can increase lithium concentrations; when treatment with such a diuretic is stopped, the clinician may need to increase the person's daily lithium dose. Osmotic and loop diuretics, carbonic anhydrase inhibitors, and xanthines (including caffeine) may reduce lithium concentrations below therapeutic concentrations. Angiotensin-converting enzyme inhibitors may cause an increase in lithium concentrations, whereas the AT_1 angiotensin II receptor inhibitors losartan (Cozaar) and irbesartan (Avapro) do not alter lithium concentrations. A wide range of nonsteroidal antiinflammatory drugs can decrease lithium clearance, thereby increasing lithium concentrations. These drugs include indomethacin (Indocin), phenylbutazone (Azolid), diclofenac (Voltaren), ketoprofen (Orudis), oxyphenbutazone (Oxalid), ibuprofen (Motrin, Advil, Nuprin), piroxicam (Feldene), and naproxen (Naprosyn). Aspirin and sulindac (Clinoril) do not affect lithium concentrations.

Coadministration of lithium and quetiapine (Seroquel) may cause somnolence but is otherwise well tolerated. Coadministration of lithium and ziprasidone (Geodon) may modestly increase the incidence of tremor. Coadministration of lithium and calcium channel inhibitors should be avoided because of potentially fatal neurotoxicity.

A person taking lithium who is about to undergo ECT should discontinue taking lithium 2 days before beginning ECT, to reduce the risk of delirium resulting from the coadministration of these two treatments.

LABORATORY INTERFERENCES

Lithium is not known to interfere with any laboratory tests. However, lithium treatment does affect a number of commonly obtained laboratory values.

DOSAGE AND CLINICAL GUIDELINES

Initial Medical Workup

Before a clinician administers lithium, the patient should have a routine laboratory workup and physical examination. The laboratory tests should include serum creatinine concentration (or a 24-hour urine creatinine if the clinician has any reason to be concerned about renal function), electrolytes, thyroid function (TSH, triiodothyronine [T_3], and thyroxine [T_4]), a complete blood count (CBC), ECG, and a pregnancy test in women of child-bearing age.

If a person has previously been treated with lithium and the previous dosage is known, then the same dosage should be used for the current episode unless changes in the person's pharmacokinetic parameters have affected lithium clearance. The starting dosage for most adults is 300 mg of the regular-release formulation three times daily. The starting dosage for elderly persons or persons with renal impairment should be 300 mg once or twice daily. An eventual dosage between 900 and 1,200 mg a day usually produces a therapeutic plasma concentration of 0.6 to 1 mEq/L, and a daily dose of 1,200 to 1,800 mg usually produces a therapeutic concentration of 0.8 to 1.2 mEq/L. Maintenance dosing can be given either in two or three divided doses of the regular-release formulation or in a single dose of the sustained-release formulation equivalent to the combined daily dose of the regular-release formulation. The use of divided doses reduces gastric upset and avoids single high-peak lithium concentrations. No data show a difference in clinical efficacy between the regular- and sustained-release formulations.

Serum and Plasma Concentrations

Serum and plasma concentrations of lithium are the standard methods of assessing lithium concentrations, and they serve as the basis for titrating the dosages. Lithium concentrations should be determined routinely every 2 to 6 months and promptly in persons suspected to be noncompliant with the prescribed dosages, in persons who exhibit signs of toxicity, and during dosage adjustments. Although reports have noted the measurement of lithium concentrations in saliva, tears, and red blood cells, these methods have no clinical superiority to analysis of serum or plasma.

The most common guidelines are 1.0 to 1.5 mEq/L for the treatment of acute mania and 0.4 to 0.8 mEq/L for maintenance treatment. Biological variations in regulation of mood and in lithium metabolism bolster the universal maxim "treat the patient, not the laboratory results." A small number of persons will not achieve therapeutic benefit with a lithium concentration of 1.5 mEq/L yet will have no signs of toxicity. For such persons, titration of the lithium dosage to achieve a concentration above 1.5 mEq/L may be warranted. If there is no response after 2 weeks at a concentration that is beginning to cause adverse effects, then the person should taper off lithium use over 1 to 2 weeks and should try other mood-stabilizing drugs. Other therapeutic options include carbamazepine, valproate, other anticonvulsants, thyroid hormones, ECT, calcium channel inhibitors, monoamine oxidase inhibitors (MAOIs), dopamine receptor antagonists, and SDAs.

Discontinuation

Lithium use is discontinued if it is ineffective or not tolerated. Patients may stop the drug for other reasons, such as a perceived or real loss in creativity, feeling cured, or a dislike for feeling controlled by a medicine. After a period of stability with maintenance therapy, a trial off lithium may be considered, although the risk of recurrence is considerable (especially if there have been several prior episodes), and there have been reports of failure to respond to lithium when treatment is reinstituted. Discontinuation should be gradual over many weeks, because more abrupt discontinuation appears to be associated with a higher likelihood of early recurrence of mania or depression. Teaching patients and significant others to recognize early signs of recurrence is an important part of the discontinuation process.

Patient Education

Persons taking lithium should be advised that changes in the body's water and salt content can affect the amount of lithium excreted, resulting in either increased or decreased lithium concentrations. Excessive sodium intake (e.g., a dramatic dietary change) lowers lithium concentrations. Conversely, too little sodium (e.g., fad diets) can lead to potentially toxic concentrations of lithium. Decreases in body fluid (e.g., excessive perspiration) can lead to dehydration and lithium intoxication.

▲ 32.3.19 Mirtazapine

Mirtazapine (Remeron) is an effective medication used to treat depression. It lacks the annoying anticholinergic effects of the tricyclic antidepressants.

PHARMACOLOGICAL ACTIONS

Mirtazapine is rapidly and completely absorbed from the gastrointestinal (GI) tract. Peak concentration is achieved within 2 hours of ingestion. Plasma clearance may be slowed up to 30 percent in persons with impaired hepatic function and up to 50 percent in those with impaired renal function. Clearance may be up to 40 percent slower in elderly males and up to 10 percent slower in elderly females. The mean elimination half-life is 20 to 40 hours, and steady-state levels are achieved within approximately 5 days. A clinical response may require 2 to 4 weeks.

Mirtazapine acts as an antagonist of central presynaptic α_2-adrenergic receptors within the central nervous system (CNS), where it has a net effect of increasing synaptic levels of noradrenaline and serotonin. It is a potent antagonist of serotonin 5-HT$_2$ and 5-HT$_3$ receptors but has little effect on 5-HT$_1$ receptors. This appears to bias the activation of serotonin receptors in favor of the 5-HT$_1$ family, whose activation is thought to reduce anxiety and depression. Mirtazapine is a potent antagonist of histamine H$_1$ receptors and is a moderately potent antagonist at α_1-adrenergic and muscarinic-cholinergic receptors.

EFFECTS ON SPECIFIC ORGANS AND SYSTEMS

Mirtazapine exerts most of its effects in the CNS, and the principal non-CNS effects are in the GI system (e.g., weight gain, increased appetite).

THERAPEUTIC INDICATIONS

Mirtazapine is effective for the treatment of depression. It is highly sedating, in the same range as amitriptyline (Elavil, Endep), clomipramine (Anafranil), and trazodone (Desyrel), and is thus useful for treatment of sleep disturbances. However, some of the sedating effects generally lessen within the first week of treatment. In direct comparison, it causes somewhat less somnolence, weight gain, and constipation than amitriptyline and less headache and nausea than fluoxetine (Prozac). It also appears to reduce somatic and psychological symptoms of anxiety and agitation.

PRECAUTIONS AND ADVERSE REACTIONS

The most common adverse effect of mirtazapine is somnolence, which may occur in more than 50 percent of persons. Therefore, when persons start to take mirtazapine, they should exercise caution when driving or operating dangerous machinery. This adverse effect may be minimized by giving the dose before sleep. Mirtazapine also causes dizziness in 7 percent of persons. It does not appear to increase the risk for seizures. Mania or hypomania occurred in 0.2 percent of persons in clinical trials, a rate similar to that of other antidepressant drugs. Mirtazapine potentiates the sedative effects of alcohol.

Mirtazapine increases appetite in approximately 15 percent of patients. Mirtazapine may also increase serum cholesterol concentration to 20 percent or more above the upper limit of normal in 15 percent of persons and increase triglycerides to 500 mg/dL or more in 6 percent of persons. Elevations of alanine transaminase (ALT) levels to more than three times the upper limit of normal were seen in 2 percent of mirtazapine-treated persons, as opposed to 0.3 percent of placebo controls.

A small number of persons experience orthostatic hypotension while taking mirtazapine. Although no human data exist regarding effects on fetal development, mirtazapine should be used with caution during pregnancy. Because the drug may be excreted in breast milk, it should not be taken by nursing mothers. There may be a risk of agranulocytosis associated with mirtazapine use; thus, persons should be attuned to signs of infection. Because of the sedating effects of mirtazapine, persons should determine the degree to which they are affected before driving or engaging in other potentially dangerous activities. Other potentially sedating prescription or over-the-counter drugs and alcohol should be avoided during use of mirtazapine.

DRUG–DRUG INTERACTIONS

Mirtazapine can potentiate the sedation of alcohol and benzodiazepines. Mirtazapine should not be used within 14 days of a monoamine oxidase inhibitor (MAOI).

LABORATORY INTERFERENCES

No laboratory interferences have been described for mirtazapine.

DOSAGE AND ADMINISTRATION

Mirtazapine is available in 15-, 30-, and 45-mg scored tablets. If persons fail to respond to an initial dose of mirtazapine of 15 mg before sleep, the dose may be increased in 15-mg increments every 5 days to a maximum of 45 mg before sleep. Lower dosages may be necessary in elderly persons or those with renal or hepatic insufficiency.

▲ 32.3.20 Monoamine Oxidase Inhibitors

The monoamine oxidase (MAO) inhibitors (MAOIs) are highly effective antidepressants and anxiolytics, but they are used less frequently than other antidepressants because of the dietary precautions that must be followed to avoid tyramine-induced hypertensive crises. MAOIs increase biogenic amine neurotransmitter levels by inhibiting their degradation. The degradation of the biogenic amines—serotonin, norepinephrine, and dopamine—occurs by only two mechanisms. The more important pathway involves the presynaptic reuptake of these neurotransmitters through specific transporter molecules, followed by deamination in mitochondria by the enzyme MAO. MAOIs, however, are generally considered equal in efficacy to other antidepressant drugs. The transporters may be inhibited, for example, by the tricyclic antidepressants and the selective serotonin reuptake inhibitors (SSRIs), which form the mainstay of current antidepressant drugs.

The currently available MAOIs include phenelzine (Nardil), isocarboxazid (Marplan), tranylcypromine (Parnate), and selegiline (Eldepryl). Selegiline is a selective inhibitor of type B MAO (MAO_B) used for the treatment of parkinsonism. A newer class of reversible inhibitors of MAO_A (RIMAs), not available

in the United States (e.g., moclobemide [Aurorix, Manerix] and befloxatone), requires few dietary restrictions. Some clinicians believe that MAOIs are underused as effective antidepressant treatment.

PHARMACOLOGICAL ACTIONS

Phenelzine, tranylcypromine, and isocarboxazid are readily absorbed through the gastrointestinal (GI) tract and reach peak plasma concentrations within 2 hours. Their plasma half-lives are in the range of 2 to 3 hours; tissue half-lives are considerably longer. Because they irreversibly inactivate MAOs, the therapeutic effect of a single dose of irreversible MAOIs may persist for as long as 2 weeks. The RIMA moclobemide is rapidly absorbed and has a half-life of 0.5 to 3.5 hours. Because it is a reversible inhibitor, moclobemide has a much briefer clinical effect after a single dose than irreversible MAOIs have.

MAO is an enzyme found intracellularly on the outer mitochondrial membrane, which degrades cytoplasmic monoamines, including norepinephrine, serotonin, dopamine, epinephrine, and tyramine. There are two types of MAOs: MAO_A and MAO_B. MAO_A primarily metabolizes norepinephrine, serotonin, and epinephrine; dopamine and tyramine are metabolized by both MAO_A and MAO_B. MAOIs act in the central nervous system (CNS), the sympathetic nervous system, the liver, and the GI tract. At dosages above 60 mg per day, tranylcypromine may inhibit the reuptake or increase the release of dopamine and norepinephrine and, to a lesser extent, serotonin.

When GI metabolism of dietary tyramine by MAOs is inactivated by an irreversible MAOI, intact tyramine can enter the circulation and exert a potent pressor effect, resulting in a hypertensive crisis. Tyramine-containing foods must therefore be avoided for 2 weeks after the last dose of an irreversible MAOI to permit resynthesis of adequate concentrations of MAOs. In contrast, RIMAs have relatively little inhibitory activity for MAO_B, and because they are reversible, normal activity of existing MAO_A returns within 16 to 48 hours of the last dose of a RIMA. Therefore, the dietary restrictions are less stringent for RIMAs, applying only to foods containing high concentrations of tyramine, which need be avoided for only 3 days after the last dose of a RIMA.

EFFECTS ON SPECIFIC ORGANS AND SYSTEMS

The primary effects of the MAOIs in psychiatry are on the CNS. In addition to their effects on depressed mood, the MAOIs are associated with potentially clinically significant disturbances in sleep and sleep architecture. MAOI use is frequently associated with decreased sleep and insomnia and sometimes results in daytime drowsiness. Furthermore, the sleep of MAOI-treated patients is characterized by significantly less rapid eye movement (REM) sleep. RIMAs lack an effect on, or may improve, sleep.

The other principal concerns when treating patients with MAOIs are the cardiovascular system and the liver. MAOIs are commonly associated with hypotension because of their effects on vascular tone, which may be mediated both centrally and peripherally. In rare cases, MAOI use alone (without tyramine) is associated with episodes of acute hypertension. With regard to the liver, phenelzine and isocarboxazid are associated with a significant liability for hepatotoxicity.

THERAPEUTIC INDICATIONS

The indications for MAOIs are similar to those for tricyclic and tetracyclic drugs. MAOIs may be particularly effective in panic disorder with agoraphobia, posttraumatic stress disorder, eating disorders, social phobia, and pain disorder. Some investigators have reported that MAOIs may be preferable to tricyclic drugs in the treatment of atypical depression characterized by hypersomnia, hyperphagia, anxiety, and the absence of vegetative symptoms. Patients with this symptom pattern are often less severely depressed than patients with classic symptoms of depression, which is often evidenced by less functional impairment. The failure of a patient to improve after treatment with an SSRI and a tricyclic or tetracyclic drug may be the most common reason that a patient is given a therapeutic trial of an MAOI.

Although depression is not an approved indication for selegiline, some positive results have been reported. A possible advantage of selegiline is that its primary effect in low dosages is on MAO_B; thus, the risk of an MAO_A-associated, tyramine-induced hypertensive crisis is lessened. Unfortunately, many of the positive results with selegiline for depression have been at higher dosages (20 to 60 mg a day) than the dosages used to treat Parkinson's disease (10 mg a day). At these higher dosages, selegiline loses a significant amount of its specificity for MAO_B and requires that patients follow the guidelines for a restricted tyramine diet.

PRECAUTIONS AND ADVERSE REACTIONS

The most frequent adverse effects of MAOIs are orthostatic hypotension, insomnia, weight gain, edema, and sexual dysfunction. The initial appearance of signs of orthostatic hypotension in the course of a cautious upward tapering of the dosage determines the maximum tolerable dosage. Treatment for orthostatic hypotension includes avoidance of caffeine, intake of 2 L of fluid per day, addition of dietary salt or adjustment of antihypertensive drugs (if applicable), support stockings, and in severe cases, treatment with fludrocortisone (Florinef), a mineralocorticoid, 0.1 to 0.2 mg a day. Orthostatic hypotension associated with tranylcypromine use can usually be relieved by dividing the daily dose.

A rare adverse effect of MAOIs, most commonly of tranylcypromine, is a spontaneous, non–tyramine-induced hypertensive crisis occurring shortly after the first exposure to the drug. Persons experiencing such a crisis should avoid MAOIs altogether. Insomnia and behavioral activation can be treated by dividing the dose, not giving the medication after dinner, and using trazodone (Desyrel) or a benzodiazepine hypnotic if necessary. Weight gain, edema, and sexual dysfunction often do not respond to any treatment and may warrant switching to another agent. When switching from one MAOI to another, the clinician should taper and stop use of the first drug for 10 to 14 days before beginning use of the second drug.

Paresthesias, myoclonus, and muscle pains are occasionally seen in persons treated with MAOIs. Paresthesias may be secondary to MAOI-induced pyridoxine deficiency, which may respond to supplementation with pyridoxine, 50 to 150 mg orally each day. Occasionally, persons complain of feeling drunk or confused, perhaps indicating that the dosage should be

reduced and then increased gradually. Reports that the hydrazine MAOIs are associated with hepatotoxic effects are relatively uncommon. MAOIs are less cardiotoxic and less epileptogenic than the tricyclic and tetracyclic drugs.

The most common adverse effects of the RIMA moclobemide are dizziness, nausea, and insomnia or sleep disturbance. RIMAs cause fewer GI adverse effects than SSRIs. Moclobemide does not have adverse anticholinergic or cardiovascular effects, and it has not been reported to interfere with sexual function.

MAOIs should be used with caution by persons with renal disease, cardiovascular disease, or hyperthyroidism. MAOIs may alter the dosage of a hypoglycemic agent required by diabetic persons. MAOIs have been particularly associated with inducing mania in persons in the depressed phase of bipolar I disorder and triggering psychotic decompensation in persons with schizophrenia. MAOIs are contraindicated during pregnancy, although data on their teratogenic risk are minimal. MAOIs should not be taken by nursing women because the drugs can pass into the breast milk.

Tyramine-Induced Hypertensive Crisis

Foods rich in tyramine (Table 32.3.20–1) or other sympathomimetic amines should be avoided by persons who are taking irreversible MAOIs to avoid significant risk of potentially life-threatening hypertension. Persons should be warned about the

Table 32.3.20–1
Tyramine-Rich Foods to Be Avoided in Planning MAOI Diets

High tyramine content[a] (≥2 mg of tyramine a serving)
  Cheese: English Stilton; blue cheese; white (3 years old); extra old; old cheddar; Danish blue; mozzarella; cheese snack spreads
  Fish, cured meats, sausage; pates and organs; salami; mortadella; air-dried sausage
  Alcoholic beverages[b]: Liqueurs and concentrated after-dinner drinks
  Marmite (concentrated yeast extract)
  Sauerkraut (Krakus)

Moderate tyramine content[a] (0.5–1.99 mg of tyramine a serving)
  Cheese: Swiss Gruyere; Muenster; feta; parmesan; gorgonzola; blue cheese dressing; Black Diamond
  Fish, cured meats, sausage, pates, and organs: Chicken liver (5 days old); bologna; aged sausage; smoked meat; salmon mousse
  Alcoholic beverages: Beer and ale (12 oz per bottle)—Amstel, Export Draft, Blue Light, Guinness Extra Stout, Old Vienna, Canadian, Miller Light, Export, Heineken, Blue Wines (per 4 oz glass)—Rioja (red wine)

Low tyramine content[b] (0.01 ta >0.49 mg of tyramine a serving)
  Cheese: Brie, Camembert, Cambozola with or without rind
  Fish, cured meat, sausage, organs, and pates: Pickled herring; smoked fish; kielbasa sausage; chicken livers, liverwurst (<2 days old)
  Alcoholic beverages: red wines; sherry; scotch[c]
  Others: Banana or avocado (ripe or not); banana peel

[a]Any food left out to age or spoil can spontaneously develop tyramine through fermentation.
[b]Alcohol can produce profound orthostasis interacting with MAOIs, but cannot produce direct hypertensive reactions.
[c]White wines, gin, and vodka have no tyramine content.
Table by Jonathan M. Himmelhoch, M.D.

Table 32.3.20–2
Available Preparations and Typical Dosages of MAOIs

Generic Name	Trade Name	Preparations	Usual Daily Dose (mg)	Usual Maximum Daily Dose (mg)
Isocarboxazid[a]	Marplan	10-mg tablets	20–40	60
Moclobemide[b]	Manerix	100-, 150-mg tablets	300–600	600
Phenelzine	Nardil	15-mg tablets	30–60	90
Selegiline	Eldepryl, Atapryl	5-mg capsules, 5-mg tablets	10	30
Tranylcypromine	Parnate	10-mg tablets	20–60	60

[a]Available directly from the manufacturer.
[b]Not available in the United States.

dangers of ingesting tyramine-rich foods while taking MAOIs, and they should be advised to continue the dietary restrictions for 2 weeks after they stop MAOI treatment, to allow the body to resynthesize the enzyme. Patients should also be warned that bee stings may cause a hypertensive crisis. The prodromal signs and symptoms of a hypertensive crisis may include headache, stiff neck, sweating, nausea, and vomiting. If these signs and symptoms occur, the patient should seek immediate medical treatment. An MAOI-induced hypertensive crisis should be treated with α-adrenergic antagonists—for example, phentolamine (Regitine) or chlorpromazine (Thorazine)—which lower blood pressure within 5 minutes. A diuretic to reduce fluid load and a β-adrenergic receptor antagonist to control tachycardia may also be necessary. Acute lowering of blood pressure with use of nifedipine (Procardia) is not recommended, because a person who mistakes a headache resulting from the rebound of MAOI-induced orthostatic hypotension for a hypertensive crisis–related headache and therefore takes nifedipine runs a high risk of causing signs and symptoms of hypotensive shock. MAOIs should not be used by persons with thyrotoxicosis or pheochromocytoma. The risk of tyramine-induced hypertensive crises is relatively low for persons who are taking RIMAs, such as moclobemide and befloxatone. A reasonable dietary recommendation for persons taking RIMAs is not to eat tyramine-containing foods for a period from 1 hour before to 2 hours after taking a RIMA.

Withdrawal

Persons taking regular doses of MAOIs who cease administration abruptly may experience a self-limited discontinuation syndrome consisting of arousal, mood disturbances, and somatic symptoms. To avoid these symptoms when discontinuing use of an MAOI, dosages should be gradually tapered over several weeks.

DRUG–DRUG INTERACTIONS

The inhibition of MAO can cause severe and even fatal interactions with various other drugs. In particular, because MAOIs serve to increase intrasynaptic concentrations of biogenic amine neurotransmitters, they should never be administered simultaneously with drugs with a similar effect on these neurotransmitters. This includes most antidepressants as well as precursor agents. Persons should be instructed to tell any other physicians or dentists who are treating them that they are taking

an MAOI. MAOIs may potentiate the action of CNS depressants, including alcohol and barbiturates. MAOIs should not be coadministered with serotonergic drugs such as SSRIs and clomipramine (Anafranil) because this combination can trigger a serotonin syndrome. The initial symptoms of a serotonin syndrome can include tremor, hypertonicity, myoclonus, and autonomic signs, which can then progress to hallucinosis, hyperthermia, and even death. Fatal reactions have occurred when MAOIs were combined with meperidine (Demerol) or fentanyl (Sublimaze).

As mentioned, when switching from an irreversible MAOI to any other type of antidepressant drug, persons should wait at least 14 days after the last dose of the MAOI before beginning use of the next drug, to allow replenishment of the body's MAOs. When switching from an antidepressant to an irreversible MAOI, persons should wait 10 to 14 days (or 5 weeks for fluoxetine [Prozac]) before starting use of the MAOI, to avoid drug–drug interactions. In contrast, MAO activity recovers completely 24 to 48 hours after the last dose of a RIMA.

Cimetidine (Tagamet) and fluoxetine significantly reduce the elimination of moclobemide. Modest doses of fluoxetine and moclobemide administered concurrently may be well tolerated, with no significant pharmacodynamic or pharmacokinetic interactions.

LABORATORY INTERFERENCES

The MAOIs are associated with lowering blood glucose concentrations, which are accurately reflected by laboratory analysis. MAOIs artificially raise urinary metanephrine concentrations and may cause a false-positive test result for pheochromocytoma or neuroblastoma. MAOIs have been reported to be associated with a minimal false elevation in thyroid function test results.

DOSAGE AND CLINICAL GUIDELINES

Table 32.3.20–2 lists MAOI preparations and typical dosages. There is no definitive rationale for choosing one of the currently available irreversible MAOIs over another, although some clinicians recommend tranylcypromine because of its activating qualities, possibly associated with a fast onset of action, and its low hepatotoxic potential. Elderly persons may be more sensitive to MAOI adverse effects than younger adults. MAO activity increases with age, so MAOI dosages for elderly persons are the same as those required for younger adults. The use of MAOIs in children has had minimal study.

▲ 32.3.21 Nefazodone

Nefazodone (Serzone) has antidepressant and antianxiety effects. It is structurally related to trazodone (Desyrel) and unrelated to the classic tricyclic and tetracyclic drugs, the monoamine oxidase inhibitors (MAOIs), selective serotonin reuptake inhibitors (SSRIs), and other available antidepressant drugs. Although trazodone is distinctive in having more marked sedative effects than most other antidepressants, nefazodone is relatively free of this adverse effect and generally well tolerated. Nefazodone is less likely than the SSRIs to adversely affect sexual functioning.

PHARMACOLOGICAL ACTIONS

Nefazodone is rapidly and completely absorbed but is then extensively metabolized, so the bioavailability of active compounds is approximately 20 percent of the oral dose. Its half-life is 2 to 4 hours. Steady-state concentrations of nefazodone and its principal active metabolite, hydroxynefazodone, are achieved within 4 to 5 days. Metabolism of nefazodone in the elderly, especially women, is approximately half that seen in younger persons, so that lowered doses are recommended for elderly persons. An important metabolite of nefazodone is methchlorophenylpiperazine (mCPP), which has some serotonergic effects and may cause migraine, anxiety, and weight loss.

Nefazodone is an inhibitor of serotonin uptake and, more weakly, of norepinephrine reuptake. Its antagonism of type 2A serotonin 5-HT$_{2A}$ receptors is thought to lessen anxiety and depression. By both inhibiting serotonin reuptake, which raises synaptic serotonin concentrations, and blocking 5-HT$_{2A}$ receptors, nefazodone may selectively activate 5-HT$_{1A}$ receptors, which gives additional antidepressant and anxiolytic effects. Nefazodone is a mild antagonist of the α_1-adrenergic receptors, which predisposes some persons to orthostatic hypotension but is not sufficiently potent to produce priapism. There is no significant direct activity at α_2- and β-adrenergic, 5-HT$_{1A}$, cholinergic, opioid, dopaminergic, or benzodiazepine receptors.

EFFECTS ON SPECIFIC ORGANS AND SYSTEMS

The main effects of nefazodone are on the central nervous system (CNS). The main extra-CNS effects are related to α_1-adrenergic antagonism, which may cause orthostatic hypotension. Unlike its structural relative trazodone, nefazodone has not been reported to cause priapism. There have been reports of liver failure in some patients taking nefazodone, prompting warnings about this risk factor.

Cardiovascular Effects

In premarketing trials, 5.1 percent of patients taking nefazodone experienced a significant drop in blood pressure, compared with 2.5 percent of patients receiving placebo. Although there was no increase in true syncopal events, symptoms of postural hypotension were experienced by 2.8 percent of patients treated with nefazodone. This rate compares with postural hypotension in 0.8 percent of placebo-treated, 1.1 percent of SSRI-treated, and 10.8 percent of tricyclic antidepressant–

treated patients. Sinus bradycardia was seen in 1.5 percent of nefazodone-treated patients and 0.4 percent of placebo-treated patients. Nefazodone should thus be used with caution in patients with underlying cardiac conditions, history of stroke or heart attack, dehydration, and hypovolemia and in patients under treatment with antihypertensive medications.

Activation of Mania

In patients with known bipolar illness, 1.6 percent of those treated with nefazodone experienced mania, compared with 5.1 percent of tricyclic-treated patients and 0 percent of placebo-treated patients. The activation of mania in unipolar illness patients was no higher with nefazodone than with placebo. Therefore, nefazodone may be a drug to try earlier in the treatment of patients with a history of manic episodes. Electroconvulsive therapy (ECT) and the antidepressant lithium (Eskalith) are least likely to activate mania.

THERAPEUTIC INDICATIONS

Nefazodone has been approved for the treatment of depression on the basis of data from several large clinical trials. Nefazodone has been shown to be as efficacious as imipramine (Tofranil), fluoxetine (Prozac), and paroxetine (Paxil) for treatment of moderate, severe, melancholic, nonmelancholic, chronic, and recurrent depression. Clinical reports indicate that nefazodone is also an effective treatment for depression accompanied by anxiety, such as panic disorder and panic with comorbid depression or depressive symptoms, for obsessive-compulsive disorder, for premenstrual dysphoric disorder, and for the management of chronic pain of neuropathic or nonneuropathic origin. Nefazodone also may help reduce obsessive thoughts in obsessive-compulsive disorders; however, one case report documents the initial appearance of obsessive thoughts during nefazodone treatment, which ceased when the drug was discontinued. More data are needed to establish whether nefazodone is as effective for obsessive-compulsive disorder as the SSRIs and clomipramine.

PRECAUTIONS AND ADVERSE REACTIONS

The most common adverse reactions to nefazodone use are nausea, dizziness, insomnia, weakness, and agitation. Patients with any degree of liver function impairment should not take nefazodone.

Cardiovascular Effects

Some patients taking nefazodone may experience a drop in blood pressure that can cause episodes of postural hypotension. Nefazodone should therefore be used with caution by persons with underlying cardiac conditions, history of stroke or heart attack, dehydration, or hypovolemia or by persons being treated with antihypertensive medications.

Activation of Mania

Some 1.6 percent of persons with known bipolar disorder treated with nefazodone experienced mania, compared with 5.1 percent of tricyclic-treated persons. The activation of mania in persons with unipolar depression was no higher with nefazodone than with placebo. Nonetheless, nefazodone, like other antidepressant medications, should be used with caution in persons with a history of manic episodes.

Other Precautions

The effects of nefazodone in human mothers are not yet as well understood as those of the SSRIs. Nefazodone should thus be used during pregnancy only if the potential benefit to the mother outweighs the potential risks to the fetus. It is not known whether nefazodone is excreted in human breast milk. Therefore, it should be used with caution by lactating mothers. As mentioned above, because of the risk of liver failure, nefazodone should not be used in persons with hepatic disease, but no adjustment is necessary for persons with renal disease.

DRUG–DRUG INTERACTIONS

Nefazodone should not be given concomitantly with MAOIs. In addition, nefazodone has particular drug–drug interactions with the triazolobenzodiazepines triazolam (Halcion) and alprazolam (Xanax) because of the inhibition of cytochrome P450 isoenzyme 3A4 (CYP 3A4) by nefazodone. Potentially elevated levels of each of these drugs can develop after administration of nefazodone, whereas the levels of nefazodone are generally not affected. The manufacturer recommends lowering the dose of triazolam by 75 percent and the dose of alprazolam by 50 percent when given concomitantly with nefazodone.

Nefazodone may slow the metabolism of digoxin (Lanoxin); therefore, digoxin levels should be monitored carefully in persons taking both medications. Nefazodone also slows the metabolism of haloperidol (Haldol), so that the dosage of haloperidol should be reduced in persons taking both medications. Addition of nefazodone may also exacerbate the adverse effects of lithium.

LABORATORY INTERFERENCES

There are no known laboratory interferences associated with nefazodone.

DOSAGE AND CLINICAL GUIDELINES

Nefazodone is available in 50-, 200-, and 250-mg unscored tablets and 100- and 150-mg scored tablets. The recommended starting dosage of nefazodone is 100 mg twice a day, but 50 mg twice a day may be better tolerated, especially by elderly persons. To limit the development of adverse effects, the dosage should be slowly tapered up in increments of 100 to 200 mg a day at intervals of no less than 1 week per increase. The optimal dosage is 300 to 600 mg daily in two divided doses. However, some studies report that nefazodone is effective when taken once a day, especially at bedtime. Geriatric persons should receive dosages approximately two-thirds of the usual nongeriatric dosages, with a maximum of 400 mg a day. In common with other antidepressants, clinical benefit of nefazodone usually appears after 2 to 4 weeks of treatment. Patients with premenstrual syndrome are treated with a flexible dosage that averages approximately 250 mg a day.

▲ 32.3.22 Opioid Receptor Agonists: Methadone, Levomethadyl, and Buprenorphine

Opioid receptor agonists are used in psychiatry for detoxification from heroin and other opioids and in maintenance opioid detoxification programs. Maintenance therapy is used in addicted patients who are unable to remain abstinent from opioids. Persons who switch from use of heroin to one of these drugs continue to satisfy their acute physical craving for opioids but are gradually weaned from their crippling psychological dependence on heroin. The drugs in this class include methadone (Dolophine), buprenorphine (Buprenex), and levomethadyl acetate (ORLAAM), also called L-α-acetylmethadol or LAAM. The most clinical experience is available for methadone; levomethadyl and buprenorphine are relatively new and are still being evaluated in various clinical and research settings.

PHARMACOLOGICAL ACTIONS

Methadone, levomethadyl, and buprenorphine are absorbed rapidly from the gastrointestinal (GI) tract. Hepatic first-pass metabolism significantly affects the bioavailability of each of the drugs but in markedly different ways. For methadone, hepatic enzymes reduce the bioavailability of an oral dosage by approximately half, an effect that is easily managed with dosage adjustments. For levomethadyl, hepatic enzymes metabolize an oral dosage into normethyl-LAAM and dinormethyl-LAAM, which are actually several times more potent μ-opioid receptor agonists than levomethadyl itself. For buprenorphine, in contrast, first-pass intestinal and hepatic metabolism eliminates oral bioavailability almost completely; thus, for use in opioid detoxification, buprenorphine is given sublingually, in either a liquid or a tablet formulation.

The peak plasma concentrations of oral methadone are reached within 2 to 6 hours, and the plasma half-life initially is 4 to 6 hours in opioid-naive persons and 24 to 36 hours after steady dosing of any type of opioid. Methadone is highly protein bound and equilibrates widely throughout the body, which ensures little postdosage variation in steady-state plasma concentrations. The peak plasma concentrations of oral levomethadyl are reached within 1.5 to 2 hours, and the plasma half-lives of levomethadyl and its active metabolites range from 2 to 4 days. Elimination of a sublingual dosage of buprenorphine occurs in two phases, an initial phase with a half-life of 3 to 5 hours and a terminal phase with a half-life of more than 24 hours. Buprenorphine dissociates from its receptor binding site slowly, which permits an every-other-day dosing schedule.

EFFECTS ON ORGANS AND SYSTEMS

The relative safety of long-term methadone maintenance has been established through prospective and retrospective studies. No evidence of methadone toxicity for organ systems has been found during three decades of widespread clinical use. Less information is available regarding the long-term safety of levomethadyl acetate or buprenorphine. Levomethadyl acetate prolongs the QT interval in some patients, so patients entering methadone maintenance programs need careful monitoring, since many suffer from a number of chronic diseases, including (most commonly) human immunodeficiency virus (HIV) infection, hepatitis, tuberculosis, other infectious diseases, and cardiac or renal disorders. Methadone maintenance is associated with improved health and decreased risk of HIV transmission, largely as a result of reducing drug use and facilitating appropriate use of medical services.

THERAPEUTIC INDICATIONS

Methadone

Methadone is used for short-term detoxification (7 to 30 days), long-term detoxification (up to 180 days), and maintenance (treatment beyond 180 days) of opioid-dependent individuals. For these purposes, it is only available through designated clinics called *methadone maintenance treatment programs* (MMTPs) and in hospitals and prisons. Methadone is a Schedule II drug, which means that its administration is tightly governed by specific federal laws and regulations.

Enrollment in a methadone program reduces the risk of death by 70 percent; reduces illicit use of opioids and other substances of abuse; reduces criminal activity; reduces the risk of infectious diseases of all types, most importantly HIV and hepatitis B and C infection; and, in pregnant women, reduces the risk of fetal and neonatal morbidity and mortality. The use of methadone maintenance frequently requires lifelong treatment.

Some opioid-dependence treatment programs use a stepwise detoxification protocol in which a person addicted to heroin switches first to the strong agonist methadone, then to the weaker agonist buprenorphine, and finally to maintenance on an opioid receptor antagonist, such as naltrexone (ReVia). This approach minimizes the appearance of opioid withdrawal effects, which, if they occur, are mitigated with clonidine (Catapres). However, compliance with opioid receptor antagonist treatment is poor outside settings using intensive cognitive-behavioral techniques. In contrast, noncompliance with methadone maintenance precipitates opioid withdrawal symptoms, which serve to reinforce use of methadone and make cognitive-behavioral therapy less than essential. Thus, some well-motivated, socially integrated former heroin addicts are able to use methadone for years without participation in a psychosocial support program.

Data pooled from many reports indicate that methadone is more effective when taken at dosages in excess of 60 mg a day. The analgesic effects of methadone are sometimes used in the management of chronic pain when less addictive agents are ineffective.

Pregnancy. Methadone maintenance, combined with effective psychosocial services and regular obstetrical monitoring, significantly improves obstetrical and neonatal outcomes for women addicted to heroin. Enrollment of a heroin-addicted pregnant woman in such a maintenance program reduces the risk of malnutrition, infection, preterm labor, spontaneous abortion, preeclampsia, eclampsia, abruptio placenta, and septic thrombophlebitis.

The dosage of methadone during pregnancy should be the lowest effective dosage, and no withdrawal to abstinence should be attempted during pregnancy. Methadone is metabolized more rapidly in the third trimester, which may necessitate higher dosages. To avoid potentially sedating postdose peak plasma concentrations, the daily dose can be administered in two divided doses during the third trimester. Methadone treatment has no known teratogenic effects.

Neonatal Methadone Withdrawal Symptoms. Withdrawal symptoms in newborns frequently include tremor, high-pitched cry, increased muscle tone and activity, poor sleep and eating, mottling, yawning, perspiration, and skin excoriation. Convulsions that require aggressive anticonvulsant therapy may also occur. Withdrawal symptoms may be delayed in onset and prolonged in neonates because of their immature hepatic metabolism. Women taking methadone are sometimes counseled to initiate breast-feeding as a means of gently weaning their infants from methadone dependence, but they should not breast-feed their babies while still taking methadone.

Levomethadyl

Levomethadyl is used only for maintenance treatment of opioid-dependent patients. It is not used for detoxification treatment or for analgesia. Thrice-weekly levomethadyl dosing, consisting of 100 mg on Monday, 100 mg on Wednesday, and 140 mg on Friday, is more effective for opioid maintenance than smaller doses. Daily dosing of levomethadyl may cause overdosage.

Buprenorphine

Buprenorphine is an analgesic approved only for treatment of moderate to severe pain. Buprenorphine at a dosage of 8 to 16 mg a day appears to reduce heroin use. Buprenorphine also is effective in thrice-weekly dosing because of its slow dissociation from opioid receptors. The analgesic effects of buprenorphine are sometimes used in the management of chronic pain when less addictive agents are ineffective. There are some reports of depressed patients responding to buprenorphine when other agents have failed.

PRECAUTIONS AND ADVERSE REACTIONS

The most common adverse effects of opioid receptor agonists are lightheadedness, dizziness, sedation, nausea, constipation, vomiting, perspiration, weight gain, decreased libido, inhibition of orgasm, and insomnia or sleep irregularities. Opioid receptor agonists can induce tolerance and can produce physiological and psychological dependence. Other central nervous system (CNS) adverse effects include dizziness, depression, sedation, euphoria, dysphoria, agitation, and seizures. Delirium and insomnia have also been reported in rare cases. Occasional non-CNS adverse effects include peripheral edema, urinary retention, rash, arthralgia, dry mouth, anorexia, biliary tract spasm, bradycardia, hypotension, hypoventilation, syncope, antidiuretic hormone–like activity, pruritus, urticaria, and visual disturbances. Menstrual irregularities are common in women, especially in the first 6 months of use. Various abnormal endo-

tions seen in psychiatric practice. Like valproate (Depakene) and carbamazepine (Tegretol), they represent possible alternatives or adjuncts for the treatment of bipolar disorders, anxiety disorders, agitation, pain, and substance abuse.

The newer antiepileptic agents are structurally diverse and have multiple central nervous system (CNS) effects. They differ in metabolism, drug interactions, and adverse effects. The clinical significance of the neurochemical mechanisms associated with these drugs is not fully understood. None of them has an identical combination of neurochemical actions.

Two congeners of gabapentin—tiagabine (Gabatril) and pregabalin have been developed for use in generalized anxiety disorder and have been shown to be effective in some cases.

PHARMACOLOGICAL ACTIONS

Gabapentin

Gabapentin is absorbed by the neutral amino acid membrane transporter system in the gut, and it crosses the blood–brain barrier. Bioavailability of 300- or 600-mg doses is 60 percent, whereas bioavailability of a 1,600-mg dose is 35 percent. Because higher amounts are not absorbed, doses should not exceed 1,800 mg per single dose or 5,400 mg a day. Food has no effect on gabapentin absorption, and it does not bind to plasma proteins. The steady-state half-life of 5 to 9 hours is reached in 2 days if thrice-daily dosing is used. Gabapentin is not metabolized and is excreted unchanged in the urine.

Lamotrigine

Lamotrigine is completely absorbed, and its steady-state plasma half-life is 25 hours. However, the rate of lamotrigine's metabolism varies over a sixfold range, depending on which other drugs are administered concomitantly. Dosing is escalated slowly to twice-a-day maintenance dosing. Food does not affect its absorption, and it is 55 percent protein bound in the plasma; 94 percent of lamotrigine and its inactive metabolites is excreted in the urine. Lamotrigine has an anticonvulsant profile similar to that of carbamazepine and phenytoin (Dilantin). Lamotrigine inhibits dihydrofolate reductase, the enzyme responsible for generation of folic acid, which is necessary for proper fetal development. Lamotrigine increases plasma serotonin concentrations modestly and is a weak inhibitor of serotonin 5-HT$_3$ receptors.

Topiramate

Topiramate is rapidly and completely absorbed, and its steady-state half-life is 21 hours. Food does not affect its absorption. It is 15 percent protein bound in the plasma, and 70 percent of an oral dose of topiramate is excreted unchanged in the urine, together with small amounts of several inactive metabolites. Topiramate is an inhibitor of state-dependent sodium channels. It potentiates the action of γ-aminobutyric acid (GABA) at a nonbenzodiazepine-, nonbarbiturate-sensitive GABA$_A$ receptor.

Tiagabine and Pregabalin

The pharmacological actions are poorly understood. They are congeners of gabapentin and presumably have similar pharma-

codynamics. No withdrawal syndromes have been reported with either drug.

THERAPEUTIC INDICATIONS

Gabapentin, lamotrigine, and topiramate are indicated by the Food and Drug Administration (FDA) in the treatment of seizure disorders. Gabapentin is also widely used to treat chronic pain, particularly that of polyneuropathy. Many prescriptions for these drugs are written for the nonepileptic indications listed below.

Bipolar Disorder

Each of these drugs has been used as monotherapy and adjunctive medication for treatment-refractory persons with bipolar disorders, including bipolar I, bipolar II, cyclothymic disorder, and bipolar disorder not otherwise specified. Except for lamotrigine, they are most effective when used as adjunctive therapy rather than when used alone.

Chronic Pain

Gabapentin is effective for treatment of postherpetic neuralgia and painful diabetic neuropathy, and lamotrigine has been shown to be effective for treatment of human immunodeficiency virus (HIV)–associated peripheral neuropathy and reduction of postoperative analgesic use. Other conditions responsive to gabapentin and lamotrigine include trigeminal neuralgia; central pain syndromes; compression neuropathies, such as carpal tunnel syndrome, radiculopathies, and meralgia paresthetica; and painful neuropathies due to other causes. The pain-reduction response for these conditions is similar to that with selective serotonin reuptake inhibitors (SSRIs) and tricyclic antidepressants and superior to that with intravenous (IV) and topical lidocaine (Xylocaine), carbamazepine, topical aspirin, mexiletine (Mexitil), phenytoin, topical capsaicin (Double Cap Cream), oral nonsteroidal anti-inflammatory drugs (NSAIDs), opioids, propranolol (Inderal), lorazepam (Ativan), and phentolamine (Regitine). Because of their distinct mechanisms of action and absence of interactions, gabapentin and antidepressants are often used in combination for treatment of neuropathic pain.

Other Indications

Gabapentin appears to reduce the frequency and intensity of explosive outbursts in persons with dyscontrol disorders, including children, persons with dementia, and persons with traumatic brain injury. It is also an effective treatment for social phobia and panic disorder in some persons. Because of its mildly sedating properties, gabapentin can treat insomnia and agitation due to withdrawal from benzodiazepines, alcohol, and cocaine. Gabapentin is also an effective treatment for tremor and parkinsonism. Tiagabine and pregabalin have been shown to reduce anxiety in generalized anxiety disorder in some cases.

Lamotrigine has antipsychotic effects in persons with epilepsy. This is important for those comorbid for epilepsy and psychosis, because many antipsychotic medications lower the seizure threshold. Lamotrigine may reduce intrusive and avoidance or numbing symptoms of posttraumatic stress disorder.

Topiramate can markedly reduce appetite and may have other metabolic properties. It is being used as a treatment for obesity, binge eating, and migraine prophylaxis.

PRECAUTIONS AND ADVERSE REACTIONS

Gabapentin

Gabapentin is well tolerated, and the dosage can be escalated to the maintenance range within 2 to 3 days. There are almost no dose-related adverse effects, even at doses of 5 g per day, which far exceeds the absorptive capacity of the intestines. The most frequent adverse effects of gabapentin, like other antiepileptic drugs, are somnolence, dizziness, ataxia, fatigue, and nystagmus, which are usually transient.

Lamotrigine

The most common adverse effects associated with use of lamotrigine, especially when used in combination with other antiepileptic drugs for the treatment of epilepsy, are dizziness, ataxia, somnolence, headache, diplopia, blurred vision, nausea, vomiting, and rash. Lamotrigine accumulates in melanin-rich tissues including the pigmented retina. The long-term effect on vision is unknown.

Skin Conditions. Lamotrigine is significantly associated with development of potentially life-threatening skin conditions, such as toxic epidermal necrolysis and Stevens-Johnson syndrome, in 0.1 percent of adults and 1 to 2 percent of children. These are more likely to appear if the starting dosage is too high, if the dosage is escalated too rapidly, or during concomitant administration of valproic acid. Most cases appear after 2 to 8 weeks of therapy, but cases have been reported in the absence of any of the above risk factors. The character of the rash is not a clue to the severity of the condition. Thus, lamotrigine use should be discontinued immediately upon development of any rash or other sign of hypersensitivity reaction. This may not prevent subsequent development of life-threatening rash or permanent disfiguration.

Topiramate

The most common non–dose-related adverse effects of topiramate used in combination with other antiepileptic drugs include psychomotor slowing, speech and language problems (especially word-finding difficulties), somnolence, dizziness, ataxia, nystagmus, and paresthesias. The most common dose-related adverse effects are fatigue, nervousness, poor concentration, confusion, depression, anorexia, visual problems, mood problems, weight loss, and tremor. Some 1.5 percent of persons taking topiramate develop renal calculi, a rate ten times that associated with placebo. Patients at risk for calculi should be encouraged to drink plenty of fluids. There is also a black box warning about glaucoma with topiramate. Doctors should report changes in visual acuity or eye pain.

DRUG–DRUG INTERACTIONS

Gabapentin

Gabapentin has no significant hepatic cytochrome P450 or pharmacodynamic interactions. Antacids containing aluminum hydroxide and magnesium hydroxide (Maalox) decrease gabapentin absorption by 20 percent if administered concurrently but negligibly if administered 2 hours prior to the dose of gabapentin. Tiagabine and pregabalin require further study.

Lamotrigine

Lamotrigine has significant, well-characterized drug interactions involving other anticonvulsants. Lamotrigine decreases the plasma concentration of valproic acid by 25 percent; may increase the concentration of the epoxide metabolite of carbamazepine; and may increase the incidence of carbamazepine-induced dizziness, diplopia, ataxia, and blurred vision. It has no effect on phenytoin concentrations. Lamotrigine concentrations are decreased 40 to 50 percent with concomitant administration of carbamazepine, phenytoin, or phenobarbital, whereas lamotrigine concentration is at least doubled with concurrent administration of valproic acid. Sertraline (Zoloft) also increases plasma lamotrigine concentrations, but to a lesser extent than valproic acid does. Combinations of lamotrigine and other anticonvulsants have complex effects on the time of peak plasma concentration and the plasma half-life of lamotrigine.

Topiramate

Topiramate has a few well-characterized drug interactions with other anticonvulsant drugs. Topiramate may increase phenytoin concentrations up to 25 percent and valproic acid concentrations, 11 percent; it does not affect the concentrations of carbamazepine or its epoxide, phenobarbital (Luminal) or primidone (Mysoline). Topiramate concentrations are decreased by 40 to 48 percent with concomitant administration of carbamazepine or phenytoin and by 14 percent with concurrent administration of valproic acid. Topiramate also slightly decreases digoxin (Lanoxin) bioavailability and the efficacy of estrogenic oral contraceptives. Addition of topiramate, a weak inhibitor of carbonic anhydrase, to other inhibitors of carbonic anhydrase, such as acetazolamide (Diamox) or dichlorphenamide (Daranide), may promote development of renal calculi and should be avoided.

LABORATORY INTERFERENCES

Gabapentin can cause false-positive readings with the Ames N-Multistix SG dipstick test for urinary protein. Lamotrigine and topiramate do not interfere with any laboratory tests.

DOSAGE AND CLINICAL GUIDELINES

Gabapentin

Gabapentin is available as 100-, 300-, and 400-mg capsules and as 600- and 800-mg tablets. The starting dose of gabapentin is 300 mg three times a day, and the dose can be rapidly titrated to a maximum of 1,800 mg three times a day over a period of a few days. Efficacy is broadly dose dependent, and most persons achieve satisfactory benefit within the range of 600 to 900 mg three times a day. Rapid advancement of the dosage and high doses are limited by sedation, which is usually mild. Although abrupt discontinuation of gabapentin does not cause withdrawal effects, use of all anticonvulsant drugs should be gradually tapered. Tiagabine is prescribed at 4 mg per day to 56 mg per day (the latter dosage use in epilepsy). Pregabalin is used in dosages up to 450 mg per day. Both drugs require future study for use in psychiatric disorders.

Lamotrigine

Lamotrigine is available as unscored 25-, 100-, 150-, and 200-mg tablets. The major determinant of lamotrigine dosing is minimization of the risk of rash. Lamotrigine should not be taken by anyone under the age of 16 years. Because valproic acid markedly slows the elimination of lamotrigine, concomitant administration of these two drugs necessitates a much slower titration. Persons with renal insufficiency should aim for a lower maintenance dosage. Appearance of any type of rash necessitates immediate discontinuation of lamotrigine use. Lamotrigine should usually be discontinued gradually, over 2 weeks, unless a rash emerges, in which case it should be discontinued over 1 to 2 days.

Topiramate

Topiramate is available as unscored 25-, 100-, and 200-mg tablets. To reduce the risk of adverse cognitive and sedating effects, topiramate dosage is titrated gradually over 8 weeks to a maximum of 200 mg twice a day. Higher doses are not associated with increased efficacy. Persons with renal insufficiency should reduce doses by half.

▲ 32.3.25 Reboxetine

Reboxetine (Vestra) is an effective antidepressant of a novel pharmacological class that selectively inhibits norepinephrine reuptake but has little effect on serotonin reuptake. It is thus the pharmacodynamic mirror image of the selective serotonin reuptake inhibitors (SSRIs), which inhibit the reuptake of serotonin but not of norepinephrine. Reboxetine is used in Europe but is not marketed in the United States.

PHARMACOLOGICAL ACTIONS

Reboxetine is rapidly absorbed and reaches peak plasma concentrations in 2 hours. Food does not affect the rate of absorption. The half-life is 13 hours, which permits twice-daily dosing. Steady-state concentrations are achieved in 5 days. Reboxetine is extensively metabolized in the liver (primarily via the cytochrome P450 3A4 isoenzyme [CYP 3A4]) and mostly excreted in the urine.

Reboxetine has a low affinity for muscarinic or cholinergic receptors and does not interact with α_1-, α_2-, or β-adrenergic; serotonergic; dopaminergic; or histaminic receptors.

THERAPEUTIC INDICATIONS

Reboxetine is effective for treatment of acute and chronic depressive disorders, such as major depression and dysthymia. Reboxetine is as effective as imipramine (Tofranil) and may be more effective than fluoxetine (Prozac) for treatment of persons with severe (melancholic) depression. Reboxetine promotes sleep but is not associated with daytime somnolence. Patients show improved energy, interest, and concentration and decreased anxiety. Reboxetine can also produce relatively rapid improvement in symptoms of social phobia. Social impairments, particularly those revolving around negative self-percep-

tion and a low level of social activity, appear to respond positively to reboxetine.

PRECAUTIONS AND ADVERSE REACTIONS

Reboxetine is overall as well tolerated as SSRIs. The most common adverse effects are urinary hesitancy, headache, constipation, nasal congestion, perspiration, dizziness, dry mouth, decreased libido, and insomnia. Urinary hesitancy may respond to augmentation with doxazosin (Cardura). Hypertension and tachycardia may be of clinical relevance, especially at higher doses. Reboxetine is less likely than SSRIs to cause anxiety or nausea or to inhibit sexual functioning.

Reboxetine should not be taken by women who are pregnant or breast-feeding.

DRUG–DRUG INTERACTIONS

Reboxetine has few significant drug interactions and does not inhibit hepatic metabolic enzymes.

LABORATORY INTERFERENCE

Reboxetine is not known to interfere with any clinical laboratory tests.

DOSAGE AND CLINICAL GUIDELINES

Reboxetine is available in 4-mg scored tablets. The usual starting dosage is 4 mg twice a day. Most patients do not require an increase in dosage; however, if needed, the dosage may be increased to a total of 10 mg a day in two divided doses after 3 weeks. In elderly persons and persons with severe renal impairment, therapy may be initiated at 2 mg twice a day and increased to a maximum of 6 mg a day in two divided doses after 3 weeks.

▲ 32.3.26 Selective Serotonin Reuptake Inhibitors

Selective serotonin reuptake inhibitors (SSRIs) are first-line agents for treatment of depression, obsessive-compulsive disorder (OCD), and panic disorder, as well as many other disorders. Currently, six SSRIs are available: (1) fluoxetine (Prozac), which was introduced in 1988; (2) sertraline (Zoloft); (3) paroxetine (Paxil); (4) fluvoxamine (Luvox); (5) citalopram (Celexa); and (6) escitalopram (Lexapro), a congener of citalopram.

Although depressive disorders were the initial indications for these drugs, they are effective in a wide range of disorders, including eating disorders, panic disorder, OCD, and borderline personality disorder. These drugs are called SSRIs because they share the pharmacodynamic property of specifically inhibiting serotonin reuptake by presynaptic neurons, with relatively little effect on the reuptake of norepinephrine and almost no effect on the reuptake of dopamine.

Clomipramine (Anafranil) is another serotonin-specific drug sometimes considered in the same category as SSRIs. However, because its structure and adverse effect profile are more similar to those of the tricyclic antidepressant drugs, it is discussed with the tricyclic and tetracyclic drugs (see Section 32.3.30).

PHARMACOLOGICAL ACTIONS

The major differences among the available SSRIs lie primarily in their pharmacokinetic profiles, specifically their half-lives. Fluoxetine has the longest half-life, 2 to 3 days; its active metabolite has a half-life of 7 to 9 days. The half-lives of the other SSRIs are much shorter, approximately 20 to 25 hours, and these SSRIs have no major active metabolites. All SSRIs are well absorbed after oral administration and reach their peak concentrations in 4 to 8 hours. All SSRIs are metabolized in the liver mainly by cytochrome P450 (CYP) isoenzyme CYP 2D6, a specific subtype of the enzyme, which may indicate that clinicians should be careful in the coadministration of other drugs that are also metabolized by CYP 2D6. In general, food does not have a large effect on the absorption of SSRIs; in fact, administration of SSRIs with food often reduces the incidence of the nausea and diarrhea commonly associated with SSRI use.

SSRIs have specific activity in the inhibition of serotonin reuptake without effects on norepinephrine and dopamine reuptake. Clinical efficacy is associated with 70 to 80 percent occupancy of the serotonin transporters. Inhibition of reuptake raises synaptic concentrations of serotonin.

At least 90 percent of clinical response to the SSRIs occurs at the starting doses, and higher doses tend mainly to increase adverse effects, without much additional clinical benefit. In clinical use, sertraline is most commonly raised above its usual starting dosage (50 mg a day, raised to 150 to 200 mg a day), followed by fluoxetine (starting dosage 20 mg a day, raised to 40 to 80 mg a day). The others are most likely to be continued at their starting dosages (20 mg a day). Although the available compounds differ in their specific potencies, the differences do not result in any meaningful clinical differences.

SSRIs have very mild anticholinergic effects in some patients, usually minimal and far less than the tricyclic and tetracyclic drugs.

THERAPEUTIC INDICATIONS

Depression

Fluoxetine, sertraline, paroxetine, escitalopram, and citalopram are indicated for treatment of depression. SSRIs are first-line agents for depression in the general population, the elderly, the medically ill, and those who are pregnant. SSRIs are as effective as any other class of antidepressants for mild and moderate depression. For severe depression and melancholia, several studies have found that the efficacy of serotonin-norepinephrine reuptake inhibitors, such as venlafaxine (Effexor), mirtazapine (Remeron), or tricyclic drugs, often exceeds that of SSRIs. However, sertraline may be more effective than the other SSRIs for treatment of severe depression with melancholia. It is appropriate to initiate antidepressant therapy with SSRIs for all degrees of depression.

Direct comparison of the benefits of specific SSRIs has not shown any one to be generally superior to the others. However, a given individual can exhibit considerable diversity in response to the various SSRIs. More than 50 percent of persons who respond poorly to one SSRI will respond favorably to another. Thus, before shifting to non-SSRI antidepressants, one should try other agents in the SSRI class for persons who did not respond to the first SSRI.

Studies have shown that SSRIs have a similar efficacy but markedly more favorable adverse effect profile than the tricyclic antidepressants. These studies have also shown that some nervousness or agitation, sleep disturbances, gastrointestinal (GI) symptoms, and sexual adverse effects are more common in SSRI-treated patients than in tricyclic-treated patients.

Augmentation Strategies.   In depressed persons with a partial response to an SSRI, augmentation strategies have generally not proved superior to simply increasing the SSRI dosage. However, one such drug combination, an SSRI plus bupropion (Wellbutrin), has marked added benefits. The noradrenergic and dopaminergic actions of bupropion dovetail nicely with the serotonergic actions of the SSRIs and pose a low risk of pharmacodynamic interactions. Bupropion has the additional advantage of tending to counteract the antiorgasmic adverse effects of SSRIs. Some evidence indicates that lithium (Eskalith), levothyroxine (Synthroid), sympathomimetics, pindolol (Visken), or olanzapine (Zyprexa) and risperidone (Risperdal) can also augment the antidepressant effects of SSRIs.

Suicide.   When first introduced, a widely publicized report suggested an association between fluoxetine use and violent acts, including suicide, but many subsequent reviews have clearly refuted this association. A few patients, however, become especially anxious and agitated when given fluoxetine. The appearance of these symptoms in suicidal persons could conceivably aggravate the seriousness of the suicidal ideation. In addition, suicidal persons may attempt to act out their suicidal thoughts more effectively as they rise out of their depression. Thus, potentially suicidal persons should be closely monitored during the first few weeks they are taking SSRIs.

Depression during Pregnancy and Postpartum. Many studies, including one that followed children into their early school years, have failed to find any perinatal complications, congenital fetal anomalies, decreases in global intelligence quotient (IQ), language delays, or specific behavioral problems attributable to the use of SSRIs during pregnancy.

Prospective studies have found that the risk of relapse into depression when a newly pregnant mother is taken off SSRI use is severalfold higher than the risk to the fetus of exposure to SSRIs. Since maternal depression is an independent risk factor for fetal morbidity, the clinician may want to continue the SSRI without interruption during pregnancy. SSRIs may produce a self-limited neonatal withdrawal syndrome that consists of jitteriness and mild tachypnea; it begins several hours after birth and may persist for days to a few weeks. The syndrome is rare and does not interfere with feeding.

Postpartum depression (with or without psychotic features) affects a small percentage of mothers. Some clinicians start administering SSRIs if the postpartum blues extend beyond a few weeks or if a woman becomes depressed during pregnancy. The head start afforded by starting SSRI administration during pregnancy if a woman is at risk for postpartum depression also protects the newborn, toward whom the woman may have harmful thoughts after parturition.

Whether or not SSRIs appear in the plasma of babies breast-feeding from mothers who are taking them is controversial.

Depression in the Elderly and Medically Ill.
Behavioral disturbances in the elderly, particularly those with medical illnesses, require a thorough diagnostic evaluation to rule out delirium or dementia. Diagnosis and treatment of depression significantly reduce the risk of excessive physical morbidity, myocardial infarction, prolonged hospitalization, and death. The ideal antidepressant in this population would have no cognitive, cardiotoxic, anticholinergic, antihistaminergic, or α-adrenergic adverse effects. Of the SSRIs, only paroxetine has some anticholinergic activity, though this is clinically relevant only at higher doses. All SSRIs are useful for elderly, medically frail persons. They are less well tolerated by persons with preexisting GI symptoms.

Chronic Depression.
Several studies have shown that nortriptyline (Aventyl, Pamelor) and monthly interpersonal psychotherapy markedly reduced the rate of relapse of depression over a 3-year period. Similar results have been reported with sertraline and would be expected with other SSRIs. The natural history of major depression consists of waxing and waning of symptoms over periods lasting several months. Many studies indicate that discontinuation of SSRI use only 6 months after a depressive episode is associated with a high rate of relapse. It is therefore prudent for a person with chronic depression to continue taking SSRIs for at least 1 year and preferably longer. SSRIs are well tolerated in long-term use.

Depression in Children.
Children of depressed adults are at increased risk of depression. Case reports and small series have reported that SSRIs reduce childhood depressive symptoms and may prevent efforts by children and adolescents to self-medicate their sadness with alcohol or illicit drugs. The adverse effect profile of SSRIs in children includes GI symptoms, insomnia, motor restlessness, social disinhibition, and hypomania or mania. It is therefore critical to determine that the child is truly depressed and to initiate SSRI use with small doses. There are anecdotal reports of successful treatment of children with depression together with another disorder (e.g., attention-deficit/hyperactivity disorder [ADHD]) when SSRIs are combined with other psychotropic drugs. Paroxetine should not be used in children. It may cause agitation with suicidal thoughts.

Anxiety Disorders

Obsessive-Compulsive Disorder.
Fluvoxamine, paroxetine, sertraline, and fluoxetine are indicated for treatment of OCD in persons over the age of 18. Fluvoxamine and sertraline have also been approved for treatment of pediatric OCD (ages 6 to 17). Approximately 50 percent of persons with OCD begin to show symptoms in childhood or adolescence, and more than half of these respond favorably to medication. Beneficial responses can be dramatic. Long-term data support the model of OCD as a genetically determined, lifelong condition that is best treated continuously with drugs and cognitive-behavioral therapy from the onset of symptoms in childhood throughout the life span.

In general, effective SSRI dosages for OCD are higher than those required to treat depression. Fluoxetine is effective for OCD at 20, 40, and 60 mg a day, with a dose-dependent gradation of response. The 60-mg dose is significantly more effective than the 20-mg dose. Response of OCD to sertraline is less clearly dose dependent, with efficacy demonstrated at dosages from 50 to 200 mg a day. Paroxetine is effective at 40 and 60 mg; 20 mg is not better than placebo. Response can be seen in the first few weeks of treatment, but 15 to 20 percent of persons respond only after prolonged treatment.

Comorbid depressive symptoms respond significantly better to SSRIs than to clomipramine, nortriptyline, or amitriptyline (Elavil, Endep). Comorbid tics, as in tic disorders and Tourette's syndrome, respond to the addition of dopamine receptor antagonists or serotonin-dopamine receptor antagonists such as risperidone (Risperdal). In contrast, clozapine (Clozaril) and buspirone (BuSpar) can worsen tics. There appears to be no role for lithium augmentation for OCD treatment. The combination of SSRIs and clomipramine is potentially hazardous because of the potential for cardiotoxicity.

Panic Disorder.
The SSRIs are effective for treatment of panic disorder, with or without agoraphobia. These agents work less rapidly than the benzodiazepines alprazolam (Xanax) or clonazepam, but they are better tolerated in long-term use and do not cause dependence. Citalopram, fluvoxamine, and fluoxetine also may reduce spontaneous or induced panic attacks. Because fluoxetine can initially heighten anxiety symptoms, persons with panic disorder must begin taking small dosages (5 mg a day) and raise the dosage slowly. SSRIs are far superior to benzodiazepines for treatment of panic disorder with comorbid depression.

SSRIs are effective for childhood panic symptoms. If it is well tolerated, SSRI treatment of childhood panic disorder should be continued at least for 1 year. Additional benefit and maintenance of remission would be expected well into adulthood after treatment with medication for at least 1 year.

Social Phobia.
Paroxetine is an effective agent in the treatment of social phobia. Paroxetine reduces both symptoms and disability. This response rate was comparable to that seen with the monoamine oxidase inhibitor (MAOI) phenelzine (Nardil), the previous standard treatment. SSRIs are safer to use than MAOIs or benzodiazepines. All SSRIs are probably effective for social phobia.

Posttraumatic Stress Disorder.
Pharmacotherapy for posttraumatic stress disorder (PTSD) must target specific symptoms in three clusters: reexperiencing, avoidance, and hyperarousal. For long-term treatment, SSRIs appear to have a broader spectrum of therapeutic effects on specific PTSD symptom clusters than tricyclic antidepressants and MAOIs do. Benzodiazepine augmentation is useful in the acute symptomatic state. SSRIs are associated with marked improvement of both intrusive and avoidant symptoms.

Other Anxiety Disorders.
SSRIs may be useful for the treatment of specific phobias, generalized anxiety disorder, and separation anxiety disorder. A thorough, individualized evaluation is the first approach, with particular attention to identifying

conditions amenable to drug therapy. Cognitive-behavioral or other psychotherapies can be added for greater efficacy.

Bulimia Nervosa and Other Eating Disorders

Fluoxetine is indicated for treatment of bulimia, which is best done in the context of psychotherapy. Doses of 60 mg a day are significantly more effective than 20 mg a day. In several well-controlled studies, fluoxetine 60 mg a day was superior to placebo in reducing binge eating and induced vomiting. Some experts recommend an initial course of cognitive-behavioral therapy alone. If there is no response in 3 to 6 weeks, then fluoxetine administration is added. The appropriate duration of treatment with fluoxetine and psychotherapy has not been determined.

Fluvoxamine was not effective at a statistically significant level in one double-blind, placebo-controlled trial for inpatients with bulimia.

Anorexia Nervosa.   Fluoxetine has been used in inpatient treatment of anorexia nervosa to attempt to control comorbid mood disturbances and obsessive-compulsive symptoms. However, at least two careful studies, one of 7 months and one of 24 months, failed to find that fluoxetine affected the overall outcome and the maintenance of weight. Effective treatments for anorexia include cognitive-behavioral, interpersonal, psychodynamic, and family therapies in addition to a trial with SSRIs.

Obesity.   Fluoxetine, in combination with a behavioral program, has only a modest benefit for weight loss. A significant percentage of all persons who take SSRIs, including fluoxetine, lose weight initially, but later they may gain weight. However, all SSRIs may cause initial weight gain.

Premenstrual Dysphoric Disorder

Premenstrual dysphoric disorder is characterized by debilitating mood and behavioral changes in the week preceding menstruation that interfere with normal functioning. Sertraline, paroxetine, fluoxetine, and fluvoxamine have been reported to reduce the symptoms of premenstrual dysphoric disorder. Controlled trials of fluoxetine and sertraline administered either throughout the cycle or only during the luteal phase (the 2-week period between ovulation and menstruation) showed both schedules to be equally effective.

An additional observation of unclear significance was that fluoxetine was associated with changing the duration of the menstrual period by more than 4 days, either lengthening or shortening. The effects of SSRIs on menstrual cycle length are mostly unknown and may warrant careful monitoring in women of reproductive age.

Premature Ejaculation

The antiorgasmic effects of SSRIs make them useful as a treatment for men with premature ejaculation. SSRIs permit intercourse for a significantly longer period and are reported to improve sexual satisfaction in couples in which the man has premature ejaculation. Fluoxetine and sertraline have been shown to be effective for this purpose.

Paraphilias

SSRIs reduce obsessive-compulsive behavior in persons with paraphilias. SSRIs diminish unconventional total sexual activity and average time per day spent in unconventional sexual fantasies, urges, and activities. Evidence suggests a greater response for sexual obsessions than for paraphilias. The data support the hypothesis that paraphilias and related disorders are on the impulsive rather than the compulsive end of the obsessive-compulsive spectrum.

Attention-Deficit/Hyperactivity Disorder

Sympathomimetic drugs are the first-line agents for ADHD in children, followed by bupropion, then SSRIs. In adults, sympathomimetics and antidepressants are reported to be equally effective.

Autistic Disorder

Obsessive-compulsive behavior, poor social relatedness, and aggression are prominent autistic features that respond to serotonergic agents such as SSRIs and clomipramine. Sertraline and fluvoxamine have been shown in controlled and open-label trials to mitigate aggressiveness, self-injurious behavior, repetitive behaviors, some degree of language delay, and (rarely) lack of social relatedness in adults with autistic spectrum disorders. These agents were generally well tolerated. In contrast, a controlled trial of fluvoxamine in autistic children found it to be less well tolerated in this group. Fluoxetine has been reported to be effective for features of autism in children, adolescents, and adults.

Chronic Pain Syndromes

Neuropathic Pain.   Pain due to nerve damage, typically described as tingling, numb, or burning pain, responds to SSRIs and other antidepressants. The most common causes of neuropathic pain are diabetes, trauma, herpes zoster, and chronic nerve compression.

Fibromyalgia.   Pain syndromes in which the complaints of pain and distress appear excessive for the amount of demonstrable tissue injury are highly associated with comorbid affective disorders. SSRIs and older antidepressants have been reported to reduce subjective complaints of chronic pain.

Headache.   Tricyclic drugs have long been used to reduce the frequency and intensity of both migrainous and nonmigrainous headaches. More recently, studies have shown that SSRIs are equally efficacious, with a more favorable adverse effect profile. In addition, persons with chronic or recurrent headaches have a high incidence of comorbid depression and may require antidepressant drug therapy specifically to treat depression.

Concomitant use of SSRIs and drugs in the triptan class (sumatriptan [Imitrex], naratriptan [Amerge], rizatriptan [Maxalt], and zolmitriptan [Zomig]) may (rarely) result in development of a reversible serotonin syndrome (see "Precautions Adverse Reactions"). However, many persons use while taking a low dose of an SSRI for headache without adverse reaction.

Psychosomatic Conditions

Mood and the propensity for panic regulate the autonomic nervous system and may trigger paroxysmal somatic events. SSRIs modulate the incidence of psychogenic symptoms. Some patients with chronic fatigue syndrome have benefited from long-term use of SSRIs, particularly fluoxetine.

Syncope.   Excessive vagal tone may cause bradycardia, hypotension, and syncope. This sequence is called *neurocardiogenic syncope*. Medical causes of syncope to be ruled out include acute dehydration, excessive caffeine intake, overly aggressive treatment of hypertension, parkinsonism and related neurodegenerative disorders, and inadequate fluid and salt intake. Sertraline has been reported to reduce the risk of idiopathic and neurocardiogenic syncope in some persons. Other SSRIs are also effective for neurocardiogenic symptoms such as dizziness.

Respiratory Conditions.   The use of psychotropic medications for pulmonary disorders in persons without psychiatric illness has received little attention. Airway reactivity is closely modulated by fear and panic in individuals with asthma or chronic obstructive airway disease (COPD). As many as one-fourth of persons with COPD also meet criteria for panic disorder. Increased carbon dioxide (CO_2) sensitivity and dyspnea are cardinal features of both panic attacks and COPD. Persons with COPD often must use daily steroids and bronchodilators, which can have serious adverse effects.

In a small case series of persons with COPD, sertraline use was reported to significantly decrease subjective breathlessness after 3 to 4 weeks of treatment, even in persons who did not meet criteria for diagnosable psychiatric illness. SSRIs are much better tolerated than steroids and bronchodilators. In contrast to the results with SSRIs, results have been mixed or contradictory with buspirone and tricyclic drugs in persons with obstructive airway disease.

PRECAUTIONS AND ADVERSE REACTIONS

Three-fourths of persons experience no side effects at low starting dosages of SSRIs, and dosages may be increased relatively rapidly (i.e., on the order of an increase every 1 to 2 weeks) in this group. In the remaining one-fourth of patients, most of the adverse effects of the SSRIs appear within the first 1 to 2 weeks, and they generally subside or resolve spontaneously if the drugs are continued at the same dosage. However, 10 to 15 percent of persons will not be able to tolerate even a low dosage of a particular SSRI and may discontinue taking the drug after only a few doses. One approach for such individuals is to fractionate the dosage over a week, with one dose every 2, 3, or 4 days. Some persons may tolerate a different SSRI or another class of antidepressant, such as a tricyclic drug or one of the other newer agents. Some persons appear unable to tolerate even tiny doses of any antidepressant drug.

Because of the unfortunate possibility that adverse effects may reduce compliance, some clinicians administer a low dosage for the first 3 to 6 weeks of therapy and then increase it gradually once a therapeutic benefit is seen. Because of the ong half-life of the SSRIs, especially fluoxetine, and the even 'ger time it may take for the full benefit of a particular dose

to be appreciated, steep increases in dose are to be avoided. For example, the lowest dosage may provide more than 90 percent of the benefit of the highest dosage, if enough time is allowed. On the other hand, adverse effects are much more predictably dose dependent, and increasing the dosage too rapidly may provoke an aversive response in a sensitive person.

Sexual Dysfunction

Sexual inhibition is the most common adverse effect of SSRIs, with an incidence between 50 and 80 percent. All SSRIs appear to be equally likely to cause sexual dysfunction. The most common complaints are inhibited orgasm and decreased libido, which are dose dependent. Unlike most of the other adverse effects of SSRIs, sexual inhibition does not resolve in the first few weeks of use but usually continues as long as the drug is taken.

Treatment for SSRI-induced sexual dysfunction includes decreasing the dosage and switching to drugs that cause much less sexual dysfunction such as bupropion; specific drugs such as yohimbine (Yocon), cyproheptadine (Periactin), or dopamine receptor agonists may antagonize the sexual side effect.

Reports have described successful treatment of SSRI-induced sexual dysfunction with sildenafil (Viagra). It is not immediately obvious why sildenafil, which works in the excitement phase of the sexual cycle, would counteract the orgasm-phase inhibition of SSRIs. Possibly, the positive reinforcement of robust sexual excitement due to sildenafil permits a mental state more conducive to orgasm. Amphetamine (5 mg) has also been reported to reverse anorgasmia. Alprostadil (Caverject) injections are also effective.

Gastrointestinal Adverse Effects

All SSRIs may cause GI adverse effects. The most common GI complaints are nausea, diarrhea, anorexia, vomiting, and dyspepsia. Data indicate that the nausea and loose stools are dose related and transient, resolving usually within a few weeks. Anorexia is most common with fluoxetine, but some persons gain weight while taking fluoxetine. Fluoxetine-induced appetite loss and weight loss begin as soon as the drug is taken and peak at 20 weeks, after which weight often returns to baseline.

Weight Gain.   Although most patients initially lose weight, up to one-third of persons taking SSRIs will gain weight, sometimes more than 20 pounds. Paroxetine has anticholinergic activity and is the SSRI most often associated with weight gain. In some cases, weight gain results from the drug use itself or the increased appetite associated with better mood.

Headaches.   The incidence of headache in SSRI trials was 18 to 20 percent, only 1 percentage point higher than the placebo rate. Fluoxetine is the most likely to cause headache. On the other hand, all SSRIs are effective prophylaxis against both migraine and tension-type headaches in many persons.

Central Nervous System Adverse Effects

Anxiety.   Fluoxetine is the SSRI most likely to cause anxiety, particularly in the first few weeks; however, these initial effects usually give way to an overall reduction in anxiety after a few weeks. Increased anxiety is caused considerably less frequently by the other SSRIs, which may be a better choice if sedation is desired, as in mixed anxiety and depressive disorders.

Insomnia and Sedation. The major effect SSRIs exert in the area of insomnia and sedation is improved sleep resulting from treatment of depression and anxiety. However, as many as one-fourth of persons taking SSRIs note either trouble sleeping or excessive somnolence. Fluoxetine is the most likely to cause insomnia, for which reason it is often taken in the morning. The other SSRIs are about equally likely to cause insomnia as to cause somnolence, and citalopram, escitalopram, and paroxetine are more likely to cause somnolence than insomnia. With the latter agents, persons usually report that taking the dose before retiring to bed helps them sleep better, without residual daytime somnolence.

SSRI-induced insomnia can be treated with benzodiazepines, trazodone (Desyrel) (clinicians must explain the risk of priapism), or other sedating medicines. Significant SSRI-induced somnolence often requires switching to use of another SSRI or bupropion.

Vivid Dreams and Nightmares. A minority of persons taking SSRIs report recalling extremely vivid dreams or nightmares. An individual experiencing such dreams with one SSRI may get the same therapeutic benefit without the disturbing dream images by switching to use of another SSRI. This adverse effect often resolves spontaneously over several weeks.

Seizures. Seizures have been reported in 0.1 to 0.2 percent of patients treated with SSRIs, an incidence comparable to that reported with other antidepressants and not significantly different from that with placebo. Seizures are more frequent at the highest doses of SSRIs (e.g., fluoxetine 100 mg a day or higher).

Extrapyramidal Symptoms. Tremor is seen in 5 to 10 percent of persons taking SSRIs, a frequency 2 to 4 times that seen with placebo. SSRIs may rarely cause akathisia, dystonia, tremor, cogwheel rigidity, torticollis, opisthotonos, gait disorders, and bradykinesia. Rare cases of tardive dyskinesia have been reported. Persons with well-controlled Parkinson's disease may experience acute worsening of their motor symptoms when they take SSRIs. Extrapyramidal adverse effects are most closely associated with use of fluoxetine, particularly at dosages in excess of 40 mg per day, but may occur at any time during the course of therapy. Bruxism has also been reported, which responds to small doses of buspirone.

Anticholinergic Effects

Although not considered to have anticholinergic activity, the SSRIs are associated with dry mouth in 15 to 20 percent of patients. However, the anticholinergic activity of SSRIs is perhaps only one-fifth that of tricyclic drugs.

Hematological Adverse Effects

SSRIs affect platelet function and may increase bruisability. Paroxetine and fluoxetine are (rarely) associated with develop-

ment of reversible neutropenia, particularly if administered concurrently with clozapine.

Electrolyte and Glucose Disturbances

SSRIs are (rarely) associated with a decrease in glucose concentrations; therefore, diabetic patients should be carefully monitored. Rare cases of SSRI-associated hyponatremia and the secretion of inappropriate antidiuretic hormone (SIADH) have been seen in patients treated with diuretics who are also water deprived.

Endocrine and Allergic Reactions

SSRIs can increase prolactin levels and cause mammoplasia and galactorrhea in both men and women. Breast changes are reversible upon discontinuation of the drug, but this may take several months to occur.

Various types of rashes appear in approximately 4 percent of all patients; in a small subset of these patients, the allergic reaction may generalize and involve the pulmonary system, resulting rarely in fibrotic damage and dyspnea. SSRI treatment may have to be discontinued in patients with drug-related rashes.

Serotonin Syndrome

Concurrent administration of an SSRI with an MAOI, L-tryptophan, or lithium can raise plasma serotonin concentrations to toxic levels, producing a constellation of symptoms called the *serotonin syndrome*. This serious and possibly fatal syndrome of serotonin overstimulation comprises, in order of appearance as the condition worsens, (1) diarrhea; (2) restlessness; (3) extreme agitation, hyperreflexia, and autonomic instability with possible rapid fluctuations in vital signs; (4) myoclonus, seizures, hyperthermia, uncontrollable shivering, and rigidity; and (5) delirium, coma, status epilepticus, cardiovascular collapse, and death.

Treatment of the serotonin syndrome consists of removing the offending agents and promptly instituting comprehensive supportive care with nitroglycerine, cyproheptadine (Periactin), methysergide (Sansert), cooling blankets, chlorpromazine (Thorazine), dantrolene (Dantrium), benzodiazepines, anticonvulsants, mechanical ventilation, and paralyzing agents.

SSRI Withdrawal

The abrupt discontinuation of SSRI use, especially one with a shorter half-life, such as paroxetine or fluvoxamine, has been associated with a withdrawal syndrome that may include dizziness, weakness, nausea, headache, rebound depression, anxiety, insomnia, poor concentration, upper respiratory symptoms, paresthesias, and migraine-like symptoms. It usually does not appear until after at least 6 weeks of treatment and usually resolves spontaneously in 3 weeks. Persons who experienced transient adverse effects in the first weeks of taking an SSRI are more likely to experience discontinuation symptoms.

Fluoxetine is the SSRI least likely to be associated with this syndrome, because the half-life of its metabolite is more than 1 week and it effectively tapers itself. Fluoxetine has therefore been used in some cases to treat the discontinuation syndrome caused by termination of other SSRIs.

DRUG–DRUG INTERACTIONS

SSRIs do not interfere with most other drugs. A serotonin syndrome can develop with concurrent administration of MAOIs, tryptophan, lithium, or other antidepressants that inhibit reuptake of serotonin. Fluoxetine, sertraline, and paroxetine can raise plasma concentrations of tricyclic antidepressants, which can cause clinical toxicity. A number of potential pharmacokinetic interactions have been described on the basis of in vitro analyses of the CYP enzymes, but clinically relevant interactions are rare.

LABORATORY INTERFERENCES

SSRIs do not interfere with any laboratory tests.

DOSAGE AND CLINICAL GUIDELINES

Fluoxetine

Fluoxetine is available in 10- and 20-mg capsules, in a scored 10-mg tablet, and as a liquid (20 mg/5 mL). There is also a 90-mg long-acting tablet used for once-a-week dosing that delivers the equivalent of once-daily dosing with 20 mg. For depression, the initial dosage is usually 10 or 20 mg orally each day, usually given in the morning, because insomnia is a potential adverse effect of the drug. Fluoxetine should be taken with food to minimize the possible nausea. The long half-lives of the drug and its metabolite contribute to a 4-week period to reach steady-state concentrations. As with all available antidepressants, the antidepressant effects of fluoxetine may be seen in the first weeks, but the clinician should wait until the patient has been taking the drug for 4 to 6 weeks before definitively evaluating its antidepressant activity. Several studies indicate that 20 mg is often as effective as higher doses for treating depression. The maximum dosage recommended by the manufacturer is 80 mg a day, and higher dosages may cause seizures. A reasonable strategy is to maintain a patient with 20 mg a day for 3 weeks. If the patient shows no signs of clinical improvement at that time, an increase to 40 mg may be warranted, although at least one study has found that continuing use of 20 mg a day is as effective as increasing the dosage.

To minimize the early side effects of anxiety and restlessness, some clinicians initiate fluoxetine use at 5 to 10 mg a day, either with the scored 10-mg tablet or by using the liquid preparation. Alternatively, because of the long half-life of fluoxetine, its use can be initiated with an every-other-day administration schedule.

At least 2 weeks should elapse between the discontinuation of MAOI use and the administration of fluoxetine. Fluoxetine use must be discontinued at least 5 weeks before the initiation of MAOI treatment.

The dosage of fluoxetine that is effective in other indications may differ from the 20 mg a day that is generally used for depression. A dosage of 60 mg a day has been reported to be the most effective for the treatment of OCD, obesity, and bulimia nervosa. Fluoxetine is also marketed as Sarafem for premenstrual dysphoric disorder.

Sertraline

Sertraline is available in scored 25-, 50-, and 100-mg tablets. For the initial treatment of depression, sertraline use should be initiated with a dose of 50 mg once daily. To limit the GI effects, some clinicians begin treatment using 25 mg a day and increase to 50 mg a day after 3 weeks. Patients who do not respond after 1 to 3 weeks may benefit from dosage increases of 50 mg every week up to a maximum of 200 mg, given once daily. Sertraline generally is given in the evening, because it is slightly more likely to cause sedation than insomnia. However, it can be administered in the morning or the evening. Administration after eating may reduce the GI adverse effects. Sertraline concentrate is now available (1 mL = 20 mg).

Guidelines regarding the logic of dosage increases for sertraline are similar to those for fluoxetine. Several studies suggest that maintaining the dosage at 50 mg a day for many weeks may be as beneficial as rapidly increasing the dosage. Nevertheless, many clinicians maintain their patients on doses of 100 to 200 mg a day.

Paroxetine

Paroxetine is available in scored 20-mg tablets, in unscored 10-, 30-, and 40-mg tablets, and as an orange-flavored 10 mg/5 mL oral suspension. It is also available in a controlled-release preparation (CR) in doses of 12.5 and 25 mg. Paroxetine use for the treatment of depression is usually initiated at a dosage of 10 or 20 mg a day. An increase in the dosage should be considered when an adequate response is not seen in 1 to 3 weeks. The CR preparation is also taken once daily. At that point, the clinician can initiate upward dose titration in 10-mg increments at weekly intervals to a maximum of 50 mg a day. Dosages of 60, 70, and 80 mg a day have been tolerated by certain individuals but have not been studied in controlled trials. Persons who experience GI upset may benefit from taking the drug with food. Paroxetine should be taken initially as a single daily dose in the evening; higher dosages may be divided into two doses per day. Patients with melancholic features may require dosages exceeding 20 mg a day. The suggested therapeutic dosage range for elderly patients is 10 to 20 mg a day, as the elderly have been found to have higher mean plasma concentrations than younger adults.

Paroxetine is the SSRI most likely to produce a discontinuation syndrome, because plasma concentrations drop rapidly in the absence of continuous dosing. To limit the development of symptoms of abrupt discontinuation, paroxetine use should be tapered gradually in increments of 10 mg a day each week until the daily dose is 10 mg, at which point its use may be stopped either directly or after an additional increment of 5 mg a day.

This drug should not be used in children who may develop agitation and suicidal ideation as a result.

Fluvoxamine

Fluvoxamine is available in unscored 25-mg tablets and scored 50- and 100-mg tablets. The effective daily dosage range is 50 to 300 mg a day. A usual starting dosage is 50 mg once a day at bedtime for the first week, after which the dosage can be adjusted according to the adverse effects and clinical response. Dosages above 100 mg a day may be divided into twice-daily dosing. A temporary dosage reduction or slower upward titration may be necessary if nausea develops over the first 2 weeks of therapy. Fluvoxamine can also be administered as a single evening dose to minimize its adverse effects. Tablets should be swallowed with food, without chewing the tablet. Fluvoxamine is relatively likely to cause a discontinuation syndrome.

Citalopram

Citalopram is available in 20- and 40-mg tablets and as a liquid (10 mg/5 mL). The usual starting dosage is 20 mg a day for the first week, after which it usually is increased to 40 mg a day. Some persons may require 60 mg a day, but there are no controlled trials supporting this dose. For elderly persons or persons with hepatic impairment, 20 mg a day is recommended, with an increase to 40 mg a day only if there is no response to 20 mg a day. Tablets should be taken once daily, in either the morning or the evening, with or without food.

Escitalopram

Escitalopram (Lexapro) is the newest SSRI antidepressant approved by the Food and Drug Administration (FDA) for the treatment of major depressive disorder. It has a broad spectrum of anxiolytic effects as well, as indicated by its efficacy in clinical trials of panic disorder, generalized anxiety disorder, social anxiety disorder, and in relieving the anxiety symptoms associated with depression. The usual therapeutic dose of escitalopram is 10 mg per day, which can be increased to 20 mg per day if a response is not seen within 2 weeks. It is available in 10-mg and 20-mg tablets. An oral liquid formulation, 5 mg/tsp, is also available.

Loss of Efficacy

Some patients report a lessened response to SSRIs with recurrence of depressive symptoms after a period of time (e.g., 4 to 6 months). The exact mechanism is unknown; however, data from an open-label trial suggest that persons with moderate to severe depression who respond rapidly to fluoxetine use are unlikely to experience recurrence of depression while taking fluoxetine, whereas one-third of those with milder depression whose initial response to fluoxetine was slower and less robust experienced recurrence of depression within 3 months.

Potential responses to the attenuation of response to SSRIs include increasing or decreasing the dosage; tapering drug use, then rechallenging with the same medication; switching to another SSRI or non-SSRI antidepressant; and augmenting with bupropion, sympathomimetics, buspirone, lithium, anticonvulsants, naltrexone (ReVia), or another non-SSRI antidepressant. A change in response to an SSRI should be explored in psychotherapy, which may reveal the underlying conflicts causing an increase in depressive symptoms.

▲ 32.3.27 Serotonin-Dopamine Antagonists: Second-Generation Antipsychotics

The serotonin-dopamine antagonists (SDAs) are also referred to as *second-generation*, *novel* or *atypical antipsychotic drugs* and include risperidone (Risperdal), olanzapine (Zyprexa), quetiapine (Seroquel), clozapine (Clozaril), and ziprasidone (Zel-

dox). A new atypical antipsychotic, aripiprazole (Abilify), with a different mechanism of action, a partial dopamine agonist, has an efficacy and safety profile very similar to the SDAs. These drugs improve two classes of disabilities typical of schizophrenia: (1) positive symptoms such as hallucinations, delusions, disordered thoughts, and agitation and (2) negative symptoms such as withdrawal, flat affect, anhedonia, poverty of speech, catatonia, and cognitive impairment. SDAs carry a smaller risk of extrapyramidal symptoms than the dopamine receptor antagonists, which eliminates the need for concurrent anticholinergic drug use with their annoying adverse effects.

SDAs are also effective for the treatment of mood disorders with psychotic or manic features and for behavioral disturbances associated with dementia. Olanzapine is indicated for short-term treatment of acute manic episodes associated with bipolar I disorders. All these agents are considered first-line drugs except clozapine, which causes adverse hematological effects that require weekly blood sampling.

PHARMACOLOGICAL ACTIONS

Risperidone

Between 70 and 85 percent of risperidone is absorbed from the gastrointestinal (GI) tract, and it undergoes extensive first-pass hepatic metabolism to 9-hydroxyrisperidone, a metabolite with comparable biological activity. The combined half-life of risperidone and 9-hydroxyrisperidone averages 20 hours, so that it is effective in once-daily dosing. Risperidone is an antagonist of the serotonin and dopamine receptors. Although it is as potent an antagonist of dopamine receptors as haloperidol (Haldol) is, risperidone is much less likely than haloperidol to cause extrapyramidal symptoms.

Olanzapine

Approximately 85 percent of olanzapine is absorbed from the GI tract, and approximately 40 percent of the dosage is inactivated by first-pass hepatic metabolism. Peak concentrations are achieved within 6 hours, and the half-life averages 30 hours. Therefore, it is effective in once-daily dosing.

Quetiapine

Quetiapine is rapidly absorbed from the GI tract. Peak plasma concentrations are reached in 1 to 2 hours. Steady-state half-life is approximately 6 hours, and optimal dosing is two or three times per day. Quetiapine is an antagonist of serotonin and dopamine.

Clozapine

Clozapine is rapidly absorbed from the GI tract, and peak plasma levels are reached in 1 to 4 hours. The steady-state half-life of 10 to 16 hours is usually reached in 3 to 4 days if twice-daily dosing is used. The two major metabolites have minimal pharmacological activity. Clozapine is an antagonist of serotonin and dopamine.

Ziprasidone

Peak plasma concentrations of ziprasidone are reached in 2 to 6 hours. The steady-state half-life of 5 to 10 hours is reached by the third day, and twice-daily dosing is necessary. Ziprasidone is an antagonist of serotonin and dopamine. Ziprasidone also has agonist activity at the serotonin 5-HT$_{1A}$ receptors and is a norepinephrine reuptake inhibitor. This suggests that it could possess antidepressant effects.

Aripiprazole

Aripiprazole is not an SDA; rather, it is a partial agonist at the dopamine D$_2$ receptor. Peak plasma concentration occurs within 3 to 5 hours.

THERAPEUTIC INDICATIONS

Psychotic Disorders

SDAs are effective for treating acute and chronic psychoses such as schizophrenia and schizoaffective disorders in both adults and adolescents. They are also effective for treating psychotic depression and for psychosis secondary to head trauma, dementia, or treatment drugs. SDAs are as good as, or better than, typical antipsychotics (dopamine receptor antagonists) for the treatment of positive symptoms in schizophrenia and clearly superior to dopamine receptor antagonists for the treatment of negative symptoms. Compared with persons treated with dopamine receptor antagonists, those treated with SDAs have fewer relapses and require less frequent hospitalization, fewer emergency room visits, less phone contact with mental health professionals, and less treatment in day programs.

Because clozapine has potentially life-threatening adverse effects, it is now appropriate only for patients with schizophrenia resistant to all other antipsychotics, and it retains a therapeutic niche for patients who are treatment resistant. Other indications for clozapine include treatment of persons with severe tardive dyskinesia and those with a low threshold for extrapyramidal symptoms. Persons who tolerate clozapine have done well on long-term therapy.

The studies done for the regulatory approval of aripiprazole were done with patients with schizophrenia and schizoaffective disorder. Studies using aripiprazole in other disorders are under way.

Mood Disorders

SDAs are useful for the initial control of agitation during a manic episode, but they are less effective for long-term control of bipolar disorders than traditional mood stabilizers. Olanzapine is Food and Drug Administration (FDA)–approved for treatment of acute mania at dosages of 10 or 15 mg a day. Olanzapine and risperidone can be used to augment antidepressants in the short-term management of major depression with psychotic features. SDAs are effective in the treatment of schizoaffective disorder, although risperidone has been reported to precipitate mania in persons with schizoaffective disorder. Olanzapine and clozapine augmentation can improve up to two-thirds of persons with refractory bipolar disorder, and risperidone has been used to reduce mood swings in persons with rapid-cycling bipolar disorder.

Other Indications

SDAs are effective for treatment of acquired immune deficiency syndrome (AIDS), dementia, autistic spectrum disorders, dementia-related psychosis, Tourette's disorder, Huntington's disease, and Lesch-Nyhan syndrome. Risperidone and olanzapine have been used to control aggression and self-injury in children. These drugs have also been coadministered with sympathomimetics, such as methylphenidate (Ritalin) or dextroamphetamine (Dexedrine, Dextrostat), to children with attention-deficit/hyperactivity disorder (ADHD) who are comorbid for either opposition-defiant disorder or conduct disorder. SDAs, especially olanzapine, quetiapine, and clozapine, are useful in persons who have severe tardive dyskinesia. SDA treatment suppresses the abnormal movements of tardive dyskinesia but does not appear to worsen the movement disorder.

Treatment with olanzapine and ziprasidone decreases depressive symptoms in persons with schizophrenia to a greater extent than haloperidol does. In depressed persons without psychotic features who respond only partially to antidepressants, augmentation with olanzapine can improve treatment efficacy.

Treatment with SDAs, particularly clozapine, decreases the risk of suicide in patients with schizophrenia. Patients with treatment-resistant obsessive-compulsive disorder (OCD) have responded to SDA augmentation of SSRIs; however, a few persons treated with SDAs have noted treatment-emergent symptoms of OCD. Some patients with borderline personality disorder may improve with SDAs.

ADVERSE EFFECTS

Risperidone

Weight gain, anxiety, nausea and vomiting, rhinitis, erectile dysfunction, and orgasmic dysfunction are associated with risperidone use. The most common drug-related reasons for discontinuation of risperidone use are extrapyramidal symptoms, dizziness, hyperkinesia, somnolence, and nausea.

Olanzapine

Somnolence, dry mouth, dizziness, constipation, dyspepsia, increased appetite, and tremor are associated with olanzapine use. Olanzapine is somewhat more likely than risperidone to cause weight gain.

Quetiapine

The most common adverse effects of quetiapine are somnolence, postural hypotension, and dizziness, which are usually transient and are best managed with initial gradual upward titration of the dosage. Quetiapine appears not to cause extrapyramidal symptoms. Quetiapine is associated with modest transient weight gain in 23 percent of persons, small increases in heart rate, constipation, and a transient rise in liver transaminases.

Clozapine

The most common drug-related adverse effects are sedation, dizziness, syncope, tachycardia, hypotension, electrocardiogram (ECG) changes, nausea, and vomiting. Leukopenia, granulocytopenia, agranulocytosis, and fever occur in approximately 1 percent of patients. Other common adverse effects include fatigue, sialorrhea, weight gain, various GI symptoms (most commonly, constipation), anticholinergic effects, and subjective muscle weakness. Changes in insulin metabolism have been reported. The risk of seizures is approximately 4 percent in patients taking dosages above 600 mg a day. Myocarditis and cardiomyopathy are also adverse events reported.

Ziprasidone

The most common adverse effects in patients taking ziprasidone were somnolence, headache, dizziness, nausea, and lightheadedness. Ziprasidone has almost no significant effects outside the central nervous system (CNS) and is associated with almost no weight gain; however, QT prolongation is potentially fatal in patients with a history of cardiac arrhythmia.

Aripiprazole

Aripiprazole appears to be associated with low risk of extrapyramidal symptoms, low sedation, minimal weight gain, no QT prolongation, and no prolactin elevation. Additional information about adverse effects is needed. The most commonly associated side effects include headache, anxiety, and insomnia.

Neuroleptic Malignant Syndrome

Although rare with use of SDAs, all antipsychotic drugs may cause neuroleptic malignant syndrome. This syndrome consists of muscular rigidity, fever, dystonia, akinesia, mutism, shifting between obtundation and agitation, diaphoresis, dysphagia, tremor, incontinence, labile blood pressure, leukocytosis, and elevated creatine phosphokinase (CPK). Neuroleptic malignant syndrome has been reported with clozapine, risperidone, and olanzapine and must be considered in the differential diagnosis of fever in a clozapine-treated person.

Tardive Dyskinesia

SDAs are much less likely than dopamine receptor antagonists to be associated with treatment-emergent tardive dyskinesias. Moreover, SDAs ameliorate the symptoms of tardive dyskinesias and are especially indicated for psychotic persons with preexisting tardive dyskinesias. Tardive dyskinesias can occur in persons treated with dopamine receptor antagonists for as little as 1 month. Therefore, use of dopamine receptor antagonists for long-term maintenance of patients with psychosis has become a questionable practice. SDAs should replace dopamine receptor antagonists for long-term treatment.

Orthostatic Hypotension, Syncope, and Tachycardia

All SDAs, but most frequently quetiapine, are associated with orthostatic hypotension, particularly if dosages are escalated rapidly. SDAs should be used with caution in persons with hypotension, diabetes mellitus, or myocardial infarction and those who are taking antihypertensive medications. Clozapine is associated with paradoxical hypertension in 4 percent of persons.

Cardiac Changes

Potential ECG changes include nonspecific ST-T wave changes, T wave flattening, or T wave inversions, although these changes are usually not clinically significant. Olanzapine, quetiapine, ziprasidone, and clozapine are not associated with significant changes in QT or PR intervals; however, ziprasidone may have clinically significant QT prolon-

gation in susceptible patients. Because of the variety of cardiac changes associated with SDA use, the drugs should be used with caution by persons with preexisting cardiac disease or in combination with drugs that prolong the QT interval significantly, such as quinidine (Cardioquin).

Agranulocytosis

Agranulocytosis is a potentially fatal condition defined as a decrease in the absolute neutrophil count that occurs most commonly in clozapine-treated persons. Agranulocytosis can appear precipitously or gradually and most often develops in the first 6 months of treatment. Clozapine should not be used by persons with white blood cell (WBC) counts below 3,500, a history of a bone marrow disorder, or a history of clozapine-induced agranulocytosis.

Seizures

Persons with preexisting seizure disorders or histories of significant head trauma are at greatest risk for seizures while taking clozapine, compared to other drugs in this section. If seizures develop, clozapine use should be temporarily stopped. Anticonvulsant treatment can be initiated, and clozapine use can be resumed at approximately 50 percent of the previous dosage, then gradually raised again.

Hyperprolactinemia

The D_2 receptor antagonist activity of antipsychotic drugs causes a rise in prolactin levels for the duration of the therapy. Of the SDAs, risperidone is most strongly associated with hyperprolactinemia, followed by olanzapine and ziprasidone. Clozapine and quetiapine do not increase prolactin secretion. Hyperprolactinemia can cause galactorrhea, amenorrhea, gynecomastia, and impotence. Aripiprazole does not increase prolactin release.

Cognitive and Motor Impairment

All currently available SDAs cause sedation. Therefore, persons who take SDAs should exercise caution when driving or operating dangerous machinery. This adverse effect may be minimized by giving most of the dosage before sleep.

Body Temperature Regulation

Because SDAs alter the ability of the body to regulate temperature, persons taking them should avoid strenuous exercise, exposure to extreme heat, concomitant administration of anticholinergic drugs, and dehydration.

Extrapyramidal Symptoms

All SDAs are much less likely than dopamine receptor antagonists to produce extrapyramidal symptoms, such as acute dystonia, parkinsonism, rabbit syndrome, and akinesia.

Weight Gain

Risperidone, olanzapine, quetiapine, and clozapine are associated with weight gain, which can be controlled with strict adherence to a planned diet. Clozapine and olanzapine in particular may be associated with a gain of as much as 30 to 50 pounds with short-term use. Significant weight gain may induce or exacerbate diabetes mellitus, and olanzapine and clozapine should therefore be used with caution by persons who have, or are at risk for, diabetes. Ziprasidone and aripiprazole appear not to cause significant weight gain.

Sialorrhea

Clozapine can cause sialorrhea, which may place the patient at risk for aspiration of saliva and gagging, particularly during sleep. Clozapine is thought to produce sialorrhea by inhibiting swallowing rather than by increasing salivation. Treatment options include the clonidine patch, 0.1 or 0.2 mg each week, or amitriptyline (Elavil, Endep) or clomipramine (Anafranil), 75 to 100 mg, before sleep. Anticholinergic drugs, such as atropine, should not be used because they can exacerbate the anticholinergic activity of clozapine. Clozapine-induced sialorrhea may resolve spontaneously in a small number of patients after several months.

Obsessive-Compulsive Symptoms

Treatment-emergent obsessive-compulsive symptoms have been reported in patients with a favorable antipsychotic response to clozapine, risperidone, and olanzapine. Controlled trials have not established a clear causal relationship. When used by persons with a prior diagnosis of OCD, on the other hand, SDAs have been successful in augmenting the antiobsessional effects of serotonin reuptake inhibitors.

Priapism

The α-receptor antagonism of SDAs can induce priapism. There are a few isolated case reports of priapism during treatment with risperidone, olanzapine, quetiapine, and clozapine.

Genitourinary Symptoms

Enuresis, urinary frequency or urgency, and urinary hesitancy or retention have been seen with use of clozapine. These problems may respond to desmopressin (DDAVP), oxybutynin (Ditropan), or timed interruption of sleep.

Dysphagia

Antipsychotic drug use is infrequently associated with esophageal dysmotility and aspiration, which can cause aspiration pneumonia.

Transaminase Elevations and Hepatic Dysfunction

Approximately 6 percent of persons who take quetiapine and 2 percent of those who take olanzapine have serum transaminase concentrations more than three times the upper limit of normal in the first 3 weeks of treatment. This has no clinical significance and is transient; however, quetiapine and olanzapine should be used with caution by persons with underlying liver disease. Clozapine is also associated with hepatic toxicity.

Cholesterol and Triglyceride Elevations

Quetiapine and olanzapine use may increase serum cholesterol and triglyceride concentrations by 11 to 17 percent.

Hypothyroidism

A small number of persons taking higher dosages of quetiapine have decreased serum concentrations of total and free thyroxine. This usually has no clinical significance.

Use in Pregnancy and Lactation

SDA use by pregnant women has not been studied, but consideration should be given to the potential of risperidone to raise prolactin concentrations, sometimes to three to four times the upper limit of the normal range. Because the drugs can be excreted in breast milk, they should not be taken by nursing mothers.

DRUG–DRUG INTERACTIONS

CNS depressants, alcohol, or tricyclic drugs coadministered with SDAs may increase the risk for seizures, sedation, and cardiac effects. Antihypertensive medications may potentiate the orthostatic hypotension caused by SDAs. Coadministration of benzodiazepines and SDAs may be associated with an increased incidence of orthostasis, syncope, and respiratory depression. Risperidone, olanzapine, quetiapine, and ziprasidone can antagonize the effects of levodopa (Larodopa) and dopamine agonists. Long-term use of SDAs with drugs that induce cytochrome P450 isoenzymes, such as carbamazepine, barbiturates, omeprazole (Prilosec), rifampin (Rifadin, Rifamate), or glucocorticoids, may increase the clearance of the SDAs by 50 percent or more.

DOSAGE AND CLINICAL GUIDELINES

Risperidone, olanzapine, quetiapine, and ziprasidone are appropriate for the management of an initial psychotic episode, whereas clozapine is reserved for persons refractory to all other antipsychotic drugs. If a person does not respond to the first SDA, other SDAs or aripiprazole should be tried. Olanzapine and clozapine have some initial calming effects due to their anticholinergic activity. The SDAs are less effective sedatives for treatment of acute psychosis than dopamine receptor antagonists or benzodiazepines. It is thus sometimes necessary to augment an SDA with a high-potency dopamine receptor antagonist or benzodiazepine in the first few weeks of use. Lorazepam 1 to 2 mg orally or intramuscularly (IM) can be used as needed for acute agitation. SDAs usually require 4 to 6 weeks to reach full effectiveness. Once effective, dosages can be lowered as tolerated. Clinical improvement may take 6 months of treatment with SDAs in some particularly treatment-refractory persons.

Risperidone

Risperidone is available in 1-, 2-, 3-, and 4-mg tablets, and a 1-mg/mL oral solution. The initial dosage is usually 1 to 2 mg at night. The dosage can then be raised gradually (1 mg per dose every 2 or 3 days) to 4 to 6 mg at night. Risperidone was initially given twice a day, but several studies have shown equal efficacy with once-a-day dosing. Dosages above 6 mg a day are associated with a higher incidence of adverse effects. Dosages below 6 mg a day have generally not been associated with extrapyramidal symptoms, but dystonic reactions have been seen at dosages from 4 to 16 mg a day.

Olanzapine

Olanzapine is available in 2.5-, 5-, 7.5-, 10-, and 15-mg tablets. The initial dosage for treatment of psychosis is usually 5 or 10 mg and for treatment of acute mania is usually 10 or 15 mg, given once daily. A starting daily dose of 5 mg is recommended for elderly and medically ill persons and those with hepatic impairment or hypotension; after 1 week the dosage can be raised to 10 mg a day. Given the long half-life, 1 week must be allowed to achieve each new steady-state blood level. Dosages in clinical use range from 5 to 20 mg a day, but a beneficial response usually occurs at dosages of 10 mg a day. The higher dosages are associated with increased extrapyramidal and other adverse effects. The manufacturer recommends "periodic" assessment of transaminases during treatment with olanzapine.

Olanzapine will shortly be available in the United States as an IM formulation for administration in acute care situations.

Quetiapine

Quetiapine is available in 25-, 100-, and 200-mg tablets. Dosing should begin at 25 mg twice daily, and dosages can be raised by 25 to 50 mg per dose every 2 to 3 days up to a target of 300 to 400 mg a day, divided into two or three daily doses. Studies have shown efficacy in the range of 300 to 800 mg a day, with most persons receiving maximum benefit at 300 to 500 mg a day.

Clozapine

Clozapine is available in 25- and 100-mg tablets. The initial dosage is usually 25 mg one or two times daily, although a conservative initial dosage is 12.5 mg twice daily. The dosage can then be raised gradually (25 mg a day every 2 or 3 days) to 300 mg a day in divided dosages, usually two or three times daily. Dosages up to 900 mg a day can be used.

Weekly WBC counts are indicated to monitor the patient for the development of agranulocytosis. Although monitoring is expensive, early indication of agranulocytosis can prevent a fatal outcome. If the WBC count is below 2,000 cells per mm^3 or the granulocyte count is below 1,000 per mm^3, clozapine use should be discontinued, a hematological consultation should be obtained, and obtaining a bone marrow sample should be considered. Persons with agranulocytosis should not be reexposed to the drug. Persons can obtain the WBC count through any laboratory. Proof of monitoring must be presented to the pharmacist to obtain the medication.

Ziprasidone

Ziprasidone dosing should be initiated at 40 mg a day, divided into two daily doses. Studies have shown efficacy in the range of 80 to 160 mg a day, divided twice daily. Ziprasidone is expected to be the first SDA to be available in both oral and long-acting (depot) injectable formulations.

Aripiprazole

Aripiprazole tablets are available in 10-, 15-, 20-, and 30-mg tablets. Aripiprazole has been shown to be effective in a dose range of 10 to 30 mg a day; doses higher than 10 or 15 mg a day, the lowest doses in these trials, were not more effective than 10 or 15 mg a day.

Switching from Typical to Atypical Antipsychotic Drugs

Although the transition from a dopamine receptor antagonist to an SDA may be made abruptly, it is probably wiser to taper off use of the dopamine receptor antagonist slowly while titrating up the SDA. Clozapine and olanzapine both have anticholinergic effects, and the transition from one to the other can usually be accomplished with little risk of cholinergic rebound. The transition from risperidone to olanzapine is best accomplished by tapering off risperidone use over 3 weeks while simultaneously beginning olanzapine use directly at 10 mg a day. Risperidone, quetiapine, and ziprasidone lack anticholinergic effects, and the abrupt transition from a dopamine receptor antagonist, olanzapine, or clozapine to one of these agents may cause cholinergic rebound, which consists of excessive salivation, nausea, vomiting, and diarrhea. The risk of cholinergic rebound can be mitigated by initially augmenting risperidone, quetiapine, or ziprasidone with an anticholinergic drug, which is then tapered off slowly. Any initiation and termination of SDA use should be accomplished gradually.

It is wise to overlap administration of the new drug with the old drug. Of interest, some persons have a more robust clinical response while taking the two agents during the transition, then regress on monotherapy with the newer drug. Little is known about the effectiveness and safety of a strategy of combining the use of one SDA with another SDA or with a dopamine receptor antagonist.

Persons receiving regular injections of depot formulations of a dopamine receptor antagonist who are to switch to SDA use are given the first dose of the SDA on the day the next injection is due. At present, SDAs are only available in oral formulations.

Persons who developed agranulocytosis while taking clozapine can safely switch to olanzapine use, although initiation of olanzapine use in the midst of clozapine-induced agranulocytosis can prolong the time of recovery from the usual 3 to 4 days up to 11 to 12 days. It is prudent to wait for resolution of agranulocytosis before initiating olanzapine use. Emergence or recurrence of agranulocytosis has not been reported with olanzapine, even in persons who developed it while taking clozapine.

▲ 32.3.28 Sympathomimetics and Related Drugs

Sympathomimetic drugs cause the stimulation of α- and β-adrenergic receptors directly as agonists and, indirectly, cause the release of dopamine and norepinephrine from presynaptic terminals. They are variously referred to as *stimulants*, *psychostimulants*, or *analeptics*. While these drugs act specifically on symptoms of poor concentration and hyperactivity in children and adults, as well as increasing alertness in narcolepsy, they are also used to maintain wakefulness, alertness, and energy. Because of their rapid onset, immediate behavioral effects, and the propensity to develop tolerance, which leads to the risk of abuse and dependence in vulnerable individuals, they have been classified as controlled drugs, and their manufacture, distribution, and use are regulated by state and federal agencies.

Despite these caveats, they are valuable agents and their use persists and may be increasing in medicine and psychiatry in specific clinical situations. Stimulants can be of great help, if appropriately prescribed and monitored, because of their effectiveness in disorders in which no other drug has been helpful. Sympathomimetics have been widely used in attention-deficit/hyperactivity disorder (ADHD) and narcolepsy because no other equally effective agent exists. They are effective in medical or surgical disorders that result in secondary depression or profound apathy (e.g., acquired immune deficiency syndrome [AIDS]) and also are used to augment antidepressant medications in treatment-refractory depressions.

The sympathomimetics used in psychiatry include methylphenidate (Ritalin, Concerta), dexmethylphenidate (Focalin), dextroamphetamine (Dexedrine), a combination of amphetamine and dextroamphetamine (Adderall), methamphetamine (Desoxyn), and pemoline (Cylert), the last now considered a second-line agent, because of rare but potentially fatal hepatic toxicity. The drugs are indicated for the treatment of attention deficit/hyperactivity disorder (ADHD) and narcolepsy and are also effective in the treatment of depressive disorders in special populations (e.g., the medically ill).

Both amphetamine and nonamphetamine sympathomimetics have been used as appetite suppressants. Other sympathomimetics used for appetite suppression include methamphetamine (Desoxyn), benzphetamine (Didrex), phentermine (Adipex-P, Fastin, Ionamin), diethylpropion (Tenuate), phenmetrazine (Preludin), phendimetrazine (Bontril, Adipost), and mazindol (Sanorex, Mazanor). A novel stimulant approved for treatment of narcolepsy in the United States, modafinil (Provigil), is discussed at the end of this section. Also discussed is atomoxetine (Strattera), a selective norepinephrine inhibitor used in the treatment of ADHD.

PHARMACOLOGICAL ACTIONS

All of these drugs are well absorbed from the gastrointestinal (GI) tract. Dextroamphetamine reaches peak plasma concentrations in 2 to 3 hours and has a half-life of approximately 6 hours, thereby necessitating twice- or thrice-daily dosing.

Methylphenidate is available in immediate-release (Ritalin), sustained-release (Ritalin SR), and extended-release (Concerta) formulations. Immediate-release methylphenidate reaches peak plasma concentrations in 1 to 2 hours and has a short half-life of 2 to 3 hours, thereby necessitating multiple daily dosing. The sustained-release formulation reaches peak plasma concentrations in 4 to 5 hours and doubles the effective half-life of methylphenidate. The extended-release formulation reaches peak plasma concentrations in 6 to 8 hours and is designed to be effective for 12 hours in once-daily dosing. Dexmethylphenidate reaches peak plasma level in approximately 7 hours and is given twice daily.

Pemoline reaches peak plasma concentrations in 2 to 4 hours and has a half-life of approximately 12 hours, and modafinil reaches peak plasma concentrations in 2 to 4 hours and has a half-life of 15 hours, thereby allowing once-daily dosing of these two agents.

Dextroamphetamine (Adderall) is available in immediate-release and sustained-release (Adderall XR) formulations. The immediate-release drug reaches peak plasma concentrations in approximately 3 hours. The time to peak concentration for the extended-release drug is approximately 7 hours and provides effective full-day symptom control in a single morning dose; the immediate-release preparation requires multiple dosing.

Methylphenidate, dexmethylphenidate, dextroamphetamine, and amphetamine are indirectly acting sympathomimetics, with the primary effect of causing the release of catecholamines from presynaptic neurons. Clinical effectiveness is associated with increased release of both dopamine and norepinephrine. Dextroamphetamine and methylphenidate are also weak inhibitors of catecholamine reuptake and inhibitors of monoamine oxidase. Pemoline may indirectly stimulate dopaminergic activity by a poorly understood mechanism, but it has little actual sympathomimetic activity.

EFFECTS ON SPECIFIC ORGANS AND SYSTEMS

Central Nervous System

Amphetamine stimulates the medullary respiratory center and has excitatory effects on cortical function. Depending on personality and contextual factors, amphetamine in adults can increase wakefulness, energy, alertness, initiative, self-confidence, and physical and mental performance, lessen fatigue, and produce euphoria. These effects occur shortly after dosing.

Cardiovascular System

Amphetamines can raise blood pressure (particularly in patients with hypertension), and high doses can lead to cardiac arrhythmias (especially in patients with cardiovascular disease). Such effects are not likely at usual clinical doses in a patient without cardiovascular disease or hypertension. Amphetamine is more potent in producing cardiovascular effects than dextroamphetamine because of stronger effects on norepinephrine.

Endocrine Effects

Early reports suggested that both dextroamphetamine and methylphenidate might suppress growth in children. A recent controlled study of children and young adolescents found small but significant height differences evident in early (but not late) adolescent children with ADHD, unrelated to the use of psychotropic medications. This study concluded that the effects on growth seemed to be related to the disorder, not its treatment.

THERAPEUTIC INDICATIONS

Attention-Deficit/Hyperactivity Disorder

Sympathomimetics are the first-line drugs for treatment of ADHD in children and are effective approximately 75 percent of the time. Methylphenidate and dextroamphetamine are equally effective and work within 15 to 30 minutes. Pemoline requires 3 to 4 weeks to reach its full efficacy, which nevertheless may be less than that of methylphenidate and dextroamphetamine. The drugs decrease hyperactivity, increase attentiveness, and reduce impulsivity. They may also reduce comorbid oppositional behaviors associated with ADHD. Many persons take these drugs throughout their schooling and beyond. In responsive persons, use of a sympathomimetic may be a critical determinant of scholastic success.

Sympathomimetics improve the core ADHD symptoms of hyperactivity, impulsivity, and inattentiveness and permit improved social interactions with teachers, family, other adults, and peers. The success of long-term treatment of ADHD with sympathomimetics, which are efficacious for most of the various constellations of ADHD symptoms present from childhood to adulthood, supports a model in which ADHD results from a genetically determined neurochemical imbalance that requires lifelong pharmacological management.

Methylphenidate is the most commonly used initial agent, at a dosage of 5 to 10 mg every 3 to 4 hours. Dosages may be increased to a maximum of 20 mg four times daily or 1 mg/kg a day. Use of the 20-mg sustained-release formulation to achieve 6 hours of benefit and eliminate the need for dosing at school is supported by many experts, although other authorities feel it is less effective than the immediate-release formulation. Dexmethylphenidate is prescribed at an initial dose of 2.5 mg and increased in 2.5- to 5-mg increments to a maximum of 10 mg twice a day.

Dextroamphetamine is approximately twice as potent as methylphenidate on a per-milligram basis and provides 6 to 8 hours of benefit. Some 70 percent of nonresponders to one sympathomimetic may benefit from another. All the sympathomimetic drugs should be tried before switching to drugs of a different class. The previous dictum that sympathomimetics worsen tics and therefore should be avoided by persons with comorbid ADHD and tic disorders has been questioned more recently because of reports that small to moderate dosages of sympathomimetics may be well tolerated without causing an increase in the frequency and severity of the tics. Alternatives to sympathomimetics for ADHD include bupropion (Wellbutrin), venlafaxine (Effexor), guanfacine (Tenex), clonidine (Catapres), and tricyclic drugs.

Short-term use of the sympathomimetics induces a euphoric feeling; however, tolerance can develop for both the euphoric feeling and the sympathomimetic activity. Tolerance does not develop for the therapeutic effects in ADHD.

Narcolepsy

Narcolepsy consists of sudden sleep attacks, sudden loss of postural tone (cataplexy), loss of voluntary motor control going into (hypnagogic) or coming out of (hypnopompic) sleep (sleep paralysis), and hypnagogic or hypnopompic hallucinations. Sympathomimetics reduce narcoleptic sleep attacks and also improve wakefulness in other types of hypersomnolent states. Sympathomimetics are used to maintain wakefulness and accuracy of motor performance in persons subject to sleep deprivation, such as pilots and military personnel. Persons with narcolepsy, unlike persons with ADHD, may develop tolerance for the therapeutic effects of the sympathomimetics.

Depressive Disorders

Sympathomimetics may be used for treatment-resistant depressive disorders, usually to augment standard antidepressant drug therapy. Possible indications for use of sympathomimetics as monotherapy include depression in the elderly, who are at increased risk for adverse effects from standard antidepressant drugs; depression in medically ill persons, especially persons with AIDS; obtundation due to chronic use of opioids; and clinical situations in which a rapid response is important but electroconvulsive therapy (ECT) is contraindicated. Depressed patients with abulia and anergia may also benefit.

Dextroamphetamine may be useful in differentiating pseudodementia of depression from dementia. A depressed person generally responds to a 5-mg dose with increased alertness and improved cognition. Sympathomimetics are thought to provide only short-term benefit (2 to 4 weeks) for depression, because most persons rapidly develop tolerance for the antidepressant effects of the drugs. However, some clinicians report that long-term treatment with sympathomimetics can benefit some persons.

Encephalopathy Due to Brain Injury

Sympathomimetics increase alertness, cognition, motivation, and motor performance in persons with neurological deficits caused by strokes, trauma, tumors, or chronic infections. Treatment with sympathomimetics may permit earlier and more robust participation in rehabilitative programs. Poststroke lethargy and apathy may respond to long-term use of sympathomimetics.

Obesity

Sympathomimetics are used in the treatment of obesity because of their anorexia-inducing effects. Because tolerance develops for the anorectic effects and because of the drugs' high abuse potential, their use for this indication is limited. Of the sympathomimetic drugs, phentermine is the most widely used for appetite suppression.

Careful limitation of caloric intake and judicious exercise are at the core of any successful weight loss program. Sympathomimetic drugs facilitate loss of, at most, an additional fraction of a pound per week. Sympathomimetic drugs are effective appetite suppressants only for the first few weeks of use; then the anorexigenic effects tend to decrease.

Other Disorders

As mentioned above, patients suffering from abulia or anergia as part of a depressive syndrome may benefit from sympathomimetics. These symptoms are also found in other conditions such as chronic fatigue syndrome, neurasthenia, fibromyalgia, dysthymia, and depressive personality disorder. In each of these conditions, psychostimulants have benefited individual patients. A daily dose of dextroamphetamine (5 to 15 mg) may enable patients to overcome their lethargy and engage in constructive activity. When using these medications, the potential development of tolerance and dependence must be considered and discussed with the patient, and drug use must be closely monitored. When prescribed appropriately, many patients are able to maintain the use of amphetamine at a daily stable dosage level for long periods.

PRECAUTIONS AND ADVERSE REACTIONS

The most common adverse effects associated with amphetamine-like drugs are stomach pain, anxiety, irritability, insomnia, tachycardia, cardiac arrhythmias, and dysphoria. Sympathomimetics decrease appetite, although tolerance usually develops for this effect. The treatment of common adverse effects in children with ADHD is usually straightforward. Use of these drugs can also increase the heart rate and the blood pressure and may cause palpitations. Less common adverse effects include the induction of movement disorders, such as tics, Tourette's disorder–like symptoms, and dyskinesias, which are often self-limited over 7 to 10 days. If a person taking a sympathomimetic develops one of these movement disorders, a correlation between the dose of the medication and the severity of the disorder must be firmly established prior to adjustments in the medication dosage. In severe cases, augmentation with risperidone (Risperdal), clonidine, or guanfacine is necessary. Methylphenidate may worsen tics in one-third of persons; these persons fall into two groups: those whose methylphenidate-induced tics resolve immediately upon metabolism of the dosage and a smaller group in whom methylphenidate appears to trigger tics that persist for several months but eventually resolve spontaneously.

Longitudinal studies do not indicate that sympathomimetics cause growth suppression. Sympathomimetics may exacerbate glaucoma, hypertension, cardiovascular disorders, hyperthyroidism, anxiety disorders, psychotic disorders, and seizure disorders.

High dosages of sympathomimetics can cause dry mouth, pupillary dilation, bruxism, formication, excessive ebullience, restlessness, and emotional lability. Long-term use of high dosages can cause a delusional disorder that resembles paranoid schizophrenia. Overdoses of sympathomimetics result in hypertension, tachycardia, hyperthermia, toxic psychosis, delirium, and occasionally seizures. Overdoses of sympathomimetics can also result in death, often due to cardiac arrhythmias. Seizures can be treated with benzodiazepines, cardiac effects with β-adrenergic receptor antagonists, fever with cooling blankets, and delirium with dopamine receptor antagonists.

The most limiting adverse effect of sympathomimetics is their association with psychological and physical dependence. At the doses used for treatment of ADHD, psychological dependence virtually never develops. A larger concern is the presence of adolescent or adult cohabitants who might confiscate the supply of sympathomimetics for abuse or sale.

The use of sympathomimetics should be avoided during pregnancy, especially during the first trimester. Dextroamphetamine and methylphenidate pass into the breast milk, and it is not known whether pemoline and modafinil do.

A review of postmarketing experience with pemoline from 1975 to 1996 found 13 cases of acute hepatic failure, 10 of which were in children. This prompted the Food and Drug Administration (FDA) to change the package insert to recommend that pemoline no longer be considered first-line therapy for ADHD.

DRUG–DRUG INTERACTIONS

Coadministration of sympathomimetics and tricyclic or tetracyclic antidepressants, warfarin (Coumadin), primidone (Mysoline), phenobarbital (Luminal), phenytoin (Dilantin), or phenylbutazone (Butazolidin) decreases the metabolism of these compounds, resulting in increased plasma levels. Sympathomimetics decrease the therapeutic efficacy of many antihypertensive drugs, especially guanethidine (Esimil, Ismelin). The sympathomimetics should be used with extreme caution with monoamine oxidase inhibitors (MAOIs).

LABORATORY INTERFERENCES

Dextroamphetamine may elevate plasma corticosteroid levels and interfere falsely with some assay methods for urinary corticosteroids.

DOSAGE AND ADMINISTRATION

The dosage ranges and the available preparations for some common sympathomimetics are presented in Table 32.3.28–1.

Pretreatment evaluation should include an evaluation of the person's cardiac function, with particular attention to the presence of hypertension or tachyarrhythmias. The clinician should also examine the person for the presence of movement disorders, such as tics and dyskinesia, because these conditions can be exacerbated by the use of sympathomimetics. If tics are present, many experts will not use sympathomimetics, but will instead choose clonidine or an antidepressant. However, recent data indicate that sympathomimetics may cause only a mild increase in motor tics and may actually suppress vocal tics. Liver function and renal function should be assessed, and dosages of sympathomimetics should be reduced for persons with impaired metabolism. In the case of pemoline, any elevation of liver enzymes is a compelling reason to discontinue use of the medication.

Persons with ADHD can take immediate-release methylphenidate at 8 AM, 12 noon, and 4 PM. Sustained-released amphetamine, sustained-release methylphenidate, or extended-release methylphenidate may be taken once at 8 AM. The starting dosage of methylphenidate ranges from 2.5 to 20 mg daily. If this is inadequate, the dosage may be increased to a maximum of 80 mg. Dexmethylphenidate is given twice daily, starting at 5 mg per day and increasing to 20 mg per day. The dosage of dextroamphetamine is 2.5 to 40 mg a day. Pemoline is given in dosages of 18.75 to 112.5 mg a day. Liver function tests should be monitored when using pemoline. Although it is not clear that routine liver screening can predict acute liver failure due to pemoline, it is certainly necessary to stop pemoline use if screening tests give any hint of hepatic dysfunction. Children are generally more sensitive to adverse effects than adults are. Dosing for treatment of narcolepsy and depression is comparable to that for treatment of ADHD.

Many psychiatrists believe that amphetamine use has been overly regulated by governmental authorities. Amphetamines are listed as Schedule II drugs by the U.S. Drug Enforcement Agency (DEA). In some states, physicians must use official prescriptions for such drugs, with a copy filed with a state government agency. Such mandates worry both patients and physicians about breaches in confidentiality, and physicians are concerned that their prescribing practices may be misinterpreted by official agencies. Consequently, some physicians may withhold prescriptions of sympathomimetics, even from persons who may benefit from the medications.

MODAFINIL

Modafinil (Provigil) is a unique compound among the currently approved psychostimulant drugs. Modafinil is approved for use in improving wakefulness in patients with excessive daytime sleepiness associated with narcolepsy. The mechanism of action is unknown, but the novel effects of modafinil are prompting clinicians to use the drug to treat daytime sleepiness in other neurologic and psychiatric conditions.

Pharmacological Actions

Modafinil is rapidly absorbed from the gastrointestinal (GI) tract and reaches peak plasma concentrations in 2 to 4 hours, has a half-life of approximately 15 hours, and reaches steady state after

Table 32.3.28–1
Sympathomimetics Commonly Used in Psychiatry

Generic Name	Trade Name	Preparations	Initial Daily Dose	Usual Daily Dose for ADHD[a]	Usual Daily Dose for Narcolepsy	Maximum Daily Dose
Amphetamine-dextro-amphetamine	Adderall	5-, 10-, 20-, 30-mg tablets; 10-, 20-, 30-mg extended-release (ER) tablets	5–10 mg	20–30 mg	5–60 mg	Children: 40 mg Adults: 60 mg
Dextroamphet-amine	Dexedrine, DextroStat	5-, 10-, 15-mg ER capsules; 5-, 10-mg tablets	5–10 mg	20–30 mg	5–60 mg	Children: 40 mg Adults: 60 mg
Modafinil	Provigil	100-, 200-mg tablets	100 mg	Not used	400 mg	400 mg
Methamphetamine	Desoxyn	5-mg tablets; 5-, 10-, 15-mg ER tablets	5–10 mg	20–25 mg	Not generally used	45 mg
Methylphenidate	Ritalin, Methi-date, Methy-lin, Attenade	5-, 10-, 15-, 20-mg tablets; 10-, 20-mg SR tablets	5–10 mg	5–60 mg	20–30 mg	Children: 80 mg Adults: 90 mg
	Concerta	18-, 36-, 54-mg ER tablets	18 mg	18–54 mg	Not yet estab-lished	54 mg
Dexmethylpheni-date	Focalin	2.5-, 5-, 10-mg tablets	2.5 mg	5–20 mg	Not yet estab-lished	60 mg
Pemoline	Cylert	18.75-, 37.5-, 75-mg tablets; 37.5 mg chewable tablets	37.5 mg	56.25–75 mg	Not used	112.5 mg

[a]For children 6 years of age or older.

2 to 4 days of daily dosing. Food does not affect the bioavailability of modafinil, but may delay its rate of absorption, which could be clinically meaningful if the patient is in need of therapeutic effects early in the morning. Modafinil is metabolized in the liver, and the metabolites are secreted primarily through the kidney.

The mechanism of action for the wakefulness-inducing properties of modafinil is not known. One possibility is that modafinil acts as a weak inhibitor of dopamine reuptake. This is supported in in vitro models by the observation of an increase in extracellular dopamine levels without an increase in dopamine release.

Therapeutic Indications

The only approved indication for modafinil is to reduce the daytime sleepiness in patients with narcolepsy. Since its introduction, however, clinicians have used modafinil to treat daytime sedation in other neurological and psychiatric disorders. The fatigue associated with depression has also been reported to be improved with the use of modafinil. Because of the effect on alertness, modafinil has been studied in children with ADHD, and some of the preliminary studies in this disorder have been positive.

Effects on Specific Organs and Systems

Central Nervous System.   Modafinil has been reported to be associated with euphoric effects and alterations in mood, perception, and thinking.

Cardiovascular System.   There were a small number of cardiovascular-related adverse effects in the narcolepsy clinical studies; therefore, it is currently not recommended that modafinil be used in combination with sympathomimetic drugs in patients who are at increased risk of cardiovascular disorders (e.g., his-

tory of left ventricular hypertrophy, ischemic electrocardiographic [ECG] changes, recent history of myocardial infarction).

Precautions and Adverse Effects

The most common adverse effects associated with modafinil use are headache and nausea. Modafinil is not associated with changes in vital signs, ECG measurements, or weight. In general, modafinil is a well-tolerated drug.

Abuse Potential.   Because modafinil has some properties somewhat similar to the sympathomimetic drugs, use of modafinil in patients with a history of stimulant abuse should be avoided or carefully monitored if prescribed. In clinical studies, no withdrawal symptoms were seen related to the discontinuation of modafinil use.

Pregnancy.   As with most other psychoactive drugs, modafinil should not be used in women who are pregnant. It is not known whether modafinil is excreted in human milk; therefore, nursing mothers should not be prescribed modafinil at this time.

Drug–Drug Interactions

Modafinil is metabolized by cytochrome P450 (CYP) isoenzyme 2C9 and also causes a modest induction of CYP 3A4 with chronic administration. An important result of the CYP 3A4 induction is that plasma concentrations of low-dose steroidal contraceptives may be reduced to levels below therapeutic effectiveness. Upward adjustment of the dose of low-dose steroidal contraceptives and some other drugs metabolized by CYP 3A4 (e.g., cyclosporine, theophylline) might be warranted. The competitive effects of modafinil on the enzyme CYP 2C9 could result in increased plasma concentrations of other CYP 2C9 substrates such as diazepam, phenytoin, and propranolol.

Laboratory Interferences

There have been no laboratory interferences reported for modafinil.

Dosage and Administration

Modafinil is supplied as 100- and 200-mg tablets. The starting dosage is 200 mg a day given once in the morning. Some patients may require 300 to 400 mg a day, also given once in the morning. These doses are for the approved indication in narcolepsy, but these are also the range of doses that have been used by clinicians in other indications as well.

ATOMOXETINE

Atomoxetine (Strattera) is a selective norepinephrine reuptake inhibitor used in the treatment of ADHD.

Pharmacological Actions

Atomoxetine is thought to be related to selective inhibition of the presynaptic norepinephrine transporter. It is well absorbed after oral administration and is minimally affected by food. It is eliminated primarily by oxidative metabolism through the cytochrome P450 2D6 (CYP 2D6) enzymatic pathway and subsequent glucuronidation.

Atomoxetine is excreted mainly in the urine (greater than 80 percent of the dose) and, to a lesser extent, in the feces (less than 17 percent of the dose). Atomoxetine has a half-life of approximately 5 hours.

Therapeutic Indications

Atomoxetine is indicated for the treatment of ADHD. Long-term use and effectiveness have not been systematically evaluated in controlled trials. Therefore, physicians should periodically reevaluate the long-term effects after 2 to 3 months of use.

Precautions and Adverse Reactions

Atomexetine should not be taken with a MAOI, or within 2 weeks after discontinuing an MAOI. There have been reports of serious, sometimes fatal, reactions when sympathomimetics are taken in combination with an MAOI. Such reactions may occur when these drugs are given concurrently or in close proximity.

In clinical trials, atomoxetine use was associated with an increased risk of mydriasis, and, therefore, its use is not recommended in patients with narrow angle glaucoma. Although uncommon, allergic reactions, including angioneurotic edema, urticaria, and rash, have been reported.

Atomoxetine should be used with caution in patients with hypertension, tachycardia, or cardiovascular disease because it can increase blood pressure and heart rate. Some persons have experienced orthostatic hypotension; therefore, the drug should be used with caution in patients predisposed to low blood pressure. In adults using the drug, urinary retention and urinary hes-

itation were increased; thus, urinary complaints should be considered potentially related to atomoxetine.

Drug–Drug Interactions

This medication should be administered with caution to patients being treated with systemically administered (oral or intravenous) albuterol (and other β_2 agonists) or pressor agents. The actions of those drugs on the cardiovascular system can be potentiated when used with atomoxetine.

Atomoxetine is primarily metabolized by the CYP 2D6 pathway to 4-hydroxyatomoxetine. Drugs that inhibit CYP 2D6, such as fluoxetine, paroxetine, and quinidine, cause increases in plasma levels. Atomoxetine should not be used during pregnancy or in lactating women.

Dosage and Clinical Guidelines

Atomoxetine should be initiated at a total daily dose of 40 mg and increased after a minimum of 3 days to a total daily dose of approximately 80 mg administered either as a single daily dose in the morning or as evenly divided doses in the morning and late afternoon or early evening. After 2 to 4 additional weeks, the dose may be increased to a maximum of 100 mg in patients who have not achieved an optimal response. There are no data that support increased effectiveness at higher doses. The maximum recommended total daily dose in children and adolescents over 70 kg and in adults is 100 mg. For those ADHD patients who have hepatic insufficiency, dosage adjustment should be reduced to 50 percent of the normal dose.

Atomoxetine is available in capsules of 10-, 18-, 25-, 40-, and 60-mg strengths. The drug can be discontinued without being tapered, as no withdrawal syndrome has been reported.

▲ 32.3.29 Trazodone

Trazodone (Desyrel) is effective in the treatment of depressive disorders. It is structurally unrelated to the tricyclic and tetracyclic drugs used to treat depressive disorders, the monoamine oxidase inhibitors (MAOIs), selective serotonin reuptake inhibitors (SSRIs), and other currently available antidepressant drugs. Trazodone may have benefit in anxiety disorders such as panic disorder and obsessive-compulsive disorder (OCD). It is chemically related to nefazodone (Serzone), which is discussed in Section 32.3.21.

Trazodone is a weak inhibitor of serotonin reuptake and has a half-life of 14 hours. It has no anticholinergic effects.

EFFECTS ON SPECIFIC ORGANS AND SYSTEMS

Aside from its effects on the central nervous system (CNS), trazodone has relatively few effects on organs and systems. The effects it does have are primarily the result of its α_1-adrenergic antagonism, which can affect vascular tone and result in orthostatic hypotension. The drug is also associated with gastric irritation. Relatively rare among the antidepressants is trazodone's association with priapism, which is also probably a result of its α_1-adrenergic antagonist activity. Trazodone has weak activity as a relaxer of skeletal muscles.

THERAPEUTIC INDICATIONS

Depressive Disorders

The primary indication for the use of trazodone is major depressive disorder. Trazodone is as effective as the standard antidepressants in short-term and long-term treatment of major depressive disorder. The drug is particularly effective at improving sleep quality—increasing total sleep time, decreasing the number and duration of nighttime awakenings, and decreasing the amount of rapid eye movement (REM) sleep. Unlike tricyclic drugs, trazodone does not decrease stage 4 sleep. Trazodone may be less likely than tricyclic drugs to precipitate mania.

Insomnia

The marked sedative qualities of trazodone and its favorable effects on sleep architecture have suggested to many clinicians that it would be effective as a hypnotic, and a number of clinicians have used trazodone effectively for this purpose. A recent controlled study confirmed that trazodone is superior to placebo for treatment of insomnia. It has also been used effectively as a hypnotic in combination with less sedating psychotropic drugs. Trazodone has been reported to be useful in treating fluoxetine (Prozac)-induced insomnia. The usual dosage is 50 to 100 mg at bedtime.

Other Indications

Some data indicate that trazodone may be useful in low dosages (50 mg a day) for controlling severe agitation in elderly patients, particularly those with personality change due to a general medical condition. A few case reports and uncontrolled trials of trazodone have indicated its usefulness in the treatment of depression with marked anxiety symptoms, of posttraumatic stress disorder (PTSD), and of panic disorder with agoraphobia. Because it does not worsen psychotic symptoms, trazodone is preferable to tricyclic drugs as adjunctive treatment for schizophrenia. Limited data support an adjunctive role for trazodone in treatment of alcohol-induced tremor, alcohol-induced depressive disorder, and alcohol-induced anxiety disorder; anxiety; OCD; eating disorders; chronic pain; autistic disorder; male erectile disorder; and paraphilias. The final evaluation of the use of trazodone in the treatment of these disorders requires further research.

PRECAUTIONS AND ADVERSE REACTIONS

The most common adverse effects associated with trazodone are sedation, orthostatic hypotension, dizziness, headache, and nausea. As a result of α_1-adrenergic blockade, dry mouth is present in some patients. Trazodone may also cause gastric irritation. The drug is not associated with the usual anticholinergic adverse effects, such as urinary retention and constipation. A few case reports have noted an association between trazodone and arrhythmias in patients with preexisting premature ventricular contractions or mitral valve prolapse. Neutropenia, usually not clinically significant, may develop and should be considered if patients have fever or sore throat.

Trazodone is relatively safe in overdose attempts. No fatalities from trazodone overdoses have been reported when the drug was taken alone, but there have been fatalities when trazodone was taken with other drugs. The symptoms of overdose include priapism, loss of muscle coordination, nausea and vomiting, and drowsiness. Trazodone does not have the quinidine-like antiarrhythmic effects of imipramine (Tofranil).

As mentioned above, trazodone is associated with the rare occurrence of priapism, prolonged erection in the absence of sexual stimuli. Patients should be advised to tell their clinicians if erections are gradually becoming frequent or prolonged. Physicians should strongly consider switching these patients to another antidepressant medication. Other forms of sexual dysfunction may also occur with trazodone treatment. The use of trazodone is contraindicated in pregnant and nursing women, and it should be used with caution in patients with hepatic and renal diseases.

DRUG–DRUG INTERACTIONS

Trazodone potentiates the CNS depressant effects of other centrally acting drugs and alcohol. The combination of MAOIs and trazodone should be avoided. Trazodone concentrations are increased by fluoxetine, and trazodone increases concentrations of digoxin (Lanoxin) and phenytoin (Dilantin). Concurrent use of trazodone and antihypertensives may cause hypotension. Electroconvulsive therapy (ECT) concurrent with trazodone administration should also be avoided.

LABORATORY INTERFERENCES

No known laboratory interferences are associated with the use of trazodone.

DOSAGE AND ADMINISTRATION

The sedative effects of trazodone appear within 1 hour of administration, whereas the antidepressant effects usually appear after 2 to 4 weeks of treatment. Trazodone is available in tablets that can be divided into 50-, 100-, 150-, and 300-mg amounts. The usual starting dose is 50 mg orally the first day. The dosage can be increased to 50 mg orally twice daily on the second day and possibly 50 mg orally three times daily on the third and fourth days if sedation or orthostatic hypotension does not become a problem. The therapeutic range for trazodone is 200 to 600 mg a day in divided doses. Some reports indicate that dosages of 400 to 600 mg a day are required for maximal therapeutic effects; other reports indicate that 300 to 400 mg a day is sufficient. The dosage may be titrated up to 300 mg a day; then the patient can be evaluated for the need for further dosage increases on the basis of the presence or the absence of signs of clinical improvement.

▲ 32.3.30 Tricyclics and Tetracyclics

The tricyclic antidepressants and the tetracyclic antidepressants (commonly abbreviated TCAs) are effective treatments for persons with a wide range of disorders, including depression, panic disorder, generalized anxiety disorder, posttraumatic stress disorder (PTSD), obsessive-compulsive disorder (OCD), eating disorders, and pain syndromes. With the current availability of several less toxic alternatives, including the selective serotonin reuptake inhibitors (SSRIs), bupropion (Wellbutrin), nefazodone (Serzone), venlafaxine (Effexor), trazodone (Desyrel), and mirtazapine (Remeron), the TCAs are no longer widely used for these indications.

PHARMACOLOGICAL ACTIONS

Most TCAs are completely absorbed from oral administration, and there is significant metabolism from the first-pass effect. Peak plasma concentrations occur within 2 to 8 hours, and the half-lives of the TCAs vary from 10 to 70 hours; nortriptyline (Pamelor, Aventyl), maprotiline, and particularly protriptyline (Vivactil) can have longer half-lives. The long half-lives allow all these compounds to be given once daily; 5 to 7 days are needed to reach steady-state plasma concentrations. Imipramine pamoate is a depot form of the drug for intramuscular (IM) administration; indications for the use of this preparation are limited. TCAs block the reuptake of norepinephrine and serotonin and are competitive antagonists at the muscarinic acetylcholine, histamine H_1, and α_1- and β_2-adrenergic receptors.

EFFECTS ON SPECIFIC ORGANS AND SYSTEMS

The major effects of the TCAs are on the central nervous system (CNS), although the anticholinergic effects of these drugs produce a diverse range of adverse effects mediated by the autonomic nervous system. In addition to these effects, the TCAs have significant effects on the cardiovascular system. In therapeutic dosages, the drugs are classified as type 1A antiarrhythmic drugs, as they terminate ventricular fibrillation and can increase the collateral blood supply to an ischemic heart. In overdoses, however, the drugs are highly cardiotoxic and cause decreased contractility, increased myocardial irritability, hypotension, and tachycardia.

THERAPEUTIC INDICATIONS

Major Depressive Disorder

The treatment of a major depressive episode and the prophylactic treatment of major depressive disorder are the principal indications for using TCAs. The drugs are also effective in treating depression in patients with bipolar I disorder. Melancholic features, previous major depressive episodes, and a family history of depressive disorders increase the likelihood of a therapeutic response. The treatment of a major depressive episode with psychotic features almost always requires coadministration of an antipsychotic drug and an antidepressant.

Mood Disorder Due to a General Medical Condition with Depressive Features

Depression associated with a general medical condition (secondary depression) may respond to TCA treatment. Depression is associated with dementias and with movement disorders such as Parkinson's disease. Depression associated with acquired immune deficiency syndrome (AIDS) may respond to the drugs.

Panic Disorder with Agoraphobia

Imipramine (Tofranil) is the tricyclic most studied for panic disorder with agoraphobia, but other TCAs are also effective. Early reports indicated that small dosages of imipramine (50 mg a day) were often effective; recent studies, however, indicate that the usual antidepressant dosages are usually required. In the past few years, SSRIs, especially paroxetine (Paxil), have become additional agents for treatment of panic disorder.

Generalized Anxiety Disorder

The use of doxepin (Adapin, Sinequan) to treat anxiety disorders is approved by the U.S. Food and Drug Administration (FDA). Some research data show that imipramine may also be useful, and some clinicians use a drug containing a combination of chlordiazepoxide and amitriptyline (Limbitrol) for mixed anxiety and depressive disorders.

Obsessive-Compulsive Disorder

Obsessive-compulsive disorder is classified as an anxiety disorder. The disorder appears to respond specifically to clomipramine and SSRIs. None of the other TCAs appears to be nearly as effective as clomipramine for the disorder. Multicenter, placebo-controlled trials found clomipramine to be superior to SSRIs, and another controlled trial found paroxetine to be equal in efficacy to clomipramine for treatment of OCD.

Eating Disorders

Both anorexia nervosa and bulimia nervosa have been treated successfully with imipramine and desipramine (Norpramin, Pertofane), although other TCAs may also be effective.

Pain Disorder

Chronic pain disorder, including headache (such as migraine), is often treated with TCAs.

Other Disorders

Childhood enuresis is often treated with imipramine. Peptic ulcer disease can be treated with doxepin, which has marked antihistaminergic effects. Other indications for tricyclics and tetracyclics are narcolepsy, nightmare disorder, and PTSD. The drugs are sometimes used for children and adolescents with attention-deficit/hyperactivity disorder (ADHD), sleepwalking disorder, separation anxiety disorder, and sleep terror disorder. Clomipramine has been used to treat premature ejaculation, movement disorders, and compulsive behavior in children with autistic disorder.

PRECAUTIONS AND ADVERSE REACTIONS

Psychiatric Effects

A major adverse effect of all TCAs and other antidepressants is the possibility of inducing a manic episode in patients with and without a history of bipolar I disorder. Clinicians should watch for this effect in patients with bipolar I disorder, especially if substance-induced mania has been a problem in the past. It is prudent to use low dosages of TCAs in such patients or to use an agent such as fluoxetine (Prozac) or bupropion, which may be less likely to induce a manic episode. TCAs have also been reported to exacerbate psychotic disorders in susceptible patients.

Anticholinergic Effects

Clinicians should warn patients that anticholinergic effects are common but that patients may develop a tolerance for these effects with continued treatment. Amitriptyline (Elavil, Endep), imipramine, trimipramine (Surmontil), and doxepin are the most anticholinergic drugs; amoxapine (Asendin), nortriptyline, and maprotiline are less anticholinergic; and desipramine may be the least anticholinergic. Anticholinergic effects include dry mouth, constipation, blurred vision, and urinary retention. Sugarless gum, candy, or fluoride lozenges can alleviate the dry mouth. Bethanechol (Urecholine), 25 to 50 mg three or four times a day, may reduce urinary hesitancy and may help patients with impotence if the drug is taken 30 minutes before sexual intercourse. Narrow-angle glaucoma can also be aggravated by anticholinergic drugs, and precipitation of glaucoma requires emergency treatment with a miotic agent. TCAs can be used in patients with narrow-angle glaucoma, provided pilocarpine eyedrops are administered concurrently. Severe anticholinergic effects can lead to a CNS anticholinergic syndrome with confusion and delirium, especially if TCAs are administered with antipsychotics or anticholinergic drugs. Some clinicians have used intramuscular (IM) or intravenous (IV) physostigmine (Antilirium) as a diagnostic tool to confirm the presence of anticholinergic delirium.

Sedation

Sedation is a common effect of TCAs and may be welcomed if sleeplessness has been a problem. The sedative effect of TCAs results from serotonergic, cholinergic, and histaminergic (H_1) activities. Amitriptyline, trimipramine, and doxepin are the most sedating agents; imipramine, amoxapine, nortriptyline, and maprotiline have some sedating effects; and desipramine and protriptyline are the least sedating agents.

Autonomic Effects

The most common autonomic effect, partly because of α_1-adrenergic blockade, is orthostatic hypotension, which can result in falls and injuries in affected patients. Nortriptyline may be the drug least likely to cause the problem, and some patients respond to fludrocortisone (Florinef), 0.05 mg twice a day. Other possible autonomic effects are profuse sweating, palpitations, and increased blood pressure.

Cardiac Effects

When administered in their usual therapeutic dosages, the TCAs may cause tachycardia, flattened T waves, prolonged QT intervals, and depressed ST segments on electrocardiograms (ECGs). Imipramine has a quinidine-like effect at therapeutic plasma concentrations and may reduce the number of premature ventricular contractions. Because the drugs prolong conduction time, their use in patients with preexisting conduction defects is contraindicated. In patients with cardiac histories, TCAs should be initiated at low dosages, with gradual increases in dosage and monitoring of cardiac functions. At high plasma concentrations, as occur in overdoses, the drugs become arrhythmogenic. The agents should be discontinued several days before elective surgery because of the occurrence of hypertensive episodes during surgery in patients receiving TCAs.

Neurological Effects

In addition to the sedation induced by TCAs and the possibility of anticholinergic-induced delirium, two tricyclics—desipramine and protriptyline—are associated with psychomotor stimulation. Myoclonic twitches and tremors of the tongue and the upper extremities are common. Rare effects include speech blockage, paresthesia, peroneal palsies, and ataxia.

Amoxapine is unique in causing parkinsonian symptoms, akathisia, and even dyskinesia because of the dopaminergic blocking activity of one of its metabolites. Amoxapine may also cause neuroleptic malignant syndrome in rare cases. Maprotiline may cause seizures when the dosage is increased too quickly or is kept at high levels for too long. Clomipramine and amoxapine may lower the seizure threshold more than other drugs in the class. As a class, however, the TCAs have a relatively low risk for inducing seizures, except in patients who are at risk for seizures (e.g., patients with epilepsy or brain lesions). Although TCAs can still be used in such patients, the initial dosages should be lower than usual, and subsequent dosage increases should be gradual.

Allergic and Hematological Effects

Exanthematous rashes are seen in 4 to 5 percent of all patients treated with maprotiline. Jaundice is rare. Agranulocytosis, leukocytosis, leukopenia, and eosinophilia are rare complications of tetracyclic drug treatment. A patient who has a sore throat or a fever during the first few months of TCA treatment, however, should have a complete blood count (CBC) done immediately.

Other Adverse Effects

Weight gain, primarily an effect of the blockade of histamine type 2 (H_2) receptors, is common. If weight gain is a major problem, changing to a different class of antidepressants may help. Impotence, an occasional problem, is perhaps most often associated with amoxapine because of the drug's blockade of dopamine receptors in the tuberoinfundibular tract. Amoxapine can also cause hyperprolactinemia, galactorrhea, anorgasmia, and ejaculatory disturbances. Other TCAs have also been associated with gynecomastia and amenorrhea. Inappropriate secretion of antidiuretic hormone has also been reported with TCAs. Other effects include nausea, vomiting, and hepatitis.

Precautions

The TCAs should be avoided during pregnancy. The drugs pass into breast milk and can potentially cause serious adverse reactions in nursing infants. A case series suggested, however, that clomipramine at therapeutic concentrations in women who are breast-feeding does not produce detectable concentrations in the infant. The drugs should be used with caution in patients with hepatic and renal diseases. TCAs should not be administered during a course of electroconvulsive therapy (ECT), primarily because of the risk of serious adverse cardiac effects.

DRUG–DRUG INTERACTIONS

Antihypertensives

TCAs block the neuronal reuptake of guanethidine (Ismelin), which is required for antihypertensive activity. The antihypertensive effects of β-adrenergic receptor antagonists (e.g., propranolol [Inderal]) and clonidine (Catapres) may also be blocked by TCAs. Coadministration of a TCA and methyldopa (Aldomet) may cause behavioral agitation.

Antipsychotics

The plasma concentrations of TCAs and antipsychotics are increased by their coadministration. Antipsychotics also add to the anticholinergic and sedative effects of the TCAs.

Central Nervous System Depressants

Opioids, alcohol, anxiolytics, hypnotics, and over-the-counter cold medications have additive effects by causing CNS depression when coadministered with TCAs.

Sympathomimetics

Tricyclic drug use with sympathomimetic drugs may cause serious cardiovascular effects.

Oral Contraceptives

Birth control pills may decrease TCA plasma concentrations via the induction of hepatic enzymes.

Other Interactions

TCA plasma concentrations may also be increased by acetazolamide (Diamox), aspirin, cimetidine, thiazide diuretics, fluoxetine, and sodium bicarbonate. Decreased plasma concentrations may be caused by ascorbic acid, ammonium chloride, barbiturates, cigarette smoking, chloral hydrate, lithium (Eskalith), and primidone (Mysoline). Tricyclic drugs that are metabolized by cytochrome P450 (CYP) 2D6 may interfere with the metabolism of other drugs metabolized by the hepatic enzyme.

LABORATORY INTERFERENCES

Laboratory interferences with the TCAs have not been reported.

DOSAGE AND CLINICAL GUIDELINES

Persons who intend to take TCAs should undergo routine physical and laboratory examination, including a CBC, a white blood cell (WBC) count with differential, and serum electrolytes with liver function tests. An ECG should be obtained for

Table 32.3.30–1
General Information for the Tricyclic and Tetracyclic Antidepressants

Generic Name	Trade Name	Usual Adult Dosage Range (mg a day)	Therapeutic Plasma Concentrations (mg per mL)
Imipramine	Tofranil	150–300	150–300[a]
Desipramine	Norpramin, Pertofrane	150–300	150–300[a]
Trimipramine	Surmontil	150–300	?
Amitriptyline	Elavil, Endep	150–300	100–250[b]
Nortriptyline	Pamelor, Aventyl	50–150	50–150[a] (maximum)
Protriptyline	Vivactil	15–60	75–250
Amoxapine	Asendin	150–400	?
Doxepin	Adapin, Sinequan	150–300	100–250[a]
Maprotiline	Ludiomil	150–230	150–300[a]
Clomipramine	Anafranil	130–250	?

[a]Exact range may vary among laboratories.
[b]Includes parent compound and desmethyl metabolite.

all persons, especially women over 40 and men over 30. TCAs are contraindicated in persons with a QTc above 450 milliseconds. The initial dose should be small and should be raised gradually. Because of the availability of highly effective alternatives to TCAs, a newer agent should be used if there is any medical condition that may interact adversely with the TCAs. Elderly persons and children are more sensitive to TCA adverse effects than are young adults. In children, the ECG should be monitored regularly during use of a TCA. The available preparations of TCAs and their dosage ranges are presented in Table 32.3.30–1.

Persons with chronic pain may be particularly sensitive to adverse effects when TCA use is started. Therefore, treatment should begin with low dosages that are raised in small increments. However, persons with chronic pain may experience relief on long-term low-dosage therapy, such as amitriptyline or nortriptyline at 10 to 75 mg a day.

TCAs should be avoided in children, except as a last resort. Dosing guidelines in children for imipramine include initiation at 1.5 mg/kg a day. The dosage can be titrated to no more than 5 mg/kg a day. In enuresis, the dosage is usually 50 to 100 mg a day taken at bedtime. Clomipramine use can be initiated at 50 mg a day and increased to no more than 3 mg/kg a day or 200 mg a day.

Overdose Attempts

Overdose attempts with TCAs are serious and can often be fatal. Prescriptions for these drugs should be nonrefillable and for no longer than a week at a time for patients at risk for suicide. Amoxapine may be more likely than the other TCAs to result in death when taken in overdose. The newer antidepressants are safer in overdose.

Symptoms of overdose include agitation, delirium, convulsions, hyperactive deep tendon reflexes, bowel and bladder paralysis, dysregulation of blood pressure and temperature, and mydriasis. The patient then progresses to coma and perhaps respiratory depression. Cardiac arrhythmias may not respond to treatment. Because of the long half-lives of TCAs, the patients are at risk of cardiac arrhythmias for 3 to 4 days after the overdose, so they should be monitored in an intensive care medical setting.

Monoamine Oxidase Inhibitors (MAOIs).

MAOIs should be discontinued for 2 weeks before initiating treatment with a TCA. A minimum of a 1-week washout is needed when switching from a TCA tetracyclic to an MAOI.

Termination of Short-Term Treatment

TCAs effectively resolve the acute symptoms of depression. If treatment is stopped prematurely, symptoms are likely to reemerge. To minimize the risk for recurrence or relapse, clinicians should continue the TCA at the same treatment dosage throughout the course of treatment. When treatment is discontinued, clinicians may reasonably reduce the dosage to three-fourths of the maximal dosage for another month. At this time, if no symptoms are present, the drug can be tapered by 25 mg (5 mg for protriptyline) every 2 to 3 days. The slow tapering process is indicated for most psychotherapeutic drugs; in the case of most TCAs, slow tapering avoids a cholinergic rebound syndrome, consisting of nausea, upset stomach, sweating, headache, neck pain, and vomiting. This syndrome can be treated by reinstituting a small dosage of the drug and tapering use more slowly than before. Several case reports note the appearance of rebound mania or hypomania after abrupt discontinuation of TCAs. If a patient has been treated with lithium augmentation, the clinician should probably taper and stop use of the lithium first and then the tricyclic or tetracyclic drug. But clinical studies supporting this approach are lacking, and the guidelines may change as more physicians report their experience with this drug combination.

▲ 32.3.31 Valproate

Valproate (Depakene), also called *valproic acid* (because it is rapidly converted to the acid form in the stomach) and *divalproex* (Depakote), has been shown to be effective for absence seizures, generalized epilepsy, and partial epilepsy with or without secondary generalization and for prophylaxis against migraine headaches. In addition, valproate and two other anticonvulsant drugs, carbamazepine (Tegretol) and clonazepam (Klonopin), have been shown to be effective in treating bipolar I disorder.

PHARMACOLOGICAL ACTIONS

All valproate formulations are rapidly and completely absorbed after oral administration. The steady-state half-life of valproate is about 8 to 17 hours, and clinically effective plasma concentrations can usually be maintained with dosing one to four times a day. Protein binding becomes saturated and concentrations of therapeutically effective free valproate increase at serum concentrations above 50 to 100 mg/mL.

The therapeutic effects of valproate in bipolar I disorder may be mediated by as-yet-undefined effects of the drug on the γ-aminobutyric acid (GABA) neurotransmitter system.

THERAPEUTIC INDICATIONS

Bipolar I Disorder

Acute Episodes.   Valproate controls manic symptoms in approximately two-thirds of persons with acute mania. Valproate also reduces overall psychiatric symptoms and the need for supplemental doses of benzodiazepines or dopamine receptor antagonists. Persons with mania usually respond 1 to 4 days after valproate serum concentrations rise above 50 mg/mL. Using gradual dosing strategies, this serum concentration may be achieved within 1 week of initiation of dosing, but newer, rapid oral-loading strategies achieve therapeutic serum concentrations in 1 day and can control manic symptoms within 5 days. The short-term antimanic effects of valproate can be augmented with addition of lithium, carbamazepine, or dopamine receptor antagonists. Serotonin-dopamine antagonists (SDAs) and gabapentin (Neurotonin) may also potentiate the effects of valproate, albeit less rapidly. Because of its more favorable profile of cognitive, dermatological, thyroid, and renal adverse effects, valproate is preferred to lithium (Eskalith) for treatment of acute mania in children and elderly persons.

Valproate alone is less effective for the short-term treatment of depressive episodes in bipolar I disorder than for treatment of manic episodes. Among depressive symptoms, valproate is more effective for treatment of agitation than dysphoria.

Prophylaxis.   Valproate is effective in the prophylactic treatment of bipolar I disorder, resulting in fewer, less severe, and shorter manic episodes. In direct comparison, valproate is at least as effective as lithium and is better tolerated than lithium. Compared with lithium, valproate may be particularly effective in persons with rapid-cycling and ultrarapid-cycling bipolar disorders, dysphoric or mixed mania, and mania due to a general medical condition and in persons who have comorbid substance abuse or panic attacks or who have not had completely favorable responses to lithium treatment. Addition of valproate to lithium may be more effective than use of lithium alone.

In persons with bipolar I disorder, maintenance valproate treatment markedly reduces the frequency and severity of manic episodes but is only mildly to moderately effective in the prophylactic treatment of depressive episodes. The prophylactic effectiveness of valproate can be augmented by addition of lithium, carbamazepine, dopamine receptor antagonists, SDAs, antidepressant drugs, gabapentin, or lamotrigine (Lamictal).

Schizoaffective Disorder

Valproate is effective in treating the short-term phase of the bipolar type of schizoaffective disorder, but valproate alone is generally less effective in schizoaffective disorder than in bipolar I disorder. Valproate may be an effective adjunct agent for use with lithium, carbamazepine, or a SDA by persons with schizoaffective disorder. Valproate alone is ineffective for treatment of psychotic symptoms.

Other Mental Disorders

Valproate can be effective for treatment of intermittent explosive disorder, kleptomania, and other behavioral dyscontrol syndromes, particularly if these disorders are comorbid with bipolar symptoms. Valproate can control physical aggression, restlessness, agitation, and (to a lesser degree) verbal aggression associated with dementia, organic brain diseases, or traumatic brain injury, although it should be considered for use only after therapeutic trials of benzodiazepines and SDAs have failed. Valproate may be effective alone or in combination with other psychotropic drugs in treatment of other mental disorders, including major depressive disorder; panic disorder; posttraumatic stress disorder (PTSD); obsessive-compulsive disorder (OCD); bulimia nervosa; alcohol and sedative, hypnotic, or anxiolytic (particularly benzodiazepine) withdrawal; symptoms of borderline personality disorder; and cocaine detoxification.

PRECAUTIONS AND ADVERSE REACTIONS

The common adverse effects associated with valproate are those affecting the gastrointestinal (GI) system, such as nausea, vomiting, dyspepsia, and diarrhea. Other common adverse effects involve the nervous system, such as sedation, ataxia, dysarthria, and tremor. Valproate-induced tremor may respond well to treatment with β-adrenergic receptor antagonists or gabapentin. Treatment of the other neurological adverse effects usually requires lowering the valproate dosage.

Weight gain is a common adverse effect, especially in long-term treatment, and can best be treated by strict limitation of caloric intake. Hair loss may occur in 5 to 10 percent of all persons treated, and rare cases of complete loss of body hair have been reported. The two most serious adverse effects of valproate treatment affect the pancreas and the liver. Risk factors for potentially fatal hepatotoxicity include young age (less than 3 years), concurrent use of phenobarbital (Luminal, Solfoton), and the presence of neurological disorders, especially inborn errors of metabolism. The rate of fatal hepatotoxicity in persons who have been treated with only valproate is 0.85 per 100,000 persons; no persons over the age of 10 years are reported to have died from fatal hepatotoxicity. Therefore, the risk of this adverse reaction in adult psychiatric persons seems low. Nevertheless, if symptoms of lethargy, malaise, anorexia, nausea and vomiting, edema, and abdominal pain occur in a person treated with valproate, the clinician must consider the possibility of severe hepatotoxicity. A modest increase in liver function test results does not correlate with the development of serious hepatotoxicity. Rare cases of pancreatitis have been reported; they occur most often in the first 6 months of treatment, and the condition occasionally results in death. Pancreatic function can be assessed and followed with serum amylase determinations.

Valproate should not be used by pregnant or nursing women. The drug is associated with neural tube defects (e.g., spina bifida) in approximately 1 to 2 percent of all women who take valproate during the first trimester of the pregnancy. Women who require valproate therapy should therefore inform their physicians if they intend to become pregnant. Infants breast-fed by mothers taking valproate develop serum valproate concentrations 1 to 10 percent of maternal serum concentrations. No data suggest that this poses a risk to the infant; however, valproate is relatively contraindicated in nursing mothers. Rare cases of polycystic ovary disease have been reported in women using valproate.

EFFECTS ON SPECIFIC ORGANS AND SYSTEMS

Although the principal effects of valproate are on the central nervous system (CNS), the drug also affects the GI and hematopoietic systems. The effects on the GI system lead both to common adverse effects (e.g., nausea) and to serious but rare effects (e.g., fatal hepatotoxicity).

DRUG–DRUG INTERACTIONS

Valproate is commonly coadministered with lithium, carbamazepine, and dopamine receptor antagonists. The only consistent drug interaction with lithium, if both drugs are maintained in their respective therapeutic ranges, is the exacerbation of drug-induced tremors, which can usually be treated with β-receptor antagonists. Plasma concentrations of valproate may be decreased when the drug is coadministered with carbamazepine and may be increased when coadministered with amitriptyline or fluoxetine (Prozac). Valproate can be displaced from plasma proteins by carbamazepine, diazepam, and aspirin. Persons who are treated with anticoagulants (e.g., aspirin and warfarin [Coumadin]) should also be monitored when valproate use is initiated, to detect the development of any undesired augmentation of the anticoagulation effects.

LABORATORY INTERFERENCES

Valproate use has been reported to cause an overestimation of serum free fatty acids in almost half of the patients tested. Valproate use has also been reported to elevate urinary ketone estimations falsely and to result in falsely abnormal thyroid function test results.

DOSAGE AND ADMINISTRATION

Prior to administration of valproate, hepatic and pancreatic disease should be ruled out by a combination of clinical and laboratory evaluations. Valproate is available in a number of formulations and dosages (Table 32.3.31–1). It is best to initiate drug treatment gradually to minimize the common adverse effects of nausea, vomiting, and sedation. The dose on the first day should be 250 mg administered with a meal. The dosage can be raised to 250 mg orally three times daily over the course of 3 to 6 days. Plasma concentrations can be assessed in the morning before the first daily dose of the drug is administered. Therapeutic plasma concentrations for the control of seizures range between 50 and 100 mg/mL, although some physicians use 125 or even 150 mg/mL if the drug is well tolerated. It is reasonable to use the same range for the treatment of mental disorders; most of the controlled studies have used 50 to 100 mg/mL. Most patients attain therapeutic plasma concentrations on a daily dose between 1,200 and 1,500 mg in divided doses. The mood-stabilizing effects of valproate appear between 5 and 15 days after initiation of treatment.

Table 32.3.31–1
Valproate Preparations Available in the United States

Generic Name	Trade Name, Form (doses)	Time to Peak
Valproate sodium injection	Depacon injection (100 mg valproic acid/mL)	1 h
Valproic acid	Depakene, syrup (250 mg/5 mL)	1–2 h
	Depakene, capsules (250 mg)	1–2 h
Divalproex sodium	Depakote, delayed-released tablets (125, 250, 500 mg)	3–8 h
Divalproex sodium-coated particles in capsules	Depakote, sprinkle capsules (125 mg)	Compared with divalproex tablets, divalproex sprinkle has earlier onset and slower absorption, with slightly lower peak plasma concentration

▲ 32.3.32 Venlafaxine

Venlafaxine (Effexor) is an effective antidepressant drug that may have a faster onset of action than other antidepressant drugs when the dosage is increased rapidly. Venlafaxine is among the most efficacious drugs for treatment of severe depression with melancholic features. Venlafaxine has also been approved by the Food and Drug Administration (FDA) for treatment of generalized anxiety disorder. A related drug, duloxetine (Cymbalta), is discussed at the end of this section.

PHARMACOLOGICAL ACTIONS

Venlafaxine is well absorbed from the gastrointestinal (GI) tract. The immediate-release formulation of venlafaxine and the sustained-release formulation reach peak plasma concentrations in 5.5 hours and 9 hours, respectively. Venlafaxine has a half-life of approximately 3.5 hours, and the sustained-release form has a half-life of 9 hours.

Venlafaxine is a potent inhibitor of serotonin and norepinephrine reuptake and a weak inhibitor of dopamine reuptake. Venlafaxine does not have activity at muscarinic, nicotinic, histaminergic, opioid, or adrenergic receptors, and it is not active as a monoamine oxidase inhibitor (MAOI). It is metabolized in the liver by cytochrome P450 isoenzyme 2D6 (CYP 2D6).

THERAPEUTIC INDICATIONS

Depression

Venlafaxine is used for the treatment of major depressive disorder. Severely depressed persons may respond within 2 weeks to 200 mg a day of venlafaxine, which is somewhat faster than the 2 to 4 weeks usually required for the selective serotonin reuptake inhibitors (SSRIs). Therefore, high-dosage venlafaxine may become a preferred drug to use for seriously ill persons when a rapid response is desired. In studies directly comparing fluoxetine (Prozac) with venlafaxine for the treatment of seriously depressed persons with melancholic features, venlafaxine has consistently been superior in terms of rate of response, percentage response, and completeness of response. No direct comparisons of venlafaxine and sertraline (Zoloft), one of the most effective SSRI for treatment of seriously depressed persons with melancholic features, have been described.

Generalized and Social Anxiety Disorders

The extended-release formulation of venlafaxine is approved for treatment of generalized and social anxiety disorders. In clinical trials, dosages of 75 to 225 mg a day were effective against insomnia, poor concentration, restlessness, irritability, and excessive muscle tension related to generalized anxiety disorder.

Other Indications

Case reports and uncontrolled studies have indicated that venlafaxine may be beneficial in the treatment of obsessive-compulsive disorder (OCD), panic disorder, agoraphobia, social phobia, and attention-deficit/hyperactivity disorder (ADHD). It has also been used in chronic pain syndromes with good effect.

PRECAUTIONS AND ADVERSE REACTIONS

Venlafaxine has generally been reported to be well tolerated. The most common adverse reactions are nausea, somnolence, dry mouth, dizziness, nervousness, constipation, asthenia, anxiety, anorexia, blurred vision, abnormal ejaculation or orgasm, erectile disturbances, and impotence. The incidence of nausea is reduced considerably with use of the extended-release capsules. Abrupt discontinuation of venlafaxine use may produce a discontinuation syndrome consisting of nausea, somnolence, and insomnia. Therefore, venlafaxine use should be tapered gradually over 2 to 4 weeks.

The most potentially worrisome adverse effect associated with venlafaxine is an increase in blood pressure in some persons, particularly those who are treated with more than 300 mg a day. In clinical trials, a mean increase of 7.2 mm Hg in diastolic blood pressure was observed in persons who were receiving 375 mg a day of venlafaxine, in contrast to no significant change in persons receiving 75 or 225 mg a day.

No information concerning use of venlafaxine by pregnant and nursing women is available at this time. Clinicians should avoid the use of venlafaxine by pregnant and nursing women until more clinical experience has been gained.

DRUG–DRUG INTERACTIONS

Cimetidine (Tagamet) appears to inhibit the first-pass hepatic metabolism of venlafaxine and to raise the levels of the unmetabolized drug. However, since the metabolite is mainly responsible for the therapeutic effect, this interaction is of concern only in persons with preexisting hypertension or hepatic disease, in whom this combination should be avoided. Venlafaxine may raise plasma concentrations of concurrently administered haloperidol (Haldol). Like all antidepressant medications, venlafaxine should not be used within 14 days of use of MAOIs, and it may potentiate the sedative effects of other drugs that act on the central nervous system (CNS).

LABORATORY INTERFERENCES

Data are not currently available on laboratory interferences with venlafaxine.

DOSAGE AND ADMINISTRATION

Venlafaxine is available in 25-, 37.5-, 50-, 75-, and 100-mg tablets and 37.5-, 75-, and 150-mg extended-release capsules. The tablets should be given in two or three daily doses, and the extended-release capsules are to be taken in a single dose before sleep, up to a maximum of 225 mg a day. The tablets and the extended-release capsules are equally potent, and persons stabilized with one can switch to an equivalent dosage of the other. The usual starting dosage in depressed persons is 75 mg a day, given as tablets in two to three divided doses or as extended-release capsules in a single dose before sleep. Some persons require a starting dosage of 37.5 mg for 4 to 7 days to minimize adverse effects, particularly nausea, prior to titration up to 75 mg a day. In persons with depression, the dosage can be raised to 150 mg a day, given as tablets in two or three divided doses or as extended-release capsules once at night, after an appropriate period of clinical assessment at the lower dosage (usually 2 to 3 weeks). The dosage can be raised in increments of 75 mg a day every 4 or more days. The maximum dosage of immediate-release venlafaxine is 375 mg a day and extended-release is 225 mg a day. The dosage of venlafaxine should be halved in persons with significantly diminished hepatic or renal function. If discontinued, venlafaxine use should be gradually tapered over 2 to 4 weeks.

DULOXETINE

Duloxetine hydrochloride (Cymbalta) is a dual reuptake inhibitor of serotonin and norepinephrine that acts as an antidepressant. It is chemically unrelated to venlafaxine. Duloxetine has minimal receptor affinity for dopamine, histamine, or other receptor types. Limited information is available about its clinical profile. Doses used in clinical trials ranged from 60 mg once a day to 60 mg twice a day. At lower doses, duloxetine is used once a day, but at higher doses it is used twice a day. In clinical trials, duloxetine demonstrates a similar side effect profile to SSRIs. Discontinuation due to adverse events was similar to SSRIs (15 percent for fluoxetine versus 5 percent for placebo). The most common side effects are nausea, dry mouth, fatigue, dizziness, constipation, somnolence, and sweating. Duloxetine is a moderate inhibitor of CYP450 2D6 enzyme.

▲ 32.4 Electroconvulsive Therapy

More than 75 years after it was developed, electroconvulsive therapy (ECT) remains an important, effective, and safe treatment for a variety of neuropsychiatric disorders. Major depression, especially in the elderly, is presently the most common indication for the treatment; however, it is used in other serious mental disorders such as schizophrenia and bipolar I illness.

INDICATIONS

Major Depressive Disorder

The most common indication for ECT is major depressive disorder, for which ECT is the fastest and most effective available therapy. ECT should be considered for use in patients who have failed medication trials, have not tolerated medications, have severe or psychotic symptoms, are acutely suicidal or homicidal, or have marked symptoms of agitation or stupor. Controlled studies have shown that up to 70 percent of patients who fail to respond to antidepressant medications may respond positively to ECT.

ECT is effective for depression in both major depressive disorder and bipolar I disorder. Delusional or psychotic depression has long been considered particularly responsive to ECT; but recent studies have indicated that major depressive episodes with psychotic features are no more responsive to ECT than nonpsychotic depressive disorders. Nevertheless, because major depressive episodes with psychotic features respond poorly to antidepressant pharmacotherapy alone, ECT should be considered much more often as the first-line treatment for patients with the disorder. Major depressive disorder with melancholic features (such as markedly severe symptoms, psychomotor retardation, early morning awakening, diurnal variation, decreased appetite and weight, and agitation) is considered likely to respond to ECT. ECT is particularly indicated for persons who are severely depressed, who have psychotic symptoms, who show suicidal intent, or who refuse to eat. Depressed patients less likely to respond to ECT include those with somatization disorder. Elderly patients tend to respond to ECT more slowly than young patients. ECT is a treatment for major depressive episode and does not provide prophylaxis unless it is administered on a long-term maintenance basis.

Manic Episodes

ECT is at least equal to lithium (Eskalith) in the treatment of acute manic episodes. The pharmacological treatment of manic episodes, however, is so effective in the short term and for prophylaxis that the use of ECT to treat manic episodes is generally limited to situations with specific contraindications to all available pharmacological approaches. The relative rapidity of the ECT response indicates its usefulness for patients whose manic behavior has produced dangerous levels of exhaustion. ECT should not be used for a patient who is receiving lithium, because lithium may lower the seizure threshold and cause a prolonged seizure.

Schizophrenia

ECT is an effective treatment for the symptoms of acute schizophrenia but not for those of chronic schizophrenia. Patients with schizophrenia who have marked positive symptoms, catatonia, or affective symptoms are considered most likely to respond to ECT. In such patients, the efficacy of ECT is approximately equal to that of antipsychotics, but improvement may occur faster.

Other Indications

ECT is effective in the treatment of catatonia, a symptom associated with mood disorders, schizophrenia, and medical and neurological disorders. ECT is also reportedly useful to treat episodic psychoses, atypical psychoses, obsessive-compulsive disorder (OCD), and delirium and such medical conditions as neuroleptic malignant syndrome, hypopituitarism, intractable seizure disorders, and the on–off phenomenon of Parkinson's disease. ECT may also be the treatment of choice for depressed suicidal pregnant women who require treatment and cannot take medication, for geriatric and medically ill patients who cannot take antidepressant drugs safely, and perhaps even for severely depressed and suicidal children and adolescents who may be less likely to respond to antidepressant drugs than are adults. ECT is not effective in somatization disorder (unless accompanied by depression), personality disorders, and anxiety disorders.

CLINICAL GUIDELINES

Patients and their families are often apprehensive about ECT; therefore, clinicians must explain both beneficial and adverse effects and alternative treatment approaches. The informed-consent process should be documented in the patient's medical records and should include a discussion of the disorder, its natural course, and the option of receiving no treatment. Printed literature and videotapes about ECT may be useful in attempting to obtain a truly informed consent. The use of involuntary ECT is rare today and should be reserved for patients who urgently need treatment and who have a legally appointed guardian who has agreed to its use. Clinicians must know local, state, and federal laws about the use of ECT.

Pretreatment Evaluation

Pretreatment evaluation should include standard physical, neurological, and preanesthesia examinations and a complete medical history. Laboratory evaluations should include blood and urine chemistries, a chest X-ray, and an electrocardiogram (ECG). A dental examination to assess the state of patients' dentition is advisable for elderly patients and patients who have had inadequate dental care. An X-ray of the spine is needed if there is other evidence of a spinal disorder. Computed tomography (CT) or magnetic resonance imaging (MRI) should be performed if a clinician suspects the presence of a seizure disorder or a space-occupying lesion. Practitioners of ECT no longer consider even a space-occupying lesion to be an absolute contraindication to ECT, but with such patients the procedure should be performed only by experts.

Concomitant Medications. Patients' ongoing medications should be assessed for possible interactions with the induc-

tion of a seizure, for effects (both positive and negative) on the seizure threshold, and for drug interactions with the medications used during ECT. The use of tricyclic and tetracyclic drugs, monoamine oxidase inhibitors (MAOIs), and antipsychotics is generally considered acceptable. Benzodiazepines used for anxiety should be withdrawn because of their anticonvulsant activity; lithium should be withdrawn because it can result in increased postictal delirium and can prolong seizure activity; clozapine (Clozaril) and bupropion (Wellbutrin) should be withdrawn because they are associated with the development of late-appearing seizures. Lidocaine (Xylocaine) should not be administered during ECT because it markedly increases the seizure threshold; theophylline (Theo-Dur) is contraindicated because it increases the duration of seizures. Reserpine (Serpasil) is also contraindicated because it is associated with further compromise of the respiratory and cardiovascular systems during ECT.

Premedications, Anesthetics, and Muscle Relaxants

Patients should not be given anything orally for 6 hours before treatment. Just before the procedure, the patient's mouth should be checked for dentures and other foreign objects, and an intravenous (IV) line should be established. A bite block is inserted in the mouth just before the treatment is administered to protect the patient's teeth and tongue during the seizure. Except for the brief interval of electrical stimulation, 100 percent oxygen is administered at a rate of 5 L a minute during the procedure until spontaneous respiration returns. Emergency equipment for establishing an airway should be immediately available in case it is needed.

Muscarinic Anticholinergic Drugs. Muscarinic anticholinergic drugs are administered before ECT to minimize oral and respiratory secretions and to block bradycardias and asystoles, unless the resting heart rate is above 90 beats a minute. Some ECT centers have stopped the routine use of anticholinergics as premedications, although their use is still indicated for patients taking β-adrenergic receptor antagonists and those with ventricular ectopic beats. The most commonly used drug is atropine, which can be administered 0.3 to 0.6 mg intramuscularly (IM) or subcutaneously (SC) 30 to 60 minutes before the anesthetic or 0.4 to 1.0 mg IV 2 or 3 minutes before the anesthetic. An option is to use glycopyrrolate (Robinul) (0.2 to 0.4 mg IM, IV, or SC), which is less likely to cross the blood–brain barrier and less likely to cause cognitive dysfunction and nausea, although it is thought to have less cardiovascular protective activity than does atropine.

ECT Anesthesia. Administration of ECT requires general anesthesia and oxygenation. The depth of anesthesia should be as light as possible, not only to minimize adverse effects but also to avoid elevating the seizure threshold associated with many anesthetics. Methohexital (Brevital) (0.75 to 1.0 mg/kg IV bolus) is the most commonly used anesthetic because of its shorter duration of action and lower association with postictal arrhythmias than thiopental (Pentothal) (usual dose 2 to 3 mg/kg IV), although this difference in cardiac effects is not universally accepted. Four other anesthetic alternatives are etomidate (Amidate), ketamine (Ketalar), alfentanil (Alfenta), and propofol (Diprivan). Etomidate (0.15 to 0.3 mg/kg IV) is sometimes used because it does not increase the seizure threshold; this effect is particularly useful for elderly patients, because the seizure threshold increases with age. Ketamine (6 to 10 mg/kg IM) is sometimes used because it does not increase the seizure threshold, although its use is limited by the frequent association of psychotic symptoms with emergence from anesthesia with this drug. Alfentanil (2 to 9 mg/kg IV) is sometimes coadministered with barbiturates to allow the use of low doses of the barbiturate anesthetics and thus reduce the seizure threshold less than usual, although its use may be associated with an increased incidence of nausea. Propofol (0.5 to 3.5 mg/kg IV) is less useful because of its strong anticonvulsant properties.

Muscle Relaxants.   After the onset of the anesthetic effect, usually within a minute, a muscle relaxant is administered to minimize the risk of bone fractures and other injuries resulting from motor activity during the seizure. The goal is to produce profound relaxation of the muscles, not necessarily to paralyze them, unless the patient has a history of osteoporosis or spinal injury or has a pacemaker and is, therefore, at risk for injury related to motor activity during the seizure. Succinylcholine, an ultrafast-acting depolarizing blocking agent, has gained virtually universal acceptance for the purpose. Succinylcholine is usually administered in a dose of 0.5 to 1 mg/kg as an IV bolus or drip. Because succinylcholine is a depolarizing agent, its action is marked by the presence of muscle fasciculations, which move in a rostrocaudal progression. The disappearance of these movements in the feet or the absence of muscle contractions after peripheral nerve stimulation indicates maximal muscle relaxation. In some patients, tubocurarine (3 mg IV) is administered to prevent myoclonus and increases in potassium and muscle enzymes; these reactions may be a problem in patients with musculoskeletal or cardiac disease. To monitor the duration of the convulsion, a blood pressure cuff may be inflated at the ankle to a pressure in excess of the systolic pressure before infusion of the muscle relaxant, to allow observation of relatively innocuous seizure activity in the foot muscles.

If a patient has a known history of pseudocholinesterase deficiency, atracurium (Tracrium) (0.5 to 1 mg/kg IV) or curare can be used instead of succinylcholine. In such a patient, the metabolism of succinylcholine is disrupted, and prolonged apnea may necessitate emergency airway management. In general, however, because of the short half-life of succinylcholine, the duration of apnea after its administration is generally shorter than the delay in regaining consciousness caused by the anesthetic and the postictal state. Table 32.4–1 summarizes medications used in ECT.

Electrode Placement

ECT can be conducted with either bilaterally or unilaterally placed electrodes. Bilateral placement usually yields a more rapid therapeutic response, and unilateral placement results in less marked cognitive adverse effects in the first week or weeks after treatment, although this difference between placements is absent 2 months after treatment. In bilateral placement, which was introduced first, one stimulating electrode is placed several centimeters apart over each hemisphere of the brain. In unilateral ECT, both electrodes are placed several centimeters apart over the nondominant hemisphere, almost always the right hemisphere. Some attempts have been made to vary the loca-

Table 32.4–1
Medications Used in the Administration of ECT

Drug	Dose
Anticholinergics	
Atropine	0.4–1.0 mg IV or IM
Glycopyrrolate	0.2–0.4 mg IV or IM
Anesthetics	
Methohexital	0.5–1.0 mg/kg IV
Thiopental	1.5–2.5 mg/kg IV
Etomidate	0.1–0.3 mg/kg IV
Alfentanil	0.2–0.3 mg/kg IV
Ketamine	0.5–1.0 mg/kg IV
Propofol	0.75–1.5 mg/kg IV
Midazolam	0.15–0.3 mg/kg IV
Muscle relaxants	
Depolarizing	
Succinylcholine	0.75–1.5 mg/kg IV
Nondepolarizing	
Mivacurium	0.1–0.2 mg/kg IV
Atracurium	0.3–0.4 mg/kg IV
Antihypertensives	
Esmolol	0.05–0.1 mg/kg IV
Labetalol	0.04–0.2 mg/kg IV
Nifedipine	10–30 mg PO

Table by K. E. Isenberg, M.D., and C. F. Zorumski, M.D.

tion of the electrodes in unilateral ECT, but these attempts have not obtained the rapidity of response seen with bilateral ECT or further reduced the cognitive adverse effects. The most common approach is to initiate treatment with unilateral ECT because of its more favorable adverse effect profile. If a patient does not improve after four to six unilateral treatments, bilateral placement is used. Initial bilateral placement of the electrodes may be indicated in the following situations: severe depressive symptoms, marked agitation, immediate suicide risk, manic symptoms, catatonic stupor, and treatment-resistant schizophrenia. Some patients are particularly at risk for anesthetic-related adverse effects, and these patients may also be treated with bilateral placement from the beginning to minimize the number of treatments and exposure to anesthetics.

In traditional bilateral ECT, the electrodes are placed bifrontotemporally with the center of each electrode approximately 1 inch above the midpoint of an imaginary line drawn from the tragus to the external canthus. With unilateral ECT, one stimulus electrode is typically placed over the nondominant frontotemporal area. Although several locations for the second stimulus electrode have been proposed, placement on the nondominant centroparietal scalp, just lateral to the midline vertex, appears to provide the most effective configuration.

Which cerebral hemisphere is dominant can generally be determined by a simple series of performance tasks (e.g., for handedness and footedness) and stated preference. Right body responses correlate highly with left brain dominance. If the responses are mixed or if they clearly indicate left body dominance, clinicians should alternate the polarity of unilateral stimulation during successive treatments. Clinicians should also monitor the time that it takes for patients to recover consciousness and to answer simple orientation and naming questions. The side of stimulation associated with less rapid recovery and return of function is considered dominant. The left hemisphere is dominant in most persons; therefore, unilateral electrode placement is almost always over the right hemisphere.

Electrical Stimulus

The electrical stimulus must be strong enough to reach the seizure threshold (the level of intensity needed to produce a seizure). The electrical stimulus is given in cycles, and each cycle contains a positive and a negative wave. Old machines use a sine wave; however, this type of machine is now considered obsolete because of the inefficiency of that wave shape. When a sine wave is delivered, the electrical stimulus in the sine wave before the seizure threshold is reached and after the seizure is activated is unnecessary and excessive. Modern ECT machines use a brief pulse waveform that administers the electrical stimulus usually in 1 to 2 ms at a rate of 30 to 100 pulses a second. Machines that use an ultrabrief pulse (0.5 ms) are not as effective as brief pulse machines.

Establishing a patient's seizure threshold is not straightforward. A 40-fold variability in seizure thresholds occurs among patients. In addition, during the course of ECT treatment, a patient's seizure threshold may increase 25 to 200 percent. The seizure threshold is also higher in men than in women and higher in older than in younger adults. A common technique is to initiate treatment at an electrical stimulus that is thought to be below the seizure threshold for a particular patient and then to increase this intensity by 100 percent for unilateral placement and by 50 percent for bilateral placement until the seizure threshold is reached. A debate in the literature concerns whether a minimally suprathreshold dose, a moderately suprathreshold dose ($1^1/2$ times the threshold), or a high suprathreshold dose (three times the threshold) is preferable. The debate about stimulus intensity resembles the debate about electrode placement. Essentially, the data support the conclusion that doses of three times the threshold are the most rapidly effective and that minimal suprathreshold doses are associated with the fewest and least severe cognitive adverse effects.

Induced Seizures

A brief muscular contraction, usually strongest in a patient's jaw and facial muscles, is seen concurrently with the flow of stimulus current, regardless of whether a seizure occurs. The first behavioral sign of the seizure is often a plantar extension, which lasts 10 to 20 seconds and marks the tonic phase. This phase is followed by rhythmic (i.e., clonic) contractions that decrease in frequency and finally disappear. The tonic phase is marked by high-frequency, sharp electroencephalographic (EEG) activity on which a higher-frequency muscle artifact may be superimposed. During the clonic phase, bursts of polyspike activity occur simultaneously with the muscular contractions but usually persist for at least a few seconds after the clonic movements stop.

Monitoring Seizures.   A physician must have an objective measure that a bilateral generalized seizure has occurred after the stimulation. The physician should be able to observe either some evidence of tonic-clonic movements or electrophysiological evidence of seizure activity from the EEG or electromyogram (EMG). Seizures with unilateral ECT are asymmetrical, with higher ictal EEG amplitudes over the stimulated hemisphere than over the nonstimulated hemisphere. Occasionally, unilateral seizures are induced; for this reason, at least a single pair of EEG electrodes should be placed over the contralateral hemisphere when using unilateral ECT. For a seizure to be effective in the course of ECT, it should last at least 25 seconds.

Number and Spacing of ECT Treatments

ECT treatments are usually administered two to three times a week; twice-weekly treatments are associated with less memory impairment than thrice-weekly treatments. In general, the course of treatment of major depressive disorder can take 6 to 12 treatments (although up to 20 sessions are possible); the treatment of manic episodes can take 8 to 20 treatments; the treatment of schizophrenia can take more than 15 treatments; and the treatment of catatonia and delirium can take as few as 1 to 4 treatments. Treatment should continue until the patient achieves what is considered the maximum therapeutic response. Further treatment does not yield any therapeutic benefit but increases the severity and duration of the adverse effects. The point of maximal improvement is usually thought to occur when a patient fails to continue to improve after two consecutive treatments. If a patient is not improving after 6 to 10 sessions, bilateral placement and high-density treatment (three times the seizure threshold) should be attempted before ECT is abandoned.

Maintenance Treatment

A short-term course of ECT induces a remission in symptoms but does not, of itself, prevent a relapse. Post-ECT maintenance treatment should always be considered. Maintenance therapy is generally pharmacological, but maintenance ECT treatments (weekly, biweekly, or monthly) have been reported to be effective relapse prevention treatments, although data from large studies are lacking. Indications for maintenance ECT treatments may include rapid relapse after initial ECT, severe symptoms, psychotic symptoms, and the inability to tolerate medications. If ECT was used because a patient was unresponsive to a specific medication, then, after ECT, the patient should be given a trial of a different medication.

ADVERSE EFFECTS
Contraindications

ECT has no absolute contraindications, only situations in which a patient is at increased risk and has an increased need for close monitoring. Pregnancy is not a contraindication for ECT, and fetal monitoring is generally considered unnecessary unless the pregnancy is high risk or complicated. Patients with space-occupying central nervous system (CNS) lesions are at increased risk for edema and brain herniation after ECT. But if the lesion is small, pretreatment with dexamethasone (Decadron) is given, and hypertension is controlled during the seizure, the risk of serious complications can be minimized for these patients. Patients who have increased intracerebral pressure or are at risk for cerebral bleeding (e.g., those with cerebrovascular diseases and aneurysms) are at risk during ECT because of the increased cerebral blood flow during the seizure. This risk can be lessened, although not eliminated, by control of the patient's blood pressure during the treatment. Patients with recent myocardial infarctions are another high-risk group, although the risk is greatly diminished 2 weeks after the myocardial infarction and is even further reduced 3 months after the infarction. Patients with hypertension should be stabilized on their antihypertensive medications before ECT is administered. Propranolol (Inderal) and sublingual nitroglycerin can also be used to protect such patients during treatment.

Mortality

The mortality rate with ECT is approximately 0.002 percent per treatment and 0.01 percent for each patient. These numbers compare favorably with the risks associated with general anesthesia and childbirth. ECT death is usually from cardiovascular complications and is most likely to occur in patients whose cardiac status is already compromised.

Central Nervous System Effects

Common adverse effects associated with ECT are headache, confusion, and delirium shortly after the seizure while the patient is coming out of anesthesia. Marked confusion may occur in up to 10 percent of patients within 30 minutes of the seizure and can be treated with barbiturates and benzodiazepines. Delirium is usually most pronounced after the first few treatments and in patients who receive bilateral ECT or who have coexisting neurological disorders. The delirium characteristically clears within days or a few weeks at the longest.

Memory.   The greatest concern about ECT is the association between ECT and memory loss. Approximately 75 percent of all patients given ECT say that the memory impairment is the worst adverse effect. Although memory impairment during a course of treatment is almost the rule, follow-up data indicate that almost all patients are back to their cognitive baselines after 6 months. Some patients, however, complain of persistent memory difficulties. For example, a patient may not remember the events leading up to the hospitalization and ECT, and such autobiographical memories may never be recalled. The degree of cognitive impairment during treatment and the time it takes to return to baseline are related in part to the amount of electrical stimulation used during treatment. Memory impairment is most often reported by patients who have experienced little improvement with ECT. In spite of the memory impairment, which usually resolves, there is no evidence of brain damage caused by ECT. This subject has been the focus of several brain-imaging studies, using a variety of modalities; virtually all concluded that permanent brain damage is not an adverse effect of ECT. Neurologists and epileptologists generally agree that seizures that last less than 30 minutes do not cause permanent neuronal damage.

Other Adverse Effects of ECT

Fractures often accompanied treatments in the early days of ECT. With routine use of muscle relaxants, fractures of long bones or vertebrae should not occur. However, some patients may break teeth or experience back pain because of contractions during the procedure. Muscle soreness may occur in some individuals but often results from the effects of muscle depolarization by succinylcholine and is most likely to be particularly troublesome after the first session in a series. This soreness can be treated with mild analgesics, including nonsteroidal antiinflammatory drugs (NSAIDs). A significant minority of patients experience nausea, vomiting, and headaches after an ECT treatment. Nausea and vomiting can be prevented by treatment with antiemetics at the time of ECT (e.g., metoclopramide [Reglan], 10 mg IV, or prochlorperazine [Compazine], 10 mg IV; ondansetron [Zofran] is an acceptable alternative if adverse effects preclude use of dopamine receptor antagonists).

ECT can be associated with headaches, although this effect is usually readily manageable. Headaches often respond to NSAIDs given in the ECT recovery period. In patients with severe headaches, pretreatment with ketorolac (Toradol) (30 to 60 mg IV), an NSAID approved for brief parenteral use, can be helpful. Acetaminophen (Tylenol), tramadol (Ultram), propoxyphene (Darvon), and more potent analgesia provided by opioids can be used individually or in various combinations (e.g., pretreatment with ketorolac and postseizure management with acetaminophen-propoxyphene) to manage more intractable headache. ECT can induce migrainous headache and related symptoms; sumatriptan (Imitrex) (6 mg SC or 25 mg orally) may be a useful addition to the agents described above. Ergot compounds can exacerbate cardiovascular changes observed during ECT and probably should not be a component of ECT pretreatment.

▲ 32.5 Other Biological and Pharmacological Therapies

TRANSCRANIAL MAGNETIC STIMULATION

Transcranial magnetic stimulation (TMS) is a noninvasive technique for stimulating cells of the cerebral cortex. It does not cause generalized seizures as in electroconvulsive therapy (ECT). TMS uses a magnet to allow focused electrical stimulation across the scalp and cranium without the pain associated with percutaneous electrical stimulation. TMS was originally used to map cortical motor control and hemisphere dominance. Stimulating the motor cortex with TMS results in a contralateral motor response. Likewise, stimulating Broca's area with TMS has resulted in speech blockage. Currently, the potential use of TMS for the treatment of neurological and psychiatric disorders is being explored actively.

A number of small, open-labeled studies have suggested that TMS may be effective in some patients with treatment-resistant major depressive disorder as well as in those with milder major depressive disorder. Recent functional imaging studies have suggested that the baseline hypofrontality associated with major depressive disorder can be reversed. In addition to major depressive disorder, TMS has shown some preliminary efficacy in obsessive-compulsive disorder (OCD) and in posttraumatic stress disorder (PTSD).

TMS has been used to map the motor cortex, help determine hemispheric dominance, and probe short-term memory. In some symptoms of Parkinson's disease, including bradykinesia, diminished reaction time has improved transiently with TMS. Finally, TMS has been used to help elucidate the pathophysiology of migraine headache, and some patients have had temporary symptomatic relief with TMS. The application of TMS to psychiatric conditions has lagged behind its neurological applications. It is used primarily as a research tool, but its clinical use is increasing steadily.

PHOTOTHERAPY

Phototherapy (light therapy) was introduced in 1984 as a treatment for seasonal affective disorder (mood disorder with seasonal pattern). In this disorder, patients typically experience depression as the photoperiod of the day decreases with advancing winter. Women represent at least 75 percent of all patients with seasonal depression, and the mean age of presentation is 40. Patients rarely present over the age of 55 with seasonal affective disorder.

Phototherapy typically involves exposing the afflicted patient to bright light in the range of 1,500 to 10,000 lux or more, typically with a light box that sits on a table or desk. Patients sit in front of the box for approximately 1 to 2 hours before dawn each day, although some patients may also benefit from exposure after dusk. Alternatively, some manufacturers have developed light visors, with a light source built into the brim of the hat. These light visors allow mobility, but recent controlled studies have questioned the use of this type of light exposure. Trials have typically lasted 1 week, but longer treatment durations may be associated with greater response.

Phototherapy tends to be well tolerated. Newer light sources tend to use lower light intensities and come equipped with filters; patients are instructed not to look directly at the light source. As with any effective antidepressant, phototherapy has on rare occasions been implicated in switching some depressed patients into mania or hypomania.

In addition to seasonal depression, the other major indication for phototherapy may be in sleep disorders. Phototherapy has been used to decrease the irritability and diminished functioning associated with shift work. Sleep disorders in geriatric patients have reportedly improved with exposure to bright light during the day. Likewise, some evidence suggests that jet lag might respond to light therapy. Preliminary data indicate that phototherapy may benefit some patients with OCD that has a seasonal variation.

VAGAL NERVE STIMULATION (VNS)

Experimental stimulation of the vagus nerve in several studies designed for the treatment of epilepsy found that patients showed improved mood. This observation led to the use of left vagal nerve stimulation (VNS) using an electronic device implanted in the skin, similar to a cardiac pacemaker. Preliminary studies have shown that a significant number of patients with chronic, recurrent major depressive disorder went into remission when treated with VNS. The mechanism of action of VNS to account for improvement is unknown. The vagus nerve connects to the enteric nervous system and, when stimulated, may cause release of peptides that act as neurotransmitters. Extensive clinical trials are being conducted to determine the efficacy of VNS.

SLEEP DEPRIVATION

Mood disorders are characterized by sleep disturbance. Mania tends to be characterized by a decreased need for sleep, whereas depression may be associated with either hypersomnia or insomnia. Sleep deprivation may precipitate mania in bipolar I patients and temporarily relieve depression in unipolar patients. Approximately 60 percent of depressive disorder patients exhibit significant but transient benefit from total sleep deprivation. The most common procedure is to keep patients awake from 2 AM to 10 PM for 1 or 2 days. The positive results last for 1 or 2 days and then are reversed by the next night of sleep.

ENDOCRINE THERAPIES

Hormones may act directly as neurotransmitters and also indirectly influence the activity of some neurotransmitters. For example, triiodothyronine (T_3) has numerous cortical receptors, and this thyroid hormone may also modulate central and peripheral noradrenergic activity. These actions may be the basis for liothyronine's (Cytomel) use to augment antidepressants. In addition to thyroid hormone, the psychotropic effects of a number of other hormones remain under investigation.

Estrogen

Estrogen has been used for many years to relieve menopausal symptoms and as hormone replacement therapy after menopause. Some evidence suggests that estrogens may have some antidepressant effects in postmenopausal women and that progesterone may be depressogenic. Estrogens appear to lower monoamine oxidase (MAO) concentrations and increase synaptic availability of monoamines. In addition, estrogen enhances the availability of serotonin. The use of estrogen is highly controversial at this time because of the increased incidence of cancer and cardiovascular disease with long-term use.

Dehydroepiandrosterone

Dehydroepiandrosterone (DHEA), a precursor hormone for both estrogens and androgens, is available over the counter. Recent years have seen an interest in DHEA for improving cognition, depression, sex drive, and general well-being in elderly adults. Some reports suggest that DHEA in dosages of 50 to 100 mg per day increases the sense of physical and social well-being in women aged 40 to 70 years. Reports also exist of androgenic effects, including irreversible hirsutism, hair loss, voice deepening, and other undesirable sequelae. In addition, DHEA has at least a theoretical potential of enhancing tumor growth in persons with latent, hormone-sensitive malignancies such as prostate, cervical, and breast cancer. Despite its significant popularity, few controlled data exist on the safety or efficacy of DHEA.

Melatonin

Melatonin is another popular over-the-counter hormone used by many Americans on a regular basis for insomnia and jet lag. Melatonin is produced by the pineal gland, and commercially available supplies are derived synthetically or from hog pineal glands. The hormone is released naturally by the pineal gland early in the sleep cycle and appears to contribute to natural sleep cycles. A number of small, brief studies have suggested that melatonin can act as a hypnotic in doses of 0.2 and 5 mg at night. Mostly anecdotal reports suggest that melatonin can also reduce the insomnia associated with jet lag. The long-term effects of melatonin use are unknown, and the efficacy of melatonin has been poorly studied at this time, given the widespread use of the drug.

Testosterone

Testosterone derivatives are anabolic-androgenic steroids that appear to have psychotropic effects in both men and women. Testosterone is sometimes given to postmenopausal women to enhance libido, since this hormone appears to have significant effects on libido in both men and women. In hypogonadal men, testosterone may improve sexual dysfunction, mood, energy, muscle-to-fat ratio, and sex drive. High doses of testosterone derivatives are sometimes abused by bodybuilders, football players, and even teenagers trying to increase muscle bulk. Anabolic steroids have also been associated with rage attacks, aggressive behavior, and untoward physical effects, including accelerated atherosclerosis, testicular atrophy, alopecia, and enhanced tumor growth. Women who use testosterone at high doses also may experience irreversible virilization. Testosterone is now available in a transdermal patch and has been marketed fairly aggressively, resulting in a recent increase in prescriptions for both men and women.

PSYCHOSURGERY

Psychosurgery involves surgical modification of the brain with the goal of reducing the symptoms of the most severely ill psychiatric patients who have not responded adequately to less radical treatments. Psychosurgical procedures focus on lesion-specific brain regions (e.g., lobotomies and cingulotomies) or their connecting tracts (e.g., tractotomies and leukotomies). Psychosurgical techniques are also used in the treatment of neurological disorders such as epilepsy and chronic pain disorder.

The interest in psychosurgical approaches to mental disorders has recently been rekindled. The renewed interest is based on several factors, including much-improved techniques that allow neurosurgeons to make exact stereotactically placed lesions, improved preoperative diagnoses, and comprehensive preoperative and postoperative psychological assessments.

The major indication for psychosurgery is the presence of a debilitating, chronic mental disorder that has not responded to any other treatment. A reasonable guideline is that the disorder should have been present for 5 years, during which a wide variety of alternative treatment approaches was attempted. Chronic intractable major depressive disorder and OCD are the two disorders reportedly most responsive to psychosurgery. Whether psychosurgery is a reasonable treatment for intractable and extreme aggression is still controversial. Psychosurgery is not indicated for the treatment of schizophrenia, and data about manic episodes are controversial.

PLACEBOS

Pharmacologically inactive substances have long been known to sometimes produce significant clinical benefits. A patient who believes that a compound is helpful may often derive considerable benefit from taking that substance, whether it is known to be pharmacologically active or not. For many psychiatric disorders, including mild to moderate depression and some anxiety disorders, well over 30 percent of patients can exhibit significant improvement or remission of symptoms on a placebo. For other conditions, such as schizophrenia, manic episodes, and psychotic depression, the placebo response rate is very low. While suggestion is undoubtedly important in the efficacy of placebos (and active drugs), placebos may produce biological effects. For example, placebo-induced analgesia may sometimes be blocked by naloxone, which suggests that endorphins may mediate the analgesia derived from taking a placebo. It is conceivable that placebos may also stimulate endogenous anxiolytic and antidepressant factors, resulting in clinical improvement in patients with depression and anxiety disorders.

Just as placebos may produce benefit, they may also have adverse effects. In many studies, some adverse effects are likely to be more common with placebos than with the active drug. Some patients will not tolerate placebos despite the fact that they are supposedly inert, and they exhibit adverse effects (called the *nocebo phenomenon*). It is easy to discount such patients as overly suggestible; however, if beneficial endogenous factors can be stimulated by placebos, perhaps toxic endogenous factors may also be produced.

Prudence is needed in contemplating the use of a placebo in clinical practice. Treating a patient with a placebo without consent can seriously undermine a patient's confidence in the physician if, and when, it is discovered.

33 ▲

Child Psychiatry: Assessment, Examination, and Psychological Testing

A comprehensive evaluation of a child includes interviews with the parents, the child, and the family; gathering of information regarding the child's current school functioning; and often, a standardized assessment of the child's intellectual level and academic achievement. In some cases, standardized measures of developmental level and neuropsychological assessments are useful. Psychiatric evaluations of children are rarely initiated by the child, so clinicians must obtain information from the family and the school to understand the reasons for the evaluation. In some cases, the court or a child protective service agency may initiate a psychiatric evaluation. Children often have difficulty with the chronology of symptoms and are sometimes reticent to report behaviors that got them into trouble. Very young children often cannot articulate their experiences verbally and are better at showing their feelings and preoccupations in a play situation.

CLINICAL INTERVIEW

To conduct a useful interview with a child of any age, clinicians must be familiar with normal development in order to place the child's responses in the proper perspective. For example, a young child's discomfort on separation from a parent and a school-age child's lack of clarity about the purpose of the interview are both perfectly normal and should not be misconstrued as psychiatric symptoms. Furthermore, behavior that is normal in a child at one age, such as temper tantrums in a 2-year-old, takes on a different meaning, for example, in a 17-year-old.

The interviewer's first task is to engage the child and to develop a rapport, so that the child is comfortable. The interviewer should inquire about the child's concept of the purpose of the interview and should ask what the parents have told the child. If the child appears to be confused about the reason for the interview, the examiner may opt to summarize the parents' concerns in a developmentally appropriate and supportive manner. During the interview with the child, the clinician seeks to learn about the child's relationships with family members and peers, academic achievement and peer relationships in school, and the child's pleasurable activities.

The extent of confidentiality in child assessment is correlated with the age of the child. School-age and older children are informed that if the clinician becomes concerned that any

child is dangerous to himself or herself or to others, this information must be shared with parents and at times additional adults. As part of a psychiatric assessment of a child of any age, the clinician must determine whether that child is safe in his or her environment and must develop an index of suspicion as to whether the child is a victim of abuse or neglect. Whenever there is a suspicion of child maltreatment, the local child protective service agency must be notified.

Infants and Young Children

Assessments of infants usually begin with the parents present, as very young children may be frightened by the interview situation; the interview with the parents present provides the clinician with the best way to assess the parent–infant interaction. The clinician assesses areas of functioning that include motor development, activity level, verbal communication, ability to engage in play, problem-solving skills, adaptation to daily routines, relationships, and social responsiveness.

The child's developmental level of functioning is determined by combining observations made during the interview with standardized developmental measures. Observations of play reveal a child's developmental level and reflect the child's emotional state and preoccupations.

School-Age Children

Some school-age children are at ease when conversing with an adult; others are hampered by fear, anxiety, poor verbal skills, or oppositional behavior. School-age children can usually tolerate a 45-minute session. The room should be spacious enough for the child to move around in, but not large enough to reduce intimate contact between the examiner and the child. Part of the interview can be reserved for unstructured play, and various toys can be made available to capture the child's interest and to elicit themes and feelings. Children in lower grades may be more interested in the toys in the room, whereas by the sixth grade, children may be more comfortable with the interview process and less likely to show spontaneous play.

The initial part of the interview explores the child's understanding of the reasons for the meeting. Techniques that can facilitate the disclosure of feelings include asking the child to draw peers, family members, a house, or anything else that comes to mind. The child can then be questioned about the drawings. Games such as Winnicott's "squiggle," in which the examiner draws a curved line and then the child and the examiner take turns continuing the drawing, may facilitate conversation.

Questions that are partially open-ended with some multiple choices may elicit the most complete answers in school-age children, whereas simple, closed (yes/no) questions may not elicit enough information. Incidentally, completely open-ended questions can overwhelm a school-age child who is not able to construct a chronological narrative. The use of indirect commentary—such as, "I once knew a child who felt very sad when he moved away from all his friends"—is helpful, although the clinician must be careful not to lead the child into confirming what the child thinks the clinician wants to hear. School-age children respond well to clinicians who help them compare moods or feelings by asking them to rate feelings on a scale of 1 to 10.

Adolescents

Adolescents usually have distinct ideas about why the evaluation was initiated. Adolescents can usually give a chronological account of the recent events leading to the evaluation, although some may disagree with the need for the evaluation. The clinician should clearly communicate the value of hearing the story from an adolescent's point of view and must be careful to reserve judgment and not assign blame. Adolescents may be concerned about confidentiality, and clinicians can assure them that permission will be requested from them before any specific information is shared with parents, except situations involving danger to the adolescent or others, in which case confidentiality must be sacrificed. Adolescents can be approached in an open-ended manner; however, when silences occur during the interview, the clinician should attempt to reengage the patient. Clinicians can explore what the adolescent believes the outcome of the evaluation will be (change of school, hospitalization, removal from home, removal of privileges).

Clinicians must be aware of their own responses to adolescents' behavior (countertransference) and stay focused on the therapeutic process even in the face of defiant, angry, or difficult teenagers. Clinicians should set appropriate limits and should postpone or discontinue an interview if they feel threatened or if patients become destructive to property or engage in self-injurious behavior. Every interview should include an exploration of suicidal thoughts, assaultive behavior, psychotic symptoms, substance use, and knowledge of safe sexual practices along with a sexual history. Once rapport has been established, many adolescents appreciate the opportunity to tell their side of the story and may reveal things that they have not disclosed to anyone else.

Family Interview

Sometimes an interview with the entire family, including siblings, can be enlightening. The purpose is to observe the attitudes and behavior of the parents toward the patient and the responses of the children to their parents. The clinician's job is to maintain a nonthreatening atmosphere in which each member of the family can speak freely without feeling that the clinician is taking sides with any particular member. Although child psychiatrists generally function as advocates for the child, the clinician must validate each family member's feelings in this setting, because lack of communication often contributes to the patient's problems.

Parents

The interview with the patient's parents or caretakers is necessary to get a chronological picture of the child's growth and development. Parents are usually the best informants about the child's early development and previous psychiatric and medical illnesses. In some cases, especially with older children and adolescents, the parents may be unaware of significant current symptoms or social difficulties of the child. Clinicians elicit the parents' formulation of the causes and nature of their child's problems and ask about expectations about the current assessment.

DIAGNOSTIC INSTRUMENTS

The two main types of diagnostic instruments used by clinicians and researchers are diagnostic interviews and questionnaires. Diagnostic interviews are administered to either children or their parents and are often designed to elicit enough information on numerous aspects of functioning in order to determine whether criteria are met from the text revision of the fourth edition of the *Diagnostic and Statistical Manual of Mental Disorders* (DSM-IV-TR). A few are described below.

Kiddie Schedule for Affective Disorders and Schizophrenia for School-Age Children (K-SADS)

K-SADS can be used for children ranging from 6 to 18 years of age. It presents multiple items with some space for further clarification of symptoms. It elicits information on current diagnosis and those present in the last year. There is also a version that can ascertain lifetime diagnoses.

Child and Adolescent Psychiatric Assessment (CAPA)

The CAPA is an "interviewer-based" interview that can be used for children ranging from 9 to 17 years of age. It comes in modular form so that certain diagnostic entities can be administered without having to give the entire interview. It covers disruptive behavior disorders, mood disorders, anxiety disorders, eating disorders, sleep disorders, elimination disorders, substance-use disorders, tic disorders, schizophrenia, posttraumatic stress disorder (PTSD), and somatization symptoms.

Diagnostic Interview for Children and Adolescents (DICA)

The current version of the DICA was developed in 1997 to assess information resulting in diagnoses according to either DSM-IV or DSM-III-R. Although it was originally designed to be a highly structured interview, it can now be used in a semistructured format. It covers externalizing behavior disorders, anxiety disorders, depressive disorders, substance abuse disorders, among others.

Child Behavior Checklist

The parent and teacher versions of the Child Behavior Checklist were developed to cover a broad range of symptoms and several positive attributes related to academic and social competence. The checklist presents items related to mood, frustration tolerance, hyperactivity, oppositional behavior, anxiety, and various other behaviors. The parent version consists of 118 items rated on a scale of 0 (not true), 1 (sometimes true), and 2 (very true). The teacher version is similar but without the items that apply only to home life. Profiles were developed that are based on normal children of three different age groups (4 to 5, 6 to 11, and 12 to 16).

Such a checklist identifies specific problem areas that may otherwise be overlooked, and it may point out areas in which the child's behavior is deviant, compared with normal children of the same age group. The checklist is not used specifically to make diagnoses.

COMPONENTS OF THE CHILD PSYCHIATRIC EVALUATION

Psychiatric evaluation of a child includes a description of the reason for the referral, the child's past and present functioning, and any test results.

Identifying Data

To understand the clinical problems to be evaluated, the clinician must first identify the patient and keep in mind the family constellation surrounding the child. The clinician must also pay attention to the source of the referral—that is, whether it is the child's family, school, or another agency, as this fact influences the family's attitude toward the evaluation. Finally, many informants contribute to the child's evaluation, and identifying each of them is important in gaining insight into the child's functioning in different settings.

History

A comprehensive history contains information about the child's current and past functioning, from the child's report as well as based on clinical and structured interviews with the parents, along with information from teachers and previous treating clinicians. The chief complaint and the history of the present illness are generally obtained from both the child and from the parents. The developmental history is more accurately obtained from the parents. Psychiatric and medical histories, current physical examination findings, and immunization histories can be augmented with reports from psychiatrists and pediatricians who have treated the child in the past. The child's report is critical in understanding the current situation regarding peer relationships and adjustment to school. Adolescents are the best informants regarding knowledge of safe sexual practices, drug or alcohol use, and suicidal ideation. The family's psychiatric and social histories and family function are best obtained from the parents.

Mental Status Examination

A detailed description of the child's current mental functioning can be obtained through observation and specific questioning.

Physical Appearances.   The examiner should note and document the child's size, grooming, nutritional state, bruising, head circumference, physical signs of anxiety, facial expressions, and mannerisms.

Parent–Child Interaction.   The examiner can observe the interactions between parents and child in the waiting area before the interview and in the family session. The manner in which parents and child converse and the emotional overtones are pertinent.

Separation and Reunion.   The examiner should note both the manner in which the child responds to the separation from a parent for an individual interview and the reunion behavior. Either lack of affect at separation and reunion or severe distress on separation or reunion can indicate the presence of problems in the parent–child relationship or other psychiatric disturbances.

Orientation to Time, Place, and People.   Impairments in orientation can reflect organic damage, low intelligence, or a thought disorder. The age of the child must be kept in mind, however, because very young children are not expected to know the date, other chronological information, or the name of the interview site.

Speech and Language.   The examiner should note the presence of a level of speech and language acquisition appropriate for the child's age. An observable disparity between expressive language use and receptive language is notable. The examiner should also note the child's rate of speech, rhythm, latency to answer, spontaneity of speech, intonation, articulation of words, and prosody. Echolalia, repetitive stereotypical phrases, and unusual syntax are important psychiatric findings. Children who do not use words by age 18 months or who do not use phrases by age 2 ½ to 3 years, but who have a history of normal babbling and responding appropriately to nonverbal cues are probably developing normally. The examiner should consider the possibility that a hearing loss is contributing to a speech and language deficit.

Mood.   A child's sad expression, lack of appropriate smiling, tearfulness, anxiety, euphoria, and anger are valid indicators of mood, as are verbal admissions of feelings. Persistent themes in play and fantasy also reflect the child's mood.

Affect.   The examiner should note the child's range of emotional expressivity, appropriateness of affect to thought content, ability to move smoothly from one affect to another, and sudden labile emotional shifts.

Thought Process and Content.   In evaluating a thought disorder in a child, the clinician must always consider what is developmentally expected for the child's age and what is deviant for any age group. The evaluation of the form of thought considers loosening of associations, excessive magical thinking, preservation, echolalia, the child's ability to distinguish fantasy from reality, sentence coherence, and the ability to reason logically. The evaluation of the content of thought considers delusions, obsessions, themes, fears, wishes, preoccupations, and interests.

Suicidal ideation is always a part of the mental status examination for children who are sufficiently verbal to understand the questions and old enough to understand the concept. Children of average intelligence older than 4 years of age usually have some understanding of what is real and what is make-believe and may be asked about suicidal ideation, although a firm concept of the permanence of death may not be present until several years later.

Aggressive thoughts and homicidal ideation are assessed here. Perceptual disturbances, such as hallucinations, are also assessed.

Transient visual and auditory hallucinations in very young children do not necessarily represent major psychotic illnesses, but they do deserve further investigation.

Social Relatedness. The examiner assesses the appropriateness of the child's response to the interviewer, general level of social skills, eye contact, and degree of familiarity or withdrawal in the interview process. Overly friendly or familiar behavior may be as troublesome as extremely retiring and withdrawn responses. The examiner assesses the child's self-esteem, general and specific areas of confidence, and success with family and peer relationships.

Motor Behavior. This part of the mental status examination includes observations of the child's activity level, ability to pay attention and to carry out developmentally appropriate tasks, coordination, involuntary movements, tremors, motor overflow, and any unusual focal asymmetries of muscle movement.

Cognition. The examiner assesses the child's intellectual functioning, problem-solving abilities, and memory. An approximate level of intelligence can be estimated by the child's general information, vocabulary, and comprehension. For a specific assessment of the child's cognitive abilities, the examiner can use a standardized test.

Memory. School-age children should be able to remember three objects after 5 minutes and to repeat five digits forward and three digits backward. Anxiety may interfere with the child's performance, but an obvious inability to repeat digits or to add simple numbers together may reflect brain damage, mental retardation, or learning disabilities.

Judgment and Insight. The child's view of the problems, reactions to them, and potential solutions suggested by the child may give the clinician a good idea of the child's judgment and insight. In addition, the child's understanding of what he or she can realistically do to help and what the clinician can do adds to the assessment of the child's judgment.

Neuropsychiatric Assessment

A neuropsychiatric assessment is appropriate for children who are suspected of having a neurological disorder, a psychiatric impairment that coexists with neurological signs, or psychiatric symptoms that may be due to neuropathology. The neuropsychiatric evaluation combines information from neurological, physical, and mental status examinations. The neurological examination can identify asymmetrical abnormal signs (hard signs) that may indicate lesions in the brain. A physical examination can evaluate the presence of physical stigmata of particular syndromes in which neuropsychiatric symptoms or developmental aberrations play a role (for example, fetal alcohol syndrome, Down syndrome).

Part of the neuropsychiatric examination is the assessment of neurological soft signs and minor physical anomalies. The term *neurological soft signs* was first noted by Loretta Bender in the 1940s in reference to nondiagnostic abnormalities in the neurological examinations of children with schizophrenia. Soft signs are not indicative of focal neurological disorders, but they are associated with a wide variety of developmental disabilities and occur frequently in children with low intelligence, learning disabilities, and behavioral disturbances. Soft signs may refer to both behavioral symptoms (which are sometimes associated with brain damage, such as severe impulsivity and hyperactivity), physical findings (including contralateral overflow movements), and a variety of nonfocal signs (such as mild choreiform move-

ments, poor balance, mild incoordination, asymmetry of gait, nystagmus, and the persistence of infantile reflexes). The Physical and Neurological Examination for Soft Signs (PANESS) is an instrument used with children up to the age of 15 years. It consists of 15 questions about general physical status and medical history and 43 physical tasks (for example, touch your finger to your nose, hop on one foot to the end of the line, tap quickly with your finger). Neurological soft signs are important to note, but they are not specific in making a psychiatric diagnosis.

Minor physical anomalies or dysmorphic features occur with a higher-than-usual frequency in children with developmental disabilities, learning disabilities, speech and language disorders, and hyperactivity. As with soft signs, the documentation of minor physical anomalies is part of the neuropsychiatric assessment, but it is rarely helpful in the diagnostic process and does not imply a good or bad prognosis. Minor physical anomalies include a high-arched palate, epicanthus folds, hypertelorism, low-set ears, transverse palmar creases, multiple hair whorls, a large head, a furrowed tongue, and partial syndactyly of several toes.

When a seizure disorder is being considered in the differential diagnosis or a structural abnormality in the brain is suspected, an electroencephalogram (EEG), computed tomography (CT), or magnetic resonance imaging (MRI) may be indicated.

Developmental, Psychological, and Educational Testing

Psychological tests are not always required to assess psychiatric symptoms, but they are valuable in determining a child's developmental level, intellectual functioning, and academic difficulties. A measure of adaptive functioning (including the child's competence in communication, daily living skills, socialization, and motor skills) is a prerequisite when a diagnosis of mental retardation is being considered.

Development Tests for Infants and Preschoolers.
The Gesell Infant Scale, the Cattell Infant Intelligence Scale, Bayley Scales of Infant Development, and the Denver Developmental Screening Test include developmental assessments of infants as young as 2 months of age. When used with very young infants, the tests focus on sensorimotor and social responses to a variety of objects and interactions. When these instruments are used with older infants and preschoolers, emphasis is placed on language acquisition. The Gesell Infant Scale measures development in four areas: motor, adaptive functioning, language, and social.

An infant's score on one of these developmental assessments is not a reliable way to predict a child's future intelligence quotient (IQ) in most cases. Infant assessments are valuable, however, in detecting developmental deviation and mental retardation and in raising suspicions of a developmental disorder.

Whereas infant assessments rely heavily on sensorimotor functions, intelligence testing in older children and adolescents includes later-developing functions, including verbal, social, and abstract cognitive abilities.

Intelligence Tests for School-Age Children and Adolescents.
The most widely used test of intelligence for school-age children and adolescents is the third edition of the Wechsler Intelligence Scale for Children (WISC-III). It can be given to children from 6 to 17 years old, yields a verbal IQ, a performance IQ, and a

combined full-scale IQ. WISC-III consists of verbal and performance subtests, of which the scores are not included in the IQ computation.

An average full-scale IQ is 100; 70 to 80 represents borderline intellectual function; 80 to 90 is in the low average range; 90 to 109 is average; 110 to 119 is high average; and above 120 is in the superior or very superior range. The multiple breakdowns of the performance and verbal subscales allow a great flexibility in identifying specific areas of deficit and scatter in intellectual abilities. Because a large part of intelligence testing measures abilities used in academic settings, the breakdown of the WISC-III can also be helpful in pointing out skills in which a child is weak and may benefit from remedial education.

The Stanford-Binet Intelligence Scale covers an age range from 2 to 24 years. It relies on pictures, drawings, and objects for very young children and on verbal performance for older children and adolescents. This intelligence scale is the earliest version of an intelligence test of its kind and leads to a mental age score as well as an IQ.

LONG-TERM STABILITY OF INTELLIGENCE.   Although a child's intelligence is relatively stable throughout the school-age years and adolescence, some factors can influence intelligence and a child's score on an intelligence test. The intellectual functions of children with severe mental illnesses and of those from low socioeconomic levels may decrease over time, whereas the IQs of children whose environments have been enriched may increase over time. Factors that influence a child's score on a given test of intellectual functioning and thus affect the accuracy of the test are motivation, emotional state, anxiety, and cultural milieu.

Perceptual and Perceptual Motor Tests.   The Bender Visual Motor Gestalt test can be given to children between the ages of 4 and 12 years. The test consists of a set of spatially related figures that the child is asked to copy. The scores are based on the number of errors. Although not a diagnostic test, it is useful in identifying developmentally age-inappropriate perceptual performances.

Personality Tests.   Personality tests are not of much use in making diagnoses, and they are less satisfactory than intelligence tests in regard to norms, reliability, and validity, but they can be helpful in eliciting themes and fantasies.

The Rorschach test is a projective technique in which ambiguous stimuli—a set of bilaterally symmetrical inkblots—are shown to a child, who is then asked to describe what he or she sees in each. The hypothesis is that the child's interpretation of the vague stimuli reflects basic characteristics of personality. The examiner notes the themes and patterns. Two sets of norms have been established for the Rorschach test, one for children between 2 and 10 years and one for adolescents between 10 and 17 years.

A more structured projective test is the Children's Apperception Test (CAT), which is an adaptation of the Thematic Apperception Test (TAT). The CAT consists of cards with pictures of animals in scenes that are somewhat ambiguous but are related to parent–child and sibling issues, caretaking, and other relationships. The child is asked to describe what is happening and to tell a story about the scene. Animals are used because it was hypothesized that children may respond more readily to animal images than to human figures.

Educational Tests.   Achievement tests measure the attainment of knowledge and skills in a particular academic curriculum. The Wide-Range Achievement Test–Revised (WRAT–R) consists of tests of knowledge and skills and timed performances of reading, spelling, and

mathematics. It is used with children ranging from 5 years to adulthood. The test yields a score that is compared with the average expected score for the child's chronological age and grade level.

The Kaufman Test of Educational Achievement, the Gray Oral Reading Test–Revised (GORTt-R), and the Sequential Tests of Educational Progress (STEP) are achievement tests that determine whether a child has achieved the educational level expected for the child's grade level.

Biopsychosocial Formulation.   The clinician's task is to integrate all of the information obtained into a formulation that takes into account the biological predisposition, psychodynamic factors, environmental stressors, and life events that have led to the child's current level of functioning. Psychiatric disorders and any specific physical, neuromotor, or developmental abnormalities must be considered in the formulation of etiologic factors for current impairment. The clinician's conclusions are an integration of clinical information along with data from standardized psychological and developmental assessments. The psychiatric formulation includes an assessment of family function as well as the appropriateness of the child's educational setting. A determination of the child's overall safety in his or her current situation is made, and a judgment regarding suspicion of any maltreatment is made, with a report to the local child protective service agency when suspicion is present. The child's overall well-being regarding growth, development, and academic and play activities is considered.

Diagnosis

The clinician's task includes making all appropriate diagnoses according to DSM-IV-TR. Some clinical situations do not fulfill criteria for DSM-IV-TR diagnoses but cause impairment and require psychiatric attention and intervention. Clinicians who evaluate children are frequently in the position of determining the impact of behavior of family members on the child's well-being. In many cases, a child's level of impairment will be related to factors extending beyond a psychiatric diagnosis, such as the child's adjustment to his or her family life, peer relationships, and educational placement.

RECOMMENDATIONS AND TREATMENT PLAN

Recommendations and a treatment plan following an evaluation of a child most often include the cooperation of family members. As part of the treatment for a given psychiatric disorder in a child, direct family and environmental interventions are often included. The safety of the child is always a consideration when devising a set of recommendations. The clinician must communicate the recommendations and proposed treatment plan to both the parents and the child because, without the parents' cooperation, treatment may be compromised or not obtained.

A clinician seeks to give feedback to whomever has referred the child for the evaluation, with appropriate permission. Thus, when a child is referred for evaluation by an outside agency, such as a school, therapist, or protective service agency, permission is generally obtained to provide information to the persons who have made the referral.

Mental Retardation

Mental retardation is not a disease; rather, it is the result of a pathological process in the brain characterized by limitations in intellectual and adaptive function. The cause of mental retardation is often unidentified, and the consequences become evident by a person's difficulties intellectually and in living skills.

Since the passage of Public Law 94-142 (the Education for all Handicapped Children Act) in 1975, the public school system has been mandated to provide appropriate educational service to all children with disabilities. The Individuals with Disabilities Act of 1990 provides extensions and modification of the above legislation. Currently, provision of public education for all children, including those with disabilities, is mandated by law and is to be provided "within the least restrictive environment."

CLASSIFICATION

According to the text revision of the fourth edition of the *Diagnostic and Statistical Manual of Mental Disorders* (DSM-IV-TR), mental retardation is defined as significantly subaverage general intellectual functioning resulting in or associated with concurrent impairments in adaptive behavior and manifested during the developmental period, before the age of 18. The diagnosis is made regardless of whether the person has a coexisting physical disorder or other mental disorder. Table 34–1 presents an overview of developmental levels in communication, academic functioning, and vocational skills expected of people with various degrees of mental retardation.

General intellectual functioning is determined by the use of standardized tests of intelligence, and the term *significantly subaverage* is defined as an intelligence quotient (IQ) of approximately 70 or below or two standard deviations below the mean for the particular test. Adaptive functioning can be measured by using a standardized scale, such as the Vineland Adaptive Behavior Scale. In this scale, communications, daily living skills, socialization, and motor skills (up to 4 years, 11 months) are scored and generate an adaptive behavior composite that is correlated with the expected skills at a given age.

Approximately 85 percent of people who are mentally retarded fall within the mild mental retardation category. Mental retardation is influenced by genetic, environmental, and psychosocial factors, and in past years, the development of mild retardation has often been attributed to severe psychosocial deprivation. More recently, however, researchers have increasingly recognized the likely contribution of a host of subtle biological factors, including chromosomal abnormalities, subclinical lead intoxications, and prenatal exposure to drugs, alcohol, and other toxins. Furthermore, there is increasing evidence that subgroups of people who are

mentally retarded, such as those with fragile X syndrome, Down syndrome, and Prader-Willi syndrome, have characteristic patterns of social, linguistic, and cognitive development and typical behavior manifestations.

The DSM-IV-TR has included in its text on mental retardation additional information regarding etiological factors and their association with mental retardation syndromes (e.g., fragile X syndrome).

EPIDEMIOLOGY

The prevalence of mental retardation at any one time is estimated to be approximately 1 percent of the population. The incidence of mental retardation is difficult to calculate because mental retardation sometimes goes unrecognized until middle childhood when it is mild. In some cases, even when intellectual function is limited, good adaptive skills are not challenged until late childhood or early adolescence, and the diagnosis is not made until that time. The highest incidence is in school-age children, with the peak at ages 10 to 14 years. Mental retardation is approximately 1.5 times more common among men than among women. In older people, prevalence is less; those with severe or profound mental retardation have high mortality rates resulting from the complications of associated physical disorders.

COMORBIDITY

Prevalence

Epidemiological surveys indicate that up to two-thirds of children and adults with mental retardation have comorbid mental disorders; this rate is several times higher than that in non–mentally retarded community samples. The prevalence of psychopathology seems to be correlated with the degree of mental retardation. A recent epidemiological study found that 40.7 percent of intellectually disabled children between 4 and 18 years of age met criteria for at least one psychiatric disorder. The severity of retardation affected the type of psychiatric disorder. Those with profound mental retardation were less likely to exhibit psychiatric symptoms.

Neurological Disorders

In a recent review of psychiatric disorders in children and adolescents with mental retardation and epilepsy, approximately one-third also had autistic disorder or an autistic-like condition. The combination of mental retardation, active epilepsy, and

Table 34–1
Developmental Characteristics of Mentally Retarded Persons

Degree of Mental Retardation	Preschool Age (0–5) Maturation and Development	School Age (6–20) Training and Education	Adult (21 and Over) Social and Vocational Adequacy
Profound	Gross retardation; minimal capacity for functioning in sensorimotor areas; needs nursing care; constant aid and supervision required	Some motor development present; may respond to minimal or limited training in self-help	Some motor and speech development; may achieve very limited self-care; needs nursing care
Severe	Poor motor development; speech minimal; generally unable to profit from training in self-help; little or no communication skills	Can talk or learn to communicate; can be trained in elemental health habits; profits from systematic habit training; unable to profit from vocational training	May contribute partially to self-maintenance under complete supervision; can develop self-protection skills to a minimal useful level in controlled environment
Moderate	Can talk or learn to communicate; poor social awareness; fair motor development; profits from training in self-help; can be managed with moderate supervision	Can profit from training in social and occupational skills; unlikely to progress beyond second-grade level in academic subjects; may learn to travel alone in familiar places	May achieve self-maintenance in unskilled or semiskilled work under sheltered conditions; needs supervision and guidance when under mild social or economic stress
Mild	Can develop social and communication skills; minimal retardation in sensorimotor areas; often not distinguished from normal until later age	Can learn academic skills up to approximately sixth-grade level by late teens; can be guided toward social conformity	Can usually achieve social and vocational skills adequate to minimum self-support but may need guidance and assistance when under unusual social or economic stress

Adapted from *Mental Retarded Activities of the U.S. Department of Health, Education and Welfare.* Washington, DC: US Government Printing Office; 1989:2. Used with permission. DSM-IV-TR criteria are adapted essentially from this chart.

autism or an autistic-like condition occurs at a rate of 0.07 percent in the general population.

Genetic Syndromes

Some evidence indicates that genetically based syndromes such as fragile X syndrome, Prader-Willi syndrome, and Down syndrome (discussed below) are associated with comorbid specific behavioral manifestations. People with fragile X syndrome are known to have extremely high rates (up to three-fourths of those studied) of attention-deficit/hyperactivity disorders (ADHDs). High rates of aberrant interpersonal behavior and language function often meet the criteria for autistic disorder and avoidant personality disorder. Prader-Willi syndrome is almost always associated with compulsive eating disturbances, hyperphagia, and obesity.

Psychosocial Syndromes

Communication difficulties increase mentally retarded person's vulnerability to feelings of ineptness and frustration. Inappropriate behaviors, such as withdrawal, are common. The perpetual sense of isolation and inadequacy has been linked to feelings of anxiety, anger, dysphoria, and depression.

ETIOLOGY

Etiological factors in mental retardation may be primarily genetic, developmental, acquired, or a combination of factors. Genetic causes include chromosomal and inherited conditions; developmental factors include chromosomal changes such as trisomies or prenatal exposure to infections and toxins; and acquired syndromes include perinatal trauma (such as prematurity) and socio-

cultural factors. Among chromosomal and metabolic disorders, Down syndrome, fragile X syndrome, and phenylketonuria (PKU) are the most common disorders that usually produce at least moderate mental retardation. Those with mild mental retardation sometimes have a familial pattern apparent in parents and siblings. Deprivation of nutrition, nurturance, and social stimulation may contribute to the development of mental retardation. Current knowledge suggests that genetic, environmental, biological, and psychosocial factors work additively in mental retardation.

Genetic Factors

Abnormalities in autosomal chromosomes are associated with mental retardation, although aberrations in sex chromosomes are not always associated with mental retardation (such as Turner's syndrome with XO and Klinefelter's syndrome with XXY, XXXY, and XXYY variations).

Down Syndrome. Despite a plethora of theories and hypotheses advanced in the past 100 years, the cause of Down syndrome is still unknown. The problem of cause is complicated even further by the recent recognition of three types of chromosomal aberrations in Down syndrome:

1. Patients with trisomy 21 (three of chromosome 21, instead of the usual two) represent the overwhelming majority; they have 47 chromosomes, with an extra chromosome 21.
2. Nondisjunction occurring after fertilization in any cell division results in mosaicism, a condition in which both normal and trisomic cells are found in various tissues.
3. In translocation, there is a fusion of two chromosomes, mostly 21 and 15, resulting in a total of 46 chromosomes,

despite the presence of an extra chromosome 21. The disorder, unlike trisomy 21, is usually inherited.

Mental retardation is the overriding feature of Down syndrome. Most people with the syndrome are moderately or severely retarded, with only a minority having an IQ above 50. Mental development seems to progress normally from birth to 6 months of age; IQ scores gradually decrease from near normal at 1 year of age to approximately 30 at older ages. The decline in intelligence may be real or apparent: Infantile tests may not reveal the full extent of the defect, which may become manifest when sophisticated tests are used in early childhood. According to many sources, children with Down syndrome are placid, cheerful, and cooperative and adapt easily at home. With adolescence, the picture changes: Youngsters may experience various emotional difficulties, behavior disorders, and (rarely) psychotic disorders.

The diagnosis of Down syndrome is made with relative ease in an older child but is often difficult in newborn infants. The most important signs in a newborn include general hypotonia, oblique palpebral fissures, abundant neck skin, a small, flattened skull, high cheekbones, and a protruding tongue. The hands are broad and thick, with a single palmar transversal crease, and the little fingers are short and curved inward. Moro reflex is weak or absent. More than 100 signs or stigmata are described in Down syndrome, but rarely are all found in one person. Life expectancy was once approximately 12 years; with the advent of antibiotics, few young patients succumb to infections, but many do not live beyond the age of 40. Life expectancy is increasing, however.

People with Down syndrome tend to show a marked deterioration in language, memory, self-care skills, and problem solving in their 30s. Postmortem studies of those with Down syndrome over the age of 40 have shown a high incidence of senile plaques and neurofibrillary tangles, as seen in Alzheimer's disease. Neurofibrillary tangles are known to occur in a variety of degenerative diseases, whereas senile plaques seem to be found most often in Alzheimer's disease and in Down syndrome. Thus, the two disorders may share some degree of pathophysiology.

Fragile X Syndrome.   Fragile X syndrome is the second most common single cause of mental retardation. The syndrome results from a mutation on the X chromosome at what is known as the *fragile site* (Xq27.3). The behavioral profile of people with the syndrome includes a high rate of ADHD, learning disorders, and pervasive developmental disorders, such as autism.

Prader-Willi Syndrome.   Prader-Willi syndrome is postulated to be the result of a small deletion involving chromosome 15, usually occurring sporadically. Its prevalence is less than 1 in 10,000. Persons with the syndrome exhibit compulsive eating behavior and often obesity, mental retardation, hypogonadism, small stature, hypotonia, and small hands and feet. Children with the syndrome often have oppositional and defiant behavior.

Phenylketonuria.   PKU is transmitted as a simple recessive autosomal mendelian trait. Most patients with PKU are severely retarded, but some are reported to have borderline or normal intelligence. Although the clinical picture varies, typical children

with PKU are hyperactive; they exhibit erratic, unpredictable behavior and are difficult to manage. Their behavior sometimes resembles that of children with autism or schizophrenia.

Rett's Disorder.   Rett's disorder is hypothesized to be an X-linked dominant mental retardation syndrome that is degenerative and affects only females. Deterioration in communications skills, motor behavior, and social functioning starts at approximately 1 year of age. Autistic-like symptoms are common, as are ataxia, facial grimacing, teeth grinding, and loss of speech.

Lesch-Nyhan Syndrome.   Lesch-Nyhan syndrome is a rare disorder caused by a deficiency of an enzyme involved in purine metabolism. The disorder is X-linked; patients have mental retardation, microcephaly, seizures, choreoathetosis, and spasticity. The syndrome is also associated with severe compulsive self-mutilation by biting of the mouth and the fingers. Lesch-Nyhan syndrome is another example of a genetically determined syndrome with a specific, predictable behavioral pattern.

OTHER ENZYME DEFICIENCY DISORDERS

Thirty important disorders with inborn errors of metabolism, hereditary transmission patterns, defective enzymes, clinical signs, and relation to mental retardation are listed in Table 34–2.

Acquired and Developmental Factors

Prenatal Period.   Maternal infections during pregnancy, especially viral infections, have been known to cause fetal damage and mental retardation. The degree of fetal damage depends on such variables as the type of viral infection, the gestational age of the fetus, and the severity of the illness.

Rubella (German Measles).   Rubella has replaced syphilis as the major cause of congenital malformations and mental retardation caused by maternal infection. The children of affected mothers may show several abnormalities, including congenital heart disease, mental retardation, cataracts, deafness, microcephaly, and microphthalmia. Timing is crucial, as the extent and the frequency of the complications are inversely related to the duration of the pregnancy at the time of the maternal infection. Maternal rubella can be prevented by immunization.

Acquired Immune Deficiency Syndrome (AIDS). Many fetuses of mothers with AIDS never come to term because of stillbirth or spontaneous abortion. In those who are born infected with the human immunodeficiency virus (HIV), up to half have progressive encephalopathy, mental retardation, and seizures within the first year of life. Children born infected with HIV often live only a few years; however, most babies born to HIV-infected mothers are not infected with the virus.

Fetal Alcohol Syndrome.   Fetal alcohol syndrome results in mental retardation and a typical phenotypic picture of facial dysmorphism that includes hypertelorism, microcephaly, short palpebral fissures, inner epicanthal folds, and a short, turned-up nose. Often, the affected children have learning disorders, ADHD, and mental retardation without the facial dysmorphism.

Table 34–2
Thirty Impairment Disorders with Inborn Errors of Metabolism

Disorder	Hereditary Transmission[a]	Enzyme Defect	Prenatal Diagnosis	Mental Retardation	Clinical Signs
I. LIPID METABOLISM					
Niemann-Pick disease					
Group A, infantile		Unknown			Hepatomegaly
Group B, adult	A.R.	Sphingomyelinase	+	±	Hepatosplenomegaly
Groups C and D, intermediate		Unknown	−	+	Pulmonary infiltration
Infantile Gaucher's disease	A.R.	β-Glucosidase	+	±	Hepatosplenomegaly, pseudobulbar palsy
Tay-Sachs disease	A.R.	Hexosaminidase A	+	+	Macular changes, seizures, spasticity
Generalized gangliosidosis	A.R.	β-Galactosidase	+	+	Hepatosplenomegaly, bone changes
Krabbe's disease	A.R.	Galactocerebroside β-Galactosidase	+	+	Stiffness, seizures
Metachromatic leukodystrophy	A.R.	Cerebroside sulfatase	+	+	Stiffness, developmental failure
Wolman's disease	A.R.	Acid lipase	+	−	Hepatosplenomegaly, adrenal calcification, vomiting, diarrhea
Farber's lipogranulomatosis	A.R.	Acid ceramidase	+	+	Hoarseness, arthropathy, subcutaneous nodules
Fabry's disease	X.R.	α-Galactosidase	+	−	Angiokeratomas, renal failure
II. MUCOPOLYSACCHARIDE METABOLISM					
Hurler's syndrome MPS I	A.R.	Iduronidase	+	+	?
Hurler's disease II	X.R.	Iduronate sulfatase	+	+	?
Sanfilippo's syndrome III	A.R.	Various sulfatases (types A–D)	+	+	Varying degrees of bone changes, hepatosplenomegaly, joint restriction, etc.
Morquio's disease IV	A.R.	N-Acetylgalactosamine-6-sulfate sulfatase	+	−	?
Maroteaux-Lamy syndrome VI	A.R.	Arylsulfatase B	+	±	?
III. OLIGOSACCHARIDE AND GLYCOPROTEIN METABOLISM					
I-cell disease	A.R.	Glycoprotein N-acetylglucosaminyl-phosphotransferase	+	+	Hepatomegaly, bone changes, swollen gingivae
Mannosidosis	A.R.	Mannosidase	+	+	Hepatomegaly, bone changes, facial coarsening
Fucosidosis	A.R.	Fucosidase	+	+	Same as above
IV. AMINO ACID METABOLISM					
Phenylketonuria	A.R.	Phenylalanine hydroxylase	−	+	Eczema, blonde hair, musty odor
Hemocystinuria	A.R.	Cystathionine β-synthetase	+	+	Ectopia lentis, Marfan-like phenotype, cardiovascular anomalies
Tyrosinosis	A.R.	Tyrosine amine transaminase	−	+	Hyperkeratotic skin lesions, conjunctivitis
Maple syrup urine disease	A.R.	Branched-chain ketoacid decarboxylase	+	+	Recurrent ketoacidosis
Methylmalonic acidemia	A.R.	Methylmalonyl-CoA mutase	+	+	Recurrent ketoacidosis, hepatomegaly, growth retardation
Propionic acidemia	A.R.	Propionyl-CoA carboxylase	+	+	Same as above
Nonketotic hyperglycinemia	A.R.	Glycine cleavage enzyme	+	+	Seizures
Urea cycle disorders	Mostly A.R.	Urea cycle enzymes	+	+	Recurrent acute encephalopathy, vomiting
Hartnup disease	A.R.	Renal transport disorder	−	−	None consistent

(continued)

Table 34–2 (*continued*)

Disorder	Hereditary Transmission[a]	Enzyme Defect	Prenatal Diagnosis	Mental Retardation	Clinical Signs
V. OTHERS					
Galactosemia	A.R.	Galactose-1-phosphate uridyltransferase	+	+	Hepatomegaly, cataracts, ovarian failure
Wilson's hepatolenticu- lar degeneration	A.R.	Unknown factor in copper metabolism	−	±	Liver disease, Kayser-Fleischer ring, neurological problems
Menkes' kinky-hair dis- ease	X.R.	Same as above	+	−	Abnormal hair, cerebral degener- ation
Lesch-Nyhan syndrome	X.R.	Hypoxanthine guanine phosphoribosyltrans- ferase	+	+	Behavioral abnormalities

[a]A.R., autosomal recessive transmission; X.R., X-linked recessive transmission.
Adapted from Leroy JC. Hereditary, development, and behavior. In: Levine MD, Carey WB, Crocker AC, eds. *Developmental-Behavioral Pediatrics*. Phila- delphia: WB Saunders; 1983:315.

Prenatal Drug Exposure.   Prenatal exposure to opiates, such as heroin, often results in infants who are small for their ges- tational age, with a head circumference below the 10th percentile and withdrawal symptoms that are manifest within the first 2 days of life. The withdrawal symptoms of infants include irritability, hypertonia, tremor, vomiting, a high-pitched cry, and an abnormal sleep pattern. Seizures are unusual, but the withdrawal syndrome can be life threatening to infants if it is untreated. Diazepam (Valium), phenobarbital (Luminal), chlorpromazine (Thorazine), and paregoric have been used to treat neonatal opiate withdrawal.

Complications of Pregnancy.   Toxemia of pregnancy and uncontrolled maternal diabetes present hazards to the fetus and sometimes result in mental retardation. Maternal malnutrition during pregnancy often results in prematurity and other obstetri- cal complications. Vaginal hemorrhage, placenta previa, prema- ture separation of the placenta, and prolapse of the cord may damage the fetal brain by causing anoxia. The potential terato- genic effect of pharmacological agents administered during preg- nancy was widely publicized after the thalidomide tragedy (the drug produced a high percentage of deformed babies when given to pregnant women). The use of lithium (Eskalith) during preg- nancy was recently implicated in some congenital malforma- tions, especially of the cardiovascular system (e.g., Ebstein's anomaly).

Perinatal Period.   Some evidence indicates that premature infants and infants with low birth weight are at high risk for neuro- logical and intellectual impairments that are manifest during their school years. Recent studies have documented that, among chil- dren with very low birth weight (less than 1,000 grams), 20 percent were found to have significant disabilities, including cerebral palsy, mental retardation, autism, and low intelligence with severe learning problems.

Acquired Childhood Disorders.   Occasionally, a child's developmental status changes dramatically as a result of a spe- cific disease or physical trauma. In retrospect, it is sometimes difficult to ascertain the full picture of the child's developmen- tal progress before the insult, but the adverse effects on the child's development or skills are apparent afterward.

Infection.   The most serious infections affecting cerebral integrity are encephalitis and meningitis. Most episodes of encephalitis are caused by viral organisms. Meningitis that was diagnosed late, even when followed by antibiotic treatment, can seriously affect a child's cognitive development.

Head Trauma.   The best-known causes of head injury in chil- dren that produce developmental handicaps, including seizures, are motor vehicle accidents, but more head injuries are caused by household accidents, such as falls from tables, from open win- dows, and on stairways. Child abuse is also a cause of head injury.

Other Issues.   One cause of complete or partial brain dam- age is asphyxia associated with near drowning. Long-term exposure to lead is a well-established cause of compromised intelligence and learning skills. Intracranial tumors of various types and origins, surgery, and chemotherapy can also adversely affect brain function.

Environmental and Sociocultural Factors

Mild retardation may occur as a result of significant deprivation of nutrition, nurturance, and appropriate stimulation. Children who have endured these conditions are subject to long-lasting damage to their physical and emotional development. Prenatal environment compromised by poor medical care and poor maternal nutrition can be contributing factors in the develop- ment of mild mental retardation. Teenage pregnancies are risk factors and are associated with obstetrical complications, pre- maturity, and low birth weight. Poor postnatal medical care, malnutrition, exposure to such toxic substances as lead, and physical trauma are risk factors for mild mental retardation. Family instability, frequent moves, and multiple but inadequate caretakers may deprive an infant of necessary emotional rela- tionships, leading to failure to thrive and potential risk to the developing brain.

DIAGNOSIS

The diagnosis of mental retardation can be made after the history, a standardized intellectual assessment, and a measure of adaptive

Table 34–3
DSM-IV-TR Diagnostic Criteria for Mental Retardation

A. Significantly subaverage intellectual functioning: an IQ of approximately 70 or below on an individually administered IQ test (for infants, a clinical judgment of significantly subaverage intellectual functioning).

B. Concurrent deficits or impairments in present adaptive functioning (i.e., the person's effectiveness in meeting the standards expected for his or her age by his or her cultural group) in at least two of the following areas: communication, self-care, home living, social/interpersonal skills, use of community resources, self-direction, functional academic skills, work, leisure, health, and safety.

C. The onset is before age 18 years.

Code based on degree of severity reflecting level of intellectual impairment:

Mild mental retardation:	IQ level 50–55 to approximately 70
Moderate mental retardation:	IQ level 35–40 to 50–55
Severe mental retardation:	IQ level 20–25 to 35–40
Profound mental retardation:	IQ level below 20 or 25
Mental retardation, severity unspecified:	When there is strong presumption of mental retardation but the person's intelligence is untestable by standard tests

From American Psychiatric Association. *Diagnostic and Statistical Manual of Mental Disorders.* 4th ed. Text rev. Washington, DC: American Psychiatric Association; copyright 2000, with permission.

function indicate that a child's current behavior is significantly below the expected level (Table 34–3). The diagnosis itself does not specify either the cause or the prognosis. Laboratory tests can be used to ascertain the cause and prognosis.

History

The history is most often taken from the parents or the caretaker, with particular attention to the mother's pregnancy, labor, and delivery; the presence of a family history of mental retardation; consanguinity of the parents; and hereditary disorders. As part of the history, the clinician assesses the overall level of functioning and the intellectual capacity of the parents and the emotional climate of the home.

Psychiatric Interview

Two factors are of paramount importance when interviewing the patient: the interviewer's attitude and the manner of communicating with the patient. The interviewer should not be guided by the patient's mental age, which cannot fully characterize the person.

The patient's verbal abilities, including receptive and expressive language, should be assessed as soon as possible by observing the verbal and nonverbal communication between the caretakers and the patient and by taking the history. Leading questions should be avoided, as retarded people may be suggestible and wish to please others. Subtle direction, structure, and reinforcement may be necessary to keep them on the task or topic.

In general, the psychiatric examination of a retarded person should reveal how the patient has coped with the stages of development.

Physical Examination

Various parts of the body may have certain characteristics that have prenatal causes and are commonly found in people who are mentally retarded. Table 34–4 lists the multiple handicaps associated with mental retardation syndromes. The clinician should bear in mind during the examination that mentally

Table 34–4
Representative Sample of Mental Retardation Syndromes and Behavioral Phenotypes

Disorder	Pathophysiology	Clinical Features and Behavioral Phenotype
Down syndrome	Trisomy 21, 95% nondisjunction, approx. 4% translocation; 1/1,000 live births: 1:2,500 in women less than 30 years old, 1:80 over 40 years old, 1:32 at 45 years old; possible overproduction of β-amyloid due to defect at 21q 21.1	Hypotonia, upward-slanted palpebral fissures, midface depression, flat wide nasal bridge, simian crease, short stature, increased incidence of thyroid abnormalities and congenital heart disease Passive, affable, hyperactivity in childhood, stubborn; verbal > auditory processing, increased risk of depression, and dementia of the Alzheimer type in adulthood
Fragile X syndrome	Inactivation of *FMR-1* gene at X q27.3 due to CGG base repeats, methylation; recessive; 1:1,000 male births, 1:3,000 female; accounts for 10–12% of mental retardation in males	Long face, large ears, midface hypoplasia, high arched palate, short stature, macroorchidism, mitral valve prolapse, joint laxity, strabismus Hyperactivity, inattention, anxiety, stereotypies, speech and language delays, IQ decline, gaze aversion, social avoidance, shyness, irritability, learning disorder in some females; mild mental retardation in affected females, moderate to severe in males; verbal IQ > performance IQ
Prader-Willi syndrome	Deletion in 15q12 (15q11–15q13) of paternal origin; some cases of maternal uniparental disomy; dominant 1/10,000 live births; 90% sporadic; candidate gene: small nuclear ribonucleoprotein polypeptide (SNRPN)	Hypotonia, failure to thrive in infancy, obesity, small hands and feet, microorchidism, cryptorchidism, short stature, almond-shaped eyes, fair hair and light skin, flat face, scoliosis, orthopedic problems, prominent forehead and bitemporal narrowing Compulsive behavior, hyperphagia, hoarding, impulsivity, borderline to moderate mental retardation, emotional lability, tantrums, excess daytime sleepiness, skin picking, anxiety, aggression

(continued)

Table 34–4 (continued)

Disorder	Pathophysiology	Clinical Features and Behavioral Phenotype
Angelman syndrome	Deletion in 15q12 (15q11–15q13) of maternal origin; dominant; frequent deletion of GABA B-3 receptor subunit, prevalence unknown but rare, estimated 1/20,000–1/30,000	Fair hair and blue eyes (66%); dysmorphic faces including wide smiling mouth, thin upper lip, and pointed chin; epilepsy (90%) with characteristic EEG; ataxia; small head circumference, 25% microcephalic Happy disposition, paroxysmal laughter, hand flapping, clapping; profound mental retardation; sleep disturbance with nighttime waking; possible increased incidence of autistic features; anecdotal love of water and music
Cornelia de Lange syndrome	Lack of pregnancy associated plasma protein A (PAPPA) linked to chromosome 9q33; similar phenotype associated with trisomy 5p, ring chromosome 3; rare (1/40,000–1/100,000 live births); possible association with 3q26.3	Continuous eyebrows, thin downturning upper lip, microcephaly, short stature, small hands and feet, small upturned nose, anteverted nostrils, malformed upper limbs, failure to thrive Self-injury, limited speech in severe cases, language delays, avoidance of being held, stereotypic movements, twirling, severe to profound mental retardation
Williams syndrome	1/20,000 births; hemizygous deletion that includes elastin locus chromosome 7q11–23; autosomal dominant	Short stature, unusual facial features including broad forehead, depressed nasal bridge, stellate pattern of the iris, widely spaced teeth, and full lips; elfin-like facies; renal and cardiovascular abnormalities; thyroid abnormalities; hypercalcemia Anxiety, hyperactivity, fears, outgoing, sociable, verbal skills > visual spatial skills
Cri-du-chat syndrome	Partial deletion 5p; 1/50,000; region may be 5p15.2	Round face with hypertelorism, epicanthal folds, slanting palpebral fissures, broad flat nose, low-set ears, micrognathia; prenatal growth retardation; respiratory and ear infections; congenital heart disease; gastrointestinal abnormalities Severe mental retardation, infantile catlike cry, hyperactivity, stereotypies, self-injury
Smith-Magenis syndrome	Incidence unknown, estimated 1/25,000 live births; complete or partial deletion of 17p11.2	Broad face; flat midface; short, broad hands; small toes; hoarse, deep voice Severe mental retardation; hyperactivity; severe self-injury including hand biting, head banging, and pulling out finger- and toenails; stereotyped self-hugging; attention seeking; aggression; sleep disturbance (decreased REM)
Rubinstein-Taybi syndrome	1/250,000, approx. male = female; sporadic; likely autosomal dominant; documented microdeletions in some cases at 16p13.3	Short stature and microcephaly, broad thumb and big toes, prominent nose, broad nasal bridge, hypertelorism, ptosis, frequent fractures, feeding difficulties in infancy, congenital heart disease, EEG abnormalities, seizures Poor concentration, distractible, expressive language difficulties, performance IQ > verbal IQ; anecdotally happy, loving, sociable, responsive to music, self-stimulating behavior; older patients have mood lability and temper tantrums
Tuberous sclerosis complex 1 and 2	Benign tumors (hamartomas) and malformations (hamartias) of CNS, skin, kidney, heart; dominant; 1/10,000 births; 50% TSC 1, 9q34; 50% TSC 2, 16p13	Epilepsy, autism, hyperactivity, impulsivity, aggression; spectrum of mental retardation from none (30%) to profound; self-injurious behaviors, sleep disturbances
Neurofibromatosis type 1 (NF1)	1/2,500–1/4,000; male = female; autosomal dominant; 50% new mutations; more than 90% paternal NF1 allele mutated; NFI gene 17q11.2; gene product is neurofibromin thought to be tumor suppressor gene	Variable manifestations; café au lait spots, cutaneous neurofibromas, Lisch nodules; short stature and macrocephaly in 30–45% Half with speech and language difficulties; 10% with moderate to profound mental retardation; verbal IQ > performance IQ; distractible, impulsive, hyperactive, anxious; possibly associated with increased incidence of mood and anxiety disorders
Lesch-Nyhan syndrome	Defect in hypoxanthine guanine phosphoribosyltransferase with accumulation of uric acid; Xq26–27; recessive; rare (1/10,000–1/38,000)	Ataxia, chorea, kidney failure, gout Often severe self-biting behavior; aggression; anxiety; mild to moderate mental retardation
Galactosemia	Defect in galactose-1-phosphate uridyltransferase or galactokinase or empiramase; autosomal recessive; 1/62,000 births in the U.S.	Vomiting in early infancy, jaundice, hepatosplenomegaly; later cataracts, weight loss, food refusal, increased intracranial pressure and increased risk for sepsis, ovarian failure, failure to thrive, renal tubular damage Possible mental retardation even with treatment, visuospatial deficits, language disorders, reports of increased behavioral problems, anxiety, social withdrawal, and shyness

(continued)

Table 34–4 (continued)

Disorder	Pathophysiology	Clinical Features and Behavioral Phenotype
Phenylketon-uria	Defect in phenylalanine hydroxylase (PAH) or cofactor (biopterin) with accumulation of phenylalanine; approximately 1/11,500 births; varies with geographical location; gene for PAH, 12q22–24.1; autosomal recessive	Symptoms absent neonatally, later development of seizures (25% generalized), fair skin, blue eyes, blond hair, rash Untreated: mild to profound mental retardation, language delay, destructiveness, self-injury, hyperactivity
Hurler's syndrome	1/100,000; deficiency in α-ʟ-iduronidase activity; autosomal recessive	Early onset; short stature, hepatosplenomegaly; hirsutism, corneal clouding, death before age 10 years, dwarfism, coarse facial features, recurrent respiratory infections Moderate-to-severe mental retardation, anxious, fearful, rarely aggressive
Hunter's syndrome	1/100,000, X-linked recessive; iduronate sulfatase deficiency; X q28	Normal infancy; symptom onset at age 2–4 years; typical coarse faces with flat nasal bridge, flaring nostrils; hearing loss, ataxia, hernia common; enlarged liver and spleen, joint stiffness, recurrent infections, growth retardation, cardiovascular abnormality Hyperactivity, mental retardation by 2 years; speech delay; loss of speech at 8–10 years; restless, aggressive, inattentive, sleep abnormalities; apathetic, sedentary with disease progression
Fetal alcohol syndrome	Maternal alcohol consumption (trimester III>II>I); 1/3,000 live births in Western countries; 1/300 with fetal alcohol effects	Microcephaly, short stature, midface hypoplasia, short palpebral fissure, thin upper lip, retrognathia in infancy, micrognathia in adolescence, hypoplastic long or smooth philtrum Mild to moderate mental retardation, irritability, inattention, memory impairment

Table by B. H. King, M.D., R. M. Hodapp, Ph.D., and E. M. Dykens, Ph.D.

retarded children, particularly those with associated behavioral problems, are at increased risk for child abuse.

Neurological Examination

Skull X-rays are usually taken routinely but are illuminating in only a relatively few conditions, such as craniosynostosis, hydrocephalus, and other disorders that result in intracranial calcifications (for example, toxoplasmosis, tuberous sclerosis, cerebral angiomatosis, and hypoparathyroidism). Computed tomography (CT) scans and magnetic resonance imaging (MRI) have become important tools for uncovering central nervous system (CNS) pathology associated with mental retardation. The occasional findings of internal hydrocephalus, cortical atrophy, or porencephaly in a severely retarded, brain-damaged child are not considered important to the general picture.

CLINICAL FEATURES

Surveys have identified several clinical features that occur with greater frequency in people who are mentally retarded than in the general population. These features, which may occur in isolation or as part of a mental disorder, include hyperactivity, low frustration tolerance, aggression, affective instability, repetitive, stereotypic motor behaviors, and various self-injurious behaviors. Self-injurious behaviors seem to be more frequent and more intense with increasingly severe mental retardation. It is often difficult to decide whether these clinical features are comorbid mental disorders or direct sequelae of the developmental limitations imposed by mental retardation.

LABORATORY EXAMINATION

Laboratory tests used to elucidate the causes of mental retardation include chromosomal analysis, testing of the urine and blood for metabolic disorders, and neuroimaging. Chromosome abnor-

malities are the single most common cause of mental retardation found in those individuals for whom a cause can be identified.

Chromosome Studies

The determination of the karyotype in a genetic laboratory is considered whenever a chromosomal disorder is suspected or when the cause of the mental retardation is unidentified.

Amniocentesis, in which a small amount of amniotic fluid is removed from the amniotic cavity transabdominally at approximately the 15th week of gestation, has been useful in diagnosing prenatal chromosomal abnormalities. It is often considered when there is an increased fetal risk, such as with increased maternal age, of Down syndrome. Many serious hereditary disorders can be predicted with amniocentesis, and it should be considered by pregnant women over the age of 35.

Chronic villi sampling (CVS) is a screening technique to determine fetal chromosomal abnormalities. If the result is abnormal, the decision to terminate the pregnancy can be made within the first trimester.

Urine and Blood Analysis

Lesch-Nyhan Syndrome, galactosemia, PKU, Hurler syndrome, and Hunter syndrome are examples of disorders that include mental retardation and can be identified through assays of the appropriate enzyme or organic or amino acids. Enzymatic abnormalities in chromosomal disorders, particularly Down syndrome, promise to become useful diagnostic tools. Unexplained growth abnormality, seizure disorder, poor muscle tone, ataxia, bone or skin abnormalities, and eye abnormalities are some indications for obtaining tests of metabolic function.

Psychological Assessment

Psychological testing, performed by an experienced psychologist, is a standard part of an evaluation for mental retardation. The Gesell and Bayley scales and the Cattell Infant Intelligence Scale are most commonly used with infants. For children, the Stanford-

Binet Intelligence Scale and the third edition of the Wechsler Intelligence Scale for Children (WISC-III) are the most widely used in the United States.

COURSE AND PROGNOSIS

In most cases of mental retardation, the underlying intellectual impairment does not improve, yet the affected person's level of adaptation can be positively influenced by an enriched and supportive environment. In general, people with mild and moderate mental retardation have the most flexibility in adapting to various environmental conditions.

Differential Diagnosis

By definition, mental retardation must begin before the age of 18. Several sensory disabilities, especially deafness and blindness, may be mistaken for mental retardation if, during testing, no compensation is allowed. Speech deficits and cerebral palsy often make a child seem retarded, even in the presence of borderline or normal intelligence. Chronic, debilitating diseases of any kind may depress a child's functioning in all areas. Convulsive disorders may give an impression of mental retardation, especially in the presence of uncontrolled seizures. Chronic brain syndromes may result in isolated handicaps—failure to read (alexia), failure to write (agraphia), failure to communicate (aphasia), and several other handicaps—that may exist in a person of normal and even superior intelligence. Children with learning disorders, which can coexist with mental retardation, experience a delay or a failure of development in a specific area, such as reading or mathematics, but the children develop normally in other areas. In contrast, children with mental retardation show general delays in most areas of development.

Mental retardation and pervasive developmental disorders often coexist. Because of their general level of functioning, children with pervasive developmental disorders have more problems with social relatedness and more deviant language than do those with mental retardation.

Children under the age of 18 years who meet the diagnostic criteria for dementia and who manifest an IQ of less than 70 are given the diagnoses of dementia and mental retardation. Those whose IQs drop to less than 70 after the age of 18 years and who have new onsets of cognitive disorders are not given the diagnosis of mental retardation but only the diagnosis of dementia.

TREATMENT

Mental retardation is associated with a variety of comorbid psychiatric disorders and most often requires a multitude of psychosocial supports. The treatment of individuals with mental retardation is based on an assessment of social and environmental needs as well as attention to comorbid conditions. The optimal treatment of conditions that could lead to mental retardation is primary, secondary, and tertiary prevention.

Primary Prevention

Primary prevention concerns actions taken to eliminate or reduce the conditions that lead to developing of the disorders associated with mental retardation. Such measures include education to increase the general public's knowledge and awareness of mental retardation; continuing efforts of health professionals to ensure and upgrade public health policies; legislation to provide optimal maternal and child health care; and eradication of the known disorders associated with CNS damage.

Secondary and Tertiary Prevention

Once a disorder associated with mental retardation has been identified, the disorder should be treated to shorten the course of the illness (secondary prevention) and to minimize the sequelae or consequent disabilities (tertiary prevention). Hereditary metabolic and endocrine disorders, such as PKU and hypothyroidism, can be effectively treated in an early stage by dietary control or hormone replacement therapy. Mentally retarded children frequently have emotional and behavioral difficulties requiring psychiatric treatment. Their limited cognitive and social capabilities require modified psychiatric treatment modalities based on the children's level of intelligence.

Education for the Child.   Educational settings for children who are mentally retarded should include a comprehensive program that addresses adaptive skills training, social skills training, and vocational training. Particular attention should be focused on communication and efforts to improve the quality of life. Group therapy has often been a successful format in which mentally retarded children can learn and practice hypothetical real-life situations and receive supportive feedback.

Behavioral, Cognitive, and Psychodynamic Therapies.   Behavior therapy has been used for many years to shape and enhance social behaviors and to control and minimize people's aggressive and destructive behaviors. Cognitive therapy, such as dispelling false beliefs and relaxation exercises with self-instruction, has also been recommended for those mentally retarded people who are able to follow the instructions. Psychodynamic therapy has been used with patients and their families to decrease conflicts about expectations that result in persistent anxiety, rage, and depression.

Family Education.   One of the most important areas that a clinician can address is that of educating the family of a mentally retarded patient about ways to enhance competence and self-esteem while maintaining realistic expectations for the patient. The parents may benefit from continuous counseling or family therapy and should be allowed opportunities to express their feelings of guilt, despair, anguish, recurring denial, and anger about their child's disorder and future. The psychiatrist should be prepared to give the parents all the basic and current medical information regarding causes, treatment, and other pertinent areas (such as special training and the correction of sensory defects).

Social Intervention.   Special Olympics International is the largest recreational sports program geared for this population. In addition to providing a forum to develop physical fitness, Special Olympics also enhances social interactions, friendships, and, it is hoped, general self-esteem.

Pharmacology.   Pharmacological approaches to the treatment of comorbid mental disorders in mentally retarded patients are much the same as for patients who are not mentally retarded. Increasing data support the use of a variety of psychotropic medications for patients with mental disorders who are mentally retarded.

35 ▲

Learning Disorders

Learning disorders refer to a child's or adolescent's deficits in acquiring expected skills in reading, writing, speaking, use of listening, reasoning, or mathematics, compared to other children of the same age and intellectual capacity. Learning disorders are not uncommon, affecting at least 5 percent of school-age children. The fourth edition of *Diagnostic and Statistical Manual of Mental Disorders* (DSM-IV) introduced the term *learning disorders*, formerly called *academic skills disorders*. All of the current learning disorder diagnoses require that the child's achievement in that particular learning disorder is significantly lower than expected, and that the learning problems interfere with academic achievement or activities of daily living.

The text revision of DSM-IV (DSM-IV-TR) includes four diagnostic categories in the chapter on learning disorders: reading disorder, mathematics disorder, disorder of written expression, and learning disorder not otherwise specified. Children with a learning disorder, such as reading disorder, for example, can be identified in two different ways: those children who read poorly compared to most other children of the same age; and children whose achievement in reading is significantly lower than their overall intelligence quotient (IQ) would predict. DSM-IV-TR criteria for learning disorders requires a substantial IQ–achievement discrepancy and significantly poor achievement in reading compared to most children of the same age.

READING DISORDER

In DSM-IV-TR, reading disorder (once called *dyslexia*) is defined as reading achievement that is below the expected level for a child's age, education, and intelligence; and the impairment significantly interferes with academic success or the daily activities that involve reading. It is characterized by an impaired ability to recognize words, slow and inaccurate reading, and poor comprehension. In addition, children with attention-deficit/hyperactivity disorder (ADHD) are at high risk for reading disorder.

Epidemiology

An estimated 4 percent of school-age children in the United States have reading disorder; prevalence studies find rates ranging between 2 and 8 percent. Three to four times as many boys as girls are reported to have reading disability in clinically referred samples. Careful epidemiological studies have found closer to equal rates of reading disorder among boys and girls. Boys with reading disorder may be referred for evaluation more often than girls due to frequently associated behavior problems.

Comorbidity

Children with reading disorder are at higher-than-average risk for attentional problems, disruptive behavior disorders (e.g., conduct disorder), and depressive disorders, particularly in older children and adolescents. Data suggest that up to 25 percent of children with reading disorder also have ADHD. Family studies indicate that there may be some common genetic factors producing both reading disorder and attentional syndromes. Children with reading disorders have higher-than-average rates of depression on self-report measures and experience higher levels of anxiety symptoms than children without learning disorders. Furthermore, children with reading disorders tend to have difficulties with peer relationships, with less skill in responding sensitively in ambiguous social situations.

Etiology

There is no single etiology identified as the cause of reading disorder; genetic factors, developmental factors, and environmental factors may contribute to the core deficits in reading disorder. Current research on reading disorder indicates that in most cases, children who struggle with reading have a deficit in phonological processing skills. These children are unable to effectively identify the parts of words that denote specific sounds, which leads to grave difficulty in recognizing and sounding out words. Children with reading disorder have been found to be slower than average in naming letters and numbers, even when controlling for IQ. Thus, the core deficit for children with reading disorder lie within the domain of language use.

Many studies support the hypothesis that genetic factors play a major role in the presence of reading disorder. Studies indicate that 35 to 40 percent of first-degree relatives of children with reading disorder also have some degree of reading disability. Several recent studies suggested that phonological awareness (i.e., the ability to decode sounds and sound out words) is linked to chromosome 6. Furthermore, the ability for single-word identification has been linked to chromosome 15.

A higher-than-average incidence of reading disorder occurs among children of normal intelligence who have cerebral palsy. A slightly increased incidence of reading disorder appears among epileptic children. Complications during pregnancy; prenatal and perinatal difficulties, including prematurity; and low birth weight are common in the histories of children with reading disorder. Children with postnatal brain lesions in the left occipital lobe, which results in right visual-field blindness, may have secondary reading disorder, as may children with lesions in the splenium of the corpus callosum that block the transmission of visual information from the intact right hemisphere to the language areas of the left hemisphere.

Diagnosis

Reading disorder is diagnosed when a child's reading achievement is significantly below that expected of a child of the same age and intellectual capacity. Characteristic diagnostic features include difficulties with recalling, evoking, and sequencing printed letters and words; processing sophisticated grammatical constructions; and making inferences.

Clinical Features

Children who have reading disorder can usually be identified by the age of 7 years (second grade). Reading difficulty may be apparent among students in classrooms where reading skills are expected as early as the first grade. Children can sometimes compensate for reading disorder in the early elementary grades by the use of memory and inference, particularly when the disorder is associated with high intelligence. In such instances, the disorder may not be apparent until the age of 9 years (fourth grade) or later. Associated problems include language difficulties, shown often as impaired sound discrimination and difficulties in properly sequencing words.

Most children with reading disorder dislike and avoid reading and writing. Many children with the disorder who do not receive remedial education have a sense of shame and humiliation because of their continuing failure and subsequent frustration. Older children tend to be angry and depressed, and they exhibit poor self-esteem.

Pathology and Laboratory Examination

No specific physical signs or laboratory measures are helpful in the diagnosis of reading disorder. The diagnosis of reading disorder is made after collecting data from a standardized intelligence test and an educational assessment of achievement. The diagnostic battery generally includes a standardized spelling test, written composition, processing and using oral language, and design copying—a judgment of the adequacy of pencil use. The reading subtests of the Woodcock-Johnson Psycho-Educational Battery–Revised, and the Peabody Individual Achievement Test–Revised are useful in identifying reading disability. A screening projective battery may include human-figure drawings, picture-story tests, and sentence completion. The evaluation should also include a systematic observation of behavior variables.

Course and Prognosis

Many children with reading disorder gain some knowledge of printed language during their first 2 years in grade school, even without any remedial assistance. When remediation is instituted early, in milder cases, it is no longer necessary by the end of the first or second grade. In severe cases and depending on the pattern of deficits and strengths, remediation may be continued into the middle and high school years.

Differential Diagnosis

Reading disorder is often accompanied by comorbid disorders, such as expressive language disorder, disorder of written expression (see below), and ADHD. A recent study indicates that children with reading disorder consistently present difficulties with linguistic abilities, whereas children with ADHD do not. Deficits in expressive language and speech discrimination present in reading disorder may be severe enough to warrant the additional diagnosis of expressive language disorder or mixed receptive-expressive language disorder. Reading disorder must be differentiated from mental retardation syndromes in which reading, along with other skills, is below the achievement expected for a child's chronological age. Intellectual testing helps to differentiate global deficits from more specific reading difficulties. Hearing and visual impairments should be ruled out with screening tests.

B.C. was a 12-year-old male student who presented for evaluation of problems in school. He attended an academic preschool and was presently enrolled in a regular sixth-grade class at a public school.

Current evaluation revealed no history of neurological, visual, or hearing problems that could explain B.C.'s school difficulties. Intelligence testing revealed high-average scores in both the verbal and performance subtests of the third edition of the Wechsler Intelligence Scale for Children (WISC-III). Reading and mathematical scores on standardized tests of academic performance were consistent with his intelligence and chronological age; however, spelling scores were significantly below the predicted level of performance. Multiple misspellings occurred. Although the examiner noted adequate handwriting, B.C. appeared unable to express thoughts in complete sentences. His sentences were short and failed to state intended points clearly. Careful study of B.C.'s written paragraphs revealed numerous grammatical and syntactic errors as well as errors in punctuation and capitalization.

The clinical picture of an inability to compose, poor spelling, and grammatical errors in the absence of low intelligence, problems with reading or mathematics, or pervasive attentional problems led to a diagnosis of disorder of written expression. (Courtesy of Michael E. Spagna, Ph.D., Dennis P. Cantwell, M.D., and Lorian Baker, Ph.D.)

Treatment

Many effective remediation programs begin with teaching a given child to make accurate associations between letters and sounds. After those skills have been mastered, remediation can target larger components of reading, such as syllables and words. The exact focus of any reading program can only be determined after an accurate assessment of a child's specific deficits and weaknesses. Positive coping strategies include small, structured reading groups that offer individual attention and make it easier for a child to ask for help.

Reading instruction programs begin by concentrating on individual letters and sounds, then advance to the mastery of simple phonetic units, followed by the blending of these units into words and sentences. Other reading remediation programs, such as the Merill program and the SRA Basic Reading Program, begin by introducing whole words first and then teach children how to break them down and recognize the sounds of the syllables and the individual letters in the word. Another approach, such as the Bridge Reading Program, teaches children with reading disorder to recognize whole words through the use of visual aids and to bypass the "sounding out" process. The Fernald Method uses a multisensory approach that combines teaching whole words with a tracing technique so that the child has kinesthetic stimulation while learning to read the words.

MATHEMATICS DISORDER

Children with mathematics disorder have difficulty learning and remembering numerals, are unable to remember basic facts about numbers, and are slow and inaccurate in computation. Poor achievement in four groups of skills have been identified in mathematics disorder: linguistic skills (those related to understanding mathematical terms and to converting written problems into mathematical symbols), perceptual skills (the ability to recognize and understand symbols and to order clusters of numbers), mathematical skills (basic addition, subtraction, multiplication, division, and following sequencing of basic operations), and attentional skills (copying figures correctly and observing operational symbols correctly).

Epidemiology

The prevalence of mathematics disorder alone is estimated to occur in approximately 1 percent of school-age children, that is, approximately one out of every five children with learning disorders. Epidemiologic studies have indicated that up to 6 percent of school-aged children have some difficulty with mathematics. Mathematics disorder may occur with greater frequency in girls.

Comorbidity

Mathematics disorder is commonly found comorbid with reading disorder and disorder of written expression. Children with mathematics disorder may also be at higher risk for expressive language disorder, mixed receptive-expressive language disorder, and developmental coordination disorder.

Etiology

The emergence of mathematics disorder, similar to other learning disorders, is likely to be due at least in part to genetic factors. An early theory proposed a neurological deficit in the right cerebral hemisphere, particularly in the occipital lobe areas. These regions are responsible for processing visual-spatial stimuli that, in turn, are responsible for mathematical skills.

Currently, the cause is thought to be multifactorial, so that maturational, cognitive, emotional, educational, and socioeconomic factors account in varying degrees and combinations for mathematics disorder.

Diagnosis

The diagnosis of mathematics disorder is made when a child's skills in mathematics fall significantly below what is expected for that child's age, intellectual ability, and education. A definitive

diagnosis can be made only after a child takes an individually administered standardized arithmetic test and scores markedly below the level expected, in view of the child's schooling and intellectual capacity as measured by a standardized intelligence test. A pervasive developmental disorder and mental retardation should also be ruled out before confirming the diagnosis of mathematics disorder.

Clinical Features

Common features of mathematics disorder include difficulty with various components of mathematics such as learning number names, remembering the signs for addition and subtraction, learning multiplication tables, translating word problems into computations, and doing calculations at the expected pace.

Mathematics disorder often coexists with other disorders affecting reading, expressive writing, coordination, and expressive and receptive language. Spelling problems, deficits in memory or attention, and emotional or behavioral problems may be present. Young grade-school children often first show other learning disorders and should be checked for mathematics disorder. Children with cerebral palsy may have mathematics disorder with normal overall intelligence.

The relation between mathematics disorder and other communication and learning disorders is not clear. Although children with mixed receptive-expressive language disorder and expressive language disorder are not necessarily affected by mathematics disorder, the conditions often coexist, as they are associated with impairments in both decoding and encoding processes.

Pathology and Laboratory Examination

No physical signs or symptoms indicate mathematics disorder, but educational testing and standardized measure of intellectual function are necessary to make this diagnosis. The Keymath Diagnostic Arithmetic Test measures several areas of mathematics, including knowledge of mathematical content, function, and computation. It is used to assess abilities in mathematics for children in grades 1 to 6.

Course and Prognosis

A child with a mathematics disorder can usually be identified by the age of 8 years (third grade). In some children, the disorder is apparent as early as 6 years (first grade); in others it may not occur until age 10 (fifth grade) or later. Thus far, few longitudinal study data are available to predict clear patterns of developmental and academic progress of children classified as having mathematics disorder in early school grades. On the other hand, children with a moderate mathematics disorder who do not receive intervention may have complications, including continuing academic difficulties, shame, poor self-concept, frustration, and depression. These complications may lead to reluctance to attend school, truancy, and eventual hopelessness about academic success.

Differential Diagnosis

Mathematics disorder must be differentiated from global causes of impaired functioning such as mental retardation syndromes. Arithmetic difficulties in mental retardation are accompanied by a generalized impairment in overall intellectual functioning. In unusual cases of mild mental retardation, arithmetic skills may be significantly below the level expected, on the basis of a person's schooling and level of mental retardation. In such cases, an additional diagnosis of mathematics disorder should be made; treatment of the arithmetic difficulties can be particularly helpful for a child's chances for employment in adulthood. Inadequate schooling can often affect a child's poor arithmetic performance on a standardized arithmetic test. Conduct disorder or ADHD may occur with mathematics disorder, and in these cases both diagnoses should be made.

Treatment

Currently, the most effective treatments for mathematics disorder combine teaching of mathematics concepts along with continuous practice in solving math problems. Social skills deficits may contribute to a child's hesitation in asking for help, so a child identified with a mathematics disorder may benefit from gaining positive problem-solving skills in a social arena as well as in mathematics.

DISORDER OF WRITTEN EXPRESSION

Disorder of written expression is characterized by writing skills that are significantly below the expected level for a child's age and intellectual capacity. These difficulties interfere with the child's academic performance and with the demands for writing in everyday life. The many components of disorder of written expression include poor spelling, errors in grammar and punctuation, and poor handwriting.

Epidemiology

The prevalence of disorder of written expression alone has not been studied, but like reading disorder, it is estimated to occur in approximately 4 percent of school-age children. It is thought that the gender ratio in disorder of written expression is similar to that of reading disorder, occurring in about three times as many boys. Disorder of written expression often occurs along with reading disorder, but not always.

Comorbidity

Children with disorder of written expression are at higher risk for a variety of other learning and language disorders, including reading disorder, mathematics disorder, and expressive and receptive language disorders. ADHD occurs with greater frequency in children with disorder of written expression than in the general population. Finally, children with disorder of written expression are believed to be at higher risk for social skills difficulties, and some go on to develop poor self-esteem and depressive symptoms.

Etiology

Causes of disorder of written expression are believed to be similar to those of reading disorder—that is, a deficit in the use of the components of language related to letter sounds. It is likely that genetic factors play a role in the development of disorder of written expression. Hereditary predisposition to the disorder is supported by findings that most children with disorder of written expression have first-degree relatives with the disorder.

Children with limited attention spans and high levels of distractibility may find writing an arduous task.

Diagnosis

A diagnosis of disorder of written expression is based on a child's poor performance on composing written text, including handwriting and impaired ability to spell and to place words sequentially in coherent sentences, compared to most other children of the same age and intellectual ability.

Clinical Features

Children with disorder of written expression have difficulties early in grade school in spelling words and in expressing their thoughts according to age-appropriate grammatical norms. Common features of the disorder of written expression are spelling errors, grammatical errors, punctuation errors, poor paragraph organization, and poor handwriting. Associated features of disorder of written expression include refusal or reluctance to go to school and to do assigned written homework, poor academic performance in other areas (e.g., mathematics), general avoidance of school work, truancy, attention deficit, and conduct disturbance.

Many children with disorder of written expression become frustrated and angry because of their feelings of inadequacy and failure in their academic performance. In severe cases, depressive disorders may develop as a result of a growing sense of isolation, estrangement, and despair.

Ryan was a 9-year-old boy who was referred by his teacher for an evaluation of his poor classwork production. The teacher reported to Ryan's parents that he was not disruptive in class, but he never seemed to know exactly what was going on. He often seemed to be preoccupied or day dreaming. He had good ideas when he spoke up in class but did not volunteer to answer questions verbally most of the time. When he was given written assignments in class, he rushed through them and could not remember how to spell even simple words correctly. His stories often did not make sense, since he often left out important verbs, the names of the main subjects, or critical parts of the plot. Ryan's teacher reported that she used to get frustrated with Ryan because she felt that he wasn't paying attention because he just didn't care, but even after she moved his seat to the very front of the room, his work did not improve. Ryan always did well on assignments that involved drawing, which he did quickly and effortlessly.

Ryan was administered a standardized test of intelligence (third edition of the Wechsler Intelligence Scale for Children [WISC-III]), the Test of Written Language, (TOWL), the Diagnostic Evaluation of Writing Skills (DEWS), and a clinical psychiatric interview with a child and adolescent psychiatrist. Ryan's full-scale IQ was in the superior range, 122, with a verbal scale of 112, and a performance scale of 128. His tests of written language revealed that he had significant deficits in spelling, use of punctuation, and in applying grammatical rules. A diagnosis of disorder of written expression was made. Ryan's psychiatric interview revealed that he also met criteria for ADHD.

Ryan was referred for resource room remediation in writing for one period each day in school and was given a trial of stimulant medication. Ryan's attention improved modestly in the classroom, and he began to demonstrate more motivation to write more carefully, especially while he was with his resource room teacher. His self-esteem improved as his problems were being addressed.

Pathology and Laboratory Examination

Although there are no physical stigmata of a writing disorder, educational testing is used in making a diagnosis of disorder of written expression. Tests of written language that are now available include the TOWL, the DEWS, and Test of Early Written Language (TEWL). A child suspected of having disorder of written expression should first be given a standardized intelligence test, such as WISC-III or the revised Wechsler Adult Intelligence Scale (WAIS-R) to determine the child's overall intellectual capacity.

Course and Prognosis

In severe cases, a disorder of written expression is apparent by age 7 (second grade); in less severe cases, the disorder may not be apparent until age 10 (fifth grade) or later. Most people with mild and moderate disorder of written expression fare well if they receive timely remedial education early in grade school. Severe disorder of written expression requires continual, extensive remedial treatment through the late part of high school and even into college.

The prognosis depends on the severity of the disorder, the age or grade when the remedial intervention is started, the length and continuity of treatment, and the presence or absence of associated or secondary emotional or behavioral problems.

Differential Diagnosis

One must determine whether another disorder such as ADHD or a depressive disorder is preventing a child from being able to concentrate on writing tasks, in the absence of disorder of written expression itself. If this is the case, treatment for the above disorder should improve a child's writing performance. Disorder of written expression may also occur along with a variety of other language and learning disorders. Common associated disorders are reading disorder, mixed receptive-expressive language disorder, expressive language disorder, mathematics disorder, developmental coordination disorder, and disruptive behavior and attention-deficit disorders (ADDs).

Treatment

Remedial treatments for disorder of written expression include direct practice of spelling and sentence writing, as well as a review of grammatical rules. Intensive and continuous administration of individually tailored, one-to-one expressive and creative writing therapy appears to effect favorable outcome.

LEARNING DISORDER NOT OTHERWISE SPECIFIED

Learning disorder not otherwise specified is a new category in DSM-IV-TR for disorders that do not meet the criteria for any specific learning disorder but that cause impairment and reflect learning abilities below those expected for a person's intelligence, education, and age. An example of a disability that could be placed in this category is a spelling skills deficit.

36 ▲

Motor Skills Disorder: Developmental Coordination Disorder

Developmental coordination disorder is a condition characterized by performance in daily activities requiring coordination that is below what is expected for a child's age and intellectual level. According to the text revision of the fourth edition of *Diagnostic and Statistical Manual of Mental Disorders* (DSM-IV-TR), the disorder may present with delays in achieving motor milestones such as sitting, crawling, and walking. Developmental coordination disorder is the sole disorder in the DSM-IV-TR category of motor skills disorder.

Developmental coordination disorder may also be manifested by clumsy gross and fine motor skills resulting in poor performance in sports and even in poor handwriting. A child with developmental coordination disorder may bump into things more often than siblings or drop things.

EPIDEMIOLOGY

The prevalence of developmental coordination disorder has been estimated at approximately 5 percent of school-age children. The male-to-female ratio in referred populations tends to show increased rates of the disorder in males, but schools refer boys more often for testing and special education evaluations. Reports in the literature of the male-to-female ratio have ranged from 2 to 1 to as much as 4 to 1. These rates may be inflated also due to a bias toward increased scrutiny of motor behaviors in male compared to female children.

COMORBIDITY

Developmental coordination disorder is strongly associated with speech and language disorders. Developmental coordination disorder is also associated with reading disorders, mathematics disorder, and disorder of written expression. Higher-than-expected rates of attention-deficit/hyperactivity disorder (ADHD) have also been found to be associated with developmental coordination disorder.

ETIOLOGY

The causes of developmental coordination disorder are unknown and are believed to include both "organic" and "developmental" factors. Risk factors postulated to contribute to this disorder include prematurity, hypoxia, perinatal malnutrition, and low birth weight. Developmental coordination disorder and communication disorders have strong associations, although the specific causative agents are unknown for both. Coordination problems are also more frequently found in children with hyperactivity syndromes and learning disorders. Developmental coordination disorder probably has a multifactorial cause.

DIAGNOSIS

The diagnosis of developmental coordination disorder is dependent on poor performance in activities requiring coordination for a given child's age and intellectual level. Diagnosis is based on a history of the child's delay in achieving early motor milestones as well as through direct observation of current deficits in coordination.

The diagnosis may be associated with below-normal scores on performance subtests of standardized intelligence tests and by normal or above-normal scores on verbal subtests. Specialized tests of motor coordination can be useful, such as the Bender Visual Motor Gestalt Test, the Frostig Movement Skills Test Battery, and the Bruininks-Oseretsky Test of Motor Development.

CLINICAL FEATURES

The clinical signs suggesting the existence of developmental coordination disorder are evident in some cases, as early as infancy, when a child begins to attempt tasks requiring motor coordination. The essential clinical feature is significantly impaired performance in motor coordination. The difficulties in motor coordination may vary with a child's age and developmental stage.

> Johnny, age 8, was brought to a clinic for evaluation by his mother, who said, "There is something wrong with his brain." When asked to be more specific, she replied with a vague litany of complaints that were frequently self-contradictory.
>
> He was always slow to learn things, slower than any of my other children. But I know he's really very smart. Sometimes

he just amazes me with what he remembers or can figure out. He doesn't do much, for example, at school or with activities outside school. Sometimes I think it's because he's lazy, and other times I think he's depressed, and other times I think maybe it's because he is sick a lot. He gets a lot of stomachaches. He's really such a sweet boy. I mean, he's so nice with his four sisters and our pets. But sometimes he's so nasty I get afraid. For example, he gets frustrated with some of his toys, and then he gets destructive. He's broken more toys than all of my other three children put together. He seems to like people, but he only has one friend at school. He refuses to try out for soccer or anything like that where he could play with the other boys. Sometimes I think he just doesn't care about anything. He's always dropping dishes and things around the house.

A more detailed history revealed that the pregnancy, birth, and early medical history had been unremarkable, but minor problems had appeared in his first year of life. These included being slow to sit up, crawl, and walk. Because Johnny was the fourth child in the family, the mother had not "had time" to record the actual ages when these milestones were reached. She could only pinpoint that "he was much older than any of the other children when he did finally manage to do those things," adding that the pediatrician had nonetheless assured her that Johnny was not retarded. "A good thing he did," she laughed, "because later when Johnny had so much trouble learning to use the knife and fork, and to tie his shoelaces, and to button his shirts, I did worry about that."

Asked if there were any remaining concerns along these lines, the mother replied "none at all." Apparently, Johnny excelled in reading and did well in all his school subjects except handwriting and physical education.

His medical history was also unremarkable. During the preschool years, there had been only "the normal childhood illnesses" (chicken pox, earaches, and flu) and "an awful lot of bruises and scraped knees." The stomachaches had started "sometime around age 7," but again, the pediatrician had assured the mother that they were not cause for concern.

Examination revealed a pleasant but rather quiet boy with appropriate affect, good concentration, and apparently normal cognitive skills. Although quiet and reserved, Johnny did not appear apathetic; indeed, he became quite enthusiastic when describing a book he had just read. During the interview, Johnny denied any problems in school or with peers. When specifically asked, he did admit to occasional stomachaches and to nonparticipation in group activities, which he attributed to simply "not liking that stuff."

Psychological testing performed in the school setting revealed above-average intelligence and academic performance. However, Johnny scored well below the norm on a test of motor development requiring tasks involving running, balancing, coordination, and motor speed. The psychologist noted that he showed good concentration and attention during the testing.

DISCUSSION

Many features of this case are typical of developmental coordination disorder. These include late gross motor milestones (standing, sitting, walking), early history of bruises (from bumping into things) and falls, reported "destructiveness"

(dropping things or breaking toys when trying to manipulate them), difficulty with tasks requiring fine motor coordination (buttoning clothes, tying shoelaces, and handwriting), and difficulty with sports, such as ball games.

The stomachaches, "laziness," "depression," and "apathy" probably represent Johnny's efforts to avoid physical education class, tests in which handwriting is necessary, and the embarrassment of repeated failures in team sports situations. Similarly, Johnny's "bad temper" and "frustration" are probably not evidence of disturbed attention or conduct, but rather a manifestation of his motor difficulties. As often happens, it is these secondary problems that have brought him to professional attention.

One may wonder why a disorder of physical coordination appears in a classification of mental disorders. It is true that the defining features of the disorder are more physical than behavioral or psychological, and therefore one could argue that the disorder is more properly a physical, not a mental, disorder. However, it seems reasonable to classify it with the other developmental disorders of childhood because of the absence of a specific known cause and because the behavioral consequences of the disorder (e.g., irritability and avoidance behavior) are treated by mental health professionals. (From *DSM-IV Casebook*.)

DIFFERENTIAL DIAGNOSIS

The differential diagnosis includes medical conditions that produce coordination difficulties (such as cerebral palsy and muscular dystrophy), pervasive developmental disorders, and mental retardation. In mental retardation and in the pervasive developmental disorders, coordination usually does not stand out as a significant deficit compared with other skills. Children with neuromuscular disorders may exhibit more global muscle impairment rather than clumsiness and delayed motor milestones. In cases of neurological conditions, neurologic examination and workups usually reveal more extensive deficits than are present in developmental coordination disorder. Extremely hyperactive and impulsive children may be physically careless because of their high levels of motor activity. Clumsy gross and fine motor behavior and ADHD seem to be associated.

COURSE AND PROGNOSIS

Few data are available on the prospective longitudinal outcomes of both treated and untreated children with developmental coordination disorder. For the most part, although clumsiness may continue, some children are able to compensate by developing interests in other skills. Clumsiness generally persists into adolescence and adult life. Commonly associated features include delays in nonmotor milestones, expressive language disorder, and mixed receptive-expressive language disorder.

TREATMENT

The treatments of developmental coordination disorder generally include versions of sensory-integration programs and modified physical education. Sensory integration programs are usually administered by occupational therapists and consist of physical activities that increase awareness of motor and sensory function.

37 ▲

Communication Disorders

Spoken language is an essential part of communicating ideas, social interactions, and academic understanding. Effective communication for a child or adolescent includes proficiency in both language and speech skills. The text revision of the fourth edition of *Diagnostic and Statistical Manual of Mental Disorders* (DSM-IV-TR) includes four specific communication disorders and one residual category. Two of the communication disorders (expressive and mixed receptive-expressive communication disorder) are language disorders, whereas the other two (phonological disorder and stuttering) are speech disorders. A child with a language disorder may have a limited vocabulary, speak in short, simple sentences, and may tell stories in a disorganized and incomplete manner. A child with a speech disorder may attempt to use appropriate descriptive words but has difficulty pronouncing the speech sounds correctly and may either omit sounds or pronounce sounds in an unusual way. A child with stuttering generally has acquired a normal vocabulary but his or her speech fluency is disrupted by pauses, sound repetitions, or sound prolongations.

EXPRESSIVE LANGUAGE DISORDER

Expressive language disorder is present when a child's skills are below the expected level in vocabulary, the use of correct tenses, the production of complex sentences, and the recall of words. Children with expressive language disorder alone have courses and prognoses that differ from children with mixed receptive-expressive language disorder.

Epidemiology

The prevalence of expressive language disorder is estimated to be between 3 and 5 percent of all school-age children. There have been some estimates of combined language disorders of up to 10 percent. According to DSM-IV-TR, it can be as high as 15 percent in children under age 3. The disorder is two to three times more common in boys than in girls and is most prevalent among children whose relatives have a family history of phonological disorder or other communication disorders.

Etiology

The specific cause of developmental expressive language disorder is unknown. Subtle cerebral damage and maturational lags in cerebral development have been postulated as underlying causes. Left-handedness and ambilaterality appear to be associated with expressive language problems. There is good evidence showing that language disorders occur with higher frequency in certain families. Genetic factors have been suspected to play a role, and several studies of twins show significant concordance for monozygotic twins for communication disorders. Environmental and educational factors are also postulated to make a contribution to the presence of developmental language disorders.

Diagnosis

Expressive language disorder is present when a child has a selective deficit in language skills and is functioning well in nonverbal areas and in receptive skills. Markedly below-age-level verbal or sign language, accompanied by a low score on standardized expressive verbal tests, is diagnostic of expressive language disorder (Table 37–1).

To confirm the diagnosis, a child is given standardized expressive language and nonverbal intellectual tests. Observations of children's verbal and sign language patterns in various settings (e.g., in the school yard, classroom, home, and playroom) and during interactions with other children help ascertain the severity and the specific areas of a child's impairment and aid in early detection of behavioral and emotional complications. Family history should include the presence or absence of expressive language disorder among relatives.

Clinical Features

The essential feature of expressive language disorder is a marked impairment in the development of age-appropriate expressive language that results in the use of verbal or sign language markedly below the expected level in view of a child's nonverbal intellectual capacity. Language understanding (decoding) skills remain relatively intact. When severe, the disorder becomes recognizable by approximately the age of 18 months, when a child fails to utter spontaneously or even to echo single words or sounds.

When a child with expressive language disorder begins to speak, the language impairment gradually becomes apparent. Articulation is often immature; numerous articulation errors occur but are inconsistent.

By the age of 4 years, most children with expressive language disorder can speak in short phrases, but they may have difficulty retaining new words. After beginning to speak, they acquire language more slowly than do normal children.

Jennifer was a sociable, active 5-year-old who was diagnosed with expressive language disorder. She often played with her best friend, Sarah. One day, in the course of pretend play, each girl told the story of Little Red Riding Hood to her doll. Sarah's story began: "Little Red Riding Hood was taking a basket of food to her grandmother who was sick. A bad wolf stopped Riding Hood in the forest. He tried to get the basket away from her but she wouldn't give it to him." By contrast, Jennifer's story illustrated her marked difficulties in verbal expression: "Riding Hood going to grandma house. Her taking food. Bad wolf in a bed. Riding Hood say, 'What big ears, grandma?' 'Hear you, dear.' 'What big eyes, grandma?' 'See you, dear.' 'What big mouth, grandma?' 'Eat you all up!'"

Many features of Jennifer's story were characteristic of children with expressive language disorder, including the short, incomplete sentences, simple sentence structure, omission of grammatical function words (e.g., is, the) and endings (e.g., possessives, present tense verbs), problems in question formation, and incorrect use of pronouns (e.g., her for she). Nonetheless, testing by methods that did not require verbal responding showed clearly that Jennifer understood the details and plot of the Riding Hood tale as well as Sarah did. Jennifer also demonstrated adequate comprehension skills in her kindergarten classroom, where she readily followed the teacher's complex, multistep verbal instructions (e.g., "Before you get ready for recess, make sure that you draw a green circle around all the animals, put your library books under your chair, and line up at the back of the room."). (Courtesy of Carla J. Johnson, Ph.D., and Joseph H. Beitchman, M.D.)

Differential Diagnosis

In mental retardation, patients have an overall impairment in intellectual functioning, but the nonverbal intellectual capacity and functioning of children with expressive language disorder are within normal limits. In mixed receptive-expressive language disorder, comprehension of language (decoding) is markedly below the expected age-appropriate level, whereas in expressive language disorder, language comprehension remains within normal limits.

In pervasive developmental disorders, affected children have no inner language or appropriate use of gesture and show little or no frustration with the inability to communicate verbally. In contrast, all these characteristics are present in children with expressive language disorder.

Children with acquired aphasia or dysphasia have a history of early normal language development; the disordered language had its onset after a head trauma or other neurological disorder (e.g., a seizure disorder). Children with selective mutism have a history of normal language development.

Course and Prognosis

The rapidity and degree of recovery depend on the severity of the disorder, the child's motivation to participate in therapies, and the timely institution of speech and other therapeutic interventions. The presence or absence of other factors—such as moderate to

Table 37–1
DSM-IV-TR Diagnostic Criteria for Expressive Language Disorder

A. The scores obtained from standardized individually administered measures of expressive language development are substantially below those obtained from standardized measures of both nonverbal intellectual capacity and receptive language development. The disturbance may be manifest clinically by symptoms that include having a markedly limited vocabulary, making errors in tense, or having difficulty recalling words or producing sentences with developmentally appropriate length or complexity.

B. The difficulties with expressive language interfere with academic or occupational achievement or with social communication.

C. Criteria are not met for mixed receptive-expressive language disorder or a pervasive developmental disorder.

D. If mental retardation, a speech-motor or sensory deficit, or environmental deprivation is present, the language difficulties are in excess of those usually associated with these problems.

Coding note: If a speech-motor or sensory deficit or a neurological condition is present, code the condition on Axis III.

From American Psychiatric Association. *Diagnostic and Statistical Manual of Mental Disorders.* 4th ed. Text rev. Washington, DC: American Psychiatric Association; copyright 2000, with permission.

severe hearing loss, mild mental retardation, and severe emotional problems—also affects the prognosis for recovery. As many as 50 percent of children with mild expressive language disorder recover spontaneously without any sign of language impairment, but children with severe expressive language disorder may later display features of mild to moderate language impairment.

Treatment

Various techniques have been used to help a child improve the use of parts of speech such as pronouns, correct tenses, and question forms. Direct interventions use a speech and language pathologist who works directly with a child. Mediated interventions, in which a speech and language professional teaches a child's teacher or parent to promote therapeutic language techniques, have also been shown to be efficacious. Language therapy is often aimed at improving communication strategies and social interactions as well, through using words.

Psychotherapy may be useful for children whose language impairment has affected self-esteem, insofar as it can be used as a positive model for more effective communication and broadening social skills. Supportive parental counseling may be indicated in some cases. Parents may need help to reduce intrafamilial tensions arising from difficulties in rearing language-disordered children and to increase their awareness and understanding of the disorder.

MIXED RECEPTIVE-EXPRESSIVE LANGUAGE DISORDER

In mixed receptive-expressive language disorder, children are impaired in both understanding and expressing language. DSM-IV-TR combines receptive and expressive language disorder. The implication is that clinically significant receptive language impairment is believed to be accompanied by expressive language dysfunction. With DSM-IV-TR, it is impossible to code receptive language disorder in the absence of expressive language disorder.

The essential features of mixed receptive-expressive language disorder are shown by scores on standardized tests; both receptive (comprehension) and expressive language development scores fall substantially below those obtained from standardized measures of nonverbal intellectual capacity. Language difficulties must be severe enough to impair academic achievement or daily social communication. A patient with this disorder must not meet the criteria for a pervasive developmental disorder, and the language dysfunctions must be in excess of those usually associated with mental retardation and other neurological and sensory-deficit syndromes.

Epidemiology

It is believed that mixed receptive-expressive language disorder occurs in approximately 3 percent of school-age children, and the combination is less common than expressive language disorder alone. Mixed receptive-expressive language disorder is believed to be at least twice as prevalent in boys as in girls.

Etiology

The cause of mixed receptive-expressive language disorder is unknown. As with expressive language disorder alone, there is evidence of familial aggregation of mixed receptive-expressive language disorder. Genetic contribution to this disorder is implicated by twin studies, but modes of genetic transmission are not yet proven. Cognitive deficits, particularly slower processing of tasks involving naming objects as well as fine motor tasks, have been shown in some studies of children with various speech and language disorders. Slower myelinization of neural pathways has been hypothesized to account for the slow processing found in children with developmental language disorders. Several studies suggest the presence of underlying impairment of auditory discrimination, as most children with the disorder are more responsive to environmental sounds than to speech sounds.

Diagnosis

Children with mixed receptive-expressive language disorder develop language more slowly than their peers and have trouble understanding conversations that peers can follow. In mixed receptive-expressive language disorder, receptive dysfunction coexists with expressive dysfunction. Therefore, standardized tests for both receptive and expressive language abilities must be given to anyone suspected of having mixed receptive-expressive language disorder.

A markedly below-expected level of comprehension of verbal or sign language with intact age-appropriate nonverbal intellectual capacity, the confirmation of language difficulties by standardized receptive language tests, and the absence of pervasive developmental disorders confirm the diagnosis of mixed receptive-expressive language disorder (Table 37–2).

Clinical Features

The essential clinical feature of the disorder is significant impairment in both language comprehension and language expression. In

Table 37–2
DSM-IV-TR Diagnostic Criteria for Mixed Receptive-Expressive Language Disorder

A. The scores obtained from a battery of standardized individually administered measures of both receptive and expressive language development are substantially below those obtained from standardized measures of nonverbal intellectual capacity. Symptoms include those for expressive language disorder as well as difficulty understanding words, sentences, or specific types of words, such as spatial terms.

B. The difficulties with receptive and expressive language significantly interfere with academic or occupational achievement or with social communication.

C. Criteria are not met for a pervasive developmental disorder.

D. If mental retardation, a speech-motor or sensory deficit, or environmental deprivation is present, the language difficulties are in excess of those usually associated with these problems.

Coding note: If a speech-motor or sensory deficit or a neurological condition is present, code the condition on Axis III.

From American Psychiatric Association. *Diagnostic and Statistical Manual of Mental Disorders.* 4th ed. Text rev. Washington, DC: American Psychiatric Association; copyright 2000, with permission.

the mixed disorder, the expressive impairments are similar to those of expressive language disorder but can be more severe. The clinical features of the receptive component of the disorder typically appear before the age of 4 years. Children with mixed receptive-expressive language disorder show markedly delayed and below-normal ability to comprehend (decode) verbal or sign language, although they have age-appropriate nonverbal intellectual capacity. The clinical features of mixed receptive-expressive language disorder in children between the ages of 18 and 24 months are the results of a child's failure to make spontaneous utterances of a single phoneme or to mimic another person's words.

Differential Diagnosis

Children with significant mixed receptive-expressive language disorder have a deficit in language comprehension. In expressive language disorder alone, comprehension of spoken language (decoding) remains within age norms. Children with phonological disorder or stuttering have normal expressive and receptive language competence, despite the speech impairments. Mental retardation, selective mutism, acquired aphasia, and pervasive developmental disorders should be ruled out. Hearing impairment should also be ruled out. Hearing impairment, pervasive developmental disorders, and severe environmental deprivation may contribute significantly to language impairment.

Course and Prognosis

The overall prognosis for mixed receptive-expressive language disorder is less favorable than for expressive language disorder alone. Over the long run, some children with mixed receptive-expressive language disorder achieve close-to-normal language functions. The prognosis for children who acquire mixed receptive-expressive language disorder is widely variable and depends on the nature and severity of the damage.

Treatment

A comprehensive speech and language evaluation is recommended for children with mixed receptive-expressive language disorder before embarking on a speech and language remediation program. Often, a child with mixed receptive-expressive language disorder will benefit from a small, special educational setting that allows more individualized learning.

Psychotherapy may be helpful for children with mixed receptive-expressive language disorder who have associated emotional and behavioral problems. Family counseling in which parents and children can develop more effective, less frustrating means of communicating may be beneficial.

PHONOLOGICAL DISORDER

Phonological disorder includes poor sound production, substitutions of one sound for another, and omissions of sounds that are part of words. The diagnosis of a phonological disorder is made by comparing the skills of a given child with the expected skill level of others of the same age. The disorder results in errors in whole words due to incorrect pronunciation of consonants, substitutions of one sound for another, omission of entire phonemes, and, in some cases, dysarthria (slurred speech due to incoordination of speech muscles) or dyspraxia (difficulty in planning and executing speech).

Epidemiology

The reported prevalence rates of phonological disorders in children have been variable, due to the age of the children surveyed and the methods used to identify the disorder. The disorder is 2 to 3 times more common in boys than in girls. It is also more common among first-degree relatives of patients with the disorder than in the general population. According to DSM-IV-TR, the prevalence falls to 0.5 percent by mid-to-late adolescence.

Etiology

The causes of phonological disturbance are likely to include multiple variables, such as perinatal problems, genetic factors, auditory processing problems, hearing impairment, and structural abnormalities related to speech. Genetic factors are implicated by data from twin studies that show concordance rates for monozygotic twins that are higher than chance.

Diagnosis

The essential feature of phonological disorder is a child's delay or failure to produce developmentally expected speech sounds, especially consonants, resulting in sound omissions, substitutions, and distortions of phonemes. A rough guideline for clinical assessment of children's articulation is that normal 3-year-olds correctly articulate *m, n, ng, b, p, h, t, k, q,* and *d*; normal 4-year-olds correctly articulate *f, y, ch, sh,* and *z*; and normal 5-year-olds correctly articulate *th, s,* and *r.*

Phonological disorder cannot be attributed to structural or neurological abnormalities, and it is accompanied by normal language development. The DSM-IV-TR diagnostic criteria for phonological disorder are given in Table 37–3.

Table 37–3
DSM-IV-TR Diagnostic Criteria for Phonological Disorder

A. Failure to use developmentally expected speech sounds that are appropriate for age and dialect (e.g., errors in sound production, use, representation, or organization such as, but not limited to, substitutions of one sound for another [use of /t/ for target /k/ sound] or omissions of sounds such as final consonants).

B. The difficulties in speech sound production interfere with academic or occupational achievement or with social communication.

C. If mental retardation, a speech-motor or sensory deficit, or environmental deprivation is present, the speech difficulties are in excess of those usually associated with these problems.

Coding note: If a speech-motor or sensory deficit or a neurological condition is present, code the condition on Axis III.

From American Psychiatric Association. *Diagnostic and Statistical Manual of Mental Disorders.* 4th ed. Text rev. Washington, DC: American Psychiatric Association; copyright 2000, with permission.

Clinical Features

Children with phonological disorder are delayed in, or incapable of, producing speech sounds that are expected for their age, intelligence, and dialect. The sounds are often substitutions—for example, the use of *t* instead of *k*—and omissions, such as leaving off the final consonants of words. Phonological disorder can be recognized in early childhood. A child's articulation is judged when it is significantly behind the abilities of most children at the same age level, intellectual level, and educational level.

Children with phonological disorder are unable to articulate certain phonemes correctly and may distort, substitute, or even omit the affected phonemes. With omissions, the phonemes are absent entirely—for example, *bu* for *blue, ca* for *car,* or *whaa*? for *what*? With substitutions, difficult phonemes are replaced with incorrect ones—for example, *wabbit* for *rabbit, fum* for *thumb,* or *whath dat*? for *what's that*? With distortions, the correct phoneme is approximated but is articulated incorrectly. Rarely, additions (usually of the vowel *uh*) occur—for example, *puhretty* for *pretty, what's uh that uh*? for *what's that*?

Omissions are thought to be the most serious type of misarticulation, with substitutions the next most serious type, and distortions the least serious type. Omissions are most frequently found in the speech of young children and usually occur at the ends of words or in clusters of consonants (*ca* for *car, scisso* for *scissors*). Distortions, which are found mainly in the speech of older children, result in a sound that is not part of the speaker's dialect.

Most children eventually outgrow phonological disorder, usually by the third grade. After the fourth grade, however, spontaneous recovery is unlikely, and so it is important to try to remediate the disorder before the development of complications. Often, beginning kindergarten or school precipitates the improvement when recovery from phonological disorder is spontaneous. Speech therapy is clearly indicated for children who have not shown spontaneous improvement by the third or fourth grade. Speech therapy should be initiated at an early age for children whose articulation is significantly unintelligible and who are clearly troubled by their inability to speak clearly.

Children with phonological disorder may have various concomitant social, emotional, and behavioral problems, particularly when there are comorbid expressive language problems. Children with expressive language disorder and a severe degree of articulation impairment or whose disorder is chronic and nonremitting are the ones most likely to suffer from psychiatric problems.

Sasha was a talkative, likable 3-year-old whose speech was virtually unintelligible. He had normal hearing and language comprehension skills. No firm conclusion about his level of expressive language development could be made because he was so difficult to understand. He did, however, seem to be producing multiword utterances. Sasha produced only a small number of early-developing consonants (|m|, |n|, |d|, |t|, |b|, |h|, |w|), vowels (|ee|, |ah|, |oo|), and syllable shapes (V, CV, CVCV). As a result, many of his spoken words were indistinguishable from each other (e.g., he said "bahbah" for *baby bottle* and *bubble*; he used "nee" for *knee, need*, and *Anita* [his sister]). Moreover, he never produced consonant sounds at the end of words or used consonant cluster sequences (e.g., |tr-|, |st-|, |-ntl|, |-mpl|). On occasion, Sasha reacted with frustration and tantrums to his difficulties in making himself understood. (Courtesy of Carla J. Johnson, Ph.D., and Joseph H. Beitchman, M.D.)

Differential Diagnosis

The differential diagnosis of phonological disorder includes a careful determination of the severity of the symptoms and possible medical conditions that may be producing the symptoms. First, the clinician must determine that the misarticulations are severe enough to be considered impairing, rather than a normative developmental process of learning to speak. Second, the clinician must determine that no physical abnormalities account for the articulation errors and must rule out neurological disorders that may cause dysarthria, hearing impairment, mental retardation, and pervasive developmental disorders. Third, the clinician must obtain an evaluation of receptive and expressive language to determine that the speech difficulty is not solely attributable to the above disorders.

Neurological, oral structural, and audiometric examinations may be necessary to rule out physical factors that cause certain types of articulation abnormalities. Children with dysarthria, a disorder caused by structural or neurological abnormalities, differ from children with developmental phonological disorder in that dysarthria is less likely to spontaneously remit and may be more difficult to remediate. Drooling, slow or uncoordinated motor behavior, abnormal chewing or swallowing, and awkward or slow protrusion and retraction of the tongue are indications of dysarthria. A slow rate of speech is another indication of dysarthria.

Course and Prognosis

Spontaneous remission of symptoms is common in children whose misarticulations involve only a few phonemes. Children who persist in exhibiting articulation problems after the age of

5 years may be experiencing a myriad of other speech and language impairments, so that a comprehensive evaluation may be indicated at this time. Children older than age 5 years with articulation problems are at higher risk for auditory perceptual problems. Spontaneous recovery is rare after the age of 8 years.

Treatment

Speech therapy provided by a speech and language therapist is considered the most successful treatment for most phonological errors. Speech therapy is indicated when a child's articulation intelligibility is poor; when an affected child is older than 8 years; when a speech problem apparently causes problems with peers, learning, and self-image; when the disorder is so severe that many consonants are misarticulated; and when errors involve omissions and substitutions of phonemes, rather than distortions.

Parental counseling and monitoring of child–peer relationships and school behavior can be useful in minimizing the social impairment with speech and language disorder.

STUTTERING

Stuttering is a condition characterized by involuntary disruptions in the flow of speech. Various speech–motor events may occur that result in dysfluency in speaking. Stuttering may consist of one or more of the following phenomena: sound repetitions, prolongations, interjections, pauses within words, observable word substitutions to avoid blocking, and audible or silent blocking. In cases of severe stuttering, there are typically secondary features that may include disordered breathing, lip pursing, and tongue clicking. It is not uncommon for additional behaviors such as facial grimacing, head jerks, or abnormal body movements to occur during the disrupted speech. The disorder usually originates in childhood.

Epidemiology

Stuttering tends to be most common in young children and has often resolved spontaneously in older children. The typical age of onset is 2 to 7 years with a peak at age 5. It has been estimated that up to 3 to 4 percent of individuals may have stuttered at some time in their lives. Approximately 80 percent of young children who stutter are likely to have a spontaneous remission over time. Stuttering affects approximately 3 to 4 males for every female. The disorder is significantly more common among family members of affected children compared to the general population. According to DSM-IV-TR, for male persons who stutter, 20 percent of their male children and 10 percent of their female children will also stutter.

Etiology

The precise cause of stuttering is unknown, and various theories have been proposed.

Theories about the cause of stuttering include organic models and learning models. Organic models include those that focus on incomplete lateralization or abnormal cerebral dominance. Several studies using electroencephalography (EEG) found that stuttering males had right-hemispheric alpha suppression across stimulus words and tasks; nonstutterers had left-hemispheric suppression. An overrepresentation of left-handedness and ambidexterity has been noted in some studies of stutterers. Twin studies and striking gender differences in stuttering indicate that stuttering has some genetic basis.

Learning theories about the cause of stuttering include the semanto-genic theory, in which stuttering is basically a learned response to normative early childhood dysfluencies. Another learning model focuses on classical conditioning, in which the stuttering becomes conditioned to environmental factors. In the cybernetic model, speech is viewed as a process that depends on appropriate feedback for regulation; stuttering is hypothesized to occur because of a breakdown in the feedback loop. The observations that stuttering is reduced by white noise and that delayed auditory feedback produces stuttering in normal speakers increase the potential validity of the feedback theory.

The motor functioning of some children who stutter appears to be delayed or slightly abnormal. The observation of difficulties in speech planning exhibited by some children who stutter suggests that higher-level cognitive dysfunction may contribute to stuttering. Although children who stutter do not routinely exhibit other speech and language disorders, family members of these children often reveal an increased incidence of a variety of speech and language disorders. Stuttering is most likely to be caused by a set of interacting variables that include both genetic and environmental factors.

Diagnosis

The diagnosis of stuttering is not difficult when the clinical features are apparent and well-developed and each of the four phases, as described in the next section, can be readily recognized. Diagnostic difficulties may arise when trying to determine the existence of stuttering in young children, as some preschool children experience transient dysfluency. It may not be clear whether the nonfluent pattern is part of normal speech and language development or whether it represents the initial stage in the development of stuttering. If incipient stuttering is suspected, referral to a speech pathologist is indicated. Table 37–4 presents the DSM-IV-TR diagnostic criteria for stuttering.

Clinical Features

Stuttering appears in most cases between the ages of 18 months and 9 years, with two sharp peaks of onset between the ages of 2 to 3 1/2 years and 5 to 7 years. Some, but not all, stutterers have other speech and language problems, such as phonological disorder and expressive language disorder. Stuttering does not suddenly begin; it typically develops over a period of weeks or months with a repetition of initial consonants, whole words that are usually the first words of a phrase, or long words. As the disorder progresses, the repetitions become more frequent, with consistent stuttering on the most important words or phrases. Even after it develops, stuttering may be absent during oral readings, singing, and talking to pets or inanimate objects.

Stutterers may have associated clinical features: vivid, fearful anticipation of stuttering, with avoidance of particular words, sounds, or situations in which stuttering is anticipated; eye blinks; tics; and tremors of the lips or jaw. Frustration, anxiety, and depression are common among those with chronic stuttering.

Table 37–4
DSM-IV-TR Diagnostic Criteria for Stuttering

A. Disturbance in the normal fluency and time patterning of speech (inappropriate for the individual's age), characterized by frequent occurrences of one or more of the following:
   (1) sound and syllable repetitions
   (2) sound prolongations
   (3) interjections
   (4) broken words (e.g., pauses within a word)
   (5) audible or silent blocking (filled or unfilled pauses in speech)
   (6) circumlocutions (word substitutions to avoid problematic words)
   (7) words produced with an excess of physical tension
   (8) monosyllabic whole-word repetitions (e.g., "I-I-I-I see him")
B. The disturbance in fluency interferes with academic or occupational achievement or with social communication.
C. If a speech-motor or sensory deficit is present, the speech difficulties are in excess of those usually associated with these problems.
Coding note: If a speech-motor or sensory deficit or a neurological condition is present, code the condition on Axis III.

From American Psychiatric Association. *Diagnostic and Statistical Manual of Mental Disorders.* 4th ed. Text rev. Washington, DC: American Psychiatric Association; copyright 2000, with permission.

Differential Diagnosis

Normal speech dysfluency in preschool years is difficult to differentiate from incipient stuttering. In stuttering, there are more nonfluencies, part-word repetitions, sound prolongations, and disruptions in voice airflow through the vocal track. Children who stutter can be observed to be tense and uncomfortable with their speech pattern in contrast to young children who are nonfluent in their speech but seem to be at ease. Spastic dysphonia is a stuttering-like speech disorder and is distinguished from stuttering by the presence of an abnormal breathing pattern.

Cluttering is a speech disorder characterized by erratic and dysrhythmic speech patterns of rapid and jerky spurts of words and phrases. In cluttering, those affected are usually unaware of the disturbance, whereas, after the initial phase of the disorder, stutterers are aware of their speech difficulties. Cluttering is often an associated feature of expressive language disorder.

Course and Prognosis

The course of stuttering is usually long term, with some periods of partial remission lasting for weeks or months and exacerbations occurring most frequently when a stutterer is under pressure to communicate. Fifty to 80 percent of all children who stutter, mostly those with mild cases, recover spontaneously.

Treatment

Treatment entails breathing exercises, relaxation techniques, and speech therapy to help children slow the rate of speaking and modulate speech volume.

Most modern treatments of stuttering are based on the view that stuttering is essentially a learned form of behavior not necessarily associated with a basic mental disorder or neurological abnormality. The approaches work directly with the speech difficulty to minimize the issues that maintain and strengthen stuttering, to modify or decrease the severity of stuttering by eliminating the secondary symptoms, and to encourage stutterers to speak, even when stuttering, in a relatively easy and effortless fashion that thereby avoids fears and blocks.

One example of this approach is the self-therapy proposed by the Speech Foundation of America. Self-therapy is based on the premise that stuttering is not a symptom but a behavior that can be modified. The approach includes desensitizing, reducing the emotional reaction to and fears of stuttering, and substituting positive action to control the moment of stuttering.

Classic psychoanalysis, insight-oriented psychotherapy, group therapy, and other psychotherapeutic modalities have not been successful in treating stuttering. But if stutterers have a poor self-image, are anxious or depressed, or show evidence of an established emotional disorder, individual psychotherapy is indicated and effective for the associated condition. In one study, the reaction of nonstuttering listeners to stutterers who acknowledged their stuttering was much more positive than to stutterers who did not acknowledge their stuttering. Family therapy should also be considered if there is evidence of family dysfunction, family contribution to a stutterer's symptoms, or family stress caused by trying to cope with or help the stutterer.

Recently developed therapies focus on restructuring fluency. The entire speech production pattern is reshaped, with emphasis on a variety of target behaviors, including rate reduction, easy or gentle onset of voicing, and smooth transitions between sounds, syllables, and words.

Psychopharmacologic intervention such as treatment with haloperidol (Haldol) has been used in an attempt to induce increased relaxation. There are no data to accurately assess the efficacy of this approach. Whichever therapeutic approach is

Table 37–5
DSM-IV-TR Diagnostic Criteria for Communication Disorder Not Otherwise Specified

This category is for disorders in communication that do not meet criteria for any specific communication disorder; for example, a voice disorder (i.e., an abnormality of vocal pitch, loudness, quality, tone, or resonance).

From American Psychiatric Association. *Diagnostic and Statistical Manual of Mental Disorders.* 4th ed. Text rev. Washington, DC: American Psychiatric Association; copyright 2000, with permission.

used, individual and family assessments and supportive interventions may be helpful. A team assessment of a child or adolescent and his or her family should be made before any approaches to treatment are begun.

COMMUNICATION DISORDER NOT OTHERWISE SPECIFIED

Disorders that do not meet the diagnostic criteria for any specific communication disorder fall into the category of communication disorder not otherwise specified. An example is voice disorder, in which the patient has an abnormality in pitch, loudness, quality, tone, or resonance. To be coded as a disorder, the voice abnormality must be severe enough to cause an impairment in academic achievement or social communication (Table 37–5).

Cluttering is not listed as a disorder in DSM-IV-TR, but it is an associated speech abnormality in which the disturbed rate and rhythm of speech result in impaired speech intelligibility. Speech is erratic and dysrhythmic and consists of rapid, jerky spurts that are inconsistent with normal phrasing patterns. The disorder usually occurs in children between 2 and 8 years of age; in two-thirds of the cases, the patient spontaneously recovers by early adolescence. Cluttering is associated with learning disorders and other communication disorders.

Pervasive Developmental Disorders

The pervasive developmental disorders include a group of conditions in which there is a delay and deviance in the development of social skills, language and communication, and behavioral repertoire. Children with pervasive developmental disorders often exhibit idiosyncratic intense interest in a narrow range of activities, resist change, and are not appropriately responsive to the social environment. These disorders affect multiple areas of development, are manifested early in life, and cause persistent dysfunction. The text revision of the fourth edition of *Diagnostic and Statistical Manual of Mental Disorders* (DSM-IV-TR) includes five pervasive developmental disorders: autistic disorder, Rett's disorder, childhood disintegrative disorder, Asperger's disorder, and pervasive developmental disorder not otherwise specified.

AUTISTIC DISORDER

Autistic disorder (historically called *early infantile autism, childhood autism,* or *Kanner's autism*) is characterized by deviant reciprocal social interaction, delayed and aberrant communication skills, and a restricted repertoire of activities and interests.

Epidemiology

Prevalence. Autistic disorder is believed to occur at a rate of approximately 5 cases per 10,000 children (0.05 percent). Reports of the rate of autistic disorder have ranged from 2 to 20 cases per 10,000. By definition, the onset of autistic disorder is before the age of 3 years, although in some cases, it is not recognized until a child is much older.

Sex Distribution. Autistic disorder is 4 to 5 times more frequent in boys than in girls. Girls with autistic disorder are more likely to have more severe mental retardation.

Etiology and Pathogenesis

Autistic disorder is a developmental behavioral disorder. Although autistic disorder was initially hypothesized by Kanner to be due to emotionally unresponsive "refrigerator" mothers, there is no validity to this hypothesis. On the other hand, much evidence has accumulated to support a biological substrate for this disorder.

Psychosocial and Family Factors. Children with autism, as with children with other disorders, can respond with an exacerbation of symptoms to psychosocial stressors including family dis-

cord, the birth of a new sibling, or a family move. Some children with autistic disorder may be excruciatingly sensitive to even small changes in their families and immediate environments.

Biological Factors. The high rate of mental retardation among children with autistic disorder and the higher-than-expected rates of seizure disorders suggest a biological basis for autistic disorder. Approximately 75 percent of children with autistic disorder have mental retardation. Approximately one-third of these children have mild to moderate mental retardation, and close to half of these children are severely or profoundly mentally retarded. Children with autistic disorder and mental retardation typically show more marked deficits in abstract reasoning, social understanding, and verbal tasks compared to performance tasks such as block design and digit recall, in which details can be remembered without reference to the "gestalt" meaning.

Four to 32 percent of people with autism have grand mal seizures at some time, and approximately 20 to 25 percent show ventricular enlargement on computed tomography (CT) scans. Various electroencephalogram (EEG) abnormalities are found in 10 to 83 percent of autistic children, and, although no EEG finding is specific to autistic disorder, there is some indication of failed cerebral lateralization. Recently, one magnetic resonance imaging (MRI) study revealed hypoplasia of cerebellar vermal lobules VI and VII, and another MRI study revealed cortical abnormalities, particularly polymicrogyria, in some autistic patients. Those abnormalities may reflect abnormal cell migrations in the first 6 months of gestation. An autopsy study revealed decreased Purkinje's cell counts, and another study found increased diffuse cortical metabolism during positron emission tomography (PET) scanning.

Autistic disorder is also associated with neurological conditions, notably congenital rubella, phenylketonuria (PKU), tuberous sclerosis, and Rett's disorder. Autistic children show more evidence of perinatal complications than do comparison groups of normal children and those with other disorders. The finding that autistic children have significantly more minor congenital physical anomalies than expected suggests abnormal development within the first trimester of pregnancy.

Genetic Factors. In several surveys, between 2 and 4 percent of siblings of autistic children also had autistic disorder, a rate 50 times greater than in the general population. The concordance rate of autistic disorder in twin studies was 40 to 90 percent in monozygotic pairs versus 0 to 25 percent in dizygotic pairs.

Clinical reports suggest that the nonautistic members of families with autistic members have higher rates of less pronounced language or other cognitive problems. Fragile X syndrome, a genetic disorder in which a portion of the X chromosome fractures, appears to be associated with autistic disorder. Approximately 1 percent of children with autistic disorder also have fragile X syndrome. Tuberous sclerosis, a genetic disorder characterized by multiple benign tumors with autosomal dominant transmission is found with greater frequency among children with autistic disorder. Up to 2 percent of children with autistic disorder may also have tuberous sclerosis.

Recently, researchers screened the DNA of more than 150 pairs of siblings with autism. They found extremely strong evidence that two regions on chromosomes 2 and 7 contain genes that are involved with autism. Likely locations for autism-related genes were also found on chromosomes 16 and 17, although the strength of the correlation was somewhat weaker.

Immunological Factors.   There have been several reports suggesting that immunological incompatibility (i.e., maternal antibodies directed at the fetus) may contribute to autistic disorder. The lymphocytes of some autistic children react with maternal antibodies, a fact that raises the possibility that embryonic neural or extraembryonic tissues may be damaged during gestation.

Perinatal Factors.   A higher-than-expected incidence of perinatal complications seems to occur in infants who are later diagnosed with autistic disorder. Maternal bleeding after the first trimester and meconium in the amniotic fluid have been reported in the histories of autistic children more often than in the general population. In the neonatal period, autistic children have a high incidence of respiratory distress syndrome and neonatal anemia.

Neuroanatomical Factors.   MRI studies comparing autistic subjects and normal controls have shown that the total brain volume was increased in those with autism, although those autistic children with severe mental retardation generally have smaller heads. The greatest average percentage increase in size occurred in the occipital lobe, parietal lobe, and temporal lobe. The increased volume can arise from three different possible mechanisms: increased neurogenesis, decreased neuronal death, and increased production of nonneuronal brain tissue such as glial cells or blood vessels. Brain enlargement has been suggested as a possible biological marker for autistic disorder.

The temporal lobe is believed to be a critical area of brain abnormality in autistic disorder. This suggestion is based on reports of autistic-like syndromes in some people with temporal lobe damage.

Biochemical Factors.   In some autistic children, increased cerebrospinal fluid (CSF) homovanillic acid (the major dopamine metabolite) is associated with increased withdrawal and stereotypes. Some evidence indicates that symptom severity decreases as the ratio of CSF 5-hydroxyindoleacetic acid (5-HIAA, metabolite of serotonin) to CSF homovanillic acid increases. CSF 5-HIAA may be inversely proportional to blood serotonin levels; these levels are increased in one-third of autistic disorder patients, a nonspecific finding that also occurs in mentally retarded persons.

Diagnosis and Clinical Features

The DSM-IV-TR diagnostic criteria for autistic disorder are given in Table 38–1.

Table 38–1
DSM-IV-TR Diagnostic Criteria for Autistic Disorder

A. A total of six (or more) items from (1), (2), and (3), with at least two from (1), and one each from (2) and (3):
  (1) qualitative impairment in social interaction, as manifested by at least two of the following:
   (a) marked impairment in the use of multiple nonverbal behaviors such as eye-to-eye gaze, facial expression, body postures, and gestures to regulate social interaction
   (b) failure to develop peer relationships appropriate to developmental level
   (c) a lack of spontaneous seeking to share enjoyment, interests, or achievements with other people (e.g., by a lack of showing, bringing, or pointing out objects of interest)
   (d) lack of social or emotional reciprocity
  (2) qualitative impairments in communication as manifested by at least one of the following:
   (a) delay in, or total lack of, the development of spoken language (not accompanied by an attempt to compensate through alternative modes of communication such as gesture or mime)
   (b) in individuals with adequate speech, marked impairment in the ability to initiate or sustain a conversation with others
   (c) stereotyped and repetitive use of language or idiosyncratic language
   (d) lack of varied, spontaneous make-believe play or social imitative play appropriate to developmental level
  (3) restricted repetitive and stereotyped patterns of behavior, interests, and activities, as manifested by at least one of the following:
   (a) encompassing preoccupation with one or more stereotyped and restricted patterns of interest that is abnormal either in intensity or focus
   (b) apparently inflexible adherence to specific, nonfunctional routines or rituals
   (c) stereotyped and repetitive motor mannerisms (e.g., hand or finger flapping or twisting, or complex whole-body movements)
   (d) persistent preoccupation with parts of objects
B. Delays or abnormal functioning in at least one of the following areas, with onset prior to age 3 years: (1) social interaction, (2) language as used in social communication, or (3) symbolic or imaginative play.
C. The disturbance is not better accounted for by Rett's disorder or childhood disintegrative disorder.

From American Psychiatric Association. *Diagnostic and Statistical Manual of Mental Disorders.* 4th ed. Text rev. Washington, DC: American Psychiatric Association; copyright 2000, with permission.

Physical Characteristics.   Children with autistic disorder are often described as attractive, and, on first glance, do not show any physical signs indicating autistic disorder. They do have high rates of minor physical anomalies, such as ear malformations. The minor physical anomalies may be a reflection of the particular fetal developmental period in which the abnormalities arose, since ear formation occurs at approximately the same time as portions of the brain.

Autistic children also have a higher incidence of abnormal dermatoglyphics (e.g., fingerprints) than do the general population. This finding may suggest a disturbance in neuroectodermal development.

Behavioral Characteristics

QUALITATIVE IMPAIRMENTS IN SOCIAL INTERACTION.   Autistic children fail to show the subtle signs of social relatedness to their parents and other people. Less frequent or poor eye contact is a common finding. The social development of autistic children is characterized by impaired, but not usually a total absence of, attachment behavior. Autistic children often do not acknowledge or differentiate the most important people in their lives—parents, siblings, and teachers—and may show extreme anxiety when their usual routine is disrupted, but they may not react overtly to being left with a stranger. There is a notable deficit in ability to play with peers and to make friends; their social behavior is awkward and may be inappropriate. Cognitively, children with autistic disorder are more skilled in visual-spatial tasks, as opposed to tasks requiring skill in verbal reasoning.

One description of the cognitive style of children with autism is that they are unable to make attributions about the motivation or intentions of others, and thus cannot develop empathy. This lack of a "theory of mind" leaves them unable to interpret the social behavior of others and leads to a lack of social reciprocation.

DISTURBANCES OF COMMUNICATION AND LANGUAGE.   Deficits in language development and difficulty using language to communicate ideas are among the principal criteria for diagnosing autistic disorder. In contrast to normal and mentally retarded children, autistic children have significant difficulty putting meaningful sentences together even when they have large vocabularies.

STEREOTYPED BEHAVIOR.   In the first years of an autistic child's life, much of the expected spontaneous exploratory play is absent. Toys and objects are often manipulated in a ritualistic manner, with few symbolic features. Autistic children generally do not show imitative play or use abstract pantomime. The activities and play of these children are often rigid, repetitive, and monotonous. Many autistic children, especially those who are severely mentally retarded, exhibit movement abnormalities. Stereotypies, mannerisms, and grimacing are most frequent when a child is left alone and may decrease in a structured situation. Autistic children are generally resistant to transition and change.

ASSOCIATED BEHAVIORAL SYMPTOMS.   Hyperkinesis is a common behavior problem in young autistic children. Hypokinesis is less frequent; when present, it often alternates with hyperactivity. Aggression and temper tantrums are observed, often prompted by change or demands. Self-injurious behavior includes head banging, biting, scratching, and hair pulling. Short attention span, poor ability to focus on a task, insomnia, feeding and eating problems, and enuresis are also common among children with autism.

ASSOCIATED PHYSICAL ILLNESS.   Young children with autistic disorder have a higher-than-expected incidence of upper respiratory infections and other minor infections. Gastrointestinal (GI) symptoms commonly found among children with autistic disorder include excessive burping, constipation, and loose bowel movements. There is also an increased incidence of febrile seizures in children with autistic disorder. Some autistic children do not show temperature elevations with minor infectious illnesses and may not show the typical malaise of ill children. In some cases, behavior problems and relatedness seem to improve to a

noticeable degree in children during a minor illness, and in some cases such changes are a clue to physical illness.

A standardized instrument that can be very helpful in eliciting comprehensive information regarding developmental disorders is the Autism Diagnostic Observation Schedule–Generic (ADOS–G).

Roy, a 6-year-old boy, was referred for a psychiatric evaluation by his first-grade teacher, who reported that Roy was disruptive in class, was unable to follow directions, had not really made any friends, and, at unpredictable times, was hyperactive and aggressive. Roy had never had a psychiatric evaluation, but his mother suspects that, like his older brother, he probably has attention-deficit/hyperactivity disorder (ADHD). Roy has had trouble following directions since he started preschool at age 3, but he had never been described as aggressive until this year. According to his teacher, Roy is picked on often by his classmates, who think he is "weird."

Roy was the product of a normal pregnancy but was treated for 10 days with antibiotics in the neonatal intensive care unit after birth because he developed bacterial meningitis after delivery. Fortunately, it was caught early, and the doctors had assured his mother that there was no permanent damage. He was healthy after being discharged from the hospital.

Roy's parents began to get concerned about his language development because he could only say "dada" at 18 months. The pediatrician was very reassuring, stating that some children develop language later than others and that there were no signs of any neurological disease. Roy's mother had his hearing tested, since she had read that babies who were treated with antibiotics as newborns might develop hearing loss. Roy's hearing was normal, but his mother continued to notice that he did not usually turn his head toward her when she spoke to him. Roy's mother assumed that he had a poor attention span, like his older brother, and was not too worried about his lack of attention to adults. She continued to be concerned that his language was not developing appropriately.

When Roy started preschool, it became clear that he did not play with toys the same way as the other children. He did not seem to understand how to use the toys and would use a truck, for example, to bang on the floor. He had acquired more words by now, but his sentences were often incomprehensible. He often said "You" when he meant "I" and repeated verbatim phrases that he had heard earlier in the day. He was unable to share toys and never joined in group activities that required the class to sit in a circle. Instead, he stayed in the corner of the room playing by himself. He would not let the teacher know when he was thirsty or had to go to the bathroom. He would not answer questions; sometimes he became overly excited and hyperactive and ran around the room with no apparent goal. Most of the time he did not make eye contact and was isolated from others. Roy usually did not do much with the other children, so the teacher only had difficulty managing him when he became hyperactive and resisted sitting down. The teacher did mention that Roy was a creature of habit—he played with the same toy every single day and would get extremely upset if any other child tried to touch his favorite toy.

By the time Roy reached first grade, it was clear that he was not socializing with any of his classmates, and his language was still poor. He also did not seem to understand what was expected of him in class, and he often appeared distracted and distant.

An evaluation was initiated with psychological testing. On intellectual testing, Roy's full-scale intelligence quotient (IQ) was 68, with a verbal IQ of 61 and a performance IQ of 75, placing him in the range of probable mild mental retardation. Roy's language skills were an area of major weakness. Although Roy had now learned many words, he exhibited great difficulty making himself understood and responding to his peers. Roy's language problems included pronoun reversals, echolalia, and unusual syntax. Roy's social problems were as much a problem as his language. He had few interests and was rejected by his peers. He seemed fixated on running water and would spend up to an hour, if allowed, watching water run out of the faucet. Roy did not understand his schoolwork and continued to have periods of overactivity in which he would run around the classroom aimlessly.

DISCUSSION

Given the combination of aberrant language development, significant inability to relate to peers or adults, and a very restricted range of interests, a diagnosis of autistic disorder was made. In addition, after evaluating his "living skills," such as dressing himself and communicating with others, along with his intellectual testing, it was determined that Roy also had mild mental retardation. Furthermore, he also had frequent periods of hyperactivity, poor attention, and distractibility in school and at home, causing significant problems for him, which led to a diagnosis of ADHD. It was recommended that Roy's family request initiation of an Individualized Educational Plan by his school so that he could be placed in a smaller, more structured special education classroom. A referral was made for a behavioral program to reinforce both appropriate social and task-oriented behaviors. A trial of methylphenidate (Ritalin) was recommended to target Roy's hyperactivity and poor attention.

Intellectual Functioning.

Unusual or precocious cognitive or visuomotor abilities occur in some autistic children. The abilities, which may exist even in the overall retarded functioning, are referred to as *splinter functions* or *islets of precocity*. Perhaps the most striking examples are idiot or autistic savants, who have prodigious rote memories or calculating abilities, usually beyond the capabilities of normal peers. Other precocious abilities in young autistic children include hyperlexia, an early ability to read well (although they are not able to understand what they read), memorizing and reciting, and musical abilities (singing or playing tunes or recognizing musical pieces).

Differential Diagnosis

The major differential diagnoses are schizophrenia with childhood onset, mental retardation with behavioral symptoms, mixed receptive-expressive language disorder, congenital deaf-

ness or severe hearing disorder, psychosocial deprivation, and disintegrative (regressive) psychoses. Because children with a pervasive developmental disorder usually have many concurrent problems, Michael Rutter and Lionel Hersov suggested a stepwise approach to use in the differential diagnosis.

Schizophrenia with Childhood Onset.

Schizophrenia is rare in children under the age of 5. It is accompanied by hallucinations or delusions, with a lower incidence of seizures and mental retardation and a more even IQ than in autistic children. Table 38–2 compares autistic disorder and schizophrenia with childhood onset.

Mental Retardation with Behavioral Symptoms.

It is not uncommon for retarded children to have behavior symptoms that include autistic features; thus, when both disorders are present, both should be diagnosed. The main differentiating features between autistic disorder and mental retardation are the following: Mentally retarded children usually relate to adults and other children in accordance with their mental age; they use the language they do have to communicate with others; and they have a relatively even profile of impairments without splinter functions.

Acquired Aphasia with Convulsion.

Acquired aphasia with convulsion is a rare condition that is sometimes difficult to differentiate from autistic disorder and childhood disintegrative disorder. Children with the condition are normal for several years before losing both their receptive and their expressive language over a period of weeks or months. Most have a few seizures and generalized EEG abnormalities at the onset, but these signs usually do not persist. A profound language comprehension disorder then follows, characterized by a deviant speech pattern and speech impairment.

Congenital Deafness or Severe Hearing Impairment.

Because autistic children are often mute or show a selective disinterest in spoken language, they are often thought to be deaf. Differentiating factors include the following: Autistic infants may babble only infrequently, whereas deaf infants have a history of relatively normal babbling that then gradually tapers off and may stop from 6 months to 1 year of age. Deaf children respond only to loud sounds, whereas autistic children may ignore loud or normal sounds and respond to soft or low sounds. Most important, audiogram or auditory-evoked potentials indicate significant hearing loss in deaf children. Unlike autistic children, deaf children usually relate to their parents, seek their affection, and, as infants, enjoy being held.

Course and Prognosis

Autistic disorder is generally a life-long disorder with a guarded prognosis. Those autistic children with IQs above 70 and those who use communicative language by the age of 5 to 7 years tend to have the best prognoses.

The symptom areas that did not seem to improve over time were those related to ritualistic and repetitive behaviors. In general, adult-outcome studies indicate that approximately two-thirds of autistic adults remain severely handicapped and live in complete dependence or semidependence, either with their relatives or in long-term institutions. The prognosis is improved if the environment or the home is supportive and capable of meeting the extensive needs of such a child. Although a decrease of symptoms is noted in many cases, severe self-mutilation or aggressiveness and regression may develop in others.

Table 38–2
Autistic Disorder versus Schizophrenia with Childhood Onset

Criteria	Autistic Disorder	Schizophrenia (with Onset before Puberty)
Age of onset	Before 38 months	Not under 5 years of age
Incidence	2–5 in 10,000	Unknown, possibly same or even rarer
Sex ratio (M:F)	3–4:1	1.67:1 (nearly equal, or slight preponderance of males)
Family history of schizophrenia	Not raised or probably not raised	Raised
Socioeconomic status (SES)	Overrepresentation of upper SES groups (artifact)	More common in lower SES groups
Prenatal and perinatal complications and cerebral dysfunction	More common in autistic disorder	Less common in schizophrenia
Behavioral characteristics	Failure to develop relatedness; absence of speech or echolalia; stereotyped phrases; language comprehension absent or poor; insistence on sameness and stereotypies	Hallucinations and delusions; thought disorder
Adaptive functioning	Usually always impaired	Deterioration in functioning
Level of intelligence	In majority of cases subnormal, frequently severely impaired (70% ≤70)	Usually within normal range, mostly dull normal (15% ≤ 70)
Pattern of IQ	Marked unevenness	More even
Grand mal seizures	4–32%	Absent or lower incidence

Courtesy of Magda Campbell, M.D., and Wayne Green, M.D.

Treatment

The goals of treatment for children with autistic disorder are to increase socially acceptable and prosocial behavior, to decrease odd behavioral symptoms, and to improve verbal and nonverbal communication. Language remediation as well as academic remediation is often required. Children with mental retardation need intellectually appropriate behavioral interventions to reinforce socially acceptable behaviors and encourage self-care skills. In addition, parents, often distraught, need support and counseling. Insight-oriented individual psychotherapy has proved to be ineffective. Educational and behavioral interventions are currently considered the treatments of choice. Structured classroom training in combination with behavioral methods is the most effective treatment method for many autistic children.

Careful training of parents in the concepts and skills of behavior modification and the resolution of the parents' concerns may yield considerable gains in children's language, cognitive, and social areas of behavior.

There are no specific medications to treat the core symptoms of autistic disorder; however, psychopharmacotherapy is a valuable adjunctive treatment to ameliorate associated behavioral symptoms. Medication has been reported to improve associated symptoms, including aggression, severe temper tantrums, self-injurious behaviors, hyperactivity, and obsessive-compulsive behaviors and stereotypies. The administration of antipsychotic medication may reduce aggressive or self-injurious behavior.

Serotonin-dopamine antagonists (SDAs) have a decreased risk of causing extrapyramidal side effects, although some sensitive individuals are not able to tolerate the extrapyramidal or anticholinergic side effects of the atypical antipsychotic agents. The SDAs include risperidone (Risperdal), olanzapine (Zyprexa), quetiapine (Seroquel), clozapine (Clozaril), and ziprasidone (Geodon).

RETT'S DISORDER

Rett's disorder is described by DSM-IV-TR as a development of several specific deficits following a period of normal functioning after birth. In 1965, Andreas Rett, an Australian physician, identified a syndrome in 22 girls who appeared to have had normal development for a period of at least 6 months, followed by devastating developmental deterioration. Although few surveys have been done, those available indicate a prevalence of 6 to 7 cases of Rett's disorder per 100,000 girls.

Etiology

The cause of Rett's disorder is unknown, although the progressive deteriorating course after an initial normal period is compatible with a metabolic disorder. It is likely that Rett's disorder has a genetic basis. It has been seen only in girls, and case reports so far indicate complete concordance in monozygotic twins.

Diagnosis and Clinical Features

At 6 months to 2 years of age, children develop a progressive encephalopathy with a number of characteristic features. The signs often include the loss of purposeful hand movements, which are replaced by stereotypic motions such as hand-wringing, the loss of previously acquired speech, psychomotor retardation, and ataxia. Other stereotypical hand movements may occur, such as licking or biting the fingers and tapping or slapping. The head-circumference growth decelerates and produces microcephaly. All language skills are lost, and both receptive and expressive communicative and social skills seem to plateau at developmental levels between 6 months and 1 year. Poor muscle coordination and an apraxic gait develop; the gait has an unsteady and stiff quality. All these clinical features are diagnostic criteria for the disorder (Table 38–3).

Table 38–3
DSM-IV-TR Diagnostic Criteria for Rett's Disorder

A. All of the following:
   (1) apparently normal prenatal and perinatal development
   (2) apparently normal psychomotor development through the first 5 months after birth
   (3) normal head circumference at birth
B. Onset of all of the following after the period of normal development:
   (1) deceleration of head growth between ages 5 and 48 months
   (2) loss of previously acquired purposeful hand skills between ages 5 and 30 months with the subsequent development of stereotyped hand movements (e.g., hand wringing or hand washing)
   (3) loss of social engagement early in the course (although often social interaction develops later)
   (4) appearance of poorly coordinated gait or trunk movements
   (5) severely impaired expressive and receptive language development with severe psychomotor retardation

From American Psychiatric Association. *Diagnostic and Statistical Manual of Mental Disorders*. 4th ed. Text rev. Washington, DC: American Psychiatric Association; copyright 2000, with permission.

Differential Diagnosis

Some children with Rett's disorder receive initial diagnoses of autistic disorder because of the marked disability in social interactions in both disorders, but the two disorders have some predictable differences. In Rett's disorder, a child shows a deterioration of developmental milestones, head circumference, and overall growth; in autistic disorder, aberrant development in most cases is present from early on. In Rett's disorder, specific and characteristic hand motions are always present; in autistic disorder, hand mannerisms may or may not appear. Poor coordination, ataxia, and apraxia are predictably part of Rett's disorder; many persons with autistic disorder have unremarkable gross motor function. In Rett's disorder, verbal abilities are usually lost completely; in autistic disorder, patients use characteristically aberrant language. Respiratory irregularity is characteristic of Rett's disorder, and seizures often appear early on. In autistic disorder, no respiratory disorganization is seen, and seizures do not develop in most patients; when seizures do develop, they are more likely in adolescence than in childhood.

Course and Prognosis

Rett's disorder is progressive. The prognosis is not fully known, but those patients who live into adulthood remain at a cognitive and social level equivalent to that in the first year of life.

Treatment

Treatment is aimed at symptomatic intervention. Physiotherapy has been beneficial for the muscular dysfunction, and anticonvulsant treatment is usually necessary to control the seizures. Behavior therapy, along with medication, may be helpful to control self-injurious behaviors, as it is in the treat-

ment of autistic disorder, and it may help regulate the breathing disorganization.

CHILDHOOD DISINTEGRATIVE DISORDER

According to DSM-IV-TR, childhood disintegrative disorder is characterized by marked regression in several areas of functioning after at least 2 years of apparently normal development. Childhood disintegrative disorder, also known as *Heller's syndrome* and *disintegrative psychosis*, was described in 1908 as a deterioration over several months of intellectual, social, and language function occurring in 3- and 4-year-olds with previously normal functions. After the deterioration, the children closely resembled children with autistic disorder.

Epidemiology

Epidemiological data have been complicated by the variable diagnostic criteria used, but childhood disintegrative disorder is estimated to be at least one-tenth as common as autistic disorder, and the prevalence has been estimated to be approximately one case in 100,000 boys. The ratio of boys to girls is estimated to be between 4 and 8 boys to 1 girl.

Etiology

The cause of childhood disintegrative disorder is unknown, but it has been associated with other neurological conditions, including seizure disorders, tuberous sclerosis, and various metabolic disorders.

Diagnosis and Clinical Features

The diagnosis is made on the basis of features that fit a characteristic age of onset, clinical picture, and course. Cases reported have ranged in onset from ages 1 to 9 years, but in the vast majority the onset is between 3 and 4 years; according to DSM-IV-TR, the minimum age of onset is 2 years (Table 38–4). The core features of the disorder include a loss of communication skills, marked regression of reciprocal interactions, and the onset of stereotyped movements and compulsive behavior. Affective symptoms are common, particularly anxiety, as is the regression of self-help skills, such as bowel and bladder control.

To receive the diagnosis, a child must exhibit a loss of skills in two of the following areas: language, social or adaptive behavior, bowel or bladder control, play, and motor skills. Abnormalities must be present in at least two of the following categories: reciprocal social interaction, communication skills, and stereotyped or restricted behavior. The main neurological associated feature is seizure disorder.

Bob's early history was within normal limits. By age 2, he was speaking in sentences, and his development appeared to be proceeding appropriately. At age 40 months, he abruptly exhibited a period of marked behavioral regression shortly after the birth of a sibling. He lost previously acquired skills in communication and was no longer toilet trained. He became uninterested in social interaction, and various unusual self-stimulatory behaviors became evident. Comprehensive medical examination failed to reveal any conditions that might account for this developmental regression. Behaviorally, he exhibited features of autistic disorder. At follow-up at age 12, he spoke only an occasional single word and was severely retarded. (Reprinted with permission from Volkmar F. Autism and the pervasive developmental disorders. In: Lewis M, ed. *Child and Adolescent Psychiatry: A Comprehensive Approach.* 2nd ed. Baltimore: Williams & Wilkins; 1996.)

Differential Diagnosis

The differential diagnosis of childhood disintegrative disorder includes autistic disorder and Rett's disorder. In many cases, the clinical features overlap with autistic disorder, but childhood disintegrative disorder is distinguished from autistic disorder by the loss of previously acquired development. Before the onset of childhood disintegrative disorder (occurring at 2 years or older), language has usually progressed to sentence formation. This skill is strikingly different from the premorbid history of even high-functioning autistic disorder patients, in whom language generally does not exceed single words or phrases before the diagnosis of the disorder. Once the disorder occurs, however, those with childhood disintegrative disorder are more likely to have no language abilities than are high-func-

Table 38–4
DSM-IV-TR Diagnostic Criteria for Childhood Disintegrative Disorder

A. Apparently normal development for at least the first 2 years after birth as manifested by the presence of age-appropriate verbal and nonverbal communication, social relationships, play, and adaptive behavior.

B. Clinically significant loss of previously acquired skills (before age 10 years) in at least two of the following areas:
   (1) expressive or receptive language
   (2) social skills or adaptive behavior
   (3) bowel or bladder control
   (4) play
   (5) motor skills

C. Abnormalities of functioning in at least two of the following areas:
   (1) qualitative impairment in social interaction (e.g., impairment in nonverbal behaviors, failure to develop peer relationships, lack of social or emotional reciprocity)
   (2) qualitative impairments in communication (e.g., delay or lack of spoken language, inability to initiate or sustain a conversation, stereotyped and repetitive use of language, lack of varied make-believe play)
   (3) restricted, repetitive, and stereotyped patterns of behavior, interests, and activities, including motor stereotypies and mannerisms

D. The disturbance is not better accounted for by another specific pervasive developmental disorder or by schizophrenia.

From American Psychiatric Association. *Diagnostic and Statistical Manual of Mental Disorders.* 4th ed. Text rev. Washington, DC: American Psychiatric Association; copyright 2000, with permission.

tioning autistic disorder patients. In Rett's disorder, the deterioration occurs much earlier than in childhood disintegrative disorder, and the characteristic hand stereotypies of Rett's disorder do not occur in childhood disintegrative disorder.

Course and Prognosis

The course of childhood disintegrative disorder is variable, with a plateau reached in most cases, a progressive deteriorating course in rare cases, and some improvement in occasional cases to the point of regaining the ability to speak in sentences. Most patients are left with at least moderate mental retardation.

Treatment

Because of the clinical similarity to autistic disorder, the treatment of childhood disintegrative disorder includes the same components available in the treatment of autistic disorder.

ASPERGER'S DISORDER

According to DSM-IV-TR, those with Asperger's disorder show severe, sustained impairment in social interaction and restricted, repetitive patterns of behavior, interests, and activities. Unlike autistic disorder, in Asperger's disorder, there are no significant delays in language, cognitive development, or age-appropriate self-help skills. In 1944, Hans Asperger, an Austrian physician, described a syndrome that he named *autistic psychopathy.* His original description of the syndrome applied to persons with normal intelligence who exhibit a qualitative impairment in reciprocal social interaction and behavioral oddities without delays in language development. Since that time, a person with mental retardation but without language delay has received a diagnosis of Asperger's disorder, and a person with language delay but without mental retardation has also been given that diagnosis.

Etiology

The cause of Asperger's disorder is unknown, but family studies suggest a possible relationship to autistic disorder. The similarity of Asperger's disorder to autistic disorder supports the presence of genetic, metabolic, infectious, and perinatal contributing factors.

Diagnosis and Clinical Features

The clinical features include at least two of the following indications of qualitative social impairment: markedly abnormal nonverbal communicative gestures, the failure to develop peer relationships, the lack of social or emotional reciprocity, and an impaired ability to express pleasure in other people's happiness. Restricted interests and patterns of behavior are always present. According to DSM-IV-TR, the patient shows no language delay, clinically significant cognitive delay, or adaptive impairment (Table 38–5).

Differential Diagnosis

The differential diagnosis includes autistic disorder, pervasive development disorder not otherwise specified, and, in patients

Table 38–5
DSM-IV-TR Diagnostic Criteria for Asperger's Disorder

A. Qualitative impairment in social interaction, as manifested by at least two of the following:

(1) marked impairment in the use of multiple nonverbal behaviors such as eye-to-eye gaze, facial expression, body postures, and gestures to regulate social interaction

(2) failure to develop peer relationships appropriate to developmental level

(3) a lack of spontaneous seeking to share enjoyment, interests, or achievements with other people (e.g., by a lack of showing, bringing, or pointing out objects of interest to other people)

(4) lack of social or emotional reciprocity

B. Restricted repetitive and stereotyped patterns of behavior, interests, and activities, as manifested by at least one of the following:

(1) encompassing preoccupation with one or more stereotyped and restricted patterns of interest that is abnormal either in intensity or focus

(2) apparently inflexible adherence to specific, nonfunctional routines or rituals

(3) stereotyped and repetitive motor mannerisms (e.g., hand or finger flapping or twisting, or complex whole-body movements)

(4) persistent preoccupation with parts of objects

C. The disturbance causes clinically significant impairment in social, occupational, or other important areas of functioning.

D. There is no clinically significant general delay in language (e.g., single words used by age 2 years, communicative phrases used by age 3 years).

E. There is no clinically significant delay in cognitive development or in the development of age-appropriate self-help skills, adaptive behavior (other than in social interaction), and curiosity about the environment in childhood.

F. Criteria are not met for another specific pervasive developmental disorder or schizophrenia.

From American Psychiatric Association. *Diagnostic and Statistical Manual of Mental Disorders.* 4th ed. Text rev. Washington, DC: American Psychiatric Association; copyright 2000, with permission.

Table 38–6
DSM-IV-TR Diagnostic Criteria for Pervasive Developmental Disorder Not Otherwise Specified (Including Atypical Autism)

This category should be used when there is a severe and pervasive impairment in the development of reciprocal social interaction associated with impairment in either verbal or nonverbal communication skills or with the presence of stereotyped behavior, interests, and activities, but the criteria are not met for a specific pervasive developmental disorder, schizophrenia, schizotypal personality disorder, or avoidant personality disorder. For example, this category includes "atypical autism"—presentations that do not meet the criteria for autistic disorder because of late age at onset, atypical symptomatology, or subthreshold symptomatology, or all of these.

From American Psychiatric Association. *Diagnostic and Statistical Manual of Mental Disorders.* 4th ed. Text rev. Washington, DC: American Psychiatric Association; copyright 2000, with permission.

variable courses and prognoses for patients who have received diagnoses of Asperger's disorder. The factors associated with a good prognosis are a normal IQ and high-level social skills. Anecdotal reports of some adults diagnosed with Asperger's disorder as children show them to be verbal and intelligent; however, they relate in an awkward way to other adults, appear socially uncomfortable and shy, and often have illogical thinking.

Treatment

Treatment depends on the patient's level of adaptive functioning. Some of the same techniques used for autistic disorder are likely to benefit Asperger's disorder patients with severe social impairment.

PERVASIVE DEVELOPMENTAL DISORDER NOT OTHERWISE SPECIFIED

DSM-IV-TR defines pervasive disorder not otherwise specified as severe, pervasive impairment in social interaction or communication skills or the presence of stereotyped behavior, interests, and activities; however, the criteria for a specific pervasive developmental disorder, schizophrenia, and schizotypal and avoidant personality disorders are not met (Table 38–6). Some children who receive the diagnosis exhibit a markedly restricted repertoire of activities and interest. The condition usually shows a better outcome than autistic disorder.

Leslie was the oldest of two children. She had been a difficult baby who was not easy to console but whose motor and communicative development seemed appropriate. She was socially related and sometimes enjoyed interaction but was easily overstimulated. She exhibited some hand flapping. Her parents sought evaluation when she was 4 years of age because of difficulties in nursery school. Leslie had problems with peer interaction. She was often preoccupied with possible adverse events. At evaluation, she displayed

approaching adulthood, schizoid personality disorder. According to DSM-IV-TR, the most obvious distinctions between Asperger's disorder and autistic disorder are the criteria for language delay and dysfunction. The lack of language delay is a requirement for Asperger's disorder, whereas language impairment is a core feature in autistic disorder. Recent studies comparing children with Asperger's disorder and autistic disorder find that those children with Asperger's disorder were more likely to look for social interaction and sought more vigorously to make friends. More efforts seem to be made on the part of those with Asperger's disorder to engage in an activity with another child. Although significant general delay in language is an exclusionary criterion in the diagnosis of Asperger's disorder, some delay in the acquisition of language has been seen in more than one-third of clinical samples.

Course and Prognosis

Although little is known about the cohort described by the DSM-IV-TR diagnostic criteria, past case reports have shown both communicative and cognitive functions within the normal range. Although differential social relatedness was present, Leslie had difficulty using her parents as sources of support and comfort. She displayed behavioral rigidity and a tendency to impose routines on social skills. Subsequently, she was placed in a transitional kindergarten and did well academically, although problems in peer interactions and unusual affective responses persisted. As an adolescent, she describes herself as a "loner" who has difficulties with social interaction and tends to enjoy solitary activities. (Reprinted with permission from Volkmar F. Autism and the pervasive developmental disorders.

In: Lewis M, ed. *Child and Adolescent Psychiatry: A Comprehensive Approach*. 2nd ed. Baltimore: Williams & Wilkins; 1996.)

Treatment

The treatment approach is basically the same as in autistic disorder. Mainstreaming in school may be possible. Compared with autistic children, those with pervasive developmental disorder not otherwise specified generally have better language skills and more self-awareness, so they are better candidates for psychotherapy.

39 ▲

Attention-Deficit Disorders

ATTENTION-DEFICIT/HYPERACTIVITY DISORDER

Attention-deficit/hyperactivity disorder (ADHD) consists of a persistent pattern of inattention and/or hyperactive and impulsive behavior that is more severe than expected of children at a similar age and level of development. In order to meet the criteria for the diagnosis of ADHD, some symptoms must be present before the age of 7 years, although many children are not diagnosed until they are older than 7 years, when their behaviors cause problems in school and in other places. The impairment from inattention and/or hyperactivity-impulsivity must be present in at least two settings and interfere with developmentally appropriate functioning socially, academically, and in extracurricular activities. The disorder must not take place in the course of a pervasive developmental disorder, schizophrenia, or other psychotic disorder and must not be better accounted for by another mental disorder.

Epidemiology

Reports on the incidence of ADHD in the United States have varied from 2 to 20 percent of grade-school children. A conservative figure is approximately 3 to 7 percent of prepubertal elementary school children. The parents of children with ADHD show an increased incidence of hyperkinesis, sociopathy, alcohol use disorders, and conversion disorder. Symptoms of ADHD are often present by age 3 years, but the diagnosis is generally not made until the child is attending a structured school setting, such as preschool or kindergarten, when teacher information is available comparing the attention and impulsivity of the child in question with peers of the same age.

Etiology

The causes of ADHD are unknown. The suggested contributory factors for ADHD include prenatal toxic exposures, prematurity, and prenatal mechanical insult to the fetal nervous system.

Genetic Factors.   Evidence for a genetic basis for ADHD includes the greater concordance in monozygotic than in dizygotic twins. Also, siblings of hyperactive children have approximately twice the risk of having the disorder as does the general population. One sibling may predominantly have hyperactivity symptoms, and others may predominantly have inattention symptoms. Biological parents of children with the disorder have a higher risk for ADHD than do adoptive parents.

Brain Damage.   It has been speculated that some children affected by ADHD suffered subtle damage to the central nervous system (CNS) and brain development during their fetal and perinatal periods. The hypothesized brain damage may potentially be associated with circulatory, toxic, metabolic, mechanical, or physical insult to the brain during early infancy caused by infection, inflammation, and trauma. Nonfocal (soft) neurological signs are found at higher rates among children with ADHD than in the general population.

Neurochemical Factors.   The most widely studied drugs in the treatment of ADHD, the stimulants, affect both dopamine and norepinephrine, leading to neurotransmitter hypotheses that include possible dysfunction in both the adrenergic and the dopaminergic systems. Overall, no clear-cut evidence implicates a single neurotransmitter in the development ADHD, but many neurotransmitters may be involved in the process.

Neurophysiological Factors.   A physiological correlate is the presence of a variety of nonspecific abnormal electroencephalogram (EEG) patterns that are disorganized compared to normal controls.

Studies using positron emission tomography (PET) have found decreased cerebral blood flow and metabolic rates in the frontal lobe areas of children with ADHD compared with controls. PET scans have also shown that adolescent females with the disorder have globally reduced glucose metabolism compared both with normal control females and males and with males with the disorder. One theory explains these findings by supposing that the frontal lobes in children with ADHD are not adequately performing their inhibitory mechanism on lower structures, an effect leading to disinhibition.

Psychosocial Factors.   Stressful psychic events, a disruption of family equilibrium, and other anxiety-inducing factors contribute to the initiation or perpetuation of ADHD. Predisposing factors may include the child's temperament, genetic-familial factors, and the demands of society to adhere to a routinized way of behaving and performing.

Diagnosis

The principal signs of hyperactivity and impulsivity are based on detailed prenatal history of a child's early developmental patterns along with direct observation of a child, especially in situations that require attention. The diagnosis of ADHD requires persistent and impairing symptoms of either hyperactivity/impulsivity or

**Table 39–1
DSM-IV-TR Diagnostic Criteria for
Attention-Deficit/Hyperactivity Disorder**

A. Either (1) or (2):
  (1) six (or more) of the following symptoms of **inattention** have persisted for at least 6 months to a degree that is maladaptive and inconsistent with developmental level:
  Inattention
  (a) often fails to give close attention to details or makes careless mistakes in schoolwork, work, or other activities
  (b) often has difficulty sustaining attention in tasks or play activities
  (c) often does not seem to listen when spoken to directly
  (d) often does not follow through on instructions and fails to finish schoolwork, chores, or duties in the workplace (not due to oppositional behavior or failure to understand instructions)
  (e) often has difficulty organizing tasks and activities
  (f) often avoids, dislikes, or is reluctant to engage in tasks that require sustained mental effort (such as schoolwork or homework)
  (g) often loses things necessary for tasks or activities (e.g., toys, school assignments, pencils, books, or tools)
  (h) is often easily distracted by extraneous stimuli
  (i) is often forgetful in daily activities
  (2) six (or more) of the following symptoms of **hyperactivity-impulsivity** have persisted for at least 6 months to a degree that is maladaptive and inconsistent with developmental level:
  Hyperactivity
  (a) often fidgets with hands or feet or squirms in seat
  (b) often leaves seat in classroom or in other situations in which remaining seated is expected
  (c) often runs about or climbs excessively in situations in which it is inappropriate (in adolescents or adults, may be limited to subjective feelings of restlessness)
  (d) often has difficulty playing or engaging in leisure activities quietly
  (e) is often "on the go" or often acts as if "driven by a motor"
  (f) often talks excessively
  Impulsivity
  (g) often blurts out answers before questions have been completed
  (h) often has difficulty awaiting turn
  (i) often interrupts or intrudes on others (e.g., butts into conversations or games)
B. Some hyperactive-impulsive or inattentive symptoms that caused impairment were present before age 7 years.
C. Some impairment from the symptoms is present in two or more settings (e.g., at school [or work] and at home).
D. There must be clear evidence of clinically significant impairment in social, academic, or occupational functioning.
E. The symptoms do not occur exclusively during the course of a pervasive developmental disorder, schizophrenia, or other psychotic disorder and are not better accounted for by another mental disorder (e.g., mood disorder, anxiety disorder, dissociative disorder, or a personality disorder).
Code based on type:
  Attention-deficit/hyperactivity disorder, combined type: if both Criteria A1 and A2 are met for the past 6 months
  Attention-deficit/hyperactivity disorder, predominantly inattentive type: if Criterion A1 is met but Criterion A2 is not met for the past 6 months
  Attention-deficit/hyperactivity disorder, predominantly hyperactive-impulsive type: if Criterion A2 is met but Criterion A1 is not met for the past 6 months
  Coding note: For individuals (especially adolescents and adults) who currently have symptoms that no longer meet full criteria, "in partial remission" should be specified.

From American Psychiatric Association. *Diagnostic and Statistical Manual of Mental Disorders.* 4th ed. Text rev. Washington, DC: American Psychiatric Association; copyright 2000, with permission.

inattention that cause impairment in at least two different settings. The diagnostic criteria for ADHD are outlined in Table 39–1.

Other distinguishing features of ADHD are short attention span and easy distractibility. They act impulsively, show emotional lability, and are explosive and irritable.

Children who have hyperactivity as a predominant feature are more likely to be referred for treatment than are children with primarily symptoms of attention deficit. Children with the predominantly hyperactive-impulsive type are more likely to have a stable diagnosis over time and are more likely to have concurrent conduct disorder than are children with the predominantly inattentive type without hyperactivity. Disorders involving reading, arithmetic, language, and coordination may occur in association with ADHD. A child's history may give clues to prenatal (including genetic), natal, and postnatal factors that may have affected the CNS structure or function. Rates of development, deviations in development, and parental reactions to significant or stressful behavioral transitions should be ascertained, as they may help clinicians determine the degree to which parents have contributed to or reacted to a child's inefficiencies and dysfunctions.

School history and teachers' reports are important in evaluating whether a child's difficulties in learning and school behavior are primarily due to the child's attitudinal or maturational problems or to poor self-image because of felt inadequacies.

Clinicians should obtain an EEG to recognize the child with frequent bilaterally synchronous discharges resulting in short absence spells. Such a child may react in school with hyperactivity out of sheer frustration.

Clinical Features

The characteristics of children with the disorder that are most often cited are, in order of frequency, hyperactivity, perceptual motor impairment, emotional lability, general coordination deficit, attention deficit (short attention span, distractibility, perseveration, failure to finish tasks, inattention, poor concentration), impulsivity (action before thought, abrupt shifts in activity, lack of organization, jumping up in class), memory and thinking deficits, specific learning disabilities, speech and hearing deficits, and equivocal neurological signs and EEG irregularities.

School difficulties, both learning and behavioral, are common problems that often coexist with ADHD; they sometimes come from concomitant communication disorders or learning disorders or from the child's distractibility and fluctuating attention, which hampers the acquisition, retention, and display of knowledge. These difficulties are noted especially on group tests.

Sean was a 5-year-old boy who was referred for evaluation when his kindergarten teacher found that he was unable to stay on any tasks, and he would run around the room disrupting the other children. Sean was also oppositional with the teacher and unable to sit in his seat, although he was good-natured and rarely had a physical altercation with a peer. Sean was an athletic and active child who appeared to be below most of his classmates in his ability to recognize letters, numbers, and shapes. Although his teacher felt that Sean was rejected by his peers occasionally due to his impulsive nature, Sean felt that nobody liked him. At home, Sean was much more active than his two sisters, and his siblings often gave in to him in order to be left alone. He was the middle child with one sister 2 years older and the other sister 1 year younger.

Sean's mother reported that in the third month of her pregnancy with Sean, she had had some bleeding, but otherwise there were no complications. Sean was a full-term baby who seemed robust and went home from the hospital without problems. He was healthy throughout the neonatal period but had been a poor sleeper, never sleeping more than 4 hours without waking. He was usually awake between 5 and 6 o'clock in the morning, and he was just not tired. In preschool, Sean was reported to be one of the most active and impulsive children, but his teacher had taken a liking to him, and she gave him a lot of one-to-one attention to keep him under control. In spite of the extra attention, Sean seemed to be a little slower than his classmates in learning new words and his overall use of language. On intellectual testing, Sean had a full-scale intelligence quotient (IQ) of 105 with slightly higher performance than verbal score. Sean was referred for a psychiatric evaluation with a child psychiatrist who made the text revision of the fourth edition of the *Diagnostic and Statistical Manual of Mental Disorders* (DSM-IV-TR) diagnoses of ADHD, combined type; oppositional-defiant disorder; and reading disorder. It was also noted that Sean seemed to be "down on himself" and felt socially rejected. The initial treatment plan for Sean included a trial of methylphenidate (Concerta), 18 mg per day, and a therapeutic social skills group, along with a parent-training component for his parents. On medication, Sean's teacher reported significant improvement in remaining on-task and a diminished activity level.

Over time, Sean sustained his good response to the Concerta with minimal side effects that included a decreased appetite at lunchtime, but increased hunger in the evening. He was able to benefit from the practice that he had during his social skills group, and within 2 months, he was able to make a friend from school who came to his house to play. Finally, Sean's family gained competence in managing his oppositional behaviors and impulsivity by instituting a reward system for listening to them. Sean was able to follow his teacher's instructions and mastered the expected kindergarten curriculum and was recommended for a regular education class for the first grade.

Pathology and Laboratory Examination

No specific laboratory measures are pathognomonic of ADHD. Several laboratory measures often yield nonspecific abnormal results in hyperactive children, such as a disorganized, immature result on an EEG, and PET may show decreased cerebral blood flow in the frontal regions. Cognitive testing helping to confirm a child's inattention and impulsivity includes the continuous performance task, in which a child is asked to press a button each time a particular sequence of letters or numbers is flashed on a screen.

Differential Diagnosis

A temperamental constellation consisting of high activity level and short attention span, but in the normal range of expectation for a child's age, should be first considered. Differentiating these temperamental characteristics from the cardinal symptoms of ADHD before the age of 3 years is difficult, mainly because of the overlapping features of a normally immature nervous system and the emerging signs of visual-motor-perceptual impairments frequently seen in ADHD. Anxiety in a child needs to be evaluated. Anxiety may accompany ADHD as a secondary feature, and anxiety alone may be manifested by overactivity and easy distractibility.

Many children with ADHD have secondary depression in reaction to their continuing frustration over their failure to learn and their consequent low self-esteem. This condition must be distinguished from a primary depressive disorder, which is likely to be distinguished by hypoactivity and withdrawal. Mania and ADHD share many core features, such as excessive verbalization, motoric hyperactivity, and high levels of distractibility. Additionally, in children with mania, irritability seems to be more common than is euphoria. Although mania and ADHD can coexist, in children with bipolar I disorder, there is more waxing and waning of symptoms than in ADHD. ADHD in children with developed bipolar I disorder at a 4-year follow-up had a greater co-occurrence of additional disorders and a greater family history of bipolar disorders and other mood disorders than did children without bipolar disorder.

Frequently, conduct disorder and ADHD coexist, and both must be diagnosed. Learning disorders of various kinds must also be distinguished from ADHD; a child may be unable to read or to do mathematics because of a learning disorder, rather than because of inattention. ADHD often coexists with one or more learning disorders, including reading disorder, mathematics disorder, and disorder of written expression.

Course and Prognosis

The course of ADHD is variable. Symptoms may persist into adolescence or adult life; they may remit at puberty; or the hyperactivity may disappear, but the decreased attention span and impulse-control problems may persist. Overactivity is usually the first symptom to remit, and distractibility is the last. Most patients with the disorder, however, undergo partial remission and are vulnerable to antisocial behavior, substance use disorders, and mood disorders. Learning problems often continue throughout life.

Treatment

Pharmacotherapy.   Pharmacological agents shown to have significant efficacy and excellent safety records in the treatment of ADHD are the CNS stimulants, including short- and sustained-release preparations of methylphenidate, (Ritalin, Ritalin-SR, Concerta, Metadate CD, Metadate ER), dextroamphetamine (Dexedrine, Dexedrine spansules), and dextroamphetamine and amphetamine salt combinations (Adderall, Adderall XR). One additional form of methylphenidate containing only the D-enantiomer, dexmethylphenidate (Foculin), was recently placed on the market, aimed at maximizing the target effects and minimizing the side effects in individuals with ADHD who obtain partial response from methylphenidate. Second-line agents with evidence of efficacy for some children and adolescents with ADHD include antidepressants such as bupropion (Wellbutrin, Wellbutrin SR), venlafaxine (Effexor, Effexor XR), and the α-adrenergic receptor agonists clonidine (Catapres) and guanfacine (Tenex).

A novel agent, atomoxetine (Strattera), was approved in 2003 as a nonstimulant medication for the treatment of ADHD. Atomoxetine is a norepinephrine reuptake inhibitor and does not affect dopamine. It inhibits the 2D6 enzyme and may decrease the metabolism of selective serotonin reuptake inhibitors (SSRIs) as a result. The general dosage for atomoxapine is from 40 to 100 mg per day given in a single undivided dose.

Monitoring Stimulant Treatment

At baseline, in accordance with the most recent American Academy of Child and Adolescent Psychiatry (AACAP) practice parameters, before starting stimulant medications, the following work-up is recommended:

▶ Physical examination
▶ Blood pressure
▶ Pulse
▶ Weight
▶ Height

It is recommended that children and adolescents being treated with stimulants have their height, weight, blood pressure, and pulse checked on a quarterly basis, and physical examination annually.

Evaluation of Therapeutic Progress. Monitoring starts with the initiation of medication. In most patients, stimulants reduce overactivity, distractibility, impulsiveness, explosiveness, and irritability. No evidence indicates that medications directly improve any existing impairments in learning, although, when the attention deficits diminish, children can learn more effectively than in the past. In addition, medication can improve self-esteem when children are no longer constantly reprimanded for their behavior.

Psychosocial Interventions. Medication alone is often not enough to satisfy the comprehensive therapeutic needs of children with the disorder and is usually but one facet of a mul-

Table 39–2
DSM-IV-TR Diagnostic Criteria for Attention-Deficit/Hyperactivity Disorder Not Otherwise Specified

This category is for disorders with prominent symptoms of inattention or hyperactivity-impulsivity that do not meet criteria for attention-deficit/hyperactivity disorder. Examples include

1. Individuals whose symptoms and impairment meet the criteria for attention-deficit/hyperactivity disorder, predominantly inattentive type but whose age at onset is 7 years or after
2. Individuals with clinically significant impairment who present with inattention and whose symptom pattern does not meet the full criteria for the disorder but have a behavioral pattern marked by sluggishness, daydreaming, and hypoactivity

From American Psychiatric Association. *Diagnostic and Statistical Manual of Mental Disorders.* 4th ed. Text rev. Washington, DC: American Psychiatric Association; copyright 2000, with permission.

timodality regimen. Social skills groups, parent-training for parents of children with ADHD, and behavioral interventions at school and at home can often be efficacious in the overall management of children with ADHD. Evaluation and treatment of coexisting learning disorders or additional psychiatric disorders are important.

ATTENTION-DEFICIT/HYPERACTIVITY DISORDER NOT OTHERWISE SPECIFIED

DSM-IV-TR includes ADHD not otherwise specified as a residual category for disturbances with prominent symptoms of inattention or hyperactivity that do not meet the criteria for ADHD (Table 39–2).

The treatment of the disorder involves the use of amphetamines (5 to 60 mg a day) or methylphenidate (5 to 60 mg a day). Signs of a positive response are an increased attention span, decreased impulsiveness, and improved mood. Psychopharmacological therapy may need to be continued indefinitely. Because of the abuse potential of the drugs, clinicians should monitor drug response and patient compliance.

OPPOSITIONAL DEFIANT DISORDER

In oppositional defiant disorder, a child's temper outbursts, active refusal to comply with rules, and annoying behaviors exceed the expectations for these behaviors compared with others of the same age. The disorder is an enduring pattern of negativistic, hostile, and defiant behaviors in the absence of serious violations of social norms or of the rights of others.

Epidemiology

Oppositional, negativistic behavior, in moderation, is developmentally normal in early childhood. Epidemiological studies of negativistic traits in nonclinical populations found such behavior in between 16 and 22 percent of school-age children. Although oppositional defiant disorder can begin as early as 3 years of age, it typically is noted by 8 years of age and usually not later than adolescence. Oppositional defiant disorder has been reported to occur at rates ranging from 2 to 16 percent. The disorder is more prevalent in boys than in girls before puberty, and the sex ratio appears to be equal after puberty. There are no distinct family patterns, but almost all parents of children with the disorder are themselves overly concerned with issues of power, control, and autonomy.

Etiology

The ability of a child to communicate his or her own will and opposing others' wills is crucial to normal development as a route toward establishing autonomy, forming an identity, and setting inner standards and controls. Pathology begins when this developmental phase persists abnormally, authority figures overreact, or oppositional behavior recurs considerably more frequently than in most children of the same mental age.

Classic psychoanalytic theory implicates unresolved conflicts that are being expressed with all authority figures. Behaviorists have suggested that oppositionalism is a reinforced, learned behavior through which a child exerts control over authority figures; for example, by having a temper tantrum when an undesired act is requested, a child coerces the parents to withdraw their request. In addition, increased parental attention—for example, long discussions about the behavior—many reinforce the behavior.

Diagnosis and Clinical Features

Children with oppositional defiant disorder often argue with adults, lose their temper, and are angry, resentful, and easily annoyed by others. They frequently actively defy adults' requests or rules and deliberately annoy other people. They tend to blame others for their own mistakes and misbehavior. Typically, symptoms of the disorder are most evident in interactions with adults or peers whom the child knows well. Thus, the child with the disorder is likely to show little or no sign of the disorder when examined clinically. The text revision of the fourth edition of the *Diagnostic and Statistical Manual of Mental Disorders* (DSM-IV-TR) diagnostic criteria for oppositional defiant disorder are given in Table 40–1.

Robert, age 7, presented to the consultation-liaison team. He suffered from leukemia and was extremely difficult to manage. He would refuse all necessary blood work and repeatedly ran away from the clinic when asked to cooperate with requests for X-rays, blood tests, and so forth. He was sullen, argumentative, and irritable. The behavior was unchanged when his mother was used as a "filter" for the demands. He was a chronically cranky child, although his illness was in remission and he was mostly medication free at the time of consultation. His care was severely compromised. At home, his behavior was very similar and had been so for several months. He argued continuously with his single mother about any kind of request, such as cleaning up his room. Prior to his difficulties at the hospital, he began to exhibit similar problems at school. He was suspended for 1 week for being verbally abusive and out of control with his teacher. His mother had been diagnosed with acquired immune deficiency syndrome (AIDS) 2 years ago, having become infected by her drug-abusing husband who had died about 3 years ago from the effects of AIDS. She seemed dysphoric, passive, and extremely permissive with the child. She had no additional help because her own mother was also gravely ill, and she had no current social support network. Robert would often scream at his mother at the top of his voice without her evincing any reaction or making any attempt to contain him. Testing showed him to have normal intelligence, without symptoms of attention-deficit/hyperactivity disorder (ADHD) or learning disabilities. He knew of his father's death and his mother's illness. His mood remained dysphoric for many weeks when discussing this. He had never exhibited other reactions to being told about the illnesses of his parents. His mother described his early development as unremarkable except for his tendencies to have irregular sleep and eating patterns and his propensity to be cranky. His mother had intermittently taken drugs while pregnant with him, her only child. (Courtesy of Hans Steiner, M.D.)

Table 40–1
DSM-IV-TR Diagnostic Criteria for Oppositional Defiant Disorder

A. A pattern of negativistic, hostile, and defiant behavior lasting at least 6 months, during which four (or more) of the following are present:

(1) often loses temper

(2) often argues with adults

(3) often actively defies or refuses to comply with adults' requests or rules

(4) often deliberately annoys people

(5) often blames others for his or her mistakes or misbehavior

(6) is often touchy or easily annoyed by others

(7) is often angry and resentful

(8) is often spiteful or vindictive

Note: Consider a criterion met only if the behavior occurs more frequently than is typically observed in individuals of comparable age and developmental level.

B. The disturbance in behavior causes clinically significant impairment in social, academic, or occupational functioning.

C. The behaviors do not occur exclusively during the course of a psychotic or mood disorder.

D. Criteria are not met for conduct disorder, and, if the individual is age 18 years or older, criteria are not met for antisocial personality disorder.

From American Psychiatric Association. *Diagnostic and Statistical Manual of Mental Disorders.* 4th ed. Text rev. Washington, DC: American Psychiatric Association; copyright 2000, with permission.

Differential Diagnosis

Because oppositional behavior is both normal and adaptive at specific developmental stages, these periods of negativism must be distinguished from oppositional defiant disorder. Developmental-stage oppositional behavior, which is of shorter duration than oppositional defiant disorder, is not considerably more frequent or more intense than that seen in other children of the same mental age.

Oppositional defiant behavior occurring temporarily in reaction to a stress should be diagnosed as an adjustment disorder. When features of oppositional defiant disorder appear during the course of conduct disorder, schizophrenia, or a mood disorder, the diagnosis of oppositional defiant disorder should not be made. Oppositional and negativistic behaviors may also be present in ADHD, cognitive disorders, and mental retardation.

The subtype of oppositional defiant disorder that tends to progress to conduct disorder is one in which aggression is prominent. Overall, the current consensus indicates that there may be two subtypes of oppositional defiant disorder. One type is likely to progress to conduct disorder and includes certain symptoms of conduct disorder (for example, fighting, bullying). The other type is characterized by less aggression and less antisocial traits and does not progress to conduct disorder.

Course and Prognosis

The course of oppositional defiant disorder depends largely on the severity of the symptoms and the ability of the child to develop more adaptive responses to authority. The stability of oppositional defiant disorder over time is variable. Persistence of oppositional defiant symptoms poses an increased risk of additional disorders such as conduct disorder and substance use disorders. Positive outcomes are more likely for intact families who are able to modify their own expression of demands and give less attention to the child's argumentative behaviors.

The prognosis for oppositional defiant disorder in a child depends somewhat on the degree of functioning in the family and on the development of comorbid psychopathology.

Treatment

The primary treatment of oppositional defiant disorder is family intervention utilizing both direct training of the parents in child management skills, as well as a careful assessment of family interactions. Behavior therapists emphasize teaching parents how to alter their behavior to discourage the child's oppositional behavior and to encourage appropriate behavior. Behavior therapy focuses on selectively reinforcing and praising appropriate behavior and ignoring or not reinforcing undesired behavior.

Children with oppositional defiant behavior may also benefit from individual psychotherapy insofar as the child is exposed to a situation with an adult in which to "practice" more adaptive responses. In the therapeutic relationship, the child can learn new strategies to develop a sense of mastery and success in social situations with peers and families. In the safety of a more "neutral" relationship, a child may discover that he or she is capable of less provocative behaviors.

CONDUCT DISORDER

Conduct disorder is an enduring set of behaviors that evolves over time; it is characterized most often by aggression and violations of the rights of others. Conduct disorder is associated with many other psychiatric disorders, including ADHD, depression, and learning disorders, and it is also associated with several psychosocial factors such as low socioeconomic level; harsh, punitive parenting; family discord; lack of appropriate parental supervision; and lack of social competence. The DSM-IV-TR criteria state that three specific behaviors are required of the 15 listed behaviors, which include bullying, threatening, or intimidating others and staying out at night despite parental prohibitions, beginning before 13 years of age. DSM-IV-TR also specifies that truancy from school must begin before 13 years of age to be considered a symptom of conduct disorder. The disorder can be diagnosed in a person older than 18 years only if the criteria for antisocial personality disorder are not met.

Epidemiology

Conduct disturbance is common during childhood and adolescence. Estimated rates of conduct disorder among the general population range from 1 to 10 percent. The disorder is more common among boys than among girls, and the ratio ranges from 4 to 1 to as much as 12 to 1. Conduct disorder is more common in the children of parents with antisocial personality disorder and alcohol dependence than it is in the general population. The prevalence of conduct disorder and antisocial behavior is significantly related to socioeconomic factors.

Etiology

No single factor can account for a child's antisocial behavior and conduct disorder. Rather, many biopsychosocial factors contribute to the development of the disorder.

Parental Factors. Harsh, punitive parenting characterized by severe physical and verbal aggression is associated with the development of children's maladaptive aggressive behaviors. Chaotic home conditions are associated with conduct disorder and delinquency. Divorce itself is considered a risk factor, but the persistence of hostility, resentment, and bitterness between divorced parents may be the more important contributor to maladaptive behavior in children.

Sociocultural Factors. Socioeconomically deprived children are at higher risk for the development of conduct disorder, as are children and adolescents who grow up in urban environments. Unemployment among parents, lack of supportive social network, and lack of positive participation in community activities seem to predict conduct disorder.

Psychological Factors. Children brought up in chaotic, negligent conditions often express poor emotional modulation of emotions, including anger, frustration, and sadness. Poor modeling of impulse control and the chronic lack of having their own needs met leads to a less well developed sense of empathy.

Neurobiological Factors. ADHD may coexist with conduct disorder. In some children with conduct disorder, there may be decreased noradrenergic functioning. Evidence indicates that blood 5-HT levels correlate negatively with levels of the 5-HT metabolite 5-hydroxyindoleacetic acid (5-HIAA) in the cerebrospinal fluid (CSF) and that low CSF 5-HIAA correlates with aggression and violence.

Child Abuse and Maltreatment. Children chronically exposed to violence, especially those who endure physically abusive treatment, often behave aggressively. Such children may have difficulty in verbalizing their feelings, and this difficulty increases their tendency to express themselves physically. In addition, severely abused children and adolescents tend to be hypervigilant; in some cases, they misperceive benign situations and respond with violence. Not all physical behavior is synonymous with conduct disorder, but children with a pattern of hypervigilance and violent responses are likely to violate the rights of others.

Other Factors. ADHD, central nervous system (CNS) dysfunction or damage, and early extremes of temperament can predispose a child to conduct disorder. Propensity to violence correlates with CNS dysfunction and signs of severe psychopathology, such as delusional tendencies.

Diagnosis and Clinical Features

The DSM-IV-TR diagnostic criteria for conduct disorder are given in Table 40–2.

Table 40–2
DSM-IV-TR Diagnostic Criteria for Conduct Disorder

A. A repetitive and persistent pattern of behavior in which the basic rights of others or major age-appropriate societal norms or rules are violated, as manifested by the presence of three (or more) of the following criteria in the past 12 months, with at least one criterion present in the past 6 months:

Aggression to people and animals
  (1) often bullies, threatens, or intimidates others
  (2) often initiates physical fights
  (3) has used a weapon that can cause serious physical harm to others (e.g., a bat, brick, broken bottle, knife, gun)
  (4) has been physically cruel to people
  (5) has been physically cruel to animals
  (6) has stolen while confronting a victim (e.g., mugging, purse snatching, extortion, armed robbery)
  (7) has forced someone into sexual activity

Destruction of property
  (8) has deliberately engaged in fire setting with the intention of causing serious damage
  (9) has deliberately destroyed others' property (other than by fire setting)

Deceitfulness or theft
  (10) has broken into someone else's house, building, or car
  (11) often lies to obtain goods or favors or to avoid obligations (i.e., "cons" others)
  (12) has stolen items of nontrivial value without confronting a victim (e.g., shoplifting, but without breaking and entering; forgery)

Serious violations of rules
  (13) often stays out at night despite parental prohibitions, beginning before age 13 years
  (14) has run away from home overnight at least twice while living in parental or parental surrogate home (or once without returning for a lengthy period)
  (15) is often truant from school, beginning before age 13 years

B. The disturbance in behavior causes clinically significant impairment in social, academic, or occupational functioning.

C. If the individual is age 18 years or older, criteria are not met for antisocial personality disorder.

Code based on age at onset:

  Conduct disorder, childhood-onset type: onset of at least one criterion characteristic of conduct disorder prior to age 10 years

  Conduct disorder, adolescent-onset type: absence of any criteria characteristic of conduct disorder prior to age 10 years

  Conduct disorder, unspecified onset: age at onset is not known

Specify severity:

  Mild: few if any conduct problems in excess of those required to make the diagnosis **and** conduct problems cause only minor harm to others

  Moderate: number of conduct problems and effect on others intermediate between "mild" and "severe"

  Severe: many conduct problems in excess of those required to make the diagnosis **or** conduct problems cause considerable harm to others

The average age of onset of conduct disorder is younger in boys than in girls. Boys most commonly meet the diagnostic criteria by 10 to 12 years of age, whereas girls often reach 14 to 16 years of age before the criteria are met.

Children who meet the criteria for conduct disorder express their overt aggressive behavior in various forms. Aggressive antisocial behavior may take the form of bullying, physical aggression, and cruel behavior toward peers. Children may be hostile, verbally abusive, impudent, defiant, and negativistic toward adults. Persistent lying, frequent truancy, and vandalism are common. In severe cases, destructiveness, stealing, and physical violence are often present. Children usually make little attempt to conceal their antisocial behavior. Sexual behavior and the regular use of tobacco, liquor, or nonprescribed psychoactive substances begin unusually early for such children and adolescents. Suicidal thoughts, gestures, and acts are frequent.

Differential Diagnosis

Disturbances of conduct may be part of many childhood psychiatric conditions, ranging from mood disorders to psychotic disorders to learning disorders. Therefore, clinicians must obtain a history of the chronology of the symptoms to determine whether the conduct disturbance is a transient or reactive phenomenon or an enduring pattern. Isolated acts of antisocial behavior do not justify a diagnosis of conduct disorder; an enduring pattern must be present. The relation of conduct disorder to oppositional defiant disorder is still under debate. The main distinguishing clinical feature of the two disorders is that, in conduct disorder, the basic rights of others are violated, whereas, in oppositional defiant disorder, hostility and negativism fall short of seriously violating the rights of others.

Mood disorders are often present in children who have some degree of irritability and aggressive behavior. Both major depressive disorder and bipolar disorders must be ruled out, but the full syndrome of conduct disorder may occur and be diagnosed during the onset of a mood disorder. There is a substantial comorbidity of conduct disorder and depressive disorders. A recent report concludes that the high correlation between the two disorders arises from shared risk factors for both disorders, rather than one disorder causing the other. Thus, a series of factors including family conflict, negative life events, early history of conduct disturbance, level of parental involvement, and affiliation with delinquent peers contribute to the development of affective disorders and conduct disorder. This is not the case with oppositional defiant disorder, which cannot be diagnosed if it occurs exclusively during a mood disorder.

ADHD and learning disorders are commonly associated with conduct disorder. Usually, the symptoms of these disorders predate the diagnosis of conduct disorder. Substance abuse disorders are also more common in adolescents with conduct disorder than in the general population. Obsessive-compulsive disorder (OCD) also frequently seems to coexist with disruptive behavior disorders. All the disorders described here should be noted when they co-occur. Children with ADHD often exhibit impulsive and aggressive behaviors that may not meet the full criteria for conduct disorder.

Course and Prognosis

In general, the prognosis for children with conduct disorder is most guarded in those who have symptoms at a young age, exhibit the greatest number of symptoms, and express them most frequently. This finding is true partly because those with severe conduct disorder seem to be most vulnerable to comorbid disorder later in life, such as mood disorders and substance-use disorders. It stands to reason that the more concurrent mental disorders a person has, the more troublesome life will be. A good prognosis is predicted for mild conduct disorder in the absence of coexisting psychopathology, and normal intellectual functioning.

Treatment

Treatment programs have been more successful at decreasing overt symptoms of conduct disorder, rather than the covert symptoms. Multimodality treatment programs that use all the available family and community resources are likely to bring about the best results in efforts to control conduct-disordered behavior. No treatment is considered curative for the entire spectrum of behaviors that contribute to conduct disorder, but a variety of treatments may be helpful in containing symptoms and promoting prosocial behavior.

An environmental structure that provides support, along with consistent rules and expected consequences, can help control a variety of problem behaviors. The structure can be applied to family life in some cases, so that parents become aware of behavioral techniques and grow proficient at using them to foster appropriate behaviors. School settings can also use behavioral techniques to promote socially acceptable behavior toward peers and to discourage covert antisocial incidents.

Individual psychotherapy oriented toward improving problem-solving skills can be useful, as children with conduct disorder may have a long-standing pattern of maladaptive responses to daily situations. The age at which treatment begins is important, because the longer the maladaptive behaviors continue, the more entrenched they become.

Medication can be a useful adjunctive treatment for symptoms that often contribute to conduct disorder. Overt explosive aggression responds to several medications. Antipsychotics, most notably haloperidol (Haldol), have been reported to help children to control aggressive and assaultive behaviors that may be present in various disorders. Currently, the newer antipsychotics such as risperidone (Risperdal) and olanzapine (Zyprexa) have replaced haloperidol, given the decreased incidence of extrapyramidal symptoms. Lithium (Eskalith) has been reported to have efficacy for some aggressive children with or without comorbid bipolar disorders. Some trials suggest that carbamazepine (Tegretol) may help control aggression, but a double-blind, placebo-controlled study did not show the superiority of carbamazepine over placebo in decreasing aggression. Clonidine (Catapres) may also decrease aggression. The selective serotonin reuptake inhibitors (SSRIs), such as fluoxetine (Prozac), have been used in an attempt to diminish impulsivity, irritability, and lability of mood, which often occur with conduct disorder. Conduct disorder frequently coexists with ADHD, learning disorders, and, over time, mood disorders and substance-related disorders; thus, the treatment of any concurrent disorders must also be addressed.

DISRUPTIVE BEHAVIOR DISORDER NOT OTHERWISE SPECIFIED

According to DSM-IV-TR, the category of disruptive behavior disorder not otherwise specified can be used for disorders of conduct or oppositional-defiant behaviors that do not meet the diagnostic criteria for either conduct disorder or oppositional defiant disorder but in which there is notable impairment (Table 40–3).

Table 40–3
DSM-IV-TR Diagnostic Criteria for Disruptive Behavior Disorder Not Otherwise Specified

This category is for disorders characterized by conduct or oppositional defiant behaviors that do not meet the criteria for conduct disorder or oppositional defiant disorder. For example, include clinical presentations that do not meet full criteria either for oppositional defiant disorder or conduct disorder, but in which there is clinically significant impairment.

From American Psychiatric Association. *Diagnostic and Statistical Manual of Mental Disorders.* 4th ed. Text rev. Washington, DC: American Psychiatric Association; copyright 2000, with permission.

41 △

Feeding and Eating Disorders of Infancy or Early Childhood

PICA

In the text revision of the fourth edition of *Diagnostic and Statistical Manual of Mental Disorders* (DSM-IV-TR), pica is described as the persistent eating of nonnutritive substances for at least 1 month. The behavior must be developmentally inappropriate, not culturally sanctioned, and sufficiently severe to merit clinical attention. Pica is diagnosed even when these symptoms occur in the context of another disorder such as autistic disorder, schizophrenia, or Kleine-Levin syndrome. Pica appears much more frequently in young children than in adults; it also occurs in people who are mentally retarded. Among adults, certain forms of pica, including geophagia (clay eating) and amylophagia (starch eating), have been reported to occur in pregnant women.

Epidemiology

The incidence of pica is rare among older children and adolescents. Pica is more common among children and adolescents with mental retardation. It has been reported in up to 15 percent of individuals with severe mental retardation. The presence of pica appears to affect both sexes equally.

Etiology

A higher-than-expected incidence of pica seems to occur in the relatives of people with the symptoms. Nutritional deficiencies have been postulated as causes of pica; in particular circumstances, cravings for nonedible substances have been produced by dietary insufficiencies. For example, cravings for dirt and ice are sometimes associated with iron and zinc deficiencies, which are eliminated by their administration. A high incidence of parental neglect and deprivation has also been associated with cases of pica. Theories relating children's psychological deprivation and subsequent ingestion of inedible substances have been suggested as compensatory mechanisms to satisfy oral needs.

Diagnosis and Clinical Features

Eating nonedible substances repeatedly after 18 months of age is usually considered abnormal. The onset of pica is usually between ages 12 and 24 months, and the incidence declines with age. The specific substances ingested vary with their accessibil-

ity, and they increase with a child's mastery of locomotion and the resultant increased independence and decreased parental supervision. Typically, young children ingest paint, plaster, string, hair, and cloth; older children have access to dirt, animal feces, stones, and paper. The clinical implications can be benign or life-threatening, according to the objects ingested. The DSM-IV-TR diagnostic criteria for pica are given in Table 41–1.

> George, a thin, pale, 5-year-old boy, was admitted to the hospital for a nutritional anemia that seemed to result from his ingestion of paint, plaster, dirt, wood, and paste. He had had numerous hospitalizations under similar circumstances, beginning at age 19 months, when he had ingested lighter fluid.
>
> George's parents subsisted on welfare and were described as immature. He was the product of an unplanned but normal pregnancy. His mother began eating dirt when she was pregnant, at age 16. His father periodically abused drugs and alcohol.
>
> #### DISCUSSION
> Eating of nonnutritive substances may be developmentally appropriate for an infant, but its persistence up to age 5 warrants a diagnosis of pica. As in this case, it is commonly associated with a similar history in the mother and low socioeconomic status.
>
> In some cultural settings, the eating of nonnutritive substances, such as clay, may be a sanctioned practice, in which case the diagnosis would not apply, but that certainly is not the case here. In other cases, the disturbance may be associated with other disorders, such as autistic disorder, schizophrenia, or the neurological disorder Kleine-Levin syndrome. (From *DSM-IV Casebook.*)

Pathology and Laboratory Examination

No single laboratory test confirms or rules out a diagnosis of pica, but several laboratory tests are useful because pica has frequently been associated with abnormal indexes. Serum levels of iron and zinc should always be obtained; in many cases of pica, these levels are low and may contribute to the development of pica. Pica may disappear when oral iron and zinc are administered. Patients' hemoglobin level should be obtained; if the

Table 41–1
DSM-IV-TR Diagnostic Criteria for Pica

A. Persistent eating of nonnutritive substances for a period of at least 1 month.

B. The eating of nonnutritive substances is inappropriate to the developmental level.

C. The eating behavior is not part of a culturally sanctioned practice.

D. If the eating behavior occurs exclusively during the course of another mental disorder (e.g., mental retardation, pervasive developmental disorder, schizophrenia), it is sufficiently severe to warrant independent clinical attention.

From American Psychiatric Association. *Diagnostic and Statistical Manual of Mental Disorders.* 4th ed. Text rev. Washington, DC: American Psychiatric Association; copyright 2000, with permission.

level is reduced, anemia can result. In children with pica, the serum lead level should be obtained when a physician is concerned about a child; lead poisoning can result from ingesting lead. When a child's lead level is increased, this condition must be treated.

Differential Diagnosis

The differential diagnosis of pica includes iron and zinc deficiencies. Pica also may occur in conjunction with failure to thrive and several other mental and medical disorders, including schizophrenia, autistic disorder, anorexia nervosa, and Kleine-Levin syndrome. In psychosocial dwarfism, a dramatic but reversible endocrinological and behavioral form of failure to thrive, children often show bizarre behaviors, including ingesting toilet water, garbage, and other nonnutritive substances. A recent case report presented an association of pica with hypersomnolence, lead intoxication, and precocious puberty. Precocious puberty implicates the hypothalamus as a site for at least a part of the dysfunction. Lead intoxication is known to be associated with pica as well as several other neuropsychiatric abnormalities in memory and cognitive performance. A small minority of children with autistic disorder and schizophrenia may have pica. In children who exhibit pica along with another medical disorder, both disorders should be coded, according to DSM-IV-TR.

Course and Prognosis

The prognosis for pica is variable, although in children of normal intelligence it most frequently remits spontaneously. In children, pica usually resolves with increasing age; in pregnant women, pica is usually limited to the term of the pregnancy. In some adults, however, especially those who are mentally retarded, pica may continue for years. Follow-up data on these populations are too limited to permit conclusions.

Treatment

The first step in the treatment of pica is to determine the cause whenever possible. When pica is associated with situations of neglect or maltreatment, these circumstances naturally need to

be altered. Exposure to toxic substances, such as lead, must also be eliminated. No definitive treatment exists for pica; most treatment is aimed at education and behavior modification. Treatments emphasize psychosocial, environmental, behavioral, and family guidance approaches. An effort should be made to ameliorate any significant psychosocial stressors.

Several behavioral techniques have been used with some effect. The most rapidly successful technique seems to be mild aversion therapy or negative reinforcement (for example, a mild electric shock, an unpleasant noise, or an emetic drug). Positive reinforcement, modeling, behavioral shaping, and overcorrection treatment have also been used. Increasing parental attention, stimulation, and emotional nurturance may have positive results.

RUMINATION DISORDER

In DSM-IV-TR, rumination disorder is described as an infant's or a child's repeated regurgitation and rechewing of food, after a period of normal functioning. The symptoms last for at least 1 month, are not caused by a medical condition, and are severe enough to merit clinical attention. The onset of the disorder generally occurs after 3 months of age; once the regurgitation occurs, the food may be swallowed or spit out.

The diagnosis of rumination disorder can be made regardless of whether an infant has attained a normal weight for his or her age. Failure to thrive, therefore, is not a necessary criterion of this disorder, but it is sometimes a sequela. According to DSM-IV-TR, the disorder must be present for at least 1 month after a period of normal functioning, and it is not associated with gastrointestinal (GI) illness or other general medical conditions.

Epidemiology

Rumination is a rare disorder. It seems to be more common among infants between 3 months and 1 year of age and among children and adults who are mentally retarded. Adults with rumination usually maintain a normal weight. The disorder may be more common in males. No reliable figures on predisposing factors or familial patterns are available.

Etiology

Several causes of rumination have been proposed. In those who are mentally retarded, the disorder may simply be self-stimulatory behavior. In those who are nonretarded, psychodynamic theories hypothesize various disturbances in the mother–child relationship. The mothers of infants with the disorder are usually immature, involved in a marital conflict, and unable to give much attention to the baby. These factors result in insufficient emotional gratification and stimulation for the infant, who seeks gratification from within. The rumination is interpreted as the infant's attempt to recreate the feeding process and to provide gratification that the mother does not provide.

Overstimulation and tension have also been suggested as causes of rumination. A dysfunctional autonomic nervous system may be implicated. As sophisticated and accurate investigative techniques are refined, a substantial number of children classified as ruminators are shown to have gastroesophageal reflux or hiatal hernia.

Table 41–2
DSM-IV-TR Diagnostic Criteria for
Rumination Disorder

A. Repeated regurgitation and rechewing of food for a period of at least 1 month following a period of normal functioning.

B. The behavior is not due to an associated gastrointestinal or other general medical condition (e.g., esophageal reflux).

C. The behavior does not occur exclusively during the course of anorexia nervosa or bulimia nervosa. If the symptoms occur exclusively during the course of mental retardation or a pervasive developmental disorder, they are sufficiently severe to warrant independent clinical attention.

From American Psychiatric Association. *Diagnostic and Statistical Manual of Mental Disorders.* 4th ed. Text rev. Washington, DC: American Psychiatric Association; copyright 2000, with permission.

Behaviorists attribute rumination to the positive reinforcement of pleasurable self-stimulation and to the attention the baby receives from others as a consequence of the disorder.

Diagnosis and Clinical Features

The DSM-IV-TR diagnostic criteria for rumination disorder are given in Table 41–2. DSM-IV-TR notes that the essential feature of the disorder is repeated regurgitation and rechewing of food for a period of at least 1 month after a period of normal functioning. Partially digested food is brought up into the mouth without nausea, retching, disgust, or associated GI disorder. This activity can be distinguished from vomiting by the clear, purposeful movements the infant makes to induce it. The food is then ejected from the mouth or reswallowed. A characteristic position of straining and arching of the back, with the head held back, is observed. The infant makes sucking movements with the tongue and gives the impression of gaining considerable satisfaction from the activity. A usually present associated feature is the infant's irritability and hunger between episodes of rumination.

Although spontaneous remissions are common, severe secondary complications may develop, such as progressive malnutrition, dehydration, and lowered resistance to disease. Failure to thrive, with absence of growth and developmental delays in all areas, may occur. An additional complication is that the mother or caretaker is often discouraged by the failure to feed the infant successfully and may become alienated, if she is not already so. Further alienation often occurs as the noxious odor of the regurgitated material leads to avoidance of the infant.

Pathology and Laboratory Examination

No specific laboratory examination is pathognomonic of rumination disorder. Clinicians must rule out physical causes of vomiting, such as pyloric stenosis and hiatal hernia, before making the diagnosis of rumination disorder. Rumination disorder can be associated with failure to thrive and varying degrees of starvation. Thus, laboratory measures of endocrinological function (thyroid function tests, dexamethasone-suppression test), serum electrolytes, and a hematological workup help determine the severity of the effects of rumination disorder.

Differential Diagnosis

To make the diagnosis of rumination disorder, clinicians must rule out GI congenital anomalies, infections, and other medical illnesses. Pyloric stenosis is usually associated with projectile vomiting and is generally evident before 3 months of age, when rumination has its onset. Rumination has been associated with various mental retardation syndromes in which other stereotypic behaviors and eating disturbances, such as pica, are present. Rumination disorder may occur in patients with other eating disorders, such as bulimia nervosa.

Course and Prognosis

Rumination disorder is believed to have a high rate of spontaneous remission. Indeed, many cases of rumination disorder may develop and remit without ever being diagnosed. Only limited data are available about the prognosis of rumination disorder in adults.

Treatment

The treatment of rumination disorder is often a combination of education and behavioral techniques. Sometimes an evaluation of the mother–child relationship reveals deficits that can be influenced by offering guidance to the mother. Behavioral interventions, such as squirting lemon juice into the infant's mouth whenever rumination occurs, can be effective in diminishing the behavior. This practice appears to be the most rapidly effective treatment; rumination is eliminated in 3 to 5 days. In the aversive-conditioning reports on rumination disorder, infants were doing well at 9- or 12-month follow-ups, with no recurrence of the rumination and with weight gains, increased activity levels, and increased responsiveness to people. Rumination may be decreased by the technique of withdrawing attention from the child whenever this behavior occurs. The effectiveness of treatments is difficult to evaluate. Most reported are single-case studies; patients are not randomly assigned to controlled studies.

Any concomitant medical complications must also be treated. Treatments include improvement of the child's psychosocial environment, increased tender loving care from the mother or caretakers, and psychotherapy for the mother or for both parents. When anatomical abnormalities such as hiatal hernia are present, surgical repair may be necessary. Medications including metoclopramide (Reglan), cimetidine (Tagamet), and antipsychotics, such as haloperidol (Haldol) and thioridazine (Mellaril), have been tried and reported to be successful in anecdotal reports. One study showed that, when infants were allowed to eat as much as they wanted, the rate of rumination decreased.

FEEDING DISORDER OF INFANCY OR EARLY CHILDHOOD

According to DSM-IV-TR, feeding disorder of infancy or early childhood is a persistent failure to eat adequately, reflected in significant failure to gain weight or in significant weight loss over 1 month. The symptoms are not better accounted for by a medical condition or by another mental disorder and are not

Table 41–3
DSM-IV-TR Diagnostic Criteria for Feeding Disorder of Infancy or Early Childhood

A. Feeding disturbance as manifested by persistent failure to eat adequately with significant failure to gain weight or significant loss of weight over at least 1 month.

B. The disturbance is not due to an associated gastrointestinal or other general medical condition (e.g., esophageal reflux).

C. The disturbance is not better accounted for by another mental disorder (e.g., rumination disorder) or by lack of available food.

D. The onset is before age 6 years.

From American Psychiatric Association. *Diagnostic and Statistical Manual of Mental Disorders*. 4th ed. Text rev. Washington, DC: American Psychiatric Association; copyright 2000, with permission.

caused by lack of food (Table 41–3). The disorder has its onset before the age of 6 years.

Epidemiology

It is estimated that between 15 and 35 percent of infants and young children have some feeding difficulties. Data from community samples estimate a prevalence of the disorder, however, in approximately 3 percent of infants with failure to thrive syndromes, with approximately half of those infants exhibiting feeding disorders.

Differential Diagnosis

Feeding disorder of infancy must be differentiated from structural problems with the infant's GI tract that may be contributing to discomfort during the feeding process.

Course and Prognosis

Most infants exhibit feeding disorders within the first year of life and, with appropriate recognition and intervention, do not later develop failure to thrive. When feeding disorders have their onset later, in children 2 to 3 years of age, growth and development may be affected when the disorder lasts for several months. It is estimated that approximately 70 percent of infants who persistently refuse food in the first year of life continue to have some feeding problems during childhood.

Treatment

Interventions for feeding disorders are aimed at evaluating the interaction between the mother and infant during feedings and identifying any factors that may be changed in order to promote greater ingestion. The mother is helped to become more aware of the infant's stamina for length of individual feedings, the infant's biological regulation patterns, and when the infant is fatigued, with a goal of increasing the level of engagement between mother and infant during feeding.

42 ▲

Tic Disorders

Tics are defined as rapid and repetitive muscle contractions resulting in movements or vocalizations that are experienced as involuntary. Children and adolescents may exhibit tic behaviors that occur after a stimulus or in response to an internal urge. Tic disorders are a group of neuropsychiatric disorders that generally begin in childhood or adolescence and may be constant or wax and wane over time. Although tics are not volitional, in some individuals they may be suppressed for periods of time. The most widely known and most severe tic disorder is Gilles de la Tourette syndrome, also known as *Tourette's disorder*. The text revision of the fourth edition of *Diagnostic and Statistical Manual of Mental Disorders* (DSM-IV-TR) includes several other tic disorders, such as chronic motor or vocal tic disorder, transient tic disorder, and tic disorder not otherwise specified. Although tics have no particular purpose, they often consist of motions that are used in volitional movements.

TOURETTE'S DISORDER

According to DSM-IV-TR, tics in Tourette's disorder are multiple motor tics and one or more vocal tics. The tics occur many times a day for more than 1 year. Tourette's disorder causes distress or significant impairment in important areas of functioning. The disorder has an onset before the age of 18 years, and it is not caused by a substance or by a general medical condition.

Georges Gilles de la Tourette first described a patient with what was later known as Tourette's disorder in 1885, while he was studying with Jean-Martin Charcot in France. De la Tourette noted a syndrome among several patients that included multiple motor tics, coprolalia, and echolalia.

Epidemiology

The lifetime prevalence of Tourette's disorder is estimated to be 4 to 5 per 10,000. More children exhibit this disorder than adults. The onset of the motor component of the disorder generally occurs by the age of 7 years; vocal tics emerge on average by the age of 11 years. Tourette's disorder occurs approximately three times more often in boys than in girls.

Etiology

Genetic Factors. Twin studies, adoption studies, and segregation analysis studies have all supported a genetic etiology for Tourette's disorder. Twin studies have indicated that concordance for the disorder in monozygotic twins is significantly greater than in dizygotic twins. The fact that Tourette's disorder and chronic motor or vocal tic disorder are likely to occur in the same families lends support to the view that the disorders are part of a genetically determined spectrum. Evidence in some families indicates that Tourette's disorder is transmitted in an autosomal dominant fashion.

Up to half of all Tourette's disorder patients also have attention-deficit/hyperactivity disorder (ADHD). Up to 40 percent of all those with Tourette's disorder also have obsessive-compulsive disorder (OCD). In addition, first-degree relatives of people with Tourette's disorder are at high risk for the development of the disorder, of chronic motor or vocal tic disorder, and of OCD. In view of the presence of symptoms of ADHD in more than half of the people with Tourette's disorder, questions arise about a genetic relation between these two disorders.

Neurochemical and Neuroanatomical Factors. Compelling evidence of dopamine system involvement in tic disorders includes the observations that pharmacological agents that antagonize dopamine—haloperidol (Haldol)—suppress tics and that agents that increase central dopaminergic activity—amphetamines—tend to exacerbate tics. The relation of tics to the dopamine system is not simple, because in some cases antipsychotic medications, such as haloperidol, are not effective in reducing tics, and the effect of stimulants on tic disorders has been reported as variable. In some cases, Tourette's disorder has emerged during treatment with antipsychotic medications.

Endogenous opiates may be involved in tic disorders and OCD. Some evidence indicates that pharmacological agents that antagonize endogenous opiates—for example, naltrexone (ReVia)—reduce tics and attention deficits in Tourette's disorder patients. Abnormalities in the noradrenergic system have been implicated in some cases by the reduction of tics with clonidine (Catapres). This adrenergic agonist reduces the release of norepinephrine in the central nervous system (CNS), and thus may reduce activity in the dopaminergic system. Abnormalities in the basal ganglia result in various movement disorders, such as in Huntington's disease, and are implicated as possible sites of disturbance in Tourette's disorder, OCD, and ADHD.

Immunological Factors and Postinfection. An autoimmune process that is secondary to streptococcal infections has been identified as a potential mechanism causing Tourette's dis-

Table 42–1
DSM-IV-TR Diagnostic Criteria for
Tourette's Disorder

A. Both multiple motor and one or more vocal tics have been present at some time during the illness, although not necessarily concurrently. (A *tic* is a sudden, rapid, recurrent, nonrhythmic, stereotyped motor movement or vocalization.)

B. The tics occur many times a day (usually in bouts) nearly every day or intermittently throughout a period of more than 1 year, and during this period there was never a tic-free period of more than 3 consecutive months.

C. The onset is before age 18 years.

D. The disturbance is not due to the direct physiological effects of a substance (e.g., stimulants) or a general medical condition (e.g., Huntington's disease or postviral encephalitis).

From American Psychiatric Association. *Diagnostic and Statistical Manual of Mental Disorders.* 4th ed. Text rev. Washington, DC: American Psychiatric Association; copyright 2000, with permission.

order. Such a process could act synergistically with a genetic vulnerability for this disorder. The poststreptococcal syndromes have also been associated with one potential causative factor in the development of OCD, which occurs in up to 40 percent of people with Tourette's disorder.

Diagnosis and Clinical Features

To make a diagnosis of Tourette's disorder, clinicians must obtain a history of multiple motor tics and the emergence of at least one vocal tic at some point in the disorder. According to DSM-IV-TR, the tics must occur many times a day nearly every day or intermittently for more than 1 year. The average age of onset of tics is 7 years, but tics may occur as early as the age of 2 years. The onset must occur before the age of 18 years (Table 42–1).

In Tourette's disorder, the initial tics are in the face and neck. Over time, the tics tend to occur in a downward progression. The most commonly described tics are those affecting the face and head, the arms and hands, the body and lower extremities, and the respiratory and alimentary systems.

Obsessions, compulsions, attention difficulties, impulsivity, and personality problems have been associated with Tourette's disorder. Attention difficulties often precede the onset of tics, whereas obsessive-compulsive symptoms often occur after their onset. Many tics have an aggressive or sexual component that may result in serious social consequences for the patient. Phenomenologically, tics resemble a failure of censorship, both conscious and unconscious, with increased impulsivity and inability to inhibit a thought from being put into action.

Sam is a 10-year-old boy who was referred for a psychiatric inpatient admission because of persistent refusal to attend school. Sam has a past history of ADHD, diagnosed at age 7 years, and has responded well to methylphenidate, most recently Concerta, 36 mg each morning. He is in a regular class in the fifth grade, and his parents report that, since age 6 years, he has had numerous motor and vocal tics, but that they have not interfered with his social life or academic

achievement until the present time. Sam first began to have repetitive eye blinking during the first grade, but he did not seem to be aware of it, and these tics did not interfere with his friendships, sports, or social life. After several months, he experienced some jerking movements of his head and shoulder, though he no longer had the eye-blinking tic. Again, Sam did not seem to be bothered by these, and none of his friends noticed either. Sam was being treated with methylphenidate at this time, because he has always had a short attention span and would find it impossible to remain in his seat or raise his hand in class. The methylphenidate has controlled his symptoms of hyperactivity and inattention.

Sam began to refuse to attend school after he developed a repetitive complex motor tic that involved walking forward, then retracing his steps and twirling around in a circle. He did this at least once every hour, and some of his peers began to tease him. Sam reported that he "couldn't help it" and felt that he had to do this. Sam became extremely upset and decided that he would no longer attend school, since everybody was making fun of him. Examination revealed that Sam did exhibit a complex tic as he described, as well as repeated soft grunting that occurred several times per minute. Sam's tics were causing him to be self-conscious and preventing him from being able to socialize with peers. A diagnosis of Tourette's disorder was made.

Sam was admitted to the children's psychiatric inpatient unit, and a trial of risperidone (Risperdal) was started with 0.5 mg orally daily. This was increased to 0.5 mg orally twice a day and titrated upward in accordance with his ability to tolerate the medication. Initially, Sam felt sleepy during the day, but after a few days, he had adjusted to the medication and could tolerate this dose well. His risperidone dose was increased every 3 days by 0.5 mg, until he reached a dosage of 1 mg orally each morning and 2 mg orally at bedtime. Sam tolerated this dosage and did not experience any extrapyramidal symptoms. After a week at the highest dose, Sam began to feel less compelled to retrace his steps and twirl, and he started to have sessions with a behavioral psychologist who helped him become more aware of his urges to twirl around in a circle. He practiced turning that "motion" into a useful movement, so that others would be less likely to notice it. Sam continued taking Concerta, 36 mg, because he reported that, without it, he was unable to focus on any school work. After leaving the hospital, Sam returned to school and continued his medication and sessions with the psychologist. Although he still retraced his steps and twirled occasionally, the frequency of this complex behavior had diminished, and he was usually able to transform the behavior into a movement that appeared to be purposeful and useful.

Pathology and Laboratory Examination

There is no specific laboratory diagnostic test for Tourette's disorder, but many patients with Tourette's disorder have nonspecific abnormal electroencephalogram (EEG) findings. Approximately 10 percent of all patients with Tourette's disorder show some nonspecific abnormality on computed tomography (CT) scans.

Differential Diagnosis

Tics must be differentiated from other disordered movements (for example, dystonic, choreiform, athetoid, myoclonic, and hemiballismic movements) and the neurological diseases of which they are characteristic (for example, Huntington's disease, parkinsonism, Sydenham's chorea, and Wilson's disease). Tremors, mannerisms, and stereotypic movement disorder (for example, head banging or body rocking) must also be distinguished from tic disorders. Stereotypic movement disorders, including movements such as rocking, hand gazing, and other self-stimulatory behaviors, seem to be voluntary and often produce a sense of comfort, in contrast to tic disorders. Although tics in children and adolescents may or may not feel controllable, they rarely produce a sense of well-being. Compulsions are sometimes difficult to distinguish from complex tics and may be on the same continuum biologically. Tic disorders also occur comorbidly with multiple behavioral and mood disturbances. In children with Tourette's disorder and ADHD, even when the tic disorder had always been mild, a high frequency of disruptive behavior problems and mood disorder still exists. Both autistic and mentally retarded children may exhibit symptoms similar to those seen in tic disorders, including Tourette's disorder. A greater-than-expected occurrence of Tourette's disorder, autistic disorder, and bipolar disorder also is present.

Before instituting treatment with an antipsychotic medication, clinicians must make a baseline evaluation of preexisting abnormal movements; such medication can mask abnormal movements, and if the movements occur later, they can be mistaken for tardive dyskinesia. Stimulant medications (such as methylphenidate, amphetamines, and pemoline) have been reported to exacerbate preexisting tics in some cases. These effects have been reported primarily in some children and adolescents being treated for ADHD. In most but not all cases, after the drug was discontinued, the tics remitted or returned to premedication levels.

Course and Prognosis

Untreated, Tourette's disorder is usually a chronic, lifelong disease with relative remissions and exacerbations. Initial symptoms may decrease, persist, or increase, and old symptoms may be replaced by new ones. Severely afflicted people may have serious emotional problems, including major depressive disorder. Some of these difficulties appear to be associated with Tourette's disorder, whereas others result from severe social, academic, and vocational consequences, which are frequent sequelae of the disorder.

Treatment

Consideration of a child or adolescent's overall functioning is the first step in determining the most appropriate treatments for tic disorders. It is important to begin treatment with comprehensive education for families so that children are not unwittingly treated punitively for their tic behaviors. It is also important for families to understand the waxing and waning nature of many tic disorders. In mild cases, children with tic disorders who are functioning well socially and academically may not require treatment. In more severe cases, children with tic disorders may be ostracized by peers and academic work compromised by the disruptive nature of tics, and a variety of treatments must be considered.

Other behavioral techniques—including massed (negative) practice, self-monitoring, incompatible response training, presentation and removal of positive reinforcement, as well as habit reversal treatment—were reviewed by Stanley A. Hobbs. He reported that tic frequency was reduced in many cases, particularly with habit reversal treatment, but additional studies are currently under investigation to replicate the efficacy of these techniques. Behavioral techniques, including relaxation, may reduce stress that often exacerbates Tourette's disorder. It is hypothesized that behavioral techniques and pharmacotherapy together have a synergistic effect.

Pharmacotherapy. High potency, conventional antipsychotics, such as haloperidol, trifluoperazine (Stelazine), and pimozide (Orap) have been shown to have significant tic reduction effects. Discontinuation is often based on the drug's adverse effects, including extrapyramidal effects and dysphoria. Haloperidol is not approved for use in children under 3 years of age.

Clinicians must forewarn patients and families of the possibilities of acute dystonic reactions and parkinsonian symptoms when a conventional or newer "atypical" antipsychotic medication is to be initiated. The more recently marketed "atypical" antipsychotics, including risperidone and olanzapine (Zyprexa), are often chosen as a treatment option instead of the conventional antipsychotics in the hope that side effects will be less pervasive.

Even with the newer atypical antipsychotics, diphenhydramine (Benadryl) or benztropine (Cogentin) are not infrequently required to control extrapyramidal side effects.

Although not presently approved for use in Tourette's disorder, clonidine, a noradrenergic antagonist, has been reported to be efficacious in several studies; 40 to 70 percent of patients benefited from the medication. In addition to the improvement in tic symptoms, patients may experience less tension and an improved attention span. Another α-adrenergic agonist, guanfacine (Tenex), has also been used in the treatment of tic disorders.

In view of the frequent comorbidity of tic behaviors and obsessive-compulsive symptoms or OCDs, the selective serotonin reuptake inhibitor drugs (SSRIs) have been used alone or in combination with antipsychotics in the treatment of Tourette's disorder. Some data suggest that SSRIs, such as fluoxetine (Prozac), may be helpful.

Although clinicians must weigh the risks versus the benefits of using stimulants in cases of severe hyperactivity and comorbid tics, a recent study reports that methylphenidate does not increase the rate or intensity of motor or vocal tics in most children with hyperactivity and tic disorders. There was one case report that bupropion (Wellbutrin), an antidepressant of the aminoketone class, resulted in increased tic behavior in several children being treated for Tourette's disorder and ADHD. Other antidepressants, such as imipramine (Tofranil) and desipramine (Norpramin, Pertofane), may decrease disruptive behavior in children with Tourette's disorder but are no longer widely used due to the potentially serious cardiac side effects.

CHRONIC MOTOR OR VOCAL TIC DISORDER

In DSM-IV-TR, chronic motor or vocal tic disorder is defined as the presence of either motor tics or vocal tics, but not both. The other features are the same as those of Tourette's disorder, but chronic motor or vocal tic disorder cannot be diagnosed if the criteria for Tourette's disorder have ever been met. According to DSM-IV-TR criteria, the disorder must have its onset before the age of 18 years.

Epidemiology

The rate of chronic motor or vocal tic disorder has been estimated to be from 100 to 1,000 times greater than that of Tourette's disorder. School-age boys are at highest risk, but the incidence is unknown. Although the disorder was once believed to be rare, current estimates of the prevalence of chronic motor or vocal tic disorder range from 1 to 2 percent.

Etiology

Both Tourette's disorder and chronic motor or vocal tic disorder aggregate in the same families. Twin studies have found a high concordance for either Tourette's disorder or chronic motor tics in monozygotic twins. This finding supports the importance of hereditary factors in the transmission of at least some tic disorders.

Diagnosis and Clinical Features

The onset of chronic motor or vocal tic disorder appears to be in early childhood. The types of tics and their locations are similar to those in transient tic disorder. Chronic vocal tics are considerably rarer than are chronic motor tics. The chronic vocal tics are usually much less conspicuous than those in Tourette's disorder. The vocal tics are usually not loud or intense and are not primarily produced by the vocal cords; they consist of grunts or other noises caused by thoracic, abdominal, or diaphragmatic contractions. The DSM-IV-TR diagnostic criteria are given in Table 42–2.

Table 42–2
DSM-IV-TR Diagnostic Criteria for Chronic Motor or Vocal Tic Disorder

A. Single or multiple motor or vocal tics (i.e., sudden, rapid, recurrent, nonrhythmic, stereotyped motor movements or vocalizations), but not both, have been present at some time during the illness.

B. The tics occur many times a day nearly every day or intermittently throughout a period of more than 1 year, and during this period there was never a tic-free period of more than 3 consecutive months.

C. The onset is before age 18 years.

D. The disturbance is not due to the direct physiological effects of a substance (e.g., stimulants) or a general medical condition (e.g., Huntington's disease or postviral encephalitis).

E. Criteria have never been met for Tourette's disorder.

From American Psychiatric Association. *Diagnostic and Statistical Manual of Mental Disorders.* 4th ed. Text rev. Washington, DC: American Psychiatric Association; copyright 2000, with permission.

Differential Diagnosis

Chronic motor tics must be differentiated from a variety of other motor movements, including choreiform movements, myoclonus, restless legs syndrome, akathisia, and dystonias. Involuntary vocal utterances can occur in certain neurological disorders, such as Huntington's disease and Parkinson's disease.

Course and Prognosis

Children whose tics start between the ages of 6 and 8 years seem to have the best outcomes. Symptoms usually last for 4 to 6 years and stop in early adolescence. Children whose tics involve the limbs or trunk tend to do less well than those with only facial tics.

Treatment

The treatment of chronic motor or vocal tic disorder depends on the severity and the frequency of the tics; the patient's subjective distress; the effects of the tics on school, work, or job performance and socialization; and the presence of any other concomitant mental disorder. Psychotherapy may be indicated to minimize the secondary emotional problems caused by the tics. Several studies have found that behavioral techniques, particularly habit reversal treatments, have been effective in treating chronic motor or vocal tic disorder. Haloperidol has been helpful in some cases, but the risks must be weighed against the possible clinical benefits because of the drug's adverse effects, including the development of tardive dyskinesia.

TRANSIENT TIC DISORDER

DSM-IV-TR defines transient tic disorder as the presence of a single tic or multiple motor or vocal tics or both. The tics occur many times a day for at least 4 weeks but for no longer than 12 months. The other features are the same as those for Tourette's disorder, but transient tic disorder cannot be diagnosed if the criteria for Tourette's disorder or chronic motor or vocal tic disorder have ever been met. According to DSM-IV-TR, the disorder must have its onset before the age of 18 years.

Epidemiology

Transient, tic-like movements and nervous muscular twitches are common in children. Five to 24 percent of all school-age children have a history of tics. The prevalence of tics as defined here is unknown.

Etiology

Transient tic disorder probably has either organic or psychogenic origins, with some tics combining elements of both. Organic tics, which are probably most likely to progress to Tourette's disorder, have an increased family history of tics, whereas psychogenic tics are most likely to remit spontaneously. Tics that progress to chronic motor or vocal tic disorder are most likely to have components of both organic and psychogenic origins. Tics of all sorts

Table 42–3
DSM-IV-TR Diagnostic Criteria for Transient Tic Disorder

A. Single or multiple motor and/or vocal tics (i.e., sudden, rapid, recurrent, nonrhythmic, stereotyped motor movements or vocalizations)

B. The tics occur many times a day, nearly every day for at least 4 weeks, but for no longer than 12 consecutive months.

C. The onset is before age 18 years.

D. The disturbance is not due to the direct physiological effects of a substance (e.g., stimulants) or a general medical condition (e.g., Huntington's disease or postviral encephalitis).

E. Criteria have never been met for Tourette's disorder or chronic motor or vocal tic disorder.

Specify if:

Single episode or **recurrent**

From American Psychiatric Association. *Diagnostic and Statistical Manual of Mental Disorders*. 4th ed. Text rev. Washington, DC: American Psychiatric Association; copyright 2000, with permission.

Table 42–4
DSM-IV-TR Diagnostic Criteria for Tic Disorder Not Otherwise Specified

This category is for disorders characterized by tics that do not meet criteria for a specific tic disorder. Examples include tics lasting less than 4 weeks or tics with an onset after age 18 years.

From American Psychiatric Association. *Diagnostic and Statistical Manual of Mental Disorders*. 4th ed. Text rev. Washington, DC: American Psychiatric Association; copyright 2000, with permission.

are exacerbated by stress and anxiety, but no evidence is available that tics are caused by stress or anxiety.

Diagnosis and Clinical Features

The DSM-IV-TR criteria for establishing the diagnosis of transient tic disorder are as follows: The tics are single or multiple motor or vocal tics. The tics occur many times a day nearly every day for at least 4 weeks but for no longer than 12 consecutive months. The patient has no history of Tourette's disorder or chronic motor or vocal tic disorder. The onset is before age 18. The tics do not occur exclusively during substance intoxication, and they are not caused by a general medical condition. The diagnosis should specify whether a single episode or recurrent episodes are present (Table 42–3). Transient tic disorder can be distinguished from chronic motor or vocal tic disorder and Tourette's disorder only by observing the symptoms' progression over time.

Course and Prognosis

Most people with transient tic disorder do not progress to a more serious tic disorder. Their tics either disappear permanently or recur during periods of special stress. Only a small percentage develop chronic motor or vocal tic disorder or Tourette's disorder.

Treatment

Whether the tics will disappear spontaneously, progress, or become chronic is unclear at the beginning of treatment. Focusing attention on tics may exacerbate them; thus, clinicians often recommend that, at first, the family disregard the tics as much as possible. But if the tics are so severe that they impair the patient or if they are accompanied by significant emotional disturbances, complete psychiatric and pediatric neurological examinations are recommended. Treatment depends on the results of the evaluations. Psychopharmacology is not recommended unless the symptoms are unusually severe and disabling. Several studies have found that behavioral techniques, particularly habit reversal treatment, have been effective in treating transient tics.

Tic Disorder Not Otherwise Specified

According to DSM-IV-TR, tic disorder not otherwise specified refers to disorders characterized by tics but not otherwise meeting the criteria for a specific tic disorder (Table 42–4).

Elimination Disorders

Enuresis and encopresis are the two elimination disorders described in the text revision of the fourth edition of *Diagnostic and Statistical Manual of Mental Disorders* (DSM-IV-TR). These disorders are considered only when a child is chronologically and developmentally beyond the point at which it is expected that these functions can be mastered. *Encopresis* is defined as a pattern of passing feces into inappropriate places, whether the passage is involuntary or intentional. The pattern must be present for at least 3 months; the child's chronological age must be at least 4 years. *Enuresis* is the repeated voiding of urine into clothes or bed, whether the voiding is involuntary or intentional. The behavior must occur twice weekly for at least 3 months or must cause clinically significant distress or impairment socially or academically. The child's chronological or developmental age must be at least 5 years.

ENCOPRESIS

Epidemiology

In Western cultures, bowel control is established in more than 95 percent of children by their fourth birthday and in 99 percent by their fifth birthday. Thereafter, frequency decreases to virtual absence by the age of 16. After the age of 4, encopresis at all ages is three to four times as common in boys as in girls. At the ages of 7 to 8 years, frequency is approximately 1.5 percent in boys and approximately 0.5 percent in girls. By the ages of 10 to 12 years, once-a-month soiling occurs in 1.3 percent of boys and in 0.3 percent of girls. There is a significant relation between encopresis and enuresis.

Etiology

Encopresis involves an often complicated interplay between physiological and psychological factors. Inadequate training or the lack of appropriate toilet training may delay a child's attainment of continence. Evidence indicates that some encopretic children suffer from lifelong inefficient and ineffective sphincter control. Thus, encopresis may occur in children with adequate bowel control who, for a variety of emotional reasons, including anger, anxiety, fear, or some combination of these, do not deposit the feces appropriately. Other children may soil involuntarily, either because of an inability to control the sphincter adequately or because of excessive fluid caused by a retentive overflow.

Encopretic children who are clearly able to control their bowel function adequately and who deposit feces of relatively normal consistency in abnormal places usually have a psychiatric diffi-

culty. Encopresis may be associated with other neurodevelopmental problems, including easy distractibility, short attention span, low frustration tolerance, hyperactivity, and poor coordination. Occasionally, the child has a special fear of using the toilet. Encopresis may also be precipitated by life events, such as the birth of a sibling or a move to a new home. Encopresis after a long period of fecal continence sometimes appears to be a regression after such stresses as a parental separation, a change in domicile, or the start of school.

Psychogenic Megacolon. Many encopretic children also retain feces and become constipated, either voluntarily or secondarily to painful defecation. In these cases, no clear evidence indicates that preexisting anorectal dysfunction contributes to the constipation. The resulting chronic rectal distention from large, hard fecal masses may cause loss of tone in the rectal wall and desensitization to pressure. Thus, many children become unaware of the need to defecate, and overflow encopresis occurs, usually with relatively small amounts of liquid or soft stool leaking out.

Olfactory accommodation may diminish or eliminate sensory cues. Children whose parenting has been harsh and punitive and who have been severely punished for "accidents" during toilet training may also develop encopresis.

Diagnosis and Clinical Features

According to DSM-IV-TR, encopresis is diagnosed when feces are passed into inappropriate places on a regular basis (at least once a month) for 3 months (Table 43–1). Encopresis may be present in children who have bowel control and intentionally deposit feces in their clothes or other places for a variety of emotional reasons.

DSM-IV-TR breaks down the types of encopresis into with constipation and overflow incontinence and without constipation and overflow incontinence. To receive a diagnosis of encopresis, a child must have a developmental or chronological level of at least 4 years. If the fecal incontinence is directly related to a medical condition, encopresis is not diagnosed.

Henry was an 11-year-old male with almost-daily encopresis and a number of associated behaviors, including hiding the feces around the house. He resided in a specialized foster care setting, having been removed from his biological parents at age 7 because of physical and sexual abuse. Both parents were involved with substance abuse, and his early history is not well documented. However, a parent did indicate that he had not exhibited sustained bowel continence for several months. Henry had also been enuretic until age 6, but this had resolved to an occasional nocturnal episode every 4 to 6 months. Henry also qualified for a diagnosis of oppositional-defiant disorder. Although he had experienced physical and sexual abuse, he did not have flashbacks or other symptoms that would meet the criteria for posttraumatic stress disorder (PTSD). Henry also had an attention-deficit/hyperactivity disorder (ADHD) and was being treated effectively with 10 mg of methylphenidate (Ritalin) twice a day.

The foster family resided in an urban area that had access to a nationally recognized children's hospital. The Ambulatory Care Department had a specialized behavioral encopresis program that coupled the bowel training method with a psychoeducational component and psychotherapy. The psychiatric consultant to the specialized foster care program doubted that this program would be successful for Henry because he had so much associated psychopathology and the feces were often deposited around the house in a symbolic manner. Also, the encopresis was not of the retentive-overflow type, and the feces were always well formed. However, because no apparent harm could come from the referral, the consulting child psychiatrist agreed to it. Much to the surprise of the consultant, the several-week outpatient bowel training course coupled with the psychoeducational component and psychotherapy resulted in complete cessation of the encopresis. On one of her visits to the home, Henry proudly showed his case manger a diagram of the functioning of the digestive system that was part of the psychoeducational program. In retrospect, it appeared that, although there were symbolic aspects to Henry's encopretic behavior, the soiling was ego-dystonic, and he was motivated to change the behavior, although this motivation could not be prospectively detected by the treatment team because of his oppositional-defiant manner of responding to adults. (Courtesy of Edwin J. Mikkelsen, M.D.)

Pathology and Laboratory Examination

Although no specific test indicates a diagnosis of encopresis, clinicians must rule out medical illnesses, such as Hirschsprung's disease, before making a diagnosis. If it is unclear whether fecal retention is responsible for encopresis with constipation and overflow incontinence, a physical examination of the abdomen is indicated, and an abdominal X-ray can be helpful in determining the degree of constipation present. Sophisticated tests to determine whether sphincter tone is abnormal are generally not conducted in simple cases of encopresis.

Differential Diagnosis

Encopresis with constipation and overflow incontinence can be caused by faulty nutrition; structural disease of the anus, rectum, and colon; medicinal side effects; or nongastrointestinal medical (endocrine or neurological) disorders. The chief differential problem is aganglionic megacolon or Hirschsprung's disease, in which a patient may have an empty rectum and no desire to defecate but may still have an overflow of feces. The

Table 43–1
DSM-IV-TR Diagnostic Criteria for Encopresis

A. Repeated passage of feces into inappropriate places (e.g., clothing or floor) whether involuntary or intentional.

B. At least one such event a month for at least 3 months.

C. Chronological age is at least 4 years (or equivalent developmental level).

D. The behavior is not due exclusively to the direct physiological effects of a substance (e.g., laxatives) or a general medical condition except through a mechanism involving constipation.

Code as follows:

With constipation and overflow incontinence

Without constipation and overflow incontinence

From American Psychiatric Association. *Diagnostic and Statistical Manual of Mental Disorders.* 4th ed. Text rev. Washington, DC: American Psychiatric Association; copyright 2000, with permission.

disorder occurs in 1 in 5,000 children; signs appear shortly after birth.

Course and Prognosis

The outcome of encopresis depends on the cause, the chronicity of the symptoms, and coexisting behavioral problems. In many cases, encopresis is self-limiting, and it rarely continues beyond middle adolescence. Children who have contributing physiological factors, such as poor gastric motility and an inability to relax the anal sphincter muscles, are more difficult to treat than are those with constipation but normal sphincter tone.

The outcome of cases of encopresis is affected by the family's willingness and ability to participate in treatment without being overly punitive and by the child's awareness of when the passage of feces is about to occur.

Treatment

By the time a child is brought for treatment, considerable family discord and distress are common. Family tensions about the symptom must be reduced and a nonpunitive atmosphere established. Similar efforts should be made to reduce the child's embarrassment at school. Many changes of underwear with a minimum of fuss should be arranged. Education to the family and correction of misperceptions that a family may have about soiling must occur before treatment. A useful physiological approach involves a combination of daily laxatives or mineral oil along with a behavioral intervention by which the child sits on the toilet for timed intervals daily and is rewarded for successful defecation. For children who are not constipated and have good bowel control, laxatives are not necessary, but regular timed intervals on the toilet may be useful with these children as well.

Supportive psychotherapy and relaxation techniques may be useful in treating encopretic children's anxieties and other sequelae, such as low self-esteem and social isolation. In children who have bowel control but continue to deposit their feces in inappropriate locations, family interventions can be helpful. A good outcome occurs when a child feels in control of life events. Coexisting behavior problems predict a poorer outcome. In all cases, proper bowel habits may need to be taught. In some cases, biofeedback techniques have been of help.

ENURESIS

Epidemiology

The prevalence of enuresis decreases with increasing age. Prevalence rates vary, however, on the basis of the population studied and the tolerance for the symptoms in various cultures and socioeconomic groups.

The Isle of Wight study reported that 15.2 percent of 7-year-old boys were enuretic occasionally and that 6.7 percent of them were enuretic at least once a week. The study reported that 3.3 percent of girls at the age of 7 years were enuretic at least once a week. By age 10, the overall prevalence of enuresis has been reported to be 3 percent. The rate drops drastically for teenagers, in whom a prevalence of 1.5 percent has been reported for 14-year-olds. Enuresis affects approximately 1 percent of adults.

Mental disorders are present in only approximately 20 percent of enuretic children; they are most common in enuretic girls, in children with symptoms during the day and night, and in children who maintain the symptoms into older childhood.

Etiology

Most children are not enuretic with intention or even with awareness until after they are wet. Physiological factors are likely to play a major role in most cases of enuresis. Normal bladder control, which is acquired gradually, is influenced by neuromuscular and cognitive development, socioemotional factors, toilet training, and possible genetic factors. Difficulties in one or more of these areas may delay urinary continence.

Although a specific organic cause precludes a diagnosis of enuresis, the correction of an anatomical defect or the cure of an infection does not always cure the enuresis. A child's risk for enuresis has been found to be more than seven times greater if the father was enuretic. The concordance rate is higher in monozygotic twins than in dizygotic twins. There is a strong suggestion of a genetic component; much can be accounted for by tolerance for enuresis in some families and by other psychosocial factors.

Enuresis does not appear to be related to a specific stage of sleep or time of night; rather, bed-wetting appears randomly. In most cases, the quality of sleep is normal. Little evidence indicates that enuretic children sleep more soundly than do other children.

Psychosocial stressors appear to precipitate some cases of enuresis. In young children, the disorder has been particularly associated with the birth of a sibling, hospitalization between the ages of 2 and 4, the start of school, the breakup of a family because of divorce or death, and a move to a new domicile.

Diagnosis and Clinical Features

Enuresis is the repeated voiding of urine into a child's clothes or bed; the voiding may be involuntary or intentional. For the diagnosis to be made, a child must exhibit a developmental or chronological age of at least 5 years. According to DSM-IV-

Table 43–2
DSM-IV-TR Diagnostic Criteria for Enuresis

A. Repeated voiding of urine into bed or clothes (whether involuntary or intentional).
B. The behavior is clinically significant as manifested by either a frequency of twice a week for at least 3 consecutive months or the presence of clinically significant distress or impairment in social, academic (occupational), or other important areas of functioning.
C. Chronological age is at least 5 years (or equivalent developmental level).
D. The behavior is not due exclusively to the direct physiological effect of a substance (e.g., a diuretic) or a general medical condition (e.g., diabetes, spina bifida, a seizure disorder).
Specify type:
Nocturnal only
Diurnal only
Nocturnal and diurnal

From American Psychiatric Association. *Diagnostic and Statistical Manual of Mental Disorders.* 4th ed. Text rev. Washington, DC: American Psychiatric Association; copyright 2002, with permission.

TR, the behavior must occur twice weekly for a period of at least 3 months or must cause distress and impairment in functioning to meet the diagnostic criteria. Enuresis is diagnosed only if the behavior is not due to a medical condition. DSM-IV-TR breaks down the disorder into three types: nocturnal only, diurnal only, and nocturnal and diurnal (Table 43–2).

Pathology and Laboratory Examination

No single laboratory finding is pathognomonic of enuresis, but clinicians must rule out organic factors, such as the presence of urinary tract infections, that may predispose a child to enuresis. Structural obstructive abnormalities may be present in up to 3 percent of children with apparent enuresis. Sophisticated radiographic studies are usually deferred in simple cases of enuresis with no signs of repeated infections or other medical problems.

Differential Diagnosis

Possible organic causes of bed-wetting must be ruled out. Organic features occur most often in children with both nocturnal and diurnal enuresis combined with urinary frequency and urgency. The organic features include genitourinary pathology—structural, neurological, and infectious—such as obstructive uropathy, spina bifida occulta, and cystitis; other organic disorders that may cause polyuria and enuresis, such as diabetes mellitus and diabetes insipidus; disturbances of consciousness and sleep, such as seizures, intoxication, and sleepwalking disorder, during which a child urinates; and side effects from treatment with antipsychotics—for example, thioridazine (Mellaril).

Course and Prognosis

Enuresis is usually self-limited, and a child can eventually remain dry without psychiatric sequelae. Most enuretic children find their symptoms ego-dystonic and enjoy enhanced self-esteem and improved social confidence when they become continent. Enuresis after at least 1 dry year usually begins between the ages of 5 and 8 years; if it occurs much later, especially during adulthood, organic causes must be investigated. Some evidence indicates that late onset of enuresis in children is more frequently associated with a concomitant psychiatric difficulty than is enuresis without at least 1 dry year. Relapses occur in enuretic children who are becoming dry spontaneously and in those who are being treated. The significant emotional and social difficulties of enuretic children usually include poor self-image, decreased self-esteem, social embarrassment and restriction, and intrafamilial conflict.

Treatment

Treatment modalities that have been used successfully for enuresis include behavioral and pharmacological interventions. A relatively high rate of spontaneous remission over long periods also occurs. The first step in any treatment plan is to review appropriate toilet training. Other useful techniques include restricting fluids before bed and night lifting to toilet train the child.

Behavioral Therapy.   Classic conditioning with the bell (or buzzer) and pad apparatus is generally the most effective treatment for enuresis, with dryness resulting in more than 50 per-

cent of all cases. Difficulties may include child and family noncompliance, improper use of the apparatus, and relapse. Bladder training—encouragement or reward for delaying micturition for increasing times during waking hours—has also been used. Although sometimes effective, this method is decidedly inferior to the bell and pad.

Pharmacotherapy.   Medication is not the first line of treatment for enuresis and is often not warranted at all. When the problem is so troubling as to significantly interfere with a child's functioning, several medications can be considered, although the problem often recurs as soon as medications are withdrawn. Imipramine (Tofranil) is efficacious and has been approved for use in treating childhood enuresis, primarily on a short-term basis. Desmopressin (DDAVP), an antidiuretic compound that is available as an intranasal spray, has shown some initial success in reducing enuresis.

Psychotherapy.   Although many psychological and psychoanalytic theories regarding enuresis have been advanced, controlled studies have found that psychotherapy alone is not an effective treatment of enuresis. Psychotherapy, however, may be useful in dealing with the coexisting psychiatric problems and the emotional and family difficulties that arise secondary to the disorder.

44

Other Disorders of Infancy, Childhood, and Adolescence

▲ 44.1 Separation Anxiety Disorder

Separation anxiety is a universal human developmental phenomenon emerging in infants at less than 1 year of age and marking the child's awareness of a separation from his or her mother or primary caregiver. Separation anxiety, or *stranger anxiety* as it has been termed during infancy, is an expected part of normal development and most likely evolved as a human response that has survival value. Separation anxiety disorder, however, is diagnosed when developmentally inappropriate and excessive anxiety emerges related to separation from the major attachment figure.

EPIDEMIOLOGY

The prevalence of separation anxiety disorder is estimated to be approximately 4 percent in children and young adolescents. Separation anxiety disorder is more common in young children than in adolescents and has been reported to occur equally in boys and girls. The onset may occur during preschool years, but its onset is most common in 7- to 8-year-old children.

ETIOLOGY

Biopsychosocial Factors

Young children, immature and dependent on a mothering figure, are particularly prone to excessive anxiety related to separation. The relation between temperamental traits and the predisposition to develop anxiety symptoms has been investigated. The temperamental tendency to be unusually shy or to withdraw in unfamiliar situations seems to be an enduring response pattern, and young children with this propensity are at higher risk of developing anxiety disorders during their next few years of life.

There is a neurophysiological correlation of *behavioral inhibition* (extreme shyness): Children with this constellation are shown to have a higher resting heart rate and acceleration of heart rate with tasks requiring cognitive concentration. Additional physiological correlates of behavioral inhibition include elevated salivary cortisol levels, elevated urinary catecholamines, and larger pupil-

lary dilation during cognitive tasks. The quality of maternal attachment also appears to play a role in the development of anxiety disorder in children. Mothers with anxiety disorders who are observed to show insecure attachment to their children tend to have children with higher rates of anxiety disorders. External life stresses often coincide with the development of the disorder. The death of a relative, a child's illness, a change in a child's environment, or a move to a new neighborhood or school is frequently noted in the histories of children with separation anxiety disorder. In a vulnerable child, these changes probably intensify anxiety.

Learning Factors

Phobic anxiety may be communicated from parents to children by direct modeling. Some parents appear to teach their children to be anxious by overprotecting them from expected dangers or by exaggerating the dangers. Conversely, a parent who becomes angry at a child during an incipient phobic concern about animals may inculcate a phobic concern in the child by the very intensity of the anger expressed.

Genetic Factors

The temperamental constellation of behavioral inhibition, excessive shyness, the tendency to withdraw from unfamiliar situations, and separation anxiety are all likely to have a genetic contribution. Family studies have shown that the biological offspring of adults with anxiety disorders are prone to suffer from separation anxiety disorder in childhood. Parents who have panic disorder with agoraphobia appear to have an increased risk of having a child with separation anxiety disorder. Separation anxiety disorder and depression in children overlap, and some clinicians view separation anxiety disorder as a feature of a depressive disorder. Recently, a presumptive gene was located for shyness, which is related to separation anxiety.

DIAGNOSIS AND CLINICAL FEATURES

Separation anxiety disorder is the most common anxiety disorder in childhood. To meet the diagnostic criteria, according to the text revision of the fourth edition of the *Diagnostic and Statistical Manual of Mental Disorders* (DSM-IV-TR), the disorder must be characterized by three of the following symptoms for at least 4

Table 44.1–1
DSM-IV-TR Diagnostic Criteria for Separation Anxiety Disorder

A. Developmentally inappropriate and excessive anxiety concerning separation from home or from those to whom the individual is attached, as evidenced by three (or more) of the following:

(1) recurrent excessive distress when separation from home or major attachment figures occurs or is anticipated

(2) persistent and excessive worry about losing, or about possible harm befalling, major attachment figures

(3) persistent and excessive worry that an untoward event will lead to separation from a major attachment figure (e.g., getting lost or being kidnapped)

(4) persistent reluctance or refusal to go to school or elsewhere because of fear of separation

(5) persistently and excessively fearful or reluctant to be alone or without major attachment figures at home or without significant adults in other settings

(6) persistent reluctance or refusal to go to sleep without being near a major attachment figure or to sleep away from home

(7) repeated nightmares involving the theme of separation

(8) repeated complaints of physical symptoms (such as headaches, stomachaches, nausea, or vomiting) when separation from major attachment figures occurs or is anticipated

B. The duration of the disturbance is at least 4 weeks.

C. The onset is before age 18 years.

D. The disturbance causes clinically significant distress or impairment in social, academic (occupational), or other important areas of functioning.

E. The disturbance does not occur exclusively during the course of a pervasive developmental disorder, schizophrenia, or other psychotic disorder and, in adolescents and adults, is not better accounted for by panic disorder with agoraphobia.

Specify if:

Early onset: if onset occurs before age 6 years

From American Psychiatric Association. *Diagnostic and Statistical Manual of Mental Disorders.* 4th ed. Text rev. Washington, DC: American Psychiatric Association; copyright 2000, with permission.

weeks: persistent and excessive worry about losing, or possible harm befalling, major attachment figures; persistent and excessive worry that an untoward event can lead to separation from a major attachment figure; persistent reluctance or refusal to go to school or elsewhere because of fear of separation; persistent and excessive fear or reluctance to be alone or without major attachment figures at home or without significant adults in other settings; persistent reluctance or refusal to go to sleep without being near a major attachment figure or to sleep away from home; repeated nightmares involving the theme of separation; repeated complaints of physical symptoms, including headaches and stomachaches, when separation from major attachment figures is anticipated; and recurrent excessive distress when separation from home or major attachment figures is anticipated or involved. According to DSM-IV-TR, the disturbance must also cause significant distress or impairment in functioning (Table 44.1–1).

Associated features include fear of the dark and imaginary, bizarre worries. Symptoms emerge when separation from an important parent figure becomes necessary. If separation is threatened, many children with the disorder do not experience interpersonal difficulties. They frequently experience gastrointestinal (GI) symptoms of nausea, vomiting, and stomachaches and have pains in various parts of the body, sore throats, and flu-like symptoms. In older children, typical cardiovascular and respiratory symptoms of palpitations, dizziness, faintness, and strangulation are reported. The most common anxiety disorder that coexists with separation anxiety disorder is specific phobia, which occurs in approximately one-third of all referred cases of separation anxiety disorder.

Tony was a 6-year-old boy referred by his school because of persistent refusal to attend school. He had always been a somewhat "clingy" child, but his difficulties had intensified in the past 4 months. He would follow his parents around the house and refuse to leave their sides in playgrounds or other situations where separating would be age appropriate. That behavior was worse if he could not keep them in clear sight. He said that he might be kidnapped or lost if he ever got out of their sight. He would tantrum whenever they would try to go out for the evening, saying that they were not coming back. When forced to engage in any of the distressing activities, he would complain of various somatic symptoms until one of his parents remained.

He was the product of a pregnancy marred by caesarean section for premature rupture of membranes at 34 weeks' gestation. The perinatal course was complicated by moderate respiratory distress necessitating hospitalization for more than 3 weeks. Evaluation of the recent somatic symptoms revealed a child who was normal except for the psychiatric complaints.

His early development had been normal. He attempted preschool, but his mother had removed him because he cried at the beginning of each day, followed by aggression toward smaller peers. She participated as a parent aide in his kindergarten classroom, stating that she was trying to help him adjust to school. He was in grade school with peers who were after-school playmates in his home but would only go to their homes with a parent.

Family history was positive for maternal recurrent major depressive disorder, in remission, and a history of panic disorder in Tony's maternal grandmother. His maternal grandfather and a paternal uncle had alcoholism. Tony's parents were both in their early 30s, with some college education. His father worked as an assistant manager in a small service firm; his mother had worked as a bookkeeper until Tony was born. They said that his mother would have returned to work if he had liked preschool. His difficulties were straining their marriage, as he frequently insisted on sleeping in their bed. His mother insisted that she wanted to return to the workforce and that Tony's separation anxiety prevented it. There was no suggestion of domestic violence.

Mental status examination revealed a thin, nicely attired boy who had great difficulty allowing his mother to go beyond a chair outside the office door. He insisted on checking twice to see if she was there. He was fidgety and admitted feeling very worried about his mother leaving. He said that kind of worry was bad enough that he has trouble thinking. He denied depressed mood or symptoms including irritability. He denied hallucinations and did not voice any delusional ideas. He said that he enjoyed his friends and that his teacher was "nice" but that he worried about his mother when he was away from her.

Further exploration of the family situation revealed that his maternal grandfather had died 2 years earlier. His grandmother, who lived nearby, had been very agoraphobic until recently and had depended on the patient's mother, which had caused significant marital friction. Tony's father had hoped that the mother would return to work so that he could complete college and leave a job he hated. When she tried to force Tony to go to school, grandmother would come to the home to help and would then encourage mother to "go easy on the child." Mother would become angry, relent, and feel guilty about her interactions with her mother and her child. Grandmother further lectured mother that she needed to stay at home to care for her needy and delicate child because he had been premature.

Treatment focused on bringing the adults together to develop a supportive program for the child and to enlist grandmother in an appropriate role helping her daughter and son-in-law move forward with their lives. Grandmother supported Tony's return to the classroom once she understood the issues and approach. That was accomplished without directly addressing or interpreting her significant identification with her separation-anxious grandchild. Mother returned to work, with grandmother providing after-school care. Tony also responded well to a simple reward program for sleeping in his own room. Unfortunately, he presented again 7 years later as a popular, very good student and athlete who developed major depressive disorder. He responded well to fluoxetine (Prozac) and cognitive therapy. (Courtesy of Carrie Sylvester, M.D.)

DIFFERENTIAL DIAGNOSIS

Some degree of separation anxiety is a normal phenomenon, and clinical judgment must be used in distinguishing that normal anxiety from separation anxiety disorder. In generalized anxiety disorder, anxiety is not focused on separation. In pervasive developmental disorders and schizophrenia, anxiety about separation may occur but is viewed as caused by these conditions rather than as a separate disorder. In depressive disorders occurring in children, the diagnosis of separation anxiety disorder should also be made when the criteria for both disorders are met; the two diagnoses often coexist. Panic disorder with agoraphobia is uncommon before 18 years of age; the fear is of being incapacitated by a panic attack rather than of separation from parental figures. In some adult cases, however, many symptoms of separation anxiety disorder may be present. In conduct disorder, truancy is common, but children stay away from home and do not have anxiety about separation. School refusal is a frequent symptom in separation anxiety disorder but is not pathognomonic of it. Children with other diagnoses, such as phobias, also show evidence of school refusal; in these disorders, the age of onset may be later and the school refusal may be more severe than in separation anxiety disorder. Common characteristics of selected anxiety disorders that occur in children are presented in Table 44.1–2.

COURSE AND PROGNOSIS

The course and the prognosis of separation anxiety disorder are variable and are related to the age of onset, the duration of the

Table 44.1–2
Common Characteristics of Selected Anxiety Disorders That Occur in Children

Criteria	Separation Anxiety Disorder	Social Phobia	Generalized Anxiety Disorder
Minimum duration to establish diagnosis	At least 4 weeks	No minimum	At least 6 months
Age of onset	Preschool to 18 years	Not specified	Not specified
Precipitating stresses	Separation from significant parental figures, other losses, travel	Pressure for social participation with peers	Unusual pressure for performance, damage to self-esteem, feelings of lack of competence
Peer relationships	Good when no separation is involved	Tentative, overly inhibited	Overly eager to please, peers sought out and dependent relationships established
Sleep	Reluctance or refusal to go to sleep, fear of dark, nightmares	Difficulty in falling asleep at times	Difficulty in falling asleep
Psychophysiological symptoms	Complaints of stomachaches, nausea, vomiting, flu-like symptoms, headaches, palpitations, dizziness, faintness	Blushing, body tension	Stomachaches, nausea, vomiting, lump in the throat, shortness of breath, dizziness, palpitations
Differential diagnosis	Generalized anxiety disorder, schizophrenia, depressive disorders, conduct disorder, pervasive developmental disorders, major depressive disorder, panic disorder with agoraphobia	Adjustment disorder with depressed mood, generalized anxiety disorder, separation anxiety disorder, major depressive disorder, dysthymic disorder, avoidant personality disorder, borderline personality disorder	Separation anxiety disorder, attention-deficit/hyperactivity disorder, social phobia, adjustment disorder with anxiety, obsessive-compulsive disorder, psychotic disorders, mood disorders

Adapted from Sidney Werkman, M.D.

symptoms, and the development of comorbid anxiety and depressive disorders. Young children who experience the disorder but are able to maintain attendance in school generally have a better prognosis than adolescents with the disorder who refuse to attend school for long periods. Most children who recovered did so within the first year. Early age of onset and later age at diagnosis were factors that predicted slower recovery. Close to one-third of the group studied, however, had developed another psychiatric disorder within the follow-up period, and 50 percent of these children developed another anxiety disorder. Reports have indicated a significant overlap of separation anxiety disorder and depressive disorders. In these complicated cases, the prognosis is guarded.

TREATMENT

A multimodal treatment plan—including cognitive-behavioral therapy, family education, and family psychosocial intervention—is recommended in the initial management of separation anxiety disorder. Pharmacologic interventions are recommended when additional strategies are needed to control the symptoms. Cognitive-behavioral therapy is currently widely recommended as a first-line treatment for a variety of anxiety disorders for children, including separation anxiety disorder. Specific cognitive strategies and relaxation exercises are also components of treatment for some children to provide them with mechanisms that they can incorporate to control their anxiety. Family interventions can be critical in the management of separation anxiety disorder, especially in children who refuse to attend school, so that firm encouragement of school attendance is maintained while appropriate support is also provided.

Pharmacotherapy with selective serotonin reuptake inhibitors (SSRIs) has been demonstrated to be efficacious in the treatment of anxiety disorders in children. [Paroxetine (Paxil) should not be used in children.] β-Adrenergic receptor antagonists, such as propranolol (Inderal) and buspirone (BuSpar), have been used clinically in children with anxiety disorders, but there are currently no data to support their efficacy. Diphenhydramine (Benadryl) may be used in the short-term to control sleep disturbances in children with anxiety disorders. Alprazolam (Xanax), a benzodiazepine, may also be helpful in controlling anxiety symptoms in separation anxiety disorder. Clonazepam (Klonopin) may be useful in controlling symptoms of panic and other anxiety.

School refusal associated with separation anxiety disorder may be viewed as a psychiatric emergency. A comprehensive treatment plan involves the child, the parents, and the child's peers and school. The child should be encouraged to attend school, but when a return to a full school day is overwhelming, a program should be arranged for the child to progressively increase his or her time spent at school. Graded contact with an object of anxiety is a form of behavior modification that can be applied to any type of separation anxiety. In some severe cases of school refusal, hospitalization is required. Cognitive-behavioral modalities can be used in psychotherapy, including exposure to feared separations and cognitive strategies such as coping self-statements aimed at increasing a sense of autonomy and mastery.

▲ 44.2 Selective Mutism

Selective mutism is a childhood condition in which a child remains completely silent, or near silent, in social situations, most typically in school. Most children with the disorder are completely silent during the stressful situations, whereas others whisper or use single-syllable words. Children with selective mutism have the full ability to speak competently when not in a socially stressful situation. Some children with the disorder communicate with eye contact or nonverbal gestures. These children speak fluently in other situations, such as at home and in certain familiar settings. Selective mutism is believed to be a form of social phobia, due to its expression in selective social situations.

EPIDEMIOLOGY

The prevalence of selective mutism has been estimated to range between 3 and 8 per 10,000 children. More recent surveys indicate that it may be more common, emerging in more than 0.5 percent of school children in the community. Young children are more vulnerable to the disorder than older children. Selective mutism appears to be more common in girls than in boys.

ETIOLOGY

Although selective mutism is a psychologically determined inhibition or refusal to speak, many children with the disorder have histories of delayed onset of speech or speech abnormalities that may be contributory. In a recent survey, 90 percent of children with selective mutism met diagnostic criteria for social phobia. These children showed high levels of social anxiety without notable psychopathology in other areas, according to parent and teacher ratings. Thus, selective mutism may not represent a distinct disorder but may be better conceptualized as a subtype of social phobia. Similar to families with children who exhibit other anxiety disorders, maternal anxiety, depression, and heightened dependence needs are often noted in families of children with selective mutism. These factors may result in maternal overprotection and an overly close but ambivalent relationship between a mother and her selectively mute child. Children with selective mutism usually speak freely at home; they have no significant biological disability. Some children seem predisposed to selective mutism after early emotional or physical trauma; therefore, some clinicians refer to the phenomenon as *traumatic mutism* rather than selective mutism.

DIAGNOSIS AND CLINICAL FEATURES

The diagnosis of selective mutism is not difficult to make after it is clear that a child has adequate language skills in some environments but not in others (Table 44.2–1). The mutism may have developed gradually or suddenly after a disturbing experience. The age of onset can range from 4 to 8 years. Mute periods are most commonly manifested in school or outside the home; in rare cases, a child is mute at home but not in school. Children who exhibit selective mutism may also have symp-

Table 44.2–1
DSM-IV-TR Diagnostic Criteria for
Selective Mutism

A. Consistent failure to speak in specific social situations (in which there is an expectation for speaking, e.g., at school) despite speaking in other situations.

B. The disturbance interferes with educational or occupational achievement or with social communication.

C. The duration of the disturbance is at least 1 month (not limited to the first month of school).

D. The failure to speak is not due to a lack of knowledge of, or comfort with, the spoken language required in the social situation.

E. The disturbance is not better accounted for by a communication disorder (e.g., stuttering) and does not occur exclusively during the course of a pervasive developmental disorder, schizophrenia, or other psychotic disorder.

From American Psychiatric Association. *Diagnostic and Statistical Manual of Mental Disorders*. 4th ed. Text rev. Washington, DC: American Psychiatric Association; copyright 2000, with permission.

including selective mutism, remit with or without treatment. With recent data suggesting that fluoxetine (Prozac) may influence the course of selective mutism, recovery may be enhanced. Most cases last for only a few weeks or months, but some cases persist for years. Children who do not improve by age 10 appear to have a long-term course and a worse prognosis than those who do improve by age 10. As many as one-third of children with selective mutism, with or without treatment, may develop other psychiatric disorders, particularly other anxiety disorders and depression.

TREATMENT

A multimodal approach using individual, cognitive-behavioral, behavioral, and family interventions is recommended. Preschool children may also benefit from a therapeutic nursery. For school-age children, individual cognitive-behavioral therapy is recommended as a first-line treatment. Family education and cooperation are beneficial. Selective serotonin reuptake inhibitor (SSRI) medication is now an accepted component of treatment when psychosocial interventions are not sufficient to manage symptoms.

toms of separation anxiety disorder, school refusal, and delayed language acquisition. Because social anxiety is almost always present in children with selective mutism, behavioral disturbances, such as temper tantrums and oppositional behaviors, may also occur in the home.

DIFFERENTIAL DIAGNOSIS

Shy children may exhibit a transient muteness in new, anxiety-provoking situations. These children often have histories of not speaking in the presence of strangers and of clinging to their mothers. Most children who are mute upon entering school improve spontaneously and may be described as having transient adaptational shyness. Selective mutism must also be distinguished from mental retardation, pervasive developmental disorders, and expressive language disorder. In these disorders, the symptoms are widespread, and there is not one situation in which the child communicates normally; the child may have an inability, rather than a refusal, to speak. In mutism secondary to conversion disorder, the mutism is pervasive. Children introduced into an environment in which a different language is spoken may be reticent to begin using the new language. Selective mutism should be diagnosed only when children also refuse to converse in their native language and when they have gained communicative competence in the new language but refuse to speak it.

COURSE AND PROGNOSIS

Although children with selective mutism are often abnormally shy during preschool years, the onset of the disorder is usually at age 5 or 6. The most common pattern is that children speak almost exclusively at home with the nuclear family but not elsewhere, especially not at school. Consequently, they may have academic difficulties and even failure. Children with selective mutism are generally shy, anxious, and vulnerable to the development of depression. Most children with mild forms of anxiety disorder,

▲ 44.3 Reactive Attachment Disorder of Infancy or Early Childhood

According to the text revision of the fourth edition of *Diagnostic and Statistical Manual of Mental Disorders* (DSM-IV-TR), reactive attachment disorder of infancy or early childhood is marked by an inappropriate social relatedness that occurs in most contexts. The disorder appears before the age of 5 years and is associated with "grossly pathological care." It is not accounted for solely by a developmental delay and does not meet the criteria for pervasive developmental disorder. The pattern of care may exhibit lasting disregard for a child's emotional or physical needs or repeated changes of caregivers, as when a child is frequently relocated during foster care. The pathological care pattern is believed to cause the disturbance in social relatedness.

The disorder has two subtypes: the inhibited type, in which the disturbance takes the form of constantly failing to initiate and respond to most social interactions in a developmentally normal way; and the disinhibited type, in which the disturbance takes the form of undifferentiated, unselective social relatedness.

The disorder may result in a picture of failure to thrive, in which an infant shows physical signs of malnourishment and does not exhibit the expected developmental motor and verbal milestones. When this is the case, the failure to thrive is coded on Axis III.

EPIDEMIOLOGY

No specific data on the prevalence, sex ratio, or familial pattern are currently available. Although patients with reactive attachment disorder of infancy or early childhood come from all socioeconomic groups, studies of some patients (such as infants with failure to thrive) indicate an increased vulnerability among those from low socioeconomic levels.

ETIOLOGY

The cause of reactive attachment disorder of infancy or early childhood is included in the disorder's definition. Reactive attachment disorder is linked to maltreatment, including neglect and possible physical abuse as well. In evaluating a patient for whom such a diagnosis is appropriate, however, clinicians should consider the contributions of each member of the caregiver–child dyad and their interactions. Clinicians should weigh such things as infant or child temperament, deficient or defective bonding, a developmentally disabled or sensorially impaired child, and a particular caregiver–child mismatch. The likelihood of neglect increases with parental mental retardation; lack of parenting skills because of personal upbringing, social isolation, or deprivation and lack of opportunities to learn about caregiving behavior; and premature parenthood (during early and middle adolescence), in which parents are unable to respond to and care for an infant's needs and in which the parents' own needs take precedence over their infant's or child's needs.

DIAGNOSIS AND CLINICAL FEATURES

Children with reactive attachment disorder of infancy or early childhood often first come to the attention of a pediatrician. The clinical picture varies greatly according to a child's chronological and mental ages, but expected social interaction and liveliness are not present. Perhaps the most typical clinical picture of an infant with the disorder is the nonorganic failure to thrive. They may exhibit delayed responsiveness to a stimulus that would elicit fright or withdrawal from a normal infant (Table 44.3–1). Most infants appear significantly malnourished, and many have protruding abdomens. Occasionally, foul-smelling, celiac-like stools are reported. In unusually severe cases, a clinical picture of marasmus appears.

An infant's weight is often below the third percentile and markedly below the appropriate weight for his or her height. Laboratory findings are usually within normal limits, except for abnormal findings coincident with any malnutrition, dehydration, or concurrent illness. Growth hormone levels are usually normal or elevated, a finding suggesting that growth failure in these children is secondary to caloric deprivation and malnutrition. The children improve physically and gain weight rapidly after they are hospitalized.

Classic psychosocial dwarfism or psychosocially determined short stature is a syndrome that usually is first manifest in children 2 to 3 years of age. The children are typically unusually short and have frequent growth hormone abnormalities and severe behavioral disturbances. All of these symptoms are the result of an inimical caregiver–child relationship.

A 26-month-old girl, recently placed in foster care, was referred by state child protective services with her biological and foster families to assist with long-term case management. Her history included two admissions for failure to thrive in the first year of life and a third admission at 13 months that revealed retinal hemorrhage and a subdural hematoma from suspected shaken baby syndrome. No perpetrator was conclusively identified. When seen with her biological mother in a comfortable, toy-filled room, she stood completely still and maintained little facial expression. She complied completely and in rote fashion with her mother's often-angry instructions, maintaining no sustained eye contact with either her mother or the examiner. When briefly separated from her mother, she showed little reaction, looking up briefly with an odd grimace when her mother returned to the room. Her mother confirmed that her behavior had been similar when she had lived in her home; the child spoke infrequently and rarely sought comfort when distressed. When seen with her foster mother of 3 months, she was markedly more animated, although frequently irritable. She engaged in play freely and referenced both her foster mother and the examiner during play. She stopped playing and stared blankly when separated from her foster mother, although she actively reengaged her foster mother upon her return. The biological mother's parental rights were eventually terminated, and, although the child was placed in two more homes, she showed the capacity to engage with her new caregivers each time. The girl was diagnosed with reactive attachment disorder, inhibited type. (Courtesy of Neil W. Boris, M.D., and Charles H. Zeanah, M.D.)

Pathology and Laboratory Examination

Although no single specific laboratory test is used to make a diagnosis, many children with the disorder have disturbances of growth and development. Therefore, establishing a growth curve and examining the progression of developmental milestones may be helpful in determining whether associated phenomena, such as failure to thrive, are present.

DIFFERENTIAL DIAGNOSIS

Metabolic disorders, pervasive developmental disorders, mental retardation, various severe neurological abnormalities, and psychosocial dwarfism are the primary considerations in the differential diagnosis. Children with autistic disorder are typically well nourished and of age-appropriate size and weight; they are generally alert and active, despite their impairments in reciprocal social interactions. Moderate, severe, or profound mental retardation is present in approximately 50 percent of children with autistic disorder, whereas most children with reactive attachment disorder of infancy or early childhood are only mildly retarded or have normal intelligence. No evidence indicates that autistic disorder is caused by parental pathology, and most parents of autistic children do not differ significantly from the parents of normal children. Unlike most children with reactive attachment disorder, children with autistic disorder do not improve rapidly if they are removed from their homes and placed in a hospital or other favorable environment. Mentally retarded children may show delays in all social skills. Such children, unlike children with reactive attachment disorder, are usually adequately nourished, their social relatedness is appropriate to their mental age, and they show a sequence of development similar to that seen in normal children.

Table 44.3–1
DSM-IV-TR Diagnostic Criteria for Reactive Attachment Disorder of Infancy or Early Childhood

A. Markedly disturbed and developmentally inappropriate social relatedness in most contexts, beginning before age 5 years, as evidenced by either (1) or (2):

(1) persistent failure to initiate or respond in a developmentally appropriate fashion to most social interactions, as manifest by excessively inhibited, hypervigilant, or highly ambivalent and contradictory responses (e.g., the child may respond to caregivers with a mixture of approach, avoidance, and resistance to comforting, or may exhibit frozen watchfulness)

(2) diffuse attachments as manifest by indiscriminate sociability with marked inability to exhibit appropriate selective attachments (e.g., excessive familiarity with relative strangers or lack of selectivity in choice of attachment figures)

B. The disturbance in Criterion A is not accounted for solely by developmental delay (as in mental retardation) and does not meet criteria for a pervasive developmental disorder.

C. Pathogenic care as evidenced by at least one of the following:

(1) persistent disregard of the child's basic emotional needs for comfort, stimulation, and affection

(2) persistent disregard of the child's basic physical needs

(3) repeated changes of primary caregiver that prevent formation of stable attachments (e.g., frequent changes in foster care)

D. There is a presumption that the care in Criterion C is responsible for the disturbed behavior in Criterion A (e.g., the disturbances in Criterion A began following the pathogenic care in Criterion C).

Specify type:

Inhibited type: if Criterion A1 predominates in the clinical presentation

Disinhibited type: if Criterion A2 predominates in the clinical presentation

From American Psychiatric Association. *Diagnostic and Statistical Manual of Mental Disorders.* 4th ed. Text rev. Washington, DC: American Psychiatric Association; copyright 2000, with permission.

COURSE AND PROGNOSIS

The course and prognosis of reactive attachment disorder depend on the duration and severity of the neglectful and pathogenic parenting and on associated complications such as failure to thrive. Constitutional and nutritional factors interact in children who may either respond resiliently to treatment or continue to fail to thrive. Outcomes range from the extremes of death to the developmentally healthy child. In general, the longer a child remains in the adverse environment without adequate intervention, the more the physical and emotional damage and the worse the prognosis. For children who have multiple problems stemming from pathogenic caregiving, their physical recovery may be faster and more complete than their emotional well-being.

TREATMENT

The first consideration in treating reactive attachment disorder is a child's safety. The first decision is often whether to hospitalize the child or to attempt treatment while the child remains in the home. Usually, the severity of the child's physical and emotional state or the severity of the pathological caregiving determines the strategy. A determination must be made regarding the nutritional status of the child and whether there is ongoing physical abuse or threat. For cases in which malnourishment has occurred, hospitalization is necessary.

Along with an assessment of the child's physical well-being, an evaluation of the child's emotional condition is important. The treatment team must begin to alter the unsatisfactory relationship between the caregiver and the child. Doing so usually requires extensive and intensive intervention and education with the mother or with both parents when possible. Possible interventions include, but are not limited to, the following: psychosocial support services, including hiring a homemaker, improving the physical condition of the apartment or obtaining more adequate housing, improving the family's financial status and decreasing the family's isolation; psychotherapeutic interventions, including individual psychotherapy, psychotropic medications, and family or marital therapy; educational counseling services, including mother–infant or mother–toddler groups, and counseling to increase awareness and understanding of the child's needs and to increase parenting skills; and provisions for close monitoring of the progression of the patient's emotional and physical well-being.

▲ 44.4 Stereotypic Movement Disorder and Disorder of Infancy, Childhood, or Adolescence Not Otherwise Specified

STEREOTYPIC MOVEMENT DISORDER

According to the text revision of the fourth edition of *Diagnostic and Statistical Manual of Mental Disorders* (DSM-IV-TR), stereotypic movement disorder is repetitive, nonfunctional motor behavior that seems to be compulsive. The behavior significantly interferes with normal activities or produces self-inflicted bodily injuries severe enough to need medical care unless the child is protected. For children with mental retardation, the injurious behavior is dangerous enough to become the focus of treatment.

Epidemiology

The prevalence of stereotypic movement disorder is unknown. Deciding which cases are severe enough to confirm a diagnosis of stereotypic movement disorder may be difficult.

The diagnosis is a compilation of many symptoms, and various behaviors must be studied separately to obtain data about prevalence, sex ratio, and familial patterns. It is clear, however, that stereotypic movement disorder is more prevalent in boys than in girls. Stereotypic behaviors are common among children who are mentally retarded; 10 to 20 percent are affected.

Self-injurious behaviors occur in some genetic syndromes, such as Lesch-Nyhan syndrome, and are also present in some patients with Tourette's disorder. Self-injurious stereotypic behaviors are increasingly common in people with severe mental retardation. Stereotypic behaviors are also common in children with sensory impairments such as blindness and deafness.

Etiology

The cause of stereotypic movements is unknown and is likely to be multidetermined because of the wide range of behaviors that fall under this category. The progression from what are perhaps vicissitudes of normal development to stereotypic movement disorder is believed to reflect disordered development, as in mental retardation or a pervasive developmental disorder. Genetic factors are likely to play a role in some stereotypic movements such as in the X-linked recessive deficiency of enzymes leading to Lesch-Nyhan syndrome. In this syndrome, there are predictable features, including mental retardation, hyperuricemia, spasticity, and self-injurious behaviors. Other stereotypic movements (such as nail biting), although often causing minimal or no impairment, seem to run in the families. Some stereotypic behaviors seem to emerge or become exaggerated in situations of neglect or deprivation. Such behaviors as head banging have been associated with psychosocial deprivation.

Stereotypic movements seem to be associated with dopamine activity. Neurobiological factors may contribute to the development of stereotypic movement disorders. Dopamine agonists induce or increase stereotypic behaviors, whereas dopamine antagonists decrease them. Endogenous opioids also have been implicated in the production of self-injurious behaviors.

Diagnosis and Clinical Features

Affected people may suffer from one or more symptoms of stereotypic movement disorder; thus, the clinical picture varies considerably. Most commonly, one symptom predominates. The presence of several severe symptoms tends to occur among those most severely afflicted with mental retardation or a pervasive development disorder. Patients frequently have other significant mental disorders, especially disruptive behavior disorders.

In extreme cases, severe mutilation and life-threatening injuries may result, and secondary infection and septicemia may follow self-inflicted trauma. The DSM-IV-TR diagnostic criteria for stereotypic movement disorder are listed in Table 44.4–1.

Head Banging.   Head banging is an example of a stereotypic movement disorder that can result in functional impairment. Typically, head banging begins during infancy, between 6 and 12 months of age. The head banging is often transitory but sometimes persists into middle childhood.

Head banging that is a component of temper tantrums is different from stereotypic head banging and ceases after the tantrums and their secondary gains have been controlled.

Nail Biting.   Nail biting begins as early as 1 year of age and increases in incidence until 12 years of age. All of the nails are usually bitten. Most cases are not sufficiently severe to meet the DSM-IV-TR diagnostic criteria. Nail biting seems to occur or increase in intensity when a person is either anxious or bored.

Table 44.4–1
DSM-IV-TR Diagnostic Criteria for Stereotypic Movement Disorder

A. Repetitive, seemingly driven, and nonfunctional motor behavior (e.g., hand shaking or waving, body rocking, head banging, mouthing of objects, self-biting, picking at skin or bodily orifices, hitting own body).

B. The behavior markedly interferes with normal activities or results in self-inflicted bodily injury that requires medical treatment (or would result in an injury if preventive measures were not used).

C. If mental retardation is present, the stereotypic or self-injurious behavior is of sufficient severity to become a focus of treatment.

D. The behavior is not better accounted for by a compulsion (as in obsessive-compulsive disorder), a tic (as in tic disorder), a stereotypy that is part of a pervasive developmental disorder, or hair pulling (as in trichotillomania).

E. The behavior is not due to the direct physiological effects of a substance or a general medical condition.

F. The behavior persists for 4 weeks or longer.

Specify if:

   With self-injurious behavior: if the behavior results in bodily damage that requires specific treatment (or that would result in bodily damage if protective measures were not used)

From American Psychiatric Association. *Diagnostic and Statistical Manual of Mental Disorders.* 4th ed. Text rev. Washington, DC: American Psychiatric Association; copyright 2000, with permission.

Some of the most severe nail biting occurs in those who are severely and profoundly mentally retarded and in some patients with paranoid schizophrenia. Some nail biters, however, have no obvious emotional disturbance.

Differential Diagnosis

The differential diagnosis of stereotypic movement disorder includes obsessive-compulsive disorder (OCD) and tic disorders, both of which are exclusionary criteria in DSM-IV-TR. Although stereotypic movements are voluntary and not spasmodic, it is difficult to differentiate these features from tics in all cases. Stereotypic movements are likely to be comforting, whereas tics are often associated with distress. In OCD, the compulsions must be ego-dystonic, although it, too, is difficult to discern in young children.

Differentiating dyskinetic movements from stereotypic movements can be difficult. Because antipsychotic medications can suppress stereotypic movements, clinicians must note any stereotypic movements before initiating treatment with an antipsychotic agent. Stereotypic movement disorder may be diagnosed concurrently with substance-related disorders (for example, amphetamine use disorders), severe sensory impairments, central nervous system (CNS) and degenerative disorders (for example, Lesch-Nyhan syndrome), and severe schizophrenia.

Course and Prognosis

The duration and course of stereotypic movement disorder are variable, and the symptoms may wax and wane. As many as 80 percent of normal children show rhythmic activities that seem to

Table 44.4–2
DSM-IV-TR Diagnostic Criteria for Disorder of Infancy, Childhood, or Adolescence Not Otherwise Specified

This category is a residual category for disorders with onset in infancy, childhood, or adolescence that do not meet criteria for any specific disorder in the classification.

From American Psychiatric Association. *Diagnostic and Statistical Manual of Mental Disorders.* 4th ed. Text rev. Washington, DC: American Psychiatric Association; copyright 2000, with permission.

be purposeful and comforting and tend to disappear by 4 years of age. When stereotypic movements are present or emerge more severely later in childhood or in a noncomforting manner, they range from brief episodes occurring under stress to an ongoing pattern in the context of a chronic condition, such as mental retardation or a pervasive developmental disorder. Even in chronic conditions, the emergence of stereotypic behaviors may come and go. In some cases, stereotypic movements are prominent in early childhood and diminish as a child gets older.

The severity of the dysfunction caused by stereotypic movements also varies with the associated frequency, amounts, and degree of self-injury. Children who exhibit frequent, severe, self-injurious stereotypic behaviors have the poorest prognosis. Although chronic stereotypic movement disorders can severely impair daily functioning, several treatments help control the symptoms.

Treatment

Treatment should be related to the specific symptom or symptoms being treated, their causes, and the patient's mental age.

Treatment modalities yielding the most promising effects have been behavioral and pharmacological, sometimes used in combination. In extreme situations in which environmental deprivation is deemed a factor, the psychosocial environment must be adjusted. Behavioral techniques, including reinforcement and behavioral shaping, are successful in some cases. For instances in which severe physical damage occurs, especially in people who are severely retarded, psychopharmacology must be considered.

The dopamine antagonists are the most commonly used medications for treating stereotypic movements and self-injurious behavior. Phenothiazines have been the most frequently used drugs. Opiate antagonists have reduced self-injurious behaviors in some patients without exposing them to tardive dyskinesia or impaired cognition.

Additional pharmacological agents that have been tried in the treatment of stereotypic movement disorder include fenfluramine (Pondimin), clomipramine (Anafranil), and fluoxetine (Prozac). In some reports, fenfluramine diminished stereotypic behaviors in children with autistic disorder; in other studies, the results were less encouraging. Open trials indicate that both clomipramine and fluoxetine may decrease self-injurious behaviors and other stereotypic movements in some patients. Trazodone (Desyrel) and buspirone (BuSpar) have also been tried with unclear results.

DISORDER OF INFANCY, CHILDHOOD, OR ADOLESCENCE NOT OTHERWISE SPECIFIED

DSM-IV-TR describes disorder of infancy, childhood, or adolescence not otherwise specified as a category including disorders with onset in infancy, childhood, or adolescence that do not meet the criteria for any specific disorder. The DSM-IV-TR diagnostic criteria are shown in Table 44.4–2.

45

Mood Disorders and Suicide in Children and Adolescents

MOOD DISORDERS

Mood disorders appear in children of all ages, consisting of enduring patterns of disturbed mood; diminished enthusiasm in play activities, sports, friendships, or school; and a general feeling of worthlessness. The core features of major depression are similar in children, adolescents, and adults, with the expression of these features modified to match the age and maturity of the individual.

Two criteria for mood disorders in childhood and adolescence are a disturbance of mood, such as depression or elation, and irritability. Mood disorders in adults are reviewed in detail in Chapter 12. Only those issues that pertain specifically to children and adolescents are discussed here.

Although the text revision of the fourth edition of the *Diagnostic and Statistical Manual of Mental Disorders* (DSM-IV-TR) diagnostic criteria for mood disorders are almost identical across all age groups, the expression of disturbed mood varies in children according to their ages. Young, depressed children commonly show symptoms that appear less often as they grow older, including mood-congruent auditory hallucinations, somatic complaints, withdrawn, sad appearance, and poor self-esteem. Symptoms that are more common among depressed youngsters in late adolescence than in young childhood are pervasive anhedonia, severe psychomotor retardation, delusions, and a sense of hopelessness. Symptoms that appear with the same frequency regardless of age and developmental status include suicidal ideation, depressed or irritable mood, insomnia, and diminished ability to concentrate.

Epidemiology

Mood disorders increase with increasing age, and prevalence in any age group is drastically higher in psychiatrically referred groups than in the general population. Mood disorders in preschool-age children are extremely rare. Depression is more common in boys than in girls among school-age children. Some bias may be present in the clinic reports, as boys outnumber girls in psychiatric clinics. Among hospitalized children and adolescents, the rates of major depressive disorder are much higher than in the general community. Dysthymic disorder is estimated to be more common than major depressive disorder among school-age children. For school-age children with dysthymic disorder, there is a high likelihood that major depressive disorder will develop at some point after 1 year of the dysthy-

mic disorder. In adolescents, as in adults, dysthymic disorder is less common than major depressive disorder.

The rate of bipolar I disorder is exceedingly low in prepubertal children and may take years to be diagnosed, because mania typically appears for the first time in adolescence.

Etiology

Considerable evidence indicates that the mood disorders in childhood are the same fundamental diseases experienced by adults.

Genetic Factors. Mood disorders in children, adolescents, and adult patients tend to cluster in the same families. An increased incidence of mood disorders is generally found among children of parents with mood disorders and relatives of children with mood disorders. Having two depressed parents probably quadruples the risk of a child's having a mood disorder before age 18 when compared with the risk for children with two unaffected parents.

Other Biological Factors. Studies of prepubertal major depressive disorder and adolescent mood disorder have revealed biological abnormalities. Prepubertal children in an episode of depressive disorder secrete significantly more growth hormone during sleep than normal children and those with nondepressed mental disorders. These children also secrete significantly less growth hormone in response to insulin-induced hypoglycemia than nondepressed patients. Both abnormalities have been found to persist for at least 4 months of full, sustained clinical response, the last month in a drug-free state.

The dexamethasone-suppression test is used in childhood and adolescence but not as frequently or as reliably as in adults. Sleep studies are inconclusive in depressed children and adolescents. Polysomnography shows either no change or changes characteristic of adults with major depressive disorder: reduced rapid eye movement (REM) latency and an increased number of REM periods. A recent study evaluating magnetic resonance imaging (MRI) scans in more than 100 psychiatrically hospitalized children with mood disturbances showed a decrease in frontal lobe volume and an increase in ventricular volume. These results are consistent with MRI findings in adults with major depression.

Although values of thyroid function remain in the normative range, there is a slight downward shift in thyroid hormone in some children, possibly contributing to the clinical manifestations of depression. The evidence for adolescents is still only speculative, but dysfunction of the hypothalamic pituitary axis may also contribute to the development and maintenance of depression in certain teenagers.

Social Factors.   The psychosocial deficits in depressed children improve after sustained recovery from the depression. These deficits seem to be secondary to the depression itself and may be compounded by the long duration of most dysthymic or depressive episodes, during which poorly accomplished or unaccomplished developmental tasks accumulate. Among preschoolers in whom depressive clinical presentations are described, the role of environmental influences probably will receive experimental support in the future.

Diagnosis and Clinical Features

Major Depressive Disorder.   Major depressive disorder in children is diagnosed most easily when it is acute and occurs in a child without previous psychiatric symptoms. In many cases, however, the onset is insidious, and the disorder occurs in a child who has had several years of difficulties with hyperactivity, separation anxiety disorder, or intermittent depressive symptoms.

According to the DSM-IV-TR diagnostic criteria for major depressive episode, at least five symptoms must be present for a period of 2 weeks, and there must be a change from previous functioning (see Table 12.1–2). Among the necessary symptoms is either a depressed or irritable mood or a loss of interest or pleasure. Other symptoms from which the other four diagnostic criteria are drawn include a child's failure to make expected weight gains, daily insomnia or hypersomnia, psychomotor agitation or retardation, daily fatigue or loss of energy, feelings of worthlessness or inappropriate guilt, diminished ability to think or concentrate, and recurrent thoughts of death. These symptoms must produce social or academic impairment. To meet the diagnostic criteria for major depressive disorder, the symptoms cannot be the direct effects of a substance (for example, alcohol) or a general medical condition. A diagnosis of major depressive disorder is not made within 2 months of the loss of a loved one, except when marked functional impairment, morbid preoccupation with worthlessness, suicidal ideation, psychotic symptoms, or psychomotor retardation is present.

A major depressive episode in a prepubertal child is likely to be manifest by somatic complaints, psychomotor agitation, and mood-congruent hallucinations. Anhedonia is also frequent, but anhedonia, as well as hopelessness, psychomotor retardation, and delusions, are more common in adolescent and adult major depressive episodes than in those of young children. In adolescence, negativistic or frankly antisocial behavior and the use of alcohol or illicit substances may occur and may justify the additional diagnoses of oppositional defiant disorder, conduct disorder, and substance abuse or dependence. Feelings of restlessness, grouchiness, aggression, sulkiness, reluctance to cooperate in family ventures, withdrawal from social activities, and a desire to leave home are all common in adolescent depression.

Mood disorders tend to be chronic if they begin early. Childhood onset may be the most severe form of mood disorder and tends to appear in families with a high incidence of mood disorders and alcohol abuse. The children are likely to have such secondary complications as conduct disorder, alcohol and other substance abuse, and antisocial behavior. Functional impairment associated with a depressive disorder in childhood extends to practically all areas of a child's psychosocial world; school performance and behavior, peer relationships, and family relationships all suffer.

Children and adolescents with major depressive disorder may have hallucinations and delusions. Depressive hallucinations usually consist of a single voice speaking to the person from outside his or her head, with derogatory or suicidal content. Depressive delusions center on themes of guilt, physical disease, death, nihilism, deserved punishment, personal inadequacy, and sometimes persecution. These delusions are rare in prepuberty, probably because of cognitive immaturity, but are present in approximately one-half of all psychotically depressed adolescents.

Adolescent onset of a mood disorder may be difficult to diagnose when first seen if the adolescent has attempted self-medication with alcohol or other illicit substances. Only after detoxification could the psychiatric symptoms be assessed properly and the mood disorder diagnosed correctly.

Dysthymic Disorder.   Dysthymic disorder in children and adolescents consists of a depressed or irritable mood for most of the day, for more days than not, over a period of at least 1 year. DSM-IV-TR notes that, in children and adolescents, irritable mood can replace the depressed mood criterion for adults and that the duration criterion is not 2 years but 1 year for children and adolescents. According to the DSM-IV-TR diagnostic criteria, at least three of the following symptoms must accompany the depressed or irritable mood: poor self-esteem, pessimism or hopelessness, loss of interest, social withdrawal, chronic fatigue, feelings of guilt or brooding about the past, irritability or excessive anger, decreased activity or productivity, and poor concentration or memory. During the year of the disturbance, these symptoms do not resolve for more than 2 months at a time. In addition, no major depressive episode is present during the first year of the disturbance. To meet the DSM-IV-TR diagnostic criteria for dysthymic disorder, a child must not have a history of a manic or hypomanic episode. Dysthymic disorder is also not diagnosed if the symptoms occur exclusively during a chronic psychotic disorder or if they are the direct effects of a substance or a general medical condition. DSM-IV-TR provides for the specification of early onset (before 21 years of age) or late onset (after 21 years of age) (see Table 12.2–1).

A child or adolescent with dysthymic disorder may have had a previous major depressive episode before the onset of dysthymic disorder, but it is much more common for a child with dysthymic disorder for more than 1 year to have major depressive disorder. In this case, both depressive diagnoses are given (*double depression*). Dysthymic disorder in children is known to have an average age of onset that is several years earlier than the age of onset of major depressive disorder.

Bipolar I Disorder.   Bipolar I disorder is being diagnosed with increasing frequency in prepubertal children with the caveat that "classic" manic episodes are uncommon in this age group, even when depressive symptoms have already appeared. Since prepubertal children with features of depression and mania or hypomania do not usually exhibit discrete mood "cycles," it remains controversial whether these children actually meet diagnostic criteria for bipolar illness. Features of the mood and behavior disturbances among prepubertal children who are currently diagnosed with bipolar disorder by some clinicians include extreme mood variability, intermittent aggressive behavior, high levels of distractibility, and poor attention span. The group of children who are currently diagnosed by some clinicians with bipolar disorder function poorly, often requiring hospitalization, exhibit symptoms of depression, and often have a history of attention-deficit/hyperactivity disorder (ADHD). It remains under investigation whether these children will develop more discrete mood cycling as they mature, or whether their clinical pictures will remain the same over time. Long-term studies of children with a diagnosis are under way to see if they are bipolar when they reach adulthood.

According to DSM-IV-TR, the diagnostic criteria for a manic episode are the same for children and adolescents as for adults (see Table 12.1–3). The diagnostic criteria for a manic episode include a distinct period of an abnormally elevated, expansive, or irritable mood that lasts at least 1 week or for any duration if hospitalization is necessary. In addition, during periods of mood disturbance, at least three of the following significant and persistent symptoms must be present: inflated self-esteem or grandiosity, decreased need for sleep, pressure to talk, flight of ideas or racing thoughts, distractibility, an increase in goal-directed activity, and excessive involvement in pleasurable activities that may result in painful consequences.

When mania appears in an adolescent, there is a higher incidence than in adults of psychotic features, and hospitalization is often necessary. Delusions and hallucinations of adolescents may involve grandiose notions about their power, worth, knowledge, family, or relationships. Persecutory delusions and flight of ideas are common. Overall, gross impairment of reality testing is common in adolescent manic episodes. In adolescents with major depressive disorder destined for bipolar I disorder, those at highest risk have family histories of bipolar I disorder and exhibit acute severe depressive episodes with psychosis, hypersomnia, and psychomotor retardation.

Bereavement.   Bereavement is a state of grief related to the death of a loved one that may occur with symptoms characteristic of a major depressive episode. Typical depressive symptoms associated with bereavement include feelings of sadness, insomnia, diminished appetite, and in some cases, weight loss. Grieving children may become withdrawn and appear sad, and they are not easily drawn into even favorite activities.

In DSM-IV-TR, bereavement is not a mental disorder but is in the category of additional conditions that may be a focus of clinical attention. Children in the midst of a typical bereavement period may also meet the criteria for major depressive disorder when the symptoms persist longer than 2 months after the loss. In some instances, severe depressive symptoms within 2 months of the loss are considered to be beyond the scope of normal grieving, and a diagnosis of major depressive disorder is warranted.

Pathology and Laboratory Examination.   No single laboratory test is useful in making a diagnosis of a mood disorder. A screening test for thyroid function can rule out the possibility of an endocrinological contribution to a mood disorder. Dexamethasone-suppression tests may be performed serially in cases of major depressive disorder to document whether an initial nonsuppressor

becomes a suppressor with treatment or with resolution of the symptoms.

Differential Diagnosis

Psychotic forms of depressive and manic episodes must be differentiated from schizophrenia. Substance-induced mood disorder can sometimes be differentiated from other mood disorders only after detoxification. Anxiety symptoms and conduct-disordered behavior can coexist with depressive disorders and frequently can pose problems in differentiating those disorders from nondepressed emotional and conduct disorders.

Of particular importance is the distinction between agitated depressive or manic episodes and ADHD, in which the persistent excessive activity and restlessness can cause confusion. Prepubertal children do not show classic forms of agitated depression, such as hand wringing and pacing. Instead, an inability to sit still and frequent temper tantrums are the most common symptoms. Sometimes, the correct diagnosis becomes evident only after remission of the depressive episode. If a child has no difficulty concentrating, is not hyperactive when recovered from a depressive episode, and is in a drug-free state, ADHD probably is not present.

Course and Prognosis

The course and prognosis of mood disorders in children and adolescents depend on the age of onset, the severity of the episode, and the presence of comorbid disorders; a young age of onset and multiple disorders predict a poorer prognosis. The mean length of an episode of major depression in children and adolescents is approximately 9 months; the cumulative probability of recurrence is 40 percent by 2 years and 70 percent by 5 years. It has been reported that depressed children who live in families with high levels of chronic conflict are more likely to have relapses. Clinical characteristics of the depressive episode that are suggestive of the highest risk of developing bipolar I disorder include delusionality and psychomotor retardation in addition to a family history of bipolar illness. Dysthymic disorder has an even more protracted recovery than major depression; the mean episode length is approximately 4 years. Early-onset dysthymic disorder is associated with significant risks of comorbidity with major depression (70 percent), bipolar disorder (13 percent), and eventual substance abuse (15 percent). The risk of suicide, which represents 12 percent of mortalities in the adolescent age range, is significant among adolescents with depressive disorders.

Treatment

Hospitalization.   The important immediate consideration is often whether hospitalization is indicated to keep the child or adolescent safe or whether it is the only setting in which it is possible to initiate treatment. When a patient is suicidal, hospitalization is indicated to provide maximum protection against the patient's own self-destructive impulses and behavior. Hospitalization also may be needed when a child or adolescent has coexisting substance abuse or dependence.

Psychotherapy.   Cognitive-behavioral therapy is now widely recognized as an efficacious intervention for the treatment of moderately severe depression in children and adolescents. Cognitive-behavioral therapy aims to challenge maladaptive beliefs and enhance problem-solving abilities and social competence. Other "active" treatments, including relaxation techniques, were also shown to be helpful as adjunctive treatment for mild to moderate depression. Factors that seem to interfere with treatment responsiveness include the presence of comorbid anxiety disorder that probably was present before the depressive episode.

Family education and participation are necessary components of treatment for children with depression, especially to promote more effective conflict resolution. As depressed children's psychosocial function may remain impaired for long periods, even after the depressive episode has remitted, long-term social support from families and, in some cases, social skills interventions are helpful. Modeling and role-playing techniques can be useful in fostering good problem-solving skills.

Pharmacotherapy. The selective serotonin reuptake inhibitors (SSRIs) are widely accepted as first-line pharmacological intervention for moderate to severe depressive disorders in children and adolescents. The available SSRI medications, including fluoxetine (Prozac), sertraline (Zoloft), fluvoxamine (Luvox), and citalopram (Celexa), are favorable choices in the treatment of depression for children and adolescents. Paroxetine (Paxil) should not be used in children because it can produce agitation and suicidal impulses. Starting doses for prepubertal children are lower than doses recommended for adults, and adolescents are generally treated at the same dosages recommended for adults.

Other antidepressants, such as bupropion (Wellbutrin), a dopamine agonist, have stimulant properties as well as antidepressant efficacy, and have been used for youth with both ADHD and depression. Venlafaxine (Effexor), which blocks both serotonin and norepinephrine uptake, is also used clinically in the treatment of depression in adolescents. Mirtazapine (Remeron) is also a serotonin and norepinephrine uptake inhibitor with a relatively safe side effect profile, but it has not been used as frequently due to its side effect of sedation.

Bipolar I disorder and bipolar II disorder in childhood and adolescence are treated with lithium (Eskalith) with good results. Children with early-onset bipolar disorder and preexisting disruptive behavior disorders (for example, conduct disorder and ADHD) who experience bipolar disorders early in adolescence are less likely to respond well to lithium than those without the behavior disorders.

Electroconvulsive Therapy. Electroconvulsive therapy (ECT) has been used for a variety of psychiatric illnesses in adults, primarily severe depressive and manic mood disorders and catatonia. ECT rarely is used for adolescents, although there have been published case reports of its efficacy in adolescents with depression and mania. Currently, case reports suggest that ECT may be a relatively safe and useful treatment for adolescents with severe, treatment-resistant affective disorders with psychosis, catatonic symptoms, and persistent suicidality.

SUICIDE

Suicidal ideation, gestures, and attempts frequently are associated with depressive disorders, and these suicidal phenomena, particularly in adolescence, are a growing public mental health problem.

Suicidal ideation occurs in all age groups and with greatest frequency when the depressive disorder is severe. More than 12,000 children and adolescents are hospitalized in the United States each year because of suicidal threats or behavior, but completed suicide is rare in children younger than 12 years of age. A young child is hardly capable of designing and carrying out a realistic suicide plan. Cognitive immaturity seems to play a protective role in preventing even children who wish they were dead from committing suicide. Suicidal ideation is not a static phenomenon; it may wax and wane with time. The decision to engage in suicidal behavior may be made impulsively, without much forethought, or the decision may be the culmination of prolonged rumination.

Diagnosis and Management

Direct questioning of children and adolescents about suicidal thoughts is necessary, because studies have consistently shown that parents are frequently unaware of such ideas in their children. Suicidal thoughts (that is, children's talking about wanting to harm themselves) and suicidal threats (that is, children's statements that they want to jump in front of a car) are more common than suicide completion.

The characteristics of adolescents who attempt suicide and those who complete suicide are similar, and approximately one-third of those who completed suicide had made previous attempts. Mental disorders in some persons who attempt or complete suicide include major depressive disorder, manic episodes, and psychotic disorders. Those with mood disorders in combination with substance abuse and a history of aggressive behavior are particularly high-risk adolescents. Those without mood disorders who are violent, aggressive, and impulsive may be prone to suicide during family or peer conflicts.

Adolescents who attempt suicide must be evaluated before the decision is made regarding hospitalization or return to home. Those who fall into high-risk groups should be hospitalized until the suicidality is no longer present. High-risk persons include those who have made previous suicide attempts; those who have made an attempt with a lethal method, such as a gun or a toxic ingested substance; those with major depressive disorder characterized by social withdrawal, hopelessness, and a lack of energy; and any person who exhibits persistent suicidal ideation. A child or an adolescent with suicidal ideation must be hospitalized if a clinician has any doubt about the family's ability to supervise the child or to cooperate with treatment in an outpatient setting. In such a situation, child protective services must be involved before the child can be discharged. When adolescents with suicidal ideation report that they are no longer suicidal, discharge can be considered only after a complete discharge plan is in place. The plan must include psychotherapy, pharmacotherapy, and family therapy as indicated. A written contract with the adolescent, outlining the adolescent's agreement not to engage in suicidal behavior and providing an alternative if suicidal ideation reoccurs, should be in place. In addition, a follow-up outpatient appointment should be made before the discharge, and a telephone hot-line number should be provided to the adolescent and the family in case suicidal ideation reappears before treatment begins.

The reader is referred to Chapter 30 for a further discussion on suicide.

Early-Onset Schizophrenia

Schizophrenia usually has its onset in late adolescence or early adulthood, but it does rarely present in children 10 years of age or younger. Schizophrenia with childhood onset is conceptually the same as schizophrenia in adolescence and adulthood. When schizophrenia occurs in prepubertal children, it more commonly occurs in males. It is well known that psychosocial stressors may influence the course of schizophrenia, and it is possible that the same stressors may interact with biological risk factors in the emergence of the disorder.

EPIDEMIOLOGY

Schizophrenia in prepubertal children is exceedingly rare; it is estimated to occur less frequently than autistic disorder. In adolescents, the prevalence of schizophrenia is estimated to be 50 times greater than in younger children, with probable rates of 1 to 2 per 1,000. Boys seem to have a slight preponderance among children with schizophrenia, with an estimated ratio of approximately 1.67 boys to 1 girl. Boys often become symptomatic at a younger age than girls. Schizophrenia rarely is diagnosed in children younger than 5 years of age. The symptoms usually emerge insidiously, and the diagnostic criteria are met gradually over time. Occasionally, the onset of schizophrenia is sudden and occurs in a previously well-functioning child. Schizophrenia also may be diagnosed in a child who has had chronic difficulties and then experiences a significant exacerbation.

Schizotypal personality disorder is similar to schizophrenia in its inappropriate affects, excessive magical thinking, odd beliefs, social isolation, ideas of reference, and unusual perceptual experiences, such as illusions. Schizotypal personality disorder, however, does not have psychotic features; still, the disorder seems to aggregate in families with adult-onset schizophrenia. Therefore, there is an unclear relation between the two disorders.

ETIOLOGY

Although family and genetic studies provide substantial evidence of a biological contribution to the development of schizophrenia, no specific biological markers have been identified, and the precise mechanisms of transmission of schizophrenia are not understood. Schizophrenia is significantly more prevalent among first-degree relatives of those with schizophrenia than in the general population. Adoption studies of patients with adult-onset schizophrenia have shown that schizophrenia occurs in the biological relatives, not the adoptive relatives.

Additional genetic evidence is supported by the higher concordance rates for schizophrenia in monozygotic twins than in dizygotic twins.

Higher-than-expected rates of neurological soft signs and impairments in sustaining attention and in strategies for information processing appear among high-risk groups of children. Increased rates of disturbed communication styles are found in families with a patient with schizophrenia. High expressed emotion, characterized by overly critical responses in families, negatively affects the prognosis of patients with schizophrenia.

Various abnormal, nonspecific results on computed tomography (CT) scans and electroencephalograms (EEGs) have been noted in patients with schizophrenia. Children and adolescents with schizophrenia are more apt to have a premorbid history of social rejection, poor peer relationships, clingy withdrawn behavior, and academic trouble than those with adult-onset schizophrenia. Some children with schizophrenia that is first seen in middle childhood have early histories of motor milestones and delayed language acquisition that are similar to some symptoms of autistic disorder. The mechanisms of biological vulnerability and environmental influences producing manifestations of schizophrenia remain under investigation.

DIAGNOSIS AND CLINICAL FEATURES

All of the symptoms included in adult-onset schizophrenia may be manifest in children with the disorder. The onset is frequently insidious; after first exhibiting inappropriate affects of unusual behavior, a child may take months or years to meet all of the diagnostic criteria for schizophrenia. Children who eventually meet the criteria often are socially rejected and clingy and have limited social skills.

According to the text revision of the fourth edition of the *Diagnostic and Statistical Manual of Mental Disorders* (DSM-IV-TR), a child with schizophrenia may experience a deterioration of function, along with the emergence of psychotic symptoms, or the child may never achieve the expected level of functioning (see Table 10–2). Auditory hallucinations are commonly manifest in children with schizophrenia. They may hear several voices making an ongoing critical commentary, or command hallucinations may tell children to kill themselves or others. Visual hallucinations are experienced by a significant number of children with schizophrenia and often are frightening; the children may see the devil, skeletons, scary faces, or space creatures. Transient phobic visual hallucinations also occur in traumatized children who do not eventually have a major psychotic disorder.

Delusions are present in more than one-half of all children with schizophrenia; the delusions take various forms, including persecutory, grandiose, and religious. Delusions increase in frequency with increased age. Blunted or inappropriate affects are almost universally present in children with schizophrenia. Children with schizophrenia may giggle inappropriately or cry without being able to explain why. Formal thought disorders, including loosening of associations and thought blocking, are common features among children with schizophrenia. Illogical thinking and poverty of thought are also often present. Unlike adults with schizophrenia, children with schizophrenia do not have poverty of content of speech, but they speak less than other children of the same intelligence and are ambiguous in the way they refer to people, objects, and events. The communication deficits observable in children with schizophrenia include unpredictably changing the topic of conversation without introducing the new topic to the listener (loose associations). Children with schizophrenia also exhibit illogical thinking and speaking and tend to underuse self-initiated repair strategies to aid in their communication. Therefore, when an utterance is unclear or vague, normal children attempt to clarify their communication with repetitions, revision, and more detail. Children with schizophrenia, on the other hand, fail to aid in communication with revision, fillers, or starting over. These deficits may be conceptualized as negative symptoms in childhood schizophrenia.

DSM-IV-TR delineates five types of schizophrenia: paranoid, disorganized, catatonic, undifferentiated, and residual.

Tom was a 10-year-old boy who was referred for evaluation after he was found repeatedly dressing in his mother's clothing and demanding that he be taken to nightclubs that he believed wanted him to perform. Tom had always been a talkative child with few friends his own age, but his parents believed he was highly intelligent. As a young child, he had been socially rejected by peers but was able to relate to his teachers and other adults. When he entered the fourth grade, he began to be actively teased by his classmates, who considered him strange. Tom could still attend school, but his grades started to deteriorate because he was not as attentive as he used to be. At home, he became more and more obsessed with being a nightclub performer and seemed to be deep in thought most of the time.

Tom began to warn his mother not to go outside and believed that he and his mother were being followed. He increasingly resisted leaving his mother and began to refuse to go to school. He explained that he had been communicating with God and that he was here for a larger purpose. He admitted to hearing several voices that would argue and warn him when there was danger. He began to mistrust everyone, including his mother, but at the same time, he would not "allow" her to go to work. Tom was admitted to the children's psychiatric inpatient unit because of his inability to be separated from his mother and his persistent school refusal.

He was started on a trial of risperidone (Risperdal), 0.5 mg twice daily, which was increased to 1 mg twice daily. Tom seemed to be responding over a period of 10 days, the voices were less predominant, and he seemed to be less paranoid. He still seemed to be responding to internal stimuli and held on to the belief that he was a nightclub performer. He had developed troubling akathisia and required benztropine (Cogentin), 0.5 mg twice daily, in addition to the risperidone. After continuing his titration of risperidone and benztropine for approximately 2 weeks, Tom developed a severe dystonic reaction. After the dystonic reaction, Tom's mother refused to allow him to receive risperidone again and requested that another medication be tried. The treatment team agreed that Tom was unable to tolerate a therapeutic dose of risperidone, and use of olanzapine (Zyprexa) was started at 2.5 mg per day. Tom did well on olanzapine, which was increased over time to 7.5 mg per day with good response and virtually no adverse effects aside from mild sedation. Given Tom's deterioration in function over the last year, persistence of auditory hallucinations, and the delusion that he was a performer for more than a 6-month period, a diagnosis of schizophrenia was made. Tom was referred to attend a small, structured, therapeutic day-treatment school program in which he received more individualized educational programming and social skills interventions. Tom was able to attend this school, since he liked the staff, and over time, he improved his social skills with his classmates.

DIFFERENTIAL DIAGNOSIS

Children with schizotypal personality disorder have some traits in common with children who meet diagnostic criteria for schizophrenia. Blunted affect, social isolation, eccentric thoughts, ideas of reference, and bizarre behavior may be seen in both disorders; however, in schizophrenia, overt psychotic symptoms such as hallucinations, delusions, and incoherence must be present at some point. When they are present, they exclude a diagnosis of schizotypal personality disorder. Hallucinations alone, however, are not evidence of schizophrenia; patients must show either a deterioration of function or an inability to meet an expected developmental level to warrant the diagnosis of schizophrenia.

Psychotic phenomena are common among children with major depressive disorder, in which both hallucinations and, less commonly, delusions may occur. The congruence of mood with psychotic features is most pronounced in depressed children, although children with schizophrenia may also seem sad. The hallucinations and delusions of schizophrenia are more likely to have a bizarre quality than those of children with depressive disorders. In children and adolescents with bipolar I disorder, it often is difficult to distinguish a first episode of mania with psychotic features from schizophrenia if the child has no history of previous depressions. Grandiose delusions and hallucinations are typical of manic episodes, but clinicians often must follow the natural history of the disorder to confirm the presence of a mood disorder. Pervasive developmental disorders, including autistic disorder with normal intelligence, may share some features with schizophrenia. Most notably, difficulty with social relationships, an early history of delayed language acquisition, and ongoing communication deviance are manifest in both disorders; however, hallucinations, delusions, and formal thought disorder are core features of schizophrenia and are not expected features of pervasive developmental disorders. Pervasive developmental disorders usually are diagnosed by 3 years of age, but schizophrenia with childhood onset is rarely diagnosable before 5 years of age.

The abuse of alcohol and other substances sometimes can result in a deterioration of function, psychotic symptoms, and paranoid delusions. Amphetamines, lysergic acid diethylamide (LSD), and phencyclidine (PCP) may lead to a psychotic state. A sudden, flagrant onset of paranoid psychosis is more suspicious of substance-induced psychotic disorder than an insidious onset.

Medical conditions that may induce psychotic features include thyroid disease, systemic lupus erythematosus, and temporal lobe disease.

COURSE AND PROGNOSIS

Important predictors of the course and outcome of childhood-onset schizophrenia include the child's level of functioning before the onset of schizophrenia, the age of onset, the child's degree of functioning regained after the first episode, and the degree of support available from the family. Children with developmental delays, learning disorders, and premorbid behavioral disorders, such as attention-deficit/hyperactivity disorder (ADHD) and conduct disorder, seem to be poor responders to medication treatment of schizophrenia and are likely to have the most guarded prognoses.

No clear-cut data are available regarding childhood schizophrenia, but the degree of supportiveness, as opposed to critical and overinvolved family responses, probably influences the prognosis. In general, schizophrenia with childhood onset seems to be less medication-responsive than adult-onset and adolescent-onset schizophrenia, and the prognosis may be poorer. Positive symptoms—that is, hallucinations and delusions—are likely to be more responsive to medication than are negative symptoms such as withdrawal.

TREATMENT

The treatment of schizophrenia with childhood onset involves a multimodality approach. Antipsychotic medications are indicated, given the degree of impairment in both social relationships and academic function exhibited by children with schizophrenia. Children with schizophrenia seem to have less robust responses to antipsychotic medications compared to adolescents and adults with the same disorder. Family education and ongoing family interventions are critical in order to maximize the level of support that the family can give the patient. The proper educational setting for the child is also important, because social skills deficits, attention deficits, and academic difficulties often accompany childhood schizophrenia.

Pharmacotherapy

Dopamine receptor antagonists have been largely replaced by the newer atypical antipsychotics as first-line treatments for children and adolescents with schizophrenia given their more favorable side effect profiles. These serotonin-dopamine agonists, including risperidone (Risperdal), olanzapine (Zyprexa), and clozapine (Clozaril), differ from the conventional antipsychotics in that they are serotonin receptor agonists with some dopamine type 2 (D_2) receptor activity but do not have a predominance of D_2 receptor antagonism. Additional atypical antipsychotics, such as quetiapine (Seroquel) and ziprasidone (Geodon), are also serotonin-dopamine antagonist agents and are being used in clinical practice for children and adolescents with psychotic disorders who do not respond to other atypical antipsychotics.

Psychotherapy

Psychotherapists who work with children with schizophrenia must take into account a child's developmental level. They must continually support the child's good reality testing and must have sensitivity to the child's sense of self. Long-term intensive and supportive psychotherapy combined with pharmacotherapy is the most effective approach to this disorder.

47 ▲

Adolescent Substance Abuse

Adolescent substance use and abuse remain a serious concern regarding today's youth. Estimates of nearly 25 percent have been made of illicit drug use among adolescents from 12 to 17 years of age. Approximately one-third of adolescents have used cigarettes by age 17 years. Studies of alcohol use among adolescents in the United States have shown that, by 13 years of age, one-third of boys and almost one-fourth of girls have tried alcohol.

During the past decade, several risk factors have been identified for adolescent substance abuse. These include high levels of family conflict, academic difficulties, comorbid psychiatric disorders such as conduct disorder and depression, parental and peer substance use, impulsivity, and early onset of cigarette smoking. The greater the number of risk factors, the more likely it is that an adolescent will be a substance user. Emergency room visits for substance use by teenagers have risen dramatically in this century.

EPIDEMIOLOGY

Alcohol

In a recent survey, drinking was shown to be a significant problem for 10 to 20 percent of adolescents. In the age range of 13 to 17 years, in the United States, there are 3 million problem drinkers and 300,000 adolescents with alcohol dependence. The gap between male and female alcohol consumers is narrowing. By the 12th grade, 88 percent of high school students reported drinking, and 77 percent drank within the past year.

Marijuana

Marijuana is the most widely used illicit drug among high school students. It has been termed a "gateway drug," because the strongest predictor of future cocaine use is frequent marijuana use during adolescence. Of 8th-grade, 10th-grade, and 12th-grade students, 10 percent, 23 percent, and 36 percent, respectively, report using marijuana, a slight decrease from the year preceding the survey. Of 8th-grade, 10th-grade, and 12th-grade students, 0.2 percent, 0.8 percent, and 2 percent, respectively, report daily marijuana use. Prevalence rates for marijuana are highest among Native American males and females; these rates are nearly as high in white males and females and Mexican-American males. The lowest annual rates are reported by Latin-American females, African-American females, and Asian-American males and females. Among juvenile arrests for illicit drug use in 2000, marijuana was the most commonly used drug by both males (55 percent) and females (60 percent).

Cocaine

The annual cocaine use reported by high school seniors decreased more than 30 percent between 1990 and 2000. One-tenth of a percent of high school students reported daily use of cocaine. The prevalence rates for crack cocaine use are approximately one-half those for cocaine. The prevalence rates for crack cocaine use, however, are increasing and are most common among those between the ages of 18 and 25.

Lysergic Acid Diethylamide (LSD)

Lysergic acid diethylamide (LSD) is reportedly used by 2.7 percent of 8th-grade students, 5.6 percent of 10th-grade students, and 8.8 percent of 12th-grade students. Of 12th-grade students, 0.1 percent report daily use. The current LSD rates are lower than rates of LSD use during the past 2 decades.

Inhalants

The use of inhalants in the form of glue, aerosols, and gasoline is relatively more common among younger than older adolescents. Among 8th-grade, 10th-grade, and 12th-grade students, 17.6 percent, 15.7 percent, and 17.6 percent, respectively, report using inhalants; 0.2 percent of 8th-grade students, 0.1 percent of 10th-grade students, and 0.2 percent of 12th-grade students report daily use of inhalants.

Among adolescents enrolled in substance abuse treatment programs, 96 percent are polydrug users; 97 percent of adolescents who abuse drugs also use alcohol.

ETIOLOGY

Genetic Factors

The concordance for alcoholism has been reported to be higher among monozygotic than dizygotic twins. Considerably fewer studies have been conducted of families of drug abusers. Studies of children of alcoholics reared away from their biological homes have shown that these children have approximately a 25 percent chance of becoming alcoholics.

Psychosocial Factors

A recent study concluded that children in families with the lowest measures of parental supervision and monitoring initiated alcohol, tobacco, and other drug use earlier than children from families with more supervision. The risk was greatest for children younger than 11 years of age. With more rigorous parental monitoring, young adolescents might be delayed in or prevented from initiating drug and alcohol use. Furthermore, increased supervision during middle childhood years may diminish drug and alcohol sampling and ultimately diminish the risk of using marijuana, cocaine, or inhalants in the future.

Comorbidity

Rates of alcohol and drug use are reportedly higher in relatives of children with depression and bipolar disorders. On the other hand, mood disorders are common among those with alcoholism. There is evidence of a strong link between early antisocial behavior, conduct disorder, and substance abuse. Substance abuse may be viewed as one form of behavioral deviance that, unsurprisingly, is associated with other forms of social and behavioral deviance. Early intervention with children who show early signs of social deviance and antisocial behavior may conceivably impede the processes that contribute to later substance abuse.

Comorbidity, that is, the occurrence of more than one substance use disorder or the combination of a substance use disorder and another psychiatric disorder, is common. It is important to know about all comorbid disorders, which may show differential responses to treatment.

DIAGNOSIS AND CLINICAL FEATURES

According to the text revision of the fourth edition of *Diagnostic and Statistical Manual of Mental Disorders* (DSM-IV-TR), substance-related disorders include the disorders of substance dependence, substance abuse, substance intoxication, and substance withdrawal. *Substance dependence* refers to a cluster of cognitive, behavioral, and physiological symptoms indicating that a person continues the use of a substance despite significant substance-related problems. A pattern of repeated self-administration may result in tolerance, withdrawal, and compulsive drug-taking behavior. It requires the presence of at least three symptoms of the maladaptive pattern, which can occur at any time during the same 12-month period.

Substance abuse refers to a maladaptive pattern of substance use leading to clinically significant impairment or distress, as manifest by one or more of the following symptoms within a 12-month period: recurrent substance use in situations that cause physical danger to the user, recurrent substance use in the face of obvious impairment in school or work situations, recurrent substance use despite resulting legal problems, or recurrent substance use despite social or interpersonal problems. To meet the criteria for substance abuse, the symptoms must not, now or in the past, have met the criteria for substance dependence for this class of substance.

Substance intoxication refers to the development of a reversible, substance-specific syndrome caused by use of a substance. Clinically significant maladaptive behavioral or psychological changes must be present.

Substance withdrawal refers to a substance-specific syndrome caused by the cessation of, or reduction in, prolonged substance use. The substance-specific syndrome causes clinically significant distress or impairment in social or occupational functioning.

The diagnosis of alcohol or drug use in adolescents is made through careful interview, observations, laboratory findings, and history provided by reliable sources. Many nonspecific signs may point to alcohol or drug use, and clinicians must be careful to corroborate hunches before jumping to conclusions.

TREATMENT

Treatment settings that serve adolescents with alcohol or drug use disorders include inpatient units, residential treatment facilities, halfway houses, group homes, partial hospital programs, and outpatient settings. Basic components of adolescent alcohol or drug use treatment include individual psychotherapy, drug-specific counseling, self-help groups (Alcoholics Anonymous [AA], Narcotics Anonymous [NA], Alateen, Al-Anon), substance abuse education and relapse prevention programs, and random urine drug testing. Family therapy and psychopharmacological intervention may be added.

Before deciding on the most appropriate treatment setting for a particular adolescent, a screening process must take place in which structured and unstructured interviews help to determine the types of substances being used and the quantities and frequencies. Rating scales are typically used to document pretreatment and posttreatment severity of abuse. The Teen Addiction Severity Index (T-ASI), the Adolescent Drug and Alcohol Diagnostic Assessment (ADAD), and the Adolescent Problem Severity Index (APSI) are several severity-oriented rating scales. The T-ASI is broken down into dimensions that include family function, school or employment status, psychiatric status, peer–social relationships, and legal status.

After most of the information about substance use and the patient's overall psychiatric status has been obtained, a treatment strategy must be chosen and an appropriate setting must be decided on. Two very different approaches to the treatment of substance abuse are embodied in the Minnesota model and the multidisciplinary professional model. The Minnesota model is based on the premise of AA; it is an intensive 12-step program with a counselor who functions as the primary therapist. The multidisciplinary professional model consists of a team of mental health professionals that usually is led by a physician. Following a case-management model, each member of the team has specific areas of treatment for which he or she is responsible. Interventions may include cognitive-behavioral therapy, family therapy, and pharmacological intervention. This approach usually is suited for adolescents with comorbid psychiatric diagnoses.

Cognitive-behavioral approaches to psychotherapy for adolescents with substance use generally require that adolescents be motivated to participate in treatment and refrain from further substance use. The therapy focuses on relapse prevention and maintaining abstinence.

Psychopharmacological interventions for adolescent alcohol and drug users are still in their early stages. When mood disorders are present, there are clear indications for antidepressants, and generally, the serotonin reuptake inhibitors are the first line of treatment. In certain instances, administration of a medication has been used to block the reinforcing effect of the illicit drug, for instance, giving naltrexone (ReVia) for opioid abuse. Some medications mitigate the craving or withdrawal symptoms for a drug that is no longer being used. Clonidine (Catapres) has been used transiently during heroin withdrawal. Occasionally, an intervention is made to substitute the illicit drug with another drug that is more amenable to the treatment situation, for example, using methadone instead of heroin. Adolescents are required to have two documented attempts at detoxification and consent from an adult before they can enter such a treatment program.

Efficacious treatments for cigarette smoking cessation include nicotine-containing gum, patches, or nasal spray or inhaler. Bupropion (Zyban) has been shown to aid in diminishing cravings for nicotine and is beneficial in the treatment of smoking cessation.

Because comorbidity influences treatment outcome, it is important to pay attention to other disorders such as mood disorders, anxiety disorders, conduct disorder, or attention-deficit/hyperactivity disorder (ADHD) during the treatment of substance use disorders.

Fred is a 16-year-old male admitted to substance abuse treatment for the second time, following a relapse and threats of suicide. He was initially admitted to an inpatient program after a serious suicide attempt. He reported a long history of disruptive behavior and academic failure since childhood. He was increasingly truant and difficult for his family to control. During his first treatment episode, he reported an onset of substance use at age 11 years, rapid progression in substance involvement since age 13 years, then current use of marijuana on a daily basis, drinking alcohol up to several times a week, frequent trips on LSD, and experimentation with a variety of substances. Fred attended group sessions focusing on his initial denial of a substance use problem and then learned the process of recovery while attending other groups and AA and NA meetings. Family group sessions showed him and his parents the need for better communication and more adaptive interactions. Fred gradually responded to the structure of the treatment program, although he had frequent problems with anger control when confronted by peers or staff or when frustrated. Depressive symptoms failed to remit after 2 weeks of abstinence, and Fred was given fluoxetine (Prozac). He showed rapid improvement in mood and treatment compliance. Upon discharge, he was attending NA meetings and outpatient therapy. However, family conflict soon recurred, and Fred became noncompliant with outpatient treatment, medication, and meetings. He resumed old relationships with deviant peers and relapsed into daily marijuana use and occasional alcohol use. (Courtesy of Oscar G. Bukstein, M.D.)

48 ◢◣

Child Psychiatry: Additional Conditions That May Be a Focus of Clinical Attention

BORDERLINE INTELLECTUAL FUNCTIONING

The intellectual functioning of a child plays a major role in his or her adjustment to school, social relationships, and family function. A child who is not quite able to understand classwork and may also be slow in understanding rules of games and the "social" rules of his or her peer group is often bitterly rejected. Some children with borderline intellectual functioning are able to mingle socially better than they are able to keep up academically in class. In these cases, the strengths of these children may be peer relationships, especially if they excel at sports, but eventually, their academic struggles will take a toll on self-esteem, if they are not appropriately remediated.

According to the text revision of the fourth edition of *Diagnostic and Statistical Manual of Mental Disorders* (DSM-IV-TR), a child with borderline intellectual functioning has an intelligence quotient (IQ) in the range of 71 to 84. Impaired adaptive functioning accompanies the disorder, which is diagnosed when difficulties in academic, social, or vocational areas pertaining to borderline intellectual functioning become the focus of clinical attention.

Clinicians must assess a patient's intellectual level and current and past levels of adaptive functioning to diagnose borderline intellectual functioning.

Etiology

Genetic factors are increasingly found to play a role in intellectual deficits. Environmental deprivation and infectious and toxic exposures can also contribute to cognitive impairments. Twin and adoption studies support hypotheses that many genes contribute to the development of a particular IQ. Specific infectious processes (such as congenital rubella), prenatal exposures (such as fetal alcohol syndrome), and specific chromosomal abnormalities (such as fragile X syndrome) result in mental retardation.

Diagnosis

In DSM-IV-TR, the following statement about borderline intellectual functioning appears:

This category can be used when the focus of clinical attention is associated with borderline intellectual functioning, that is, an IQ in the 71 to 84 range. Differential diagnosis between Borderline Intellectual Functioning and Mental Retardation (an IQ of 70 or below) is especially difficult when the coexistence of certain mental disorders (e.g., Schizophrenia) is involved. *Coding note: This is coded on Axis II.*

Treatment

The main focus of treatment is to improve practical adaptive skills, social skills, and self-esteem. The goal is to improve the match between the person's capabilities and lifestyle. After the underlying problem becomes known to the therapist, psychiatric treatment can be useful. Many people with borderline intellectual functioning are able to function at a superior level in some areas while being markedly deficient in other areas. By directing such persons to appropriate areas of endeavor, by pointing out socially acceptable behavior, and by teaching them living skills, the therapist can help improve their self-esteem.

ACADEMIC PROBLEM

The editors of DSM-IV-TR refer to *academic problem* as a problem that is not caused by a mental disorder or, if caused by a mental disorder, is severe enough to warrant clinical attention.

This diagnostic category is used when a child or adolescent is having significant academic difficulties that are not deemed to be due to a specific learning disorder or communication disorder or directly related to a psychiatric disorder. Nevertheless, intervention is necessary because the child's achievement is significantly impaired in school.

Etiology

Academic problems have many contributing factors and may arise at any time during a child's school years. School is the major occupation of children and adolescents and is their main social and educational instrument. Adjustment and success in the school setting depend on children's physical, cognitive, social, and emotional adjustment.

Anxiety may play a major role in interfering with children's academic performances. Anxiety may hamper their abilities to

585

perform well on tests, to speak in public, and to ask questions when they do not understand something. Some children are so concerned about the way others view them that they are unable to attend to their academic tasks. For some children, conflicts about success and fears of the consequences imagined to accompany the attainment of success may hamper academic success.

Depressed children also may withdraw from academic pursuits; they require specific interventions to improve their academic performances and to treat their depression. Children who do not have major depressive disorder but who are consumed by family problems such as financial troubles, marital discord in their parents, and mental illness in family members may be distracted and unable to attend to academic tasks.

Cultural and economic background can play a role in how well accepted a child feels in school and can affect the child's academic achievement. Familial socioeconomic level, parental education, race, religion, and family functioning can influence a child's sense of fitting in and can affect preparation to meet school demands.

Schools, teachers, and clinicians can share insights about how to foster productive and cooperative environments for all students in a classroom. Teacher's expectations about their students' performance influence these performances. Therefore, a teacher's affective response to a child can prompt the appearance of an academic problem.

Diagnosis

DSM-IV-TR contains the following statement about academic problem:

> This category can be used when the focus of clinical attention is an academic problem that is not due to a mental disorder or, if due to a mental disorder, is sufficiently severe to warrant independent clinical attention. An example is a pattern of failing grades or of significant underachievement in a person with adequate intellectual capacity in the absence of a Learning or Communication Disorder or any other mental disorder that would account for the problem.

A 17-year-old student who had been getting As and Bs was active on the school football team and had a steady girlfriend. His parents were pleased when he obtained a part-time job, but, after 3 months, he was failing math. Psychiatric evaluation uncovered no evidence of depression, adjustment disorder, or other psychiatric condition. Family assessment revealed a history of financial difficulties and strong imperatives to earn money. The student modified his work schedule and repeated math in summer school; he went on to attend college without difficulty. (Courtesy of James J. McGough, M.D.)

Treatment

The initial step in determining a useful intervention for an academic problem is a comprehensive diagnostic evaluation. After it has been determined that another disorder is not directly influencing academic performance, an appropriate intervention can be developed. Psychotherapeutic techniques can be used successfully for scholastic difficulties related to poor motivation, poor self-concept, and underachievement. Early efforts to relieve the problem are critical: Sustained problems in learning and school performance frequently are compounded and precipitate severe difficulties. Generally, children with academic problems require either school-based intervention or individual attention.

Tutoring is an effective technique in dealing with academic problems and should be considered in most cases. Tutoring is of proven value in preparing for objective multiple choice examinations, such as the Scholastic Aptitude Test (SAT) and Medical College Aptitude Test (MCAT). Taking such examinations repetitively and using relaxation skills are two behavioral techniques of great value in diminishing anxiety.

CHILDHOOD OR ADOLESCENT ANTISOCIAL BEHAVIOR

According to DSM-IV-TR, child or adolescent antisocial behavior refers to behavior that is not caused by a mental disorder and includes isolated antisocial acts, not a pattern of behavior. This category covers many acts by children and adolescents that violate the rights of others, such as overt acts of aggression and violence and covert acts of lying, stealing, truancy, and running away from home. The DSM-IV-TR definition of conduct disorder requires a repetitive pattern of at least three antisocial behaviors for at least 6 months, but childhood or adolescent antisocial behavior may consist of isolated events that do not constitute a mental disorder but do become the focus of clinical attention. The emergence of occasional antisocial symptoms is common among children who have a variety of mental disorders, including psychotic disorders, depressive disorders, impulse-control disorders, and disruptive behavior and attention-deficit disorders, such as attention-deficit/hyperactivity disorder (ADHD) and oppositional defiant disorder.

A child's age and developmental level affect the manifestations of disturbed conduct and influence the child's likelihood to meet the diagnostic criteria for a conduct disorder, as opposed to childhood antisocial behavior. The term *juvenile delinquent* is defined by the legal system as a youth who has violated the law in some way, but the term does not imply that the youth meets the criteria for a mental disorder.

Epidemiology

Estimates of antisocial behavior range from 5 to 15 percent of the general population and somewhat less among children and adolescents. Reports have documented the increased frequency of antisocial behaviors in urban settings, compared with rural areas. In one report, the risk of coming into contact with the police for an antisocial behavior was estimated to be 20 percent for teenage boys and 4 percent for teenage girls.

Etiology

Antisocial behaviors may occur in the context of a mental disorder or in its absence. Antisocial behavior is multidetermined and occurs most frequently in children or adolescents with many risk factors. Among the most common risk factors are harsh and physically abusive parenting, parental criminality, and a child's tendency toward impulsive and hyperactive behavior.

Psychological Factors.   If their parenting experience is poor, children experience emotional deprivation, which leads to low self-esteem and unconscious anger. When children are not given any limits, their consciences are deficient because they have not internalized parental prohibitions that account for superego formation. Therefore, they have so-called superego lacunae, which allow them to commit antisocial acts without guilt. At times, such children's antisocial behavior is a vicarious source of pleasure and gratification for parents who act out their own forbidden wishes and impulses through their children. A consistent finding in people who perform repeated acts of violent behavior is a history of physical abuse.

Diagnosis and Clinical Features

In DSM-IV-TR, the following statement about childhood or adolescent antisocial behavior appears:

> This category can be used when the focus of clinical attention is antisocial behavior in a child or adolescent that is not due to a mental disorder (e.g., Conduct Disorder or an Impulse-Control Disorder). Examples include isolated antisocial acts of children or adolescents (not a pattern of antisocial behavior).

The childhood behaviors most associated with antisocial behavior are theft, incorrigibility, arrests, school problems, impulsiveness, promiscuity, oppositional behavior, lying, suicide attempts, substance abuse, truancy, running away, associating with undesirable people, and staying out late at night. The greater the number of symptoms present in childhood, the greater is the probability of adult antisocial behavior; however, the presence of many symptoms also indicates the development of other mental disorders in adult life.

Differential Diagnosis

Substance-related disorders (including alcohol, cannabis, and cocaine use disorders), bipolar I disorder, and schizophrenia in childhood often manifest themselves as antisocial behavior.

Treatment

Disturbances of conduct frequently accompany the onset of various other psychiatric disorders. The first step in determining the appropriate treatment for a child or an adolescent who is manifesting antisocial behavior is to evaluate the need to treat any coexisting mental disorder, such as bipolar I disorder, a psychotic disorder, or a depressive disorder that may be contributing to the antisocial behavior. The treatment of antisocial behavior usually involves behavioral management, which is most effective when the patient is in a controlled environment or when the child's family members cooperate in maintaining the behavioral program. Schools can help modify antisocial behavior in classrooms. Rewards for prosocial behaviors and positive reinforcement for the control of unwanted behaviors have merit.

In cases of rare or occasional antisocial behaviors, medications generally are not used. When repetitive episodes of explosive behavior, aggression, or violent outbursts ensue, medications have been used with some success. Lithium (Eskalith) and haloperidol (Haldol) may reduce explosive behavior and rage outbursts. When hyperactivity and impulsivity are a contributing factor, methylphenidate (Ritalin) may be helpful to reduce impulsivity and decrease aggression in some cases.

It is more difficult to treat children and adolescents with long-term patterns of antisocial behavior, particularly covert behaviors such as stealing and lying. Group therapy has been used to treat these behaviors, and cognitive problem-solving approaches are potentially helpful.

Identity Problem

According to DSM-IV-TR, identity problem refers to uncertainty about issues relating to identity, such as goals, career choice, friendships, sexual behavior, moral values, and group loyalties. An identity problem can cause severe distress for a young person and can lead a person to seek psychotherapy or guidance. Identity problem, however, is not recognized as a mental disorder in DSM-IV-TR. It is sometimes manifest in the context of such mental disorders as mood disorders, psychotic disorders, and borderline personality disorder.

Epidemiology

No reliable information is available regarding predisposing factors, familial pattern, sex ratio, or prevalence, but problems with identity formation seem to be a result of life in modern society. Today, children and adolescents often experience great instability in family life, problems with identity formation, conflicts between adolescent peer values and the values of parents and society, and exposure through the media and education to various moral, behavioral, and lifestyle possibilities.

Etiology

The causes of identity problems often are multifactorial and include the pressures of a highly dysfunctional family and the influences of coexisting mental disorders. In general, adolescents who suffer from major depressive disorder, psychotic disorders, and other mental disorders report feeling alienated from family members and experience a degree of turmoil. Children who have had difficulties in mastering expected developmental tasks all along are likely to have difficulties with the pressure to establish a well-defined identity during adolescence. Erik Erikson used the term *identity versus role diffusion* to describe the developmental and psychosocial tasks challenging adolescents to incorporate past experiences and present goals into a coherent sense of self.

Diagnosis and Clinical Features

In DSM-IV-TR, the following statement about identity problem appears:

> This category can be used when the focus of clinical attention is uncertainty about multiple issues relating to identity such as long-term goals, career choice, friendship patterns, sexual orientation and behavior, moral values, and group loyalties.

Differential Diagnosis

Identity problem must be differentiated from a mental disorder (such as borderline personality disorder, schizophreniform disorder, schizophrenia, or a mood disorder). At times, what initially seems to be an identity problem may be the prodromal manifestations of one of these disorders. Intense but normal conflicts associated with maturing, such as adolescent turmoil and midlife crisis, may be confusing, but they usually are not associated with marked deterioration in school, vocational, or social functioning or with severe subjective distress. Considerable evidence indicates that adolescent turmoil often is not a phase that is outgrown but an indication of true psychopathology.

Course and Prognosis

The onset of identity problem is most frequently in late adolescence, as teenagers separate from the nuclear family and attempt to establish an independent identity and value system. The onset usually is manifest by a gradual increase in anxiety, depression, regressive phenomena (such as loss of interest in friends, school, and activities), irritability, sleep difficulties, and changes in eating habits. The course usually is relatively brief, as developmental lags are responsive to support, acceptance, and the provision of a psychosocial moratorium.

An extensive prolongation of adolescence with continued identity problem may lead to the chronic state of role diffusion that may indicate a disturbance of early developmental stages and the presence of borderline personality disorder, a mood disorder, or schizophrenia. An identity problem usually resolves by the mid-20s. If it persists, the person with the identity problem may be unable to make career commitments or lasting attachments.

Treatment

Individual psychotherapy directed toward encouraging growth and development usually is considered the therapy of choice. Adolescents with identity problems often feel developmentally unprepared to deal with the increasing demands for social, emotional, and sexual independence. Issues of separation and individuation from their families can be challenging and overwhelming. Treatment is aimed at helping these adolescents develop a sense of competence and mastery about necessary social and vocational choices. A therapist's empathic acknowledgment of an adolescent's struggle can be helpful in the process.

49

Psychiatric Treatment of Children and Adolescents

▲ 49.1 Individual Psychotherapy

To approach a child therapeutically, one must have a sense of normal development for a child of a given age as well as an understanding of the life story of the particular child. Wide normal variation exists with respect to how facile children are at describing their emotions in words and the level of motivation they engage in this process. Individual psychotherapy with children focuses on improving children's adaptive skills in and outside the family setting. Treatment reflects an understanding of children's developmental levels and shows sensitivity toward families and environments in which children live.

Children can disclose their own thoughts, feelings, moods, and perceptual experiences better than others; however, even when external behavior problems have been identified by others, children's internal experiences may be largely unknown. Children often can describe their feelings in a particular situation but cannot make changes without an advocate's help. Thus, child psychotherapists function as advocates for their child patients in interactions with schools, legal agencies, and community organizations. Child psychotherapists may be called on to make recommendations that affect various aspects of children's lives.

TYPES OF PSYCHOTHERAPIES

Developing a psychotherapeutic intervention for a particular child includes evaluation of the child's age, developmental level, type of problem, and communication style. Whichever style or combination of techniques a therapist chooses to use in psychotherapy, the relationship between child and therapist is a critical element. The relationship itself often is the primary, if not the sole, ingredient in psychotherapy.

Cognitive-behavioral therapy is an amalgam of behavioral therapy and cognitive psychology. It emphasizes how children may use thinking processes and cognitive modalities to reframe, restructure, and solve problems. A child's distortions are addressed by generating alternative ways of dealing with problematic situations. Cognitive-behavioral strategies have been useful in the treatment of mood disorders and anxiety disorders.

Remedial, educational, and patterning psychotherapy is focused on teaching new attitudes and patterns of behavior to children who persist in using immature and inefficient patterns that are often presumed to be due to a maturational lag. Supportive psychotherapy is particularly helpful in enabling a well-adjusted youngster to cope with emotional turmoil engendered by a crisis. It also is used with disturbed youngsters whose less-than-adequate ego functioning may be seriously disrupted by an expressive-exploratory mode or by other forms of therapeutic intervention.

Release therapy, described initially by David Levy, facilitates the abreaction of pent-up emotions. It is indicated primarily for preschool-age children who have a distorted emotional reaction to an isolated trauma.

Preschool-age children are sometimes treated through the parents, a process called *filial therapy*. Therapists using this strategy should be alert to the possibility that apparently successful filial treatment can obscure a significant diagnosis because patients are not treated directly. The first case of filial therapy was that of Little Hans, reported by Freud in 1905. Hans was a 5-year-old phobic child who was treated by his father under Freud's supervision.

Child psychoanalysis, an intensive, uncommon form of psychoanalytic psychotherapy, works on unconscious resistance and defenses during three to four sessions a week. Under these circumstances, therapists anticipate unconscious resistance and allow transference manifestations to mature to a full transference neurosis, through which neurotic conflicts are resolved. Interpretations of dynamically relevant conflicts are emphasized in psychoanalytic descriptions, and elements that are predominant in other types of psychotherapies are not overlooked.

Cognitive therapy has been used with children, adolescents, and adults. The approach attempts to correct cognitive distortions, particularly negative conceptions of self, and is used mainly in depressive disorders.

DIFFERENCES BETWEEN CHILDREN AND ADULTS

Logic suggests that psychotherapy with children, who generally are more flexible than adults and who have simpler defenses and other mental mechanisms, should consume less time than comparable treatment of adults. Experience usually does not

589

confirm this expectation, because children usually lack some elements that contribute to successful treatment. A child, for example, typically does not seek help. As a consequence, one of a therapist's first tasks is to stimulate a child's motivation for treatment. Although parents may want their children to be helped or changed, the desire often is generated by frustrated anger toward the children. Typically, the anger is accompanied by relative insensitivity to what therapists perceive as the children's needs and the basis for a therapeutic alliance. Therefore, whereas adult patients frequently perceive advantages in getting well, children may envision therapeutic change as nothing more than conforming to a disagreeable reality, an attitude that heightens the likelihood of their perceiving a therapist as the parent's punitive agent. This is hardly the most fertile soil in which to nurture a therapeutic alliance.

Children tend to externalize internal conflicts in search of alloplastic adaptations, and they find it difficult to conceive of problem resolution except by altering an obstructing environment. The tendency of children to reenact their feelings in new situations facilitates the early appearance of spontaneous and global transference reactions that may be troublesome. Concurrently, children's eagerness for new experiences, coupled with their natural developmental fluidity, tends to limit the intensity and therapeutic usefulness of subsequent transference developments.

Children have a limited capacity for self-observation, with the notable exception of some obsessive children who resemble adults in this ability. Such obsessive children, however, usually isolate the vital emotional components. In exploratory-interpretative psychotherapies, the development of a capacity for ego splitting—that is, simultaneous emotional involvement and self-observation—is most helpful. Only by identifying with a trusted adult and in alliance with this adult can children approach such an ideal.

Regressive behavioral and communicative modes can be wearing on child therapists. Typically motor-minded, even when they do not require external controls, children may demand a physical stamina that is not a significant factor in therapy with adults. The age appropriateness of such primitive mechanisms as denial, projection, and isolation hinders the process of working through, which relies on a patient's synthesizing and integrating capacities, both of which are immature in children. Environmental pressures on therapists are also generally greater in psychotherapeutic work with children than in work with adults.

Although children compare unfavorably with adults in many qualities that are generally considered desirable in therapy, children have the advantage of their active maturational and developmental forces. The history of psychotherapy for children is punctuated by efforts to harness these assets and to overcome the liabilities. Recognition of the importance of play constituted a major forward stride in these efforts.

PLAYROOM

The structure, design, and furnishing of the playroom are important. Some therapists maintain that the toys should be few, simple, and carefully selected to facilitate the communication of fantasy. Other therapists suggest that a wide variety of playthings should be available to increase the range of feelings that children can express. These contrasting recommendations have been attributed to differences in therapeutic methods. Some therapists tend to avoid interpretation, even of conscious ideas, whereas others recommend the interpretation of unconscious content directly and quickly.

Therapists tend to change their preferences in equipment as they accumulate experience and develop confidence in their abilities. Although special equipment—such as genital dolls, amputation dolls, and see-through anatomically complete (except for genitalia) models—has been used in therapy, many therapists have observed that the unusual nature of such items risks making children wary and suspicious of a therapist's motives. Until the dolls available to children in their own homes include genitalia, the psychological content that special dolls are designed to elicit may be more available at the appropriate time with conventional dolls.

Although the choices of play materials vary among therapists, the following equipment can constitute a well-balanced playroom or play area: multigenerational families of flexible but sturdy dolls of various races; additional dolls representing special roles and feelings, such as police officer, doctor, and soldier; dollhouse furnishings with or without a dollhouse; toy animals; puppets; paper, crayons, paint, and blunt-ended scissors; a sponge-like ball; clay or something comparable; tools such as rubber hammers, rubber knives, and guns; building blocks, cars, trucks, and airplanes; and eating utensils. The way the child uses the toys enables the therapist to understand how the child communicates through play. Therapists should avoid toys and materials that are fragile, break easily, or that can result in physical injury.

Each child should have a special drawer or box, if space is available, in which to store items the child brings to the therapy session or to store projects, such as drawings and stories, for future retrieval. Limits must be set so that the private storage area is not used to hoard communal play equipment and thus deprive the other patients. Some therapists assert that absence of such arrangements evokes material about sibling rivalry; others believe that this assertion is a rationalization for not respecting children's privacy, since sibling feelings can be expressed in other ways.

INITIAL APPROACH

Various approaches are associated with each therapist's individual style and perception of children's needs, from approaches in which a therapist endeavors to direct children's thought content and activity (release therapy, some behavior therapy, and certain educational patterning techniques) to exploratory methods in which a therapist endeavors to follow children's leads. Even though children determine the focus, therapists structure the situation. Encouraging children to say whatever they wish and to play freely, as in exploratory psychotherapy, establishes a definite structure. Therapists create an atmosphere in which they get to know all about a child—the good side as well as the bad side, as children would put it.

THERAPEUTIC INTERVENTIONS

Psychotherapy with children and adolescents generally is more directed and active than it often is with adults. Children usually cannot synthesize histories of their own lives, but they are excellent reporters of their current internal states. Even with adolescents, a therapist often takes an active role, is somewhat less open-ended than with adults, and offers more direction and advocacy than with adults. A therapist may use interpretations, designed to expand patients' conscious awareness of themselves, by making explicit the elements that have previously been expressed implicitly in the patient's thoughts, feelings, and behavior.

PARENTS

Psychotherapy with children requires parental involvement, which does not necessarily reflect parental culpability for a youngster's emotional difficulties but is a reality of a child's dependent state. This fact cannot be stressed too much because of an occupational hazard shared by many who work with children—the urge to rescue children from their parents' negative influences, a desire that sometimes is related to an unconscious competitive desire to be a better parent than the child's or the therapist's own parents.

Parents are involved in child psychotherapy to varying degrees. Probably the most frequent parental arrangements are those developed in child guidance clinics—that is, parent guidance focused on the child or the parent–child interaction and therapy for the parents' own individual needs concurrent with the child's therapy. Parents may be seen by their child's therapist or by someone else. Recently, there have been increasing efforts to shift the focus from the child as the primary patient to the child as the family's emissary to the clinic. In such family therapy, all or selected members of the family are treated simultaneously as a family group. Although the preferences of specific clinics and practitioners for either an individual or a family therapeutic approach may be unavoidable, the final decision regarding which therapeutic strategy or combination to use should be derived from the clinical assessment.

CONFIDENTIALITY

The issue of confidentiality takes on greater meaning as children grow older. Very young children are unlikely to be as concerned about this issue as adolescents are. Confidentiality usually is preserved unless a child is believed to be in danger or to be a danger to someone else. In other situations, a child's permission usually is sought before a specific issue is raised with parents.

The therapist should try to enlist parents' cooperation in respecting the privacy of children's therapeutic sessions. The respect is not always readily honored, because parents are naturally curious about what transpires, and they may be threatened by a therapist's apparently privileged position.

Routinely reporting to a child the essence of communications with third parties about the child underscores the therapist's reliability and respect for the child's autonomy. In certain treatments, the report may be combined with soliciting the child's guesses about these transactions. A therapist also may find it fruitful to invite children, particularly older children, to participate in discussions about them with third parties.

INDICATIONS

Psychotherapy usually is indicated for children with emotional disorders that seem to be permanent enough to impede maturational and developmental forces. Psychotherapy also may be indicated when a child's development is not impeded but is inducing reactions in the environment that are considered pathogenic. Such disharmonies ordinarily are dealt with by the child with parental assistance; however, when these efforts are

persistently inadequate, psychotherapeutic interventions may be indicated.

Psychotherapy should be limited to instances in which positive indicators point to its potential usefulness. For a child to benefit from psychotherapy, the home situation must provide a certain amount of nurturance, stability, and motivation for therapy. A child must have adequate cognitive resources to participate in the process and profit from it. Psychotherapy must be judged with common sense. If a psychotherapy situation is not effective, one must determine whether the therapist and patient are poorly matched, whether the type of psychotherapy is inappropriate to the nature of the problems, and whether the child is cognitively inappropriate for the treatment.

▲ 49.2 Group Psychotherapy

Group therapy is an effective modality that can be structured in a variety of ways to address issues of interpersonal competence, peer relationships, and social skill. Group psychotherapy can be modified to suit groups of children of various age groups and can focus on behavioral, educational, and social skills and psychodynamic issues. The mode in which the group functions depends on children's developmental levels, intelligence, and problems to be addressed. In behaviorally oriented groups, the group leader is a directive, active participant who facilitates prosocial interactions and desired behaviors. In groups using psychodynamic approaches, the leader may monitor interpersonal interactions less actively than in behavior therapy groups. The children selected for group treatment have a common social hunger and need to be like their peers and be accepted by them. Selected children usually include those with phobias, effeminate boys, shy and withdrawn children, and children with disruptive behavior disorders.

Modifications of these criteria have been used in group psychotherapy for autistic children, parent group therapy, and art therapy. A modification of group psychotherapy has been used for toddlers with physical disabilities who show speech and language delays.

Groups are highly effective in providing peer feedback and support to children who are either socially isolated or unaware of their effects on their peers. Groups with very young children generally are highly structured by the leader and use imagination and play to foster socially acceptable peer relationships and positive behavior. Therapists must be keenly aware of the level of children's attention span and the need for consistency and limit setting.

Johnny was a high-functioning, 14-year-old boy diagnosed with autistic disorder. He had been in individual and family therapy for several months before he was considered ready for group therapy. Johnny was an awkward-looking adolescent who looked and acted younger than his chronological age. His academic level was above average, but his social development was very limited. A supercilious, hypermoralistic attitude of more recent development contributed considerably to his social isolation, particularly after starting seventh grade. He was assigned to an established group of early adolescents with a mixture of clinical conditions, meeting once weekly for 75 minutes. Initially Johnny limited his participation to monosyllabic answers to direct questions, then he would go back to reading a book on the history of Napoleon, his favorite subject and object of fascination. Group members chose to ignore him after a while. Over a period of several weeks, his interest in the book seemed to abate. Johnny brought it, but it remained unopened on his lap. He would make an occasional remark, mostly to criticize another group member for his "vulgarity." The group laughed at his remarks but scapegoating could be avoided. They seemed to respect his "differentness." Two months later, Peter, a very shy schizoid 13-year-old boy, joined the group. After a few sessions, Johnny developed an unexpected interest in Peter and sat by him and encouraged him to interact with the group. Soon Johnny was not bringing a book any longer and was more actively involved with group members. He responded to social cues in a more age-typical and appropriate manner, and though he continued having morbid preoccupations with power and a fascination with Napoleon, the intensity was considerably diminished. Johnny's growing interest in people was clinically evident. Group therapy was used in combination with individual and family therapy and psychotropic medication over 18 months. Although the group experience was only one component of the treatment plan, it became a most significant tool to help Johnny with his interpersonal deficits. (Courtesy of Alberto C. Serrano, M.D.)

PRESCHOOL-AGE AND EARLY SCHOOL-AGE GROUPS

Work with a preschool-age group usually is structured by a therapist through the use of a particular technique such as puppets or artwork or is coached in terms of a permissive play atmosphere. In therapy with puppets, children project their fantasies onto the puppets in a way not unlike ordinary play. The main value lies in the cathexis afforded children, especially if they show difficulty expressing their feelings. Here, the group aids the child less by interaction with other members than by action with the puppets.

In play group therapy, the emphasis rests on children's interactional qualities with each other and with the therapist in the permissive playroom setting. A therapist should be a person who can allow children to produce fantasies verbally and in play but who can also use active restraint when children undergo excessive tension. The toys are the traditional ones used in individual play therapy. The children use the toys to act out aggressive impulses and to relive their home difficulties with group members and with the therapist.

The experience of twice-weekly group activities involves mothers and children in a mutual teaching–learning setting. This experience has proved effective for mothers who received supportive psychotherapy in the group experience; their formerly hidden fantasies about their children emerged and were dealt with therapeutically.

SCHOOL-AGE GROUPS

Activity group psychotherapy is based on the idea that poor, divergent experiences have led to deficits in children's appropriate personality development; therefore, corrective experiences in a therapeutically conditioned environment modify them. Because some latency-age children have deep disturbances involving fears, high anxiety levels, and guilt, a modification of activity-interview group psychotherapy has evolved. The format uses interview techniques, verbal explanations of fantasies, group play, work, and other communications. In this type of group psychotherapy, children verbalize in a problem-oriented manner, with the awareness that problems brought them together and that the group aims to change them. They report dreams, fantasies, daydreams, and traumatic and unpleasant experiences. Open discussion includes both the experiences and the group behavior.

PUBERTAL AND ADOLESCENT GROUPS

Group therapy methods similar to those used in younger age groups can be modified to apply to pubertal children, who are often grouped monosexually. Their problems resemble those of late latency-age children, but they (especially the girls) are also beginning to feel the effects and pressures of early adolescence. Groups offer help during a transitional period; they seem to satisfy the social appetite of preadolescents, who compensate for feelings of inferiority and self-doubt by forming groups. This therapy takes advantage of the influence of the socialization process during these years. Because pubertal children experience difficulties in conceptualizing, pubertal therapy groups tend to use play, drawing, psychodrama, and other nonverbal modes of expression. The therapist's role is active and directive.

OTHER GROUP SITUATIONS

Groups are also helpful in more focused treatments, such as specific social skills training for children with attention-deficit/hyperactivity disorder (ADHD) and cognitive-behavioral group interventions for depressed children and children with bereavement problems or eating disorders. In these more specialized groups, the issues are more specific, and actual tasks (as in social skills groups) may be practiced within the group.

INDICATIONS

Many indications exist for the use of group psychotherapy as a treatment modality. Some indications are situational; a therapist may work in a reformatory setting, in which group psychotherapy seems to reach adolescents better than individual treatment does. Another indication is time economics; more patients can be reached in a given time by the use of groups than by individual therapy. Group therapy best helps a child at a given age and developmental stage and with a given type of problem.

PARENT GROUPS

In group psychotherapy, as in most treatment procedures for children, parental difficulties present obstacles. Sometimes, uncooperative parents refuse to bring a child or to participate in their own therapy. The extreme of this situation reveals itself when severely disturbed parents use a child as their channel of communication to work out their own needs. In such circumstances, a child is in the intolerable position of receiving positive group experiences that seem to create havoc at home.

Parent groups, therefore, can be a valuable aid to group psychotherapy for their children. Parents of children in therapy often have difficulty understanding their children's ailments, discerning the line of demarcation between normal and pathological behavior, relating to the medical establishment, and coping with feelings of guilt. Parent groups assist in these areas and help members formulate guidelines for action.

▲ 49.3 Residential, Day, and Hospital Treatment

RESIDENTIAL TREATMENT

More than 20,000 emotionally disturbed children are in residential treatment centers in the United States, and this number is increasing. Deteriorating social conditions, particularly in cities, often make it impossible for a child with a serious mental disorder to live at home. In these cases, residential treatment centers serve a real need. Residential treatment centers and facilities are appropriate settings for children and adolescents with mental disorders who require a highly structured and supervised setting for a substantial time. They provide a structured living environment in which children may form strong attachments to, and receive commitments from, staff members. The purpose of the center is to provide treatment and special education for children and their families.

Staff and Setting

Staffing patterns include various combinations of child-care workers, teachers, social workers, psychiatrists, pediatricians, nurses, and psychologists; therefore, residential treatment can be very expensive. The Joint Commission on the Mental Health of Children made the following structural and setting recommendations: In addition to space for therapy programs, there should be facilities for a first-rate school and a rich evening activity program, and there should be ample space for play, both indoors and out. Facilities should be small, seldom exceeding 60 patients in capacity with a limit of 100 patients, and they should make provisions for children to live in small groups. In designing residential programs, the guiding principle should be that children should be removed from their normal life settings the least possible distance in space, in time, and in the psychological texture of the experience.

Indications

Most children who are referred for residential treatment have had multiple evaluations by professionals such as school psychologists, outpatient psychotherapists, juvenile court officials, or state welfare agency staff. Attempts at outpatient treatment and foster home placement usually precede residential treatment. Many children sent to residential treatment centers have disruptive behavior problems in addition to other problems, including mood disorders and psychotic disorders. The age range of the children varies among institutions, but most children are between 5 and 15 years of age. Boys are referred more frequently than girls.

An initial review of data enables the intake staff to determine whether a particular child is likely to benefit from the treatment program; often, for every child accepted for admission, three are rejected. The next step usually is interviews with the child and the parents by various staff members, such as a therapist, a group-living worker, and a teacher. Psychological testing and neurological examinations are given, when indicated, if they have not already been performed. The child and parents should be prepared for these interviews.

Group Living

Most of a child's time in a residential treatment setting is spent in group living. The group-living staff consists of child-care workers who offer a structured environment that forms a therapeutic milieu. The environment places boundaries and limitations on the children. Tasks are defined within the limits of children's abilities; incentives, such as additional privileges, encourage them to progress rather than regress. In milieu therapy, the environment is structured, limits are set, and a therapeutic atmosphere is maintained.

The children often select one or more staff members with whom to form a relationship; through this relationship, they express, consciously and unconsciously, many of their feelings about their parents. The child-care staff should be trained to recognize such transference reactions and to respond to them in a way that differs from the children's expectations, which are based on their previous or even current relationships with their parents.

To maintain consistency and balance, the group-living staff members must communicate freely and regularly with each other and with the other professional and administrative staff members of the residential setting, particularly the children's teachers and therapists.

The structured setting should offer a corrective emotional experience and opportunities for facilitating and improving children's adaptive behavior, particularly when such problems as speech and language deficits, intellectual retardation, inadequate peer relationships, bed-wetting, poor feeding habits, and attention deficits are present. Some attention deficits are the basis of a child's poor academic performance and unsocialized behavior, including temper tantrums, fighting, and withdrawal.

Education

Children in residential treatment frequently have severe learning disorders, disruptive behavior, and attention-deficit disorders. Usually, the children cannot function in a regular community school and consequently need a special on-grounds school. A major goal of the on-grounds school is to motivate children to learn. The educational process in residential treatment is complex; Table 49.3–1 shows some of its components.

Table 49.3–1
Education Process in Residential Treatment

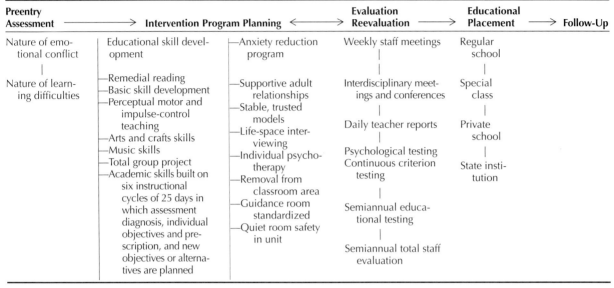

Preentry Assessment	Intervention Program Planning		Evaluation Reevaluation	Educational Placement	Follow-Up
Nature of emotional conflict	Educational skill development	—Anxiety reduction program	Weekly staff meetings	Regular school	
Nature of learning difficulties	—Remedial reading —Basic skill development —Perceptual motor and impulse-control teaching —Arts and crafts skills —Music skills —Total group project —Academic skills built on six instructional cycles of 25 days in which assessment diagnosis, individual objectives and prescription, and new objectives or alternatives are planned	—Supportive adult relationships —Stable, trusted models —Life-space interviewing —Individual psychotherapy —Removal from classroom area —Guidance room standardized —Quiet room safety in unit	Interdisciplinary meetings and conferences Daily teacher reports Psychological testing Continuous criterion testing Semiannual educational testing Semiannual total staff evaluation	Special class Private school State institution	

Courtesy of Melvin Lewis, M.B., B.S. (London), F.R.C.Psych., D.C.H.

Therapy

Most residential facilities use a basic behavior modification program to set guidelines and to give the residents a concrete sense of how to earn privileges. These behavioral programs range in detail and intensity. Most programs include basic tasks of living as well as specific therapeutic goals for the residents.

Psychotherapy offered in the program generally is supportive and oriented toward reunion with the family when possible. Insight-oriented psychotherapy is included when it can be used by a resident.

Parents

Concomitant work with parents is essential. Children usually have a strong tie to at least one parent, no matter how disturbed the parent may be. Sometimes, a child idealizes the parent, who repeatedly fails the child. Other times, the parent has an ambivalent or unrealistic expectation that the child will return home. In some instances, the parent must be helped to enable the child to live in another setting when it is in the child's best interest. Most residential treatment centers offer individual or group therapy for parents, couples or marital therapy, and, in some cases, conjoint family therapy.

DAY TREATMENT

The concept of daily comprehensive therapeutic experiences that do not require removing children from their homes or families is derived partly from experiences with a therapeutic nursery school. Day hospital programs for children were then developed, and the number of programs continues to grow. The main advantages of day treatment are that children remain with their families, and the families can be more involved in day treatment than they are in residential or hospital treatment. Day treatment also is much less expensive than residential treatment. At the same time, the risks of day treatment are a child's social isolation and confinement to a narrow band of social contacts in the program's disturbed peer population.

Indications

The primary indication for day treatment is the need for a more structured, intensive, and specialized treatment program than can be provided on an outpatient basis. At the same time, the home in which the child is living should be able to provide an environment that is at least not destructive to the child's development. Children who are likely to benefit from day treatment may have a wide range of diagnoses, including autistic disorder, conduct disorder, ADHD, and mental retardation. Exclusion symptoms include behavior that is likely to be destructive to the children themselves or to others under the treatment conditions.

Programs

A major function of child-care staff in day treatment for psychiatrically disturbed children is to provide positive experiences and a structure that enables the children and their families to internalize controls and to function better than in the past regarding themselves and the outside world. The methods used are essentially similar to those in full residential treatment programs.

Because the ages, needs, and range of diagnoses of children who may benefit from some form of day treatment vary, many day treatment programs have been developed. Some programs specialize in special educational and structured environmental needs of mentally retarded children. Others offer special therapeutic efforts required to treat children with autism and schizophrenia. Still other programs provide the total spectrum of treatment usually found in full residential treatment, of which they may be a part. Children may move from one part of the program to another and may be in residential treatment or day treatment according to their needs. The school program always is a major component of day treatment, and psychiatric treatment varies according to a child's needs and diagnosis.

Results

Recently, attempts have been made to analyze the treatment outcome of day treatment and partial hospitalization. There are many different dimensions to analyzing overall benefits of such programs. Assessment of level of improvement in clinical status, academic progress, peer relationships, community interactions (legal difficulties), and family relationships are some pertinent areas to measure. In a recent follow-up 1 year after discharge from a partial hospital program, comparison of patients at admission and 1 year postdischarge showed statistically significant improvement in clinical symptoms on each subscale of the Child Behavior Checklist except for sex problems. These improvements included mood symptoms, somatic complaints, attention problems, thought problems, delinquent behavior, and aggressive behavior. The assessment of long-term effectiveness of day treatment is fraught with difficulties, from the point of view of a child's maintenance of gains, a therapist's view of psychological gains, or cost-benefit ratios.

HOSPITAL TREATMENT

Psychiatric hospitalization is needed when a child or adolescent exhibits dangerous behavior, is contemplating suicide, or is experiencing an exacerbation of a psychotic disorder or another serious mental disorder. Safety, stabilization, and effective treatment are the goals of hospitalization. Recently, the length of stay for child and adolescent psychiatric patients has decreased because of financial pressures and increased availability of day treatment programs. Psychiatric hospitalization may be some children's first opportunity to experience a stable, safe environment. Hospitals often are the most appropriate places to start use of new medications, and they provide an around-the-clock setting in which to observe a child's behavior.

Beginning in the 1920s, inpatient psychiatric treatment of children includes two types of units: acute-care hospital units and long-term hospital units. Acute-care units generally accept children who exhibit dangerous (suicidal, assaultive, or psychotically disorganized) behavior. Diagnosis, stabilization, and formulation and initiation of a treatment plan are the goals of acute-care units. Disposition usually is to home, to residential treatment centers, or to long-term (usually state) hospitals for continued care. Acute-care hospitalization generally lasts from 6 to 12 weeks and often is extended because of the wait for beds in residential treatment centers and state hospitals.

Long-term hospitalization generally lasts many months to years. The staffs of inpatient units are interdisciplinary and include psychiatrists, psychologists, social workers, nurses, activity therapists, and teachers.

▲ 49.4 Biological Therapies

PHARMACOTHERAPY

Over the last decade, there have been many advances in the pharmacotherapy of psychiatric disorders in childhood, including data supporting the efficacy of selective serotonin reuptake inhibitors (SSRIs) in the treatment of depressive disorders, obsessive-compulsive disorders (OCDs), and anxiety disorders. The tricyclic antidepressants are rarely used due to the more favorable side effect profiles of SSRIs compared with tricyclic antidepressants. The management of severe aggression, disruptive behavior, and attention-deficit/hyperactivity disorders (ADHDs) remains a challenge. Newer atypical antipsychotic medications with serotonergic and dopamine antagonism such as risperidone (Risperdal), olanzapine (Zyprexa), clozapine (Clozaril), and ziprasidone (Geodone) have replaced conventional antipsychotics and have enabled a wider range of treatment-resistant patients to benefit from neuroleptic treatment.

Childhood Pharmacokinetics

Children, compared with adults, have greater hepatic capacity, more glomerular filtration, and less fatty tissue. Therefore, stimulants, antipsychotics, and tricyclic drugs are eliminated more rapidly by children than by adults. Because of children's quick elimination, the half-lives of many medications may be shorter in children than in adults.

Little evidence indicates that clinicians can predict a child's blood level from the dosage or a treatment response from the plasma level. As with serum levels, regular clinical monitoring for adverse effects is necessary.

Pharmacological Agents and Their Indications

Table 49.4–1 lists representative drugs and their indications, dosages, adverse reactions, and monitoring requirements.

Stimulants

The current belief is that any growth suppression is temporary and that children taking stimulants eventually reach their normal height.

OTHER BIOLOGICAL THERAPIES

Electroconvulsive therapy (ECT) is rarely, if ever, indicated in childhood or adolescence. Psychosurgery for severe and intransigent OCD should probably be delayed until adulthood, after all attempts at less drastic treatment have failed and when the patient can participate fully in the process of informed consent.

Little evidence indicates that food allergies or sensitivities play a role in childhood mental disorders. Diets that eliminate food additives, colorings, and sugar are difficult to maintain and usually have no effect. Megavitamin therapy usually is ineffective (unless the child has a frank vitamin deficiency) and can cause serious adverse effects.

Table 49.4–1
Common Psychoactive Drugs in Childhood and Adolescence

Drug	Indications	Dosage	Adverse Reactions and Monitoring
Antipsychotics—also known as *major tranquilizers, neuroleptics* Divided into (1) high-potency, low-dosage (e.g., haloperidol (Haldol), pimozide (Orap), trifluoperazine (Stelazine), thiothixene (Navane); (2) low-potency high-dosage (more sedating) (e.g., chlorpromazine (Thorazine); and (3) atypicals [(e.g., risperidone (Risperdal), olanzapine (Zyprexa), quetiapine (Seroquel), and clozapine (Clozaril)]	Psychoses; agitated self-injurious behaviors in MR, PDDs, CD, and Tourette's disorder—haloperidol and pimozide Atypical—refractory schizophrenia in adolescence	All can be given in two to four divided doses or combined into one dose after gradual buildup Haloperidol—child 0.5–6 mg/d, adolescent 0.5–16 mg/d Clozapine—dosage not determined in children; <600 mg/d in adolescents Risperidone—1–3 mg/d Olanzapine—2.5–10 mg/d Quetiapine—25–500 mg/d	Sedation, weight gain, hypotension, lowered seizure threshold, constipation, extrapyramidal symptoms, jaundice, agranulocytosis, dystonic reaction, tardive dyskinesia Hyperprolactinemia with atypicals except quetiapine Monitor blood pressure, CBC count, LFTs and prolactin if indicated; with thioridazine, pigmentary retinopathy is rare but dictates ceiling of 800 mg in adults and proportionally lower in children; with clozapine, weekly WBC counts for development of agranulocytosis and EEG monitoring because of lowering of seizure threshold
Stimulants Dextroamphetamine (Dexedrine) and amphetamine-dextroamphetamine (Adderall) FDA-approved for children 3 years and older Methylphenidate (Ritalin, Concerta) and pemoline (Cylert)—FDA-approved for children 6 years and older	In ADHD for hyperactivity, impulsivity, and inattentiveness Narcolepsy	Dextroamphetamine and methylphenidate are generally given at 8 AM and noon Dextroamphetamine—about half the dosage of methylphenidate Methylphenidate—10–60 mg/d or up to about 0.5 mg/kg per dose Adderall—about half the dosage of methylphenidate	Insomnia, anorexia, weight loss (possibly growth delay), rebound hyperactivity, headache, tachycardia, precipitation or exacerbation of tic disorders With pemoline, monitor LFTs, as hepatotoxicity and liver failure are possible
Mood stabilizers Lithium—considered an antimanic drug; also has anti-aggression properties	Studies support use in MR and CD for aggressive and self-injurious behaviors; can be used for same in PDD; also indicated for early-onset bipolar disorder	600–2,100 mg in two or three divided doses; keep blood levels to 0.4–1.2 mEq/L	Nausea, vomiting, polyuria, headache, tremor, weight gain, hypothyroidism Experience with adults suggests renal function monitoring
Divalproex (Depakote)	Bipolar disorder, aggression	Up to about 20 mg/kg per day; therapeutic blood level range appears to be 50–100 μg/mL	Monitor CBC count and LFTs for possible blood dyscrasias and hepatotoxicity Nausea, vomiting, sedation, hair loss, weight gain, possibly polycystic ovaries
Carbamazepine (Tegretol)—an anticonvulsant	Aggression or dyscontrol in MR or CD Bipolar disorder	Start with 10 mg/kg per day, can build to 20–30 mg/kg per day; therapeutic blood-level range appears to be 4–12 mg per day	Drowsiness, nausea, rash, vertigo, irritability Monitor CBC count and LFTs for possible blood dyscrasias and hepatotoxicity; must obtain blood concentrations
Antidepressants **Tricyclic antidepressants**—imipramine (Tofranil), nortriptyline (Pamelor), clomipramine (Anafranil)	Major depressive disorder, separation anxiety disorder, bulimia nervosa, enuresis; sometimes used in ADHD, sleepwalking disorder, and sleep terror disorder Clomipramine is effective in childhood OCD and sometimes in PDD	Imipramine—start with divided doses totaling about 1.5 mg/kg per day; can build up to not more than 5 mg/kg per day and eventually combine in one dose, which is usually 50–100 mg before sleep Clomipramine—start at 50 mg/d; can raise to not more than 3 mg/kg per day or 200 mg/d	Dry mouth, constipation, tachycardia, arrhythmia
Selective serotonin reuptake inhibitors—fluoxetine (Prozac), sertraline (Zoloft), fluvoxamine (Luvox), paroxetine (Paxil), citalopram (Celexa), escitalopram (Lexapro)	OCD; may be useful in major depressive disorder, anorexia nervosa, bulimia nervosa, repetitive behaviors in MR or PDD	Less than adult dosages	Nausea, headache, nervousness, insomnia, dry mouth, diarrhea, drowsiness, disinhibition

(continued)

Table 49.4–1 (*continued*)

Drug	Indications	Dosage	Adverse Reactions and Monitoring
Bupropion (Wellbutrin)	ADHD	Start low and titrate up to between 100 and 250 mg/d	Disinhibition, insomnia, dry mouth, gastrointestinal problems, tremor, seizures
Anxiolytics			
Benzodiazepines			
Clonazepam (Klonopin)	Panic disorder, generalized anxiety disorder	0.5–2.0 mg/d	Drowsiness, disinhibition
Alprazolam (Xanax)	Separation anxiety disorder	Up to 1.5 mg/d	Drowsiness, disinhibition
Buspirone (BuSpar)	Various anxiety disorders	15–90 mg/d	Dizziness, upset stomach
α_2-**Adrenergic receptor agonists**			
Clonidine (Catapres)	ADHD, Tourette's disorder, aggression	Up to 0.4 mg/d	Bradycardia, arrhythmia, hypertension, withdrawal hypotension
Guanfacine (Tenex)	ADHD	0.5–3.0 mg/d	Same as with clonidine plus headache, stomachache
β-**Adrenergic receptor antagonist (beta blocker)**			
Propranolol (Inderal)	Explosive aggression	Start at 20–30 mg/d and titrate	Monitor for bradycardia, hypotension, bronchoconstriction. Contraindicated in asthma and diabetes
Other agents			
Naltrexone (ReVia)	Hyperactivity or self-injurious behavior in autism or MR	0.5–1.0 mg/kg per day	Drowsiness, vomiting, anorexia, headache, nasal congestion, hyponatremic seizures
Desmopressin (DDAVP)	Nocturnal enuresis	20–40 µg intranasally	Headache, nasal congestion, hyponatremic seizures (rare)
Atomoxetine (Strattera)	ADHD	40–80 mg/d	Avoid with MAOIs, allergic reaction
Modafil (Provigil)	Narcolepsy	200–300 mg/d	Lower dose in persons with hepatic damage, headache, nausea

ADHD, attention-deficit/hyperactivity disorder; CBC, complete blood count; CD, conduct disorder; LFT, liver function test; MAOIs, monoamine oxidase inhibitors; MR, mental retardation; OCD, obsessive-compulsive disorder; PDD, pervasive development disorder; WBC, white blood cell.

▲ 49.5 Psychiatric Treatment of Adolescents

A variety of serious psychiatric disorders, including schizophrenia and bipolar disorder, have their onset during adolescence. In addition, the risk for completed suicide drastically increases in adolescence. Although some stress is virtually universal in adolescence, most teenagers without mental disorders can cope well with the environmental demands. Teenagers with preexisting mental disorders may experience exacerbations during adolescence and may become frustrated, alienated, and demoralized.

DIAGNOSIS

Adolescents can be assessed in both their specific stage-appropriate functions and their general progress in accomplishing the tasks of adolescence. For almost all adolescents in today's culture, at least until their late teens, school performance is the prime barometer of healthy functioning. Intellectually normal adolescents who are not functioning satisfactorily in some form of schooling have significant psychological problems whose nature and causes should be identified.

Questions to be asked regarding adolescents' stage-specific tasks are the following: What degree of separation from their parents have they achieved? What sort of identities are evolving? How do they perceive their past? Do they perceive themselves as responsible for their own development or only the passive recipients of their parents' influences? How do they perceive themselves with regard to the future, and how do they anticipate their future responsibilities for themselves and others? Can they think about the varying consequences of different ways of living? How do they express their sexual and affectionate interests? These tasks occupy all adolescents and normally are performed at varying times.

Adolescents' object relations must be evaluated. Do they perceive and accept both good and bad qualities in their parents? Do they see their peers and boyfriends or girlfriends as separate persons with needs and identities of their own, or do others exist only for the adolescent's own needs?

INTERVIEWS

Whenever circumstances permit, both an adolescent patient and his or her parents should be interviewed. Other family members also may be included, depending on their involvement in the teenager's life and difficulties. Clinicians should see the adolescent first, however; preferential treatment helps avoid the appearance of being the parents' agent. In psychotherapy with an older adolescent, the therapist and the parents usually have little contact after the initial part of the therapy, because ongoing contact inhibits the adolescent's desire to open up.

Interview Techniques

All patients test therapists, but adolescents often manifest these reactions crudely, intensely, provocatively, and for prolonged periods. Clinicians must establish themselves as trustworthy and helpful adults to promote a therapeutic alliance. They should encourage adolescents to tell their own stories, without interrupting to check discrepancies; such a tactic seems like correcting and expressing disbelief. Clinicians should ask patients for explanations and theories about what happened. Why did these behaviors or feelings occur? When did things change? What caused the identified problems to begin when they did?

Sessions with adolescents generally follow the adult model; the therapist sits across from the patient. In early adolescence, however, board games (such as checkers) may help to stimulate conversation in an otherwise quiet, anxious patient.

Language is crucial. Even when a teenager and a clinician come from the same socioeconomic group, their languages are seldom the same. Psychiatrists should use their own language, explain any specialized terms or concepts, and ask for an explanation of unfamiliar in-group jargon or slang. Many adolescents do not talk spontaneously about illicit substances and suicidal tendencies but do respond honestly to a therapist's questions. A therapist may need to ask specifically about each substance and the amount and frequency of its use.

The sexual histories and current sexual activities of adolescents are increasingly important pieces of information for adequate evaluation. The nature of adolescents' sexual behaviors often is a vignette of their whole personality structures and ego development, but a long time may elapse in therapy before adolescents begin to talk about their sexual behavior.

TREATMENT

Individual Psychotherapy

Individual outpatient therapy is appropriate for adolescents whose problems are manifest in conflicted emotions and nondangerous behavior, who are not too disorganized to be maintained outside a structured setting, and whose families or other living environments are not disturbed enough to negate the influence of therapy. Such therapy characteristically focuses on intrapsychic conflicts and inhibitions; on the meanings of emotions, attitudes, and behavior; and on the influence of the past and the present. Antianxiety agents can be considered in adolescents whose anxiety may be high at certain times during psychotherapy, but adolescents' potential for abusing these drugs must be weighed carefully.

A 17-year-old girl complained of episodes of rapid heartbeat, sweating, trembling, and fears of going out alone to the shopping mall. She had entered her senior year in high school, was considering her choice of colleges, and was planning to take her college entrance examination. Her parents wanted her to maintain the family tradition and go to the college from which her mother graduated. Psychoanalytically oriented outpatient treatment and treatment with a selective serotonin reuptake inhibitor (SSRI) were instituted to alleviate the panic disorder symptoms. The psychotherapy focused on the patient's conflicts with her parents, highlighting her chronic concern that she could not meet parental expectations and fears of her independence. Medication appeared to reduce symptoms of tachycardia, tremulousness, and preoccupation with lack of competence. Psychotherapy was maintained for 8 months during her last year in high school. (Courtesy of Cynthia R. Pfeffer, M.D.)

Group Psychotherapy

In many ways, group psychotherapy is a natural setting for adolescents. Most teenagers are more comfortable with peers than with adults. A group diminishes the sense of unequal power between the adult therapist and the adolescent patient. Participation varies, depending on an adolescent's readiness. Not all interpretations and confrontations should come from the parent-figure therapist; group members often are adept at noticing symptomatic behavior in each other, and adolescents may find it easier to hear and consider critical or challenging comments from their peers.

Family Therapy

Family therapy is the primary modality when adolescents' difficulties mainly reflect a dysfunctional family (e.g., teenagers with school refusal, runaways). The same may be true when developmental issues, such as adolescent sexuality and striving for autonomy, trigger family conflicts or when family pathology is severe, as in cases of incest and child abuse. In these instances, adolescents usually need individual therapy as well, but family therapy is mandatory if an adolescent is to remain in the home or return to it.

Inpatient Treatment

Long-term inpatient therapy is the treatment of choice for severe disorders that are considered wholly or largely psychogenic in origin, such as major ego deficits that are caused by early massive deprivation and that respond poorly or not at all to medication.

CLINICAL PROBLEMS

Atypical Puberty

Pubertal changes that occur 2 1/2 years earlier or later than the average age are within the normal range. However, body image is so important to adolescents that extremes of the norm may be distressing to some, either because markedly early maturation subjects them to social and sexual pressures for which they are unready or because late maturation makes them feel inferior and excludes them from some peer activities. Medical reassurance, even if based on examination and testing to rule out pathophysiology, may not suffice. An adolescent's distress may show as sexual or delinquent acting out, withdrawal, or problems at school that are serious enough to warrant therapeutic intervention. Therapy also may be prompted by similar disturbances in some adolescents who fail to achieve peer-valued stereotypes of physical development despite normal pubertal physiology.

50 ▲

Geriatric Psychiatry

Geriatric psychiatry is concerned with preventing, diagnosing, and treating psychological disorders in older adults. It is also concerned with promoting longevity; persons with a healthy mental adaptation to life are likely to live longer than those stressed with emotional problems. Mental disorders in the elderly often differ in clinical manifestations, pathogenesis, and pathophysiology from disorders of younger adults and do not always match the categories in the text revision of the fourth edition of *Diagnostic and Statistical Manual of Mental Disorders* (DSM-IV-TR). Diagnosing and treating older adults can present more difficulties than treating younger persons because older persons may have coexisting chronic medical diseases and disabilities, may take many medications, and may show cognitive impairments.

Prevalence data for mental disorders in elderly persons vary widely, but a conservatively estimated 25 percent have significant psychiatric symptoms. The number of mentally ill elderly persons was estimated to be approximately 9 million in the year 2000. That figure is expected to rise to 20 million by the middle of the century. The American Board of Psychiatry and Neurology established geropsychiatry (from the Greek *geros* ["old age"] and *iatros* ["physical"]) as a subspecialty in 1991, and today geriatric psychiatry is one of the fastest-growing fields in psychiatry.

PSYCHIATRIC EXAMINATION OF THE OLDER PATIENT

Psychiatric history-taking and the mental status examination of older adults follow the same format as those of younger adults, but because of the high prevalence of cognitive disorders in older persons, psychiatrists must determine whether a patient understands the nature and purpose of the examination. When a patient is cognitively impaired, an independent history should be obtained from a family member or caretaker. The patient still should be seen alone—even if there is clear evidence of impairment—to preserve the privacy of the doctor–patient relationship and to elicit any suicidal thoughts or paranoid ideation, which may not be voiced in the presence of a relative or nurse.

When approaching the examination of the older patient, one must remember that older adults differ markedly from one another. The approach to examining the older patient must take into account whether the person is a healthy 75-year-old who recently retired from a second career or a frail 96-year-old who just lost the only surviving relative with the death of the 75-year-old caregiving daughter.

Psychiatric History

A complete psychiatric history includes preliminary identification (name, age, sex, marital status), chief complaint, history of the present illness, history of previous illnesses, personal history, and family history. A review of medications (including over-the-counter medications) that the patient is currently using or has used in the recent past is also important.

Patients older than age 65 often have subjective complaints of minor memory impairments, such as forgetting persons' names and misplacing objects. Minor cognitive problems also may occur because of anxiety in the interview situation. These age-associated memory impairments are of no significance; the term *benign senescent forgetfulness* has been used to describe them.

A patient's childhood and adolescent history can provide information about personality organization and give important clues about coping strategies and defense mechanisms used under stress. A history of learning disability or minimal cerebral dysfunction is significant. The psychiatrist should inquire about friends, sports, hobbies, social activity, and work. The occupational history should include the patient's feelings about work, relationships with peers, problems with authority, and attitudes toward retirement. The patient also should be questioned about plans for the future. What are the patient's hopes and fears?

The family history should include a patient's description of parents' attitudes and adaptation to their old age and, if applicable, information about the causes of their deaths. Alzheimer's disease is transmitted as an autosomal-dominant trait in 10 to 30 percent of the offspring of parents with Alzheimer's disease; depression and alcohol dependence also run in families. The patient's current social situation should also be evaluated. Who cares for the patient? Does the patient have children? What are the characteristics of patient–child relationships? A financial history helps the psychiatrist to evaluate the role of economic hardship in the patient's illness and to make realistic treatment recommendations.

The marital history includes a description of the spouse and the characteristics of the relationship. If the patient is a widow or a widower, the psychiatrist should explore how grieving was handled. If the loss of the spouse occurred within the past year, the patient is at high risk for an adverse physical or psychological event.

The patient's sexual history includes sexual activity, orientation, libido, masturbation, extramarital affairs, and sexual symptoms (such as impotence and anorgasmia). Young clinicians may have to overcome their own biases about taking a sexual history: Sexuality is an area of concern for many geriatric patients, who welcome the chance to talk about their sexual feelings and attitudes.

Mental Status Examination

The mental status examination offers a cross-sectional view of how a patient thinks, feels, and behaves during the examination. With older adults, a psychiatrist may not be able to rely on a single examination to answer all of the diagnostic questions. Repeat mental status examinations may be needed because of fluctuating changes in the patient's family.

General Description.   A general description of the patient includes appearance, psychomotor activity, attitude toward the examiner, and speech activity.

Motor disturbances (e.g., shuffling gait, stooped posture, "pill rolling" movements of the fingers, tremors, and body asymmetry) should be noted. Involuntary movements of the mouth or tongue may be adverse effects of phenothiazine medication. Many depressed patients seem to be slow in speech and movement. A mask-like facies occurs in Parkinson's disease.

The patient's speech may be pressured in agitated, manic, and anxious states. Tearfulness and overt crying occur in depressive and cognitive disorders, especially if the patient feels frustrated about being unable to answer one of the examiner's questions. The presence of a hearing aid or another indication that the patient has a hearing problem (e.g., requesting repetition of questions) should be noted.

The patient's attitude toward the examiner—cooperative, suspicious, guarded, ingratiating—can give clues about possible transference reactions. Because of transference, older adults can react to younger physicians as if the physicians were parent figures, despite the age difference.

Functional Assessment.   Patients older than 65 years of age should be evaluated for their capacity to maintain independence and to perform the activities of daily life, which include toileting, preparing meals, dressing, grooming, and eating. The degree of functional competence in their everyday behaviors is an important consideration in formulating a plan of treatment for these patients.

Mood, Feelings, and Affect.   Suicide is a leading cause of death of older persons, and an evaluation of a patient's suicidal ideation is essential. Loneliness is the most common reason cited by older adults who consider suicide. Feelings of loneliness, worthlessness, helplessness, and hopelessness are symptoms of depression, which carries a high risk for suicide. Nearly 75 percent of all suicide victims suffer from depression, alcohol abuse, or both. The examiner should specifically ask the patient about any thoughts of suicide, whether the patient feels life is no longer worth living, and whether a person is better off dead or, when dead, is no longer a burden to others. Such thoughts—especially when associated with alcohol abuse, living alone, recent death of a spouse, physical illness, and somatic pain—indicate a high suicidal risk.

Disturbances in mood states, most notably depression and anxiety, may interfere with memory functioning. An expansive or euphoric mood may indicate a manic episode or may signal a dementing disorder. Frontal lobe dysfunction often produces *witzelsucht*, which is the tendency to make puns and jokes and then laugh aloud at them.

The patient's affect may be flat, blunted, constricted, shallow, or inappropriate, all of which can indicate a depressive disorder, schizophrenia, or brain dysfunction. Such affects are important abnormal findings, even though they are not pathognomonic of a specific disorder. Dominant lobe dysfunction causes dysprosody, an inability to express emotional feelings through speech intonation.

Perceptual Disturbances.   Hallucinations and illusions by older adults may be transitory phenomena resulting from decreased sensory acuity. The examiner should note whether the patient is confused about time or place during the hallucinatory episode; confusion points to an organic condition. It is particularly important to ask the patient about distorted body perceptions. Because hallucinations may be caused by brain tumors and other focal pathology, a diagnostic workup may be indicated. Brain diseases cause perceptive impairments; agnosia, the inability to recognize and interpret the significance of sensory impressions, is associated with organic brain diseases. The examiner should note the type of agnosia—the denial of illness (anosognosia), the denial of a body part (atopognosia), or the inability to recognize objects (visual agnosia) or faces (prosopagnosia).

Language Output.   This category of the geriatric mental status examination covers the aphasias, which are disorders of language output related to organic lesions of the brain. The best described are nonfluent, or Broca's aphasia; fluent, or Wernicke's aphasia; and global aphasia, a combination of fluent and nonfluent aphasias. In nonfluent, or Broca's, aphasia, the patient's understanding remains intact, but the ability to speak is impaired. The patient cannot pronounce "Methodist Episcopalian." Speech generally is mispronounced and may be telegraphic. A simple test for Wernicke's aphasia is to point to some common objects—such as a pen or a pencil, a doorknob, and a light switch—and ask the patient to name them. The patient also may be unable to demonstrate the use of simple objects, such as a key and a match (ideomotor apraxia).

Visuospatial Functioning.   Some decline in visuospatial capability is normal with aging. Asking a patient to copy figures or a drawing may be helpful in assessing the function. A neuropsychological assessment should be performed when visuospatial functioning is obviously impaired.

Thought.   Disturbances in thinking include neologisms, word salad, circumstantiality, tangentiality, loosening of associations, flight of ideas, clang associations, and blocking. The loss of the ability to appreciate nuances of meaning (abstract thinking) may be an early sign of dementia. Thinking is then described as concrete or literal.

Thought content should be examined for phobias, obsessions, somatic preoccupations, and compulsions. Ideas about suicide or homicide should be discussed. The examiner should determine whether delusions are present and how such delusions affect the patient's life. Delusions may be present in nursing home patients and may have been a reason for admission.

Ideas of reference or of influence should be described. Patients who are hard of hearing may be classified mistakenly as paranoid or suspicious.

Sensorium and Cognition.
Sensorium concerns the functioning of the special senses; cognition concerns information processing and intellect. The survey of both areas, known as the *neuropsychiatric examination*, consists of the clinician's assessment and a comprehensive battery of psychological tests.

CONSCIOUSNESS. A sensitive indicator of brain dysfunction is an altered state of consciousness in which the patient does not seem to be alert, shows fluctuations in levels of awareness, or seems to be lethargic. In severe cases, the patient is somnolescent or stuporous.

ORIENTATION. Impairment in orientation to time, place, and person is associated with cognitive disorders. Cognitive impairment often is observed in mood disorders, anxiety disorders, factitious disorders, conversion disorder, and personality disorders, especially during periods of severe physical or environmental stress. The examiner should test for orientation to place by asking the patient to describe his or her present location. Orientation to person may be approached in two ways: Does the patient know his or her own name, and are nurses and doctors identified as such? Time is tested by asking the patient the date, the year, the month, and the day of the week. The patient also should be asked about the length of time spent in a hospital, during what season of the year, and how the patient knows these facts. Greater significance is given to difficulties concerning person than to difficulties of time and place, and more significance is given to orientation to place than to orientation to time.

MEMORY. Memory usually is evaluated in terms of immediate, recent, and remote memory. Immediate retention and recall are tested by giving the patient six digits to repeat forward and backward. The examiner should record the result of the patient's capacity to remember. Persons with unimpaired memory usually can recall six digits forward and five or six digits backward. The clinician should be aware that the ability to do well on digit-span tests is impaired in extremely anxious patients. Remote memory can be tested by asking for the patient's place and date of birth, the patient's mother's name before she was married, and names and birthdays of the patient's children.

In cognitive disorders, recent memory deteriorates first. Recent memory assessment can be approached in several ways. Some examiners give the patient the names of three items early in the interview and ask for recall later. Others prefer to tell a brief story and ask the patient to repeat it verbatim. Memory of the recent past also can be tested by asking for the patient's place of residence, including the street number; the method of transportation to the hospital; and some current events. If the patient has a memory deficit such as amnesia, careful testing should be performed to determine whether it is retrograde amnesia (loss of memory before an event) or anterograde amnesia (loss of memory after the event). Retention and recall also can be tested by having the patient retell a simple story. Patients who confabulate make up new material in retelling the story.

INTELLECTUAL TASKS, INFORMATION, AND INTELLIGENCE. Various intellectual tasks may be presented to estimate the patient's fund of general knowledge and intellectual functioning. Counting and calculation can be tested by asking the patient to sub-tract 7 from 100 and to continue subtracting 7 from the result until the number 2 is reached. The examiner records the responses as a baseline for future testing. The examiner can also ask the patient to count backward from 20 to 1, and can record the time necessary to complete the exercise. The patient also can be asked to do simple arithmetic—for example, to state the number of nickels in $1.35.

The patient's fund of general knowledge is related to intelligence. The patient can be asked to name the president of the United States, to name the three largest cities in the United States, to give the population of the United States, and to give the distance from New York to Paris. The examiner must take into account the patient's educational level, socioeconomic status (SES), and general life experience in assessing the results of some of these tests.

READING AND WRITING. It may be important for the clinician to examine the patient's reading and writing and to determine whether the patient has a specific speech deficit. The examiner may have the patient read a simple story aloud or write a short sentence to test for a reading or writing disorder. Whether the patient is right-handed or left-handed should be noted.

Judgment.
Judgment is the capacity to act appropriately in various situations. Does the patient show impaired judgment? What would the patient do on finding a stamped, sealed, addressed envelope in the street? What would the patient do if he or she smelled smoke in a theater? Can the patient discriminate? What is the difference between a dwarf and a boy? Why are couples required to get a marriage license?

Neuropsychological Evaluation

A thorough neuropsychological examination includes a comprehensive battery of tests that can be replicated by various examiners and can be repeated over time to assess the course of a specific illness. The most widely used test of current cognitive functioning is the Mini-Mental State Examination (MMSE), which assesses orientation, attention, calculation, immediate and short-term recall, language, and the ability to follow simple commands. The MMSE is used to detect impairments, follow the course of an illness, and monitor the patient's treatment responses. It is not used to make a formal diagnosis. The maximum MMSE score is 30. Age and educational level influence cognitive performance as measured by the MMSE.

The assessment of intellectual abilities is performed with the Wechsler Adult Intelligence Scale—Revised (WAIS–R), which gives verbal, performance, and full-scale intelligence quotient (IQ) scores. Some test results, such as those of vocabulary tests, hold up as aging progresses; results of other tests, such as tests of similarities and digit-symbol substitution, do not. The performance part of the WAIS–R is a more sensitive indicator of brain damage than the verbal part.

Visuospatial functions are sensitive to the normal aging process. The Bender Gestalt test is one of a large number of instruments used to test visuospatial functions; another is the Halstead-Reitan battery, which is the most complex battery of tests covering the entire spectrum of information processing and cognition. Depression, even in the absence of dementia, often impairs psychomotor performance, especially visuospatial functioning and timed motor performance. The Geriatric Depression Scale is a useful screening instrument that excludes somatic complaints from its list of items. The presence of somatic complaints on a rating scale tends to confound the diagnosis of a depressive disorder.

Medical History.   Elderly patients have more concomitant, chronic, and multiple medical problems and take more medications than younger adults; many of these medications can influence their mental status. The past medical history includes all major illnesses, traumas, hospitalizations, and treatment interventions. The psychiatrist should also be alert to underlying medical illness. Infections, metabolic and electrolyte disturbances, and myocardial infarction and stroke may first be manifested by psychiatric symptoms. Depressed mood, delusions, and hallucinations may precede other symptoms of Parkinson's disease by many months. On the other hand, a psychiatric disorder can also cause such somatic symptoms as weight loss, malnutrition, and inanition of severe depression.

Careful review of medications (including over-the-counter medications, laxatives, vitamins, tonics, and lotions) and even substances recently discontinued is extremely important. Drug effects may be long lasting and may induce depression (e.g., antihypertensives), cognitive impairment (e.g., sedatives), delirium (e.g., anticholinergics), and seizures (e.g., neuroleptics). The review of medications must include sufficient detail to identify misuse (overuse, underuse) and relate medication use to special diets. A dietary history is also important; deficiencies and excesses (e.g., protein, vitamins) may influence physiological function and mental status.

MENTAL DISORDERS OF OLD AGE

The National Institute of Mental Health's Epidemiologic Catchment Area (ECA) program has found that the most common mental disorders of old age are depressive disorders, cognitive disorders, phobias, and alcohol use disorders. Older adults also have a high risk for suicide and drug-induced psychiatric symptoms. Many metal disorders of old age can be prevented, ameliorated, or even reversed. Of special importance are the reversible causes of delirium and dementia; but if not diagnosed accurately and treated in a timely fashion, these conditions can progress to an irreversible state requiring a patient's institutionalization. A comprehensive test battery is preferable for confident determination of presence and type of dementia or other cognitive disorder in elderly persons, but in some circumstances, administering a several-hour battery is not possible.

Many drugs can cause psychiatric symptoms in older adults. These symptoms can result from age-related alterations in drug absorption, a prescribed dosage that is too large, not following instructions and taking too large a dose, sensitivity to the medication, and conflicting regimens presented by several physicians. Almost the entire spectrum of mental disorders can be caused by drugs.

The reader is referred to the various sections in this book for more detailed information about the disorders mentioned above.

51

End-of-Life Care and Palliative Medicine

End-of-life refers to all those issues involved in caring for the terminally ill. It begins when curative therapy ceases and encompasses the following areas: (1) communication of prognosis to family and patient, and defining the patient's understanding of his or her illness; (2) advance directives about life-sustaining treatment; (3) the need for hospitalization and hospice care; (4) legal and ethical matters; (5) bereavement support and psychiatric care; and, finally, (6) palliative care to relieve pain and suffering. Each of these issues is discussed below.

GENERAL APPROACHES TO CARING FOR THE DYING PATIENT

The most important task for physicians caring for dying patients is to provide compassionate concern and continuing support. The hallmarks of appropriate care are predicated on a good doctor–patient relationship and include visiting patients regularly, maintaining eye contact, listening and touching appropriately, and being willing to answer questions respectfully and honestly.

Problems Facing the Physicians and Other Clinicians

Clinicians' abilities to care compassionately and effectively for patients who are dying depend largely on their own beliefs about death and dying. Indeed, some physicians are so upset by death that they are reluctant to discuss end-of-life issues with their patients; others may steadfastly refuse to use palliative care services for the terminally ill. Such terminally ill patients may be subject to unnecessary worry and discomfort if their doctors are unwilling to confront death with them.

Many physicians have been led by modern medicine and their training to unconsciously assume that they can prevent death. This false feeling of omnipotence is challenged by encounters with dying patients, because these doctors equate these patients with failure. It is no surprise, then, that these physicians may avoid their dying patients when their condition calls into question their own competence. Ultimately, their failure to accept their own inadequacies and limitations in treating disease often comes at the expense of patient care and comfort.

COMMUNICATION AND ITS IMPORTANCE

After a diagnosis and prognosis have been made, physicians need to talk to the patient and the patient's family. Formerly, doctors subscribed to a conspiracy of silence, believing that their patients' chances for recovery would improve if they knew less, because news of impending death might bring despair. The current practice is now one of honesty and openness toward patients; in fact, the question is not whether or not to tell the patient, but when and how. The American Hospital Association in 1972 drafted the Patient's Bill of Rights, declaring that patients have the "right to obtain complete, current information regarding diagnosis, treatment and prognosis in terms the patient can be reasonably expected to understand."

When breaking news of impending death to the patient, as when relating any bad news, diplomacy and compassion should be guiding principles. Often, bad news is not completely related during one meeting but rather is absorbed gradually over a series of separate conversations. Advance preparations, including scheduling enough time for the visit, researching pertinent information such as test results and facts about the case, and even arranging furniture appropriately can only make the patient feel more comfortable.

If possible, these conversations should take place in a private, suitable space with the patient on equal terms with the physician (i.e., the patient dressed and the physician seated). If it is possible and desired by the patient, the patient's spouse or partner should be present. The treating physician should explain the current situation to the patient in clear, simple language, even when speaking to highly educated patients. Information may need to be repeated or additional meetings may be necessary to communicate all of the information. A gentle, sensible approach will help modulate the patient's own denial and acceptance. At no time should physicians take their patient's angry comments personally, and they should never criticize the patient's response to the bad news.

Physicians can signal their availability for honest communication by encouraging and answering questions from patients. Estimates as to how long a patient has to live are usually inaccurate and thus should not be given. Also, physicians should make it clear to their patients that they are willing to see them through until death occurs. Ultimately, physicians must choose how much information to give and when on the basis of each patient's needs and capacities.

The same general approaches apply as physicians seek to comfort members of the patient's family. Helping family members deal with feelings about the patient's illness can be just as important as comforting the patient, because family members are often the main source of emotional support for patients. Table 51–1 lists seven promises that physicians may make to dying patients.

Table 51–1
The Seven Promises a Physician Should Make to a Dying Patient

- You will have the best of medical treatment, aiming to prevent exacerbation, improve function and survival, and ensure comfort.
- You will never have to endure overwhelming pain, shortness of breath, or other symptoms.
- Your care will be continuous, comprehensive, and coordinated.
- You and your family will be prepared for everything that is likely to happen in the course of your illness.
- Your wishes will be sought and respected, and followed whenever possible.
- We will help you consider your personal and financial resources and we will respect your choices about their use.
- We will do all we can to see that you and your family will have the opportunity to make the best of every day.

From Mitka M. Suggestions for help when the end is near. *JAMA.* 2000; 284:2441.
Adapted from National Coalition on Health Care (NCHC) and the Institute for Health-care Improvement (IHI). *Promises to Keep: Changing the Way We Provide Care at the End of Life,* released October 12, 2000, with permission.

TELLING THE TRUTH

Tactful honesty is the doctor's most important aid. Honesty, however, need not preclude hope or guarded optimism. One should always be aware that if 85 percent of patients with a particular disease die in 5 years, 15 percent are still alive after that time. The principles of doing good and not doing harm inform the decision of whether or not to tell the patient the truth. In general, most patients want to know the truth about their condition. Various studies of patients with malignancies show that 80 to 90 percent want to know their diagnosis. However, doctors should ask patients how much they want to know about the illness because some persons do not want to know the facts about their illness. Such patients, if told the truth, deny that they ever were told, and they cannot participate in end-of-life decisions such as the use of life-sustaining equipment. The patients who openly request that they not be given "bad news" are often those who most fear death. Physicians should deal with these fears directly, but if the patient still cannot bear to hear the truth, someone closely related to the patient must be informed.

TERMINAL CARE DECISIONS

Advance Directives

Advance directives are wishes and choices about medical intervention when the patient's condition is considered terminal. Advance directives are legally binding in all 50 states, and there are three types: living will, health care proxy, and do not resuscitate (DNR) and do not intubate (DNI) orders.

Living Will.   In a living will, a patient who is mentally competent gives specific instructions that doctors must follow when the patient cannot communicate them because of illness. These instructions may include rejection of feeding tubes, artificial airways, or any other measures to prolong life.

Health Care Proxy.   Also known as *durable power of attorney*, the health care proxy gives another person the power to make medical decisions if the patient cannot do so. That person, also known as the *surrogate*, is empowered to make all decisions about terminal care on the basis of what he or she thinks the patient would want.

Do Not Resuscitate and Do Not Intubate Orders. These orders prohibit doctors from attempting to resuscitate (DNR) or intubate (DNI) the patient who is in extremis. DNR and DNI orders are made by the patient who is competent to do so. They can be made part of the living will or expressed by the health care proxy. A sample advance directive that incorporates both a living will and a health care proxy is given in Table 51–2.

The *Uniform Rights of the Terminally Ill Act*, drafted by the National Conference on Uniform State Laws, was approved and recommended for enactment in all states. This act authorizes an adult to control the decisions regarding the administration of life-sustaining treatment by executing a declaration instructing a physician to withhold or to withdraw life-sustaining treatment if the person is in a terminal condition and cannot participate in medical treatment decisions. In 1991, the Federal Patients Self-Determination Act became law in the United States and required that all health care facilities (1) provide each patient admitted to a hospital with written information about the right to refuse treatment, (2) ask about advance directives, and (3) keep written records of whether the patient has an advance directive or has designated a health care proxy.

PALLIATIVE CARE

Palliative care is the most important part of end-of-life care. It refers to providing relief from the suffering caused by pain or other symptoms of terminal disease. While this is most commonly associated with analgesic drug administration, many other medical interventions and surgical procedures fall under the umbrella of palliative care because they can make the patient more comfortable. Monitors and their alarms, peripheral and central lines, phlebotomy, measurement of signs, and even supplemental oxygen are usually discontinued to allow the patient to die peacefully. Relocating the patient to a quiet, private room (as opposed to an intensive care unit) and allowing family members to be present is another very important palliative care modality.

The shift from active treatment to palliative care is sometimes the first tangible sign that the patient will die, a transition that is emotionally difficult for everyone concerned about the patient to accept. The discontinuation of machines and measurements, which up until this point have been an integral part of the hospital experience, can be extremely disconcerting to the patient, family members, and even other physicians. Indeed, if these parties are not active in planning this transition, it can easily seem that persons have given up on the patient.

Because of this difficulty, palliative care is sometimes avoided altogether (i.e., curative treatment is continued until the patient dies). This approach is likely to cause problems if it is adopted merely to avoid the reality of impending death. A well-negotiated transition to palliative care often decreases anxiety after the patient and family go through an appropriate anticipatory grief reaction. Furthermore, a positive emotional outcome is much more likely if the physician and staff project a conviction that palliative care will be an active, involved process, without hint of withdrawal or abandonment. When this does not occur or when the family cannot tolerate the transition, the ensuing stress frequently results in a need for psychiatric consultation.

Table 51–2
Advance Directive Living Will and Health Care Proxy

Death is a part of life. It is a reality like birth, growth, and aging. I am using this advance directive to convey my wishes about medical care to my doctors and other people looking after me at the end of my life. It is called an advance directive because it gives instructions in advance about what I want to happen to me in the future. It expresses my wishes about medical treatment that might keep me alive. I want this to be legally binding.

If I cannot make or communicate decisions about my medical care, those around me should rely on this document for instructions about measures that could keep me alive.

I do not want medical treatment (including feeding and water by tube) that will keep me alive if:

• I am unconscious and there is no reasonable prospect that I will ever be conscious again (even if I am not going to die soon in my medical condition), or

• I am near death from an illness or injury with no reasonable prospect of recovery.

I do want medicine and other care to make me more comfortable and to take care of pain and suffering. I want this even if the pain medicine makes me die sooner.

I want to give some extra instructions: *[Here list any special instructions, e.g., some people fear being kept alive after a debilitating stroke. If you have wishes about this, or any other condition, please write them here.]*

The legal language in the box that follows is a health care proxy. It gives another person the power to make medical decisions for me.

> I name _____,
> who lives at _____,
> phone number _____, to make medical decisions for me if I cannot make them myself. This person is called a health care "surrogate," "agent," "proxy," or "attorney in fact." This power of attorney shall become effective when I become incapable of making or communicating decisions about my medical care. This means that this document stays legal when and if I lose the power to speak for myself, for instance, if I am in a coma or have Alzheimer's disease.
>   My health care proxy has power to tell others what my advance directive means. This person also has power to make decisions for me based either on what I would have wanted, or, if this is not known, on what he or she thinks is best for me.
>   If my first choice health care proxy cannot or decides not to act for me, I name _____,
> address _____,
> phone number _____, as my second choice.

I have discussed my wishes with my health care proxy, and with my second choice if I have chosen to appoint a second person. My proxy(ies) has(have) agreed to act for me.

I have thought about this advance directive carefully. I know what it means and want to sign it. I have chosen two witnesses, neither of whom is a member of my family, nor will inherit from me when I die. My witnesses are not the same people as those I named as my health care proxies. I understand that this form should be notarized if I use the box to name (a) health care proxy(ies).

Signature _____

Date _____

Address _____

Witness's signature _____

Witness's printed name _____

Address _____

Witness's signature _____

Witness's printed name _____

Address _____

Notary [to be used if proxy is appointed] _____

Reprinted with permission from Choice in Dying, Inc.—the National Council for the Right to Die. (Choice in Dying is a national not-for-profit organization that works for the rights of patients at the end of life. In addition to this generic advance directive, Choice in Dying distributes advance directives that conform to each state's specific legal requirements and maintains a national Living Will Registry for completed documents.)

A 36-year-old physician with end-stage leukemia was seen in psychiatric consultation because he reported seeing the "angel of death" at the foot of his hospital bed. He described the experience as frightening and inexplicable. The consultant asked the patient, "Are you afraid that you are going to die?" That was the first time anyone had mentioned death or dying in any context to the patient. He welcomed the opportunity to talk openly about his fears to the medical staff and to his family and eventually died a peaceful death.

Psychiatric consultation is indicated for patients who become severely anxious, suicidal, depressed, or overtly psychotic. In each instance, appropriate psychiatric medication can be pre-

scribed to provide relief. Patients who are suicidal do not always have to be transferred to a psychiatric service. An attendant or nurse can be assigned to the patient on a 24-hour basis (one-on-one coverage). In such instances, the relationship that develops between the observer and the patient may have therapeutic overtones, especially with patients whose depression is related to a sense of abandonment. Terminal patients who are at high risk for suicide are usually in pain. When pain is relieved, suicidal ideation is likely to diminish. A careful evaluation of suicide potential is required for all patients. A premorbid history of past suicide attempts is a high risk factor for suicide in terminally ill patients. In patients who become psychotic, impaired cognitive function secondary to metastatic lesions to the brain must always be considered. Such patients respond to antipsychotic medications, and psychotherapy may also be of use.

PAIN MANAGEMENT

Types of Pain

Dying patients are subject to several different kinds of pain that call for different treatment strategies; somatic and visceral pain are more responsive to opiates, while neuropathic and sympathetically maintained pain respond better to adjuvant medications. Most advanced cancer patients, for example, have more than one kind of pain and require complex treatment regimens.

> A highly mobile and independent man with a malignant illness developed brain metastases that resulted in paralysis of his legs. His motility became markedly impaired and he was confined to a wheelchair. Having always been in control of his life circumstances, he now perceived others as "controlling his life." Subsequently, he began to accuse his wife of trying to kill him by giving him too much medicine and became highly suspicious of all persons in his household, feeling that they were plotting ways to harm him or force him into total submission. He developed outbursts of intense anger, which occurred without provocation. As his disease progressed, he became increasingly confused and disoriented and began to hear persons "talking about him" when no one was present. The patient was treated with small dosages of antipsychotic medications to control the psychotic symptoms. The family was encouraged to include him in planning activities of the household so as to increase his sense of control and participation. His wife received counseling to assist her in coping with the behavior. (From Barton D. Approaches to the clinical care of the dying person. In: Barton D, ed. *Dying and Death: A Clinical Guide for Caregivers*. Baltimore: Williams & Wilkins; 1977:87.)

Treatment of Pain

It cannot be overemphasized that pain management should be aggressive, and treatment should be multimodal. In fact, a good pain regimen may require several drugs or the same drug used in different ways and administered via different routes. For example, intravenous (IV) morphine may be supplemented by self-administered oral "rescue" doses, or a continuous epidural drip may be supplemented by bolus IV doses. Transdermal patches may provide baseline concentrations in patients for whom IV or oral intake is difficult. Patient-controlled analgesia systems for IV opiate administration result in better pain relief with lower amounts dispensed than in staff-administered dosing.

Opioids commonly cause delirium and hallucinations. A frequent mechanism of psychotoxicity is the accumulation of drugs or metabolites whose duration of analgesia is shorter than their plasma half-life (morphine, levorphanol [Levo-Dromoran], and methadone [Dolophine]). Use of drugs like hydromorphone (Dilaudid), which have half-lives closer to their analgesic duration, can relieve the problem without loss of pain control. Cross-tolerance is incomplete between opiates; hence, several should be tried in any patient with the dosage lowered when switching drugs.

The benefits of maintenance analgesia administration in terminally ill patients compared with as-needed administration cannot be overemphasized. Maintenance dosing improves pain control, increases drug efficiency, and relieves patient anxiety, whereas as-needed orders allow pain to increase while waiting for the drug to be given. Moreover, as-needed analgesia administration perversely sets up the patient for staff complaints about drug-seeking behavior. Even when maintenance treatment is used, extra doses of medication should be available for breakthrough pain, and repeated use of these medications should signal the need to raise the maintenance dose. Depending on their previous experiences with opioid analgesics and their weight, it is not unusual for some patients to require 2 g or more of morphine per day for relief of symptoms.

Knowing doses of different drugs and different routes of administration is important to avoid accidental undermedication. For example, when changing a patient from intramuscular (IM) to oral morphine use, one must multiply the IM dose by six to avoid causing the patient pain and provoking drug-seeking behavior. Many adjuvant drugs used for pain are psychotropics with which psychiatrists are familiar, but in some cases, their analgesic effect is separate from their primary psychotropic effect. Commonly used adjuvants include antidepressants, phenothiazines, butyrophenones, antihistamines, amphetamines, and steroids. They are particularly important in neuropathic and sympathetically maintained pain, for which they can be the mainstay of treatment.

Other developments in pain management include more intrusive procedures such as nerve blocks or the use of continuous epidural infusions. Additionally, radiation therapy, chemotherapy, and even surgical resection should always be considered as pain management modalities in palliative care. Short courses of radiotherapy or chemotherapy can be used to shrink tumors or manage metastatic lesions that cause pain or impairment. In patients with end-stage Hodgkin's disease, for example, systemic chemotherapy can improve the patient's quality of life by decreasing tumor burden. Surgical resection of invasive tumors, most notably breast carcinomas, can be useful for the same reason.

HOSPICE CARE

In 1967, the founding of St. Christopher's Hospice in England by Cicely Saunders launched the modern hospice movement. Several factors in the 1960s propelled the development of hospices, including concerns about inadequately trained physicians, inept terminal care, gross inequities in health care, and neglect of the elderly. Life expectancy had increased, and heart disease and cancer were becoming more common. Saunders emphasized an interdisciplinary approach to symptom control, care of the patient and family as a unit, the use of volunteers, continuity of care (including home care), and follow-up with family members after a patient's death. The first hospice in the United States, Connecticut Hospice, opened in 1974. By 2000, there were more than 3,000 hospices in the United States.

Round-the-clock pain control with opioids is an essential component of hospice management. In 1983, Medicare began reimbursing hospice care. Medicare hospice guidelines emphasize home care, with benefits provided for a broad spectrum of physician, nursing, psychosocial, and spiritual services at home or, if necessary, in a hospital or nursing home. To be eligible, the patient must be physician certified as having 6 months or less to live. By electing hospice care, patients agree to receive palliative rather than curative treatment. Many hospice programs are hospital-based, sometimes in separate units and sometimes in the form of hospice beds interspersed throughout the facility. Other program models include free-standing hospices and programs, hospital-affiliated hospices, nursing home hospice care, and home care programs. Nursing homes are the site of death for many elderly patients with incurable chronic illness, yet dying nursing home residents have limited access to palliative and hospice care. For example, in 1997, 3 percent of hospice enrollees were in nursing homes, while 87 percent were in private homes.

Hospice families generally express satisfaction with their personal involvement in hospice care. Savings with hospice care vary, but home care programs generally cost less than conventional institutional care, particularly in the final months of life. Hospice patients are less likely to receive diagnostic studies or such intensive therapy as surgery or chemotherapy. Hospice care is a proved, viable alternative for patients who elect a palliative approach to terminal care. In addition, hospice goals of dignified, comfortable death for the terminally ill and care for patient and family together have been increasingly adopted into mainstream medicine.

NEONATAL AND INFANT END-OF-LIFE CARE

Most decisions to forego life-sustaining procedures for newborns concern those whose death is imminent. Even if their future quality of life is determined to be bleak, most physicians feel that some life is better than no life at all. Those physicians who support withholding intensive care consider the following quality-of-life issues: (1) extent of bodily damage (e.g., severe neurological impairment), (2) the burden that a disabled child will place on the family, and (3) the ability of the child to derive some pleasure from existence (e.g., having an awareness of being alive and being able to form relationships).

The American Academy of Pediatrics permits nontreatment decisions for newborns when the infant is irreversibly comatose or when treatment would be futile and only prolong the process of dying. These standards do not permit the parents to have any input into the decision-making process. In a well-publicized case in England in 2000, it was decided to surgically separate conjoined twins knowing that one would die as a result of the procedure and despite the objections of the parents, who believed that nature should take its course even if that led to the death of both infants.

EUTHANASIA AND PHYSICIAN-ASSISTED SUICIDE

Euthanasia

Euthanasia is defined as a physician's deliberate act to cause a patient's death by directly administering a lethal dose of medication or other agent. Because such patients are thought of as hopelessly ill or injured, euthanasia has been called "mercy killing." On the basis of the doctor's action and the patient's condition, several types of euthanasia have been described: *active euthanasia*, in which a physician deliberately intends to kill a patient to alleviate or prevent uncontrollable suffering; *passive euthanasia*, in which a physician withholds artificial life-sustaining measures; *voluntary euthanasia*, in which the person who is to die is competent to give consent and does so; and *involuntary euthanasia*, in which the person who is to die is incompetent or incapable of giving consent. Euthanasia assumes that the intent of the physician is to aid and abet the patient's wish to die.

Physician-Assisted Suicide

Suicide is a deliberate taking of one's own life. *Assisted suicide* is the imparting of information or means to enable such an act to take place. When the assistance is provided by a physician, the suicide is *physician* assisted. Assisted suicide and euthanasia should not be confused with palliative care designed to alleviate the suffering of dying patients. Palliative care includes giving pain relief and emotional, social, and spiritual support, as well as psychiatric care if indicated. The intent of palliative care is to relieve pain and suffering, not to end a patient's life, even though death may result from palliative care.

The issue of physician-assisted suicide came to national attention in 1990 when Jack Kevorkian, a physician in Michigan, connected Janet Adkins, a victim of dementia of the Alzheimer's type, to a so-called suicide machine that enabled her to give herself an infusion of potassium chloride (KCl) that ended her life. After that, Kevorkian helped more than 100 persons take their own lives. In Michigan, where Kevorkian practiced, he was indicted for manslaughter and, in 1999, was sentenced to prison.

At one time, suicide was considered a type of murder, although no one was or is prosecuted for the crime. Assisted suicide, however, is a crime, and in some states (e.g., California) can be prosecuted as murder. More than 40 states in the United States, however, currently consider aiding and abetting suicide a crime without defining it as murder. In 1996, in both New York and California, state courts upheld the right to bring about one's own death through assisted suicide. In a 1994 landmark decision, the people of Oregon approved a referendum permitting physicians to prescribe lethal medication for terminally ill patients (the Oregon Death with Dignity Act).

In the United States, physician-assisted suicide and euthanasia have been consistently opposed by the American Psychiatric Association (APA), the American Medical Association (AMA), the American Nurses Association, the National Legal Center for the Disabled, and the Roman Catholic Church. The World Medical Association issued the following declaration on euthanasia in October 1987:

> Euthanasia, that is the act of deliberately ending the life of a patient, even at his own request or at the request of his close relatives, is unethical. This does not prevent the physician from respecting the will of a patient to allow the natural process of death to follow its course in the terminal phase of sickness.

The New York State Committee of Bioethical Issues is also opposed to euthanasia but has stated that physicians have an obligation to provide effective treatment to relieve pain and suffering, even though the treatment may on occasion hasten death. The committee stated the following:

> The principle of patient autonomy requires that physicians respect the decision of a patient who possesses decision-making

capacity to forgo life-sustaining treatment. Life-sustaining treatment is defined as any medical treatment that serves to prolong life without reversing the underlying medical condition. Life-sustaining treatment includes, but is not limited to, mechanical ventilation, renal dialysis, blood transfusions, chemotherapy, antibiotics, and artificial nutrition and hydration.

Physicians are obligated to relieve pain and suffering and to promote the dignity and autonomy of dying patients in their care. This obligation includes providing effective palliative treatment even though such treatment may occasionally hasten death. But physicians should not perform euthanasia or participate in assisted suicide. Support, comfort, respect for patient autonomy, good communication, and adequate pain control may dramatically decrease the demand for euthanasia and assisted suicide. In certain carefully defined circumstances, it is humane to recognize that death is certain and suffering is great.

52 ▲

Forensic Psychiatry

Forensic psychiatry is the branch of medicine that deals with disorders of the mind and their relation to legal principles. The word *forensic* means belonging to the courts of law. At various stages in their historical development, psychiatry and the law have converged. Today, the two disciplines often intersect, especially when dealing with the criminal who, by violating the rules of society secondary to mental disorder, adversely affects the functioning of the community. Traditionally, the psychiatrist's efforts help explain the causes and, through prevention and treatment, reduce the self-destructive elements of harmful behavior. The lawyer, as the agent of society, is concerned that the social deviant is a potential threat to the safety and security of other persons. Both psychiatry and the law seek to implement their respective goals through the application of pragmatic techniques based on empirical observations.

Thomas Gutheil, an influential forensic psychiatrist, points out that the interface between psychiatry and the law contains much complexity and potential for gross misunderstanding, as illustrated in the following example.

During a routine outpatient psychotherapy appointment, a male middle-level manager began to complain to his therapist about his boss. Feeling the freedom of expression that the therapeutic situation is intended to foster, the man worked himself up to a higher pitch than usual, and in the emotional intensity of the moment, he stated that he would like to kill his boss. He then calmed down, somewhat relieved by having let off steam, went on to discuss other subjects, and departed at the end of the session.

The therapist did not believe that the patient was anywhere near the point of seriously acting on the feelings that were expressed. However, the therapist had heard of a case in which a therapist got into trouble for not warning third parties, so he decided to take action.

On a sheet with his letterhead, he typed a warning to the employer that his patient, John Jones, had expressed the desire to kill him. He sent the letter by first-class mail—not express or registered—and he addressed it not to the employer but to the personnel department of the company.

The resulting uproar, although perhaps predictable, surprised the therapist. During the subsequent liability suit for breach of confidentiality, he was heard to sputter, "But I was only doing what the law requires of me!"

In this case, the therapist was not required to inform because he did not believe that his patient was going to act on his impulses; if he did believe so, his letter should have been addressed to the potential victim (return receipt requested) and not to the personnel department.

MEDICAL MALPRACTICE

Medical malpractice is a tort, or civil wrong. It is a noncriminal, noncontract wrong resulting from a physician's negligence. Simply put, negligence means doing something that a physician with a duty to care for the patient should not have done or failing to do something that should have been done as defined by current medical practice. Usually, the standard of care in malpractice cases is established by expert witnesses. The standard of care is also determined by reference to journal articles, professional textbooks and treatises, professional practice guidelines, and ethical practices promulgated by professional organizations.

To prove malpractice, the plaintiff (e.g., patient, family, or estate) must establish by a preponderance of the evidence that (1) a doctor–patient relationship existed that created a duty of care, (2) there was a deviation from the standard of care, (3) the patient was damaged, and (4) the deviation directly caused the damage.

These elements of a malpractice claim are sometimes referred to as the 4 Ds (duty, deviation, damage, direct causation). Proof by a preponderance of the evidence as required in a malpractice suit means simply more likely than not. Although the law does not assign a percentage, a preponderance of the evidence is akin to 51 to 49 percent, or just enough evidence to tip the scale one way or the other.

Each of the four elements of a malpractice claim must be present or there can be no finding of liability. For example, a psychiatrist whose negligence is the direct cause of harm to an individual (physical, psychological, or both) is not liable for malpractice if no doctor–patient relationship existed to create a duty of care. Psychiatrists are not likely to be sued successfully if they give negligent advice on a radio program that is harmful to a caller, particularly if a caveat was given to the caller that no doctor–patient relationship was being created. No malpractice claim will be sustained against a psychiatrist if a patient's worsening condition is unrelated to negligent care. Finally, if a psychiatrist treats a patient who is then harmed, no malpractice exists if the psychiatrist did not deviate from the standard of care.

Not every bad outcome is the result of negligence. Psychiatrists cannot guarantee correct diagnoses and treatments. When the psychiatrist provides due care, mistakes may be made without necessarily incurring liability. Most psychiatric cases are complicated. Psychiatrists make judgment calls when selecting a particular treatment course among the many options that may exist. In hindsight, the decision may prove wrong but not be a deviation in the standard of care.

In addition to negligence suits, psychiatrists can be sued for the intentional torts of assault, battery, false imprisonment, defamation, fraud or misrepresentation, invasion of privacy, and intentional infliction of emotional distress. In an intentional tort, wrongdoers are motivated by the intent to harm another person or realize or should have realized that such harm is likely to result from their actions. For example, telling a patient that sex with the therapist is therapeutic perpetrates a fraud. Most malpractice policies do not provide coverage for intentional torts. Other legal theories of liability include breach of contract and civil rights violations of the U.S. Constitution, state constitutions, or federal civil right statutes.

PRIVILEGE AND CONFIDENTIALITY

Privilege

Privilege is the right to maintain secrecy or confidentiality in the face of a subpoena. Privileged communications are statements made by certain persons within a relationship—such as husband–wife, priest–penitent, or doctor–patient—that the law protects from forced disclosure on the witness stand. The right of privilege belongs to the patient, not to the physician, and so the patient can waive the right.

Privilege has certain qualifications: (1) purely federal cases have no psychotherapist–patient privilege; (2) privilege does not exist at all in military courts; and (3) patients are said to waive the privilege by injecting their mental condition into litigation, thereby making their condition an element of their claim or defense.

Confidentiality

A long-held premise of medical ethics binds physicians to hold secret all information given by patients. This professional obligation is called *confidentiality*. Confidentiality applies to certain populations and not to others; a group that is within the circle of confidentiality shares information without receiving specific permission from a patient. Such groups include, in addition to the physician, other staff members treating the patient, clinical supervisors, and consultants. Parties outside the circle include the patient's family, attorney, and previous therapist; sharing information with such persons requires the patient's permission. Nevertheless, in numerous instances, a psychiatrist may be asked to divulge information imparted by a patient. Although a court demand for information is most worrisome to psychiatrists, demands most frequently come from sources such as insurers, who cannot compel disclosure but can withhold a benefit without it. A patient generally makes a disclosure or authorizes the psychiatrist to make disclosures to receive a benefit, such as employment, welfare benefits, or insurance.

A subpoena can force a psychiatrist to breach confidentiality, and courts must be able to compel witnesses to testify for the law to function adequately. A subpoena ("under penalty") is an order to appear as a witness in court or at a deposition. Physicians usually are served with a *subpoena duces tecum*, which requires that they also produce their relevant records and documents. Although the power to issue subpoenas belongs to a judge, they are routinely issued at the request of an attorney representing a party to an action.

Child Abuse.   In many states, all physicians are legally required to take a course on child abuse for medical licensure. All states now legally require that psychiatrists, among others, who have reason to believe that a child has been the victim of physical or sexual abuse, make an immediate report to an appropriate agency. In this situation, confidentiality is decisively limited by legal statute on the ground that potential or actual harm to vulnerable children outweighs the value of confidentiality in a psychiatric setting. Although many complex psychodynamic nuances accompany the required reporting of suspected child abuse, such reports generally are considered ethically justified.

HIGH-RISK CLINICAL SITUATIONS

Suicidal Patients

A review of the case law on suicide reveals that certain precautions should be taken with a suspected or confirmed suicidal patient. For example, failing to perform a reasonable assessment of a suicidal patient's risk for suicide or implement an appropriate precautionary plan will likely render a practitioner liable. The law tends to assume that suicide is preventable if it is foreseeable. Courts closely scrutinize suicide cases to determine if a patient's suicide was foreseeable. *Foreseeability* is a deliberately vague legal term that has no comparable clinical counterpart, a common-sense rather than a scientific construct. It does not (and should not) imply that clinicians can predict suicide. Foreseeability should not be confused with preventability, however. In hindsight, many suicides seem preventable that were clearly not foreseeable.

Violent Patients

Psychiatrists who treat violent or potentially violent patients may be sued for failure to control aggressive outpatients and for the discharge of violent inpatients. Psychiatrists may also be sued for failing to protect society from the violent acts of their patients if it was reasonable for the psychiatrist to have known about the patient's violent tendencies and if the psychiatrist could have done something that could have safeguarded the public. In the landmark case *Tarasoff v. Regents of the University of California*, the California Supreme Court ruled that mental health professionals have a duty to protect identifiable, endangered third parties from imminent threats of serious harm made by their outpatients. Since then, courts and state legislatures have increasingly held psychiatrists to a fictional standard of having to predict the future behavior (dangerousness) of their potentially violent patients. Research has consistently demonstrated that psychiatrists cannot predict future violence with any dependable accuracy.

The duty to protect patients and endangered third parties should be considered primarily a professional and moral obligation and, only secondarily, a legal duty. Most psychiatrists acted to protect both their patients and threatened others from violence long before *Tarasoff*.

If a patient threatens harm to another person, most states require that the psychiatrist perform some intervention that might prevent the harm from occurring. In states with duty-to-warn statutes, the options available to psychiatrists and psychotherapists are defined by law. In states offering no such guidance, health care providers are required to use the clinical judgment that will protect endangered third persons. Typically, a variety of options to warn and protect are clinically and legally available, including voluntary hospitalization, involuntary hospitalization (if civil commitment requirements are met), warning the intended victim of the threat, notifying the police, adjusting medication, and seeing the patient more frequently. The duty to protect allows the psychiatrist to consider a number of clinical options. Warning others of danger, by itself, is usually insufficient. Psychiatrists should consider the *Tarasoff* duty to be a national standard of care, even if they practice in states that do not have a duty to warn and protect.

HOSPITALIZATION

All states provide for some form of involuntary hospitalization. Such action usually is taken when psychiatric patients present a danger to themselves or others in their environment to the extent that their urgent need for treatment in a closed institution is evident. Certain states allow involuntary hospitalization when patients are unable to care for themselves adequately.

Procedures of Admission

Four procedures of admission to psychiatric facilities have been endorsed by the American Bar Association to safeguard civil liberties and to make sure that no person is railroaded into a mental hospital. Although each of the 50 states has the power to enact its own laws on psychiatric hospitalization, the procedures outlined here are gaining much acceptance.

Informal Admission. Informal admission operates on the general hospital model, in which a patient is admitted to a psychiatric unit of a general hospital in the same way that a medical or surgical patient is admitted. Under such circumstances, the ordinary doctor–patient relationship applies, with the patient free to enter and to leave, even against medical advice.

Voluntary Admission. In cases of voluntary admission, patients apply in writing for admission to a psychiatric hospital. They may come to the hospital on the advice of a personal physician, or they may seek help on their own. In either case, patients are admitted if an examination reveals the need for hospital treatment.

Temporary Admission. Temporary admission is used for patients who are so senile or so confused that they require hospitalization and are not able to make decisions of their own and for patients who are so acutely disturbed that they must be admitted immediately to a psychiatric hospital on an emergency basis. Under the procedure, a person is admitted to the hospital on the written recommendation of one physician. Once the patient has been admitted, the need for hospitalization must be confirmed by a psychiatrist on the hospital staff. The

procedure is temporary because patients cannot be hospitalized against their will for more than 15 days.

Involuntary Admission. Involuntary admission involves the question of whether patients are suicidal and thus a danger to themselves or homicidal and thus a danger to others. Because these persons do not recognize their need for hospital care, the application for admission to a hospital may be made by a relative or a friend. Once the application is made, the patient must be examined by two physicians, and if both physicians confirm the need for hospitalization, the patient can then be admitted.

Involuntary hospitalization involves an established procedure for written notification of the next of kin. Furthermore, the patients have access at any time to legal counsel, who can bring the case before a judge. If the judge does not think that hospitalization is indicated, the patient's release can be ordered.

Involuntary admission allows a patient to be hospitalized for 60 days. After this time, if the patient is to remain hospitalized, the case must be reviewed periodically by a board consisting of psychiatrists, nonpsychiatric physicians, lawyers, and other citizens not connected with the institution. In New York State, the board is called the Mental Health Information Service.

Persons who have been hospitalized involuntarily and who believe that they should be released have the right to file a petition for a writ of habeas corpus. Under law, a writ of habeas corpus may be proclaimed by those who believe that they have been illegally deprived of liberty. The legal procedure asks a court to decide whether a patient has been hospitalized without due process of law. The case must be heard by a court at once, regardless of the manner or the form in which the motion is filed. Hospitals are obligated to submit the petitions to the court immediately.

RIGHT TO TREATMENT

Among the rights of patients, the right to the standard quality of care is fundamental. This right has been litigated in much-publicized cases in recent years under the slogan of "right to treatment."

In 1966, Judge David Bazelon, speaking for the District of Columbia Court of Appeals in *Rouse v. Cameron*, noted that the purpose of involuntary hospitalization is treatment and concluded that the absence of treatment draws into question the constitutionality of the confinement. Treatment in exchange for liberty is the logic of the ruling. In this case, the patient was discharged on a writ of habeas corpus, the basic legal remedy to ensure liberty. Judge Bazelon further held that, if alternative treatments that infringe less on personal liberty are available, involuntary hospitalization cannot take place.

Alabama Federal Court Judge Frank Johnson was more venturesome in the decree he rendered in 1971 in *Wyatt v. Stickney*. The *Wyatt* case was a class-action proceeding brought under newly developed rules that sought not release but treatment. Judge Johnson ruled that persons civilly committed to a mental institution have a constitutional right to receive such individual treatment as will give them a reasonable opportunity to be cured or to have their mental condition improved. Judge Johnson set out minimum requirements for staffing, specified physical facilities, and nutritional standards, and required individualized treatment plans.

The new codes, more detailed than the old ones, include the right to be free from excessive or unnecessary medication; the right to privacy and dignity; the right to the least restrictive environment; the unrestricted right to be visited by attorneys, clergy, and private physicians; and the right not to be subjected to lobotomies, electroconvulsive treatments, and other procedures without fully informed consent. Patients can be required to perform therapeutic tasks but not hospital chores, unless they volunteer for them and are paid the federal minimum wage. This requirement is an attempt to eliminate the practice of peonage, in which psychiatric patients were forced to work at menial tasks, without payment, for the benefit of the state.

In a number of states today, medication or electroconvulsive therapy (ECT) cannot be forcibly administered to a patient without first obtaining court approval, which may take as long as 10 days. The right to refuse treatment is a legal doctrine that holds that, except in emergencies, persons cannot be forced to accept treatment against their will. An emergency is defined as a condition in clinical practice that requires immediate intervention to prevent death or serious harm to the patient or others or to prevent deterioration of the patient's clinical state.

In the 1976 case of *O'Connor v. Donaldson*, the Supreme Court of the United States ruled that harmless mentally ill patients cannot be confined against their will without treatment if they can survive outside. According to the Court, a finding of mental illness alone cannot justify a state's confining persons in a hospital against their will. Instead, involuntarily confined patients must be considered dangerous to themselves or others or possibly so unable to care for themselves that they cannot survive outside. As a result of the 1979 case of *Rennie v. Klein*, patients have the right to refuse treatment and to use an appeal process. As a result of the 1981 case of *Roger v. Oken*, patients have an absolute right to refuse treatment, but a guardian may authorize treatment. Questions have been raised about psychiatrists' ability to accurately predict dangerousness and about the risk to psychiatrists, who may be sued for monetary damages if persons are thereby deprived of their civil rights.

SECLUSION AND RESTRAINT

Seclusion and restraint raise complex psychiatric legal issues. Seclusion and restraint have both indications and contraindications. Seclusion and restraint have become increasingly regulated over the past decade.

Generally, courts hold, or consent decrees provide, that restraints and seclusion be implemented only when a patient creates a risk of harm to self or others and no less restrictive alternative is available. Additional restrictions include the following:

1. Restraint and seclusion can only be implemented by a written order from an appropriate medical official
2. Orders are to be confined to specific, time-limited periods
3. A patient's condition must be regularly reviewed and documented
4. Any extension of an original order must be reviewed and reauthorized

Informed Consent Form

The introduction of consent forms followed revelations of harm done to patients during clinical experimentation. Consent forms are written documents outlining a patient's informed consent to a proposed procedure.

The basic elements of a consent form should include a fair explanation of the procedures to be followed and their pur-

poses, including identification of any procedures that are experimental; a description of any attendant discomforts and risks reasonably to be expected; a description of any benefits reasonably to be expected; a disclosure of any appropriate alternative procedures that may be advantageous to the patient; an offer to answer any inquiries concerning the procedures; and an instruction that the patient is free to withdraw patient consent and to discontinue participation in the project or activity at any time without prejudice. The patient has the right to refuse treatment.

CHILD CUSTODY

The action of a court in a child-custody dispute is now predicated on the child's best interests. The maxim reflects the idea that a natural parent does not have an inherent right to be named a custodial parent, but the presumption, although a bit eroded, remains in favor of the mother in the case of young children. As a rule, the courts presume that the welfare of a child of tender years generally is best served by maternal custody when the mother is a good and fit parent. The best interest of the mother may be served by naming her as the custodial parent, because a mother may never resolve the effects of the loss of a child, but her best interest is not to be equated ipso facto with the best interest of the child. Care and protection proceedings are the court's interventions in the welfare of a child when the parents are unable to care for the child.

More fathers are asserting custodial claims. In approximately 5 percent of all cases, fathers are named custodians. The movement supporting women's rights also is enhancing the chances of paternal custody. With more women going to work outside the home, the traditional rationale for maternal custody has less force today than it did in the past.

TESTAMENTARY AND CONTRACTUAL CAPACITY AND COMPETENCE

Psychiatrists may be asked to evaluate patients' testamentary capacities and their competence to make a will. Three psychological abilities are necessary to prove this competence. Patients must know the nature and the extent of their bounty (property), the fact that they are making a bequest, and the identities of their natural beneficiaries (spouse, children, and other relatives).

When a will is being probated, one of the heirs or another person often challenges its validity. A judgment in such cases must be based on a reconstruction, using data from documents and from expert psychiatric testimony, of the testator's mental state at the time the will was written. When a person is unable to, or does not exercise the right to, make a will, the law in all states provides for the distribution of property to the heirs. If there are no heirs, the estate goes to the public treasury.

Witnesses at the signing of a will, who might include a psychiatrist, may attest that the testator was rational at the time the will was executed. In unusual cases, a lawyer may videotape the signing to safeguard the will from attack. Ideally, persons who are thinking of making a will and believe that questions might be raised about their testamentary competence hire a forensic psychiatrist to perform a dispassionate examination antemortem to validate and record their capacity.

An incompetence proceeding and the appointment of a guardian may be considered necessary when a family member spending the family's assets and property is in danger of dissipation as in the case of aged, retarded, alcohol-dependent, and psychotic persons. At issue is whether such persons are capable of managing their own affairs. A guardian appointed to take control of the property of one deemed incompetent, however, cannot make a will for the ward (the incompetent person).

Competence is determined on the basis of a person's ability to make a sound judgment—to weigh, to reason, and to make reasonable decisions. Competence is task specific, not general; the capacity to weigh decision-making factors (competence) often is best demonstrated by a person's ability to ask pertinent and knowledgeable questions after the risks and the benefits have been explained. Although physicians (especially psychiatrists) often give opinions on competence, only a judge's ruling converts the opinion into a finding; a patient is not competent or incompetent until the court so rules. The diagnosis of a mental disorder is not, in itself, sufficient to warrant a finding of incompetence. Instead, the mental disorder must cause an impairment in judgment for the specific issues involved. After they have been declared incompetent, persons are deprived of certain rights: they cannot make contracts, marry, start a divorce action, drive a vehicle, handle their own property, or practice their professions. Incompetence is decided at a formal courtroom proceeding, and the court usually appoints a guardian who will best serve a patient's interests. Another hearing is necessary to declare a patient competent. Admission to a mental hospital does not automatically mean that a person is incompetent.

Competence also is essential in contracts, because a contract is an agreement between parties to do a specific act. A contract is declared invalid, if, when it was signed, one of the parties was unable to comprehend the nature and effect of his or her act. The marriage contract is subject to the same standard and, thus, can be voided if either party did not understand the nature, duties, obligations, and other characteristics entailed at the time of the marriage. In general, however, the courts are unwilling to declare a marriage void on the basis of incompetence.

Whether competence is related to wills, contracts, or the making or breaking of marriages, the fundamental concern is a person's state of awareness and capacity to comprehend the significance of the particular commitment made.

Durable Power of Attorney

A modern development that permits persons to make provisions for their own anticipated loss of decision-making capacity is called a *durable power of attorney*. The document permits the advance selection of a substitute decision maker who can act without the necessity of court proceedings when the signatory becomes incompetent through illness, progressive dementia, or perhaps a relapse of bipolar I disorder.

CRIMINAL LAW

Competence to Stand Trial

The Supreme Court of the United States stated that the prohibition against trying someone who is mentally incompetent is fundamental to the U.S. system of justice. Accordingly, the Court, in *Dusky v. United States*, approved a test of competence. Criminal defendants must have "sufficient ability to consult with their lawyers with a reasonable degree of rational

understanding and have a rational as well as factual understanding of the proceedings against them."

Clinicians merely offer opinions about competence. The judge is free to honor, modify, or disregard these opinions, and a patient is not competent or incompetent until the judge so rules.

Competence to Be Executed

One of the new areas of competence to emerge in the interface between psychiatry and the law is the question of a person's competence to be executed. The requirement for competence in this area is believed to rest on three general principles. First, a person's awareness of what is happening is supposed to heighten the retributive element of the punishment. Punishment is meaningless unless the person is aware of it and knows the punishment's purpose. Second, a competent person who is about to be executed is believed to be in the best position to make whatever peace is appropriate with religious beliefs, including confession and absolution. Third, a competent person who is about to be executed preserves, until the end, the possibility (admittedly slight) of recalling a forgotten detail of the events or the crime that may prove exonerating.

Most medical bodies have taken the position that it is unethical for any clinician to participate, no matter how remotely, in state-mandated executions; a physician's duty to preserve life transcends all other competing requirements. Major medical societies, such as the American Medical Association (AMA), believe that doctors should not participate in the death penalty.

A psychiatrist who agrees to examine a patient slated for execution may find the person incompetent on the basis of a mental disorder and may recommend a treatment plan, which, if implemented, would ensure the person's fitness to be executed. While there is room for a difference of opinion regarding whether or not a psychiatrist should become involved, the authors of this textbook believe such involvement to be inhumane.

Criminal Responsibility

According to criminal law, committing an act that is socially harmful is not the sole criterion of whether a crime has been committed. Instead, the objectionable act must have two components: voluntary conduct (*actus reus*) and evil intent (*mens rea*). There cannot be an evil intent when an offender's mental status is so deficient, so abnormal, or so diseased as to have deprived the offender of the capacity for rational intent. The law can be invoked only when an illegal intent is implemented. Neither behavior, however harmful, nor the intent to do harm is, in itself, a ground for criminal action.

M'Naghten Rule.   The precedent for determining legal responsibility was established in 1843 in the British courts. The so-called M'Naghten rule, which has, until recently, determined criminal responsibility in most of the United States, holds that persons are not guilty by reason of insanity if they labored under a mental disease such that they were unaware of the nature, the quality, and the consequences of their acts or if they were incapable of realizing that their acts were wrong. Moreover, to absolve persons from punishment, a delusion used as evidence must be one that, if true, would be an adequate defense. If the delusional idea does not justify the crime, such persons are presumably held responsible, guilty, and punishable. The M'Naghten rule is known commonly as the *right–wrong test*.

The M'Naghten rule derives from the famous M'Naghten case of 1843. When Daniel M'Naghten murdered Edward Drummond, the private secretary of Robert Peel, M'Naghten had been suffering from delusions of persecution for several years, had complained to many persons about his "persecutors," and, finally, had decided to correct the situation by murdering Robert Peel. When Drummond came out of Peel's home, M'Naghten shot Drummond, whom he mistook for Peel. The jury, as instructed under the prevailing law, found M'Naghten not guilty by reason of insanity. In response to questions about what guidelines could be used to determine whether a person could plead insanity as a defense against criminal responsibility, the English chief judge wrote:

1. To establish a defense on the ground of insanity, it must be clearly proved that, at the time of committing the act, the party accused was laboring under such a defect of reason, from disease of the mind, as not to know the nature and quality of the act he was doing, or if he did know it, he did not know he was doing what was wrong.
2. Where a person labors under partial delusions only and is not in other respects insane and as a result commits an offense, he must be considered in the same situation regarding responsibility as if the facts with respect to which the delusion exists were real.

According to the M'Naghten rule, the question is not whether the accused knows the difference between right and wrong in general, it is whether the defendant understood the nature and the quality of the act and whether the defendant knew the difference between right and wrong with respect to the act—that is, specifically whether the defendant knew the act was wrong or perhaps thought the act was correct, a delusion causing the defendant to act in legitimate self-defense.

Irresistible Impulse. In 1922, a committee of jurists in England reexamined the M'Naghten rule. The committee suggested broadening the concept of insanity in criminal cases to include the irresistible impulse tests, which rules that a person charged with a criminal offense is not responsible for an act if the act was committed under an impulse that the person was unable to resist because of mental disease. The courts have chosen to interpret this concept in such a way that it has been called the *policeman-at-the-elbow law*. In other words, the court grants an impulse to be irresistible only when it can be determined that the accused would have committed the act even if a policeman had been at the accused's elbow. To most psychiatrists, this interpretation is unsatisfactory because it covers only a small, special group of those who are mentally ill.

Durham Rule. In the case of *Durham v. United States*, Judge Bazelon handed down a decision in 1954 in the District of Columbia Court of Appeals. The decision resulted in the product rule of criminal responsibility, namely that an accused is not

criminally responsible if his or her unlawful act was the product of mental disease or mental defect. In the Durham case, Judge Bazelon expressly stated that the purpose of the rule was to get good and complete psychiatric testimony. He sought to release the criminal law from the theoretical straitjacket of the M'Naghten rule, but judges and juries in cases using the Durham rule became mired in confusion over the terms "product," "disease," and "defect." In 1972, some 18 years after the rule's adoption, the Court of Appeals for the District of Columbia, in *United States v. Brawner*, discarded the rule. The court—all nine members, including Judge Bazelon—decided in a 143-page opinion to throw out its Durham rule and to adopt in its place the test recommended in 1962 by the American Law Institute in its model penal code, which is the law in the federal courts today.

Model Penal Code. In its model penal code, the American Law Institute recommended the following test of criminal responsibility: Persons are not responsible for criminal conduct if, at the time of such conduct, as a result of mental disease or defect, they lacked substantial capacity either to appreciate the criminality (wrongfulness) of their conduct or to conform their conduct to the requirement of the law. The term *mental disease or defect* does not include an abnormality manifest only by repeated criminal or otherwise antisocial conduct.

Subsection 1 of the American Law Institute rule contains five operative concepts: mental disease or defect, lack of substantial capacity, appreciation, wrongfulness, and conformity of conduct to the requirements of law. The rule's second subsection, stating that repeated criminal or antisocial conduct is not, of itself, to be taken as mental disease or defect, aims to keep the sociopath or psychopath within the scope of criminal responsibility.

Other Tests. The test of criminal responsibility and other tests of criminal liability refer to the time of the offense's commission, whereas the test of competence to stand trial refers to the time of the trial.

The AMA has proposed limiting the insanity exculpation to cases in which the person is so ill as to lack the necessary criminal intent (*mens rea*). This approach would all but eliminate the insanity defense and place a burden on the prisons to accept large numbers of persons who are mentally ill.

The American Bar Association and the American Psychiatric Association (APA) recommended a defense of nonresponsibility, which focuses solely on whether defendants, as a result of mental disease or defect, are unable to appreciate the wrongfulness of their conduct. These proposals would limit the evidence of mental illness to cognition and would exclude control, but apparently a defense would still be available under a not-guilty plea—such as extreme emotional disturbance, automatism, provocation, or self-defense—that would be established without psychiatric testimony about mental illness. The APA also urged that "mental illness" be limited to severely abnormal mental conditions.

All of the above proposals still are controversial and will be debated in each sensational case in which the insanity defense is used.

Ethics in Psychiatry

Ethics in psychiatry refers to the principles of conduct that govern the behavior of psychiatrists as well as other mental health professionals. Ethics as a discipline deals with what is good and what is bad, what is right and what is wrong, and moral duties, obligations, and responsibilities.

PROFESSIONAL CODES

Most professional organizations and many business groups have codes of ethics. Such codes reflect a consensus about the general standards of appropriate professional conduct. The American Medical Association's (AMA) *Principles of Medical Ethics,* the American Psychiatric Association's (APA) *Principles of Medical Ethics with Annotations Especially Applicable to Psychiatry,* and the *American College of Physicians Ethics Manual* articulate ideal standards of practice and professional virtues of practitioners. These codes include exhortations to use skillful and scientific techniques, to self-regulate misconduct within the profession, and to respect the rights and needs of patients, families, colleagues, and society. Such exhortations are reinforced by core ethical principles such as beneficence, autonomy, nonmaleficence, and justice (discussed below).

The *Principles of Medical Ethics with Annotations Especially Applicable to Psychiatry* (hereafter, *The Principles*) provides a useful and comprehensive example of a professional code geared to the psychiatric profession. The manual covers a broad array of psychiatric ethical issues, from fee splitting and sex with former patients to psychiatrists' participation in executions, all of which are unethical. Developed by the APA Ethics Committee members and consultants, it provides answers to commonly asked ethical questions. A summary of these principles is provided in Table 53–1.

IMPAIRED PHYSICIANS

A physician may become impaired as the result of psychiatric or medical disorders or the use of mind-altering and habit-forming substances (e.g., alcohol and drugs). Many organic illnesses can interfere with the cognitive and motor skills required to provide competent medical care. Although the legal responsibility to report an impaired physician varies, depending on the state, the ethical responsibility remains universal. An incapacitated physician should be reported to an appropriate authority, and the reporting physician is required to follow specific hospital, state, and legal procedures. A physician who treats an impaired physician should not be required to monitor the impaired physician's progress or fitness to return to work. This monitoring should be performed by an independent physician or group of physicians who have no conflicts of interest.

The Office of Professional Medical Conduct (OPMC) in New York State regulates the practice of medicine by investigating illegal or unethical practice by physicians and other health professionals, such as physician assistants. Similar regulatory agencies exist in other states. Professional misconduct in New York State is defined as one of the following:

1. Practicing fraudulently and with gross negligence or incompetence.
2. Practicing while the ability to practice is impaired.
3. Being habitually drunk or being dependent on, or a habitual user of, narcotics or a habitual user of other drugs having similar effects.
4. Immoral conduct in the practice of the profession.
5. Permitting, aiding, or abetting an unlicensed person to perform activities requiring a license.
6. Refusing a client or patient service because of creed, color, or national origin.
7. Practicing beyond the scope of practice permitted by law.
8. Being convicted of a crime or being the subject of disciplinary action in another jurisdiction.

Professional misconduct complaints derive mainly from the public in addition to insurance companies, law enforcement agencies, and doctors, among others.

PHYSICIANS IN TRAINING

It is unethical to delegate authority for patient care to anyone who is not appropriately qualified and experienced, such as a medical student or a resident, without adequate supervision from an attending physician. Residents are physicians in training and, as such, must provide a good deal of patient care. Within a healthy, ethical teaching environment, residents and medical students may be involved with, and responsible for, the day-to-day care of many ill patients, but they are supervised, supported, and directed by highly trained and experienced physicians. Patients have the right to know the level of training of their care providers and should be informed about the resident's or medical student's level of training. Residents and medical students should know and acknowledge their limitations and should ask for supervision from experienced colleagues as necessary.

Table 53–1
The Principles of Medical Ethics with Annotations Especially Applicable to Psychiatry

Each of the AMA principles of medical ethics printed separately (in italics) along with annotations especially applicable to psychiatry.

Preamble

The medical profession has long subscribed to a body of ethical statements developed primarily for the benefit of the patient. As a member of this profession, a physician must recognize responsibility not only to patients but also to society, to other health professionals, and to self. The following Principles, adopted by the American Medical Association, are not laws but standards of conduct, which define the essentials of honorable behavior for the physician.

Section 1

A physician shall be dedicated to providing competent medical service with compassion and respect for human dignity.[a]

1. A psychiatrist shall not gratify his/her own needs by exploiting a patient. The psychiatrist shall be ever vigilant about the impact that his/her conduct has upon the boundaries of the doctor–patient relationship and thus upon the well-being of the patient. These requirements become particularly important because of the essentially private, highly personal, and sometimes intensely emotional nature of the relationship with the psychiatrist.

2. A psychiatrist should not be a party to any type of policy that excludes, segregates, or demeans the dignity of any patient because of ethnic origin, race, sex, creed, age, socioeconomic status, or sexual orientation.

3. In accord with the requirements of law and accepted medical practice, it is ethical for a physician to submit his/her work to peer review and to the ultimate authority of the medical staff executive body and the hospital administration and its governing body.

4. A psychiatrist should not be a participant in a legally authorized execution.

Section 2

A physician shall deal honestly with patients and colleagues, and strive to expose those physicians deficient in character or competence, or who engage in fraud or deception.

1. The requirement that the physician conduct himself/herself with propriety in his/her profession and in all the actions of his/her life is especially important for the psychiatrist because the patient tends to model his/her behavior on that of his/her psychiatrist by identification. Further, the necessary intensity of the treatment relationship may tend to activate sexual and other needs and fantasies of both patient and psychiatrist, while weakening the objectivity necessary for control. Additionally, the inherent inequality in the doctor–patient relationship may lead to exploitation of the patient. Sexual activity with a current or former patient is unethical.

2. The psychiatrist should diligently guard against exploiting information furnished by the patient and should not use the unique position of power afforded by the psychotherapeutic situation to influence patients in any way not directly relevant to the treatment goals.

3. A psychiatrist who regularly practices outside his/her area of professional competence should be considered unethical. Determination of professional competence should be made by peer review boards or other appropriate bodies.

4. Special consideration should be given to psychiatrists who, due to illness, jeopardize the welfare of their patients and their own reputations and practices. It is ethical, even encouraged, for another psychiatrist to intercede in such situations.

5. Psychiatric services, like all medical services, are dispensed in the context of a contractual arrangement between the patient and the treating physician. The provisions of the contractual arrangement, which are binding on both the physician and the patient, should be explicitly established.

6. It is ethical for a psychiatrist to make a charge for a missed appointment when it falls within the terms of the specific contractual agreement with the patient. Charging for a missed appointment or for one not canceled 24 hours in advance need not, in itself, be considered unethical if a patient is fully advised that the physician will make such a charge. The practice, however, should be resorted to infrequently and always with the utmost consideration for the patient and his/her circumstances.

7. An arrangement in which a psychiatrist provides supervision or administration to other physicians or nonmedical persons for a percentage of their fees or gross income is not acceptable; this would constitute fee splitting.

Section 3

A physician shall respect the law and also recognize a responsibility to seek changes in those requirements which are contrary to the best interests of the patient.

1. It would seem self-evident that a psychiatrist who is a lawbreaker might be ethically unsuited to practice his/her profession. When such illegal activities bear directly upon his/her practice, this would obviously be the case. However, in other instances, illegal activities such as those concerning the right to protest social injustices might not bear on either the image of the psychiatrist or the ability of the specific psychiatrist to treat his/her patient ethically and well.

Section 4

A physician shall respect the rights of patients, of colleagues, and of other health professionals, and shall safeguard patient confidences within the constraints of the law.

1. Psychiatric records, including even the identification of a person as a patient, must be protected with extreme care. Confidentiality is essential to psychiatric treatment. This is based in part on the special nature of psychiatric therapy as well as on the traditional ethical relationship between physician and patient. Growing concern regarding the civil rights of patients and the possible adverse effects of computerization, duplication equipment, and data banks make the dissemination of confidential information an increasing hazard. Because of the sensitive and private nature of the information with which the psychiatrist deals, he/she must be circumspect in the information that he/she chooses to disclose to others about a patient. The welfare of the patient must be a continuing consideration.

2. A psychiatrist may release confidential information only with the authorization of the patient or under proper legal compulsion. The continuing duty of the psychiatrist to protect patients includes fully apprising him/her of the consequences of waiving the privilege of privacy. This may become an issue when the patient is being investigated by a government agency, is applying for a position, or is involved in legal action. The same principles apply to the release of information concerning treatment to medical departments of government agencies, business organizations, labor unions, and insurance companies. Information gained in confidence about patients seen in student health services should not be released without the students' explicit permission.

3. Clinical and other materials used in teaching and writing must be adequately disguised to preserve the anonymity of the individuals involved.

4. The ethical responsibility of maintaining confidentiality holds equally for consultations in which the patient may not have been present and in which the consultee was not a physician. In such instances, the physician consultant should alert the consultee to his/her duty of confidentiality.

5. Ethically, the psychiatrist may disclose only the information that is relevant to a given situation. He/she should avoid offering speculation as fact. Sensitive information such as an individual's sexual orientation or fantasy material is usually unnecessary.

(continued)

Table 53–1 (*continued*)

6. Psychiatrists are often asked to examine individuals for security purposes, to determine suitability for various jobs, and to determine legal competence. The psychiatrist must fully describe the nature, purpose, and lack of confidentiality of the examination to the examinee at the beginning of the examination.

7. Careful judgment must be exercised by the psychiatrist to include, when appropriate, the parents or guardian in the treatment of a minor. At the same time, the psychiatrist must assure the minor proper confidentiality.

8. When in the clinical judgment of the treating psychiatrist the risk of danger is deemed to be significant, the psychiatrist may reveal confidential information disclosed by the patient.

9. When the psychiatrist is ordered by the court to reveal the confidences entrusted to him/her by patients, he/she may comply or he/she may ethically hold the right to dissent within the framework of the law. When a psychiatrist is in doubt, the right of the patient to confidentiality and, by extension, to unimpaired treatment, should be given priority. The psychiatrist should reserve the right to raise the question of adequate need for disclosure. In the event the necessity for legal disclosure is demonstrated by the court, the psychiatrist may request the right to disclose only that information which is relevant to the legal question at hand.

10. With regard for the person's dignity and privacy and with truly informed consent, it is ethical to present a patient to a scientific gathering if the confidentiality of the presentation is understood and accepted by the audience.

11. When involved in funded research, the ethical psychiatrist advises human subjects of the funding source, retains his/her freedom to reveal data and results, and follows all appropriate and current guidelines relative to human subject protection.

12. Ethical considerations in medical practice preclude the psychiatric evaluation of any person charged with criminal acts prior to access to, or availability of, legal counsel. The only exception is rendering care to the person for the sole purpose of medical treatment.

13. Sexual involvement between a faculty member or supervisor and a trainee or student, in situations in which an abuse of power can occur, often takes advantage of inequalities in the working relationship and may be unethical because (a) any treatment of a patient being supervised may be deleteriously affected; (b) it may damage the trust relationship between teacher and student; and (c) teachers are important professional role models for their trainees and affect their trainees' future professional behavior.

Section 5

A physician shall continue to study, apply, and advance scientific knowledge, make relevant information available to patients, colleagues, and the public, obtain consultation, and use the talents of other health professionals when indicated.

1. Psychiatrists are responsible for their own continuing education and should remember that theirs must be a lifetime of learning.

2. In the practice of their specialty, the psychiatrists consult, associate, collaborate, or integrate their work with that of many professionals, including psychologists, psychometricians, social workers, alcoholism counselors, marriage counselors, and public health nurses. Furthermore, the nature of modern psychiatric practice extends the psychiatrist's contacts to such people as teachers, juvenile and adult probation officers, attorneys, welfare workers, agency volunteers, and neighborhood aides. Psychiatrists should ensure that the allied professionals or paraprofessionals with whom they are dealing and who refer patients for treatment, counseling, or rehabilitation are recognized members of their own discipline and are competent to carry out the therapeutic task required. Psychiatrists should have the same attitude toward members of the medical profession to whom they refer patients. Psychiatrists should not refer patients whenever they have reason to doubt the training, skill, or ethical qualifications of the allied professional.

3. When psychiatrists assume a collaborative or supervisory role with another mental health worker, they must expend sufficient time to ensure that proper care is given. It is contrary to the interests of the patient and to patient care if they allow themselves to be used as a figurehead.

4. In relationships between psychiatrists and practicing licensed psychologists, physicians should not delegate to the psychologist or, in fact, to any nonmedical person any matter requiring the exercise of professional medical judgment.

5. Psychiatrists should agree to the request of a patient for consultation or to such a request from the family of an incompetent or minor patient. Psychiatrists may suggest possible consultants, but the patient or family should be given free choice of the consultant. If psychiatrists disapprove of the professional qualifications of the consultant or if they cannot resolve a difference of opinion they may, after suitable notice, withdraw from the case. If this disagreement occurs within an institution or agency framework, the differences should be resolved by mediation or arbitration by higher professional authority within the institution or agency.

Section 6

A physician shall, in the provision of appropriate patient care, except in emergencies, be free to choose whom to serve, with whom to associate, and the environment in which to provide medical services.

1. Physicians generally agree that the doctor–patient relationship is such a vital factor in effective treatment of the patient that preservation of optimal conditions for development of a sound working relationship between the doctors and their patient should take precedence over all other considerations.

Section 7

A physician shall recognize a responsibility to participate in activities contributing to an improved community.

1. Psychiatrists should foster the cooperation of those legitimately concerned with the medical, psychological, social, and legal aspects of mental health and illness. Psychiatrists are encouraged to serve society by advising and consulting with the executive, legislative, and judiciary branches of the government. Psychiatrists should clarify whether they speak as an individual or as a representative of an organization. Furthermore, psychiatrists should avoid cloaking their public statements with the authority of the profession (e.g., "Psychiatrists know that. . . .").

2. Psychiatrists may interpret and share with the public their expertise in the various psychosocial issues that may affect mental health and illness. Psychiatrists should always be mindful of their separate roles as dedicated citizens and as experts in psychological medicine.

3. On occasion psychiatrists are asked for an opinion about individuals who are in the light of public attention or who have disclosed information about themselves through public media. In such circumstance, psychiatrists may share their expertise about psychiatric issues in general with the public. However, it is unethical for psychiatrists to offer a professional opinion about a specific individual unless they have conducted an examination and have been granted proper authorization for such a statement.

4. Psychiatrists may permit their certification to be used for the involuntary treatment of any person only after their personal examination of that person. To do so, they must find that the person, because of mental illness, cannot form a judgment about what is in his/her own best interests and that without such treatment, substantial impairment is likely to occur to that person or others.

ᵃStatements in italics are taken directly from the American Medical Association's Principles of Medical Ethics. Reprinted with permission from American Psychiatric Association. *The Principles of Medical Ethics with Annotations Especially Applicable to Psychiatry.* Washington, DC: American Psychiatric Association; 1995.

Index

Page numbers followed by *t* and *f* indicate tables and figures, respectively.

A

Abilify. *See* Aripiprazole (Abilify)
Abnormal swallowing syndrome, sleep-related, 321
Abraham, Karl, 177
Abstinence, rule of, in psychoanalysis, 397
Academic problem, 585–586
  diagnosis of, 586
  etiology of, 585–586
  treatment of, 586
Acculturation problem, 380–381
Acetylation status, culture and, 171
Acquired immunodeficiency syndrome (AIDS), 73
  mental retardation and, 514
Acting out, in personality disorders, 338
Acupressure, in psychosomatic disorders, 363
Acupuncture, in psychosomatic disorders, 363
Acute stress disorder, 232
  vs. adjustment disorder, 334
  clinical features of, 234–237
  diagnosis of, 234, 235t
Adalat. *See* Nifedipine (Procardia, Adalat)
Addiction, 77. *See also* Substance abuse; Substance dependence; Substance-related disorders
Additional conditions that may be a focus of clinical attention, 377–381
ADHD. *See* Attention-deficit/hyperactivity disorder (ADHD)
α_2-Adrenergic receptor agonists, 425
Adjustment disorder(s)
  with anxiety, 333
  course and prognosis of, 334
  with depressed mood, 333
  diagnosis and clinical features of, 333–334, 333t
  differential diagnosis of, 334
  with disturbance of conduct, 334
  epidemiology of, 332
  etiology of, 332–333
    family and genetic factors in, 333
    psychodynamic factors in, 332–333
  HIV-associated, 75
  with mixed anxiety and depressed mood, 333
  with mixed disturbance of emotions and conduct, 334
  vs. posttraumatic stress disorder, 334

  treatment of, 334–335
  unspecified, 334
β-Adrenergic receptor antagonists
  dosage and clinical guidelines for, 429
  drug–drug interactions of, 428
  effects on specific organs and systems of, 427
  pharmacological actions of, 427, 428t
  precautions and adverse reactions to, 428
  therapeutic indications for, 427–428
    in aggression and violent behavior, 428
    in akathisia, 437
    in alcohol withdrawal, 428
    as antidepression augmentation, 428
    in anxiety disorders, 427
    in lithium-induced postural tremor, 427
    in neuroleptic-induced acute akathisia, 427–428
Adolescent psychiatry
  clinical problems in, 598
  diagnosis in, 597
  interviews in, 597–598
Adrenal axis, in mood disorders, 175
Adrenal disorders
  mental disorders due to, 71
  psychological sequelae of, 359
Advance directives, 604
Advanced sleep phase syndrome, 316
Affect, 26–27
  in depressive episode, 189
  in geriatric patients, 600
  in manic episode, 189–190
  in mental status examination, 7
  in psychiatric evaluation of children, 509
  in schizophrenia, 146–147
Aggression
  in children, 426
  treatment of, 459
    β-adrenergic receptor antagonists in, 428
Agitation, severe, treatment of, 456
Agoraphobia
  clinical features of, 218
  comorbidity of, 214
  course and prognosis of, 219–220
  diagnosis of, 216t, 217, 217t
  differential diagnosis of, 219
  epidemiology of, 214
  etiology of, 214–216
    biological factors in, 214–216
    genetic factors in, 215

  psychosocial factors in, 215–216
  treatment of, 220–221
Agranulocytosis, serotonin-dopamine antagonists and, 485
AIDS. *See* Acquired immunodeficiency syndrome (AIDS)
Akathisia
  neuroleptic-induced, 424
    β-adrenergic receptor antagonists in, 427
  treatment of, 430, 431–432
    β-adrenergic receptor antagonists in, 437
Alcohol
  abuse
    in adolescents, 582
    vs. dysthymic disorder, 201
  dependence
    opioid receptor antagonists and, 472
    suicide risk in, 391–392
  metabolism, culture and, 171–172
Alcohol-related disorder(s), 80–92, 80t, 85t.
    See also specific disorders
  comorbidity of, 81–82
  effects of alcohol and, 83–84
    on absorption, 83
    on the brain, 83–84
      behavioral, 83–84
      sleep-related, 83–84
    drug interactions and, 84
    on the gastrointestinal system, 84
    lab tests of, 84
    on the liver, 84
    on metabolism, 83
  epidemiology of, 80–81
    education and, 81
    gender and, 81
    race and ethnicity in, 81
    region and urbanicity and, 81
    socioeconomic class and, 81
  etiology of, 82–83
    behavioral and learning factors of, 82
    childhood history in, 82
    genetic theories of, 82–83
    psychodynamic theories of, 82
    sociocultural theories of, 82
  intoxication, 84–85, 85t
    idiosyncratic, 89
  not otherwise specified, 89, 89t

Alcohol-related disorder(s)—*continued*
  prognosis of, 89–90
  sexual dysfunction and, 285
  treatment and rehabilitation and, 90–92
    counseling in, 91
    detoxification in, 90
    intervention in, 90
    medications in, 91–92
    self-help groups in, 92
    withdrawal in, 90–91
Alexander, Franz, 401
Alprazolam (Xanax), 435. *See also* Benzodi-
      azepines
  in depression, 437
  in major depressive disorder, 195
  in panic disorder, 220
  in social phobia, 227, 437
Amantadine (Symmetrel), 429
  dosage and clinical guidelines of, 430
  drug interactions of, 430
  effects of on specific organs and systems,
      429
  pharmacological actions of, 429
  precautions and adverse affects of, 429–430
  therapeutic indications for, 429
Ambien. *See* Zolpidem (Ambien)
γ-Aminobutyric acid (GABA)
  in anxiety, 212–213
  in schizophrenia, 137
Amitriptyline (Elavil)
  in posttraumatic stress disorder, 237–238
  tests for use of, 23
Amlodipine (Norvasc, Lotrel), 443. *See also*
      Calcium channel inhibitors
  dosage and clinical guidelines for, 444
Amnesia
  anteretrograde, 59
  dissociative. *See* Dissociative amnesia
  with electroconvulsive therapy, 61
  with head injury, 61
  retrograde, 59
  transient global
    amnestic disorder and, 61
    vs. dissociative amnesia, 267–268
Amnestic disorder(s)
  alcohol-induced persisting, 87–88
  classification of, 45–46
  clinical features and subtypes of, 59–61
    alcoholic blackouts in, 61
    cerebrovascular diseases in, 60
    electroconvulsive therapy in, 61
    head injury in, 61
    Korsakoff's syndrome in, 61
    transient global amnesia in, 61
  course and prognosis of, 62
  vs. delirium, 62
  vs. dementia, 62
  diagnosis of, 59, 59t, 60t
  differential diagnosis of, 61–62
  vs. dissociative disorders, 62
  epidemiology of, 58
  etiology of, 58–59
  vs. factitious disorders, 62
  vs. normal aging, 62
  pathology and lab exam in, 61
  persisting, in sedative-, hypnotic-, or anx-
      iolytic-related disorder, 128–129
  treatment of, 62
Amobarbital (Amytal)
  drug-assisted interview with, 24
  in narcoanalysis, 433
Amok, 169
Amotivational syndrome, cannabis-related
      disorder and, 102

Amphetamine-like substances, amphet-
      amine-related disorders and, 93
Amphetamine-related disorder(s)
  clinical features of, 95–96
    adverse effects in, 95–96
  diagnosis of, 93–95, 93t, 94t
  epidemiology of, 93
  intoxication, 94, 94t
  neuropharmacology of, 93
  preparations associated with, 92–93
  treatment and rehabilitation of, 96
Amphetamines
  clinical features of, 95–96
    adverse effects in, 95–96
  intoxication, 94, 94t
  neuropharmacology of, 93
  preparations associated with, 92–93
Amyloid precursor protein, in dementia of
      Alzheimer's type, 51
Amyotrophic lateral sclerosis, mental disor-
      ders due to, 69
Amytal. *See* Amobarbital (Amytal)
Anabolic steroid abuse, 131–132, 131t
  diagnosis and clinical features of,
      131–132
  epidemiology of, 131
  etiology of, 131
  neuropharmacology of, 131
Androstenedione, adverse effects of, 132
Anhedonia, orgasmic, 286
Anorexia nervosa
  course and prognosis of, 304
  diagnosis and clinical features of,
      303–304, 303t
    subtypes of, 303–304
  differential diagnosis of, 304
  epidemiology of, 302
  etiology of, 302–303
    biological factors in, 302
    psychological and psychodynamic fac-
        tors in, 302–303
    social factors in, 302
  treatment of, 304–305
    hospitalization in, 304–305
    selective serotonin reuptake inhibitors
        in, 479
Antabuse. *See* Disulfiram (Antabuse)
Antiandrogens
  in paraphilia, 294
  in sexual dysfunction, 289
Anticholinergics
  dosage and clinical guidelines for, 431,
      431t
  drug–drug interactions of, 431
  effects of on specific organs and systems,
      430
  pharmacological actions of, 430
  precautions and adverse reactions of,
      430–431
  in sexual dysfunction, 285
  therapeutic indications for, 430
Anticonvulsants, 473. *See also specific
      agents*
  in bipolar I disorder, 198, 474
  in intermittent explosive disorder, 325
  in posttraumatic stress disorder, 238
Antidepressants. *See also* Monoamine oxi-
      dase inhibitors (MAOIs); Selec-
      tive serotonin reuptake inhibitors
      (SSRIs); Tetracyclic antidepres-
      sants (TCAs); Tricyclic antide-
      pressants (TCAs)
  adverse effects of, 196
  in bulimia nervosa, 307–308

  drug–drug interactions of, 196
  in major depressive disorder, 195–197
  in mood disorder due to general medical
      condition, 63
  in pain disorders, 257
  in paraphilia, 294
  in postpartum psychosis, 167
  in postpsychotic depressive disorder of
      schizophrenia, 209
  in recurrent brief depressive disorder, 207
  in sexual dysfunction, 285
Antiestrogens, in sexual dysfunction, 289
Antihistamines
  dosage and clinical guidelines for, 432t,
      433
  drug–drug interactions of, 432
  effects of on specific organs of, 431
  laboratory interferences of, 432–433
  pharmacological actions of, 431
  precautions and adverse reactions to, 432
  in sexual dysfunction, 285
  therapeutic indications for, 431–432
Antihypertensives, tricyclic antidepressants
      and, 496
Antipsychotics
  in brief psychotic disorder, 165
  in delusional disorder, 163–164
  in paraphilia, 294
  in postpartum psychosis, 167
  in schizophreniform disorder, 155
  in schizotypal personality disorder, 342
  in sexual dysfunction, 284–285
  tests for use of, 23
  in Tourette's disorder, 559
  tricyclic antidepressants and, 496
  typical, 454. *See also* Dopamine receptor
      antagonists
Antisocial behavior
  adult, 378–379
    diagnosis and clinical features of,
        378–379
    epidemiology of, 378
    etiology of, 378
    treatment of, 379
  childhood or adolescent, 586–587
    diagnosis and clinical features of, 587
    differential diagnosis of, 587
    epidemiology of, 586
    etiology of, 586–587
    treatment of, 587
Anxiety
  γ-aminobutyric acid in, 212–213
  aplysia in, 213
  autonomic nervous system in, 212
  brain-imaging studies in, 213
  cerebral cortex in, 213–214
  depression and, 188, 436–437
  genetic studies in, 213
  insomnia and, 319–320, 320t
  limbic system in, 213
  neuroanatomical considerations in,
      213–214
  neurotransmitters in, 212
  norepinephrine in, 212
  pathological, 211–214
    behavior theories of, 211
    biological theories of, 212
    cognitive theories of, 211
    epidemiology of, 211
    existential theories of, 212
    psychoanalytic theories of, 211
    psychological theories of, 211–212
  separation. *See* Separation anxiety disor-
      der

serotonin in, 212–213
symptoms of, 211, 212t
treatment of
benzodiazepines in, 436
catecholamines in, 22
Anxiety disorder(s)
β-adrenergic receptor antagonists in, 427
alcohol-related disorders and, 81, 88
amphetamine-induced, 95
caffeine-induced, 99
cannabis-induced, 102
classification of, 214
cocaine-induced, 106
due to general medical condition, 64–65
clinical features of, 242–243
course and prognosis of, 64–65, 243
diagnosis and clinical features of, 64
diagnosis of, 242, 242t
differential diagnosis of, 243
epidemiology of, 64, 242
etiology of, 64, 242
treatment of, 65, 243
hallucinogen-induced, 110
HIV-associated, 74
inhalant-induced, 113
with mood disorder, 188
not otherwise specified, 244, 244t
phencyclidine-induced, 124
psychological sequelae of, 358
selective serotonin reuptake inhibitors in,
478–479, 480–481
substance-induced
clinical features of, 243
course and prognosis of, 243–244
diagnosis of, 243, 244t
differential diagnosis of, 243
epidemiology of, 243
etiology of, 243
treatment of, 244
suicide risk in, 392
treatment of, 436
buspirone in, 442
clonidine in, 425
guanfacine in, 425
Anxiolytic-related disorders, 125–131, 127t
clinical features of, 129–130
diagnosis of, 127–129, 127t
epidemiology of, 126
legal issues in, 130–131
neuropharmacology of, 126–127
not otherwise specified, 129
Anxiolytics, 125–126, 127t. See also Anxiolytic-related disorders; Benzodiazepines
in brief psychotic disorder, 165
in sexual dysfunction, 285
Aphasia, acquired, autism and, 538
Aplysia, in anxiety, 213
Appearance, in mental status examination, 6
Aricept. See Donepezil (Aricept)
Aripiprazole (Abilify), 483. See also Serotonin-dopamine antagonists (SDAs)
adverse effects of, 485
dosage and clinical guidelines for, 487
pharmacologic actions of, 484
Ariza. See Gepirone (Ariza)
Arsenic poisoning, mental disorders due to, 72
Artane. See Trihexyphenidyl (Artane)
Arthritis, rheumatoid, psychological seque-
lae of, 360
Asperger's disorder
course and prognosis of, 542
diagnosis and clinical features of, 541,
542t

differential diagnosis of, 541–542
etiology of, 541
treatment of, 542
Assertiveness training, 411
Asthma
psychological sequelae of, 358–359
sleep-related, 321
Ataque de nervios, 170
Atarax. See Hydroxyzine hydrochloride
(Atarax)
Atenolol (Tenormin), in avoidant personality
disorder, 348
Ativan. See Lorazepam (Ativan)
Atomoxetine (Strattera), 492. See also Sympathomimetics
Attention
disturbances in, 26
in mental status examination, 9
Attention-deficit disorders, 544. See also
Attention-deficit/hyperactivity
disorder (ADHD)
Attention-deficit/hyperactivity disorder
(ADHD)
clinical features of, 545–546
course and prognosis of, 546
diagnosis of, 544–545, 544t
differential diagnosis of, 546
epidemiology of, 544
etiology of, 544
brain damage in, 544
genetic factors in, 544
neurochemical factors in, 544
neurophysiological factors in, 544
psychosocial factors in, 544
not otherwise specified, 547, 547t
pathology and lab exam of, 546
treatment of, 426, 440, 546–547
atomoxetine in, 492
selective serotonin reuptake inhibitors
in, 479
sympathomimetics in, 488–489
Attitude toward examiner, in mental status
examination, 6
Autistic disorder(s)
vs. acquired aphasia with avulsion, 538
associated behavioral symptoms of, 537
associated physical illnesses of, 537
communication disturbances in, 537
vs. congenital deafness, 538
vs. congenital severe hearing impairment,
538
course and prognosis of, 538
diagnosis and clinical features of,
536–538, 536t
behavioral characteristics in, 537–538
intellectual functioning in, 538
physical characteristics in, 536–537
differential diagnosis of, 538
epidemiology of, 535
prevalence of, 535
sex distribution of, 535
etiology and pathogenesis of, 535
biochemical factors in, 536
biological factors in, 535
genetic factors in, 535–536
immunological factors in, 536
neuroanatomical factors in, 536
perinatal factors in, 536
psychosocial and family factors in, 535
vs. mental retardation with behavioral
symptoms, 538
vs. schizophrenia with childhood onset,
538
social interaction impairments in, 537

stereotyped behavior in, 537
treatment of, 539
selective serotonin reuptake inhibitors
in, 479
Autonomic nervous system, in anxiety, 212
Aversion therapy, 411–412

B

Back pain, lower, psychological sequelae of,
360–361
Balint, Michael, 401
Barbiturate-like substances
disorders related to, 126
intoxication from, 127t, 128
overdose of, 130
withdrawal from, 127t, 128
Barbiturates, 126
dosage and clinical guidelines for, 434t, 435
drug–drug reactions of, 434
effects of on specific organs and systems,
433
intoxication from, 127t, 128
overdose of, 129
pharmacological actions of, 433
precautions and adverse reactions to, 434
therapeutic indications for, 433–434
in electroconvulsive therapy, 433
in narcoanalysis, 433
in seizures, 433
in sexual dysfunction, 285
in sleep disorders, 433–434
in withdrawal from sedative hypnotics,
434
withdrawal from, 127t, 128
Basal ganglia, in schizophrenia, 138
Bateson, Gregory, 140
Battered child. See Child abuse and neglect
Bayley Scales of Infant Development, 510
Beck, Aaron, 194
Behavior
antisocial. See Antisocial behavior
change in, in psychosomatic disorders,
362
overt, in mental status examination, 6
sexual, 276
hormones and neurohormones in,
276–277
Type A, psychological sequelae of, 358
Behaviorism, 410. See also Behavior therapy
Behavior therapy
in anorexia nervosa, 305
in anxiety, 211–212
assertiveness training in, 411
aversion therapy in, 411–412
in bulimia nervosa, 307
in depression in children, 577–578
dialectical, 412
in dysthymic disorder, 201
in enuresis, 565
flooding in, 411
in kleptomania, 327
in mood disorders, 194
in obsessive-compulsive disorder, 232
in panic disorder, 215, 221
in paraphilia, 294
in phobia, 226
positive reinforcement in, 412
in posttraumatic stress disorder, 233
in schizophrenia, 152
in sexual dysfunction, 287–288
systematic desensitization in, 410–411
adjunctive use of drugs in, 410–411
desensitization of the stimulus in, 410

Behavior therapy—*continued*
    hierarchy construction in, 410
    indications for, 411
    relaxation training in, 410
    therapeutic graded exposure in, 411
    virtual reality in, 411
Belle indifférence, la, in conversion disorder, 251
Benadryl. *See* Diphenhydramine (Benadryl)
Bender Visual Motor Gestalt test, 511
Benzodiazepines, 126
    dosage and administration of, 439–440
    drug–drug interactions of, 439
    effects of on specific organs and systems, 435–436
    intoxication from, 127t, 128
    overdose of, 129
    pharmacological actions of, 435
    precautions and adverse reactions to, 438
        tolerance, dependence, and withdrawal in, 438–439
    tests for use of, 23
    therapeutic indications for, 436–437
        in akathisia, 437
        in anxiety, 436
        in bipolar I disorder, 437
        in depression, 437
        in generalized anxiety disorder, 241
        in insomnia, 437
        in mixed anxiety-depressive disorder, 436–437
        in obsessive-compulsive disorder, 437
        in panic disorder, 437
        in panic disorders, 220
        in Parkinson's disease, 437
        in posttraumatic stress disorder, 426, 437
        in social phobia, 227, 437
    withdrawal from, 127t, 128, 130t
Benztropine (Cogentin), 430. *See also* Anticholinergics
Bereavement, 377
    in children, 577
    uncomplicated, 190–191
Betel nuts, abuse of, 133
Bilis and colera, 170
Binge-eating disorder, 308, 308t
Binswanger's disease, 52
Biochemical markers, 24t, 25
    methods of, 409–410
        instrumentation in, 409
        relaxation therapy and, 409–410
Biofeedback
    methods of, autogenic training in, 410
    in psychosomatic disorders, 363
    results of, 410
    theory in, 409
Biogenic amines, in mood disorders, 174–175
Biperiden, 430. *See also* Anticholinergics
Bipolar disorder(s), 173–199
    not otherwise specified, 208t, 209
Bipolar I disorder
    with catatonic features, 185–186, 186t
    in children, 576–577
    chronic, 186, 186t
    classification of, 173–174
    course of, 192, 193f
    diagnosis of, 179t, 180–181
    differential diagnosis of, 191
    in elderly patients, 192
    epidemiology of
        age and, 174
        incidence and prevalence and, 174, 174t
        marital status and, 174

sex and, 174
    socioeconomic and cultural factors and, 174
    etiology of, 174–179
        biological factors in, 174–176
            biogenic amines and, 174–175
            brain imaging in, 176
            circadian rhythms in, 176
            kindling in, 176
            neuroanatomical considerations in, 176
            neurochemical factors in, 175
            neuroendocrine regulation in, 175–176
            neuroimmune regulation in, 176
            sleep abnormalities in, 176
        genetic factors in, 176–177
            adoption studies and, 177
            chromosome 11 and, 177
            family studies and, 177
            linkage studies and, 177
            twin studies and, 177
            X chromosome and, 177
        psychosocial factors in, 177–178
            life events and environmental stress in, 177
            personality factors in, 177
            psychodynamic factors in, 177–178
    maintenance in, 198–199
    manic episode in, 181, 182t
    vs. medical illness, 191
    not otherwise specified, 208t, 209
    with postpartum onset, 186, 186t
    prognosis of, 192–193
    with rapid cycling, 186, 186t, 198
    recurrent, 181, 182t, 183t
    vs. schizophrenia, 191
    with seasonal pattern, 186–187, 187t
    single manic episode in, 181, 182t
    specifiers for, 186–187, 186t, 187t
    treatment of, 197–199
        anticonvulsants in, 474
        benzodiazepines in, 437
        bupropion in, 440
        carbamazepine in, 197–198, 445
        clonazepam in, 435
        dopamine receptor antagonists in, 455–456
        hospitalization in, 193–194
        lithium in, 198, 459
        valproate in, 198, 497
        verapamil in, 443
Bipolar II disorder
    chronic, 186, 186t
    classification of, 173–174
    clinical features of, 188
    course and prognosis of, 193
    diagnosis of, 181, 184t
    differential diagnosis of, 191
    epidemiology of, 174
    etiology of, 174
    with postpartum onset, 186, 186t
    with rapid cycling, 186, 186t
    with seasonal pattern, 186–187, 187t
    specifiers for, 186–187, 186t, 187t
    treatment of, 199
Black-out, 170
    in alcohol-induced persisting amnestic disorder, 87–88
Bleuler, Eugen, 134
Blood dyscrasias, carbamazepine in, 446
Body dysmorphic disorder
    clinical features of, 254–255

course and prognosis of, 255
    diagnosis of, 254, 255t
    differential features of, 255
    epidemiology of, 254
    etiology of, 254
    relation to plastic surgery, 255
    treatment of, 255
Body image problems, 294
Body temperature regulation, serotonin-dopamine antagonists and, 485
Borderline intellectual functioning, 585
    diagnosis of, 585
    etiology of, 585
    treatment of, 585
Bouffée délirante, 144
Brain fag, 170
Brain-imaging studies
    in anxiety, 213
    in bipolar I disorder, 176
    in major depressive disorder, 176
    in mood disorders, 176
    in obsessive-compulsive disorder, 228
Brain tumor, mental disorders due to, 67
Brainwashing, in posttraumatic stress disorder, 236
Brevital. *See* Methohexital (Brevital)
Bromocriptine (Parlodel), 452. *See also* Dopamine receptor agonists
Bruxism, sleep-related, 319
Bulimia nervosa
    course and prognosis of, 307
    diagnosis and clinical features of, 306–307, 306t
        subtypes of, 306–307
    differential diagnosis of, 307
    epidemiology of, 305
    etiology of, 305–306
        biological factors in, 305–306
        psychological factors in, 306
        social factors in, 306
    pathology and lab exam in, 307
    treatment of, 307–308
        selective serotonin reuptake inhibitors in, 479
Buprenex. *See* Buprenorphine (Buprenex)
Buprenorphine (Buprenex), 468. *See also* Opioid receptor agonists
    dosage and clinical guidelines for, 471
    therapeutic indications for, 469
Bupropion (Wellbutrin, Zyban)
    dosage and clinical guidelines for, 441
    drug–drug reactions of, 441
    effects of on specific organs and systems, 440
    laboratory interferences in, 441
    pharmacological actions of, 440
    precautions and adverse reactions to, 441
    therapeutic indications for, 440–441
        in attention deficit/hyperactivity disorder, 440
        in bipolar disorder, 440
        in cocaine detoxification, 441
        in depression, 440
        in major depressive disorder, 195
        in smoking cessation, 441
BuSpar. *See* Buspirone (BuSpar)
Buspirone (BuSpar), 433, 442
    dosage and clinical guidelines of, 443
    drug–drug interactions of, 442
    effects of on specific organs and systems, 442
    laboratory interferences of, 442
    pharmacological actions of, 442

precautions and adverse reactions to, 442
therapeutic indications for, 442
in generalized anxiety disorder, 241
in social phobia, 227

C

Caffeine-related disorder(s)
clinical features of, 99
comorbidity of, 97
diagnosis of, 97–98, 98t
epidemiology of, 97
intoxication, 98, 98t
neuropharmacology of, 97
effect on cerebral blood flow and, 97
genetics and, 97
substance abuse and, 97
not otherwise specified, 98t, 99
treatment of, 99–100
Calan. *See* Verapamil (Calan)
Calcium channel inhibitors
dosage and clinical guidelines for, 444
drug–drug interactions of, 444
effects of on specific organs and systems, 443
pharmacological actions of, 443
precautions and adverse reactions to, 444
therapeutic indications for, 443–444
in bipolar disorder, 443
in recurrent brief depressive disorder, 443
Cannabis
abuse, 101
amotivational syndrome and, 102
dependence, 101
intoxication, 101
in sexual dysfunction, 285
Cannabis-related disorder(s)
diagnosis and clinical features of, 100–102, 102t
epidemiology of, 100
neuropharmacology of, 100
not otherwise specified, 102, 102t
treatment and rehabilitation of, 102
Cannon, Walter, 355
Capgras' syndrome, 161
Carbamazepine (Tegretol), 444
dosage and clinical guidelines for, 447
drug–drug interactions of, 446
effects of on specific organs and systems, 445
laboratory interferences of, 447
pharmacological actions of, 444
precautions and adverse reactions to, 445–446
tests for use of, 24
therapeutic indications for, 445
in alcohol and benzodiazepine withdrawal, 445
in bipolar I disorder, 197–198, 445
in impulse control disorder, 445
in posttraumatic stress disorder, 426, 445
in schizoaffective disorder, 157, 445
in schizophrenia, 445
Carbidopa-levodopa (Sinemet), 452. *See also* Dopamine receptor agonists
Cardene. *See* Nicardipine (Cardene)
Cardizem. *See* Diltiazem (Cardizem)
Catapres. *See* Clonidine (Catapres)
Catatonia, 185–186, 186t
due to general medical condition, 65–66, 65t

Catecholamines, 22
Catnip, abuse of, 133
Cattell Infant Intelligence Scale, 510
Celexa. *See* Citalopram (Celexa)
Central nervous system, carbamazepine in, 446
Central nervous system depressants, tricyclic antidepressants and, 496
Centrax. *See* Prazepam (Centrax)
Cerebral cortex, in anxiety, 213–214
Charcot, Jean-Martin, 414
Child abuse and neglect, 370, 371t
confidentiality and, 610
course and prognosis of, 373
diagnosis and clinical features of, 371–373
neglect of child in, 372–373
pathology and lab exam in, 373
physical abuse of child in, 371
sexual abuse of child in, 371–372
incest in, 372
statutory rape in, 372
differential diagnosis of, 373
epidemiology of, 370
etiology of, 370–371
treatment of, 373–374
Child and Adolescent Psychiatric Assessment (CAPA), 508
Child Behavior Checklist, 508–509
Childhood disintegrative disorder
course and prognosis of, 541
diagnosis and clinical features of, 540–541, 541t
differential diagnosis of, 541
epidemiology of, 540
etiology of, 540
treatment of, 541
Child(ren)
abuse and neglect of. *See* Child abuse and neglect
aggression in, 426
bereavement in, 577
bipolar I disorder in, 576–577
clinical interview of, 507–508
of adolescents, 508
of family, 508
of infants and young children, 507
of parents, 508
of school-age children, 507–508
components of evaluation of, 509–511
developmental, psychological, and educational testing in, 510–511
history in, 509
identifying data in, 509
mental status examination in, 509–510
neuropsychiatric assessment in, 510
day treatment for, 594–595
indications for, 594
programs in, 594–595
results in, 595
depression in, 576
treatment of, 577–578
behavior therapy in, 577–578
cognitive therapy in, 577–578
diagnostics instruments for, 508–509
dysthymic disorder in, 576
electroconvulsive therapy for, 578, 595
gender identity disorder in, 298–299
hospital treatment for, 595
major depressive disorder in, 576
pharmacotherapy, 595, 596t–597t
psychotherapy for
confidentiality in, 591

differences between children and adults in, 589–590
group, 591–593
indications for, 591
initial approach in, 590
in mood disorders, 577–578
parents in, 591
playroom in, 590
therapeutic interventions in, 590–591
types of psychotherapies in, 589
recommendations and treatment plan for, 511
residential treatment for, 593–594
education in, 593–594, 594f
group living in, 593
indications for, 593
parents in, 594
staff and setting in, 593
therapy in, 594
suicide in, 578
Children's Apperception Test (CAT), 511
Chloral hydrate, 448
Chlordiazepoxide (Librium), 435. *See also* Benzodiazepines
Chlorpromazine (Thorazine), 454. *See also* Dopamine receptor antagonists
Cholesterol elevations, serotonin-dopamine antagonists and, 485
Cholinesterase inhibitors, 448
dosage and clinical guidelines for, 450
drug–drug interactions of, 450
effects of on specific organs and systems, 449
pharmacological actions of, 449
precautions and adverse reactions of, 449–450
therapeutic indications for, 449
Chromosome 11, bipolar I disorder and, 177
Chronic fatigue syndrome
course and prognosis of, 260
diagnosis and clinical features of, 259, 260t
differential diagnosis of, 260
epidemiology of, 259
etiology of, 259
treatment of, 260
Chronic obstructive airway disease (COPD), selective serotonin reuptake inhibitors in, 480
Cigarette smoking, in schizophrenia, 135–136
Circadian rhythms, in depression, 176
Citalopram (Celexa), 476. *See also* Selective serotonin reuptake inhibitors (SSRIs)
dosage and clinical guidelines for, 483
in major depressive disorder, 195
Clomipramine (Anafranil), 476–477
in obsessive-compulsive disorder, 231
in panic disorder, 220
Clonazepam (Klonopin), 435. *See also* Benzodiazepines
in obsessive-compulsive disorder, 351
in posttraumatic stress disorder, 426
in social phobia, 227, 437
Clonidine (Catapres)
dosage and clinical guidelines for, 427
drug–drug interactions of, 426–427
effects of specific organs and systems of, 425
overdose of, 426
pharmacological actions of, 425

Clonidine (Catapres)—*continued*
  therapeutic indications for, 425–426
    in alcohol withdrawal, 425
    in benzodiazepine withdrawal, 425
    in hyperactivity and aggression in children, 426
    in nicotine withdrawal, 425
    in opioid withdrawal, 425
    in posttraumatic stress disorder, 426
    in tic disorders, 426
    in Tourette's disorder, 425–426
  withdrawal from, 426
Clorazepate, 435. *See also* Benzodiazepines
Clozapine (Clozaril), 483. *See also* Serotonin-dopamine antagonists (SDAs)
  adverse effects of, 484–485
  dosage and clinical guidelines for, 487
  pharmacological actions of, 483
  tests for use of, 23
  therapeutic indications for, 484
    in early-onset schizophrenia, 581
Clozaril. *See* Clozapine (Clozaril)
Cluster headache, sleep-related, 321
Cluttering, 534
Cobalamin deficiency, mental disorders due to, 72
Cocaine
  abuse, 104
    in adolescents, 582
  dependence, 104
  intoxication, 104–105
    treatment of, 441
Cocaine-related disorder(s), 102–107, 104t
  adverse effects of, 106
  comorbidity of, 103
  diagnosis and clinical features of, 104–106, 105t
  epidemiology of, 103
  etiology of, 103
  methods of use and, 104
  neuropharmacology of, 103–104
  not otherwise specified, 106, 106t
  treatment and rehabilitation of, 106–107
    detoxification in, 107, 441
Codependence, 78
Cogentin. *See* Benztropine (Cogentin)
Cognex. *See* Tacrine (Cognex)
Cognition
  clinical evaluation of, 46
  in depressive episode, 189
  disturbances in, in dementia, 54–55
  in geriatric patients, 601
  in manic episode, 190
  in psychiatric evaluation of children, 510
  in schizophrenia, 148
Cognitive decline, age-related, 381
Cognitive disorder(s)
  classification of, 45–46
  not otherwise specified, classification of, 46, 46t
  perceptual disturbances associated with, 31
Cognitive impairment, serotonin-dopamine antagonists and, 485
Cognitive theory
  of depression, 178, 413
  of dysthymic disorder, 200
Cognitive therapy, 413–414
  in anorexia nervosa, 305
  in anxiety, 211–212
  in bulimia nervosa, 307
  definition of, 413. *See also* Cognitive theory
  in depression in children, 577–578
  in dysthymic disorder, 201
  efficacy of, 414

in mood disorders, 194
in panic disorder, 215, 221
in paraphilia, 294
in posttraumatic stress disorder, 233
in schizophrenia, 152
strategies and techniques of, 413–414
  behavioral techniques in, 414
  cognitive techniques in, 413
  didactic aspects of, 413
  imagery and, 414
Colitis, ulcerative, psychological sequelae of, 357
Communication disorders, 528. *See also* specific disorders
  not otherwise specified, 534, 534t
Competence to be executed, 613
Competence to stand trial, 613
Computed tomography (CT), in schizophrenia, 138
Conation, 27–28
Concentration, in mental status examination, 9
Concerta. *See* Methylphenidate (Ritalin, Concerta)
Conduct disorder(s)
  course and prognosis of, 551
  diagnosis and clinical features of, 550–551, 550t
  differential diagnosis of, 551
  epidemiology of, 549–550
  etiology of, 550
  treatment of, 551–552
Confabulation, in dissociative amnesia, 267
Conjoint therapy, 408
Consciousness, 26
  in geriatric patients, 601
  in mental status examination, 8
Contamination, in obsessive-compulsive disorder, 230
Contraceptives, oral, tricyclic antidepressants and, 496
Conversion disorder
  clinical features of, 250–251
    motor symptoms in, 251
    seizure symptoms in, 251
    sensory symptoms in, 251
  comorbidity of, 250
  course and prognosis of, 252
  diagnosis of, 250, 250t
  differential diagnosis of, 251–252
  epidemiology of, 249–250
  etiology of, 250
  perceptual disturbances associated with, 31–32
  treatment of, 252
Coprophilia, 293
Coronary artery bypass graft surgery, psychological sequelae of, 358
Coronary heart disease, psychological sequelae of, 358
Corticotropin-releasing factor, in posttraumatic stress disorder, 233
Cortisol
  in depression, 175
  in mood disorders, 175
Cotard, Jules, 161
Counterphobic attitude, 223
Countertransference, in psychoanalysis, 397
Couple problems, 294
Couples therapy, 408–409
  contraindications to, 409
  goals of, 409
  indications for, 409
  types of, 408–409

Crack (cocaine), cocaine-related disorder and, 104
Creutzfeldt-Jakob disease
  mental disorders due to, 70
  variant, mental disorders due to, 70
Crisis intervention, in adjustment disorders, 334
Crohn's disease, psychological sequelae of, 357–358
Cross-dressing, 299
  treatment of, 301
Cults, 380
Culture-bound syndromes, 169–171. *See also specific syndromes*
  psychopharmacology and, 171–172
Cushing's syndrome, psychological sequelae of, 359
Cyclothymic disorder, 173
  course and prognosis of, 204
  diagnosis and clinical features of, 203–204, 203t
  differential diagnosis of, 204
  epidemiology of, 202
  etiology of, 203
    biological factors in, 203
    psychosocial factors in, 203
  signs and symptoms of, 203–204
  substance abuse in, 204
  treatment of, 204
Cylert. *See* Pemoline (Cylert)
Cymbalta. *See* Duloxetine hydrochloride (Cymbalta)
Cyproheptadine (Periactin), 431. *See also* Antihistamines
Cytochrome p450 isoenzymes, 172, 419

D

Dalmane. *See* Flurazepam (Dalmane)
Dantrium. *See* Dantrolene (Dantrium)
Dantrolene (Dantrium)
  dosage and administration of, 451
  drug–drug interactions of, 451
  effects of on specific organs and systems, 451
  pharmacological actions of, 450–451
  precautions and adverse reactions to, 451
  therapeutic indications for, 451
Deafness, congenital, autism and, 538
de Clérambault's syndrome, 160
Defense mechanisms
  in delusional disorder, 159
  in personality disorders, 337–338
Defensive Functioning Scale, 44t
Dehydroepiandrosterone, 505
  adverse effects of, 132
Delirium, 46–47
  alcohol-related, 86–87
  vs. amnestic disorder, 62
  amphetamine intoxication, 95
  cannabis-related, 101
  classification of, 45
  cocaine intoxication, 105
  cognition in, 46
  course and prognosis of, 49–50
  delusional disorders and, 162
  vs. dementia, 56
  diagnosis and clinical features of, 47–49, 48t, 49t
  differential diagnosis of, 49
  due to general medical condition, 48, 48t
  epidemiology of, 47
  etiology of, 47
  hallucinogen intoxication, 109

HIV-associated, 74
inhalant intoxication, 113
opioid intoxication, 120
phencyclidine intoxication, 124
physical and lab examinations of, 49
vs. schizophrenia, 49
sedative, hypnotic, or anxiolytic, 128
substance intoxication, 48, 48t
substance withdrawal, 48, 48t
treatment of, 50
Delusional disorder(s), 157, 158t
course and prognosis of, 162–163
diagnosis and clinical features of, 159–162
mental status in, 159–160
types in, 159–160
erotomanic type, 160–161
grandiose type, 161
jealous type, 160
mixed type, 161
persecutory type, 160
somatic type, 161
unspecified type, 161
differential diagnosis of, 162
epidemiology of, 158
etiology of, 158–159
biological factors in, 159
psychodynamic factors in, 159
shared psychotic disorder and, 161–162,
162t
treatment of, 163–164
hospitalization in, 163
pharmacotherapy in, 163–164
psychotherapy in, 163
Delusions
defined, 8, 157, 158t
in dementia, 54
of dysmorphophobia, 161
erotomanic, 160–161
of foul body odors, 161
of infestation, 161
of infidelity, 160
jealous, 160
of misidentification, 161
nonbizarre, 157
of persecution, 160
somatic, 161
substance-induced, 168–169
Dementia, 32
alcohol-induced persisting, 87
of Alzheimer's type
diagnosis of, 53t
epidemiology of, 50–51
etiology of, 51–52
genetic factors in, 51
neuropathology in, 51
neurotransmitters in, 51–52
vs. vascular dementia, 56
vs. amnestic disorder, 62
classification of, 45
course and prognosis of, 57
in Creutzfeld-Jakob disease, 70
vs. delirium, 49, 56
delusional disorders and, 162
vs. depression, 56
diagnosis and clinical features of, 53, 53t,
54t, 55t
catastrophic reaction in, 55
cognitive change in, 54–55
hallucinations and delusions in, 54
mood in, 54
personality in, 53–54
sundowner syndrome in, 55–56
differential diagnosis of, 56–57
epidemiology of, 50–51

etiology of, 51–53
vs. factitious disorder, 56
head trauma–related, 53
HIV-associated, 74
human immunodeficiency virus–related,
52–53
inhalant-induced persisting, 113
vs. normal aging, 56
pathology, physical findings, and lab
exam in, 56
persisting, in sedative-, hypnotic-, or anxiolytic related disorder, 128
vs. schizophrenia, 56
treatment of, 57–58
vascular
vs. dementia of Alzheimer's type, 56
diagnosis of, 54t
etiology of, 52
vs. transient ischemic attacks, 56
Demyelinating disorders, mental disorders
due to, 68–69
Denver Developmental Screening Test, 510
Depakene. See Valproate (Depakene)
Dependence, psychological, 77
Depersonalization disorder
course and prognosis of, 273
diagnosis and clinical features of, 272, 272t
differential diagnosis of, 273
epidemiology of, 271–272
etiology of, 272
treatment of, 273
Depression. See also Bipolar I disorder; Dysthymic disorder; Major depres-
sive disorder; Minor depressive
disorder; Mood disorder(s)
alcohol dependence and, 82, 188
antihypertensives and, 496
anxiety and, 188
atypical, 209
catecholamines and, 22
in children
treatment of, 577–578
in children and adolescents, 188, 478
clinical features of, 187–188
cognitive therapy for, 178, 413
vs. delirium, 49
vs. dementia, 56
diagnosis of, with dexamethasone-suppression test, 175
double, 201
in elderly patients, 188, 602
HIV-associated, 75
vs. hypochondriasis, 253
vs. hypothyroidism, 359
learned helplessness and, 178–179
with medical illness, 188
mental status exam in, 188–189
postpartum, 364–365, 365t
rating scales for, 189
suicide and, 391–392
treatment of
alprazolam in, 437
bupropion in, 440
mirtazapine in, 463
nefazodone in, 467
selective serotonin reuptake inhibitors
in, 477, 478
sympathomimetics in, 489
venlafaxine in, 499
unipolar, 173
Depressive disorder(s)
with anxiety, treatment of, 436–437
not otherwise specified, 204, 205t
recurrent brief, treatment of, 443

suicide risk in, 391
trazodone in, 493
Depressive episode, 459
with atypical features, 184–185, 185t
with catatonic features, 185–186, 186t
with melancholic features, 184, 184t
with postpartum onset, 186, 186t
with psychotic features, 180t, 182–184
Dermatitis
atopic, psychological sequelae of, 360
exfoliative, carbamazepine in, 446
Desensitization, systematic, 410–411
Desipramine (Norpramin), tests for use of,
23
Desoxyn. See Methamphetamine (Desoxyn)
Desyrel. See Trazodone (Desyrel)
Detoxification, rapid, 473
Developmental coordination disorder
clinical features of, 526–527
comorbidity of, 526
course and prognosis of, 527
diagnosis of, 526
differential diagnosis of, 527
epidemiology of, 526
etiology of, 526
treatment of, 527
Dexamethasone-suppression test, 21
in depression, 175
Dexedrine. See Dextroamphetamine
(Dexedrine)
Dexmethylphenidate (Focalin), 488. See also
Sympathomimetics
Dextroamphetamine (Dexedrine), 488. See
also Sympathomimetics
in attention-deficit/hyperactivity disorder,
546–547
Dhat, 170
Diabetes mellitus, psychological sequelae of,
359
Diabetic ketoacidosis, mental disorders due
to, 72
Diagnostic and Statistical Manual of Mental
Disorders (DSM-IV-TR), 33
basic features in, 33
classifications of, 34t–40t
multiaxial evaluation in, 33, 40
relation to ICD-10, 33
Diagnostic Interview for Children and Adolescents (DICA), 508
Dialectical behavior therapy, 412
Diazepam (Valium), 435. See also Benzodiazepines
in hallucinogen intoxication, 111
in paranoid personality disorder, 340
Diltiazem (Cardizem), dosage and clinical
guidelines for, 444
Diphenhydramine (Benadryl), 431. See also
Antihistamines
Disorder of infancy, childhood, or adolescence, 574, 574t
Disorder of written expression, 524–525
clinical features of, 524–525
comorbidity of, 524
course and prognosis of, 525
diagnosis of, 524
differential diagnosis of, 525
epidemiology of, 524
etiology of, 524
pathology and lab exam of, 525
treatment of, 525
Disorganized sleep–wake pattern, 316
Disruptive behavior disorders, 548. See also
specific disorders
not otherwise specified, 552, 552t

Dissociation, in personality disorders, 338
Dissociative amnesia
    clinical features of, 267
    confabulation and self-monitoring in, 267
    course and prognosis of, 268
    diagnosis of, 267, 267t
    differential diagnosis of, 267
    epidemiology of, 266
    etiology of, 266–267
    treatment of, 268
Dissociative disorder, 266. *See also specific disorders*
    vs. amnestic disorder, 62
    disturbances associated with, 31–32
    not otherwise specified, 273, 273t
Dissociative fugue
    course and prognosis of, 269
    diagnosis and clinical features of, 268–269, 269t
    differential diagnosis of, 269
    epidemiology of, 268
    etiology of, 268
    treatment of, 269
Dissociative identity disorder
    course and prognosis of, 271
    diagnosis of clinical features of, 270, 270t
    differential diagnosis of, 270–271
    epidemiology of, 269–270
    etiology of, 270
    treatment of, 271
        forensic issues in, 271
Dissociative trance disorder, 273–274, 274t
Disulfiram (Antabuse)
    dosage and administration of, 452
    drug–drug interactions of, 452
    laboratory interferences of, 452
    pharmacological actions of, 451
    precautions and adverse reactions to, 452
    therapeutic indications for, 451–452
Dolophine. *See* Methadone (Dolophine)
Donepezil, precautions and adverse reactions of, 449
Donepezil (Aricept), 448. *See also* Cholinesterase inhibitors
Do Not Intubate orders, 604
Do Not Resuscitate orders, 604
Dopamine, in mood disorders, 175
Dopamine receptor agonists
    dosage and clinical guidelines of, 454, 454t
    drug–drug interactions of, 453
    effects of on specific organs and systems, 453
    laboratory interferences of, 453–454
    pharmacological actions of, 452–453
    precautions and adverse reactions to, 453
    therapeutic indications for, 453
Dopamine receptor antagonists, 454–458, 455t
    dosage and administration of, 457–458
        choice of drug in, 457
    effects of on specific organs and systems, 454–455
    laboratory interferences of, 457
    pharmacological actions of, 454
    precautions and adverse reactions to, 456–457
    therapeutic indications for, 455–456
        in bipolar disorder, 455–456
        in primary psychotic disorders, 455
        in schizophrenia, 150, 455
        in secondary psychoses, 456
        in severe agitation, 456
        in violent behavior, 456
Doral. *See* Quazepam (Doral)

Double bind concept, of schizophrenia, 140
Double depression, vs. dysthymic disorder, 201
Doubt, pathological, in obsessive-compulsive disorder, 230
Down syndrome, 513–514
Downward drift hypothesis, of schizophrenia, 136
Dreams, interpretation of, 397
Drug-assisted interview, 24
Drug dependence, 77
DSM-IV-TR. *See Diagnostic and Statistical Manual of Mental Disorders (DSM-IV-TR)*
Dual-sex therapy, 286–287
Duloxetine hydrochloride (Cymbalta), 500
Durable power of attorney, 613
Durham rule, criminal responsibility and, 614
Durkheim, Émile, on suicide, 392
DynaCirc. *See* Isradipine (DynaCirc)
Dyslexia. *See* Reading disorder
Dyspareunia, 282, 282t
    due to general medical condition, 283
Dysphagia, serotonin-dopamine antagonists and, 485
Dysphoria, postcoital, 294
Dyssomnias, 312–317
    not otherwise specified, 316–317, 316t.
        See also specific disorders
Dysthymic disorder
    vs. alcohol abuse, 201
    in children, 576
    classification of, 173
    cognitive theory of, 200
    course and prognosis of, 201
    diagnosis and clinical features of, 200, 200t
    differential diagnosis of, 200–201
    vs. double depression, 201
    epidemiology of, 199
    etiology of, 199–200
        biological factors in, 199
        psychosocial factors in factors in, 199–200
    vs. minor depressive disorder, 201
    vs. recurrent brief depressive disorder, 201
    treatment of, 201–202
        behavior therapy in, 201
        cognitive therapy in, 201
        family therapy in, 202
        interpersonal therapy in, 202
Dystonia, acute, neuroleptic-induced, 423–424
    treatment of, 430, 431–432

E

Eating disorder(s). *See also* Anorexia nervosa; Binge-eating disorder; Bulimia nervosa
    of childhood, 553. *See also specific disorders*
    not otherwise specified, 308, 308t
    selective serotonin reuptake inhibitors in, 479
    tricyclic antidepressants in, 494
Effexor. *See* Venlafaxine (Effexor)
Elavil. *See* Amitriptyline (Elavil)
Eldepryl. *See* Selegiline (Eldepryl)
Elder abuse, 375
Electroconvulsive therapy (ECT)
    adverse effects of, 503–504
    amnestic disorder and, 61
    barbiturates in, 433
    in children, 578, 595

clinical guidelines for, 501–503
    anesthesia in, 501–502
    electrical stimulus in, 503
    electrode placement in, 502–503
    induced seizures in, 503
    maintenance treatment in, 503
    muscarinic anticholinergic drugs in, 501
    muscle relaxants in, 502
    number and spacing of treatments in, 503
    pretreatment evaluation in, 501
    contraindications to, 503–504
    indications for, 500–501
    in major depressive disorder, 195, 500
    in schizophrenia, 501
Elimination disorders, 562. *See also specific disorders*
Emergencies, psychiatric
    clinical features and diagnosis of, 383
    epidemiology of, 382
    evaluation and treatment of, 167–168, 383–384, 384t–389t
        disposition in, 383–384
        drug treatment in, 383
        restraints in, 383
    interview in, 382–383
        range of problems in, 382
        violence in, 383
Emotion, 26–27
Encephalitis, herpes simplex, mental disorders due to, 69
Encephalopathy
    alcoholic pellagra, 89
    hepatic, mental disorders due to, 71
    hypoglycemic, mental disorders due to, 71
    uremic, mental disorders due to, 71
Encephalopathy due to brain injury, sympathomimetics in, 489
Encopresis
    course and prognosis of, 563
    diagnosis and clinical features of, 562–563, 563t
    differential diagnosis of, 563
    epidemiology of, 562
    etiology of, 562
        psychogenic megacolon in, 562
    pathology and lab exam of, 563
    treatment of, 563–564
Endocrine disorders
    mental disorders due to, 71
    treatment of, 505–506
End-of-life care
    communication in, 603–604
    general approaches to, 603
    neonatal and infant, 607
    pain management in, 606
    telling the truth in, 604
    terminal care decisions in, 604, 605t
        advance directives in, 604
        Do Not Intubate orders in, 604
        Do Not Resuscitate orders in, 604
        health care by proxy in, 604
        living will in, 604
Enuresis
    course and prognosis of, 564–565
    diagnosis and clinical features of, 564, 564t
    differential diagnosis of, 564
    epidemiology of, 564
    etiology of, 564
    pathology and lab exam of, 564
    treatment of, 565
Ephedra, abuse of, 133

Epilepsy
  complex partial, schizophrenia and, 139
  mental disorders due to, 67
Epileptic seizure, sleep-related, 321
Erectile dysfunction, 279–280. *See also* Sexual dysfunction
  due to general medical condition, 282–283
Erikson, Erik, 159
Erotomania, 160–161
Escitalopram (Lexapro), 476. *See also* Selective serotonin reuptake inhibitors (SSRIs)
  dosage and clinical guidelines for, 483
  in major depressive disorder, 195
Eskalith. *See* Lithium
Estazolam (ProSom), 435. *See also* Benzodiazepines
Estrogen, 505
Ethchlorvynol (Placidyl), 435
Ethics
  impaired physicians and, 615
  for physicians in training, 615
  professional codes of, 615, 616t–617t
Ethopropazine, 430. *See also* Anticholinergics
Euthanasia, 607
Evoked potential, schizophrenia and, 139
Excoriation, psychogenic, psychological sequelae of, 360
Exelon. *See* Rivastigmine (Exelon)
Exhibitionism, 291, 291t
Existential theories, in anxiety, 212
Expressed emotion, schizophrenia and, 141
Expressive language disorder
  clinical features of, 528–529
  course and prognosis of, 529
  diagnosis of, 528, 529t
  differential diagnosis of, 529
  epidemiology of, 528
  etiology of, 528
  treatment of, 529
External control mechanism, in paraphilia, 294
Extrapyramidal symptoms
  selective serotonin reuptake inhibitors and, 481
  serotonin-dopamine antagonists and, 485
Eye movements
  desensitization and reprocessing (EMDR), 412
  smooth pursuit, in personality disorders, 337

F

Factitious disorder
  vs. amnestic disorder, 62
  comorbidity of, 261
  course and prognosis of, 264
  vs. dementia, 56
  diagnosis and clinical features of, 262, 262t
    predominantly physical signs and symptoms in, 262–263
    predominantly psychological signs and symptoms in, 262
  differential diagnosis of, 263–264
  epidemiology of, 261
  etiology of, 261–262
    biological factors on, 262
    psychosocial factors on, 261–262
  not otherwise specified, 263, 263t
  pathology and lab exam in, 263

  by proxy, 263, 263t
  schizophrenia and, 149
  treatment of, 264–265
Falling-out, 170
Familial multiple system taupathy, with presenile dementia, 52
Families, pseudomutual and pseudohostile, and schizophrenia, 141
Family therapy, 407–408
  for adolescents, 598
  in anorexia nervosa, 305
  in dysthymic disorder, 202
  goals of, 408
  modifications of, 408
  in mood disorders, 194–195
  in panic disorders, 221
  in psychosomatic disorders, 362–363
  techniques in, 407–408
  theoretical issues in, 407
Fantasy, in personality disorders, 338
Feeding disorders of infancy or early childhood, 553, 555–556, 556t. *See also specific disorders*
Feelings
  in depressive episode, 189
  in geriatric patients, 600
  in manic episode, 189–190
  in schizophrenia, 146–147
Fenichel, Otto, 223, 396
Fetal Acquired Immune Deficiency Syndrome Transmission, opioids and, 122
Fetal alcohol syndrome, 89
  mental retardation and, 514
Fetishism, 291, 291t
  transvestic, 292
Fibromyalgia, selective serotonin reuptake inhibitors in, 479
Flashbacks, cannabis-related disorder and, 102
Flooding, 411
Flumazenil (Romazicon), 435. *See also* Benzodiazepines
  for benzodiazepine overdose, 438
Fluoxetine (Prozac), 476. *See also* Selective serotonin reuptake inhibitors (SSRIs)
  dosage and clinical guidelines for, 482
  suicide and, 447
  withdrawal, 481
Fluphenazine (Prolixin), 454. *See also* Dopamine receptor antagonists
Flurazepam (Dalmane), 435. *See also* Benzodiazepines
Fluvoxamine (Luvox), 476. *See also* Selective serotonin reuptake inhibitors (SSRIs)
  dosage and clinical guidelines for, 482
  in major depressive disorder, 195
  in panic disorder, 220
Focalin. *See* Dexmethylphenidate (Focalin)
Four-way session, 408
Fragile X syndrome, 514
Free association, 396–397
Free-floating attention, in psychoanalysis, 397
Frégoli's phenomenon, 161
French, Thomas, 401
Freud, Sigmund
  on anxiety, 211
  on delusions, 159
  on depression, 177–178
  on dysthymic disorder, 199–200

  on hypnosis, 414
  on obsessive-compulsive disorder, 228
  on phobia, 222
  psychoanalytic theory, 396
  on schizophrenia, 140
  on suicide, 392
Frotteurism, 291, 291t

G

Gabapentin (Neurontin), 473
  dosage and clinical guidelines for, 475
  drug–drug interactions of, 475
  laboratory interferences of, 475
  pharmacological actions of, 474
  precautions and adverse reactions to, 475
  therapeutic indications for, 474
Galantamine (Reminyl), 448. *See also* Cholinesterase inhibitors
  precautions and adverse reactions of, 449
Gamblers Anonymous (GA), 329–330
Gambling, pathological, 328–330
  comorbidity of, 328
  course and prognosis of, 329
  diagnosis and clinical features of, 329, 329t
  differential diagnosis of, 329
  epidemiology of, 328
  etiology of, 328–329
  psychological testing and lab exam of, 329
  treatment of, 329–330
Gamma hydroxybutyrate, mental disorders related to, 132
Ganser's syndrome, 274
  vs. factitious disorder, 264
Gastroesophageal reflux, sleep-related, 321
Gastroesophageal reflux disease, psychological sequelae of, 357
Gender identity disorder
  clinical features of, 298–299
    in adolescents and adults, 299
    in children, 298–299
  course and prognosis of, 299–300
  cross-dressing and, 299
  diagnosis of, 298, 298t
  epidemiology of, 297
  etiology of, 297
  intersex conditions in, 299, 300t
  not otherwise specified, 299
  treatment of, 300–301
    hormonal, 300–301
    surgical, 300
Gender roles, in gender identity, 275–276
General adaptation syndrome, 355
Generalized anxiety disorder
  clinical features of, 239–240
  comorbidity of, 238–239
  course and prognosis of, 240
  diagnosis of, 239, 240t
  differential diagnosis of, 240
  epidemiology of, 238
  etiology of, 239
    biological factors in, 239
    psychosocial factors in, 239
  treatment of, 240–242, 442
    tricyclic antidepressants in, 494
    venlafaxine in, 499
Genitourinary symptoms, serotonin-dopamine antagonists and, 485
Gepirone (Ariza), 443

Geriatric psychiatry
and bipolar I disorder in elderly patients, 192
congenital mental disorders in, 602
and depression in elderly patients, 188, 602
elder abuse and, 375
and lithium in elderly patients, 461
neuropsychological evaluation in, 601–602
psychiatric examination in, 599–602
history in, 599–600
mental status examination in, 600–601
German measles, mental retardation and, 514
Gerstmann-Straüssler-Scheinker disease, mental disorders due to, 70
Gesell Infant Scale, 510
Ghost sickness, 170
Global Assessment of Functioning Scale (GAF), 41, 41t
Global Assessment of Relational Functioning Scale (GARF), 43t
Glutamate, in schizophrenia, 138
Glutethimide (Doriden), 435
Gray Oral Reading Test-Revised (GORT-R), 511
Group psychotherapy
for adolescents, 598
inpatient, 405
mechanisms of, 405
group formation in, 405
therapeutic factors in, 405, 406t
patient selection in, 404
authority anxiety in, 404
diagnosis of, 404
peer anxiety in, 404
preparation in, 404–405
frequency and length of sessions in, 404–405
homogeneous *versus* heterogeneous groups in, 405
open *versus* closed groups in, 405
size of group in, 404
in psychosomatic disorders, 362–363
role of the therapist in, 405
self-help groups and, 405
Group therapy
for children, 591–593
in schizophrenia, 152
in sexual dysfunction, 288
Growth hormone, in depression, 176
Guanfacine (Tenex)
dosage and clinical guidelines for, 427
drug–drug interactions of, 426–427
effects of specific organs and systems of, 425
overdose of, 426
pharmacological actions of, 425
therapeutic indications for, 425–426
in alcohol withdrawal, 425
in benzodiazepine withdrawal, 425
in hyperactivity and aggression in children, 426
in nicotine withdrawal, 425
in opioid withdrawal, 425
in posttraumatic stress disorder, 426
in tic disorders, 426
in Tourette's disorder, 425–426
withdrawal from, 426
Gulf War syndrome, 235–236

H

Halazepam (Paxipam), 435. *See also* Benzodiazepines
Halcyon. *See* Triazolam (Halcyon)
Haldol. *See* Haloperidol (Haldol)
Hallucinations
in dementia, 54
in mental status examination, 7
substance-induced, 168
types of, 31
Hallucinogen-related disorder(s), 107–111. *See also specific hallucinogens*
clinical features of, 110–111
diagnosis of, 108–110, 108t
epidemiology of, 108
neuropharmacology of, 108
not otherwise specified, 110, 110t
treatment of, 111
Hallucinogens
abuse, 108
dependence, 108
intoxication, 108, 109t
treatment of, 111
in sexual dysfunction, 285
Haloperidol (Haldol), 454. *See also* Dopamine receptor antagonists
in delirium, 50
in paranoid personality disorder, 340
in Tourette's disorder, 559
Hamilton Rating Scale for Depression, 189
Headache
cluster, psychological sequelae of, 361
psychological sequelae of, 361–362
selective serotonin reuptake inhibitors in, 479
tension, psychological sequelae of, 361–362
Head banging
sleep-related, 319
in stereotypic movement disorder, 573
Head injury
amnestic disorder and, 61
mental disorders due to, 67–68, 68t
Head trauma, mental retardation and, 516
Hearing impairment, severe, autism and, 538
Hemolysis, sleep-related, 321
Hepatic dysfunction, serotonin-dopamine antagonists and, 485
Hepatitis, carbamazepine in, 446
Heroin, withdrawal from, 120
History, psychiatric, 1–6, 2t
chief complaint in, 1–2
family history in, 3
identifying data in, 1
past illness in, 2–3
personal history in, 3–6
adulthood, 4–5
early childhood, 3
fantasies and dreams in, 6
late childhood, 4
middle childhood, 3–4
prenatal and perinatal, 3
sexual history, 5–6
values in, 6
present illness in, 2
in psychiatric report, 11–12
Homicide, in schizophrenia, 148
Homosexuality, 277
Hormones, in personality disorders, 336–337
Hormone therapy
in gender identity disorder, 300–301
in sexual dysfunction, 289
Hospice care, 606–607

Hostility, psychological sequelae of, 358
Human immunodeficiency virus (HIV)
confidentiality and, 74
counseling and, 73–74
diagnosis of, 73
psychiatric syndromes associated with, 74–75
transmission of, 73, 74t
treatment of, 75–76
Huntington's disease, 52
Hwa-byung, 170
Hydroxyzine hydrochloride (Atarax), 431. *See also* Antihistamines
Hydroxyzine pamoate (Vistaril), 431. *See also* Antihistamines
Hyperactivity in children, treatment of, 426
Hyperemesis gravidarum, 365
Hyperhidrosis, psychological sequelae of, 360
Hyperprolactinemia, serotonin-dopamine antagonists and, 485
Hypersomnia
major symptoms of, 312
primary, 313, 313t
related to other mental disorder, 320, 320t
Hypertension
crisis, tyramine-induced, 465–466, 465t
psychological sequelae of, 358
Hyperthyroidism, psychological sequelae of, 359
Hyperventilation syndrome, psychological sequelae of, 359
Hypnosis
capacity and induction of, 415
history, 414
hypnotherapy in, 415
neurophysiologic correlates of, 415
in psychosomatic disorders, 363
trance state in, 415
Hypnotherapy, in sexual dysfunction, 287
Hypnotic-related disorders, 125–131, 127t
clinical features of, 129–130
diagnosis of, 127–129, 127t
epidemiology of, 126
legal issues in, 130–131
neuropharmacology of, 126–127
not otherwise specified, 129
treatment of, 130, 434
Hypochondriasis
clinical features of, 253
course and prognosis of, 254
diagnosis of, 253, 253t
differential diagnosis of, 253–254
epidemiology of, 252
etiology of, 252–253
treatment of, 254
Hypomanic episode, 173
diagnosis of, 179t
Hypotension, orthostatic, serotonin-dopamine antagonists and, 485
Hypothalamic-pituitary-adrenal axis, in posttraumatic stress disorder, 233
Hypothyroidism
psychological sequelae of, 359
serotonin-dopamine antagonists and, 485
subclinical, psychological sequelae of, 359
Hypoventilation, central alveolar, 315
Hypoxyphilia, 293

I

ICD-10. *See International Classification of Diseases* (ICD-10)

Identification
  in conversion disorder, 251
  projective, in personality disorders, 338
Identity problem. *See also* Dissociative iden-
       tity disorder
  course and prognosis of, 588
  diagnosis and clinical features of, 587
  differential diagnosis of, 587–588
  epidemiology of, 587
  etiology of, 587
  of gender, 275
  sexual, 275
  treatment of, 588
Illusions, in schizophrenia, 147
Imipramine (Tofranil). *See also* Anticholin-
       ergics
  in posttraumatic stress disorder, 237
  tests for use of, 23
Immune disorders, mental disorders due to, 71
Impotence. *See* Erectile dysfunction
Impulse control
  in depression, 189
  disorders of. *See* Impulse-control disor-
       der(s); *specific disorders*
  in manic episode, 190
  in mental status examination, 9–10
Impulse-control disorder(s)
  classification of, 323
  etiology of, 323–324
    biological factors in, 323–324
    psychodynamic factors in, 323
    psychological factors in, 323
  features of, 323
  not otherwise specified, 331, 331t
  treatment of, carbamazepine in, 445
Incest, 372
  treatment options in, 374
Infectious diseases
  mental disorders due to, 69–70
  mental retardation and, 516
Informed consent, forensic psychiatry and, 612
Inhalant-related disorder(s), 111–114, 112t
  adverse effects of, 113
  clinical features of, 113
  diagnosis of, 112–113, 112t
  epidemiology of, 111, 112t
  neuropharmacology of, 112
  not otherwise specified, 113, 113t
  treatment of, 113–114
Inhalants
  abuse, 112
    in adolescents, 582
  dependence, 112
  intoxication, 112–113
  nitrite, mental disorders related to, 132–133
Insight, 32
  in depressive episode, 189
  in manic episode, 190
  in mental status examination, 10
  in psychiatric evaluation of children, 510
  in psychoanalytic psychotherapy, 399
  in schizophrenia, 148
Insomnia
  fatal familial, mental disorders due
      to, 71
  major symptoms of, 311–312
  primary, 312, 312t
  related to other mental disorder, 319–320,
      320t
  selective serotonin reuptake inhibitors
    and, 481
  treatment of, 437
    trazodone in, 193

Intelligence, 32
  in mental status examination, 9
Intermittent explosive disorder, 324–325
  comorbidity of, 324
  course and prognosis of, 325
  diagnosis and clinical features of, 324, 325t
  differential diagnosis of, 325
  epidemiology of, 324
  etiology of, 324
  physical findings and lab exam of, 324–325
  treatment of, 325
International Classification of Diseases
    (ICD-10), 33
Internet sex, 293
Interpersonal therapy
  in dysthymic disorder, 202
  in mood disorders, 194
Interpretation
  of dreams, in psychoanalysis, 397
  in psychoanalysis, 397
Intersex conditions, 299, 300t
  treatment of, 301
Intoxication
  alcohol, 84–85, 85t
    idiosyncratic, 89
  amphetamine, 94, 94t
  caffeine, 98, 98t
  cannabis, 101
  cocaine, 104–105
    treatment of, 441
  hallucinogen, 108, 109t
    treatment of, 111
  inhalant, 112–113
  opioid, 119t, 120
  phencyclidine, 123–124, 123t
  sedative, hypnotic, or anxiolytic, 127t, 128
In vivo exposure, in panic disorder, 221
Irresistible impulse, criminal responsibility
    and, 614
Isocarboxazid (Marplan), 464. *See also*
    Monoamine oxidase inhibitors
    (MAOIs)
Isolation, in personality disorders, 338
Isradipine (DynaCirc), 443. *See also* Cal-
    cium channel inhibitors
  dosage and clinical guidelines for, 444

J

Jactatio capitis nocturna, 319
Jackson, Donald, 140
Jealousy, delusions of, 160
Judgment, 32
  in depressive episode, 189
  in geriatric patients, 601
  in manic episode, 190
  in mental status examination, 10
  in psychiatric evaluation of children,
    510
  in schizophrenia, 148

K

Kaufman Test of Educational Achievement,
    511
Kava, abuse of, 133
Ketamine, phencyclidine-related disorders
    and, 125
Kevorkian, Jack, 607
Khat, adverse effects of, 96
Kiddie Schedule for Affective Disorders and
    Schizophrenia for School-Age
    Children (K-SADS), 508

Kindling
  in bipolar disorder, 176
  in depression, 176
  in mood disorders, 176
Kleine-Levin syndrome, 317
Kleptomania, 325–327
  comorbidity of, 326
  course and prognosis of, 326
  diagnosis and clinical features of, 326, 326t
  differential diagnosis of, 326
  epidemiology of, 325
  etiology of, 326
  treatment of, 327
Klerman, Gerald, 194
Klismaphilia, 293
Klonopin. *See* Clonazepam (Klonopin)
Koro, 170
Korsakoff's syndrome, 61
Kraepelin, Emil, 134
Kuru, mental disorders due to, 70

L

LAAM. *See* Levomethadyl acetate
    (ORLAAM)
Lamictal. *See* Lamotrigine (Lamictal)
Lamotrigine (Lamictal), 473
  dosage and clinical guidelines for, 476
  drug–drug interactions of, 475
  pharmacological actions of, 474
  precautions and adverse reactions to, 475
  therapeutic indications for, 474
Language
  in geriatric patients, 600
  in psychiatric evaluation of children, 509
Language disorder
  expressive. *See* Expressive language dis-
    order
  mixed receptive-expressive. *See* Mixed
    receptive-expressive language
    disorder
Larodopa. *See* Levodopa (Larodopa)
Latah, 170
Lead poisoning, mental disorders due to, 72
Learned helplessness, depression and,
    178–179
Learning disorders, 521. *See also specific*
    disorders
  not otherwise specified, 525
Learning theory, of conversion disorder, 250
Lesch-Nyhan syndrome, 514
Levodopa (Larodopa), 452. *See also* Dopam-
    ine receptor agonists
Levomethadyl acetate (ORLAAM), 468. *See*
    also Opioid receptor agonists
  dosage and clinical guidelines for, 471
  therapeutic indications for, 469
Lewy body disease, 52
Lexapro. *See* Escitalopram (Lexapro)
Librium. *See* Chlordiazepoxide (Librium)
Lidz, Theodore, 140
Limbic system
  in anxiety, 213
  in schizophrenia, 138
Liothyronine, antidepressants plus, 196–197
Lithium, 458–463
  dosage and clinical guidelines for,
    462–463
    discontinuation and, 463
    initial medical workup in, 462
    patient education in, 463
    serum and plasma concentrations in,
      462–463

Lithium—*continued*
  drug interactions of, 462
  effects of on specific organs and systems, 458–459
  pharmacological actions of, 458
  precautions and adverse effects of, 460–462
    in adolescents, 461
    cardiac effects in, 461
    dermatological effects in, 461
    in elderly patients, 461
    GI symptoms in, 460
    neurological effects in, 460
    during pregnancy, 462
    renal effects in, 460
    thyroid effects in, 21, 22t, 461
    toxicity and overdose in, 461
  tests for use of, 23–24
  therapeutic indications for, 459–460
    in aggressive behavior, 459
    antidepressants plus, 196
    in bipolar I disorder, 197–198, 459
    in depressive episodes, 459
    in manic episodes, 459
    in narcissistic personality disorder, 347
    in postpartum psychosis, 167
    in schizoaffective disorder, 157, 459
    in schizophrenia, 459
    in sexual dysfunction, 285
Lithobid. *See* Lithium
Lithonate. *See* Lithium
Liver function tests, 22
Living wills, 604
Locura, 170
Lorazepam (Ativan), 435. *See also* Benzodiazepines
Lotrel. *See* Amlodipine (Norvasc, Lotrel)
LSD. *See* Lysergic acid diethylamide (LSD)
Lumbar puncture, 25
Luminal. *See* Phenobarbital (Solfoton, Luminal)
Luvox. *See* Fluvoxamine (Luvox)
Lysergic acid diethylamide (LSD), 107–108
  in adolescents, 582

M

Magnetic resonance imaging (MRI), in schizophrenia, 138
Magnetic resonance spectroscopy, in schizophrenia, 138
Major depressive disorder
  alcohol dependence and, 82, 188
  with atypical features, 184, 185t
  in children, 576
  chronic, 186, 186t
  classification of, 173–174
  clinical features of, 187–188
  coexisting disorders and, 188
  course of, 191–192
  diagnosis of, 178t, 179–180, 180t
  differential diagnosis of, 190–191
    pseudodementia and, 190–191
    uncomplicated bereavement and, 190–191
  epidemiology of
    age and, 174
    incidence and prevalence and, 174, 174t
    marital status and, 174
    sex and, 173
    socioeconomic and cultural factors and, 174
  etiology of, 174–179
    biological factors in, 174–176

      biogenic amines and, 174–175
      brain imaging in, 176
      circadian rhythms in, 176
      kindling in, 176
      neuroanatomical considerations in, 176
      neurochemical factors in, 175
      neuroendocrine regulation in, 175–176
      neuroimmune regulation in, 176
      sleep abnormalities in, 176
    genetic factors in, 176–177
      adoption studies and, 177
      family studies and, 177
      linkage studies and, 177
      twin studies and, 177
    psychosocial factors in, 177–178
      life events and environmental stress in, 177
      personality factors in, 177
      psychodynamic factors in, 177–178
  medical illness and, 191
  with melancholic features, 184, 184t
  mental disorders and, 191
  with postpartum onset, 186, 186t
  prognosis of, 192
  with psychotic features, 180t, 182
  with rapid cycling, 186, 186t
  recurrent, diagnosis of, 180, 182t
  schizophrenia and, 191
  with seasonal pattern, 186–187, 187t
  single episode, diagnosis of, 179–180, 181t
  specifiers for, 186–187, 186t, 187t
  treatment of, 195–197
    behavior therapy in, 194
    cognitive therapy in, 194
    electroconvulsive therapy in, 195, 500
    family therapy in, 194–195
    hospitalization in, 193–194
    interpersonal therapy in, 194
    lithium in, 459
    pharmacotherapy in, 195–199, 197f
    phototherapy in, 195
    psychoanalytically oriented therapy in, 194
    psychosocial therapy in, 194–195
    tricyclic antidepressants in, 494
  uncomplicated bereavement and, 191
Mal de ojo, 170
Malingering, 379–380
  diagnosis and clinical features of, 379
  differential diagnosis of, 379
  epidemiology of, 379
  vs. factitious disorder, 264
  schizophrenia and, 149
  treatment of, 379–380
Malpractice, 609–610
Manganese poisoning, mental disorders due to, 72
Mania. *See also* Bipolar disorder(s)
  in adolescents, 188
  HIV-associated, 75
  nefazodone in, 467–468
  psychodynamic factors in, 178
Manic episode, 173. *See also* Bipolar disorder(s)
  clinical features of, 188
  diagnosis of, 179t, 181, 182t
  treatment of, 445, 459
    electroconvulsive therapy in, 500
MAOIs. *See* Monoamine oxidase inhibitors (MAOIs)

Marijuana
  abuse, in adolescents, 582
  medical use of, 102
Marplan. *See* Isocarboxazid (Marplan)
Marriage, unconsummated, 294
Masturbation, 276–277, 293
  pain during, 286
Mathematics disorder, 523–524
  clinical features of, 523
  comorbidity of, 523
  course and prognosis of, 523
  diagnosis of, 523
  differential diagnosis of, 523–524
  epidemiology of, 523
  etiology of, 523
  pathology and lab exam of, 523
  treatment of, 524
Medical condition, psychological factors affecting
  classification of, 355, 356t
  stress theory and, 355–356
Melatonin, 505–506
Mellaril. *See* Thioridazine (Mellaril)
Memantine, 450
Memory, 32
  in depressive episode, 189
  in geriatric patients, 601
  loss of, in electroconvulsive therapy, 504
  in mental status examination, 8–9
  in psychiatric evaluation of children, 510
  recovered, 274
  in schizophrenia, 148
Meningitis, chronic, mental disorders due to, 69
Menninger, Karl, on suicide, 392
Mens rea, 614
Menstrual-associated syndrome, 317
Mental disorder, due to general medical condition, 65, 66t
Mental retardation, 32
  autism and, 538
  classification of, 512, 513t
  clinical features in, 519
  comorbidity of, 512–513
    genetic syndromes and, 513
    neurological disorders and, 512–513
    prevalence of, 512
    psychosocial syndromes and, 513
  course and prognosis of, 520
  diagnosis in, 516–519, 517t
    history in, 517
    neurological examination in, 519
    physical examination in, 517–519, 517t–518t
    psychiatric interview in, 517
  differential diagnosis of, 520
  epidemiology of, 512
  etiology of, 513–516
    acquired and developmental factors in, 514–516
    environmental and sociocultural factors in, 516
    enzyme deficiency disorders and, 514, 515t–516t
    genetic factors in, 513–514
  lab exam in, 519–520
    chromosome studies in, 519
    psychological assessment in, 519–520
    urine and blood analysis in, 519
  treatment of, 520
Mental status examination, 6–10, 6t
  of children, 509–510
  general description in, 6
  of geriatric patients, 600–601

impulsivity in, 9–10
judgment and insight in, 10
in manic episodes, 189–190
mood and affect in, 7
in mood disorders, 188–190
in obsessive-compulsive disorder, 230
perception in, 7
in psychiatric report, 12–14
reliability in, 10
in schizophrenia, 146–148
sensorium and cognition in, 8–9
speech characteristics in, 7
thought content and mental trends in, 7–8
Mental stress, acute, psychological sequelae
     of, 358
Meperidine, withdrawal from, 120
Meprobamate, 435
Mercury poisoning, mental disorders due to, 72
Mesmer, Friedrich, 414
Metabolic disorders, mental disorders due to,
     71–72
Methadone (Dolophine), 468. *See also* Opi-
     oid receptor agonists
   dosage and clinical guidelines for, 470–471
   during pregnancy, 469
   therapeutic indications for, 469
   withdrawal from, 120, 121
Methamphetamine (Desoxyn), 488. *See also*
     Sympathomimetics
   amphetamine-related disorders and, 93
Methohexital (Brevital), in electroconvulsive
     therapy, 433
Methylphenidate (Ritalin, Concerta), 488.
     See also Sympathomimetics
   in attention-deficit/hyperactivity disorder,
     546–547
Milieu therapy, 417
   token economy in, 417
Miller, Neal, 409
Minnesota Multiphasic Personality Inven-
     tory (MMPI), 145
Minor depressive disorder, 204–206
   course and prognosis of, 205–206
   diagnosis and clinical features of, 205, 205t
   differential diagnosis of, 205
   vs. dysthymic disorder, 201
   epidemiology of, 204–205
   etiology of, 205
   treatment of, 206
Mirapex. *See* Pramipexole (Mirapex)
Mirtazapine (Remeron), 463–464
   dosage and administration of, 464
   drug interactions of, 464
   effects of on specific organs and systems,
     463
   pharmacological actions of, 463
   precautions and adverse reactions to,
     463–464
   therapeutic indications for, 463
     in major depressive disorder, 195
Mitral valve prolapse, panic disorder and, 215
Mixed anxiety-depressive disorder, 244–246
   clinical features of, 245
   course and prognosis of, 246
   diagnosis of, 245, 245t
   differential diagnosis of, 245
   epidemiology of, 245
   etiology of, 245
   treatment of, 246
     benzodiazepines in, 436–437
Mixed receptive-expressive language disor-
     der, 529
   clinical features of, 530
   course and prognosis of, 530

diagnosis of, 530, 530t
differential diagnosis of, 530
epidemiology of, 530
etiology of, 530
treatment of, 531
M'Naghten rule, criminal responsibility and,
     613–614
Modafinil (Provigil), 490–492. *See also*
     Sympathomimetics
   dosage and administration of, 492
   drug–drug interactions of, 491–492
   effects of on specific organs and systems,
     491
   pharmacological actions of, 490–491
   precautions and adverse effects of, 491
   therapeutic indications for, 491
Monoamine oxidase, platelet, in personality
     disorders, 337
Monoamine oxidase inhibitors (MAOIs),
     464–466
   dosage and clinical guidelines for, 466, 466t
   drug interactions of, 466
   effects of on specific organs and systems,
     464–465
   laboratory interferences of, 466
   pharmacological actions of, 464
   precautions and adverse reactions to,
     465–466
   tests for use of, 23
   therapeutic indications for, 465
     antidepressants plus, 197, 197f
     in major depressive disorder, 195
     in panic disorders, 220
     in posttraumatic stress disorder, 238
   tricyclic antidepressants and, 497
Mood, 27
   in dementia, 54
   in depressive episode, 189
   in geriatric patients, 600
   in manic episode, 189–190
   in mental status examination, 7
   in psychiatric evaluation of children, 509
   in schizophrenia, 146–147
Mood disorder(s). *See also* Bipolar I disor-
     der; Bipolar II disorder; Depres-
     sion; Major depressive disorder
   alcohol-induced, 88
   alcohol-related disorders and, 81, 188
   amphetamine-induced, 95
   anxiety and, 188
   with atypical features, 184, 185t
   with catatonic features, 185–186, 186t
   in children
     course and prognosis of, 577
     diagnosis and clinical features of,
       576–577
     differential diagnosis of, 577
     epidemiology of, 575
     etiology of, 575–576
       biological factors in, 575–576
       genetic factors in, 575
       social factors in, 575–576
     pathology and lab exam of, 577
     treatment of, 577–578
   chronic, 186, 186t
   classification of, 173–174
   clinical features of, 187–188
   cocaine-induced, 105–106
   course and prognosis of, 191–193
   diagnosis of, 178t, 179–187, 179t, 180t,
       181t
   differential diagnosis of, 190–191
   due to general medical condition, 62–63
     course and prognosis of, 63

diagnosis and clinical features of, 63
differential diagnosis of, 63
epidemiology of, 62
etiology of, 63, 63t
treatment of, 63
   tricyclic antidepressants in, 494
epidemiology of
   age and, 174
   incidence and prevalence and, 174,
       174t
   marital status and, 174
   sex and, 173
   socioeconomic and cultural factors
       and, 174
etiology of, 174–179
   biological factors in, 174–176
     biogenic amines and, 174–175
     brain imaging in, 176
     circadian rhythms in, 176
     kindling in, 176
     neuroanatomical considerations in,
       176
     neurochemical factors in, 175
     neuroendocrine regulation in,
       175–176
     neuroimmune regulation in, 176
     sleep abnormalities in, 176
   genetic factors in, 176–177
     adoption studies and, 177
     family studies and, 177
     linkage studies and, 177
     twin studies and, 177
   psychosocial factors in, 177–178
     life events and environmental stress
       in, 177
     personality factors in, 177
     psychodynamic factors in, 177–178
hallucinogen-induced, 110
incidence and prevalence of, 174, 174t
inhalant-induced, 113
longitudinal course specifiers in, 187, 187t
with melancholic features, 184, 184t
mental status examination in, 188–190
not otherwise specified, 210, 210t
opioid-induced, 120
phencyclidine-induced, 123, 123t
postpartum onset, 186, 186t
with psychotic features, 180t, 182
rapid cycling in, 186, 186t
recent episodes in, 186–187, 186t, 187t
schizophrenia and, 149
seasonal pattern in, 186–187, 187t
secondary, 209–210
substance-induced, 209–210
   course and prognosis of, 210
   diagnosis and clinical features of, 209t,
       210
   differential diagnosis of, 210
   epidemiology of, 210
   etiology of, 210
   treatment of, 210
treatment of, 193–199
   hospitalization in, 193–194
   pharmacotherapy in, 195–199, 197f
   psychosocial therapy in, 194–195
   serotonin-dopamine antagonists in, 484
Morning glory seeds, abuse of, 133
Morphine, withdrawal from, 120
Motor behavior, 27–28
   in psychiatric evaluation of children, 510
Motor impairment, serotonin-dopamine
     antagonists and, 485
Motor skills disorder, 526. *See also* Develop-
     mental coordination disorder

Movement disorder(s)
  medication-induced, 422–423. *See also specific disorders*
    not otherwise specified, 425
    treatment of, 453
  stereotypic
    course and prognosis of, 573–574
    diagnosis and clinical features of, 573, 573t
    differential diagnosis of, 573
    epidemiology of, 572–573
    etiology of, 573
    treatment of, 574
Multiple E4 genes, in dementia of Alzheimer's type, 51
Multiple sclerosis, mental disorders due to, 69
Münchausen syndrome, 261. *See also* Factitious disorder
Mutism, selective
  course and prognosis of, 570
  diagnosis and clinical features of, 569–570, 570t
  differential diagnosis of, 570
  epidemiology of, 569
  etiology of, 569
  treatment of, 570
Myalgic encephalomyelitis. *See* Chronic fatigue syndrome
Myoclonus, nocturnal, 316

N

Nail biting, in stereotypic movement disorder, 573
Nalmefene (Revex), 471. *See also* Opioid receptor antagonists
Naltrexone (ReVia), 471. *See also* Opioid receptor antagonists
Narcoanalysis, barbiturates in, 433
Narcolepsy, 313–314, 313t
  sympathomimetics in, 489
Nardil. *See* Phenelzine (Nardil)
National Alliance for the Mentally Ill, 152
Necrophilia, 293
Nefazodone (Serzone), 467–468
  dosage and clinical guidelines for, 468
  drug interactions of, 468
  effects of on specific organs and systems, 467
  pharmacological actions of, 467
  precautions and adverse reactions to, 467–468
  therapeutic indications for, 467
    in major depressive disorder, 195
Nervios, 170
Neurasthenia, 260
Neurocognitive disorder, mild, HIV-associated, 74
Neuroendocrine tests, 21–22
Neuroimmunology, in obsessive-compulsive disorder, 228
Neuroleptic malignant syndrome, 423
  serotonin-dopamine antagonists and, 485
Neurontin. *See* Gabapentin (Neurontin)
Neuropeptides, in schizophrenia, 138
Neurosyphilis, mental disorders due to, 69
Neurotransmitters
  in anxiety, 212
  in dementia of Alzheimer's type, 51–52
  endocrine therapies and, 505–506
  in obsessive-compulsive disorder, 228
  in personality disorders, 337

in stress theory, 356–357
in substance-related disorders, 79
Niacin deficiency, mental disorders due to, 72
Nicardipine (Cardene), 443. *See also* Calcium channel inhibitors
Nicotine
  dependence, 115
  replacement therapies, 116–117
Nicotine-related disorders, 114–117, 115t
  adverse effects of, 116
  clinical features of, 116
  diagnosis of, 115–116, 115t
  epidemiology of, 114–115
    death and, 114–115
    education and, 114
    psychiatric patients and, 114
  neuropharmacology of, 115
  not otherwise specified, 115–116, 116t
  treatment of, 116–117, 116t
    psychopharmacological therapies in, 116–117
    psychosocial therapies in, 116
Nifedipine (Procardia, Adalat), 443. *See also* Calcium channel inhibitors
  dosage and clinical guidelines for, 444
Nightmare disorder, 317, 317t
Nightmares, selective serotonin reuptake inhibitors and, 481
Nimodipine (Nimotop), 443. *See also* Calcium channel inhibitors
  dosage and clinical guidelines for, 444
Nimotop. *See* Nimodipine (Nimotop)
Nisoldipine (Sular), 443. *See also* Calcium channel inhibitors
Nitrous oxide, mental disorders related to, 133
Noncompliance with treatment, 380
Noradrenergic system
  in obsessive-compulsive disorder, 228
  in posttraumatic stress disorder, 233
Norepinephrine
  in anxiety, 212
  in mood disorders, 175
  in schizophrenia, 137
Norpramin. *See* Desipramine (Norpramin)
Nortriptyline (Pamelor), tests for use of, 23
Norvasc. *See* Amlodipine (Norvasc, Lotrel)
Nutmeg, abuse of, 133
Nutritional disorders, mental disorders due to, 72

O

Obesity
  selective serotonin reuptake inhibitors in, 479
  sympathomimetics in, 489
Obsessive-compulsive disorder (OCD)
  brain-imaging studies in, 228
  clinical features of, 229–230
    mental status examination in, 230
    symptom patterns in, 229–230
  comorbidity of, 227–228
  course and prognosis of, 231
  diagnosis of, 229, 229t
  differential diagnosis of, 230–231
  epidemiology of, 227
  etiology of, 228–229
    behavioral factors in, 228
    biological factors in, 228
    psychosocial factors in, 228–229
  serotonin-dopamine antagonists and, 485

vs. Tourette's disorder, 230
treatment of, 231–232, 437
  behavior therapy in, 232
  pharmacologic, 231
  psychotherapy in, 232
  selective serotonin reuptake inhibitors in, 478
  tricyclic antidepressants in, 494
Obstructive sleep apnea syndrome, 314–315
Occupational problem, 377–378
  career choices and changes in, 377–378
  vocational rehabilitation and, 378
OCD. *See* Obsessive-compulsive disorder (OCD)
Olanzapine (Zyprexa), 483. *See also* Serotonin-dopamine antagonists (SDAs)
  adverse effects of, 484
  dosage and clinical guidelines for, 487
  in early-onset schizophrenia, 581
  pharmacological actions of, 483
  in Tourette's disorder, 559
Olfactory reference syndrome, 161
Opioid receptor agonists, 468
  dosage and clinical guidelines for, 470–471
  drug–drug interactions of, 470
  effects of on specific organs and systems, 468–469
  overdose of, 470
  pharmacological actions of, 468
  precautions and adverse reactions to, 469–470
  therapeutic indications for, 469
Opioid receptor antagonists, 471–473
  alcohol dependence and, 472
  dosage and clinical guidelines for, 473
  drug–drug interactions of, 473
  opioid dependence and, 471–472
  pharmacological actions of, 471
  precautions and adverse reactions to, 472–473
  therapeutic indications for, 471–472
Opioid-related disorder(s), 117–122, 119t
  adverse effects of, 121
  clinical features of, 121
  comorbidity of, 118
  diagnosis of, 119–120, 119t
  epidemiology of, 117–118
  etiology of, 118–119
    biological and genetic factors in, 118–119
    psychodynamic theory in, 119
    psychosocial factors in, 118
  neuropharmacology of, 118
    tolerance and dependence in, 118
  not otherwise specified, 120, 120t
  overdose and, 121
  treatment and rehabilitation of, 121–122
    education and needle-exchange programs in, 122
    opioid antagonists in, 122
    psychotherapy in, 122
    self-help in, 122
    therapeutic communities in, 122
Opioids
  abuse, 120
    opioid receptor antagonists and, 471–472
  dependence, 120
    in pregnancy, 122
  intoxication, 119t, 120
  in sexual dysfunction, 285

withdrawal, 119t, 120
  clonidine in, 425
  guanfacine in, 425
  neonatal, 122
Opioid system, in posttraumatic stress disorder, 233
Oppositional defiant disorder
  course and prognosis of, 549
  diagnosis and clinical features of, 548–549, 549t
  differential diagnosis of, 549
  epidemiology of, 548
  etiology of, 548
  treatment of, 549
Orap. See Pimozide (Orap)
Orgasm disorders, 280–282
  female, 280, 280t
    premature orgasm in, 286
  male, 280–281
    premature ejaculation in, 281–282, 282t
Orientation
  in depressive episode, 189
  in geriatric patients, 601
  in mental status examination, 8
  in psychiatric evaluation of children, 509
ORLAAM. See Levomethadyl acetate (ORLAAM)
Orne, Martin, 414
Orphenadrine, 430. See also Anticholinergics
Othello syndrome, 160
Overdose, 422
  amantadine, 430
  antihistamine, 432
  barbiturate, 129
  barbiturate-like substance, 130
  benzodiazepine, 129
    flumazenil in, 438
  carbamazepine, 445
  clonidine, 426
  dopamine receptor antagonist, 453
  fluoxetine, 477
  guanfacine, 426
  haloperidol, 456
  lithium, 461
  opioid, 121
  opioid receptor agonist, 470
  tetracyclic antidepressant, 496–497
  thioridazine, 454
  tricyclic antidepressant, 496–497
  valproate, 498
Oxazepam (Serax), 435. See also Benzodiazepines

P

Pain, chronic
  anticonvulsants in, 474
  selective serotonin reuptake inhibitors in, 479
Pain control programs, in pain disorder, 258
Pain disorder(s)
  clinical features of, 256–257
  course and prognosis of, 257
  diagnosis of, 256, 256t
  differential diagnosis of, 257
  epidemiology of, 255–256
  etiology of, 256
  sexual, 282
  treatment of, 257–258
    selective serotonin reuptake inhibitors in, 479
    tricyclic antidepressants in, 494
Palliative care, 604–605

Pamelor. See Nortriptyline (Pamelor)
Panencephalitis, subacute sclerosing, mental disorders due to, 69
Panic attack, 214. See also Panic disorder(s)
  diagnosis of, 216, 216t
  epidemiology of, 214
  provocation with sodium lactate, 24
  psychoanalytic theories of, 215–216, 216t
Panic disorder(s)
  with agoraphobia, tricyclic antidepressants in, 494
  clinical features of, 217–218
  comorbidity of, 214
  course and prognosis if, 219
  diagnosis of, 216–217, 216t, 217t
  differential diagnosis of, 218–219, 218t
    medical disorders in, 218–219
    mental disorders in, 219
  epidemiology of, 214
  etiology of, 214–216
    biological factors in, 214–215
    genetic factors in, 215
    psychosocial factors in, 215–216
  panic-inducing substances in, 214–215
  treatment of, 220–221, 436–437
    benzodiazepines in, 437
    calcium channel inhibitors in, 443
    cognitive and behavioral therapies in, 221
    pharmacotherapy in, 220–221
    selective serotonin reuptake inhibitors in, 478
Paradoxical conduct, in delusional disorders, 160–161
Paradoxical therapy, 408
Paraldehyde (Paral), 435
Paranoia, conjugal, 160
Paranoid pseudocommunity, 159
Paraphilia
  course and prognosis of, 293
  diagnosis and clinical features of, 291–293, 291t
  differential diagnosis of, 293
  epidemiology, 290
  etiology of, 290–291
    biological factors in, 291
    psychosocial factors in, 290–291
  not otherwise specified, 292–293, 293t
  treatment of, 294
    selective serotonin reuptake inhibitors in, 479
Parasomnia, 317–319, 317t, 318t
  major symptoms of, 312
  not otherwise specified, 319, 319t
Parathyroid disorders, mental disorders due to, 71
Parkinsonism
  MTPT-induced, 121
  neuroleptic-induced, 423
    treatment of, 430, 431–432
Parkinson's disease, 52
  treatment of, 437
Parlodel. See Bromocriptine (Parlodel)
Parnate. See Tranylcypromine (Parnate)
Paroxetine (Paxil), 476. See also Selective serotonin reuptake inhibitors (SSRIs)
  dosage and clinical guidelines for, 482
  in panic disorder, 220
Paroxysmal hemicranial, chronic, 321
Partialism, 293
Passive aggression, in personality disorders, 338

Paxil. See Paroxetine (Paxil)
Paxipam. See Halazepam (Paxipam)
PCP. See Phencyclidine (PCP)
Pedophilia, 291–292, 292t
Pemoline (Cylert), 488. See also Sympathomimetics
Penal Code, criminal responsibility and, 614
Peptic ulcer disease, psychological sequelae of, 357
Perception, 31
  disturbances of, 31
    associated with cognitive disorder, 31
    associated with conversion and dissociative disorders, 31–32
    in brain tumor, 67
    in depressive episode, 189
    in manic episode, 190
  in mental status examination, 7
Perception disorder, hallucinogen persisting, 109, 109t
  treatment of, 111
Pergolide (Permax), 452. See also Dopamine receptor agonists
Periactin. See Cyproheptadine (Periactin)
Permax. See Pergolide (Permax)
Personality
  change in, due to general medical condition, 66, 66t, 353–354
    course and prognosis of, 354
    diagnosis and clinical features of, 353–354
    differential diagnosis of, 354
    etiology of, 353
    treatment of, 354
  in dementia, 53–54
Personality disorder(s)
  acting out in, 338
  antisocial, 342–343
    alcohol-related disorders and, 81
    clinical features of, 342–343
    course and prognosis of, 344
    diagnosis of, 342
    differential diagnosis of, 343–344
    epidemiology of, 342
    treatment of, 344
  avoidant, 347–348
    clinical features of, 348
    course and prognosis of, 348
    diagnosis of, 348, 348t
    differential diagnosis of, 348
    epidemiology of, 347–348
    treatment of, 348
  borderline, 344–345
    clinical features of, 344–345
    course and prognosis of, 345
    diagnosis of, 344, 344t
    differential diagnosis of, 345
    epidemiology of, 344
    treatment of, 345
  classification of, 336, 337t
  defense mechanisms in, 337–338
  dependent, 348–350
    clinical features of, 349
    course and prognosis of, 349
    diagnosis of, 349, 349t
    differential diagnosis of, 349
    epidemiology of, 349
    treatment of, 349–350
  depressive, 352–353
    course and prognosis of, 352
    diagnosis and clinical features of, 352, 353t
    differential diagnosis of, 352

Personality disorder(s)—*continued*
  epidemiology of, 352
  etiology of, 352
  treatment of, 353
 dissociation in, 338
 electrophysiology in, 337
 etiology of, 336–338
  biological factors in, 336–337
  cluster A, 336
  cluster B, 336
  cluster C, 336
  genetic factors in, 336
  psychoanalytic factors in, 337–338
 vs. factitious disorder, 264
 fantasy in, 338
 histrionic, 345–346
  clinical features of, 346
  course and prognosis of, 346
  diagnosis of, 346, 346t
  differential diagnosis of, 346
  epidemiology of, 346
  treatment of, 346
 hormones in, 336–337
 isolation in, 338
 narcissistic, 346–347
  clinical features of, 347
  course and prognosis of, 347
  diagnosis of, 347, 347t
  differential diagnosis of, 347
  epidemiology of, 347
  treatment of, 347
 neurotransmitters in, 337
 not otherwise specified, 351, 351t
 obsessive-compulsive, 350–351. *See also*
    Obsessive-compulsive disorder
    (OCD)
  clinical features of, 350
  course and prognosis of, 350–351
  diagnosis of, 350, 350t
  differential diagnosis of, 350
  epidemiology of, 350
  treatment of, 351
 paranoid, 338–340
  clinical features of, 339
  course and prognosis of, 339
  diagnosis of, 339, 339t
  differential diagnosis of, 339
  epidemiology of, 339
  treatment of, 339–340
 passive aggression in, 338
 passive-aggressive, 351–352
  clinical features of, 351–352
  course and prognosis of, 352
  diagnosis of, 351, 351t
  differential diagnosis of, 352
  epidemiology of, 351
  treatment of, 352
 platelet monoamine oxidase in, 337
 projection in, 338
 projective identification in, 337
 sadistic, 353
 sadomasochistic, 353
 schizoid, 340–341
  clinical features of, 340
  course and prognosis of, 341
  diagnosis of, 340, 340t
  differential diagnosis of, 341
  epidemiology of, 340
  treatment of, 341
 schizophrenia and, 149
 schizotypal, 341–342
  clinical features of, 341–342
  course and prognosis of, 342
  diagnosis of, 341, 341t

  differential diagnosis of, 342
  epidemiology of, 341
  treatment of, 342
 smooth pursuit eye movements in, 337
 splitting in, 338
 suicide risk in, 392
Pervasive developmental disorders, 535. *See
    also specific disorders*
 not otherwise specified, 542–543, 542t
Pharmacogenetics, culture and, 171
Pharmacotherapy. *See also* Psychopharma-
    cology; *specific drugs*
 in adjustment disorders, 334–335
 in anorexia nervosa, 305
 in antisocial personality disorder, 344
 in attention-deficit/hyperactivity disorder,
    546–547
 in avoidant personality disorder, 348
 in bipolar I disorder, 197–199
 in bipolar II disorder, 199
 in borderline personality disorder, 345
 in brief psychotic disorder, 165
 in bulimia nervosa, 307–308
 for children, 595, 596t–597t
 in delirium, 50
 in delusional disorder, 163–164
 for dementia, 58
 in dependent personality disorder, 350
 in dysthymic disorder, 202
 in early-onset schizophrenia, 581
 in enuresis, 565
 in generalized anxiety disorder, 241
 in histrionic personality disorder, 346
 for HIV/AIDS, 75
 in major depressive disorder, 195–199, 197f
 in mood disorders, 195–199, 197f
  in children, 578
 in narcissistic personality disorder, 347
 in obsessive-compulsive disorder, 231
 in obsessive-compulsive personality dis-
    order, 351
 in pain disorder, 257
 in panic disorders, 220–221
 in paranoid personality disorder, 340
 in posttraumatic stress disorder, 237–238
 in psychiatric emergencies, 383
 in schizoid personality disorder, 341
 in schizophrenia, 150–151
 in schizotypal personality disorder, 342
 in sex addiction, 295–296
 in sexual therapy, 288–289
 in Tourette's disorder, 559
Phase of life problem, 380
Phencyclidine (PCP), 122
 abuse, 123
 dependence, 123
 intoxication, 123–124, 123t
Phencyclidine-related disorder(s), 122–125,
    123t
 clinical features of, 124–125
 diagnosis of, 123–124, 123t
 differential diagnosis of, 125
 epidemiology of, 122–123
 neuropharmacology of, 123
 not otherwise specified, 124, 124t
 treatment and rehabilitation for, 125
Phenelzine (Nardil), 464. *See also* Monoam-
    ine oxidase inhibitors (MAOIs)
Phenergan. *See* Promethazine (Phenergan)
Phenobarbital (Solfoton, Luminal), in sei-
    zures, 433
Phenylketonuria, 514
Phobia
 defined, 221

etiology of
 behavioral factors in, 222
 general principles of, 222–223
 psychoanalytic factors in factors in,
    222–223
 social, 221–222
  clinical features of, 225
  comorbidity of, 222
  course and prognosis of, 226
  diagnosis of, 224–225, 224t
  differential diagnosis of, 225–226
  epidemiology of, 222
  etiology of, 222, 223
  treatment of, 226–227, 437
   β-adrenergic receptor antagonists in,
    427
   selective serotonin reuptake inhibi-
    tors in, 478
 specific, 221–222
  clinical features of, 225
  comorbidity of, 222
  course and prognosis of, 226
  diagnosis of, 223–224, 224t
  differential diagnosis of, 225–226
  epidemiology of, 222
  etiology of, 222, 223
  treatment of, 226–227
Phobic neurosis, 222
Phonological disorder
 clinical features of, 531–532
 course and prognosis of, 532
 diagnosis of, 531, 531t
 differential diagnosis of, 532
 epidemiology of, 531
 etiology of, 531
 treatment of, 532
Phototherapy, 505
 in major depressive disorder, 195
Physical abuse
 of adult, 374–375
 of child. *See* Child abuse and neglect
Physical appearance, in psychiatric evalua-
    tion of children, 509
Physical examination
 general observation in, 17–18
  hearing in, 18
  smell in, 18
  vision in, 17–18
 history of medical illness in, 15
 intercurrent illnesses and, 20
 neurological examination in, 19
 patient selection in, 18
 psychological factors in, 18–19
 review of systems in, 15–17
  cardiovascular system in, 16–17
  eye, ear, nose, and throat in, 16
  gastrointestinal system in, 17
  genitourinary system in, 17
  head in, 15–16, 16t
  menstrual history in, 17
  respiratory system in, 16
 timing of, 19
Piblokto, 170–171
Pica, 365–366
 course and prognosis of, 554
 diagnosis and clinical features of, 553,
    554t
 differential diagnosis of, 554
 epidemiology of, 553
 etiology of, 553
 pathology and lab exam of, 553–554
 treatment of, 554
Pick's disease, 52
Pimozide (Orap), in Tourette's disorder, 559

Pindolol, in antidepressant augmentation, 428

Pituitary disorders, mental disorders due to, 71

Placebos, 506

Plastic surgery, body dysmorphic disorder and, 255

Platelet function, selective serotonin reuptake inhibitors and, 481

Polysubstance abuse, 133, 133t

Porphyria, acute intermittent, mental disorders due to, 72

Positive reinforcement, 412

Positron emission tomography (PET), in schizophrenia, 138–139

Postcoital headache, 286

Postpartum depression, selective serotonin reuptake inhibitors in, 477–478

Postpartum psychosis. *See* Psychosis, postpartum

Postpsychotic depressive disorder of schizophrenia, 208–210
  diagnosis and differential diagnosis of, 208, 208t
  epidemiology of, 208
  prognostic significance of, 208
  treatment of, 209

Posttraumatic stress disorder
  vs. adjustment disorder, 334
  clinical features of, 234–237
    brainwashing and, 236
    in children and adolescents, 235
    Gulf War syndrome in, 235–236
    terrorism and, 236–237
    torture and, 236
  comorbidity of, 232–233
  course and prognosis of, 237
  diagnosis of, 234, 234t
  differential diagnosis of, 237
  epidemiology of, 232
  etiology of, 233
    biological factors in, 233–234
    cognitive-behavioral factors in, 233
    psychodynamic factors in, 233
    risk factors in, 233
    stressors in, 233
  treatment of, 237–238, 426, 437, 445
    catecholamines in, 22
    selective serotonin reuptake inhibitors in, 478
    tricyclic drugs in, 494

Postural tremor, medication-induced, 425
  β-adrenergic receptor antagonists in, 427
  from lithium, 460

Prader-Willi syndrome, 514

Pramipexole (Mirapex), 452. *See also* Dopamine receptor agonists

Prazepam (Centrax), 435. *See also* Benzodiazepines

Precox feeling, in schizophrenia, 146

Pregabalin, pharmacological actions of, 474

Pregnancy
  complications in, mental retardation and, 516
  dopamine receptor antagonists during, 457
  lithium during, 462
  methadone during, 469
  opioid dependence in, 122
  psychology of, 364–366
    grief reactions and, 366
    hyperemesis gravidarum and, 365
    maternal-fetal attachment and, 364
    parturition and, 364
    perinatal death and, 366

pica and, 365–366
    postpartum depression and psychosis in, 364–365, 365t
    pseudocyesis and, 365
  psychotherapeutic drug use during, 421
  selective serotonin reuptake inhibitors in, 477–478
  serotonin-dopamine antagonists during, 485
  tricyclic antidepressants and, 495

Premature ejaculation, 281–282, 282t
  selective serotonin reuptake inhibitors in, 479

Premenstrual dysphoric disorder
  course and prognosis of, 207
  diagnosis and clinical features of, 207, 207t
  differential diagnosis of, 207
  epidemiology of, 207
  etiology of, 207
  treatment of, 207
    selective serotonin reuptake inhibitors in, 479

Prenatal drug exposure, mental retardation and, 516

Prevention, in mental retardation, 520

Priapism, serotonin-dopamine antagonists and, 485

Primary gain, in conversion disorder, 251

Prion disease, mental disorders due to, 69–70

Procardia. *See* Nifedipine (Procardia, Adalat)

Procyclidine, 430. *See also* Anticholinergics

Projection, in personality disorders, 338

Prolactin, in depression, 176

Prolixin, Fluphenazine (Prolixin)

Promethazine (Phenergan), 431. *See also* Antihistamines

Propranol (Inderal). *See also* β-adrenergic receptor antagonists
  dosage and clinical guidelines for, 428–429
  drug–drug interactions of, 428–429
  precautions and adverse reactions to, 428
  therapeutic indications for, 427–428
    in aggression and violent behavior, 428
    in alcohol abuse, 428
    in anxiety disorders, 427
    in lithium-induced postural tremor, 427
    in social phobia, 427

ProSom. *See* Estazolam (ProSom)

Prostheses, male, in sexual dysfunction, 289

Provigil. *See* Modafinil (Provigil)

Prozac. *See* Fluoxetine (Prozac)

Pruritus vulvae, psychological sequelae of, 360

Pseudocyesis, 365

Pseudodementia, 32
  vs. major depressive disorder, 190–191

Pseudoseizures, in conversion disorder, 251

Psoriasis, psychological sequelae of, 360

Psychiatric report
  comprehensive treatment plan in, 14
  diagnosis in, 14
  further diagnostic studies in, 14
  history in, 11–12
  mental status in, 12–14
  prognosis in, 14
  psychodynamic formulation in, 14
  summary of findings in, 14

Psychiatry, forensic, 609–614
  child custody in, 612
  criminal law and, 613–614
    criminal responsibility and, 613–614

durable power of attorney in, 613
  high-risk clinical situations in, 610–611
    suicidal patients in, 610
    violent patients in, 610–611
  hospitalization in, 611
  medical malpractice and, 609–610
  privilege and confidentiality in, 610
  right to treatment and, 611–612
  seclusion and treatment in, 612
  testament and contractual capacity and competence in, 612–613

Psychoactive drugs, in sexual dysfunction, 284–285

Psychoanalysis, 396–397, 400t
  analytic process in, 397
    countertransference in, 397
    interpretation in, 397
    resistance in, 397
    therapeutic alliance in, 397
    transference in, 397
  analytic setting in, 396
  in anxiety, 211
  contraindications for treatment, 398
  dynamics of therapeutic results in, 398
  goal of, 396
  indications for treatment, 398
  insight-oriented, in dysthymic disorder, 201–202
  in mood disorders, 194
  in panic disorder, 215–216, 215t
  role of the analyst in, 396
  schizophrenia and, 140
  treatment methods of, 396–397
    free association in, 396–397
    free-floating attention in, 397
    rule of abstinence in, 397

Psychodrama, 407

Psycho-oncology, 362

Psychopharmacology. *See also* Pharmacotherapy; *specific drugs*
  adverse effects of, 421–422
  clinical guidelines for, 419–421
    choice of drug in, 420–421
      off-label use and nonapproved dosages in, 420, 420t
      therapeutic failures in, 421
  drug interactions in, 422
  intoxication and overdose in, 422
  pharmacological actions in, 418–419
    metabolism and excretion in, 419
    pharmacodynamics in, 418–419
    pharmacokinetics in, 419
      absorption in, 419
      distribution and bioavailability in, 419
  special treatment considerations in, 421
    in children, 421
    in geriatric patients, 421
    in persons with renal or hepatic insufficiency, 421
    in pregnant and nursing women, 421
  withdrawal syndromes in, 422

Psychosis
  acute delusional, 144
  autoscopic, 166
  postpartum, 166–168, 364–365, 365t
    clinical features of, 167
    course and prognosis of, 167
    diagnosis of, 167
    differential diagnosis of, 167
    epidemiology of, 166
    etiology of, 166–167
    treatment of, 167–168

Psychosis—*continued*
  secondary
    antipsychotics in, 456
    dopamine receptor antagonists in, 456
Psychosocial therapies, 415
  for dementia, 57–58
  for mood disorders, 194–195
  for schizoaffective disorder, 157
  for schizophrenia, 151–153
Psychosomatic disorder(s)
  selective serotonin reuptake inhibitors in, 480
  treatment of, 362–363
Psychosurgery, 506
Psychotherapy
  in adjustment disorders, 334
  in anorexia nervosa, 305
  in antisocial personality disorder, 344
  in avoidant personality disorder, 348
  in borderline personality disorder, 345
  brief, 401–402
    history of, 401
    outcome of, 402
    types of, 401–402
  brief focal, 401
  in brief psychotic disorder, 166
  in bulimia nervosa, 307
  combined individual and group, 405–406
  in cyclothymic disorder, 204
  in dependent personality disorder, 349
  in depressive personality disorder, 353
  in dissociative fugue, 269
  dynamic, in bulimia nervosa, 307
  in early-onset schizophrenia, 581
  in enuresis, 565
  in generalized anxiety disorder, 240–241
  group. *See* Group psychotherapy
  in histrionic personality disorder, 346
  for HIV, 76
  individual, for adolescents, 598
  insight-oriented
    in dissociative identity disorder, 271
    in panic disorder, 221
    in phobias, 226
  in intermittent explosive disorder, 325
  interpersonal, 402–404
    requirements and techniques for, 403
    results in, 404
  in mood disorders in children, 577–578
  in narcissistic personality disorder, 347
  in obsessive-compulsive disorder, 232
  in obsessive-compulsive personality disorder, 351
  in pain disorder, 257–258
  in panic disorders, 221
  in paranoid personality disorder, 339–340
  in paraphilia, 294
  in posttraumatic stress disorder, 238
  psychoanalytic, 398–399, 400t
    corrective emotional experience in, 400–401
    treatment techniques in, 399
      role of insight in, 399
      supportive psychotherapy in, 399–400
  in schizoid personality disorder, 341
  in schizophrenia, 152–153
  in schizotypal personality disorder, 342
  in sex addiction, 295
  short-term anxiety-provoking, 402
  short-term dynamic, 402
  in suicidal ideation, 395
  Tavistock-Malan, 401
  time-limited, 401–402

Psychotic disorder(s)
  alcohol-induced, 88
  amphetamine-induced, 95
  brief
    clinical features of, 164
    comorbidity of, 164
    course and prognosis of, 165, 165t
    diagnosis of, 164, 165t
    differential diagnosis of, 164–165
    epidemiology of, 164
    etiology of, 164
    schizophrenia and, 149
    treatment of, 165–166
      hospitalization in, 165
      pharmacotherapy in, 165
      psychotherapy in, 166
  cannabis-induced, 101–102
  cocaine-induced, 105
  due to general medical condition, 63–64
    course and prognosis of, 64
    diagnosis and clinical features of, 64
    differential diagnosis of, 169
    epidemiology of, 64
    etiology of, 64
    treatment of, 64, 169
  due to medical condition
    clinical features of, 168–169
    diagnosis of, 168, 168t
    epidemiology of, 168
    etiology of, 168
  hallucinogen-induced, 109–110
  HIV-associated, 75
  inhalant-induced, 113
  not otherwise specified, 166–168, 166t
  opioid-induced, 120
  phencyclidine-induced, 124
  primary, treatment of, 455
  secondary, schizophrenia and, 148–149
  serotonin-dopamine antagonists in, 484
  shared, 157, 158t, 161–162, 162t
  substance-induced
    clinical features of, 168–169
    diagnosis of, 168, 169t
    differential diagnosis of, 169
    epidemiology of, 168
    etiology of, 168
    treatment of, 169
Psychotropic drugs, tests of blood levels of, 22–24
Puberty, atypical, 598
Pyromania, 327–328
  comorbidity of, 327
  course and prognosis of, 328
  diagnosis and clinical features of, 327–328, 327t
  differential diagnosis of, 328
  epidemiology of, 327
  etiology of, 327
  treatment of, 328

Q

Qi-gong psychotic reactions, 171
Quazepam (Doral), 435. *See also* Benzodiazepines
Quetiapine (Seroquel), 483. *See also* Serotonin-dopamine antagonists (SDAs)
  adverse effects of, 484
  dosage and clinical guidelines for, 487
  pharmacological actions of, 483

R

Rabbit syndrome, 423

Rape, 375–376
  date, 376
  of men, 376
  statutory, 372
  of women, 375–376
Rapid eye movement sleep behavior disorder, 319
Raskin Depression Scale, 189
Rating scales, psychiatric, 40–44
Reactive attachment disorder of infancy or early childhood
  course and prognosis of, 572
  diagnosis and clinical features of, 571, 572t
  differential diagnosis of, 571
  epidemiology of, 570–571
  etiology of, 571
  pathology and lab exam of, 571
  treatment of, 572
Reading, in mental status examination, 9
Reading disorder, 521–523
  clinical features of, 522
  comorbidity of, 521
  course and prognosis of, 522
  diagnosis of, 522
  differential diagnosis of, 522
  epidemiology of, 521
  etiology of, 521–522
  pathology and lab exam of, 522
  treatment of, 522–523
Reboxetine (Vestra), 476
Recovered memory syndrome, 274
Recurrent brief depressive disorder
  course and prognosis of, 206
  diagnosis and clinical features of, 206, 206t
  differential diagnosis of, 206
  vs. dysthymic disorder, 201
  epidemiology of, 206
  etiology of, 206
  treatment of, 206–207, 443
Reenactment, in posttraumatic stress disorder, 235
Reexperiencing, in posttraumatic stress disorder, 235
Reframing, 408
Relational problem
  definition of, 367
  epidemiology of, 367
  not otherwise specified, 369
  parent–child, 368
  partner, 368–369
  related to general medical condition, 367–368
  related to mental disorder, 367–368
  sibling, 369
Relaxation
  applied, in panic disorder, 221
  in behavior therapy, 410
  biofeedback and, 409–410
  in psychosomatic disorders, 363
Reliability
  in depressive episode, 189
  in manic episode, 190
  in mental status examination, 10
  in schizophrenia, 148
Religious and cultural problem, 380
Remeron. *See* Mirtazapine (Remeron)
Reminyl. *See* Galantamine (Reminyl)
Renal damage, from lithium, 460
Renal function tests, 22
Requip. *See* Ropinirole (Requip)
Resistance, in psychoanalysis, 397
Respiratory training, in panic disorder, 221
Responsibility, criminal, 613–614

Restless legs syndrome, 317
Restoril. *See* Temazepam (Restoril)
Rett's disorder, 514
    course and prognosis of, 540
    diagnosis and clinical features of, 539, 540t
    differential diagnosis of, 539, 540t
    etiology of, 539
    treatment of, 540
Reunion, in psychiatric evaluation of children, 509
Revex. *See* Nalmefene (Revex)
ReVia. *See* Naltrexone (ReVia)
Risperdal. *See* Risperidone (Risperdal)
Risperidone (Risperdal), 483. *See also* Serotonin-dopamine antagonists (SDAs)
    adverse effects of, 484
    dosage and clinical guidelines for, 486–487
    in early-onset schizophrenia, 581
    pharmacological actions of, 483
    in Tourette's disorder, 559
Ritalin. *See* Methylphenidate (Ritalin, Concerta)
Rivastigmine, precautions and adverse reactions of, 449
Rivastigmine (Exelon), 448. *See also* Cholinesterase inhibitors
Romazicon. *See* Flumazenil (Romazicon)
Rootwork, 171
Ropinirole (Requip), 452. *See also* Dopamine receptor agonists
Rorschach test, 511
Rubella, mental retardation and, 514
Rumination disorder
    course and prognosis of, 555
    diagnosis and clinical features of, 555, 555t
    differential diagnosis of, 555
    epidemiology of, 554
    etiology of, 554–555
    pathology and lab exam of, 555
    treatment of, 555

S

Sangue dormido, 171
Schisms and skewed families, of schizophrenia, 140
Schizoaffective disorder
    course and prognosis of, 157
    diagnosis and clinical features of, 156–157, 156t
    differential diagnosis of, 157
    epidemiology of, 155–156
        gender and age difference in, 155–156
    etiology of, 156
    treatment of, 157, 445, 459
        electroconvulsive therapy in, 500
        lithium in, 157, 459
        psychosocial, 157
        valproate in, 497
Schizophrenia
    γ-aminobutyric acid in, 137
    basal ganglia in, 138
    vs. brief psychotic disorder, 149
    childhood onset
        autism, 538, 538t
        course and prognosis of, 581
        differential diagnosis of, 580–581
        epidemiology of, 579
        etiology of, 579
        treatment of, 581
    clinical features of, 145–148
        mental status examination in, 146–148
            impulsiveness, violence and suicide in, 147–148

perceptual disturbances in, 147
            thought in, 147
        positive and negative symptoms of, 146
        premorbid signs and symptoms of, 146
    course of, 149
    vs. delirium, 49, 191
    vs. delusional disorder, 149
    vs. dementia, 56
    diagnosis of, 141–145, 141t, 142t
        psychological testing in, 145
            intelligence testing in, 145
            projective and personality testing in, 145
        subtypes of, 141–144, 142t
            acute delusional psychosis, 144
            catatonic type, 143–144
            disorganized type, 143
            early onset, 145, 145t
            latent, 144
            late-onset, 145, 145t
            oneiroid, 144–145
            paranoid type, 142–143
            paraphrenia, 145
            postpsychotic depressive disorder of, 145, 145t
            pseudoneurotic, 145
            residual type, 144
            simple, 145
            undifferentiated type, 144
    differential diagnosis of, 148–149
    double bind concept of, 140
    downward drift hypothesis of, 136
    epidemiology of, 134–136
        gender and age in, 134–135
        geographical distribution in, 135
        infection and birth season in, 135
        medical illness in, 135
        population factors in, 136
        reproductive factors in, 135
        socioeconomic and culture factors in, 136
        substance use in, 135–136
        suicide risk in, 135
    etiology of, 136–141
        genetic factors in, 139–140
        neurobiology in, 137–139
            applied electrophysiology in, 139
            dopamine hypothesis in, 137
            eye movement dysfunction in, 139
            neurotransmitters in, 137–138
            psychoneuroendocrinology, 139
            psychoneuroimmunology in, 139
        neuroimaging in, 138–139
        neuropathology in, 138
        psychosocial factors in, 140
            family dynamics in, 140–141
            learning theories in, 140
            psychoanalytic theories in, 140
            social theories in, 141
        stress-diathesis model in, 136
    evoked potentials and, 139
    expressed emotion and, 141
    eye examination in, 148
    vs. factitious disorder, 149, 264
    history of disease, 134
    homicide in, 148
    vs. malingering, 149
    vs. mood disorders, 149
    neurological findings in, 148
    vs. personality disorders, 149
    postpsychotic depressive disorder of, 208–210, 208t
    prognosis of, 149–150
    schisms and, 140

vs. schizoaffective disorder, 149
    vs. schizophreniform disorder, 149
    vs. secondary psychotic disorders, 148–149
    sensorium and cognition in, 148
    skewed families and, 140
    social causation hypothesis, 136
    speech in, 148
    suicide risk in, 391
    treatment of, 150–153, 445, 455, 459
        biological therapies in, 150–151
        electroconvulsive therapy in, 501
        hospitalization in, 150
        psychosocial therapies in, 151–153
            assertive community treatment in, 152
            case management in, 152
            cognitive behavioral therapy in, 152
            family-oriented therapies in, 152
            group therapy in, 152
            individual psychotherapy in, 152–153
            social skills training in, 151
            vocational therapy in, 153
Schizophreniform disorder
    course and prognosis of, 155
    diagnostic and clinical features of, 154, 155t
    differential diagnosis of, 154–155
    epidemiology of, 154
    etiology of, 154
    schizophrenia and, 149
    treatment of, 155
Schreber, Daniel Paul, 159
SDAs. *See* Serotonin-dopamine antagonists (SDAs)
Secondary gain, in conversion disorder, 251
Sedation, tricyclic antidepressants and, 495
Sedative-related disorders, 125–131, 127t
    clinical features of, 129–130
    diagnosis of, 127–129, 127t
    epidemiology of, 126
    legal issues in, 130–131
    neuropharmacology of, 126–127
    not otherwise specified, 129
    treatment and rehabilitation for, 130
Seizures
    barbiturates in, 433
    selective serotonin reuptake inhibitors and, 481
    serotonin-dopamine antagonists and, 485
Selective serotonin reuptake inhibitors (SSRIs), 476–483
    dosage and clinical guidelines for, 482–483
    drug–drug interactions of, 482
    pharmacological actions of, 477
    precautions and adverse reactions to, 480–481
    therapeutic indications for, 477–480
        in anorexia nervosa, 479
        in anxiety disorders, 478–479
        in anxiety in children, 569
        in attention deficit/hyperactivity disorder, 479
        in autistic disorder, 479
        in bulimia nervosa, 479
        in chronic pain syndromes, 479
        in depression, 477–478
        in depression in children, 578
        in generalized anxiety disorder, 241–242
        in kleptomania, 327
        in major depressive disorder, 195–197
        in obsessive-compulsive disorder, 231

Selective serotonin reuptake inhibitors (SSRIs)—*continued*
  in panic disorders, 220
  in paraphilias, 479
  in posttraumatic stress disorder, 237
  in premature ejaculation, 479
  in premenstrual dysphoric disorder, 479
  in psychosomatic conditions, 480
  in sex addiction, 296
  in social phobia, 227
Selegiline (Eldepryl), 464. *See also* Monoamine oxidase inhibitors (MAOIs)
Self-help programs, 417
Selye, Hans, 355
Sensorium
  in depressive episode, 189
  in geriatric patients, 601
  in manic episode, 190
  in schizophrenia, 148
Separation, in psychiatric evaluation of children, 509
Separation anxiety disorder
  course and prognosis of, 568–569
  diagnosis and clinical features of, 566–568, 567t
  differential diagnosis of, 568, 568t
  epidemiology of, 566
  etiology of, 566
  treatment of, 569
Sequential Tests of Educational Progress (STEP), 511
Serax. *See* Oxazepam (Serax)
Seroquel. *See* Quetiapine (Seroquel)
Serotonergic system, in obsessive-compulsive disorder, 228
Serotonin
  in anxiety, 212–213
  in mood disorders, 175
  in schizophrenia, 137
Serotonin-dopamine antagonists (SDAs), 454, 483
  adverse effects of, 484–486
  dosage and clinical guidelines for, 486–487
  drug–drug interactions in, 486
  pharmacological actions of, 483–484
  therapeutic indications for, 484
    in early-onset schizophrenia, 581
    in schizophrenia, 150
Serotonin syndrome, selective serotonin reuptake inhibitors in, 481
Sertraline (Zoloft), 476. *See also* Selective serotonin reuptake inhibitors (SSRIs)
  dosage and clinical guidelines for, 482
  in panic disorder, 220
Serzone. *See* Nefazodone (Serzone)
Sex addiction, 294–296
  behavioral patterns in, 295
  comorbidity of, 295
  diagnosis of, 295
  treatment of, 295–296
Sex-reassignment surgery, in gender identity disorder, 300
Sex therapy, analytically-oriented, 288
Sexual abuse
  of adult, 375–376
  of child, 371–372, 371t
Sexual arousal disorders, 278–280
  female, 279, 279t
  hypoactive, due to general medical condition, 283
  male, 279–280

Sexual coercion, 376
Sexual desire disorders, 278, 278t
Sexual disorder, not otherwise specified, 294
Sexual dysfunction
  alcohol-induced, 89
  amphetamine-induced, 95
  cocaine-induced, 106
  due to general medical condition, 65, 282–284, 283t
  female, due to medical condition, 284
  male, due to general medical condition, 283–284
  not otherwise specified, 286, 286t
  opioid-induced, 120
  pharmacological agents implicated in, 284–285
  selective serotonin reuptake inhibitors and, 480
  substance-induced, 284
  subtypes of, 277–278
  treatment of, 286–290, 453
    behavior therapy in, 287–288
    biological treatments in, 288
    dual-sex therapy in, 286–287
    exercises in, 287
    group therapy in, 288
    hypnotherapy in, 287
    surgical therapy in, 289
Sexual harassment, 376
Sexuality
  abnormal, 277–278. *See also* Sexual dysfunction; *specific disorders*
  normal
    homosexuality and, 277
    love and intimacy in, 277
    masturbation in, 276–277
    psychosocial factors in, 275–276
    sexual orientation in, 276
Sexually transmitted diseases, blood test for, 22
Sexual masochism, 292, 292t
Sexual orientation
  in normal sexuality, 276
  persistent and marked distress about, 296
Sexual pain disorders, 282
Sexual sadism, 292, 292t
Shejing shuariu, 171
Shen-k'uei, 171
Shenkui, 171
Shin-byung, 171
Sialorrhea, serotonin-dopamine antagonists and, 485
Signs and symptoms
  of medical illness, 20
  of psychiatric illness, 26–32. *See also specific signs and symptoms*
Simple deteriorative disorder, 145
Sinemet. *See* Carbidopa-levodopa (Sinemet)
Sleep
  disorders of. *See* Sleep disorders
  electrophysiology of, 309–310, 310f
  functions of, 311
  insufficient, 317
  regulation of, 310–311
  requirements for, 311
  sleep–wake rhythm and, 311
Sleep deprivation, 311, 505
Sleep disorders, 309
  alcohol-related disorders and, 83–84, 89
  amphetamine-induced, 95
  breathing-related, 314, 314t
  caffeine-induced, 99

  circadian rhythm, 315–316, 315t
    delayed sleep phase type, 315
    jet lag type, 315
    shift work type, 315–316
  classification of, 312
  cocaine-induced, 106
  in depression, 176
  due to general medical condition, 65, 320–321, 320t
  major disorders of, 311–312
  opioid-induced, 120
  parasomnias, 317–319, 317t, 318t
  in pregnancy, 317
  related to other mental disorder, 319
  substance-induced, 321–322, 321t
  treatment of, 433–434
Sleep drunkenness, 317
Sleep paralysis, 319
Sleeptalking, 319
Sleep terror disorder, 317–318, 318t
Sleep–wake schedule disturbance, 316
  major symptoms of, 312
Sleepwalking disorder, 318–319, 318t
Smoke-free environments, nicotine-related disorders and, 117
Smoking cessation, 441
  nicotine-related disorders and, 116
Social and Occupational Functioning Assessment Scale (SOFAS), 41, 42t
Social anxiety disorder, 222. *See also* Phobia, social
  venlafaxine in, 499
Social causation hypothesis, of schizophrenia, 136
Social network therapy, 408
Social relatedness, in psychiatric evaluation of children, 510
Social skills training, 415–416
  goals of, 416
  information-processing model of, 417
  methods of, 416, 416t
  and social perception skills training, 416
Sodium lactate, provocation of panic attacks with, 24
Solfoton. *See* Phenobarbital (Solfoton, Luminal)
Somatization disorder
  clinical features, 248
  course and prognosis of, 249
  diagnosis of, 248, 248t
  differential diagnosis of, 248–249
  epidemiology of, 247
  etiology of, 247–248
    biological and genetic factors in, 247–248
    psychosocial factors in, 247
  treatment of, 249
Somatoform disorder(s)
  defined, 247
  vs. factitious disorder, 263–264
  not otherwise specified, 258, 258t
  undifferentiated, 258, 258t
Somatostatin, in depression, 176
Somniloquy, 319
Sonata. *See* Zaleplon (Sonata)
Speech, 30–31
  aphasic disturbances in, 31
  in depressive episode, 189
  in manic episode, 190
  in mental status examination, 7
  in phonological disorder, 531
  in psychiatric evaluation of children, 509
Spell, 171

Spiegel, Herbert, 414
Splitting, in personality disorders, 338
Spouse abuse, 374–375
SSRIs. *See* Selective serotonin reuptake
  inhibitors (SSRIs)
Stalking, 376
Stanford-Binet Intelligence Scale, 511
Stelazine. *See* Trifluoperazine (Stelazine)
Strattera. *See* Atomoxetine (Strattera)
Stress theory, 355–356. *See also* Acute
  stress disorder; Posttraumatic
  stress disorder
  endocrine responses in, 356
  immune response in, 356
  neurotransmitter responses in, 355–356
  vicissitudes of life in, 356, 357t
Stuttering
  clinical features of, 533
  course and prognosis of, 533
  diagnosis of, 533, 533t
  differential diagnosis of, 533
  epidemiology of, 532
  etiology of, 532–533
  treatment of, 533–534
Substance abuse, 77–78
  adolescent
    comorbidity in, 583
    diagnosis and clinical features of, 583
    epidemiology of, 582
    etiology of, 582–583
      genetic factors in, 582
      psychosocial factors in, 582–583
    treatment of, 583–584
  codependence with, 78
  comorbidity with, 79–80
  diagnosis of, 77, 78t
  etiology of, 78–79
    behavioral theories of, 79
    genetic factors in, 79
    neurochemical factors in, 79
    psychodynamic factors of, 78–79
  vs. factitious disorder, 264
  HIV-associated, 75
  neurotransmitters in, 79
  in schizophrenia, 135–136
  treatment of, 80
  urine testing for, 24t, 25
Substance dependence, 77–78, 79t
  codependence and, 78
  comorbidity with, 79–80
  diagnosis of, 77, 79t
  etiology of, 78–79
    behavioral theories in, 79
    genetic factors in, 79
    neurochemical factors in, 79
    psychodynamic factors in, 78–79
  neurotransmitters in, 79
  suicide risk in, 392
  treatment of, 80
Substance-related disorders. *See also* Sub-
    stance abuse; Substance depen-
    dence
  codependence and, 78
  comorbidity of, 79–80
  diagnosis of, 77, 78t, 79t
  etiology of, 78–79
    behavioral theories of, 79
    genetic factors in, 79
    neurochemical factors in, 79
    psychodynamic factors in, 78–79
  neurotransmitters in, 79
  terminology of, 77–78, 78t
  treatment and rehabilitation of, 80

Suggestibility, disturbances in, 26
Suicide
  alcohol-related disorders and, 82
  in children, 578
  epidemiology of, 389–392
    risk factors in, 389–392
      age, 389
      marital status, 390
      mental health, 390
      methods and, 390
      occupation, 390
      physical health, 390
      physicians and, 390
      previous suicidal behavior, 392
      psychiatric patients, 390–392
      race, 389–390
      religion, 390
      sex, 389
  etiology of, 392–393
    biological factors in, 393
    genetic factors in, 393
    psychological factors in, 392–393
    sociological factors in, 392
  in fluoxetine use, 447
  HIV-associated, 75
  parasuicidal behavior and, 393
  physician-assisted, 607–608
  prediction, of, 393–394, 394t
  in schizophrenia, 135, 147–148
  treatment of, 394–395
    inpatient *versus* outpatient, 394–395
    legal and ethical factors in, 395
    selective serotonin reuptake inhibitors
      in, 477
Sular. *See* Nisoldipine (Sular)
Sundowner syndrome, in dementia, 55–56
Susto, 171
Symmetrel. *See* Amantadine (Symmetrel)
Symmetry, in obsessive-compulsive disor-
    der, 230
Sympathomimetics, 487
  dosage and administration of, 490, 491t
  drug–drug interactions of, 490
  effects of on specific organs and systems,
    488
  laboratory interferences of, 490
  pharmacological actions of, 488
  precautions and adverse reactions to,
    489–490
  therapeutic indications for, 488–489
    in sexual dysfunction, 285
  tricyclic antidepressants and, 496
Syncope
  selective serotonin reuptake inhibitors in,
    480
  serotonin-dopamine antagonists and, 485
Systemic lupus erythematosus
  mental disorders due to, 71
  psychological sequelae of, 360

T

Tachycardia, serotonin-dopamine antago-
    nists and, 485
Tacrine (Cognex), 448. *See also* Cholinest-
    erase inhibitors
  precautions and adverse reactions of,
    449–450
  tests for use of, 24
Taijin kyofu sho, 171
Tardive dyskinesia
  neuroleptic-induced, 424–425, 424t
  serotonin-dopamine antagonists and, 485

TCAs. *See* Tetracyclic antidepressants (TCAs);
    Tricyclic antidepressants (TCAs)
Tegretol. *See* Carbamazepine (Tegretol)
Telephone scatologia, 293
Temazepam (Restoril), 435. *See also* Benzo-
    diazepines
Tenex. *See* Guanfacine (Tenex)
Tenormin. *See* Atenolol (Tenormin)
Terrorism, in posttraumatic stress disorder,
    236–237
Testosterone, 506
Tetracyclic antidepressants (TCAs),
    493–497
  dosage and clinical guidelines for,
    496–497, 497t
  drug–drug interactions of, 496
  effects of on specific organs and systems,
    494
  overdose of, 496–497
  pharmacological actions of, 494
  precautions and adverse reactions to,
    494–496
  tests for use of, 23
  therapeutic indications for, 494
    in panic disorders, 220
Thematic Apperception Test (TAT), 145, 511
Therapeutic alliance, in psychoanalysis, 397
Therapeutic graded exposure, 411
Thiamine deficiency, mental disorders due
    to, 72
Thioridazine (Mellaril), 454. *See also*
    Dopamine receptor antagonists
  in paranoid personality disorder, 340
Thorazine. *See* Chlorpromazine (Thorazine)
Thought
  abstract, 28–30, 32
    in mental status examination, 9
  concrete, 32
  content, 29–30
    in geriatric patients, 600
    in psychiatric evaluation of children,
      509
    in schizophrenia, 147
  in depressive episode, 189
  elicitation of automatic, 413
  form of, in schizophrenia, 147
  in geriatric patients, 600
  intrusive, in obsessive-compulsive disor-
    der, 230
  in manic episode, 190
  process, 28–30
    in mental status examination, 7–8
    in psychiatric evaluation of children,
      509
    in schizophrenia, 147
Thyroid axis, in mood disorders, 175–176
Thyroid disorders, mental disorders due to, 71
Thyroid function tests, 21, 22t
Tiagabine, pharmacological actions of, 474
Tic disorder, 557. *See also specific disorders*
  chronic motor or vocal, 560
    course and prognosis of, 560
    diagnosis and clinical features of, 560,
      560t
    differential diagnosis of, 560
    epidemiology of, 560
    etiology of, 560
    treatment of, 560
  not otherwise specified, 561, 561t
  transient, 560–561
    course and prognosis of, 561
    diagnosis and clinical features of, 561,
      561t

Tic disorder—*continued*
   epidemiology of, 560
   etiology of, 560–561
   treatment of, 561
   treatment of, 426
Tics. *See* Tic disorder
Tofranil. *See* Imipramine (Tofranil)
Topamax. *See* Topiramate (Topamax)
Topiramate (Topamax), 473
   dosage and clinical guidelines for, 476
   drug–drug interactions of, 475
   pharmacological actions of, 474
   precautions and adverse reactions to, 475
   therapeutic indications for, 474
Torture, in posttraumatic stress disorder, 236
Tourette's disorder
   course and prognosis of, 559
   diagnosis and clinical features of, 558, 558t
   differential diagnosis of, 559
   epidemiology of, 557
   etiology of, 557–558
     genetic factors in, 557
     immunological factors and postinfection in, 557–558
     neurochemical and neuroanatomical factors in, 557
   vs. obsessive-compulsive disorder, 230
   pathology and lab exam of, 558
   treatment of, 425–426, 559
Transaminase elevations, serotonin-dopamine antagonists and, 485
Transcranial magnetic stimulation, 504–505
Transference, in psychoanalysis, 397
Tranylcypromine (Parnate), 464. *See also* Monoamine oxidase inhibitors (MAOIs)
Trazodone (Desyrel), 492–493
   dosage and administration of, 493
   drug–drug interactions of, 493
   effects of on specific organs and systems, 492–493
   precautions and adverse reactions to, 493
   therapeutic indications for, 493
     in major depressive disorder, 195
Tremor, selective serotonin reuptake inhibitors and, 481
Triazolam (Halcyon), 435. *See also* Benzodiazepines
Trichotillomania
   comorbidity of, 330
   course and prognosis of, 331
   diagnosis and clinical features of, 330–331, 330t
   differential diagnosis of, 331
   epidemiology of, 330
   etiology of, 330
   pathology and lab exam of, 331
   treatment of, 331
Tricyclic antidepressants (TCAs), 493–497
   dosage and clinical guidelines for, 496–497, 496t
   drug–drug interactions of, 496
   effects of on specific organs and systems, 494
   overdose of, 496–497
   pharmacological actions of, 494
   precautions and adverse reactions to, 494–496

tests for use of, 23
therapeutic indications for, 494
   in panic disorders, 220
Trifluoperazine (Stelazine), in Tourette's disorder, 559
Triglyceride elevations, serotonin-dopamine antagonists and, 485
Trihexyphenidyl (Artane), 430. *See also* Anticholinergics
L-Tryptophan, antidepressants plus, 197
Tryptophan hydroxylase (TPH), suicide and, 393
Twins, monozygotic, schizophrenia in, 139
Twin studies, suicide in, 393
Tyramine, monoamine oxidase inhibitors and, 465–466, 465t

U

Urophilia, 293

V

Vacuum pump, in sexual dysfunction, 289
Vagal nerve stimulation, 505
Vaginismus, 282, 282t
Valium. *See* Diazepam (Valium)
Valproate (Depakene), 497
   dosage and administration of, 498–499, 499t
   drug–drug interactions of, 498
   effects of on specific organs and systems, 498
   laboratory interferences of, 498
   pharmacologic actions of, 497
   precautions and adverse reactions to, 498
   tests for use of, 24
   therapeutic indications for, 497–498
     in bipolar I disorder, 198
Valproic acid. *See* Valproate (Depakene)
Valvular heart disease, psychological sequelae of, 358
Venlafaxine (Effexor), 499
   dosage and administration of, 500
   drug–drug interactions of, 500
   pharmacological actions of, 499
   precautions and adverse reactions to, 499
   therapeutic indications for, 499
     in generalized anxiety disorder, 241
     in major depressive disorder, 195
     in social phobia, 227
Verapamil (Calan), 443. *See also* Calcium channel inhibitors
   dosage and clinical guidelines for, 444
Vestra. *See* Reboxetine (Vestra)
Violence
   β-adrenergic receptor antagonists in, 428
   dopamine receptor antagonists in, 456
   in schizophrenia, 147
Vistaril. *See* Hydroxyzine pamoate (Vistaril)
Visuospatial ability, in mental status examination, 9
Vocational training, 417
Voyeurism, 292

W

Watson, John B., 222, 410

Wechsler Intelligence Scale for Children (WISC-III), 510–511
Weight gain
   selective serotonin reuptake inhibitors and, 480
   serotonin-dopamine antagonists and, 485–486
Wellbutrin. *See* Bupropion (Wellbutrin, Zyban)
Wernicke-Korsakoff syndrome, 87
Wide-Range Achievement Test–Revised (WRAT–R), 511
Withdrawal
   alcohol, 85–86, 85t, 90–91
     β-adrenergic receptor antagonists in, 428
     carbamazepine in, 445
     clonidine in, 425
     guanfacine in, 425
   amphetamine, 94–95, 94t
   benzodiazepine, 130t
     carbamazepine in, 445
     clonidine in, 425
     guanfacine in, 425
   caffeine, 98–99, 98t
   cocaine, 105
   delirium in, 48, 48t
   MAOI, 466
   nicotine, 115
     clonidine in, 425
     guanfacine in, 425
   opioid, 119t, 120
     clonidine in, 425
     guanfacine in, 425
     neonatal, 122
   opioid receptor agonists, 470
   sedative, hypnotic, or anxiolytic, 127t, 128
   SSRI, 481
Wolf, P. H., 171–172
Wolpe, Joseph, 410
Worried well, HIV and, 75
Writing, in mental status examination, 9

X

Xanax. *See* Alprazolam (Xanax)
X chromosome, bipolar I disorder and, 177

Z

Zaleplon (Sonata), 433, 435. *See also* Benzodiazepines
   dosage and administration of, 440 Zar, 171 Zeldox. *See* Ziprasidone (Zeldox)
Ziprasidone (Zeldox), 483. *See also* Serotonin-dopamine antagonists (SDAs)
   adverse effects of, 485
   dosage and clinical guidelines for, 487
   pharmacological actions of, 483–484
Zoloft. *See* Sertraline (Zoloft)
Zolpidem (Ambien), 433, 435. *See also* Benzodiazepines
   dosage and administration of, 440
Zoophilia, 293
Zung Self-Rating Depression Scale, 189
Zyban. *See* Bupropion (Wellbutrin, Zyban)
Zyprexa. *See* Olanzapine (Zyprexa)